AF583884

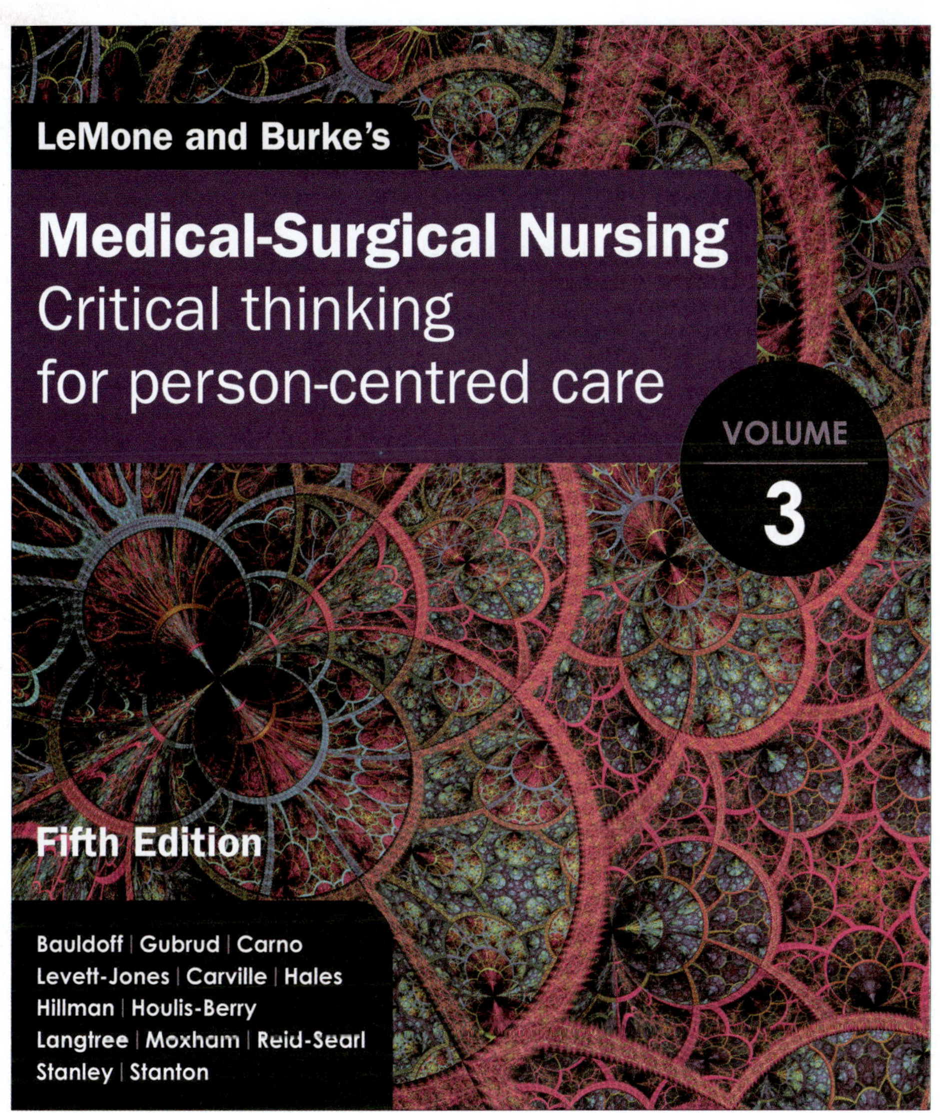
LeMone and Burke's
Medical-Surgical Nursing
Critical thinking
for person-centred care
VOLUME
3
Fifth Edition
Bauldoff | Gubrud | Carno
Levett-Jones | Carville | Hales
Hillman | Houlis-Berry
Langtree | Moxham | Reid-Searl
Stanley | Stanton

Pearson Australia
Building B, Level 1
459–471 Church Street
Richmond Victoria 3121

www.pearson.com.au

Authorised adaptation from the United States edition entitled *LeMone's Medical–Surgical Nursing: Clinical Reasoning in Patient Care*, 7th edition, by LeMone, Priscilla; Burke, Karen; Bauldoff, Gerene, Gubrud, Paula, published by Pearson Education, Inc., Copyright © 2020.

Fifth adaptation edition published by Pearson Australia Group Pty Ltd, Copyright © 2024

Pearson respects and honours Aboriginal and Torres Strait Islander Elders past, present and future. We acknowledge the stories, traditions and living cultures of the Traditional Custodians of the lands on which our company is located and where we conduct our business. Pearson is committed to honouring Australian Aboriginal and Torres Strait Islander peoples' unique cultural and spiritual relationships to the land, waters and seas and their rich contribution to society.

Aboriginal and Torres Strait Islander peoples are advised that this text may contain images, voices and names of deceased persons.

Links to National Patient Safety Standards reproduced with permission from *National Safety and Quality Health Service Standards* (second edition), developed by the Australian Commission on Safety and Quality in Health Care (ACSQHC). ACSQHC: Sydney 2021.

Senior Commercial Product Manager: Mandy Sheppard
Development Editor: Anna Carter
Senior Project Manager: Bernadette Chang
Content Producer: Linda Chryssavgis
Digital Media Production Manager: Paul Ryan
Assistant Manager Rights and Permissions: Samantha Russell-Tulip
Lead Editor/Copy Editor: Katie Millar
Indexer: Integra Software Services
Cover and internal design by Natalie Bowra
Cover image by Sabena Jane Blackbird/Alamy Stock Photo
Typeset by Integra Software Services

Printed in Malaysia (CTP-VVP)

Etext ISBN: 9780655709152
Print ISBNs: 9780655709145 (Vol 1), 9780655709275 (Vol 2), 9780655709282 (Vol 3)
ePUB ISBN: 9780655709169

1 2 3 4 5 28 27 26 25 24

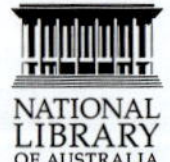

A catalogue record for this work is available from the National Library of Australia

Pearson Australia Group Pty Ltd ABN 40 004 245 943

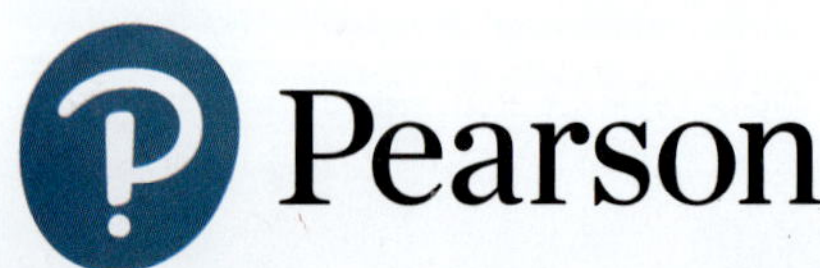

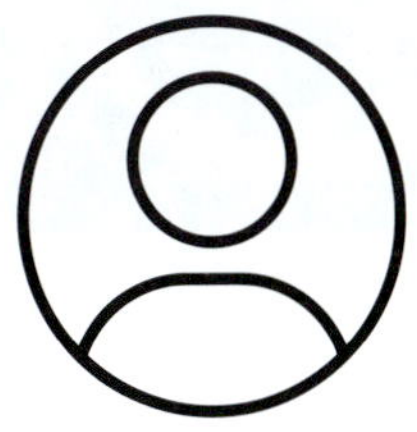

Pearson's Commitment to Diversity, Equity, and Inclusion

Pearson is dedicated to creating bias-free content that reflects the diversity, depth, and breadth of all learners' lived experiences.

We embrace the many dimensions of diversity, including but not limited to race, ethnicity, gender, sex, sexual orientation, socioeconomic status, ability, age, and religious or political beliefs.

Education is a powerful force for equity and change in our world. It has the potential to deliver opportunities that improve lives and enable economic mobility. As we work with authors to create content for every product and service, we acknowledge our responsibility to demonstrate inclusivity and incorporate diverse scholarship so that everyone can achieve their potential through learning. As the world's leading learning company, we have a duty to help drive change and live up to our purpose to help more people create a better life for themselves and to create a better world.

Our ambition is to purposefully contribute to a world where:

- Everyone has an equitable and lifelong opportunity to succeed through learning.
- Our educational content accurately reflects the histories and lived experiences of the learners we serve.
- Our educational products and services are inclusive and represent the rich diversity of learners.
- Our educational content prompts deeper discussions with students and motivates them to expand their own learning (and worldview).

Accessibility

We are also committed to providing products that are fully accessible to all learners. As per Pearson's guidelines for accessible educational Web media, we test and retest the capabilities of our products against the highest standards for every release, following the WCAG guidelines in developing new products for copyright year 2022 and beyond.

You can learn more about Pearson's commitment to accessibility at **https://www.pearson.com/us/accessibility.html**

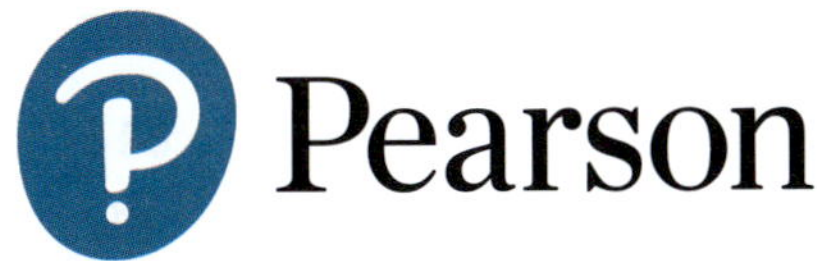

Contact Us

While we work hard to present unbiased, fully accessible content, we want to hear from you about any concerns or needs with this Pearson product so that we can investigate and address them.

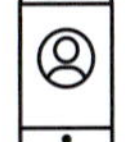

Please contact us with concerns about any potential bias at **https://www.pearson.com/report-bias.html**

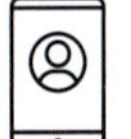

For accessibility-related issues, such as using assistive technology with Pearson products, alternative text requests, or accessibility documentation, email the Pearson Disability Support team at **disability.support@pearson.com**

Brief contents

VOLUME 3

Detailed contents

VOLUME 2

UNIT 6 Responses to altered gastrointestinal function

VOLUME 3

UNIT 9

Responses to altered respiratory function 1191

Guided tour

Key features of the Australian edition include:

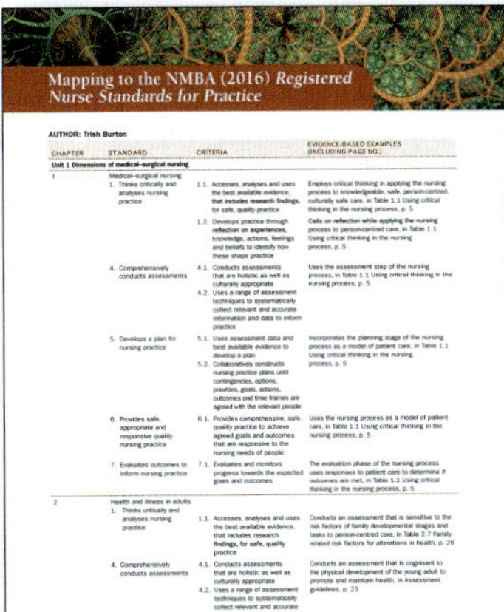

Mapping to the NMBA (2016) Registered Nurse Standards for Practice

AUTHOR: Trish Burton

Mapping to the NMBA (2016) ***Registered Nurse Standards for Practice*** *maps examples from the text to relevant* Registered Nurse Standards for Practice, *thereby aligning the content to contemporary professional practice in Australia.*

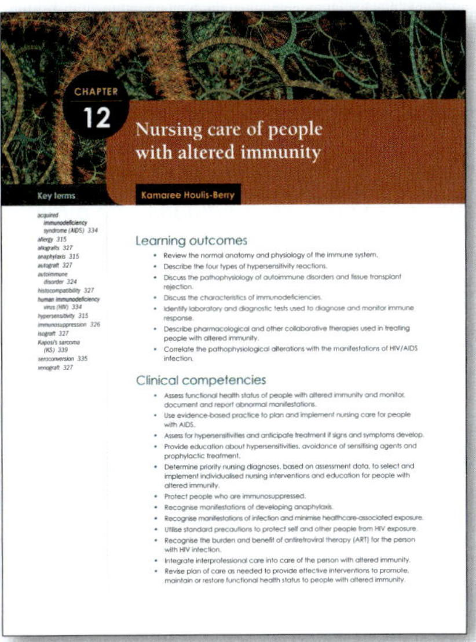

CHAPTER 12

Nursing care of people with altered immunity

Kamaree Houlis-Berry

Key terms

acquired immunodeficiency syndrome (AIDS) 334
allergy 315
allografts 327
anaphylaxis 315
autograft 327
autoimmune disorder 324
histocompatibility 327
human immunodeficiency virus (HIV) 334
hypersensitivity 315
immunosuppression 326
isograft 327
Kaposi's sarcoma (KS) 339
seroconversion 335
xenograft 327

Learning outcomes

- Review the normal anatomy and physiology of the immune system.
- Describe the four types of hypersensitivity reactions.
- Discuss the pathophysiology of autoimmune disorders and tissue transplant rejection.
- Discuss the characteristics of immunodeficiencies.
- Identify laboratory and diagnostic tests used to diagnose and monitor immune response.
- Describe pharmacological and other collaborative therapies used in treating people with altered immunity.
- Correlate the pathophysiological alterations with the manifestations of HIV/AIDS infection.

Clinical competencies

- Assess functional health status of people with altered immunity and monitor, document and report abnormal manifestations.
- Use evidence-based practice to plan and implement nursing care for people with AIDS.
- Assess for hypersensitivities and anticipate treatment if signs and symptoms develop.
- Provide education about hypersensitivities, avoidance of sensitising agents and prophylactic treatment.
- Determine priority nursing diagnoses, based on assessment data, to select and implement individualised nursing interventions and education for people with altered immunity.
- Protect people who are immunosuppressed.
- Recognise manifestations of developing anaphylaxis.
- Recognise manifestations of infection and minimise healthcare-associated exposure.
- Utilise standard precautions to protect self and other people from HIV exposure.
- Recognise the burden and benefit of antiretroviral therapy (ART) for the person with HIV infection.
- Integrate interprofessional care into care of the person with altered immunity.
- Revise plan of care as needed to provide effective interventions to promote, maintain or restore functional health status to people with altered immunity.

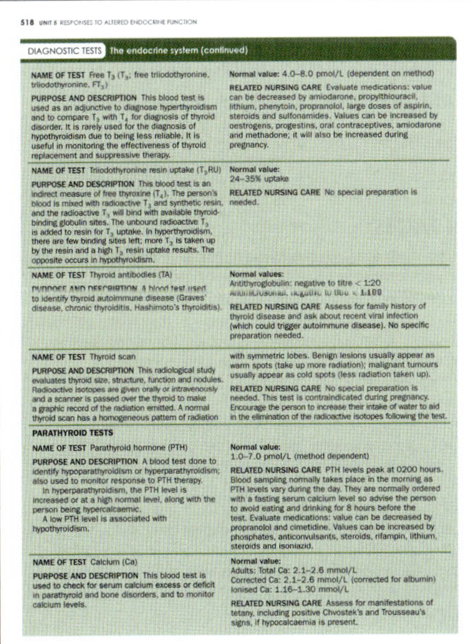

518 UNIT 5 RESPONSES TO ALTERED ENDOCRINE FUNCTION

DIAGNOSTIC TESTS The endocrine system (continued)

NAME OF TEST Free T_3 (T_3: free triiodothyronine, triiodothyronine, FT_3) **PURPOSE AND DESCRIPTION** This blood test is used as an adjunctive to diagnose hyperthyroidism and to compare T_3 with T_4 for diagnosis of thyroid disorder. It is rarely used for the diagnosis of hypothyroidism due to being less reliable. It is useful in monitoring the effectiveness of thyroid replacement and suppressive therapy.	**Normal value:** 4.0–8.0 pmol/L (dependent on method) **RELATED NURSING CARE** Evaluate medications: value can be decreased by amiodarone, propylthiouracil, lithium, phenytoin, propranolol, large doses of aspirin, steroids and sulfonamides. Values can be increased by oestrogens, progestins, oral contraceptives, amiodarone and methadone; it will also be increased during pregnancy.
NAME OF TEST Triiodothyronine resin uptake (T_3RU) **PURPOSE AND DESCRIPTION** This blood test is an indirect measure of free thyroxine (T_4). The person's blood is mixed with radioactive T_3 and synthetic resin, and the radioactive T_3 will bind with available thyroid-binding globulin sites. The unbound radioactive T_3 is added to resin for T_3 uptake. In hyperthyroidism, there are few binding sites left; more T_3 is taken up by the resin and a high T_3 resin uptake results. The opposite occurs in hypothyroidism.	**Normal value:** 24–35% uptake **RELATED NURSING CARE** No special preparation is needed.
NAME OF TEST Thyroid antibodies (TA) **PURPOSE AND DESCRIPTION** A blood test used to identify thyroid autoimmune disease (Graves' disease, chronic thyroiditis, Hashimoto's thyroiditis).	**Normal values:** Antithyroglobulin: negative to titre < 1:20 [illegible] < 1:100 **RELATED NURSING CARE** Assess for family history of thyroid disease and ask about recent viral infection (which could trigger autoimmune disease). No specific preparation needed.
NAME OF TEST Thyroid scan **PURPOSE AND DESCRIPTION** This radiological study evaluates thyroid size, structure, function and nodules. Radioactive isotopes are given orally or intravenously and a scanner is passed over the thyroid to make a graphic record of the radiation emitted. A normal thyroid scan has a homogeneous pattern of radiation	with symmetric lobes. Benign lesions usually appear as warm spots (take up more radiation); malignant tumours usually appear as cold spots (less radiation taken up). **RELATED NURSING CARE** No special preparation is needed. This test is contraindicated during pregnancy. Encourage the person to increase their intake of water to aid in the elimination of the radioactive isotopes following the test.
PARATHYROID TESTS **NAME OF TEST** Parathyroid hormone (PTH) **PURPOSE AND DESCRIPTION** A blood test done to identify hypoparathyroidism or hyperparathyroidism; also used to monitor response to PTH therapy. In hyperparathyroidism, the PTH level is increased or at a high normal level, along with the person being hypercalcaemic. A low PTH level is associated with hypothyroidism.	**Normal value:** 1.0–7.0 pmol/L (method dependent) **RELATED NURSING CARE** PTH levels peak at 0200 hours. Blood sampling normally takes place in the morning as PTH levels vary during the day. They are normally ordered with a fasting serum calcium level so advise the person to avoid eating and drinking for 8 hours before the test. Evaluate medications: value can be decreased by propranolol and cimetidine. Values can be increased by phosphates, anticonvulsants, steroids, rifampin, lithium, steroids and isoniazid.
NAME OF TEST Calcium (Ca) **PURPOSE AND DESCRIPTION** This blood test is used to check for serum calcium excess or deficit in parathyroid and bone disorders, and to monitor calcium levels.	**Normal value:** Adults: Total Ca: 2.1–2.6 mmol/L Corrected Ca: 2.1–2.6 mmol/L (corrected for albumin) Ionised Ca: 1.16–1.30 mmol/L **RELATED NURSING CARE** Assess for manifestations of tetany, including positive Chvostek's and Trousseau's signs, if hypocalcaemia is present.

Diagnostic Tests *include diagnostic test tables and a narrative summary. The tables include the name of the test, the purpose and description of the test, and related nursing care.*

Learning Outcomes *show you the knowledge you'll gain, while* **Clinical Competencies** *demonstrate how you will apply that knowledge.*

Pathophysiology Illustrated *art brings physiological processes to life.*

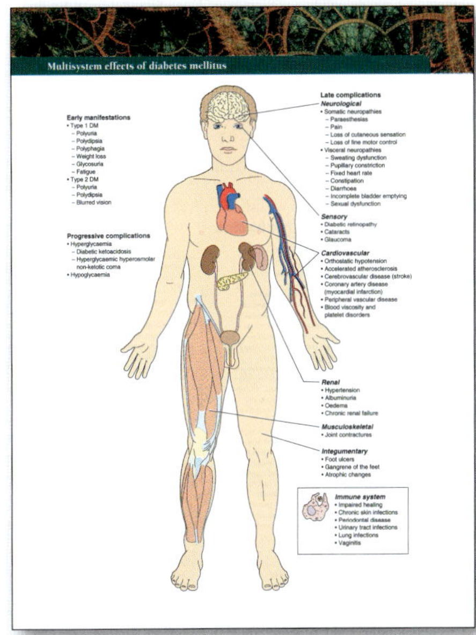

FOCUS ON CULTURAL DIVERSITY Diabetes in Aboriginal and Torres Strait Islander communities

Type 2 DM represents a serious public health problem for Aboriginal and Torres Strait Islander communities, occurring at a much higher rate than in the non-Indigenous population, and with a much earlier age of onset of the disease and its micro- and macrovascular complications. It is likely that type 2 DM is an important contributor to the considerably higher circulatory disease mortality rate among Aboriginal and Torres Strait Islander communities at younger ages. Thus, type 2 DM imposes significant financial and human costs on Australian society, which are disproportionately borne by Aboriginal and Torres Strait Islander communities.

The National Aboriginal and Torres Strait Islander Health Survey of 2018–2019 found that 8% of Aboriginal and Torres Strait Islander people reported they had DM (ABS, 2019), the most common being type 2 DM. The prevalence of DM is almost three higher in Aboriginal and Torres Strait Islander communities than in the rest of the population across all age groups. In 2021, diabetes was the second leading cause of death for Aboriginal and Torres Strait Islander people (ABS, 2022). The incidence of GDM in pregnancy is also two to three times higher among Aboriginal and Torres Strait Islander women than in the general Australian population. Living in remote areas also increases the prevalence rates for Aboriginal and Torres Strait Islander groups to six times higher than non-remote areas.

Focus on Cultural Diversity boxes *demonstrate how culture, age and gender produce differences in incidence, prevalence and mortality.*

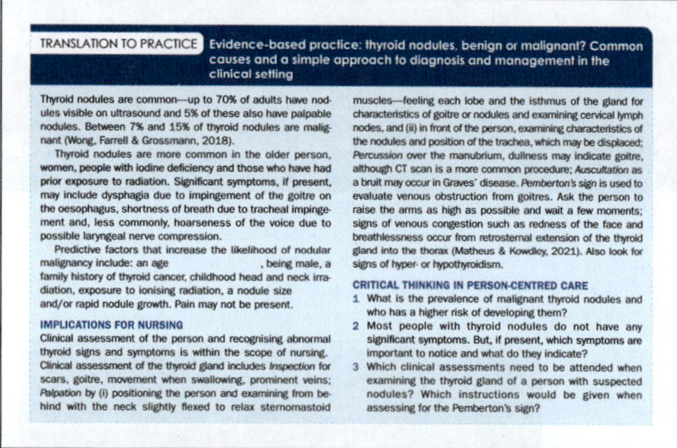

TRANSLATION TO PRACTICE **Evidence-based practice: thyroid nodules, benign or malignant? Common causes and a simple approach to diagnosis and management in the clinical setting**

Thyroid nodules are common—up to 70% of adults have nodules visible on ultrasound and 5% of these also have palpable nodules. Between 7% and 15% of thyroid nodules are malignant (Wong, Farrell & Grossmann, 2018).

Thyroid nodules are more common in the older person, women, people with iodine deficiency and those who have had prior exposure to radiation. Significant symptoms, if present, may include dysphagia due to impingement of the goitre on the oesophagus, shortness of breath due to tracheal impingement and, less commonly, hoarseness of the voice due to possible laryngeal nerve compression.

Predictive factors that increase the likelihood of nodular malignancy include: an age , being male, a family history of thyroid cancer, childhood head and neck irradiation, exposure to ionising radiation, a nodule size and/or rapid nodule growth. Pain may not be present.

IMPLICATIONS FOR NURSING

Clinical assessment of the person and recognising abnormal thyroid signs and symptoms is within the scope of nursing. Clinical assessment of the thyroid gland includes *Inspection* for scars, goitre, movement when swallowing, prominent veins; *Palpation* by (i) positioning the person and examining from behind with the neck slightly flexed to relax sternomastoid muscles—feeling each lobe and the isthmus of the gland for characteristics of goitre or nodules and examining cervical lymph nodes, and (ii) in front of the person, examining characteristics of the nodules and position of the trachea, which may be displaced; *Percussion* over the manubrium, dullness may indicate goitre, although CT scan is a more common procedure; *Auscultation* as a bruit may occur in Graves' disease. *Pemberton's sign* is used to evaluate venous obstruction from goitres. Ask the person to raise the arms as high as possible and wait a few moments; signs of venous congestion such as redness of the face and breathlessness occur from retrosternal extension of the thyroid gland into the thorax (Matheus & Kowdley, 2021). Also look for signs of hyper- or hypothyroidism.

CRITICAL THINKING IN PERSON-CENTRED CARE

1 What is the prevalence of malignant thyroid nodules and who has a higher risk of developing them?
2 Most people with thyroid nodules do not have any significant symptoms. But, if present, which symptoms are important to notice and what do they indicate?
3 Which clinical assessments need to be attended when examining the thyroid gland of a person with suspected nodules? Which instructions would be given when assessing for the Pemberton's sign?

Translation to Practice boxes *focus on how research relates to current nursing care and application of evidence in clinical settings.*

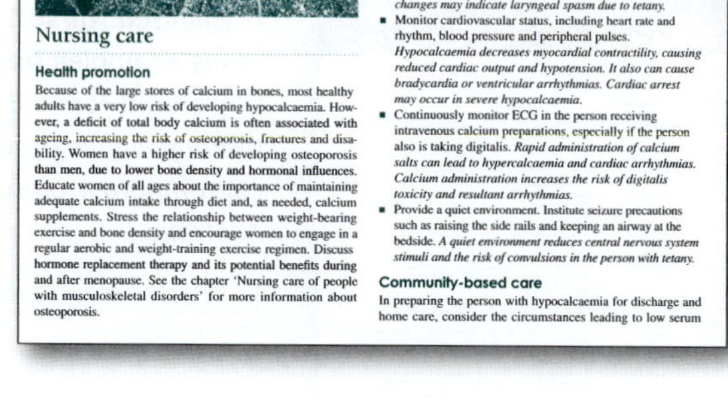

Nursing care

Health promotion

Because of the large stores of calcium in bones, most healthy adults have a very low risk of developing hypocalcaemia. However, a deficit of total body calcium is often associated with ageing, increasing the risk of osteoporosis, fractures and disability. Women have a higher risk of developing osteoporosis than men, due to lower bone density and hormonal influences. Educate women of all ages about the importance of maintaining adequate calcium intake through diet and, as needed, calcium supplements. Stress the relationship between weight-bearing exercise and bone density and encourage women to engage in a regular aerobic and weight-training exercise regimen. Discuss hormone replacement therapy and its potential benefits during and after menopause. See the chapter 'Nursing care of people with musculoskeletal disorders' for more information about osteoporosis.

inspiratory sound indicative of upper airway obstruction), or increased respiratory rate or effort, to the doctor. *These changes may indicate laryngeal spasm due to tetany.*

- Monitor cardiovascular status, including heart rate and rhythm, blood pressure and peripheral pulses. *Hypocalcaemia decreases myocardial contractility, causing reduced cardiac output and hypotension. It also can cause bradycardia or ventricular arrhythmias. Cardiac arrest may occur in severe hypocalcaemia.*
- Continuously monitor ECG in the person receiving intravenous calcium preparations, especially if the person also is taking digitalis. *Rapid administration of calcium salts can lead to hypercalcaemia and cardiac arrhythmias. Calcium administration increases the risk of digitalis toxicity and resultant arrhythmias.*
- Provide a quiet environment. Institute seizure precautions such as raising the side rails and keeping an airway at the bedside. *A quiet environment reduces central nervous system stimuli and the risk of convulsions in the person with tetany.*

Community-based care

In preparing the person with hypocalcaemia for discharge and home care, consider the circumstances leading to low serum

Nursing Care *sections detail the assessment and planning aspects relating to specific conditions and outline potential pain and risks.*

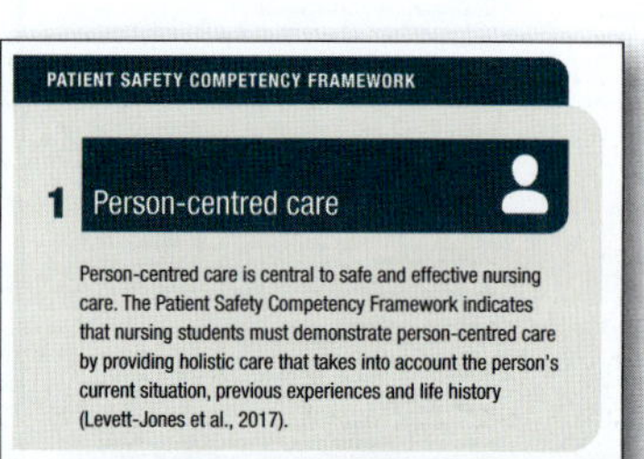

PATIENT SAFETY COMPETENCY FRAMEWORK

1 Person-centred care

Person-centred care is central to safe and effective nursing care. The Patient Safety Competency Framework indicates that nursing students must demonstrate person-centred care by providing holistic care that takes into account the person's current situation, previous experiences and life history (Levett-Jones et al., 2017).

Patient Safety Competency Framework *boxes appear in the chapters where applicable to demonstrate how concepts relate back to the skills and knowledge that underpin patient safety.*

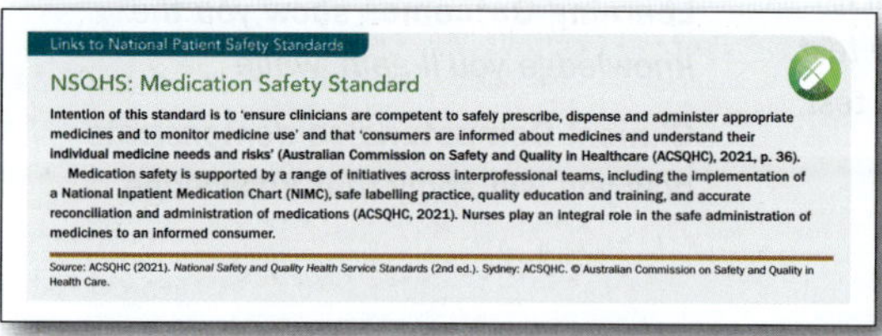

Links to National Patient Safety Standards

NSQHS: Medication Safety Standard

Intention of this standard is to 'ensure clinicians are competent to safely prescribe, dispense and administer appropriate medicines and to monitor medicine use' and that 'consumers are informed about medicines and understand their individual medicine needs and risks' (Australian Commission on Safety and Quality in Healthcare (ACSQHC), 2021, p. 36).

Medication safety is supported by a range of initiatives across interprofessional teams, including the implementation of a National Inpatient Medication Chart (NIMC), safe labelling practice, quality education and training, and accurate reconciliation and administration of medications (ACSQHC, 2021). Nurses play an integral role in the safe administration of medicines to an informed consumer.

Source: ACSQHC (2021). *National Safety and Quality Health Service Standards* (2nd ed.). Sydney: ACSQHC. © Australian Commission on Safety and Quality in Health Care.

Links to National Patient Safety Standards *boxes appear in the chapters where applicable to demonstrate how concepts relate back to patient safety standards.*

FAST FACTS

- Older people have the highest rate of illness and surgical procedures associated with pain; they also have the highest rate of complications associated with surgical interventions.
- Persistent pain is common in older adults. For those over 70 years of age, 50% of those living in the community and 80% of those in residential care suffer persistent pain.
- Musculoskeletal pain affecting major joints and back, or neuropathic pain from diabetic neuropathy and post-herpetic neuralgia have an increased prevalence in the ageing population.
- Concurrent illnesses are common in the elderly, making clinical presentation complex and sometimes difficult.
- Cognitive impairment enhances the risk of poor pain control, negatively influencing the individual's quality of life.

Sources: ANZCA (2020). *Acute pain management: Scientific evidence* (5th ed.). Melbourne: Australian and New Zealand College of Anaesthetists; Youngcharoen (2022). A cross-sectional study of factors associated with nurses' postoperative pain management practices for older patients. *Nursing Open*. https://doi.org/10.1002/nop2.1281

Fast Facts boxes *highlight and summarise important data about the prevalence and incidence of selected disorders in Australia, and of other featured content.*

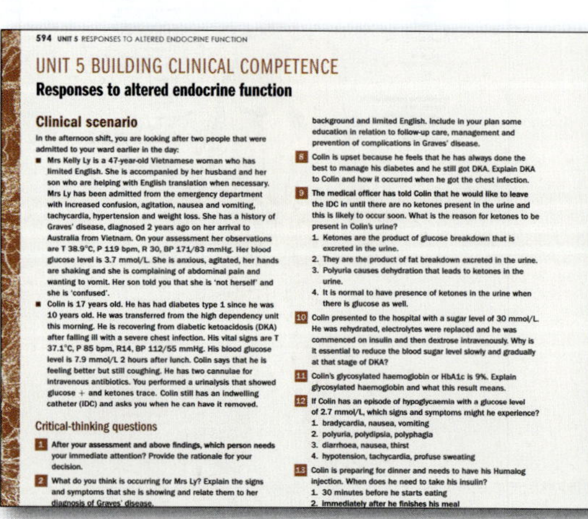

594 UNIT 5 RESPONSES TO ALTERED ENDOCRINE FUNCTION

UNIT 5 BUILDING CLINICAL COMPETENCE

Responses to altered endocrine function

Clinical scenario

In the afternoon shift, you are looking after two people that were admitted to your ward earlier in the day:

- Mrs Kelly Ly is a 47-year-old Vietnamese woman who has limited English. She is accompanied by her husband and her son who are helping with English translation when necessary. Mrs Ly has been admitted from the emergency department with increased confusion, agitation, nausea and vomiting, tachycardia, hypertension and weight loss. She has a history of Graves' disease, diagnosed 2 years ago on her arrival to Australia from Vietnam. On your assessment her observations are T 38.9°C, P 119 bpm, R 30, BP 171/83 mmHg. Her blood glucose level is 3.7 mmol/L. She is anxious, agitated, her hands are shaking and she is complaining of abdominal pain and wanting to vomit. Her son told you that she is 'not herself' and she is 'confused'.
- Colin is 17 years old. He has had diabetes type 1 since he was 10 years old. He was transferred from the high dependency unit this morning. He is recovering from diabetic ketoacidosis (DKA) after falling ill with a severe chest infection. His vital signs are T 37.1°C, P 85 bpm, R14, BP 112/55 mmHg. His blood glucose level is 7.9 mmol/L 2 hours after lunch. Colin says that he is feeling better but still coughing. He has two cannulae for intravenous antibiotics. You performed a urinalysis that showed glucose + and ketones trace. Colin still has an indwelling catheter (IDC) and asks you when he can have it removed.

Critical-thinking questions

1 After your assessment and above findings, which person needs your immediate attention? Provide the rationale for your decision.
2 What do you think is occurring for Mrs Ly? Explain the signs and symptoms that she is showing and relate them to her diagnosis of Graves' disease.

background and limited English. Include in your plan some education in relation to follow-up care, management and prevention of complications in Graves' disease.

8 Colin is upset because he feels that he has always done the best to manage his diabetes and he still got DKA. Explain DKA to Colin and how it occurred when he got the chest infection.
9 The medical officer has told Colin that he would like to leave the IDC in until there are no ketones present in the urine and this is likely to occur soon. What is the reason for ketones to be present in Colin's urine?
   1. Ketones are the product of glucose breakdown that is excreted in the urine.
   2. They are the product of fat breakdown excreted in the urine.
   3. Polyuria causes dehydration that leads to ketones in the urine.
   4. It is normal to have presence of ketones in the urine when there is glucose as well.
10 Colin presented to the hospital with a sugar level of 30 mmol/L. He was rehydrated, electrolytes were replaced and he was commenced on insulin and then dextrose intravenously. Why is it essential to reduce the blood sugar level slowly and gradually at that stage of DKA?
11 Colin's glycosylated haemoglobin or HbA1c is 9%. Explain glycosylated haemoglobin and what this result means.
12 If Colin has an episode of hypoglycaemia with a glucose level of 2.7 mmol/L, which signs and symptoms might he experience?
   1. bradycardia, nausea, vomiting
   2. polyuria, polydipsia, polyphagia
   3. diarrhoea, nausea, thirst
   4. hypotension, tachycardia, profuse sweating
13 Colin is preparing for dinner and needs to have his Humalog injection. When does he need to take his insulin?
   1. 30 minutes before he starts eating
   2. Immediately after he finishes his meal

An end-of-unit review for each of the units, called **Building Clinical Competence**, *synthesises what you have learned in the unit and applies the knowledge to specific cases. The feature includes:*

- *A* **clinical scenario** *involving a priority issue reflection piece that synthesises the underlying concepts and includes a variety of questions that allow students to apply different skills.*
- *A* **case study** *with concept map that further synthesises material using the nursing process.*

Educator support

A suite of resources is provided to assist with delivery of the text, as well as to support teaching and learning.

Solutions Manual

The Solutions Manual provides educators with detailed, accuracy-verified solutions to in-chapter and end-of-chapter problems in the text.

Test Bank

The Test Bank provides a wealth of accuracy-verified testing material. Updated for the new edition, each chapter offers a wide variety of question types, arranged by learning objective and tagged by NMBA Standards.

Questions can be integrated into Blackboard, Canvas and Moodle Learning Management Systems.

Digital Image Powerpoint slides

All the diagrams and tables from the text are available for lecturer use.

Mapping to the NMBA (2016) *Registered Nurse Standards for Practice*

AUTHOR: Trish Burton

CHAPTER	STANDARD	CRITERIA	EVIDENCE-BASED EXAMPLES (INCLUDING PAGE NO.)
Unit 9 Responses to altered respiratory function			
33 A person-centred approach to assessing the respiratory system	1. Thinks critically and analyses nursing practice	1.6. Maintains accurate, comprehensive and timely documentation of assessments, planning, decision-making, actions and evaluations	Documents a health history for a person with an alteration in respiratory function, in Sample documentation, p. 1200
	2. Engages in therapeutic and professional relationships	2.6. Uses delegation, supervision, coordination, consultation and referrals in professional relationships to achieve improved health outcomes	Consults doctor in relation to health history findings and subsequent management for a person with an alteration in respiratory function, in Sample documentation, p. 1200
	4. Comprehensively conducts assessments	4.1. Conducts assessments that are holistic as well as culturally appropriate	Conducts a health history for a person with an alteration in respiratory function, in Sample documentation, p. 1200
		4.2. Uses a range of assessment techniques to systematically collect relevant and accurate information and data to inform practice	Conducts and/or assists in the collection of respiratory secretions, blood samples, tissue samples, pleural fluid, pulse oximetry and radiographical studies, in Diagnostic tests, pp. 1203–1205
			Conducts a physical assessment for a person with an alteration in the respiratory system, in Respiratory assessments, pp. 1205–1208
	6. Provides safe, appropriate and responsive quality nursing practice	6.1. Provides comprehensive, safe, quality practice to achieve agreed goals and outcomes that are responsive to the nursing needs of people	Provides related nursing care and monitors the results of diagnostic tests, in Diagnostic tests, pp. 1203–1205
34 Nursing care of people with upper respiratory disorders	4. Comprehensively conducts assessments	4.1. Conducts assessments that are holistic as well as culturally appropriate	Provides comprehensive nursing care for a person with a total laryngectomy, in Nursing care plan, p. 1239
	5. Develops a plan for nursing practice	5.1. Uses assessment data and best available evidence to develop a plan	Provides appropriate and safe nursing management of decongestants and antihistamines medication, in Medication administration, pp. 1213–1214
			Devises a teaching plan for the person with sinusitis, in Community-based care, p. 1220
			Devises a teaching plan for the person with pharyngitis or tonsillitis, in Community-based care, p. 1222
			Plans for nursing care for a person with nasal packing, in Nursing care of the person, p. 1226
			Devises a teaching plan for the person with epistaxis, in Community-based care, p. 1227
			Devises a teaching plan for the person with a nasal fracture, in Community-based care, p. 1229

CHAPTER	STANDARD	CRITERIA	EVIDENCE-BASED EXAMPLES (INCLUDING PAGE NO.)
			Plans the preoperative care and postoperative care for a person undergoing a total laryngectomy, in Nursing care of the person, p. 1236
			Provides comprehensive nursing care for a person with a total laryngectomy, in Nursing care plan, p. 1239
			Devises a teaching plan for the person with a benign laryngeal tumour, in Community-based care, p. 1242
	6. Provides safe, appropriate and responsive quality nursing practice	6.1. Provides comprehensive, safe, quality practice to achieve agreed goals and outcomes that are responsive to the nursing needs of people	Safely and knowledgeably administers decongestant and antihistamine medications, monitors contraindications, drug interactions and adverse reactions, and provides health education, in Medication administration, pp. 1213–1214
			Provides airway management and haemastasis for a person with nasal packing, in Nursing care of the person, p. 1226
			Implements preoperative care of teaching and assessment of anxiety levels, demonstrates knowledge of the purpose and outcomes of the procedure and provides postoperative care of airway management, positioning, oxygenation, fluid balance, stoma care and person and family support for a person with a total laryngectomy, in Nursing care of the person, p. 1236
			Provides safe and effective nursing care for a person with a total laryngectomy, in Nursing care plan, p. 1239
	7. Evaluates outcomes to inform nursing practice	7.1. Evaluates and monitors progress towards the expected goals and outcomes	Evaluates pain management, respiratory status, temperature, nutrition and weight for a person with a total laryngectomy, in Nursing care plan, p. 1239
35 Nursing care of people with ventilation disorders	2. Engages in therapeutic and professional relationships	2.6. Uses delegation, supervision, coordination, consultation and referrals in professional relationships to achieve improved health outcomes	Collaborates with the social worker, community team and treating doctor in providing healthcare for the person with tuberculosis, in Nursing care plan, p. 1266
	4. Comprehensively conducts assessments	4.1. Conducts assessments that are holistic as well as culturally appropriate	Uses the nursing process and evidence-based nursing research to assess the person with pneumonia, in Nursing care plan, p. 1257
			Provides a risk assessment for tuberculosis for older adults, in Nursing care of the older adult, p. 1261
			Conducts an assessment for the person with tuberculosis, in Nursing care plan, p. 1266
			Conducts an assessment for the person with lung cancer, in Nursing care plan, p. 1288
	5. Develops a plan for nursing practice	5.1. Uses assessment data and best available evidence to develop a plan	Plans nursing care for the person with for pneumonia, in Nursing care plan, p. 1257
			Devises a teaching plan for the person with pneumonia, in Community-based care, p. 1257
			Plans health education for self-managing tuberculosis, in Nursing care of the older adult, p. 1261
			Plans the care before, during and after the procedure for a person having a thoracentesis, in Nursing care of the person, p. 1270

CHAPTER	STANDARD	CRITERIA	EVIDENCE-BASED EXAMPLES (INCLUDING PAGE NO.)
			Plans the care before, during and after the procedure for a person with chest tubes, in Nursing care of the person, p. 1274
			Plans preoperative and postoperative care for the person having lung surgery, in Nursing care of the person, p. 1287
			Plans the nursing responsibilities for the person receiving radiation, in Nursing care of the person, p. 1288
			Devises a teaching plan for the person with lung cancer, in Community-based care, p. 1291
		5.2. Collaboratively constructs nursing practice plans until contingencies, options, priorities, goals, actions, outcomes and time frames are agreed with the relevant people	Constructs a nursing care plan with the community team and treating doctor, in Nursing care plan, p. 1266
			Constructs a nursing care plan with the treating doctor, oncologist and dietitian, in Nursing care plan, p. 1289
	6. Provides safe, appropriate and responsive quality nursing practice	6.1. Provides comprehensive, safe, quality practice to achieve agreed goals and outcomes that are responsive to the nursing needs of people	Provides evidence-based practice in relation to the nursing care of the person with pneumonia, in Nursing care plan, p. 1257
			Plans and provides appropriate teaching for health promotion for a person with tuberculosis, in Nursing care of the older adult, p. 1261
			Conducts education for self-managing tuberculosis, in Nursing care plan, p. 1266
			Provides appropriate care for the person having a thoracentesis, including collecting consent, positioning and establishing a sterile field before the procedure, and during and after the procedure monitoring vital signs, applying a dressing, specimen collection, respiratory assessment and obtaining a chest x-ray, in Nursing care of the person, p. 1270
			Before the procedure, provides care including collecting consent, positioning and establishing a sterile field, and after the procedure, monitors vital signs, drainage system, position changes and occlusive dressing application for the person having chest tubes, in Nursing care of the person, p. 1274
			Provides appropriate preoperative care of assessment, emotional and psychological support and education and postoperative care of pain management, respiratory assessment, airway management, chest tube drainage, monitoring vital signs, positioning and maintaining nutrition for the person having lung surgery, in Nursing care of the person, p. 1287
			Monitors complications, fluid intake, pain levels and food intake, and provides health education for the person receiving radiation therapy, in Nursing care of the person, p. 1288
			Conducts education for the person and family in relation to the signs and symptoms of lung cancer, chemotherapy, nutrition, cessation of smoking and community support, in Nursing care plan, p. 1289

CHAPTER	STANDARD	CRITERIA	EVIDENCE-BASED EXAMPLES (INCLUDING PAGE NO.)
	7. Evaluates outcomes to inform nursing practice	7.1. Evaluates and monitors progress towards the expected goals and outcomes	Evaluates the effectiveness of nursing interventions and teaching for the person with pneumonia, in Nursing care plan, p. 1258
			Evaluates the outcomes of health teaching for the person with tuberculosis, in Nursing care plan, p. 1266
		7.3. Determines, documents and communicates further priorities, goals and outcomes with the relevant persons	Evaluates the outcomes of chemotherapy and assists the person with the next planning stage of palliative care, in Nursing care plan, p. 1289
36 Nursing care of people with gas exchange disorders	4. Comprehensively conducts assessments	4.1. Conducts assessments that are holistic as well as culturally appropriate	Assesses the person requiring medication for asthma, in Medication administration, pp. 1303–1304
			Undertakes a comprehensive health assessment for a person with COPD, in Nursing care plan, p. 1316
			Assesses the person requiring neuromuscular blocker medication, in Medication administration, p. 1335
			Includes evidence-based practice in relation to the assessment of the person with ARDS, in Nursing care plan, p. 1349
	5. Develops a plan for nursing practice	5.1. Uses assessment data and best available evidence to develop a plan	Plans the nursing management of medication for asthma, in Medication administration, pp. 1303–1304
			Devises a teaching plan for the person with asthma, in Community-based care, pp. 1307–1308
			Develops a nursing care plan for a person with COPD, in Nursing care plan, pp. 1316–1317
			Devises a teaching plan for the person with a pulmonary embolism, in Community-based care, p. 1331
			Plans for the safe nursing management of neuromuscular blocker medication, in Medication administration, p. 1335
			Uses data and knowledge of the effects of ARDS and prescribed treatment to identify priority nursing diagnoses and to plan care for a person with ARDS, in Nursing care plan, p. 1349
	6. Provides safe, appropriate and responsive quality nursing practice	6.1. Provides comprehensive, safe, quality practice to achieve agreed goals and outcomes that are responsive to the nursing needs of people	Administers prescribed oral and inhalation medications for asthma and monitors contraindications, desired effects, adverse effects, blood tests, drug therapeutic blood levels and drug interactions and provides health education in Medication administration, pp. 1303–1304
			Provides comprehensive nursing care for a person with COPD, in Nursing care plan, pp. 1316–1317
			Administers prescribed intravenous medications for the person requiring mechanical ventilation, monitors oxygenation and provides adjunct care, in Medication administration, p. 1335
			Uses evidence-based nursing research to implement individualised nursing care for individuals with ARDS, in Nursing care plan, p. 1349

CHAPTER	STANDARD	CRITERIA	EVIDENCE-BASED EXAMPLES (INCLUDING PAGE NO.)
	7. Evaluates outcomes to inform nursing practice	7.1. Evaluates and monitors progress towards the expected goals and outcomes	Evaluates the effectiveness of nursing interventions and teaching for a patient with COPD, in Nursing care plan, p. 1317 Evaluates the effectiveness of nursing interventions for a patient with ARDS, in Nursing care plan, p. 1349
Unit 10 Responses to altered musculoskeletal function			
37 A person-centred approach to assessing the musculoskeletal system	4. Comprehensively conducts assessments	4.1. Conducts assessments that are holistic as well as culturally appropriate	Conducts a health history for a person with an alteration in musculoskeletal function, in Functional health pattern interview, p. 1365
		4.2. Uses a range of assessment techniques to systematically collect relevant and accurate information and data to inform practice	Conducts and/or assists in the collection of blood samples, tissue samples, synovial fluid, radiographical studies, electrical activity and nerve conduction, in Diagnostic tests, pp. 1368–1369 Conducts a physical assessment of the musculoskeletal system, in Musculoskeletal assessments, pp. 1370–1374
	6. Provides safe, appropriate and responsive quality nursing practice	6.1. Provides comprehensive, safe, quality practice to achieve agreed goals and outcomes that are responsive to the nursing needs of people	Provides related nursing care and monitors the results of diagnostic tests, in Diagnostic tests, pp. 1368–1369
38 Nursing care of people with musculoskeletal trauma	2. Engages in therapeutic and professional relationships	2.6. Uses delegation, supervision, coordination, consultation and referrals in professional relationships to achieve improved health outcomes	Collaborates with the social worker in the development of a nursing care plan for a person with a below-the-knee amputation, in Nursing care plan, p. 1403 Coordinates the interprofessional care, including the social worker, physiotherapist, occupational therapist, prosthetist and home nurses, of the person with an amputation, in Meeting individualised needs, p. 1405
	4. Comprehensively conducts assessments	4.1. Conducts assessments that are holistic as well as culturally appropriate	When caring for a person with a hip fracture, carries out the processes involved in the assessment phase, in Nursing care plan, p. 1396 When caring for a person with a below-the-knee amputation, carries out assessment, in Nursing care plan, p. 1403 Assesses the home environment and acceptance of diagnosis of the person with an amputation, in Meeting individualised needs, p. 1405
	5. Develops a plan for nursing practice	5.1. Uses assessment data and best available evidence to develop a plan	Plans safe nursing management of a cast, in Nursing care of the person, p. 1388 Plans health education for self-prevention of falls, in Nursing care of the older adult, p. 1395 Determines priority nursing diagnoses based on assessed data for a person with a hip fracture, in Nursing care plan, p. 1396 Plans for health teaching of the person with an amputation, in Meeting individualised needs, pp. 1405–1406

CHAPTER	STANDARD	CRITERIA	EVIDENCE-BASED EXAMPLES (INCLUDING PAGE NO.)
	6. Provides safe, appropriate and responsive quality nursing practice	6.1. Provides comprehensive, safe, quality practice to achieve agreed goals and outcomes that are responsive to the nursing needs of people	Performs assessments, monitors for complications and provides health education for the person with a cast, in Nursing care of the person, p. 1388 When caring for a person with a hip fracture, carries out interventions that specifically address the person's postoperative needs, in Nursing care plan, p. 1396 Implements targeted nursing interventions that address the person with a below-the-knee amputation, in Nursing care plan, p. 1403 Provides appropriate teaching for the person with an amputation, in Meeting individualised needs, pp. 1405–1406
	7. Evaluates outcomes to inform nursing practice	7.1. Evaluates and monitors progress towards the expected goals and outcomes	When caring for a person with a hip fracture, evaluates postoperative management, in Nursing care plan, p. 1396 Evaluates postoperative management of a person with a below-the-knee amputation, in Nursing care plan, p. 1403
39 Nursing care of people with musculoskeletal disorders	2. Engages in therapeutic and professional relationships	2.6. Uses delegation, supervision, coordination, consultation and referrals in professional relationships to achieve improved health outcomes	Collaborates with the physiotherapist in providing preoperative and postoperative care, in Nursing care plan, p. 1435
	4. Comprehensively conducts assessments	4.1. Conducts assessments that are holistic as well as culturally appropriate	Conducts a health history for the person with osteoporosis, in Nursing care plan, p. 1416 When caring for a person with osteoarthritis, completes a health history and physical examination, in Nursing care plan, p. 1435 Conducts a health history and physical assessment for a person with rheumatoid arthritis, in Nursing care plan, p. 1446
	5. Develops a plan for nursing practice	5.1. Uses assessment data and best available evidence to develop a plan	Develops a plan for nursing management and health education of medication for a person with osteoporosis, in Medication administration, pp. 1415–1416 Determines nursing diagnoses, based on assessed data, to plan individualised nursing interventions for a person with osteoporosis, in Nursing care plan, p. 1416 Develops a plan for nursing management and health education of medication for a person with Paget's disease, in Medication administration, p. 1421 Develops a plan for nursing management and health education of medication for a person with gout, in Medication administration, p. 1425 Plans preoperative and postoperative care for the person having a total joint replacement, in Nursing care of the person, pp. 1433–1434 Provides a teaching plan appropriate for community-based self-care of rheumatoid arthritis, in Nursing care plan, p. 1446 Develops a plan for nursing management and health education of medication for a person requiring immunosuppressive agents for SLE, in Medication administration, p. 1453

CHAPTER	STANDARD	CRITERIA	EVIDENCE-BASED EXAMPLES (INCLUDING PAGE NO.)
			Devises a teaching plan for the person with SLE, in Community-based care, p. 1455
			Plans preoperative and postoperative care for the surgical debridement for osteomyelitis, in Nursing care of the person, p. 1458
			Provides a teaching plan appropriate for self-care of scoliosis and kyphosis, in Community-based care, p. 1470
		5.2. Collaboratively constructs nursing practice plans until contingencies, options, priorities, goals, actions, outcomes and time frames are agreed with the relevant people	Integrates interprofessional care into care of a person with osteoarthritis, in Nursing care plan, pp. 1416–1417
	6. Provides safe, appropriate and responsive quality nursing practice	6.1. Provides comprehensive, safe, quality practice to achieve agreed goals and outcomes that are responsive to the nursing needs of people	Administers topical, oral and injectable medications, monitors for adverse reactions, contraindications, adverse effects, blood levels and bone density and provides health education for the person with osteoporosis, in Medication administration, pp. 1415–1416
			When caring for a person with osteoporosis, carries out the nursing interventions that specifically address the person's needs, in Nursing care plan, pp. 1416–1417
			Administers oral and intravenous medications, monitors contraindications and adverse effects and provides health education for the person with Paget's disease, in Medication administration, p. 1421
			Administers intravenous and oral medications, monitors contraindications, adverse effects, drug interactions, blood glucose levels, kidney function, urine output and full blood count and provides health education for the person with gout, in Medication administration, p. 1425
			Provides appropriate preoperative care of assessment and education and postoperative care of monitoring vital signs, neurovascular checks, wound drainage, intravenous infusions, positioning, pain management, mobilisation, prosthesis dislocation, fluid and nutritional intake for the person a total joint replacement, in Nursing care of the person, pp. 1433–1434
			When caring for a person with osteoarthritis, carries out specific nursing interventions, in Nursing care plan, p. 1435
			Conducts education for self-managing rheumatoid arthritis, in Nursing care plan, p. 1446
			Administers oral medications, monitors full blood count, renal function, liver function, urine output, abnormal bleeding, signs of infection and adverse reactions and provides health education for the person requiring immunosuppressive agents for SLE, in Medication administration, p. 1453

CHAPTER	STANDARD	CRITERIA	EVIDENCE-BASED EXAMPLES (INCLUDING PAGE NO.)
			Provides preoperative education and postoperative care of dressing and irrigation and monitoring for infection, and conducts health education for a person undergoing a surgical debridement for osteomyelitis, in Nursing care of the person, p. 1458
	7. Evaluates outcomes to inform nursing practice	7.1. Evaluates and monitors progress towards the expected goals and outcomes	Evaluates health outcomes for the person with osteoporosis, in Nursing care plan, p. 1417 When caring for a person with osteoarthritis, evaluates nursing interventions and mobility, in Nursing care plan, p. 1435 Evaluates the effectiveness of health education for the person with rheumatoid arthritis, in Nursing care plan, pp. 1446–1447
Unit 11 Responses to altered neurological function			
40 A person-centred approach to assessing the nervous system	2. Engages in therapeutic and professional relationships	2.6. Uses delegation, supervision, coordination, consultation and referrals in professional relationships to achieve improved health outcomes	Monitors the results of diagnostic tests and reports abnormal findings, in Diagnostic tests, pp. 1490–1493
	4. Comprehensively conducts assessments	4.1. Conducts assessments that are holistic as well as culturally appropriate	Conducts a health history for a person with an alteration in neurological function, in Functional health pattern interview, pp. 1488–1489
		4.2. Uses a range of assessment techniques to systematically collect relevant and accurate information and data to inform practice	Conducts and/or assists in the collection of CSF fluid, radiographical studies, blood flow, electrical activity and nerve conduction, in Diagnostic tests, pp. 1490–1493 Conducts a physical assessment of the neurological system, in Neurological assessments, Reflex assessments and Special neurological assessments, pp. 1494–1501
	6. Provides safe, appropriate and responsive quality nursing practice	6.1. Provides comprehensive, safe, quality practice to achieve agreed goals and outcomes that are responsive to the nursing needs of people	Provides related nursing care and monitors the results of diagnostic tests, in Diagnostic tests, pp. 1490–1493
41 Nursing care of people with intracranial disorders	2. Engages in therapeutic and professional relationships	2.6. Uses delegation, supervision, coordination, consultation and referrals in professional relationships to achieve improved health outcomes	Communicates nursing assessment of the person with a migraine headache to the doctor, in Nursing care plan, p. 1524 Reports seizure activity and decreasing LOC for the person with bacterial meningitis, in Nursing care plan, p. 1544
	4. Comprehensively conducts assessments	4.1. Conducts assessments that are holistic as well as culturally appropriate	Takes a health history for the person with a migraine headache, in Nursing care plan, p. 1524 Completes a health history for the person with a seizure disorder, in Nursing care plan, p. 1529 Assesses the deteriorating patient with a subdural haematoma, in Nursing care plan, p. 1538 Conducts a nursing assessment for a person with bacterial meningitis, in Nursing care plan, p. 1544 Conducts an initial assessment of the person with a brain tumour, in Nursing care plan, p. 1550

CHAPTER	STANDARD	CRITERIA	EVIDENCE-BASED EXAMPLES (INCLUDING PAGE NO.)
	5. Develops a plan for nursing practice	5.1. Uses assessment data and best available evidence to develop a plan	Plans safe nursing management of medication for a person with increased intracranial pressure, in Medication administration, p. 1515
			Plans safe nursing management of medication for a person with headaches, in Medication administration, pp. 1521–1522
			Plans safe nursing management of medication for a person with seizures, in Medication administration, p. 1528
			Plans safe nursing management for a person with seizures who is having surgery, in Nursing care of the person, p. 1528
			Plans appropriate teaching to facilitate community-based care to promote safety and prevent injury and to provide information and support necessary long-term care of a person with a seizure disorder, in Nursing care plan, p. 1529
			Plans safe nursing management of a person with a subdural haematoma, in Nursing care plan, p. 1538
			Plans for comprehensive nursing care for a person with bacterial meningitis, in Nursing care plan, p. 1544
			Determines priority nursing diagnoses, based on assessed data, to select and implement individualised nursing interventions for a person with a brain tumour, in Nursing care plan, p. 1550
		5.2. Collaboratively constructs nursing practice plans until contingencies, options, priorities, goals, actions, outcomes and time frames are agreed with the relevant people	Integrates interprofessional care into care of a person with a migraine headache, in Nursing care plan, p. 1524
	6. Provides safe, appropriate and responsive quality nursing practice	6.1. Provides comprehensive, safe, quality practice to achieve agreed goals and outcomes that are responsive to the nursing needs of people	Administers intravenous medications safely and monitors vital signs, central venous pressure, pulmonary artery pressure, adverse effects, neurological status, renal function and electrolytes for the person who has increased intracranial pressure, in Medication administration, p. 1515
			Administers oral medications, monitors vital signs, serum glucose, full blood count, electrolytes, liver function, renal function, contraindications, adverse effects and weight and provides health education for the person with headaches, in Medication administration, pp. 1521–1522
			Conducts health education for the person with a migraine headache, in Nursing care plan, p. 1524
			Provides appropriate preoperative care of medication administration and postoperative care of administering medication for the person who has seizures and has had surgery, in Nursing care of the person, p. 1528
			Conducts education for seizure disorder, in Nursing care plan, p. 1529

CHAPTER	STANDARD	CRITERIA	EVIDENCE-BASED EXAMPLES (INCLUDING PAGE NO.)
			Provides skilled care to a person with a subdural haematoma, in Nursing care plan, p. 1538
			Provides comprehensive nursing care for a person with bacterial meningitis, in Nursing care plan, p. 1544
			Implements interventions that specifically address the person's needs, in Nursing care plan, p. 1550
	7. Evaluates outcomes to inform nursing practice	7.1. Evaluates and monitors progress towards the expected goals and outcomes	Evaluates the health education outcomes for the person with a migraine headache, in Nursing care plan, p. 1524
			Evaluates the health education outcomes for the person with a seizure disorder, in Nursing care plan, p. 1529
			Evaluates the nursing management of a person with a subdural haematoma, in Nursing care plan, p. 1538
			Evaluates the nursing care for a person with bacterial meningitis, in Nursing care plan, p. 1544
			Evaluates the preoperative care outcomes for the person with a brain tumour, in Nursing care plan, p. 1550
		7.3. Determines, documents and communicates further priorities, goals and outcomes with the relevant persons	Reports a deteriorating patient with a subdural haematoma, in Nursing care plan, p. 1538
42 Nursing care of people with cerebrovascular and spinal cord disorders	4. Comprehensively conducts assessments	4.1. Conducts assessments that are holistic as well as culturally appropriate	Conducts a health history and physical assessment for a person with a stroke, in Nursing care plan, pp. 1563–1564
			Assesses the person with an SCI, in Nursing care plan, p. 1579
	5. Develops a plan for nursing practice	5.1. Uses assessment data and best available evidence to develop a plan	Plans the safe nursing management of a person with a carotid endarterectomy, in Nursing care of the person, p. 1562
			Plans targeted nursing care for the person with a stroke, in Nursing care plan, p. 1564
			Plans nursing management of medication and health education for a person requiring antispasmodics for a spinal cord injury, in Medication administration, p. 1577
		5.2. Collaboratively constructs nursing practice plans until contingencies, options, priorities, goals, actions, outcomes and time frames are agreed with the relevant people	Determines priority nursing diagnoses, based on assessed data, to select and implement individualised nursing interventions for a person with an SCI, in Nursing care plan, p. 1579
			Plans the safe nursing management of a person having a posterior laminectomy, in Nursing care of the person, pp. 1586–1587
			Plans teaching to facilitate self-care of a ruptured intervertebral disc, in Meeting individualised needs, p. 1588

CHAPTER	STANDARD	CRITERIA	EVIDENCE-BASED EXAMPLES (INCLUDING PAGE NO.)
	6. Provides safe, appropriate and responsive quality nursing practice	6.1. Provides comprehensive, safe, quality practice to achieve agreed goals and outcomes that are responsive to the nursing needs of people	Provides postoperative care, including positioning and focused assessments for monitoring complications, for a person with a carotid endarterectomy, in Nursing care of the person, p. 1562 Provides appropriate nursing interventions for a person with a stroke, in Nursing care plan, p. 1564 Administers oral medications, assesses responses to therapy and provides health education for a person requiring antispasmodics for a spinal cord injury, in Medication administration, p. 1577 Provides care for the halo fixation device and monitors neuromuscular function and skin integrity for a person with a halo fixation device, in Nursing care of the person, p. 1579 When caring for a person with an SCI, implements nursing care that specifically address the person's needs, in Nursing care plan, p. 1579 Provides appropriate preoperative teaching and postoperative care of positioning, monitoring nerve root compression, haematoma, pain, cerebrospinal fluid, urinary retention, pain and infection and mobilisation for the person who is having a posterior laminectomy, in Nursing care of the person, pp. 1586–1587 Conducts education for self-managing a ruptured intervertebral disc, in Meeting individualised needs, p. 1588
	7. Evaluates outcomes to inform nursing practice	7.1. Evaluates and monitors progress towards the expected goals and outcomes	Evaluates functional outcomes for the person with a stroke, in Nursing care plan, p. 1564 Evaluates the expected outcomes for the person with a SCI, in Nursing care plan, pp. 1579–1580
43 Nursing care of people with neurological disorders	2. Engages in therapeutic and professional relationships	2.6. Uses delegation, supervision, coordination, consultation and referrals in professional relationships to achieve improved health outcomes	Collaborates with the community nurse in caring for a person with Alzheimer's disease, in Nursing care plan, p. 1599
	4. Comprehensively conducts assessments	4.1. Conducts assessments that are holistic as well as culturally appropriate	Assesses the person with Alzheimer's disease, in Nursing care plan, p. 1599 Assesses the person with multiple sclerosis, in Nursing care plan, p. 1610 Assesses the person with Parkinson's disease, in Nursing care plan, p. 1616 Conducts a physical examination of the person with myasthenia gravis, in Nursing care plan, p. 1629
	5. Develops a plan for nursing practice	5.1. Uses assessment data and best available evidence to develop a plan	Plans nursing management of medication for the person with Alzheimer's disease, in Medication administration, p. 1598 Plans health-education-based care for the person with Alzheimer's disease, in Nursing care plan, p. 1599 Plans risk of falls assessment and safety education for the person with Alzheimer's disease, in Meeting individualised needs, p. 1600

CHAPTER	STANDARD	CRITERIA	EVIDENCE-BASED EXAMPLES (INCLUDING PAGE NO.)
			Plans nursing management of medication for the person with multiple sclerosis, in Medication administration, p. 1608
			Uses evidence-based research to design nursing interventions specific to the needs of the person with multiple sclerosis, in Nursing care plan, p. 1610
			Plans nursing management of medication for the person with Parkinson's disease, in Medication administration, pp. 1614–1615
			Plans nursing interventions specific to the needs of the person with Parkinson's disease, in Nursing care plan, pp. 1616–1617
			Devises a teaching plan for the person with Parkinson's disease, in Community-based care, p. 1619
			Plans nursing management of medication for the person with myasthenia gravis, in Medication administration, p. 1627
			Plans the preoperative and postoperative nursing care for a person having a thymectomy, in Nursing care of the person, p. 1627
			Plans pre-procedure care and care during and after the procedure for a person having plasmapheresis, in Nursing care of the person, p. 1628
			Determines priority nursing diagnoses, based on assessed data, to select and implement individualised nursing interventions for a person with myasthenia gravis, in Nursing care plan, p. 1629
			Plans postoperative care for the person having a percutaneous rhizotomy, in Nursing care of the person, p. 1634
			Plans teaching for home care for the person with trigeminal neuralgia, in Meeting individualised needs, p. 1635
	6. Provides safe, appropriate and responsive quality nursing practice	6.1. Provides comprehensive, safe, quality practice to achieve agreed goals and outcomes that are responsive to the nursing needs of people	Administers oral medications safely, including monitoring liver function, gastrointestinal bleeding and ulcer pain, adverse reactions and response to therapy, for the person with Alzheimer's disease, in Medication administration, p. 1598
			Provides health education to the person with Alzheimer's disease and the family, in Nursing care plan, pp. 1599–1600
			Conducts safety interventions for the person with Alzheimer's disease, in Meeting individualised needs, p. 1600
			Administers oral medications safely, including monitoring adverse reactions, full blood count, liver function, contraindications, muscle strength, renal function and bleeding, and provides health teaching for the person with multiple sclerosis, in Medication administration, p. 1608

CHAPTER	STANDARD	CRITERIA	EVIDENCE-BASED EXAMPLES (INCLUDING PAGE NO.)
			Implements nursing care, including referral to the physiotherapist, occupational therapist and urologist, for the person with multiple sclerosis, in Nursing care plan, p. 1610
			Administers oral medications safely, including monitoring functional status, adverse reactions, drug interactions, blood pressure, liver function and contraindications, and provides health teaching for the person with Parkinson's disease, in Medication administration, pp. 1614–1615
			Implements nursing care, including referral to the speech therapist, dietitian, physiotherapist and occupational therapist, for the person with Parkinson's disease, in Nursing care plan, p. 1617
			Administers oral and parenteral medications safely, including monitoring functional status, response to medication and adverse reactions, and provides health teaching for the person with myasthenia gravis, in Medication administration, p. 1627
			Provides appropriate preoperative teaching and postoperative respiratory care and pain management for the person who is having a thymectomy, in Nursing care of the person, p. 1627
			Provides pre-procedure care of education and assessment and post-procedure monitoring of access site for infection and bleeding, electrolytes and full blood count for a person having plasmapheresis, in Nursing care of the person, p. 1628
			When caring for a person with myasthenia gravis, implements specific nursing interventions, in Nursing care plan, p. 1629
			Provides postoperative care of monitoring neurological function and patient education for the person who is having a percutaneous rhizotomy, in Nursing care of the person, p. 1634
			Conducts home care education for the person with trigeminal neuralgia, in Meeting individualised needs, p. 1635
	7. Evaluates outcomes to inform nursing practice	7.1. Evaluates and monitors progress towards the expected goals and outcomes	Evaluates health education outcomes for a person with Alzheimer's disease and the family, in Nursing care plan, p. 1600
			Evaluates the outcomes of multidisciplinary care for the person with multiple sclerosis, in Nursing care plan, p. 1610
			Evaluates the outcomes of multidisciplinary care for the person with Parkinson's disease, in Nursing care plan, p. 1617
			Evaluates the outcomes of nursing care for the person with myasthenia gravis, in Nursing care plan, p. 1629

CHAPTER	STANDARD	CRITERIA	EVIDENCE-BASED EXAMPLES (INCLUDING PAGE NO.)
Unit 12 Responses to altered visual and auditory function			
44 A person-centred approach to assessing the eye and ear	2. Engages in therapeutic and professional relationships	2.6. Uses delegation, supervision, coordination, consultation and referrals in professional relationships to achieve improved health outcomes	Monitors the results of visual diagnostic tests and reports abnormal findings, in Diagnostic tests, p. 1655 Monitors the results of aural diagnostic tests and reports abnormal findings, in Diagnostic tests, p. 1666
	4. Comprehensively conducts assessments	4.1. Conducts assessments that are holistic as well as culturally appropriate	Conducts a health history for a person with an alteration in visual function, in Functional health pattern interview, p. 1653 Conducts a health history for a person with an alteration in hearing function, in Functional health pattern interview, pp. 1663
		4.2. Uses a range of assessment techniques to systematically collect relevant and accurate information and data to inform practice	Conducts and/or assists in the collection of refraction, intraocular pressure and radiographical studies, in Diagnostic tests, p. 1655 Conducts a physical assessment, in Eye and vision assessments, pp. 1656–1659 Conducts and/or assists in the collection of audiometry, nerve conduction and ear pressure studies, in Diagnostic tests, p. 1666 Conducts a physical assessment, in Ear and hearing assessments, pp. 1666–1668
	6. Provides safe, appropriate and responsive quality nursing practice	6.1. Provides com-prehensive, safe, quality practice to achieve agreed goals and outcomes that are responsive to the nursing needs of people	Provides related nursing care and monitors the results of visual diagnostic tests, in Diagnostic tests, p. 1655 Provides related nursing care and monitors the results of aural diagnostic tests, in Diagnostic tests, p. 1666
45 Nursing care of people with eye and ear disorders	2. Engages in therapeutic and professional relationships	2.6. Uses delegation, supervision, coordination, consultation and referrals in professional relationships to achieve improved health outcomes	Collaborates with the social worker, in Nursing care plan, p. 1691
	4. Comprehensively conducts assessments	4.1. Conducts assessments that are holistic as well as culturally appropriate	Conducts a preoperative admission assessment for a person with glaucoma and cataracts, in Nursing care plan, p. 1690
	5. Develops a plan for nursing practice	5.1. Uses assessment data and best available evidence to develop a plan	Plans individualised evidence-based nursing interventions and education for blindness, in Nursing care of the person, pp. 1671–1672 Plans safe nursing management of a person who is having eye surgery, in Nursing care of the person, p. 1678 Plans medication management for a person with glaucoma, in Medication administration, pp. 1688–1689 Plans nursing interventions and care for a person with glaucoma and cataracts, in Nursing care plan, pp. 1690 Plans nursing management for a person who is having ear surgery, in Nursing care of the person, pp. 1704–1705 Devises a teaching plan for the person with ear disorders, in Community-based care, p. 1709

CHAPTER	STANDARD	CRITERIA	EVIDENCE-BASED EXAMPLES (INCLUDING PAGE NO.)
	6. Provides safe, appropriate and responsive quality nursing practice	6.1. Provides comprehensive, safe, quality practice to achieve agreed goals and outcomes that are responsive to the nursing needs of people	Implements nursing care for blindness, in Nursing care of the person, pp. 1671–1672 Provides preoperative care, including education, postoperative care such as wound management, positioning, pain management, monitoring complications and administering medication, and health education for the person who is having eye surgery, in Nursing care of the person, p. 1678 Administers medications via the ocular route, monitors contraindications, adverse reactions, desired effects, drug interactions, weight, eye health, vital signs and liver function and delivers health education, in Medication administration, pp. 1688–1689 Provides postoperative care, including social worker referral, for the person with glaucoma and cataracts, in Nursing care plan, pp. 1690–1691 Provides preoperative care, including education, postoperative care such as wound management, administering medication, positioning and hearing, and health education for the person who is having ear surgery, in Nursing care of the person, pp. 1704–1705
	7. Evaluates outcomes to inform nursing practice	7.1. Evaluates and monitors progress towards the expected goals and outcomes	Evaluates the postoperative outcomes for the person with glaucoma and cataracts, in Nursing care plan, p. 1691
Unit 13 Responses to altered reproductive function			
46 A person-centred approach to assessing the male and female reproductive systems	2. Engages in therapeutic and professional relationships	2.6. Uses delegation, supervision, coordination, consultation and referrals in professional relationships to achieve improved health outcomes	Monitors the results of male reproductive diagnostic tests and reports abnormal findings, in Diagnostic tests, pp. 1725–1726 Monitors the results of female reproductive diagnostic tests and reports abnormal findings, in Diagnostic tests, pp. 1736–1739
	4. Comprehensively conducts assessments	4.1. Conducts assessments that are holistic as well as culturally appropriate	Conducts a health history for a man with an alteration in the male reproductive system, in Functional health pattern interview, p. 1723 Conducts a physical assessment of the male reproductive system, in Male reproductive assessments, pp. 1726–1727 Conducts a health history for a woman with an alteration in the female reproductive system, in Functional health pattern interview, pp. 1734–1735 Conducts a physical assessment of the female reproductive system, in Female reproductive assessments, pp. 1740–1744
		4.2. Uses a range of assessment techniques to systematically collect relevant and accurate information and data to inform practice	Conducts and/or assists in the collection of blood samples and cell and tissue samples and radiographical studies for the male reproductive system, in Diagnostic tests, pp. 1725–1726 Conducts and/or assists in the collection of blood samples and cell and tissue samples and radiographical studies for the female reproductive system, in Diagnostic tests, pp. 1736–1739

CHAPTER	STANDARD	CRITERIA	EVIDENCE-BASED EXAMPLES (INCLUDING PAGE NO.)
	6. Provides safe, appropriate and responsive quality nursing practice	6.1. Provides comprehensive, safe, quality practice to achieve agreed goals and outcomes that are responsive to the nursing needs of people	Provides related nursing care and monitors the results of male reproductive diagnostic tests, in Diagnostic tests, pp. 1725–1726 Provides related nursing care and monitors the results of female reproductive diagnostic tests, in Diagnostic tests, pp. 1736–1739
47 Nursing care of men with reproductive system and breast disorders	4. Comprehensively conducts assessments	4.1. Conducts assessments that are holistic as well as culturally appropriate	Assesses the health knowledge of a man having a prostatectomy, in Nursing care of the man, p. 1761 Assesses the home environment and health management of a man with prostate cancer, in Nursing care plan, p. 1769
	5. Develops a plan for nursing practice	5.1. Uses assessment data and best available evidence to develop a plan	Develops a preoperative and postoperative plan of care for the man having a prostatectomy, in Nursing care of the man, pp. 1761–162 Plans evidence-based discharge teaching for a man after having prostate surgery, in Meeting individualised needs, p. 1763 Plans home-based health teaching for a man with prostate cancer, in Nursing care plan, p. 1769
		5.3. Documents, evaluates and modifies plans accordingly to facilitate the agreed outcomes	Revises plan of care to include a community nurse referral to restore urinary function for a man with prostate cancer post discharge, in Nursing care plan, p. 1770
	6. Provides safe, appropriate and responsive quality nursing practice	6.1. Provides comprehensive, safe, quality practice to achieve agreed goals and outcomes that are responsive to the nursing needs of people	Provides preoperative care of preoperative teaching and postoperative care of urinary irrigation, fluid balance, pain management, fluid intake post catheter removal and any specific wound management for a man undergoing prostate surgery, in Nursing care of the man, pp. 1761–1762 Conducts education using discharge instructions for men after prostate surgery for a man having a prostatectomy, in Meeting individualised needs, p. 1763 Provides focused health teaching to restore urinary function for a man with prostate cancer, in Nursing care plan, p. 1769
	7. Evaluates outcomes to inform nursing practice	7.1. Evaluates and monitors progress towards the expected goals and outcomes	Evaluates the effectiveness of home-based health teaching for a man with prostate cancer, in Nursing care plan, p. 1770
48 Nursing care of women with reproductive system and breast disorders	2. Engages in therapeutic and professional relationships	2.6. Uses delegation, supervision, coordination, consultation and referrals in professional relationships to achieve improved health outcomes	Refers the woman with cervical cancer to a social worker, in Nursing care plan, p. 1794 Refers the woman with breast cancer to a social worker, in Nursing care plan, p. 1811
	4. Comprehensively conducts assessments	4.1. Conducts assessments that are holistic as well as culturally appropriate	Conducts a physical examination and health history for a woman with cervical cancer, in Nursing care plan, p. 1794 Conducts a health history and physical examination for a woman with breast cancer, in Nursing care plan, p. 1811

CHAPTER	STANDARD	CRITERIA	EVIDENCE-BASED EXAMPLES (INCLUDING PAGE NO.)
		4.2. Uses a range of assessment techniques to systematically collect relevant and accurate information and data to inform practice	Conducts a physical assessment for a woman with endometriosis, in Nursing care plan, p. 1791
	5. Develops a plan for nursing practice	5.1. Uses assessment data and best available evidence to develop a plan	Plans the preoperative and postoperative care for a woman having a laparoscopy, in Nursing care of the woman, p. 1780
			Plans medication management for the woman with dysmenorrhoea, in Medication administration, p. 1781
			Plans the preoperative and postoperative care for a woman having a dilation and curettage, in Nursing care of the woman, p. 1782
			Plans the preoperative and postoperative care for a woman having a hysterectomy, in Nursing care of the woman, p. 1783
			Determines priority nursing diagnoses, based on assessed data, to plan individualised nursing interventions for a woman with endometriosis, in Nursing care plan, p. 1791
			Determines priority nursing diagnoses in planning individualised nursing interventions for a woman with cervical cancer, in Nursing care plan, p. 1794
			Plans medication management for a person with breast cancer, in Medication administration, p. 1808
			Plans the preoperative and postoperative care for a woman having a mastectomy, in Nursing care of the woman, p. 1809
			Plans the health education for a woman having a breast reconstruction, in Nursing care of the woman, p. 1811
			Constructs a plan of care to provide effective interventions to address the needs of a woman with breast cancer, in Nursing care plan, p. 1811
	6. Provides safe, appropriate and responsive quality nursing practice	6.1. Provides comprehensive, safe, quality practice to achieve agreed goals and outcomes that are responsive to the nursing needs of people	Provides preoperative education and postoperative care of monitoring vital signs and bleeding for a woman having a laparoscopy, in Nursing care of the woman, p. 1780
			Monitors for contraindications and provides health education for the woman with dysmenorrhoea, in Medication administration, p. 1781
			Provides preoperative education and postoperative care of monitoring bleeding and health education for a woman having a dilation and curettage, in Nursing care of the woman, p. 1782
			Provides preoperative education and nursing care, postoperative care of monitoring bleeding, vital signs, urine output, complications, wound, bowel sounds and fluid intake and health education for a woman having a hysterectomy, in Nursing care of the woman, p. 1783

CHAPTER	STANDARD	CRITERIA	EVIDENCE-BASED EXAMPLES (INCLUDING PAGE NO.)
			Implements pain management strategies and health education for the woman with endometriosis, in Nursing care plan, p. 1791
			Provides education and monitoring of intervention outcomes for the woman with cervical cancer, in Nursing care plan, p. 1794
			Administers oral medications safely, including monitoring contraindications and liver function, and provides health teaching for the woman with breast cancer, in Medication administration, p. 1808
			Provides preoperative education and nursing care and postoperative care of deep breathing, monitoring the wound, pain management, bleeding, positioning and health knowledge for a woman having a mastectomy, in Nursing care of the woman, p. 1809
			Provides health education for a woman having a breast reconstruction, in Nursing care of the woman, p. 1811
			Provides comprehensive nursing care for a woman with breast cancer, in Nursing care plan, p. 1812
	7. Evaluates outcomes to inform nursing practice	7.1. Evaluates and monitors progress towards the expected goals and outcomes	Evaluates health education outcomes and family goals for a woman with endometriosis, in Nursing care plan, p. 1791
			Evaluates the cancer treatment response, health education outcomes and psychosocial wellbeing for a woman with cervical cancer, in Nursing care plan, p. 1794
			Evaluates the cancer treatment response and health education outcomes for a woman with breast cancer, in Nursing care plan, p. 1812
49 Nursing care of people who have sexually transmitted infections	4. Comprehensively conducts assessments	4.1. Conducts assessments that are holistic as well as culturally appropriate	Conducts a health history and physical examination of the person with gonorrhoea, in Nursing care plan, p. 1831
			Conducts a health history and physical examination for the person who has syphilis, in Nursing care plan, p. 1834
	5. Develops a plan for nursing practice	5.1. Uses assessment data and best available evidence to develop a plan	Plans safe nursing management of medication for the person who has genital warts, in Medication administration, p. 1825
			Determines nursing priorities and selects and implements individualised nursing intervention for a person with gonorrhoea, in Nursing care plan, p. 1831
		5.2. Collaboratively constructs nursing practice plans until contingencies, options, priorities, goals, actions, outcomes and time frames are agreed with the relevant people	Integrates interprofessional care into care of a person with syphilis, in Nursing care plan, pp. 1834–1835

CHAPTER	STANDARD	CRITERIA	EVIDENCE-BASED EXAMPLES (INCLUDING PAGE NO.)
	6. Provides safe, appropriate and responsive quality nursing practice	6.1. Provides comprehensive, safe, quality practice to achieve agreed goals and outcomes that are responsive to the nursing needs of people	Administers topical medications as per standards, monitors mental status, vital signs and weight and provides health education to the person who has genital warts, in Medication administration, p. 1825 Provides nursing interventions for the person with gonorrhoea, in Nursing care plan, p. 1831 Provides targeted nursing care as per protocols for the person with syphilis and their sexual partners, in Nursing care plan, p. 1835
	7. Evaluates outcomes to inform nursing practice	7.1. Evaluates and monitors progress towards the expected goals and outcomes	Evaluates the response to the antibiotic and health education outcomes when caring for a person with gonorrhoea, in Nursing care plan, p. 1831 Evaluates interventions' outcomes and health education for the person who has syphilis and their sexual partners, in Nursing care plan, p. 1835
Unit 14 Special topics in medical–surgical nursing			
50 Mental healthcare in the Australian context	4. Comprehensively conducts assessments	4.1. Conducts assessments that are holistic as well as culturally appropriate	Conducts a mental state assessment of the person, in Box 50.4 Components of a mental state assessment, p. 1853
	5. Develops a plan for nursing practice	5.1. Uses assessment data and best available evidence to develop a plan	Uses an evidence-based approach to design interventions which promote Recovery, in Recovery, pp. 1850–1852
	6. Provides safe, appropriate and responsive quality nursing practice	6.1. Provides comprehensive, safe, quality practice to achieve agreed goals and outcomes that are responsive to the nursing needs of people	Implements person-centred mental health nursing care, in Recovery, pp. 1850–1852
51 Community care	4. Comprehensively conducts assessments	4.1. Conducts assessments that are holistic as well as culturally appropriate	Conducts assessments of the individual and the community, in Primary healthcare, pp. 1869–1870
	5. Develops a plan for nursing practice	5.1. Uses assessment data and best available evidence to develop a plan	Incorporates the principles of primary care in the planning of nursing care in the regional and remote setting, in Primary healthcare, pp. 1869–1870
	6. Provides safe, appropriate and responsive quality nursing practice	6.1. Provides comprehensive, safe, quality practice to achieve agreed goals and outcomes that are responsive to the nursing needs of people	Provides comprehensive nursing care for the person and the community, in Primary healthcare, pp. 1869–1870
	7. Evaluates outcomes to inform nursing practice	7.1. Evaluates and monitors progress towards the expected goals and outcomes	Evaluates health outcomes of the person and the community, in Primary healthcare, pp. 1869–1870
52 Nursing care of people in regional and remote areas of Australia	1. Thinks critically and analyses nursing practice	1.2. Practises within a professional and ethical nursing framework	Practises cultural safety, in Indigenous health considerations in regional and remote areas, p. 1883
	2. Engages in therapeutic and professional relationships	2.2. Communicates effectively and is respectful of a person's dignity, culture, values, beliefs and rights	Establishes a therapeutic relationship based on trust, in Establishing boundaries, pp. 1890–1891

CHAPTER	STANDARD	CRITERIA	EVIDENCE-BASED EXAMPLES (INCLUDING PAGE NO.)
		2.6. Uses delegation, supervision, coordination, consultation and referrals in professional relationships to achieve improved health outcomes	Consults and/or refers to specialist healthcare individuals/organisations, in Acute assessment and Emergency nursing care, pp. 1887–1890
	4. Comprehensively conducts assessments	4.1. Conducts assessments that are holistic as well as culturally appropriate	Provides culturally sensitive assessments of the person and the community as active participants, in Indigenous health considerations in regional and remote areas, p. 1883
			Conducts comprehensive assessment of the person, including referral and transfer, in Acute assessment and Emergency nursing care, pp. 1887–1890
			Provides comprehensive nursing care for a person in the community, in Establishing boundaries, pp. 1890–1891
	5. Develops a plan for nursing practice	5.1. Uses assessment data and best available evidence to develop a plan	Uses assessment findings to determine initial nursing care, referral and transfer as deemed necessary, in Acute assessment and Emergency nursing care, pp. 1887–1890
		5.2. Collaboratively constructs nursing practice plans until contingencies, options, priorities, goals, actions, outcomes and time frames are agreed with the relevant people	Plans culturally sensitive nursing care with the person and the community as active participants, in Indigenous health considerations in regional and remote areas, p. 1883
	6. Provides safe, appropriate and responsive quality nursing practice	6.1. Provides comprehensive, safe, quality practice to achieve agreed goals and outcomes that are responsive to the nursing needs of people	Provides initial nursing care as deemed necessary, in Acute assessment and Emergency nursing care, pp. 1887–1890
	7. Evaluates outcomes to inform nursing practice	7.1. Evaluates and monitors progress towards the expected goals and outcomes	Evaluates the health outcomes of the person, in Acute assessment and Emergency nursing care, pp. 1887–1890

Source: Nursing and Midwifery Board of Australia (NMBA) (2016). *Registered Nurse Standards for Practice*. © Nursing and Midwifery Board of Australia, www.nursingmidwiferyboard.gov.au/.

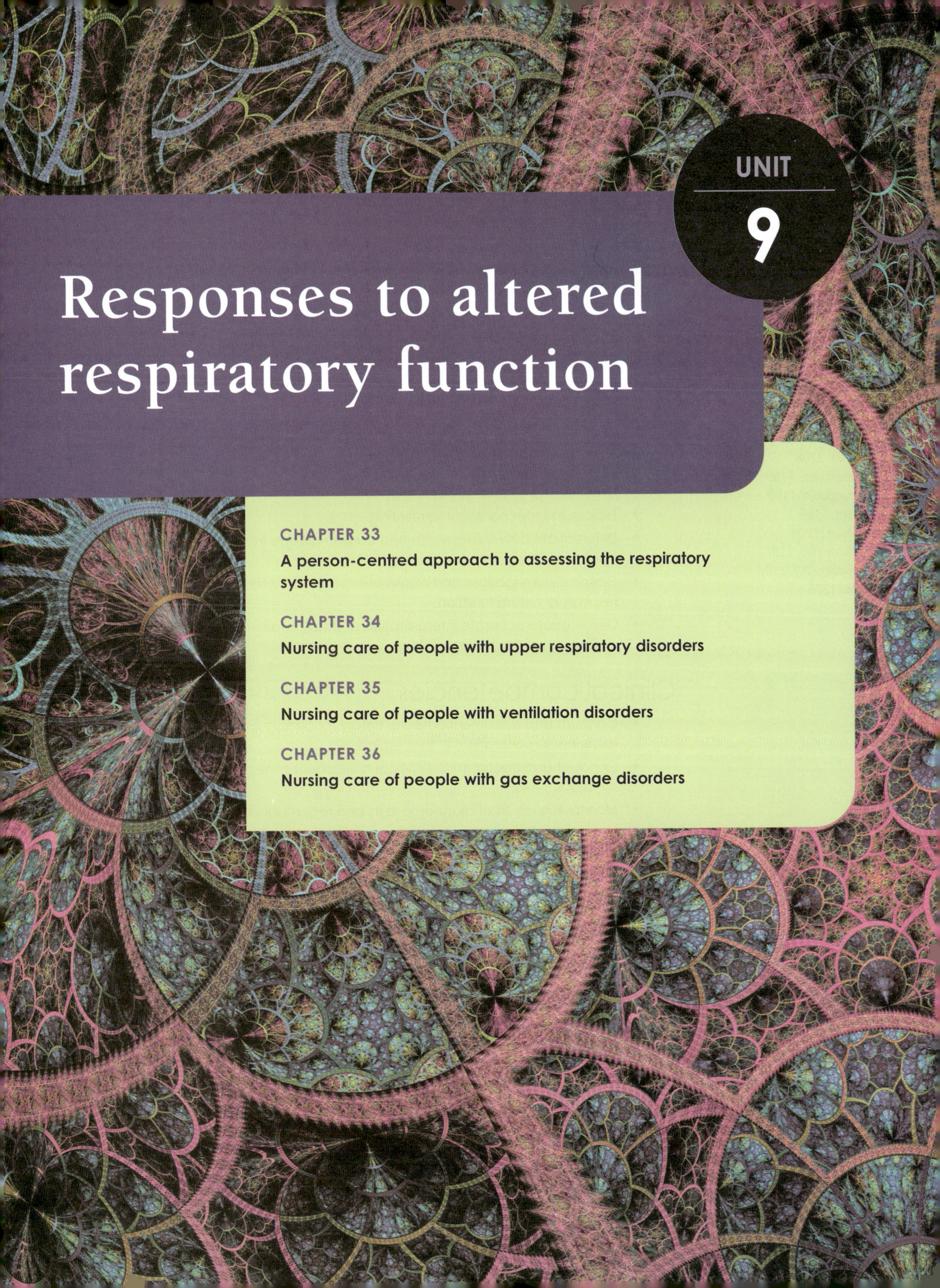

UNIT 9

Responses to altered respiratory function

CHAPTER 33

A person-centred approach to assessing the respiratory system

Allison Kloehs, Majella Hales

Key terms

Learning outcomes

- Describe the anatomy, physiology and functions of the respiratory system.
- Explain the mechanics of ventilation.
- Differentiate between oxygen and carbon dioxide transport and how affinity influences loading and unloading.
- Examine investigations and observations important for assessing a person's respiratory system function.
- Demonstrate accurate interpretation of data obtained from a person requiring review of their respiratory system.

Clinical competencies

- Conduct and document a health history for people at risk of or currently experiencing alterations in the respiratory system.
- Conduct and document a physical assessment of respiratory structures and functions.
- Monitor the results of diagnostic tests and report abnormal findings.

Equipment needed

- Tongue depressor
- Penlight
- Nasal speculum
- Metric ruler
- Marking pen
- Stethoscope with diaphragm

The respiratory system provides the cells of the body with oxygen and eliminates carbon dioxide, formed as a waste product of cellular metabolism. The events in this process, called respiration, are:

- *Pulmonary ventilation*: air is moved into and out of the lungs.
- *External respiration*: exchange of oxygen and carbon dioxide occurs between the alveoli and the blood.
- *Gas transport*: oxygen and carbon dioxide are transported to and from the lungs and the cells of the body via the blood.
- *Internal respiration*: exchange of oxygen and carbon dioxide occurs between the blood and the cells.

Anatomy, physiology and functions of the respiratory system

The respiratory system functions as a whole but is divided into the upper respiratory system and the lower respiratory system for discussion of respiratory disorders in the following chapters.

THE UPPER RESPIRATORY SYSTEM

The upper respiratory system serves as a passageway for air moving into the lungs and carbon dioxide moving out to the external environment (see Figure 33.1). As air moves through these structures, it is cleaned, humidified and warmed.

The nose

The nose is the external opening of the respiratory system. The external nose is given structure by the nasal, frontal and maxillary bones as well as by plates of hyaline cartilage. The nostrils (also called the external nares) are two cavities within the nose, separated by the nasal septum, a dividing wall that runs down the middle of the nose composed of bone and cartilage and covered by mucous membranes. These cavities open into the nasal portion of the pharynx through the internal nares. The nasal cavities just behind the nasal openings are lined with skin that contains hair follicles, sweat glands and sebaceous glands. The nasal hairs filter the air as it enters the nares. The rest of the cavity is lined with mucous membranes that contain olfactory neurons and goblet cells that secrete thick mucus. The mucus not only traps dust and bacteria but also contains lysozyme, an enzyme that destroys bacteria as they enter the nose. As mucus and debris accumulate, mucosal ciliated cells move them towards the pharynx, where they are swallowed (Dezube, 2021). The mucosa is highly vascular, warming air that moves across its surface.

Three structures project outward from the lateral wall of each nasal cavity: the superior, middle and inferior turbinates. The turbinates cause air entering the nose to become turbulent and also increase the surface area of mucosa exposed to the air. As air moves through this area, heavier particles of debris drop out and are trapped in the mucosa of the turbinates.

The sinuses

The nasal cavity is surrounded by paranasal sinuses (see Figure 33.2), located in the frontal, sphenoid, ethmoid and maxillary bones. Sinuses lighten the skull, assist in speech and produce mucus that drains into the nasal cavities to help trap debris.

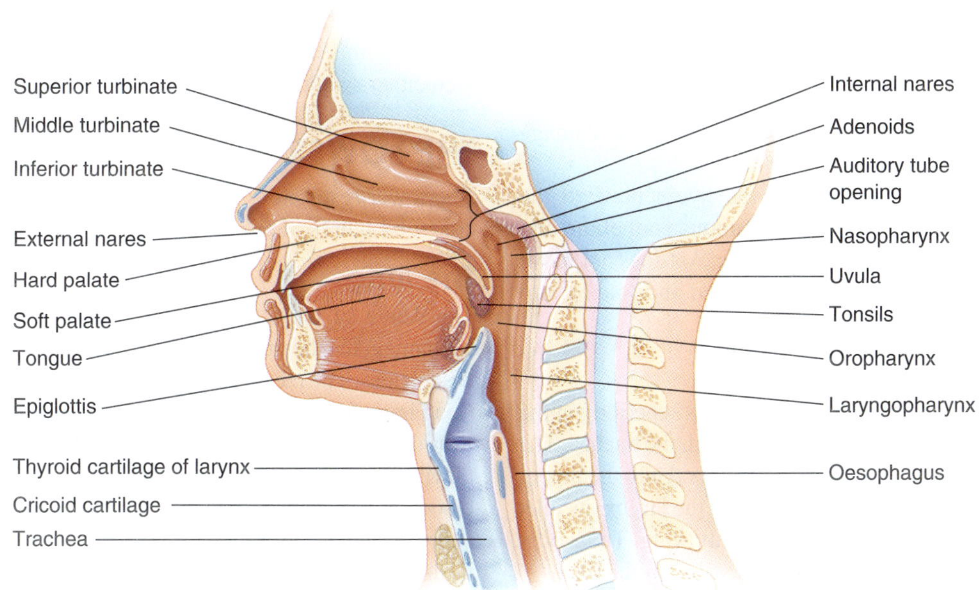

FIGURE 33.1 *The upper respiratory system*

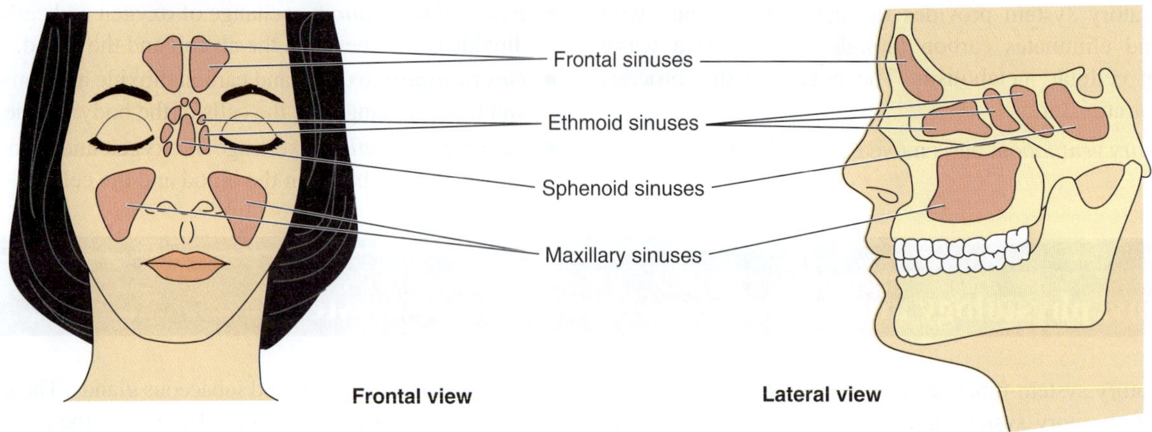

FIGURE 33.2 *Sinuses—frontal and lateral views*

The pharynx

The pharynx, a funnel-shaped passageway approximately 13 cm long, extends from the base of the skull to the level of the C6 vertebra. The pharynx serves as a passageway for both air and food. It is divided into three regions: the nasopharynx, the oropharynx and the laryngopharynx.

The nasopharynx serves only as a passageway for air. Located beneath the sphenoid bone and above the level of the soft palate, the nasopharynx is continuous with the nasal cavities. This segment is lined with ciliated epithelium, which continues to move debris from the nasal cavities to the pharynx. Masses of lymphoid tissue (the tonsils and adenoids) are located in the mucosa high in the posterior wall; these tissues trap and destroy infectious agents entering with the air (Bullock & Hales, 2019). The auditory (eustachian) tubes also open into the nasopharynx, connecting it with the middle ear.

The oropharynx lies behind the oral cavity and extends from the soft palate to the level of the hyoid bone. It serves as a passageway for both air and food. An upward rise of the soft palate prevents food from entering the nasopharynx during swallowing. The oropharynx is lined with stratified squamous epithelium that protects it from the friction of food and damage from the chemicals found in food and fluids.

The laryngopharynx extends from the hyoid bone to the larynx. It is also lined with stratified squamous epithelium and serves as a passageway for both food and air. Air does not move into the lungs while food is being swallowed and moved into the oesophagus (Marieb & Keller, 2021).

The larynx

The larynx is approximately 5 cm long. It opens superiorly at the laryngopharynx and is continuous inferiorly with the trachea. The larynx provides an airway and directs air and food into the proper passageway. As long as air is moving through the larynx, its inlet is open; however, the inlet closes during swallowing. The larynx also contains the vocal cords, necessary for voice production.

The larynx is formed by cartilages, connected by ligaments and membranes. The thyroid cartilage is formed by the fusion of two cartilages; the fusion point is visible as the Adam's apple. The cricoid cartilage lies below the thyroid cartilage; other pairs of cartilages form the walls of the larynx. The epiglottis, also a cartilage, normally projects upwards to the base of the tongue; however, during swallowing the larynx moves upwards and the epiglottis tips to cover the opening to the larynx (Tortora, 2022). If anything other than air enters the larynx, a cough reflex expels the foreign substance before it can enter the lungs. This protective reflex does not work if the person is unconscious or has a decreased level of consciousness that results in an inability to manage this reflex.

The trachea

The trachea begins at the inferior larynx and descends anteriorly to the oesophagus to enter the mediastinum, where it divides to become the right and left primary bronchi of the lungs. The trachea is approximately 12 to 15 cm long and 2.5 cm in diameter. It contains 16 to 20 C-shaped rings of cartilage joined by connective tissue. The mucosa lining the trachea consists of pseudostratified ciliated columnar epithelium-containing seromucous glands that produce thick mucus. Dust and debris in the inspired air are trapped in this mucus, moved towards the throat by the cilia and then either swallowed or coughed out through the mouth.

THE LOWER RESPIRATORY SYSTEM

The lower respiratory system includes the lungs and the bronchi (see Figures 33.3 and 33.4).

The lungs

The centre of the thoracic cavity is filled by the *mediastinum*, containing the heart, great blood vessels, bronchi, trachea and oesophagus. The mediastinum is flanked on either side by the lungs (see Figure 33.3). Each lung is suspended in its own pleural cavity, with the anterior, lateral and posterior lung surfaces lying close to the ribs. The hilus, on the mediastinal surface of each lung, is where blood vessels of the pulmonary and circulatory systems enter and exit the lungs (Tortora, 2022). The primary bronchus also enters in this area. The apex of each lung lies just below the clavicle, whereas the base of each lung rests on the diaphragm. The lungs are elastic connective tissue, called stroma, and are soft and spongy.

The two lungs differ in size and shape. The left lung is smaller and has two lobes, whereas the right lung has three

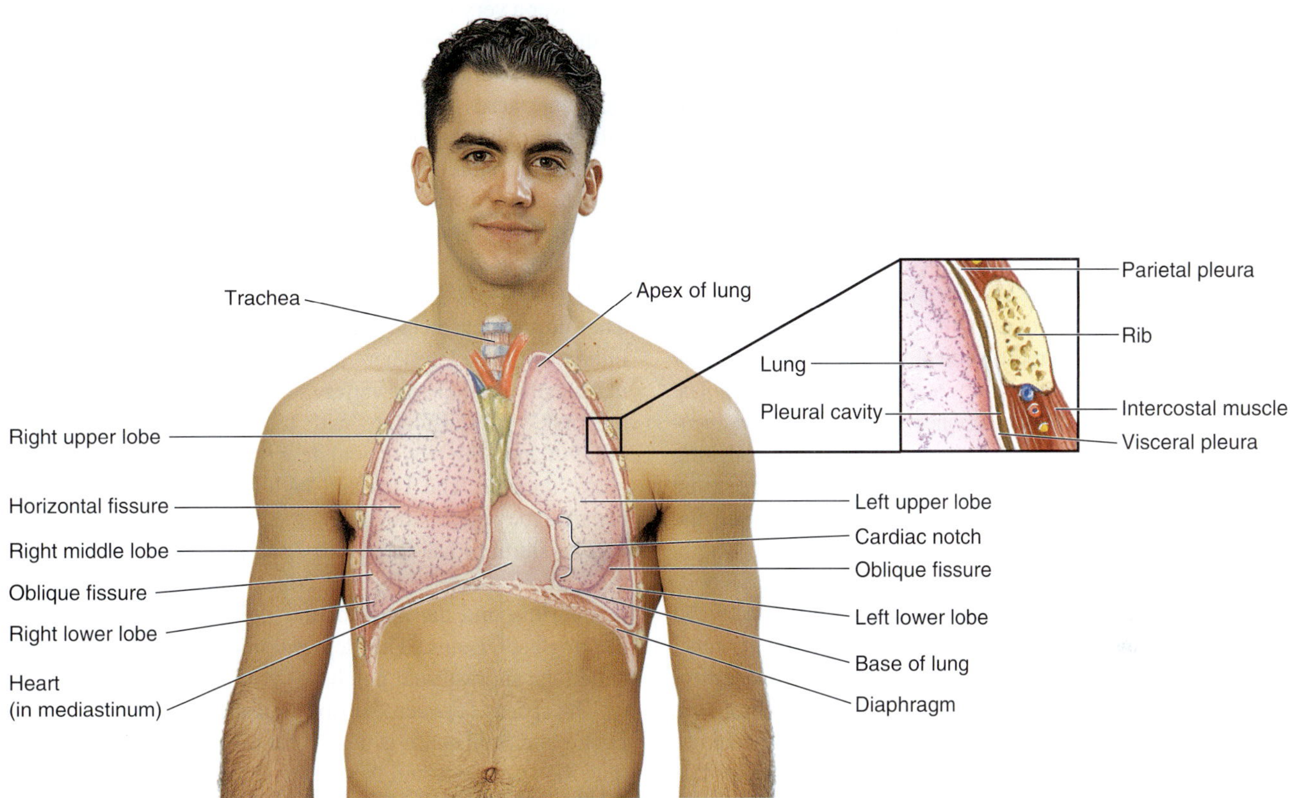

FIGURE 33.3 *The lower respiratory system, showing the location of the lungs, the mediastinum and layers of visceral and parietal pleura*

lobes. Each of the lung lobes contains a different number of bronchopulmonary segments, separated by connective tissue. There are eight segments in the two lobes of the left lung and 10 segments in the three lobes of the right lung.

The vascular system of the lungs consists of the pulmonary arteries, which deliver blood to the lungs for oxygenation, and the pulmonary veins, which deliver oxygenated blood to the heart (Tortora, 2022). Within the lungs, the pulmonary arteries branch into a pulmonary capillary network that surrounds the alveoli. Lung tissue receives its blood supply from the bronchial arteries and drains by the bronchial and pulmonary veins.

The pleura

The pleura is a double-layered membrane that covers the lungs and the inside of the thoracic cavities (see Figure 33.3). The parietal pleura lines the thoracic wall and mediastinum. It is continuous

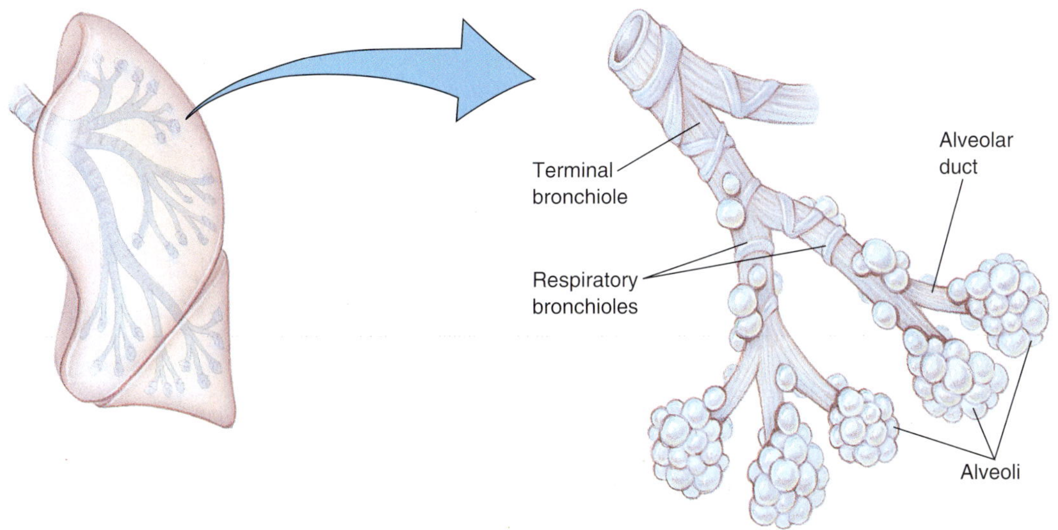

FIGURE 33.4 *Respiratory bronchi, bronchioles, alveolar ducts and alveoli*

with the *visceral pleura*, which covers the external lung surfaces. The pleura produces pleural fluid, a lubricating, serous fluid that allows the lungs to move easily over the thoracic wall during breathing. The pleura's two layers also cling tightly together and hold the lungs to the thoracic wall. The structure of the pleura creates a slightly negative pressure in the pleural space (which is a potential rather than an actual space), necessary for lung function.

The bronchi and alveoli

The trachea divides into right and left primary bronchi; in comparison to the left primary bronchus, the right primary bronchus is shorter, wider and situated more vertically (making aspiration of foreign bodies into the right primary bronchus more likely). The point where the trachea divides is innervated with sensory neurons; activities such as tracheal suctioning may induce coughing and bronchospasm from stimulation of these neurons. These main bronchi subdivide into the secondary (lobar) bronchi, with the right middle lobe bronchus being smaller in diameter and length, and sometimes bending sharply near its bifurcation. The secondary bronchi then branch into the tertiary (segmental) bronchi and then into smaller and smaller bronchioles, ending in the terminal bronchioles (see Figure 33.4). These branching passageways collectively are called the bronchial or respiratory tree. From the terminal bronchioles, air moves into the respiratory bronchioles (air sacs), which further branch into alveolar ducts that lead to alveolar sacs and then to the alveoli. During inspiration, air enters the lungs through the primary bronchus and then moves through the increasingly smaller passageways of the lungs to the alveoli, where oxygen and carbon dioxide exchange occurs in the process of external respiration. During expiration, the carbon dioxide is expelled.

Alveoli cluster around the alveolar sacs, which open into a common chamber called the atrium. The adult lung has approximately 300 million alveoli, providing an enormous surface for gas exchange (Marieb & Keller, 2021). Alveoli have extremely thin walls of a single layer of squamous epithelial cells over a very thin basement membrane. The external surface of the alveoli is covered with pulmonary capillaries. The alveolar and capillary walls form the respiratory membrane. Gas exchange across the respiratory membrane occurs by simple diffusion. The alveolar walls also contain cells that secrete a surfactant-containing fluid, necessary for maintaining a moist surface and reducing the surface tension of the alveolar fluid to help prevent collapse of the lungs.

The rib cage and intercostal muscles

The lungs are protected by the bones of the rib cage and the intercostal muscles. There are 12 pairs of ribs, which all articulate with the thoracic vertebrae (see Figure 33.5). Anteriorly, the first 7 ribs articulate with the body of the sternum. The 8th, 9th and 10th ribs articulate with the cartilage immediately above the ribs. The 11th and 12th ribs are called floating ribs because they are unattached.

The sternum has three parts: the manubrium, the body and the xiphoid process (Tortora, 2022). The junction between the manubrium and the body of the sternum is commonly called the angle of Louis. The depression above the manubrium is called the suprasternal notch.

The spaces between the ribs are called the intercostal spaces. Each intercostal space is named for the rib immediately above it (e.g. the space between the third and fourth ribs is designated as the third intercostal space). The intercostal muscles between the ribs, along with the diaphragm, are called the inspiratory muscles.

MECHANICS OF VENTILATION

Many factors affect ventilation and respiration. Those discussed here include changes in volume and capacity; air pressures; oxygen, carbon dioxide and hydrogen ion concentrations in the blood; airway resistance, lung compliance and elasticity; and alveolar surface tension.

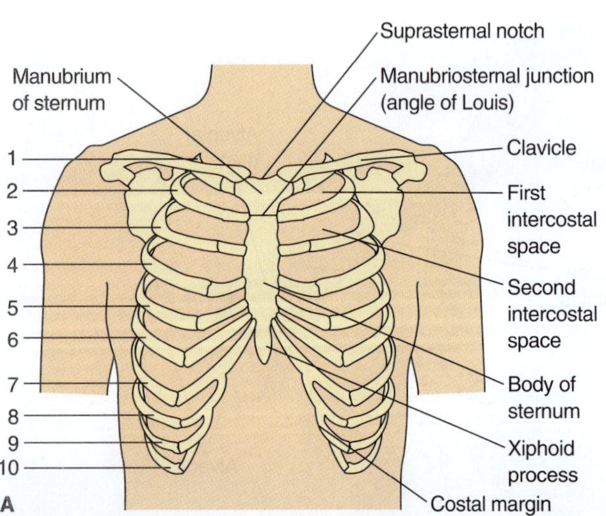

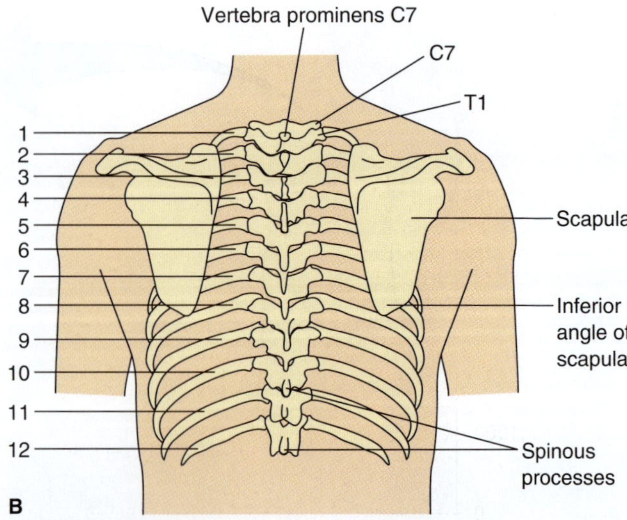

FIGURE 33.5 *A, Anterior rib cage, showing intercostal spaces. B, Posterior rib cage*

Respiratory volume and capacity

Respiratory volume and capacity are affected by gender, age, weight and health status.

- **Tidal volume (TV)** is the amount of air (approximately 500 mL) moved in and out of the lungs with each normal, quiet breath.
- *Inspiratory reserve volume (IRV)* is the amount of air (approximately 2,100 to 3,100 mL, depending on body size) that can be inhaled forcibly over the tidal volume.
- *Expiratory reserve volume (ERV)* is the volume of air (approximately 1,000 mL) that can be forced out over the tidal volume.
- The *residual volume* is the volume of air (approximately 1,100 mL) that remains in the lungs after a forced expiration.
- **Vital capacity (VC)** refers to the sum of TV + IRV + ERV and is approximately 4,500 mL in the healthy person.
- About 150 mL of air never reaches the alveoli (the amount remaining in the passageways) and is called anatomical dead space volume.

Pulmonary function tests measure these and other respiratory volumes (National Asthma Council Australia, 2020) and capacities and are discussed in Box 33.1.

BOX 33.1 Pulmonary function tests

Pulmonary function tests (PFTs) are performed in a pulmonary function laboratory. After preparing the person, a nose clip is applied and the person breathes into a spirometer or body plethysmograph, a device for measuring and recording lung volume in litres versus time in seconds. The person is instructed how to breathe for specific tests; for example, to inhale as deeply as possible and then exhale to the maximal extent possible. Using measured lung volumes, respiratory capacities are calculated to assess pulmonary status (Kaminsky, 2022). The specific values determined by PFTs and illustrated in the figure include the following.

- *Total lung capacity (TLC)* is the total volume of the lungs at their maximum inflation. Four values are used to calculate TLC:
  1. *tidal volume (TV)*, the volume inhaled and exhaled with normal quiet breathing (also called total volume)
  2. *inspiratory reserve volume (IRV)*, the maximum amount that can be inhaled over and above a normal inspiration
  3. *expiratory reserve volume (ERV)*, the maximum amount that can be exhaled following a normal exhalation
  4. *residual volume (RV)*, the amount of air remaining in the lungs after maximal exhalation.
- *Vital capacity (VC)* is the total amount of air that can be exhaled after a maximal inspiration. It is calculated by adding together the IRV, TV and ERV.
- *Inspiratory capacity* is the total amount of air that can be inhaled following a normal quiet exhalation. It is calculated by adding the TV and IRV.
- *Functional residual capacity (FRC)* is the volume of air left in the lungs after a normal exhalation. The ERV and RV are added to determine the FRC.
- *Forced expiratory volume (FEV1)* is the amount of air that can be exhaled in 1 second.
- *Forced vital capacity (FVC)* is the amount of air that can be exhaled forcefully and rapidly after maximum air intake.
- *Minute volume (MV)* is the total amount or volume of air breathed in 1 minute.

In older people, residual capacity is increased and vital capacity is decreased (Kaminsky, 2022). These age-related changes result from the following:

- calcification of the costal cartilage and weakening of the intercostal muscles, which reduce movement of the chest wall
- vertebral osteoporosis, which decreases spinal flexibility and increases the degree of kyphosis, further increasing the anterior–posterior diameter of the chest
- diaphragmatic flattening and loss of elasticity.

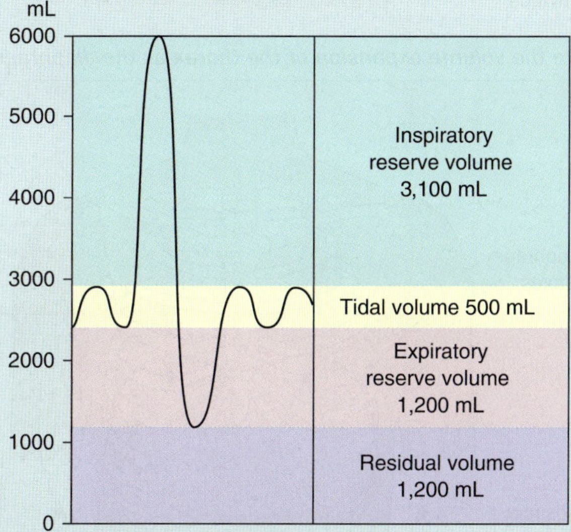

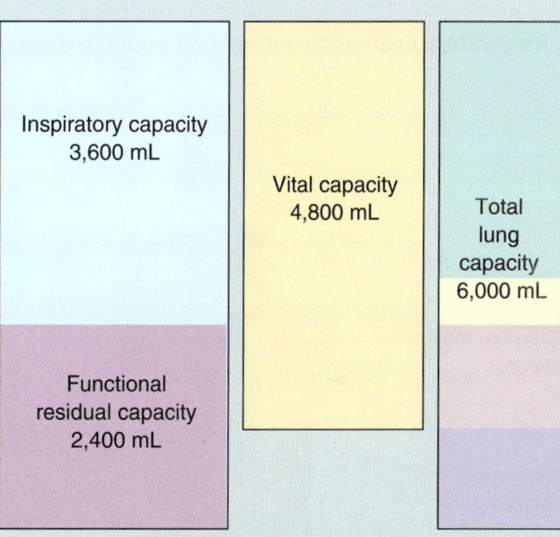

The relationship of lung volumes and capacities. Volumes (mL) shown are for an average adult male

Air pressures

Pulmonary ventilation depends on volume changes within the thoracic cavity. A change in the volume of air in the thoracic cavity leads to a change in the air pressure within the cavity. Because gases always flow along their pressure gradients, a change in pressure results in gases flowing into or out of the lungs to equalise the pressure.

The pressures normally present in the thoracic cavity are intrapulmonary and intrapleural pressure. The intrapulmonary pressure, within the alveoli of the lungs, rises and falls constantly as a result of the acts of ventilation (inhalation and exhalation). The intrapleural pressure, within the pleural space, also rises and falls with the acts of ventilation, but it is always less than (or negative to) the intrapulmonary pressure. Intrapulmonary and intrapleural pressures are necessary not only to expand and contract the lungs, but also to prevent their collapse.

Pulmonary ventilation has two phases: inspiration, during which air flows into the lungs; and expiration, during which gases flow out of the lungs. The two phases make up a single breath and normally occur from 12 to 20 times each minute (Tortora, 2022). Inspiration occurs generally in a 1:2 ratio. A single inspiration lasts for approximately 1 to 1.5 seconds, whereas an expiration lasts for approximately 2 to 3 seconds.

During inspiration, the diaphragm contracts and flattens out to increase the vertical diameter of the thoracic cavity (see Figure 33.6). The external intercostal muscles contract, elevating the rib cage and moving the sternum forward to expand the lateral and anteroposterior diameter of the thoracic cavity, decreasing intrapleural pressure. The lungs stretch and the intrapulmonary volume increases, decreasing intrapulmonary pressure slightly below atmospheric pressure. Air rushes into the lungs as a result of this pressure gradient until the intrapulmonary and atmospheric pressures equalise.

Expiration is primarily a passive process that occurs as a result of the elasticity of the lungs (see Figure 33.7). The inspiratory muscles relax, the diaphragm rises, the ribs descend and the lungs recoil. Both the thoracic and the intrapulmonary pressures increase, compressing the alveoli. The intrapulmonary pressure rises to a level greater than atmospheric pressure and gases flow out of the lungs.

Oxygen, carbon dioxide and hydrogen ion concentrations

The rate and depth of respirations are controlled by respiratory centres in the medulla oblongata and pons of the brain and by chemoreceptors located in the medulla and in the carotid

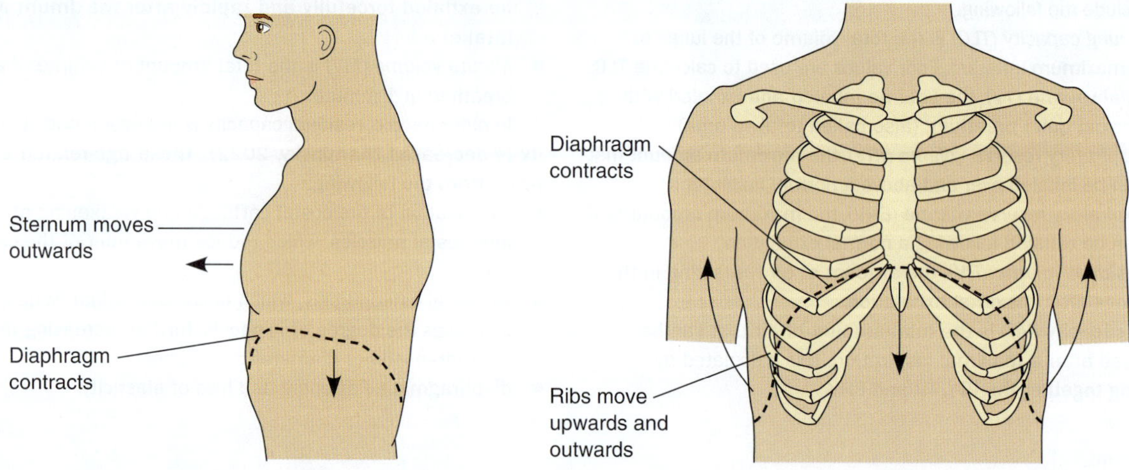

FIGURE 33.6 ***Respiratory inspiration: lateral and anterior views. Note the volume expansion of the thorax as the diaphragm flattens***

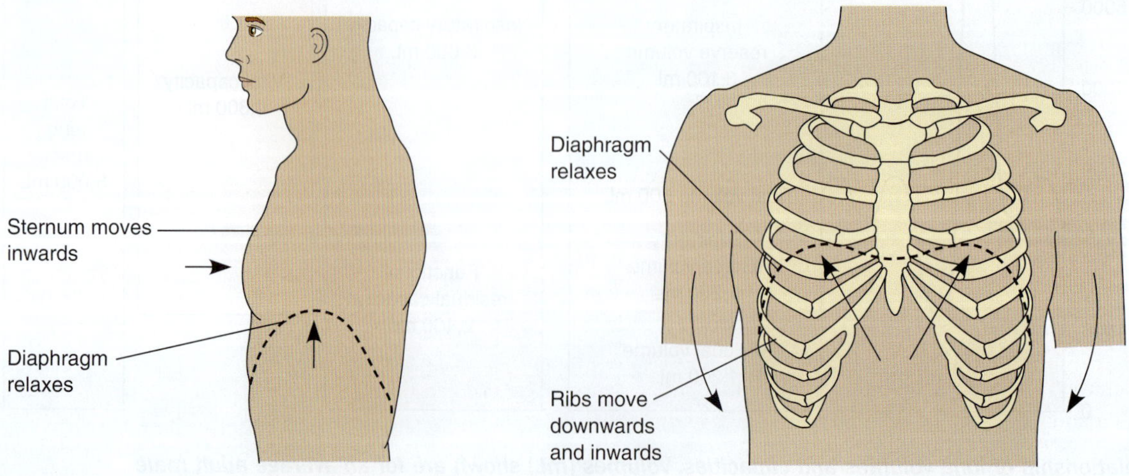

FIGURE 33.7 ***Respiratory expiration: lateral and anterior views***

and aortic bodies. The centres and chemoreceptors respond to changes in the concentration of oxygen, carbon dioxide and hydrogen ions in arterial blood. For example, when carbon dioxide concentration increases or the pH decreases, the respiratory rate increases (Patel & Mohiuddin, 2022). This process is further described in the chapter 'Nursing care of people with altered fluid, electrolyte and acid–base balance'.

Airway resistance, lung compliance and elasticity

Respiratory passageway resistance, lung compliance and lung elasticity also affect respiration.

- Respiratory passageway resistance is created by the friction encountered as gases move along the respiratory passageways, by constriction of the passageways (especially the larger bronchioles), by accumulations of mucus or infectious material, and by tumours. As resistance increases, gas flow decreases.
- **Lung compliance** depends on the elasticity of the lung tissue and the flexibility of the rib cage. Compliance is decreased by factors that decrease the elasticity of the lungs, block the respiratory passageways or interfere with movement of the rib cage.
- Lung elasticity is essential for lung distension during inspiration and lung recoil during expiration. Decreased elasticity from disease such as emphysema impairs respiration.

Alveolar surface tension

A liquid film of mostly water covers the alveolar walls. At any gas–liquid boundary, the molecules of liquid are more strongly attracted to each other than to gas molecules. This produces a state of tension, called surface tension, which draws the liquid molecules even more closely together. The water content of the alveolar film compacts the alveoli and aids in the lungs' recoil during expiration. In fact, if the alveolar film were pure water, the alveoli would collapse between breaths.

Surfactant, a lipoprotein produced by the alveolar cells, interferes with this adhesiveness of the water molecules, reducing surface tension and helping to expand the lungs. With insufficient surfactant, the surface tension forces can become great enough to collapse the alveoli between breaths, requiring tremendous energy to reinflate the lungs for inspiration.

GAS TRANSPORT AND AFFINITY

Blood gases

Gases are transported by the blood to provide cells with oxygen and to remove carbon dioxide produced during cellular activities.

Oxygen transport and unloading

Oxygen is carried in the blood either bound to haemoglobin or dissolved in the plasma. Oxygen is not very soluble in water, so almost all oxygen that enters the blood from the respiratory system is carried to the cells of the body by haemoglobin. This combination of haemoglobin and oxygen is called **oxyhaemoglobin**.

Each haemoglobin molecule is made of four polypeptide chains, with each chain bound to an iron-containing haem group (Marieb & Keller, 2021). The iron groups are the binding sites for oxygen; each haemoglobin molecule can bind with four molecules of oxygen.

Oxygen binding is rapid and reversible. It is affected by temperature, blood pH, partial pressure of oxygen (PO_2), partial pressure of carbon dioxide (PCO_2) and serum concentration of an organic chemical called 2,3-DPG (Rengasamy et al., 2021). These factors interact to ensure adequate delivery of oxygen to the cells.

The relative saturation of haemoglobin depends on the PO_2 of the blood, as illustrated in the oxygen–haemoglobin dissociation curve (see Figure 33.8).

- Under normal conditions, the haemoglobin in arterial blood is 97.4% saturated with oxygen. Haemoglobin is almost fully saturated at a PO_2 of 70 mmHg. As arterial blood flows through the capillaries, oxygen is unloaded, so that the oxygen saturation of haemoglobin in venous blood is 75% under normal conditions.
- The affinity of oxygen and haemoglobin decreases as the temperature of body tissues increases above normal. As a result, less oxygen binds with haemoglobin and oxygen unloading is enhanced. Conversely, as the body is chilled, oxygen unloading is inhibited.
- The oxygen–haemoglobin bond is weakened by increased hydrogen ion concentrations. As blood becomes more acidotic, oxygen unloading to the tissues is enhanced. The same process occurs when the partial pressure of carbon dioxide increases because this decreases the pH.
- The organic chemical 2,3-DPG is formed in red blood cells and enhances the release of oxygen from haemoglobin by binding to it during times of increased metabolism (as when body temperature increases). This binding alters the structure of haemoglobin to facilitate oxygen unloading.

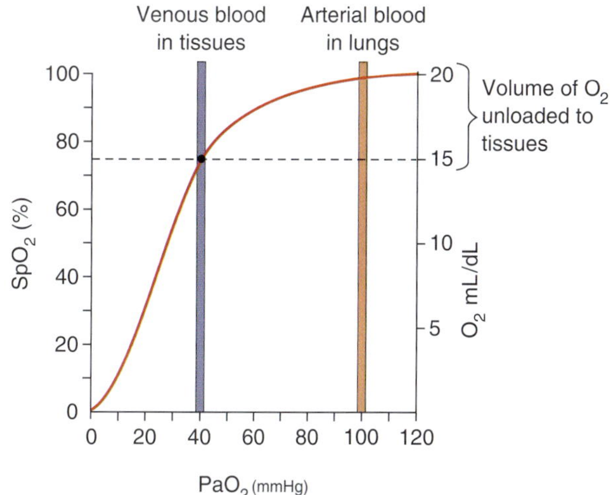

FIGURE 33.8 *Oxygen–haemoglobin dissociation curve. The percentage of O_2 saturation of haemoglobin and total blood oxygen volume are shown for different oxygen partial pressures (PO_2). Arterial blood in the lungs is almost completely saturated. During one pass through the body, about 25% of haemoglobin-bound oxygen is unloaded to the tissues. Thus, venous blood is still about 75% saturated with oxygen. The steep portion of the curve shows that haemoglobin readily off-loads or on-loads oxygen at PO_2 levels below about 50 mmHg*

Carbon dioxide transport

Active cells produce about 200 mL of carbon dioxide each minute; this amount is exactly the same as that excreted by the lungs each minute. Excretion of carbon dioxide from the body requires transport by the blood from the cells to the lungs. Carbon dioxide is transported in three forms: dissolved in plasma, bound to haemoglobin and as bicarbonate ions in the plasma (the largest amount is in this form.)

The amount of carbon dioxide transported in the blood is strongly influenced by the oxygenation of the blood. When the PO_2 decreases, with a corresponding decrease in oxygen saturation, increased amounts of carbon dioxide can be carried in the blood. Carbon dioxide entering the systemic circulation from the cells causes more oxygen to dissociate from haemoglobin, in turn allowing more carbon dioxide to combine with haemoglobin and more bicarbonate ions to be generated. This situation is reversed in the pulmonary circulation, where the uptake of oxygen facilitates the release of carbon dioxide.

ASSESSING A PERSON'S RESPIRATORY FUNCTION

Respiratory system function is assessed by findings from a health assessment interview to collect subjective data, a physical assessment to collect objective data and diagnostic tests. Sample documentation of an assessment of the respiratory system is included in the 'Sample documentation' box.

Health assessment interview

A health assessment interview to determine problems with respiratory structure and function may be conducted during a health screening, may focus on a chief complaint (such as shortness of breath) or may be part of a total health assessment. If the person has a problem with respiratory function, analyse its onset, characteristics, course, severity, precipitating and relieving factors, and any associated symptoms, noting the timing and circumstances. For example, ask the person:

- Describe the problems you are having with your breathing. Is your breathing more difficult if you lie flat? Is it painful to breathe in or out?
- When did you first notice that your cough was becoming a problem? Do you cough up mucus? What colour is the mucus?
- Have you had nosebleeds in the past?

During the interview, carefully observe the person for difficulty in breathing, pausing to breathe in the middle of a sentence, hoarseness, changes in voice quality, audible wheeze and cough. Ask about present health status, medical history, family health history and risk factors for illness.

To determine present health status, ask about pain in the nose, throat or chest. Information about cough includes what type of cough, when it occurs and how it is relieved. The person should describe the sputum colour and volume associated with the cough. Is the person experiencing any dyspnoea (difficult or laboured breathing)? How is the dyspnoea associated with activity levels and time of day? Is the person having chest pain? How is this related to activity and time of day? Note the severity, type and location of the pain. Explore problems with swallowing, smelling or taste. Also ask about nosebleeds and nasal or sinus stuffiness or pain, and about current medication use, aerosols or inhalants, and oxygen use. Gastro-oesophageal reflux disease is also known to induce a cough, so enquiry as to the proximity of the cough to meal times may assist in better understanding the person's symptomology (Khoma et al., 2022).

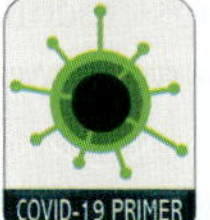

In the context of the COVID-19 pandemic, it is also important to note if the person has had any exposure to close contacts who are COVID positive. Also note if they are fully vaccinated with primary and booster doses and discuss their mask-wearing behaviours in public when they cannot adequately socially distance. (See the COVID-19 Primer regarding transmission.)

Document past medical history by asking questions about a history or family history of allergies, asthma, bronchitis, emphysema, pneumonia, tuberculosis or congestive heart failure. Other questions include a history of surgery or trauma to the respiratory structures and a history of other chronic illnesses such as cancer, kidney disease and heart disease and medications used. The person's personal lifestyle, environment and occupation may provide clues to risk factors for actual or potential health problems. Ask the person about a history of smoking and/or exposure to environmental chemicals (including smog), dust, vapours, animals, coal dust, asbestos, fumes or pollens. Other risk factors include a sedentary lifestyle and obesity. Also ask the person about use of alcohol and illicit substances.

> **SAMPLE DOCUMENTATION**
> **Assessment of respiratory function**
>
> | | |
> |---|---|
> | 14/4/2023
NURS
1100 hrs | 57-year-old male, presenting to unit with an SOB and 3-day history of increasing cough. He has smoked two packets of cigarettes/day for 45 years and continues despite previous attempts to quit. Works as a fibreglass boat builder. No family history of cancer or TB. Reports paroxysmal nocturnal dyspnoea and often sleeps on a recliner 'to breathe better'. Complains of a cough but denies sputum production. Diagnosed 3 years ago with emphysema. No central or peripheral cyanosis noted. No digital clubbing observed. Respirations 30/min, unlaboured, regular. (Respiration rate 26–32) SpO_2 91% on room air. Afebrile, heart rate 104 bpm; BP 134/78. Thoracic assessment L = R and decreased air entry in bases. Crackles present in upper lobes, not cleared by coughing. Intercostal recession and use of accessory muscles of respiration noted. Has barrel chest. Discussed with RMO. For oxygen via nasal prongs at 2 Lpm. Will review within a few hours. ______________ L Nguyen
(LILY NGUYEN, RN) |

Physical assessment

Physical assessment of the respiratory system may be performed either as part of a total assessment or alone for a person with known or suspected problems. The techniques used to assess the respiratory system are inspection, palpation, percussion and

TABLE 33.1 Age-related changes in the respiratory system

AGE-RELATED CHANGE	SIGNIFICANCE
• ↓ elastic recoil of lungs during expiration because of less elastic collagen and elastin. • Loss of skeletal muscle strength in the thorax and diaphragm. • Alveoli are less elastic, more fibrotic and have fewer functional capillaries. • Cough is less effective. • PO_2 reduces as much as 15% by age 80.	The older adult often has an increased anterior-posterior chest diameter, with kyphosis and barrel chest. There is a reduction in vital capacity and an increase in residual volume, with decreased effectiveness in coughing up phlegm or sputum. All of these changes greatly increase the risk of respiratory infections (such as pneumonia), especially if the person becomes immobile. They also mean that respiratory infections are more difficult to treat.

auscultation (Squires, 2022). In addition, note the person's level of consciousness, restlessness and anxiety level, and assess the colour of the lips and nail beds. Normal age-related findings for the older adult are summarised in Table 33.1.

The room should be warm and well lit. Ask the person to remove all clothing above the waist; give them a gown to wear during the examination. Conduct the examination with the person in the sitting position. Prior to the examination, collect all necessary equipment and explain the techniques to the person to decrease anxiety.

Diagnostic tests

The results of diagnostic tests of respiratory function are used to support the diagnosis of a specific disease, to provide information to identify or modify the appropriate medications or therapy used to treat the disease, and to help nurses monitor the person's response to treatment and nursing care interventions. Diagnostic tests to assess the structures and functions of the respiratory system are described in the 'Diagnostic tests' box and summarised in the bulleted list below. More information is included in the discussion of specific disorders in the chapters 'Nursing care of people with upper respiratory disorders', 'Nursing care of people with ventilation disorders' and 'Nursing care of people with gas exchange disorders'.

- Respiratory virus polymerase chain reaction (PCR) panel testing for people presenting with respiratory symptoms can be informative, especially in those with high risk of severe illness. Upper respiratory secretions from naso- and/or oropharyngeal mucus samples and sputum, or lower respiratory secretions from tracheal aspirates, can be tested to determine a viral cause of the presenting symptoms. Depending on the panel requested, various viruses can be detected including influenza, respiratory syncytial virus (RSV) and the SARS-CoV-2 virus (Department of Health Victoria, 2022).

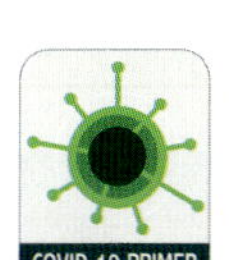

- An alternative to the PCR is an at-home rapid antigen test (RAT) for the diagnosis of a specific respiratory illness such as the SARS-CoV-2 virus. RATs are beneficial when they do identify a positive result for the respiratory illness to which they are testing; however, they are far less reliable (with sensitivity rate measured between 18.4% and 96.1%) than a healthcare-professional-sampled PCR (Jarrom et al., 2022). RATs can be carried out on naso- and/or oropharyngeal mucus samples and sputum, depending on the brand. Diagnostic accuracy should be considered in the context of the possibility of false-negative results from sampling error, sample timing and manner of viral shedding. Nevertheless, they can be valuable in the context of a positive test to inform public health and isolation requirements and help with interventions to limit respiratory virus spread, especially to individuals at severe risk for complications of contracting a respiratory virus. (See the COVID-19 Primer.)
- Sputum tests include a culture and sensitivity to identify organisms causing infections as well as the most effective antibiotic to treat the infection, an acid-fast smear and culture to identify the tuberculosis bacillus and cytology to identify malignancies (see Procedure 33.1).
- Arterial blood gases are conducted to evaluate alterations in acid–base balances and determine oxygen saturations and partial pressure for oxygen and carbon dioxide.
- Pulse oximetry is used to evaluate or monitor the oxygen saturation of the blood.
- Many different radiological examinations are used to diagnose respiratory disorders, including a chest x-ray to evaluate structures and tissues, a computed tomography (CT) scan to differentiate pathological conditions, magnetic resonance imaging (MRI) to more accurately identify abnormal masses and fluid accumulation, a positron emission tomography (PET) to identify lung cancers and a pulmonary angiogram to identify various disorders including pulmonary emboli and emphysema.
- A bronchoscopy is a direct visualisation of the larynx, trachea and bronchi. During the test, lesions can be identified, foreign bodies or mucus plugs removed, and tissue taken for biopsy. In addition, a biopsy of lung tissue may be done through an incision through the chest wall.
- A thoracentesis, when done for diagnostic purposes, is conducted to obtain a specimen of pleural fluid.

Regardless of the type of diagnostic test, the nurse is responsible for explaining the procedure and any special preparation needed, for assessing for medication use that may affect the outcome of the tests, for supporting the person during the examination as necessary, for documenting the procedures as appropriate and for monitoring the results of the tests.

Genetic considerations

When conducting a health assessment interview and a physical assessment, it is important for the nurse to consider genetic influences on the health of the adult. During the health assessment interview, ask about family members with health problems affecting respiratory function. In addition, ask about a family history of emphysema, asthma, cystic fibrosis or lung cancer (Hall, Hall & Sayers, 2019). During the physical assessment, assess for any manifestations that might indicate a genetic disorder (see the 'Genetic considerations' box). If data are found to indicate genetic risk factors or alterations, ask about genetic testing and refer for appropriate genetic counselling and evaluation. The chapter 'Genetic implications of adult health nursing' provides further information about genetics in medical–surgical nursing.

PROCEDURE 33.1 Obtaining a sputum specimen

GATHER SUPPLIES

- Sterile sputum container, specimen cup or mucus trap
- Mouth care supplies
- Sterile suction kit, if necessary
- Gloves

BEFORE THE PROCEDURE

If the person is presenting with upper respiratory symptoms, they quite possibly should be managed as having COVID-19 (depending on pandemic stage, season and local incidence). Follow institution instructions regarding the use of personal protective equipment (PPE) in relation to individuals presenting with respiratory symptoms.

If the sputum specimen is to establish the initial diagnosis, obtain the specimen before starting oxygen and/or antibiotic therapy. Antibiotics reduce the bacterial count, making it difficult to identify the infecting organism. Oxygen therapy dries mucous membranes, making it more difficult to obtain a specimen. Unless otherwise instructed, obtain the specimen early in the morning, just after awakening. Respiratory secretions tend to pool during sleep; it is easier to obtain a specimen before normal coughing and daily activity have cleared them.

Provide for privacy and explain the procedure. Emphasise the importance of coughing deeply to obtain sputum from the lower respiratory tract, avoiding expectoration of saliva. Increasing fluid intake prior to obtaining the specimen can help liquefy secretions, making them easier to expectorate.

DURING THE PROCEDURE

1. Provide for mouth care prior to obtaining the specimen to reduce contamination by oral flora.
2. Instruct to cough deeply several times, expectorating mucus into the container.
3. Close the container securely.
4. Label the container according to the institution's requirements, usually with the person's name, date of birth, hospital identification number, time and date, signature of specimen collector and any special conditions, such as antibiotic or oxygen therapy. Enclose specimen container in a specimen bag and send to the laboratory with the pathology request slip, or refrigerate as ordered to preserve the specimen.
5. To obtain a specimen by suctioning:
   - Be aware that respiratory suctioning is a highly aerosol-generating technique and significantly increases the risk of transmission of airborne infections (such as COVID-19). Full PPE should be worn for healthcare professional safety.
   - Provide mouth care.
   - Obtain a sterile mucus trap. Using aseptic technique, attach the trap to the suction apparatus between the suction catheter and tubing.
   - Pre-oxygenate for suctioning as needed.
   - Perform tracheal suctioning using aseptic technique via the nasotracheal route, endotracheal tube or tracheostomy. Lubricate the catheter with sterile normal saline. Do not apply suction as the catheter is being inserted into the trachea; apply suction for no longer than 10 seconds while withdrawing the catheter.
   - If the secretion remains in the tubing of the trap, suction sterile water into the trap to encourage the secretion into the container section.
   - Detach the mucus trap; close and label. Reattach the catheter and clear the suction catheter and tubing with normal saline after removing the mucus trap. Dispose of equipment appropriately.
   - Label the specimen as identified above before sending to the laboratory.
6. A sputum specimen also may be obtained during a bronchoscopy procedure.

AFTER THE PROCEDURE

Provide mouth care as needed. Teach the importance of completing all ordered antibiotic prescriptions to ensure complete eradication of microorganisms. Document the time and date that the specimen was obtained; and note colour, consistency and odour of sputum.

GENETIC CONSIDERATIONS
Respiratory disorders

- Deficiency of alpha-1 antitrypsin (a protein that protects the body from damage by its immune cells) is caused by a mutation of a gene located on chromosome 14. Deficiency of this protein leaves the lung susceptible to emphysema.
- Asthma is a respiratory disease which affects 11% of the population. Although mortality has declined substantially in the past 30 years, it remains high in Australia compared with international rates. Unacceptably, over 417 people died from asthma in 2020 (National Asthma Council Australia, 2021). It is an obstructive respiratory condition and is associated with inheritable factors.
- The prevalence of cystic fibrosis in Australia in 2020 was 3,538, with 74 new cases diagnosed, and mortality was 18 (Cystic Fibrosis Australia, 2021). All gene defects result in defective transport of chloride and sodium by epithelial cells. As a result, the amount of sodium chloride is increased in body secretions. Thick mucus is produced that clogs the lungs, leads to infection and blocks pancreatic enzymes from reaching the intestines to digest food.
- Lung cancer is the fifth most common cancer in Australia and accounts for almost 17.7% of all cancer deaths (Cancer Australia, 2022). A familial history of lung cancer increases the risk of developing lung cancer, and small-cell lung cancer has a definite genetic component. In addition, researchers have found that people with lung cancer who never smoked are more likely than smokers to have one of two genetic mutations linked to the disease.

FOCUS ON CULTURAL DIVERSITY

- Aboriginal and Torres Strait Islander people are 2.2 times more likely than non-Indigenous Australians to be hospitalised for respiratory diseases.
- Ten per cent of all Aboriginal and Torres Strait Islander deaths are caused by respiratory disease.
- Past medical history assessment is important. In 2018–2019, almost 30% of Aboriginal and Torres Strait Islander Australians reported having a respiratory disease lasting more than 6 months.
- Culturally safe considerations are critical when undertaking respiratory assessment, especially in relation to Indigenous ways of communication and gender such as 'women's business' and 'men's business'. Understanding barriers associated with a difference in the gender of the healthcare professional and the Indigenous person being assessed is critical in order to obtain the most complete, relevant history and assessment data, with the least distress possible.

Sources: Australian Institute of Health and Welfare: National Indigenous Australians Agency (2020). *Health Performance Framework. Tier 1—Health status and outcomes—1.04 Respiratory disease*. Retrieved from https://www.indigenoushpf.gov.au/; Meharg et al. (2022). Implementing evidence into practice to improve chronic lung disease management in Indigenous Australians: The breathe easy, walk easy, lungs for life (BE WELL) project (protocol). *BMC Pulmonary Medicine, 22*, 239. https://doi.org/10.1186/s12890-022-02033-8.

DIAGNOSTIC TESTS The respiratory system

NAME OF TEST Sputum studies

- Culture and sensitivity
- Acid-fast bacilli smear and culture
- Cytology

PURPOSE AND DESCRIPTION Culture and sensitivity of a single sputum specimen is performed to diagnose bacterial infections, identify the most effective antibiotic and evaluate treatment.

Sputum is examined for presence of acid-fast bacillus, specifically tuberculosis. A series of three early-morning sputum specimens is used.

Sputum is examined for presence of abnormal (malignant) cells. A single sputum specimen is collected in a special container of fixative solution.

RELATED NURSING CARE See Procedure 33.1 for obtaining a sputum specimen. Sputum specimens may also be obtained during bronchoscopy (described later) if the person is unable to provide a specimen.

NAME OF TEST Arterial blood gases (ABGs)

PURPOSE AND DESCRIPTION This test of arterial blood is performed to assess alterations in acid–base balance caused by a respiratory disorder, a metabolic disorder or both. A pH of less than 7.35 indicates acidosis and a pH of more than 7.45 indicates alkalosis (see the chapter 'Nursing care of people with altered fluid, electrolyte and acid–base balance'). To determine a respiratory cause, assess the $PaCO_2$: If pH is decreased and $PaCO_2$ is increased, respiratory acidosis is indicated.

Normal values:
pH: 7.35 – 7.45
$PaCO_2$: 35 – 45 mmHg
PaO_2: 75 – 100 mmHg
HCO_3^-: 22 – 26 mEq/L
BE: ±2 mEq/L

RELATED NURSING CARE Arterial blood is collected in a heparinised needle and syringe. Sample is placed on an ice bag and taken immediately to the lab. If the person is receiving oxygen, you are required to indicate this on the lab slip. Apply pressure to puncture site for 2–5 minutes post test or longer if needed. Do not collect blood from the same arm used for an IV infusion as this can make the results of the test inaccurate.

NAME OF TEST Pulse oximetry

PURPOSE AND DESCRIPTION This non-invasive test is used to evaluate or monitor oxygen saturation of the blood. A device that uses infrared light is attached to an extremity (most commonly the finger, but can also be the toe, earlobe, nose or forehead) and light is passed through the tissues or reflected off bony structures.

Normal value: 95–100%

RELATED NURSING CARE Assess for factors that may alter findings, including faulty placement, movement, dark skin colour, acrylic nails, ambient light, peripheral hypothermia, and peripheral vasoconstriction.

(continued)

DIAGNOSTIC TESTS The respiratory system (continued)

NAME OF TEST Chest x-ray

PURPOSE AND DESCRIPTION Chest x-rays are used to identify abnormalities in chest structure and lung tissue, for diagnosis of diseases and injuries of the lungs, and to monitor treatment.

RELATED NURSING CARE Remove any metal objects around area such as jewellery or brassieres containing underwire.

NAME OF TEST Computed tomography (CT)

PURPOSE AND DESCRIPTION CT of the thorax may be performed when x-rays do not show some areas well, such as the pleura and mediastinum. It is also performed to differentiate pathological conditions (such as tumours, abscesses and aortic aneurysms), to identify pleural effusion and enlarged lymph nodes and to monitor treatment. Images are shown in cross-section.

RELATED NURSING CARE Need to assess whether the person is able to lie still for extended periods and is not claustrophobic.

NAME OF TEST Magnetic resonance imaging (MRI)

PURPOSE AND DESCRIPTION An MRI of the thorax is used to diagnose alterations in lung tissue more difficult to visualise by CT scan and to identify abnormal masses and fluid accumulation.

RELATED NURSING CARE Assess for any metallic implants (such as pacemaker, pacemaker wires, implants) or history of metal shavings etc. in eyes. Also assess for any metal worn on the body. Test will not be performed if present.

NAME OF TEST Positron emission tomography (PET)

PURPOSE AND DESCRIPTION This relatively non-invasive test, when used to examine the lungs, is performed to identify lung nodules (cancers). The person is given a radioactive substance and cross-sectional images are displayed on a computer. Radiation from PET is only 25% of that from a CT scan.

RELATED NURSING CARE No alcohol, coffee or tobacco is allowed for 24 hours prior to the test. Encourage increased fluid intake post test to help eliminate the radioactive material.

NAME OF TEST Pulmonary angiography

PURPOSE AND DESCRIPTION This test is performed to identify pulmonary emboli, tumours, aneurysms, vascular changes associated with emphysema and pulmonary circulation. A catheter is inserted into the brachial or femoral artery, threaded into the pulmonary artery and dye is injected. Electrocardiograph leads are applied to the chest for cardiac monitoring. Images of the lungs are taken.

RELATED NURSING CARE Monitor injection site and pulses distal to the site after the test.

NAME OF TEST Pulmonary ventilation–perfusion scan (V/Q scan)

PURPOSE AND DESCRIPTION This test is performed to measure breathing (ventilation) and circulation (perfusion) in all parts of the lungs. A perfusion scan is performed by injecting radioactive albumin into a vein and scanning the lungs. A ventilation scan is performed by scanning the lungs as the person inhales radioactive gas. A decreased uptake of radioisotope during the perfusion scan indicates a blood flow problem, such as from a pulmonary embolus or pneumonitis. A decreased uptake of gas during the ventilation scan may indicate airway obstruction, pneumonia or chronic obstructive pulmonary disease (COPD).

RELATED NURSING CARE No special preparation is needed other than ensuring the person has a patent intravenous catheter.

NAME OF TEST Bronchoscopy

PURPOSE AND DESCRIPTION A bronchoscopy is the direct visualisation of the larynx, trachea and bronchi through a bronchoscope to identify lesions, remove foreign bodies and secretions, obtain tissue for biopsy and improve tracheobronchial drainage (see Figure 33.9). During the test, a catheter brush or biopsy forceps can be passed to obtain secretions or tissue for examination for cancer.

RELATED NURSING CARE Provide routine preoperative care as ordered. Bronchoscopy is an invasive procedure requiring conscious sedation or anaesthesia. *Care provided prior to the procedure is similar to that provided before many minor surgical procedures.*

DIAGNOSTIC TESTS **The respiratory system (continued)**

HEALTH EDUCATION FOR THE PERSON AND FAMILY

- Fibre-optic bronchoscopy requires 30 to 45 minutes to complete. It may be done at the bedside, in a special procedure room or in the surgical suite.
- The procedure usually causes little pain or discomfort because an anaesthetic is given. You will be able to breathe during the bronchoscopy.
- Some voice hoarseness and a sore throat are common following the procedure. Throat lozenges or warm saline gargles may help relieve discomfort.
- You may develop a mild fever within the first 24 hours following the procedure. This is a normal response.
- Persistent cough, bloody or purulent sputum, wheezing, shortness of breath or chest pain may indicate a complication. Notify your doctor if they develop.

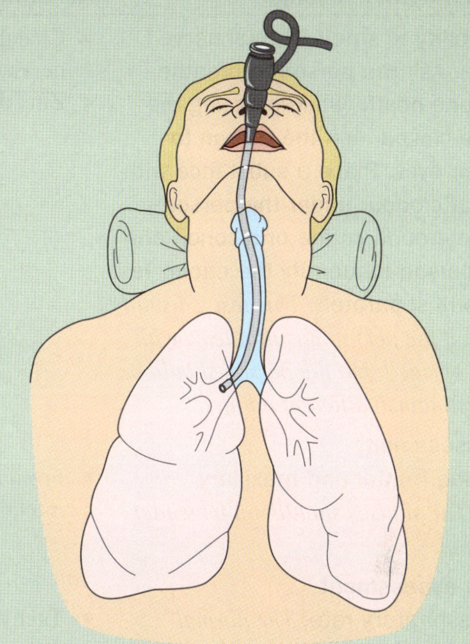

FIGURE 33.9 *Fibre-optic bronchoscopy*

NAME OF TEST Lung biopsy

PURPOSE AND DESCRIPTION Performed to obtain tissue to differentiate benign from malignant tumours of the lungs. May be performed during a bronchoscopy or by surgical procedure.

RELATED NURSING CARE Same as for bronchoscopy or the same as for a thoracotomy (incision through the chest wall) if a surgical biopsy is performed.

NAME OF TEST Thoracentesis

PURPOSE AND DESCRIPTION Performed to obtain a specimen of pleural fluid for diagnosis (and used as a procedure to remove pleural fluid or instil medication). A large-bore needle is inserted through the chest wall and into the pleural space. Following the procedure, a chest x-ray is taken to check for a pneumothorax.

RELATED NURSING CARE Nursing care of the person having a thoracentesis is provided in the chapter 'Nursing care of people with ventilation disorders'.

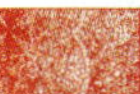

RESPIRATORY ASSESSMENTS

Technique/normal findings	Abnormal findings
Nasal assessment	
Inspect the nose for changes in size, shape or colour. *The nose should be midline in the face, of the same colour as the face and the nares should be symmetrical.*	■ The nose may be asymmetrical as a result of previous surgery or trauma. ■ The skin around the nostrils may be red and swollen with allergies or upper respiratory infections.
Inspect the nasal cavity. Use an otoscope with a broad, short speculum. Gently insert the speculum into each of the nares and assess the condition of the mucous membranes and the turbinates. *The septum should be midline with pink mucosa and without drainage.*	■ The septum may be deviated. ■ Perforation of the septum may occur with chronic cocaine abuse. ■ Red mucosa indicates infection. ■ Purulent drainage indicates nasal or sinus infection. ■ Allergies may be indicated by watery nasal drainage, pale turbinates and polyps on the turbinates.

(continued)

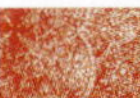

RESPIRATORY ASSESSMENTS (continued)

Technique/normal findings	Abnormal findings
Assess ability to smell (cranial nerve I, olfactory). Ask the person to breathe through one nostril while pressing the other one closed. Ask the person to close their eyes. Place a substance with an aromatic odour under the person's nose (use ground coffee or alcohol) and ask the person to identify the odour. Test each nostril separately. *This test is usually done only if the person has problems with the sense of smell, but the person should be able to distinguish different odours.*	▪ Changes in the ability to smell may be the result of damage to the olfactory nerve or to chronic inflammation of the nose. ▪ Zinc deficiency may cause a loss of the sense of smell.
Sinus assessment	
Palpate the frontal and maxillary sinuses. *The sinuses should not be tender to palpation.*	▪ Frontal and maxillary sinuses are tender to palpation with allergies or sinus infections.
Thoracic assessment	
Assess respiratory rate. *The normal respiratory rate is 12 to 20 breaths per minute.*	▪ **Tachypnoea** (rapid respiratory rate) is seen in atelectasis (collapse of lung tissue following obstruction of the bronchus or bronchioles), pneumonia, asthma, pleural effusion, pneumothorax, congestive heart failure, anxiety and in response to pain. ▪ Damage to the brainstem from a stroke or head injury may result in either tachypnoea or **bradypnoea** (low respiratory rate). ▪ Bradypnoea is seen with some circulatory disorders, lung disorders and as a side effect of some medications. ▪ **Apnoea**, cessation of breathing lasting from a few seconds to a few minutes, may occur following a stroke or head trauma, as a side effect of some medications or following airway obstruction.
Inspect the anteroposterior diameter of the chest. *The anteroposterior diameter of the chest should be less than the transverse diameter. Normal ratio is 1:2.*	▪ The anteroposterior diameter is equal to the transverse diameter in barrel chest, which typically occurs with emphysema.
Inspect for intercostal retraction or bulging. *There should be no retraction or bulging.*	▪ Retraction of intercostal spaces may be seen in asthma. ▪ Bulging of intercostal spaces may be seen in pneumothorax.
Inspect and palpate for chest expansion. Place your hands with the fingers spread apart palm down on the person's posterolateral chest. Gently press the skin between your thumbs (see Figure 33.10). Ask the person to breathe deeply. As the person inhales, watch your hands for symmetry of movement. *Chest expansion should be bilaterally symmetrical with the examiner's hands moving 5 to 10 cm apart.*	▪ Thoracic expansion is decreased on the affected side in atelectasis, pneumonia, pneumothorax and pleural effusion. ▪ Bilateral chest expansion is decreased in emphysema.

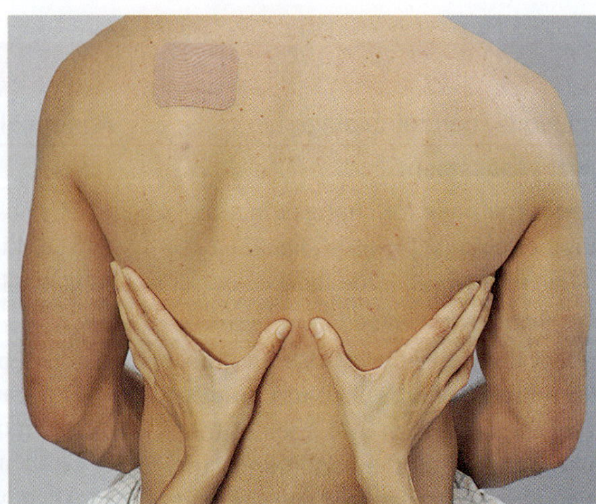

FIGURE 33.10 *Palpating for chest expansion*

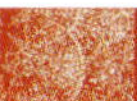

RESPIRATORY ASSESSMENTS (continued)

Technique/normal findings	Abnormal findings
Gently palpate the location and position of the trachea. *The trachea should be midline.*	■ The trachea shifts to the unaffected side in pleural effusion and pneumothorax and shifts to the affected side in atelectasis.
Palpate for tactile fremitus. Ask the person to say 'ninety-nine' as you palpate at three different levels for a vibratory sensation called tactile fremitus, which occurs as sound waves from the larynx travel through patent bronchi and lungs to the chest wall. *Fremitus is symmetrical and easily palpated in the upper regions of the lungs.*	■ Tactile fremitus is decreased in atelectasis, emphysema, asthma, pleural effusion and pneumothorax. It is increased in pneumonia if the bronchus is patent.
Percuss the lungs for dullness over shoulder apices and over anterior, posterior and lateral intercostal spaces (see Figure 33.11). *The normal percussion tone over normal lung tissue is resonance.*	■ Dullness is heard in people with atelectasis, lobar pneumonia and pleural effusion. ■ Hyperresonance is heard in those with chronic asthma, emphysema and pneumothorax.
Percuss the posterior chest for diaphragmatic excursion. Systematic percussion of the posterior chest from a level of lung resonance to the level of diaphragmatic dullness reveals *diaphragmatic excursion*, a measurement of the level of the diaphragm. First percuss downward over the posterior thorax while the person exhales fully and holds the breath. Mark the spot at which the sound changes from resonant to dull. Then ask the person to inhale and hold the breath while you percuss downward again to note the descent of the diaphragm. Again mark the spot where the sound changes. *Measure the difference in diaphragmatic excursion, which normally varies from about 3 to 5 cm (see Figure 33.12).*	■ Diaphragmatic excursion is decreased in emphysema, ascites, on the affected side in pleural effusion and in pneumothorax. ■ A high level of dullness or a lack of excursion may indicate atelectasis or pleural effusion.

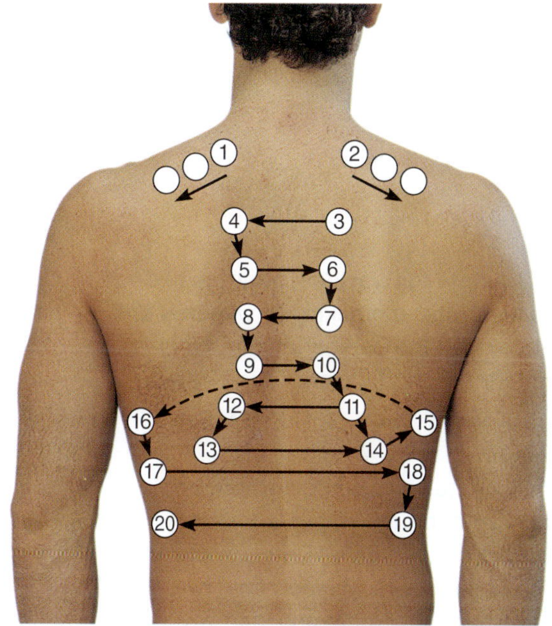

FIGURE 33.11 *Sequence for lung percussion*

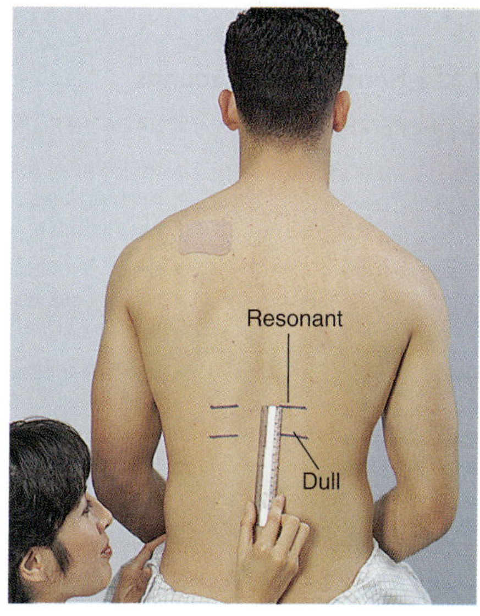

FIGURE 33.12 *Measuring diaphragmatic excursion*

(continued)

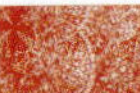

RESPIRATORY ASSESSMENTS (continued)

Technique/normal findings	Abnormal findings
Breath sound assessment **Auscultate the lungs for breath sounds with the diaphragm of the stethoscope by having the person take slow deep breaths through the mouth. Listen over anterior, posterior and lateral intercostal spaces (see Figure 33.13).** *The three different types of normal breath sounds are vesicular, bronchovesicular and bronchial (see Table 33.2).*	▪ Bronchial breath sounds (expiration > inspiration) and bronchovesicular breath sounds (inspiration = expiration) are heard over lungs filled with fluid or solid tissue. ▪ Breath sounds are decreased or diminished over atelectasis, emphysema, asthma, pleural effusion and pneumothorax. ▪ Breath sounds are increased over lobar pneumonia. ▪ Breath sounds are absent over collapsed lung, surgical removal of lung, pleural effusion and primary bronchus obstruction.
Auscultate for crackles, wheezes and friction rubs. If crackles or wheezes are heard, ask the person to cough and note if adventitious sound is cleared. *Normally, there are no crackles, wheezes or friction rubs.*	▪ **Crackles** (short, discrete, crackling or bubbling sounds) may be noted in pneumonia, bronchitis and congestive heart failure. ▪ **Wheezes** (continuous, musical sounds) may be heard in people with bronchitis, emphysema and asthma. ▪ A **friction rub** is a loud, dry, creaking sound that indicates pleural inflammation.
Auscultate voice sounds where any abnormal breath sound is noted by having the person say 'ninety-nine' (bronchophony); whisper 'one, two, three' (whispered pectoriloquy); and say 'ee' (egophony). *Normally, these sounds are heard by the examiner, but are muffled.*	▪ Voice sounds are decreased or absent over areas of atelectasis, asthma, pleural effusion and pneumothorax. ▪ Voice sounds are increased and clearer over lobar pneumonia. ▪ When testing egophony, the sound becomes louder and changes to 'a' over areas of consolidation or compression.

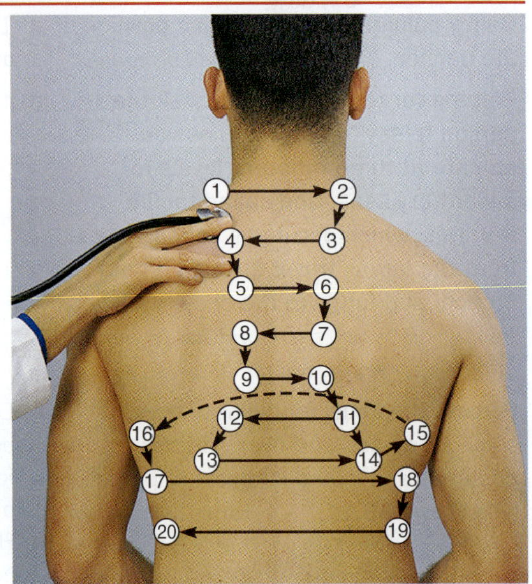

FIGURE 33.13 *Sequence for lung auscultation*

TABLE 33.2 Normal breath sounds

TYPE OF BREATH SOUND	CHARACTERISTICS
Vesicular	• Soft, low-pitched, gentle sounds • Heard over all areas of the lungs except the major bronchi • Have a 3:1 ratio for inspiration and expiration, respectively
Bronchovesicular	• Medium pitch and intensity of sounds • Have a 1:1 ratio, with inspiration and expiration being equal in duration • Heard anteriorly over the primary bronchus on each side of the sternum and posteriorly between the scapulae
Bronchial	• Loud, high-pitched sounds • Gap between inspiration and expiration • Have a 2:3 ratio for inspiration and expiration, respectively • Heard over the manubrium

TRANSLATION TO PRACTICE *The COPD-X plan: Australian and New Zealand Guidelines for the Management of Chronic Obstructive Pulmonary Disease*

Lung Foundation Australia's COPD Guidelines Committee updates evidence-based practice guidelines quarterly by evaluating current literature and research in order to remain relevant in the clinical management of COPD (Yang et al., 2021). The recommendation to cite a paper and make correlating changes to the COPD treatment guidelines includes feedback from the Thoracic Society of Australia and New Zealand through the Clinical Care and Resources Subcommittee (CCRS) and consumer representatives.

IMPLICATIONS FOR NURSING

Complete treatment plans for COPD are available on Lung Foundation Australia's website. As of December 2021, the Lung Foundation Australia's COPD Guidelines Committee recommendations should be followed as they represent the most recent, evidence-based changes needed in the care of individuals experiencing COPD:

- COPD is confirmed by persistent airflow limitation using spirometry tests post bronchodilator. Increased reliability is achieved with a repeat spirometry test if the test result is close to threshold in order to verify diagnosis.
- The use of long-acting bronchodilators can improve a patient's quality of life through reduction of symptoms and overall improvement in lung function. The use of long-acting muscarinic antagonists (LAMAs) rather than long-acting beta agonists (LABAs) to reduce exacerbations and prevent hospitalisations due to exacerbations is recommended.
- Smoking remains the most important risk factor in the development of COPD and smoking cessation the most important factor in reducing progression of COPD. Unfortunately, users of electronic cigarettes have been shown to have added risks as they are less likely to quit and often develop chronic bronchitis and exacerbations of COPD.
- Management of a chronic disease such as COPD should involve a multidisciplinary team approach based on the individual patient's needs. A speech therapist will play a key role in being able to assess dysphagia (difficulty swallowing) in individuals with COPD to prevent further exacerbations.
- Antibiotics can benefit individuals with signs of infection (increased volume and change in colour of sputum, with or without fever) experiencing an exacerbation of their COPD. However, it is important that treatment guidelines are followed to prevent overuse of intravenous antibiotics and dual antibiotic prescriptions.

CRITICAL THINKING IN PERSON-CENTRED CARE

1. This Committee uses evidence-based guidelines to determine the best plan of care for patients with COPD. The findings indicate smoking cessation remains a primary goal. How will you accommodate these findings into the health management plan of people with COPD?
2. How will the findings of this study impact on the assessment and individualised care that you provide when implementing a multidisciplinary approach to prevent further exacerbations in a patient with complex COPD?

FOCUS ON CULTURAL DIVERSITY **Are we working cooperatively with our Pacific partners to control multidrug-resistant tuberculosis at our borders?**

An article by Bainomugisa et al. (2022) confirmed that multidrug-resistant tuberculosis (MDR-TB) in Papua New Guinea (PNG) continues to pose a threat to public health for Australia's northern coast. With genotypic sequencing, they discovered that major clade in PNG has acquired a mutation to the newer antituberculosis drug even without exposure to it. Therefore, it is critical that public health workers and other healthcare professionals responsible for caring for individuals with respiratory symptoms stay hypervigilant to prevent further spread of this airborne transmitted respiratory disease.

Implications for nursing

The Department of Health and Aged Care (2022) reported that 89% of all cases of people newly diagnosed with tuberculosis (TB) in each year occurred in individuals born overseas. The rate of TB in overseas-born individuals is 19 times higher than for those born in Australia (Bright et al., 2022). In Australia in 2021, there were 1,452 new cases of TB, including seven multidrug-resistant cases (NSW Health, 2022). Although incidence and mortality is low and treatment success is high, and screening and management protocols have clearly withstood the current challenges associated with TB and MDR-TB in Papua New Guinea, care must be taken to ensure that policies support continued disease prevention and control.

Critical thinking in person-centred care

1. How could you find out more information about the epidemiology of tuberculosis within the local region?
2. How might cultural and language diversity complicate care of people requiring treatment for tuberculosis?
3. How might people with cultural and language diversity contribute to multidrug-resistant tuberculosis following discharge? Identify mechanisms and interventions to avoid this occurrence.

CHAPTER HIGHLIGHTS

- The respiratory system is divided into the upper respiratory system and the lower respiratory system.
- The upper respiratory system functions mostly as protection, filtration and the conductive section directing air to the lower respiratory system.
- The lower system has some conducting function but is largely responsible for provision of oxygen and elimination of carbon dioxide.
- Critical factors affecting ventilation and respiration include changes in volume and capacity; air pressures; oxygen, carbon dioxide and hydrogen ion concentrations in the blood; airway resistance, lung compliance and elasticity; and alveolar surface tension.
- Important components of a health history for an individual with a respiratory condition should include questions that can elicit answers to onset, characteristics, course, severity, precipitating and relieving factors, and any associated symptoms.
- Physical assessment techniques for assessing the respiratory system of an individual include inspection, palpation, percussion and auscultation. Other factors that should be noted include the person's level of consciousness, restlessness and anxiety level, and the colour of the lips and nail beds.

CONCEPT CHECK

1 Where is the apex of each lung located?
1 in the mediastinum
2 resting on the diaphragm
3 within the parietal pleura
4 just below the clavicle

2 Which physiological process is involved in gas exchange at the respiratory membrane?
1 facilitated transport
2 active transport
3 simple diffusion
4 hydrostatic pressure

3 Which structures cover the external surface of the alveoli?
1 terminal bronchioles
2 pulmonary arteries
3 pulmonary veins
4 pulmonary capillaries

4 Which process is initiated between oxygen and haemoglobin as the temperature of body tissues increases?
1 oxygen unloading is enhanced
2 oxygen unloading is inhibited
3 respiratory rate is decreased
4 lung compliance is increased

5 Which of the following questions should be included when conducting a health history to identify a genetic risk of respiratory disease?
1 'Tell me how many colds you have each year.'
2 'Has anyone in your family had a stroke or heart attack?'
3 'Has lung cancer ever been diagnosed in your family?'
4 'Do your children have trouble breathing at night?'

6 While auscultating the person's breath sounds, you note continuous musical sounds. You document these sounds as:
1 murmurs
2 wheezes
3 crackles
4 rales

7 The person you are assessing has had a lung removed. What type of breath sound would you expect to assess over the affected side?
1 resonance
2 crackles
3 bronchovesicular
4 absent

8 While assessing the person with a left pneumothorax you note decreased diaphragmatic excursion on the left. What would you do next?
1 Notify the doctor immediately.
2 Document the assessment.
3 Repeat the assessment several times.
4 Tell the person to hold their breath.

BIBLIOGRAPHY

Australian Institute of Health and Welfare: National Indigenous Australians Agency (2020). *Health Performance Framework. Tier 1—Health status and outcomes—1.04 Respiratory disease*. Retrieved from https://www.indigenoushpf.gov.au/

Bainomugisa, A., Lavu, E., Pandey, S. et al. (2022). Evolution and spread of a highly drug resistant strain of *Mycobacterium tuberculosis* in Papua New Guinea. *BMC Infectious Diseases, 22*, 437. https://doi.org/10.1186/s12879-022-07414-2

Bright, A., Denholm, J., Coulter, C., Waring, J. & Stapledon, R. (2020). Tuberculosis notifications in Australia, 2015–2018. *Communicable Disease Intelligence, 44*. https://doi.org/10.33321/cdi.2020.44.88

Bullock, S. & Hales, M. (2019). *Principles of pathophysiology*. Frenchs Forest, NSW: Pearson Australia.

Cancer Australia (2022). *Lung cancer in Australia statistics*. Retrieved from https://www.canceraustralia.gov.au/

Cystic Fibrosis Australia (2021). *The Australian Cystic Fibrosis Data Registry annual report, 2020*. Retrieved from https://www.cysticfibrosis.org.au/

Department of Health and Aged Care (2022). *World Tuberculosis (TB) Day*. Retrieved from http://www.health.gov.au/

Department of Health Victoria (2022). *Testing for respiratory pathogens—Health advisory*. Retrieved from https://www.health.vic.gov.au

Dezube, R. (2021). *Defense mechanisms of the respiratory system*. MSD Manual. Retrieved from https://www.msdmanuals.com/

Hall, R., Hall, I. & Sayers, I. (2019). Genetic risk factors for the development of pulmonary disease identified by genome-wide association. *Respirology, 24*(3), 204–214. https://doi.org/10.1111/resp.13436

Jarrom, D., Elston, L., Washington, J. et al. (2022). Effectiveness of tests to detect the presence of SARS-CoV-2 virus, and antibodies to SARS-CoV-2, to inform COVID-19 diagnosis: A rapid systematic review. *BMJ Evidence-Based Medicine, 27*, 33–45. http://dx.doi.org/10.1136/bmjebm-2020-111511

Kaminsky, D. A. (2022). *Overview of pulmonary function testing in adults*. Retrieved from https://www.uptodate.com/

Khoma, O., Park, J. O., Lee, F. M., Van der Wall, H. & Falk, G. L. (2022). Different clinical symptom patterns in patients with reflux micro-aspiration. *ERJ Open Research, 8*(00508). doi: 10.1183/23120541.00508-2021

Marieb, E. & Keller, S. (2021). *Essentials of human anatomy & physiology* (13th ed.). Harlow, Essex: Pearson.

Meharg, D., Jenkins, C., Maguire, G. et al. (2022). Implementing evidence into practice to improve chronic lung disease management in Indigenous Australians: The breathe easy, walk easy, lungs for life (BE WELL) project (protocol). *BMC Pulmonary Medicine, 22*, 239. https://doi.org/10.1186/s12890-022-02033-8

National Asthma Council Australia (2020). *Spirometry quick reference guide*. Melbourne: National Asthma Council Australia.

National Asthma Council Australia (2021). *Asthma deaths remain stubbornly high in Australia*. Retrieved from https://www.nationalasthma.org.au/

NSW Health (2022). *World TB Day 2022*. Retrieved from https://www.health.nsw.gov.au/

Patel, J. & Mohiuddin, S. (2022). *Physiology, oxygen transport and carbon dioxide dissociation curve*. StatPearls. Treasure Island (FL): StatPearls Publishing.

Rengasamy, N., Bilotta, F., Pugliese, F., Nozari, A. & Ortega, R. (2021). Administration of supplemental oxygen. *The New England Journal of Medicine, 385*(3), e9–e9. https://doi.org/10.1056/NEJMvcm2035240

Squires, E. (2022). Assessment and examination of the respiratory system. *Practice Nursing, 33*(1), 18–24. https://doi.org/10.12968/pnur.2022.33.1.18

Tortora, G. (2022). *Principles of anatomy and physiology* (3rd ed.). Brisbane: John Wiley and Sons Australia.

Yang, I., Brown, J., George, J. et al. (2021). *The COPD-X plan: Australian and New Zealand guidelines for the management of chronic obstructive pulmonary disease 2021*. Version 2.65. Retrieved from https://copdx.org.au/

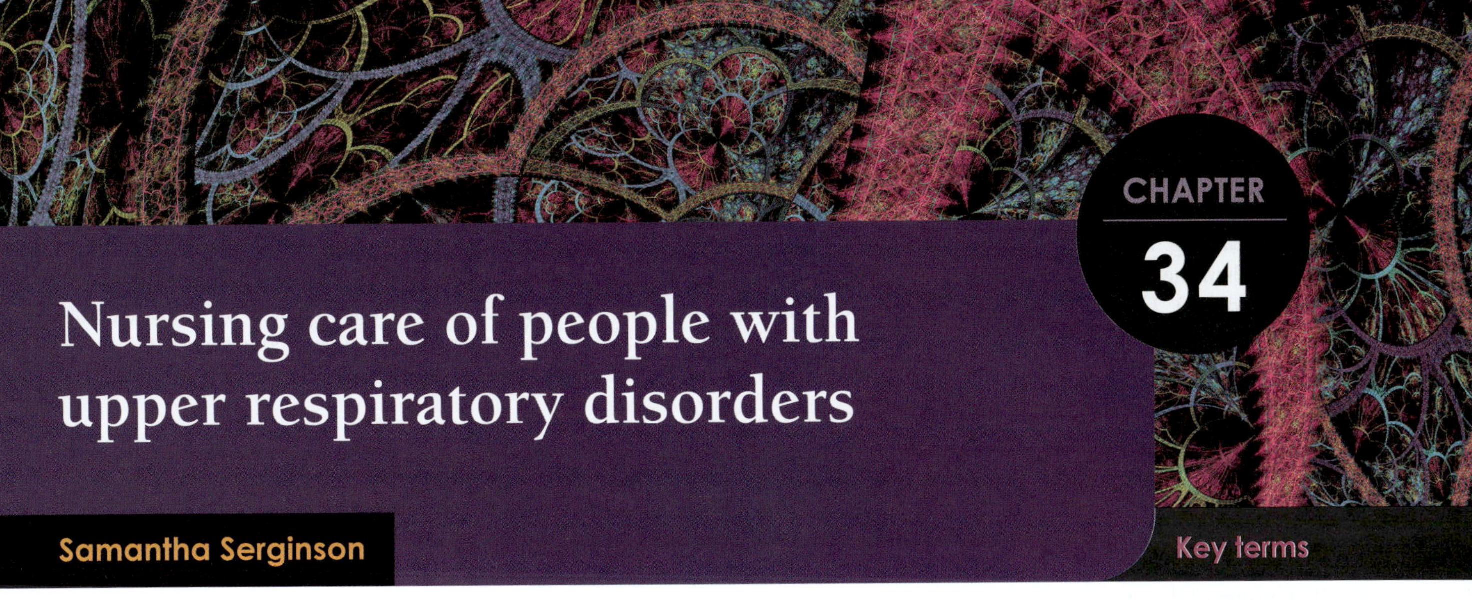

CHAPTER 34

Nursing care of people with upper respiratory disorders

Samantha Serginson

Learning outcomes

- Discuss the causes and implications of individuals experiencing selected infectious or inflammatory disorders of the upper respiratory system.
- Explore the occurrence and management of people experiencing obstructive conditions to the upper respiratory system such as trauma, epistaxis or surgery.
- Describe the critical considerations related to caring for a person with laryngeal obstruction from trauma or obstructive sleep apnoea.
- Examine the biopsychosocial implications and potential outcomes for a person with laryngeal tumour.

Clinical competencies

- Assess functional health status of people with upper respiratory tract disorders, using current data to identify and prioritise holistic nursing care needs.
- Apply nursing research and evidence-based practice to plan, implement and review nursing care for people with upper respiratory disorders.
- Provide safe, informed and effective nursing care for people having surgery involving the upper respiratory system and/or with a tracheostomy.
- Provide safe and informed administration of medications and prescribed treatments for people with disorders of the upper respiratory tract.
- Provide appropriate education for the patient and family affected by upper respiratory tract disorders.
- Evaluate the effectiveness of care, reassessing and modifying the plan of care as needed to achieve desired outcomes in alignment with patient goals.

Key terms

coryza 1213
COVID-19 1212
epistaxis 1224
influenza 1215
laryngectomy 1235
laryngitis 1223
pertussis 1223
pharyngitis 1220
rhinitis 1212
rhinoplasty 1228
sinusitis 1218
sleep apnoea 1230
tonsillitis 1220

Upper respiratory disorders can affect the nose, paranasal sinuses, tonsils, adenoids, larynx and pharynx. Upper respiratory disorders may be minor, such as the common cold, or acute if the airway is compromised. A patent upper airway is necessary for effective breathing. Acute and even life-threatening problems develop when the upper airway patency is affected (e.g. by laryngeal oedema). Upper respiratory disorders can affect breathing, communication, ability to participate in activities and body image. When breathing is compromised due to swelling, bleeding or accumulation of secretions, fear and anxiety may develop, often leading to exacerbation of the condition.

Nursing care focuses on maintaining a patent airway, managing pain and symptoms, promoting effective communication and providing psychological support for the person and family. Prior to proceeding with this chapter, a review of the anatomy and physiology, diagnostic tests and assessment of the upper respiratory system in the chapter 'A person-centred approach to assessing the respiratory system' is conducted and referred to as needed.

Infectious and inflammatory disorders of the upper respiratory system

Constant exposure of the upper respiratory tract to environmental factors such as pollution and inhalation of potentially harmful substances can make it vulnerable to a variety of infectious and inflammatory conditions. Although most upper respiratory infections and inflammations are minor, complications may result. In the older adult and other vulnerable groups, the risk of serious problems following an upper respiratory infection can be significant.

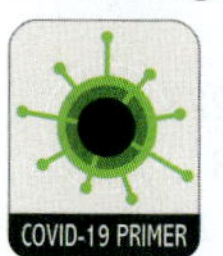

COVID-19 is a novel coronavirus not previously seen in humans.

Rhinitis, inflammation of the nasal cavities, is the most common upper respiratory disorder. Rhinitis may be either acute or chronic. *Acute viral rhinitis* is often described as the common cold. *Chronic rhinitis* includes allergic, vasomotor and atrophic rhinitis. *Allergic rhinitis*, or hay fever, results from a sensitivity reaction to allergens such as plant pollens or unidentified environmental factors. It tends to occur seasonally. *Vasomotor rhinitis* occurs when the blood vessels inside the nasal cavity dilate or expand (Ortega, Nickle & Carter, 2021). The aetiology of *vasomotor rhinitis* is unknown. Although its manifestations are similar to those of allergic rhinitis, it is not linked to allergens. *Atrophic rhinitis* is characterised by changes in the mucous membrane of the nasal cavities. Symptoms of atrophic rhinitis include excessive nasal discharge, crust formation at opening of nares due to discharge build-up, nasal obstruction due to excessive mucus production, sore throat, susceptibility to frequent nasal infections, eye watering and headaches.

FAST FACTS

- Rhinoviruses are the most common cause of viral URTIs. Colds due to rhinovirus are more common in early autumn and late spring.
- More than 100 different serotypes of rhinovirus have been identified.
- Parainfluenza viruses, respiratory syncytial virus (RSV), coronaviruses and adenoviruses can also cause URTIs (Dekker et al., 2022).
- There is no cure for the common cold. The goal is to minimise the effects of the common cold.

THE PERSON WITH VIRAL UPPER RESPIRATORY TRACT INFECTION

Viral upper respiratory tract infections (URTIs, or the common cold) are the most common respiratory tract infections and are among the most common human diseases. URTIs are highly contagious and are prevalent in environments where people are gathered such as schools, work environments, shopping centres and music festivals.

Pathophysiology

More than 200 strains of virus causes URTI, including rhinoviruses, adenoviruses, parainfluenza viruses, coronaviruses and respiratory syncytial virus. (See the section that follows for more information about RSV.) Occasionally, more than one virus may be present. Viruses causing acute URTIs are spread by aerosolised droplet nuclei during sneezing or coughing, or by direct contact with a fomite such as touching an object (e.g. a door handle) that is contaminated. The virus usually spreads when the hands and fingers pick it up from contaminated surfaces and carry it to the eyes and mucous membranes of the susceptible host. People who have been infected are highly contagious, shedding the virus for a few days prior to and after the appearance of symptoms. Although immunity is produced to the individual virus strain, the number of viruses causing URTI ensures that most people continue to experience colds throughout their lifetimes.

Viscous mucus secretions in the upper respiratory tract trap invading organisms, preventing contamination of more vulnerable areas in the lung. Cells of the upper respiratory tract are infected when the virus attaches to receptors on the cell. Local immunological defences, such as secretory IgA antibodies in respiratory secretions, then attempt to inactivate the antigen, producing a local inflammatory response. The mucous membranes of the nasal passages swell and become hyperaemic and engorged. Mucus-secreting glands become hyperactive, causing excessive mucus production. These responses to the virus produce the typical manifestation viral URTI (Wang et al., 2021).

Manifestations and complications

Acute viral URTI often presents as the common cold. Nasal mucous membranes appear red (*erythematous*) and *boggy* (swollen). Swollen mucous membranes, local vasodilation and secretions often cause nasal congestion. Clear, watery secretions lead to **coryza**, profuse nasal discharge. Sneezing and coughing are common. A sore throat is common and may be the initial and presenting symptom. Systemic manifestations of acute viral URTI may include low-grade fever, headache, malaise, muscle aches and generally feeling unwell. Symptoms generally last for a few days up to 2 weeks. Although acute viral URTI is typically mild and self-limited, its effects on the immune defences of the upper respiratory tract can increase the risk of more serious secondary bacterial infections, such as sinusitis or otitis media.

INTERPROFESSIONAL CARE

Because most acute viral URTIs are self-limiting, self-care is most appropriate and encouraged. Medical treatment is usually required only when complications such as sinusitis or otitis media develop, or a medical certificate is required to support sick leave from commitments such as work or school.

Diagnosis of acute viral URTI is usually based on the patient history, physical examination and presenting symptoms. Diagnostic testing may be indicated if a complication such as bacterial infection is suspected. A white blood count (WBC) may be ordered to assess for leucocytosis (an elevated WBC). Cultures may also be taken of the purulent nasal discharge or coughed secretions to identify the bacterium that is causing the infection. This assists in determining which class of antibiotic may be suitable.

Treatment is aimed at relieving symptoms. Adequate rest, maintaining fluid intake, managing anorexia and avoiding feeling chilled can help relieve systemic symptoms such as fever, malaise and muscle ache. People are instructed to cover the mouth and nose with tissues when coughing or sneezing, dispose of soiled tissues appropriately and wash hands thoroughly. Additionally, avoiding crowds and maintaining a distance of 1 m from others helps prevent spread of the infection to others.

Medications

Medications may be recommended to shorten the duration of the illness and relieve symptoms. Mild decongestants or over-the-counter (OTC) antihistamines may help relieve coryza and nasal congestion. Nasal sprays such as phenylephrine rapidly relieve nasal congestion but may lead to dependence and rebound congestion if used for more than a few days at a time. Warm saltwater gargles, throat lozenges or mild analgesics may be used for sore throat. Although no specific antiviral therapy has been shown to be effective in shortening the duration of a URTI, experimental vaccines to prevent acute viral URTI are in developmental stages. For the nursing implications of decongestants and common antihistamines, see the 'Medication administration' box.

MEDICATION ADMINISTRATION Decongestants and antihistamines

DECONGESTANTS

Decongestants promote vasoconstriction, reducing the inflammation and oedema of nasal mucosa and relieving nasal congestion. They are very effective when applied topically (via a nasal spray) because of their rapid onset of action. However, the duration of effect is short, and can be followed by vasodilation and rebound congestion. Because of their rapid effect and short duration, these preparations are habit forming. Chronic use may lead to rhinitis medicamentosa, a rebound phenomenon of drug-induced nasal irritation and inflammation. Caution is advised when using nasal decongestant sprays.

Nursing responsibilities

- Assess for contraindications, such as hypertension or chronic heart disease. Decongestants can stimulate the sympathetic nervous system, increasing peripheral vascular resistance, blood pressure and heart rate.
- Evaluate medication regimen for potential interactions such as antihypertensive medications and monoamine oxidase (MAO) inhibitors.
- Advise the patient to only use nasal decongestants for the recommended timeframes to avoid rhinitis medicamentosa.

Health education for the person and family

- Do not use more than the recommended dose or for longer than advised by a medical officer.
- Use nasal sprays for no more than 3 to 5 days, or as directed.
- Check with a medical officer before taking decongestants if you are taking any prescription medications or are being treated for high blood pressure or heart disease due to the known side effects of decongestants constricting blood vessels and causing an increase in heart rate.
- Increase fluid intake and use saline mouth rinses to relieve mouth dryness.
- Decongestants may cause nervousness, shakiness or difficulty sleeping. Stop the drug if these effects occur or if a person's ability to function safely is impaired.
- Read the medication information and instructions included prior to use.

ANTIHISTAMINES

Antihistamines are widely available with and without a prescription. They are frequently combined with decongestants in OTC cold and allergy preparations. Antihistamines relieve the systemic effects of histamine and dry respiratory secretions through an anticholinergic effect. Most antihistamines cause drowsiness, although non-sedating forms are less likely to interfere with alertness. Diphenhydramine is used in numerous OTC sleep aids as well as in cold and allergy preparations.

(continued)

MEDICATION ADMINISTRATION Decongestants and antihistamines (continued)

Nursing responsibilities

- Before administering or recommending these drugs, assess for possible contraindications, including the following:
  - acute asthma or lower respiratory disease that may be aggravated by antihistamines drying mucous membrane secretions; caution is advised
  - hypersensitivity or allergy to antihistamines
  - glaucoma (increased intraocular pressure). Antihistamines can cause pupils to dilate. If a person has a history of glaucoma, antihistamines may cause a further increase in intraocular pressure and should be used with caution or avoided
  - impaired gastrointestinal motility or obstruction. Some antihistamine preparations can increase the risk of constipation and steps should be taken to manage this to reduce straining when defecating
  - prostatic hypertrophy or other urinary tract obstruction
  - heart disease.
- It is recommended that for people who must remain alert while on antihistamine therapy, non-sedating forms should be used.
- Read the medication information and instructions included prior to use.

Health education for the person and family

- Do not drive or operate machinery while taking OTC or prescription forms of antihistamines known to be sedating.
- Stop the drug and notify your doctor immediately if you develop confusion, excessive sedation, chest tightness, wheezing, bleeding or easy bruising while taking antihistamines.
- Do not use alcohol or other central nervous system depressants while taking antihistamines.
- Hard lollies, chewing gum, ice chips and liquids help relieve mouth dryness caused by antihistamines.

Complementary therapies

Currently there is little published evidence to demonstrate that complementary therapies are useful in the management of respiratory infections. Herbal remedies, such as echinacea and garlic, may have some antiviral and antibiotic effects (Rouf et al., 2020). Echinacea is also thought to stimulate the immune system, improving the body's response to infection. Taken at the first sign of infection, echinacea may reduce the duration and symptoms, although clinical trials have shown no consistent benefit. Studies of the use of garlic in acute respiratory tract infections also suggest limited or uncertain effectiveness (Rouf et al., 2020).

Vitamin C is also promoted as a measure to reduce the severity and duration of URTI. Again, however, little consistent benefit is demonstrated in well-designed rigorous clinical trials (Holford et al., 2020). It is possible that zinc helps reduce the length and severity of a cold; however, it can cause nausea and other gastrointestinal issues. Patients should discuss any complementary therapies they may be utilising with their GP.

Aromatherapy with essential oils such as basil, cedarwood, eucalyptus, frankincense, lavender, marjoram, peppermint or rosemary may reduce congestion and promote comfort and recovery. Education should include that these essential oils are to be used only for inhalation and are not for internal consumption.

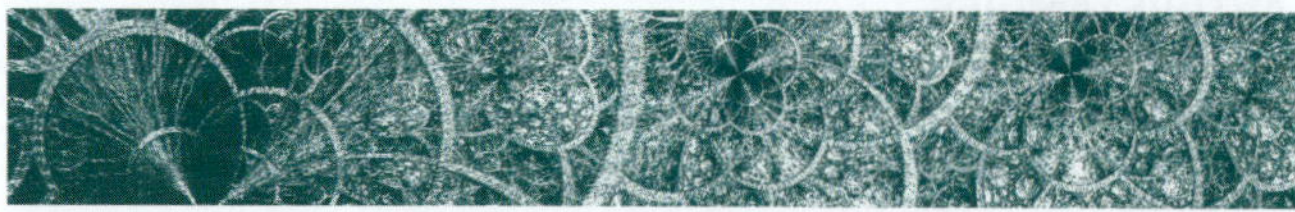

Nursing care

Health promotion

Most importantly, people can limit their incidence of acute viral URTI by frequent handwashing and avoiding exposure to crowds, especially in winter when respiratory infections are high. Maintaining good general health and stress-reducing activities support the immune system and can assist in helping to reduce the risk of an acute viral URTI. Education should include advising the patient that becoming chilled or going out in the rain does not cause colds and that URTIs are more likely to occur during periods of physical or psychological stress.

Community-based care

The primary nursing role in caring for people with acute viral URTI is educational. Education is directed towards self-management and alleviation of symptoms. Self-care is appropriate for most people unless the problem is recurrent or a complication occurs. Acute viral URTI may interfere with work and recreational activities. Unless limited by symptoms, normal daily activities and roles usually can be maintained. Additional rest, increased fluid intake and a well-balanced diet during the acute phase of illness is recommended to support the immune response and to hasten recovery.

The following recommendations can be included in teaching self-management and home care:

- using disposable tissues to cover the mouth and nose while coughing or sneezing to reduce airborne spread of the virus
- disposing of tissues after use
- blowing the nose with both nostrils open to prevent infected matter from being forced into the eustachian tubes
- washing hands frequently, especially after coughing or sneezing, to limit viral transmission
- using OTC preparations for symptomatic relief; precautions related to the sedating effects of antihistamines
- limiting use of nasal decongestants to every 4 hours for only a few days at a time to prevent rebound effect.

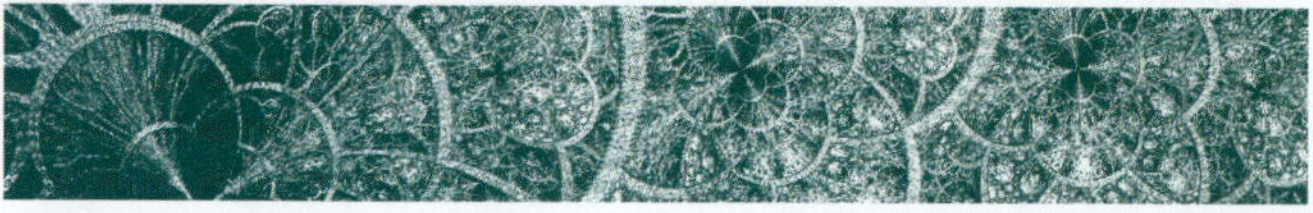

THE PERSON WITH RESPIRATORY SYNCYTIAL VIRUS

Respiratory syncytial virus (RSV) is a common virus that is the primary cause of respiratory illnesses in young children and the majority of lower respiratory disease in infants. Older children and adults are commonly and repetitively infected by RSV, but the disease is milder, usually presenting as a common cold. However, older adults and people who are immunocompromised may develop severe pneumonitis when exposed to RSV (Karron, 2021). Mortality rates for RSV are higher in older adults and people who are immunocompromised (Branche et al., 2022).

RSV is transmitted in much the same way as other URTIs: via contaminated hands or objects, and by coarse droplets in the atmosphere spread by coughing and sneezing. The incubation period is 4 to 6 days. In adults, the manifestations of RSV are those of other common URTIs, including rhinorrhoea, sore throat and cough. Headache, malaise and low-grade fever may occur. In older adults, RSV may present as lower respiratory infection with fever or pneumonia (Branche et al., 2022).While the illness also presents as URTI in infants, it is more likely to progress to pneumonia, bronchiolitis and tracheobronchiolitis in this population.

Treatment for adults with upper respiratory RSV is symptomatic (see the preceding section on URTI). When the lower respiratory tract is involved, hydration and other supportive measures to mobilise respiratory secretions are important. Intubation and mechanical ventilation may be necessary if hypoxia develops. The focus of nursing care for the adult with URTI manifestations of RSV is on teaching for self-care, identification of complications and prevention of viral spread. When lower respiratory symptoms are present, nursing care is similar to that provided for people with pneumonia (see the chapter 'Nursing care of people with ventilation disorders').

THE PERSON WITH INFLUENZA

Influenza, or *flu*, is a highly contagious viral respiratory disease characterised by coryza, fever, cough and systemic symptoms such as headache and malaise. In Australia in 2021, notifications of laboratory-confirmed influenza continued to decrease and remained lower than average compared to previous years. However, data reported may not have been an accurate reflection of influenza activity due to COVID-19 (Department of Health and Aged Care, 2022a).

Influenza usually occurs in epidemics or pandemics, although sporadic cases do occur. Localised outbreaks of influenza usually occur about every 1–3 years. Global epidemics and pandemics are less frequent, developing every 10–15 years until the past two decades. A recently identified strain of influenza A, H1N1 (swine flu), reached pandemic stage in 2009 and is currently classified in the post-pandemic stage. Influenza A demonstrated the ability to spread between humans. This strain of virus is thought to be a re-assortment of four known strains of influenza A virus subtype H1N1, with one strain originating from humans, one from birds and two from swine.

Although influenza tends to be mild and self-limited in healthy adults, older adults and people with chronic heart or pulmonary disease have a high incidence of complications (such as pneumonia) and a higher risk of mortality related to the disease and its complications (Uyeki, 2020).

Pathophysiology

Influenza virus is transmitted by airborne droplet and direct contact. Three main strains of the virus have been identified as influenza A virus, influenza B virus and influenza C virus. Influenza A is responsible for most infections and the most severe outbreaks of influenza. This is primarily due to its ability to alter its surface antigens, bypassing previously developed immune defences to the virus. New strains of influenza virus are named according to the strain, geographical origin and the year the strain was identified (e.g. A/Taiwan/89). Surface antigens of the specific virus may be used to further differentiate influenza A viruses. Outbreaks of influenza B virus are generally less extensive and less severe than those caused by influenza A virus. Illness associated with influenza C virus is mild and often goes unrecognised.

The incubation period for influenza is short, only 18 to 72 hours. The virus infects the respiratory epithelium. It rapidly replicates in infected cells and is released to infect neighbouring cells. Inflammation leads to necrosis and shedding of serous and ciliated cells of the respiratory tract. Nasally, this allows extracellular fluid to escape, producing rhinorrhoea. With recovery, serous cells are replaced more rapidly than ciliated cells, leading to continued cough and coryza. Systemic manifestations of influenza likely are caused by release of inflammatory mediators such as tumour necrosis factor alpha, interleukin-alpha and interleukin-6. The humoral and cell-mediated immune responses are activated by influenza infection and are supplemented by other local and systemic responses (such as interferons). Viral shedding lasts 5–10 days, starting just before the onset of symptoms; however, young children and immunocompromised individuals may shed for much longer.

FAST FACTS

- Type A influenza viruses are found in many animals including birds, bats, pigs, whales, horses, seals and humans (Nguyen, Rollon & Choi, 2021). Type A influenza is believed to have caused four pandemics: 1918 (Spanish flu), 1957 (Asian flu), 1968 (Hong Kong flu) and most recently the H1N1 'swine flu' in 2009 (worldwide).
- Type B influenza viruses are commonly found in humans and often are responsible for influenza outbreaks but not pandemics.
- Type C influenza viruses, found in humans, pigs and dogs, typically cause mild respiratory infections (Nguyen et al., 2021).

Manifestations

Infection with influenza virus produces one of three syndromes: uncomplicated nasopharyngeal inflammation, viral upper respiratory infection followed by bacterial infection, or viral pneumonia. The onset is rapid; profound malaise may develop in a matter of minutes.

Manifestations of influenza include sudden onset of chills and fever, malaise, muscle aches and headache. Respiratory manifestations include dry, non-productive cough, sore throat, substernal burning and coryza (see the 'Manifestations' box). Acute symptoms subside within 2 to 3 days, although fever may last as long as a week. The cough may be severe and productive. Along with fatigue and weakness, the cough can persist for days or several weeks.

MANIFESTATIONS Influenza

RESPIRATORY MANIFESTATIONS
- Coryza
- Cough, initially dry becoming productive
- Substernal burning
- Sore throat

SYSTEMIC MANIFESTATIONS
- Fever and chills
- Malaise
- Muscle aches
- Fatigue

Complications

The respiratory epithelial necrosis caused by influenza increases the risk of secondary bacterial infections. Sinusitis and otitis media are frequent complications of influenza. Tracheobronchitis, inflammation of the trachea and bronchi, may develop. Although tracheobronchitis is not a serious health risk, its manifestations may persist for up to 3 weeks.

Influenza is linked to an increased risk of pneumonia, particularly in older adults. Changes in respiratory function associated with ageing, including decreased effectiveness of cough and increased residual lung volume, pose little risk in the healthy older adult but greatly increase the risk of pneumonia associated with influenza. Primary influenza viral pneumonia, while uncommon, is a serious complication that may be fatal. It typically develops within 48 hours of the onset of influenza, often in people with pre-existing heart valve or pulmonary disease. Influenza pneumonia progresses rapidly and can cause hypoxaemia and death within a few days. Bacterial pneumonia is more likely to occur in older at-risk adults but may also affect otherwise healthy adults. It usually presents as a relapse of influenza, with a productive cough and evidence of pneumonia on the chest x-ray. See the chapter 'Nursing care of people with ventilation disorders' for more information about pneumonia.

Other respiratory complications of influenza include exacerbation of chronic obstructive pulmonary disease (COPD), chronic bronchitis or asthma. Sinusitis (discussed later in this chapter) may also develop.

Reye's syndrome is a rare but potentially fatal complication of influenza. Although it is more likely to affect children, it also has been identified in older adults. It is most often associated with influenza B virus. Reye's syndrome develops 2 to 3 weeks after the onset of influenza. It has a 30% mortality rate. Hepatic failure and encephalopathy develop rapidly in people with Reye's syndrome.

While uncommon, other potential complications of influenza include myositis (inflammation of skeletal muscles), myocarditis (inflammation of the heart muscle) and central nervous system (CNS) disorders such as encephalitis and Guillain–Barré syndrome.

INTERPROFESSIONAL CARE

Preventing community outbreaks and protecting vulnerable populations (e.g. older adults and people with chronic diseases) are the primary focus for interprofessional care related to influenza. Medical treatment of influenza focuses on establishing the diagnosis, providing symptomatic relief and preventing complications.

Prevention

Preventing influenza by immunising at-risk populations is an important aspect of care. Immunisation with polyvalent (containing antigens of several viral strains) influenza virus vaccine is largely effective in preventing influenza infection for several months to a year (Nguyen et al., 2021). Annual immunisation is recommended for at-risk people, including people over the age of 65, residents of nursing homes, adults and children with chronic cardiopulmonary disorders (e.g. asthma) or chronic metabolic diseases such as diabetes, and healthcare workers who have frequent contact with high-risk people. Additionally, family members of at-risk people should be vaccinated to reduce the person's risk of exposure. The vaccine is given in autumn, prior to the annual winter outbreak (Mohammed et al., 2021).

Diagnosis

The diagnosis of influenza is based on history, clinical findings and knowledge of an influenza outbreak in the community. A chest x-ray and WBC count may be done to rule out complications such as pneumonia. The WBC count is commonly decreased in viral influenza; bacterial infections usually cause increased WBCs.

Medications

Yearly immunisation with influenza vaccine is the single most important measure to prevent or minimise symptoms of influenza. About 5% of people experience mild symptoms of low-grade fever, malaise or myalgia for up to 24 hours after vaccination. Because the vaccine is produced using an egg-based manufacturing process, it should not be given to people who are allergic to egg protein. Serious adverse reactions to influenza vaccine are rare. *Guillain–Barré syndrome*, an acute neurological disorder characterised by muscle weakness and distal sensory loss, has been associated with the vaccine; however, this is very rare.

Over-the-counter analgesics such as aspirin, paracetamol or non-steroidal anti-inflammatory drugs (NSAIDs) provide symptomatic relief of fever and muscle ache. Antitussives may decrease cough, promoting rest. Antibiotics are not indicated unless secondary bacterial infection occurs.

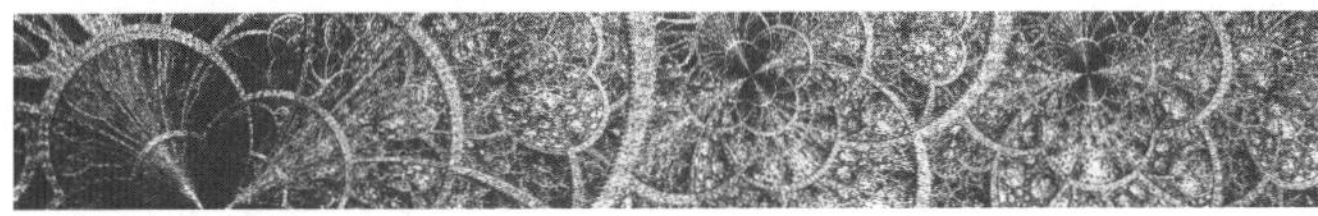

Nursing care

Health promotion

Stress the importance of yearly influenza vaccination for people in high-risk groups and their families. Teach about spread of the disease, including measures to reduce the risk of contracting influenza, such as avoiding crowds, adopting coughing and sneezing etiquette techniques, avoiding people who are ill and practising general hygiene practices such as handwashing.

Assessment

Unless there is a known outbreak of influenza in the community, it can be difficult to differentiate the manifestations of influenza from those of other URTIs.

- *Health history*: known exposure to virus; current symptoms, their onset and duration; presence of dyspnoea, chest pain, productive cough, facial pain or pressure in sinus areas; current medications, history of influenza vaccine; chronic diseases such as heart disease, asthma, COPD or diabetes; known medication allergies.
- *Physical examination*: general appearance; vital signs including temperature; skin colour; lung sounds; abdominal exam.
- *Diagnostic tests*: WBC, throat and sputum cultures, and chest x-ray for evidence of bacterial infection or pneumonia.

Nursing diagnoses and interventions

Although the symptoms of influenza are distressing, most people with the illness provide self-care and do not contact a healthcare provider. Recommendations are to rest in bed during the acute phase of the illness, manage symptoms and limit activities until recovery from influenza.

Severe disease or complications of influenza may necessitate hospitalisation for respiratory support and management. For these people, nursing care focuses on maintaining airway clearance, breathing patterns, consuming increased fluids and ensuring adequate rest.

Ineffective breathing pattern

Muscle aches, malaise and elevated temperature may increase the respiratory rate and alter the depth of respirations, decreasing effective alveolar ventilation. Shallow respirations also increase the risk of *atelectasis* (lack of ventilation in an area of lung).

> **CONSIDERATION FOR PRACTICE**
> **Monitor respiratory rate and pattern. Tachypnoea and/or rapid, shallow respirations may impair effective alveolar ventilation and gas exchange, increasing the risk of additional complications such as atelectasis.**

- Pace activities to provide for periods of rest. *Tachypnoea increases the work of breathing, causing fatigue; fatigue, in turn, can further impair ventilation and reduce the effectiveness of coughing.*
- Elevate the head of the bed. *The upright position improves lung excursion and reduces the work of breathing by lowering the diaphragm, moving abdominal contents downwards, creating less resistance to diaphragmatic excursion and slightly decreasing venous return.*

Ineffective airway clearance

Swelling and congestion of mucous membranes, extracellular fluid exudate and impaired ciliary action due to cell damage increase the risk of impaired airway clearance in influenza. The older adult is at particular risk because of reduced ciliary activity and increased lung compliance.

> **CONSIDERATION FOR PRACTICE**
> **Monitor the effectiveness of cough and ability to remove airway secretions. Fatigue and general malaise may impair the ability to cough effectively and mobilise secretions.**

- Maintain adequate hydration. Assess mucous membranes and skin turgor for evidence of dehydration. *Fever and decreased oral fluid intake may lead to dehydration and increased viscosity of secretions. Thick, viscous secretions are more difficult to expectorate, causing fatigue and the risk of infection.*
- Increase the humidity of inspired air with a bedside humidifier. *Increasing the water content of inhaled air helps loosen thick secretions and soothe mucous membranes.*
- Teach effective cough techniques. Administer analgesics as ordered. *The huff cough is effective to maintain open airways and it spares energy. (See Box 36.4 in the chapter 'Nursing care of people with gas exchange disorders' for teaching of this technique.) Relieving muscle ache increases the ability to cough effectively.*

Disturbed sleep pattern

Airway congestion, malaise, muscle aches and persistent cough may interfere with the ability to rest, increasing fatigue and prolonging recovery.

- Assess sleep patterns using subjective and objective information. *The person may appear to be sleeping but not achieving normal sleep patterns because of influenza symptoms such as coughing and sneezing. Both subjective and objective data are important to accurately assess sleep.*

> **CONSIDERATION FOR PRACTICE**
> **If necessary, request a cough suppressant for night-time use. Cough suppressants are not recommended during the day because coughing promotes airway clearance. They may, however, be necessary at night to allow rest.**

- Provide antipyretic and analgesic medications at or shortly before bedtime. *These drugs promote comfort by reducing fever and relieving muscle aches.*

Risk of infection

Infection control measures are recommended to prevent person-to-person transmission of influenza and to control influenza outbreaks in healthcare facilities.

- Use standard precautions and encourage all staff and visitors to frequently wash hands. *Handwashing is a primary infection control measure for infections transmitted via respiratory secretions.*
- Instruct people and visitors to control respiratory secretions by using tissues and to maintain a distance of at least 1.5 m from others when coughing or sneezing. Handkerchiefs are not recommended due to spread of contaminants with multiple use. Provide masks for people and visitors who are unable to control secretions. *Limiting the spread of aerosolised secretions by covering the nose and mouth and maintaining distance from other people can reduce the spread of the disease to vulnerable populations.*
- Use droplet precautions for people with suspected or confirmed influenza: private room, masks for caregivers and visitors, and a mask for the person when being transported within the facility. *These measures limit the spread of respiratory secretions.*

Community-based care

Encourage appropriate self-care for people with influenza. Discuss the following topics related to home care:

- Increase rest during the acute, febrile phase of the illness.
- Maintain an increased fluid intake even if anorexic.
- Appropriately use OTC medications for symptom relief.
- Employ hygiene measures such as using disposable tissues and frequent handwashing to reduce spread of the disease.
- Know manifestations of potential complications of influenza to report to the primary care provider.

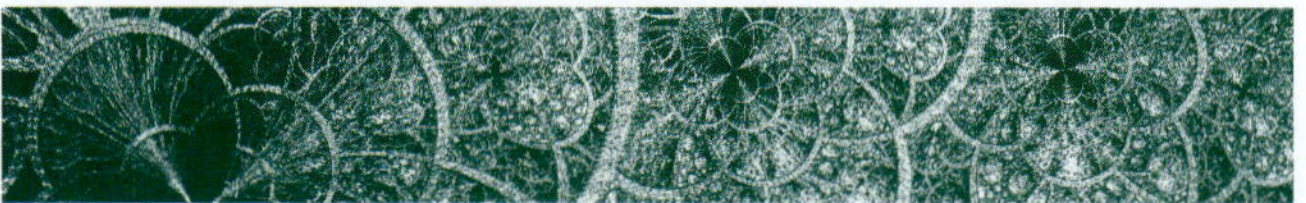

THE PERSON WITH SINUSITIS

Sinusitis is inflammation of the mucous membranes of one or more of the sinuses (see Figure 33.2 in the chapter 'A person-centred approach to assessing the respiratory system'). Sinusitis is a common condition that usually follows an upper respiratory infection such as acute viral upper respiratory infection or influenza. Common causative organisms include streptococci, *S. pneumoniae, Haemophilus influenzae* and staphylococci. The risk of sinusitis is higher when the immune system is suppressed by immunosuppressive drugs and in immune-compromised disorders such as HIV infection. Sinusitis is common and difficult to treat in people who have AIDS.

Physiology review

The sinuses (or *paranasal sinuses*) are air-filled cavities in the facial bones that open into the turbinates of the nasal cavity. They are lined with ciliated mucous membranes that help move fluid and microorganisms out of the sinuses into the nasal cavity. The sinuses normally are a sterile area. Air within the sinuses has lower oxygen content than inspired air.

Pathophysiology

Sinusitis develops when nasal mucous membranes swell or other disorders obstruct sinus openings, impairing drainage. Mucus secretions collect in the sinus cavity, serving as a medium for bacterial growth. The nasal and sinus mucous membranes are continuous; therefore, bacteria generally spread to the sinuses via the opening into the nasal turbinates. The inflammatory response provoked by bacterial invasion draws serum and leucocytes to the area to combat the infection, increasing swelling and pressure, causing discomfort and facial pain.

Any process that impairs drainage from the sinuses may precipitate sinusitis. These include nasal polyps, deviated septum, rhinitis, tooth abscess, swimming or diving trauma. In hospitalised people, sinusitis may develop following prolonged nasotracheal intubation. Usually more than one sinus is infected. The frontal and maxillary sinuses are usually involved in adults.

Sinusitis may be acute or chronic. Chronic sinusitis results when acute sinusitis is untreated or inadequately treated. With continued infection, bacteria can become isolated, producing chronic inflammation. Over time, mucous membranes become thickened. Fungal infections may cause chronic infections, especially in immunosuppressed people. Other factors that may contribute to chronic sinusitis are smoking, a history of allergy and habitual use of nasal sprays or inhalants.

Manifestations and complications

The person with acute sinusitis often looks sick. Manifestations of sinusitis include pain and tenderness across the infected sinuses, headache, fever and malaise. The pain usually increases with leaning forward. When the maxillary sinuses are involved, pain and pressure are felt over the cheek. The pain may be referred to the upper teeth. Frontal sinusitis causes pain and tenderness across the lower forehead. Infection of the ethmoid sinus produces retro-orbital pain and pain over the high lateral aspect of the nose. Sphenoid sinusitis, the rarest form, may cause pain in the occiput, vertex or middle of the head. Symptoms often worsen for 3 to 4 hours after awakening and then become less severe in the afternoon and evening as secretions drain. The intensity and location of headache pain may change as sinuses drain. In acute sinusitis, the pain is usually constant and severe. In chronic sinusitis, the pain is described as dull and may be constant or intermittent.

Other symptoms include nasal congestion, purulent nasal discharge and bad breath. The nasal mucous membrane is red and swollen. Purulent drainage may be noted at the opening to the middle turbinate. This may be the only sign of chronic sinusitis. Swallowed secretions irritate and inflame the throat and may cause nausea or vomiting.

Complications develop when the infection spreads to surrounding structures (see Box 34.1). These include periorbital abscess or cellulitis, cavernous sinus thrombosis, meningitis, brain abscess or sepsis. Eustachian tube oedema may lead to hearing loss.

BOX 34.1 Potential complications of sinusitis

Local complications

- Orbital cellulitis
- Subperiosteal abscess
- Orbital abscess
- Cavernous sinus thrombosis
- Mucocoele
- Osteomyelitis

Intracranial complications

- Meningitis
- Epidural abscess
- Subdural abscess
- Brain abscess
- Venous sinus thrombosis

INTERPROFESSIONAL CARE

Treatment of sinusitis focuses on restoring drainage of obstructed sinuses, controlling infection, relieving pain, reducing symptoms and preventing complications.

Diagnosis

The diagnosis of acute sinusitis usually can be made using the history and physical exam. Diagnostic studies such as computed tomography (CT) scan or sinus x-rays generally are done only when sinusitis is persistent, chronic or recurrent. See the chapter 'A person-centred approach to assessing the respiratory system' for more information about diagnostic studies and their nursing implications.

- *Sinus x-rays* are evaluated. Sinuses are normally translucent because they are filled with air; affected sinuses appear cloudy or opaque. A visible air–fluid level or thickening of the sinus mucosa may be seen in infected sinuses.
- *CT scan* is a more sensitive indicator of acute and chronic sinusitis and often is performed without preceding x-rays.
- *Magnetic resonance imaging (MRI)* may be ordered if malignancy of the sinus is suspected.

Medications

Antibiotic therapy directed at the usual organisms causing sinusitis typically is prescribed. Amoxicillin and Augmentin (penicillin and clavulanic acid), possibly combined with cefaclor, are commonly used antibiotics for sinusitis. Antibiotic therapy is continued for 10 to 14 days; occasionally a longer course is prescribed to prevent relapse. If the sinusitis does not respond to treatment with oral antibiotics, hospitalisation and intravenous antibiotic therapy may be required. See the chapter 'Nursing care of people with infections' for nursing care related to antibiotic therapy.

Oral or topical (in the form of nasal sprays) decongestants such as pseudoephedrine or phenylephrine are also prescribed to reduce mucosal oedema and promote sinus drainage. Antihistamines may decrease nasal congestion and facilitate sinus drainage, but they also tend to increase the viscosity of secretions and hinder drainage. For this reason, they may not be as effective as decongestants. Saline nose drops or sprays promote sinus drainage, as does inhalation of warm steam. Aerobic exercise also promotes mucus flow and may be recommended, although caution is advised with acute symptomology and infection.

CONSIDERATION FOR PRACTICE

To administer topical drugs, the person's head is tilted backwards and to the side on which the drops are to be instilled. The person may need to remain in position for 5 minutes to allow the drops to reach the posterior nares.

Surgery

People who do not respond to pharmacological measures and who experience persistent facial pain, headache or nasal congestion may require *endoscopic sinus surgery*. People who have endoscopic sinus surgery usually do not require nasal packing postoperatively. Instead, frequent nasal cleaning and irrigation with normal saline are performed. The person is instructed to sneeze with the mouth open and avoid blowing the nose, lifting or straining for a week following surgery to reduce the risk of complications such as bleeding.

Antral irrigation can be done in the doctor's office under local anaesthesia. Saline solution is instilled into the maxillary sinus to irrigate the area and wash out the sinus of purulent exudate. The person is seated with the head forward and mouth open to allow drainage of the solution through the nose and mouth. A culture of the exudate may be obtained to determine appropriate antibiotic therapy.

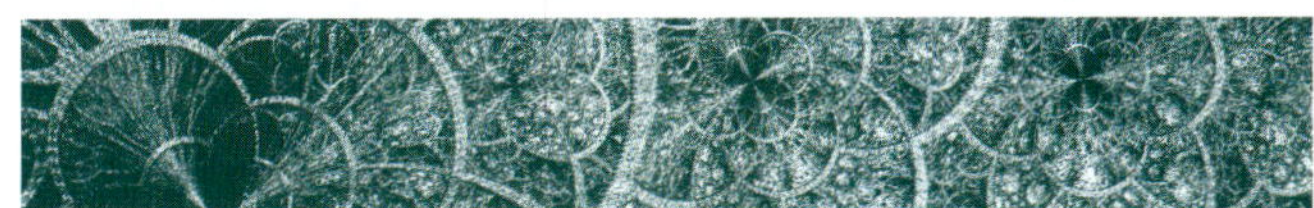

Nursing care

Health promotion

Measures to prevent sinusitis are those that promote nasal drainage: encouraging liberal fluid intake, judicious use of nasal decongestants as needed and treating any obstructive process. Encourage individuals with URTI to blow their nose with both nares open. Advise people that use of saline nasal sprays can help maintain patency of the opening to the sinuses, promoting drainage and reducing the risk of obstruction and infection.

Assessment

Focused assessment of the person with suspected sinusitis includes the following:

- *Health history*: complaints of frontal or periorbital headache, cheek, teeth or ear pain; timing of pain and changes in intensity over course of the day; nasal discharge or post-nasal drip; other symptoms; previous sinus problems; current medications, known medication allergies.
- *Physical examination*: general appearance; vital signs including temperature; inspect nasal and pharyngeal mucous membranes; percuss sinuses for tenderness.
- *Diagnostic tests*: WBC and differential, cultures of sinus drainage, sinus x-rays or other imaging studies if indicated.

Nursing diagnoses and interventions

The person with sinusitis is often acutely uncomfortable. Obstructed and congested sinuses cause pain and pressure that increase with position changes and leaning forward. Treatment usually is community based, making patient education the key nursing role. When the person is hospitalised for intravenous antibiotic therapy or sinus surgery, pain and nutritional considerations are the priority for nursing care.

Pain

Although sinus surgery is relatively minor, both the incision and postoperative swelling can cause discomfort. Nasal packing, if used, contributes to the discomfort.

- Assess pain using a standardised pain scale. Administer analgesics as ordered. *Relief of pain promotes a feeling of wellbeing and enhances recovery.*
- Apply ice packs to the nose. *Cold compresses reduce swelling, control bleeding and provide local analgesia.*
- Elevate the head of the bed to Fowler's or high-Fowler's position for 24 to 48 hours after surgery. *Elevating the operative site minimises tissue swelling and promotes comfort.*

Imbalanced nutrition

Postoperatively, the sense of smell, an appetite stimulus, is diminished by nasal packing. Mouth discomfort from the incision and numbness of the upper teeth also may affect appetite and eating.

- Provide a clear liquid diet progressing to soft foods as tolerated. High-kilojoule dietary supplements may be used. *A progressive diet is used to assess the ability to swallow without choking and allay fears. Food high in kilojoules and nutritional value provides metabolic and healing requirements.*
- Monitor intake, output and weight. *This information allows assessment of overall fluid balance and the adequacy of dietary intake.*
- Elevate the head of the bed during meals or encourage the person to sit out of bed. *The upright position facilitates swallowing and minimises risk of aspiration.*

Community-based care

Teaching for people with sinusitis and their families focuses on following through with appropriate treatment and promoting comfort. Discuss the following topics when preparing for home care:

- The importance of completing the entire course of prescribed antibiotics to achieve cure and prevent the development of antibiotic-resistant bacteria. Assist in developing a schedule that helps ensure all doses are taken. Measures to prevent superinfections (such as vaginitis or oral thrush) during the prolonged course of treatment (e.g. consume 200 g of yoghurt containing live bacterial cultures daily while on antibiotics).
- Use of systemic or topical decongestants to promote sinus drainage.
- Maintaining a liberal fluid intake to reduce the viscosity of mucus drainage.
- Use of a humidifier or steam inhalation to promote sinus drainage.
- Sleeping with the head of the bed elevated to a 45-degree angle and on the unaffected side to promote drainage of affected sinuses.
- Application of a warm, moist pack to the area of pain and tenderness to promote comfort.
- Notify the doctor if symptoms do not improve with treatment or if signs of a complication develop, such as increased pain and redness and swelling around the nose or eyes.
- Postoperative instructions to prevent bleeding, such as avoiding blowing the nose for 7 to 10 days and avoiding strenuous activity such as heavy lifting for about 2 weeks.
- Use of saline nasal sprays postoperatively to keep the nasal mucosa moist.

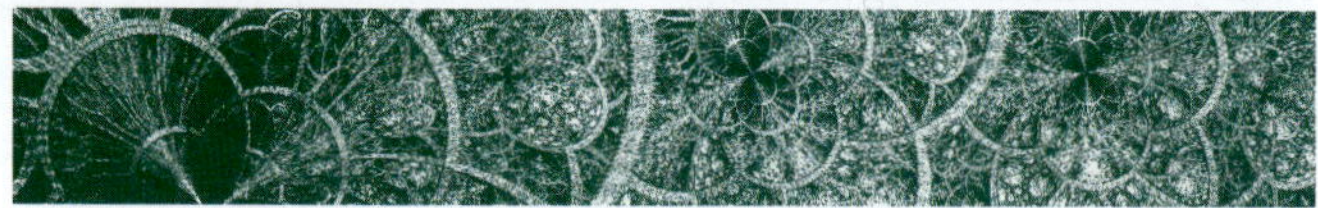

THE PERSON WITH PHARYNGITIS OR TONSILLITIS

Pharyngitis, acute inflammation of the pharynx, is one of the most identified clinical problems. Although it is usually viral in origin, pharyngitis may also be caused by bacterial infection. *Group A beta-haemolytic streptococcus* (strep throat) is the most common cause of bacterial pharyngitis. Other bacteria that may cause pharyngitis include *Neisseria gonorrhoeae*, a Gram-negative diplococcus that is sexually transmitted, *Mycoplasma* and *Chlamydia trachomatis*.

Tonsillitis is acute inflammation of the palatine tonsils. Although it is sometimes viral in origin, tonsillitis is usually due to streptococcal infection. The incidence of streptococcal infections is greatest between late autumn and spring, especially in cold climates. Viral tonsillitis may occur in epidemics in people living in crowded conditions, such as children in boarding schools, asylum seekers in refugee camps and Indigenous children in crowded living circumstances.

Pathophysiology and manifestations

Pharyngitis and tonsillitis are contagious and spread by droplet nuclei. Incubation varies from a few hours to several days, depending on the organism. Viral infections are communicable for 2 to 3 days. Symptoms usually resolve 3 to 10 days after onset.

Viral pharyngitis may be attributed to the same viruses as cause the common cold: rhinovirus, coronavirus or parainfluenza virus. Pharyngitis caused by adenovirus, influenza virus or Epstein–Barr virus (associated with infectious mononucleosis) may be particularly severe.

Acute pharyngitis causes pain and fever. The pain may vary from a scratchy sore throat to one so painful that swallowing is difficult. Streptococcal pharyngitis is usually marked by an abrupt onset, with fever of 38.3°C or higher, severe sore throat with dysphagia, malaise and often arthralgias and myalgias. Anterior lymph nodes are often enlarged and tender. Exudate (pus) may be seen on the pharynx and tonsils (see Figure 34.1). By contrast, the onset of viral pharyngitis is often gradual, with manifestations of low-grade fever, sore throat, mild hoarseness, headache and rhinorrhoea. The pharyngeal membranes appear mildly red with vascular congestion. Infectious mononucleosis, caused by the Epstein–Barr virus, often presents as acute pharyngitis, with visible patches of exudate on the pharynx or tonsils. The cervical lymph nodes are enlarged and tender as well. See the 'Manifestations' box for the manifestations of pharyngitis and tonsillitis.

In tonsillitis, the tonsils appear bright red and oedematous. White exudate is present on the tonsils; pressing on a tonsil may produce purulent drainage. The uvula may also be reddened and swollen. Cervical lymph nodes are usually tender and enlarged.

The person with tonsillitis complains of a sore throat, difficulty swallowing, general malaise, fever and otalgia (pain referred to the ear). Manifestations are often more severe in adolescents and adults than in children. Infection may extend via the eustachian tubes causing acute otitis media. This may lead to further damage such as spontaneous rupture of the eardrums and mastoiditis. See the chapter 'Nursing care of people with eye and ear disorders' for more information about otitis media.

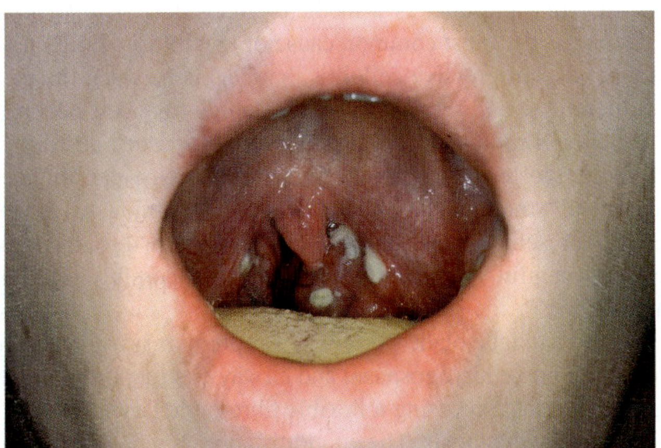

FIGURE 34.1 ***The appearance of the oral pharynx and tonsils in acute pharyngitis and tonsillitis***

Source: Scott Camazine/Alamy Stock Photo.

MANIFESTATIONS Pharyngitis and tonsillitis

LOCAL
- Sore throat
- Possible dysphagia and ear pain
- Tender, swollen anterior cervical lymph nodes
- Hoarse voice
- Red, swollen pharyngeal mucous membranes and/or tonsils
- Possible visible exudate on pharyngeal membranes and/or tonsils

GENERAL
- Fever
- General malaise
- Arthralgia, myalgia

Complications

Although bacterial pharyngitis may be mild and indistinguishable from viral pharyngitis by its signs and symptoms, it can lead to significant complications such as abscess, scarlet fever, toxic shock syndrome, rheumatic fever or acute post-streptococcal glomerulonephritis.

Peritonsillar abscess, often known as *quinsy*, is a potential complication of tonsillitis. It usually results from group A beta-haemolytic streptococcus infection extending from the tonsils to the surrounding tissue. The abscess causes pus formation behind the tonsil with marked swelling and asymmetrical deviation of the uvula. The degree of swelling may make it difficult to swallow anything other than liquids. The person may exhibit thickening of the voice, drooling and trismus (a tonic contraction of the muscles of mastication).

Rare (1–3%) but serious complications of streptococcal pharyngitis and tonsillitis include acute glomerulonephritis and rheumatic fever, abnormal immune responses to the infection. Acute glomerulonephritis generally presents with sudden onset of haematuria, proteinuria and, less commonly, hypertension and oedema within 7 to 10 days after the acute infection. Rheumatic fever typically presents 3 to 5 weeks after acute infection with fever, painful or swollen joints, rash and heart murmur. Other complications of bacterial infection include sinusitis, otitis media, mastoiditis and cervical adenitis.

INTERPROFESSIONAL CARE

Both viral and bacterial pharyngitis are usually self-limited diseases. However, because of the risk of serious complications associated with streptococcal sore throat, an effort is usually made to establish an accurate diagnosis and treat bacterial pharyngitis.

Diagnosis

A *throat swab* may be obtained and examined for streptococcus antigen. These tests allow rapid identification of the antigen but are not highly sensitive. When the test is positive, treatment for strep throat is initiated. If the test is negative, the swab is cultured to ensure that streptococcus organisms are not present. Even throat cultures are not always accurate, with approximately 10% false negative and 20% false positive results.

A *full blood count (FBC)* may be performed on patients who are severely ill or to rule out other causes of pharyngitis. The WBC count is usually normal or low in viral infections and elevated in bacterial infections.

Medications

Antipyretics and mild analgesics such as aspirin or paracetamol provide symptomatic relief for throat pain and associated myalgias. Penicillin is the drug of choice for group A streptococci. Erythromycin may be used if the person is allergic to penicillin. Antibiotic therapy is continued for at least 10 days. The person is no longer contagious after 24 hours of antibiotic therapy.

Surgery

Tonsillectomy (surgical removal of the tonsils) is indicated for recurrent or chronic infections that have not responded to antibiotic therapy, hypertrophy of the tonsils with risk of airway obstruction, peritonsillar abscess, repeated attacks of purulent otitis media and tonsil malignancy. Adenoid tissue usually is removed at the same time. Bleeding is the most significant postoperative complication of tonsillectomy and may develop up to 2 weeks following the surgery.

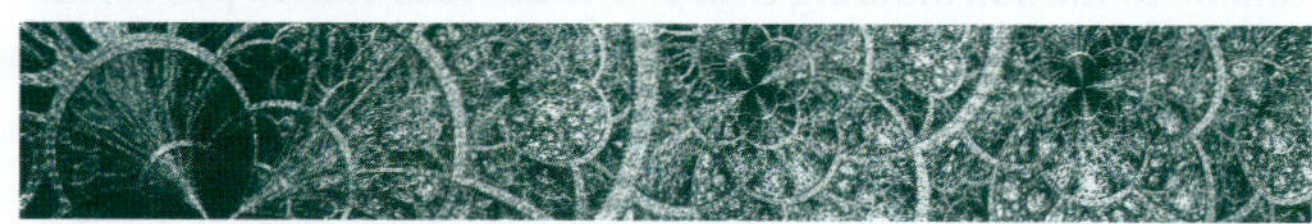

Nursing care

Because of the risk of significant complications associated with streptococcal pharyngitis, encourage all individuals with symptoms that persist for several days or that include fever, lymphadenopathy and myalgias to seek evaluation and treatment.

Home care is appropriate for acute uncomplicated pharyngitis. Treatment focuses on adequate rest and relief of symptoms. A liquid or soft diet is useful when swallowing is difficult. Increased fluid intake is encouraged, especially when febrile. Warm saline gargles, moist inhalations and application of an ice collar are soothing to the sore throat.

Following tonsillectomy, in the immediate postoperative period, ensure a patent airway by placing the person in semi-Fowler's position with the head turned to the side to allow secretions to drain from the mouth and pharynx. Keep the airway in place until the gag and swallowing reflexes have returned. Apply an ice collar to reduce swelling and pain. Notify the surgeon immediately if excessive bleeding or haemorrhage occurs. If there is no bleeding, allow water and ice chips as desired. Warm saline mouthwashes are helpful in managing thick oral secretions following tonsillectomy. A liquid or semi-liquid diet is recommended for several days.

Community-based care

Discuss the following topics when preparing the person for home care:

- the importance of completing the entire course of antibiotic therapy if prescribed
- using warm saline gargles or throat lozenges for symptomatic relief
- signs and symptoms of possible complications of streptococcal infection such as glomerulonephritis or rheumatic fever
- monitoring temperature in the morning and evening until well to ensure that the infection has not spread to deeper tissues
- proper use and disposal of tissues and frequent handwashing to prevent spreading the infection to others.

For the person who has had a peritonsillar abscess drainage or tonsillectomy, provide the following instructions:

- postoperative mouth and throat care as above
- avoiding use of aspirin for 2 weeks to reduce the risk of postoperative bleeding
- manifestations of bleeding to report to the doctor. (Delayed haemorrhage may occur for up to 1 week post surgery.)

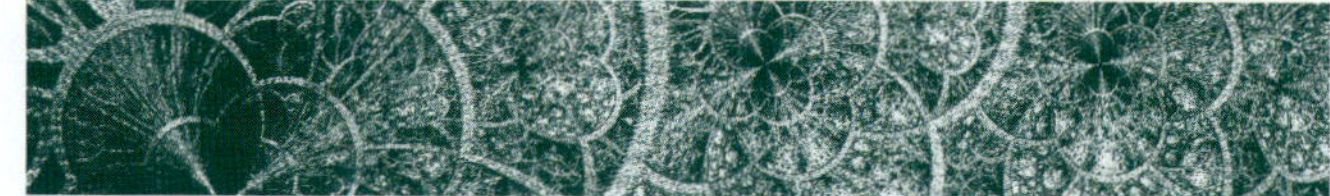

THE PERSON WITH A LARYNGEAL INFECTION

The larynx, located between the upper airways and the lungs, protects the lower respiratory tract from inhaled substances other than air and allows speech. The larynx includes the epiglottis, which covers the larynx during swallowing, and the glottis or vocal cords. Part or all of the larynx may become inflamed.

Epiglottitis

Epiglottitis, inflammation of the epiglottis, is an uncommon disorder that presents as a medical emergency. *H. influenzae* infection is the most common cause of epiglottitis. Epiglottitis is a rapidly progressive cellulitis that begins between the base of the tongue and the epiglottis. The epiglottis itself becomes swollen and inflamed; swelling of adjacent tissues pushes the epiglottis posteriorly. This swelling and oedema can threaten airway obstruction and should be treated cautiously. Adults usually present with a 1- to 2-day history of sore throat, *odynophagia* (painful swallowing), dyspnoea and possibly drooling and stridor.

Using a tongue blade to view the oropharynx is avoided; this may precipitate laryngospasm and airway obstruction. The epiglottis is visualised using a flexible fibre-optic laryngoscope to establish the diagnosis. The epiglottis appears red, swollen and oedematous. Nasotracheal intubation may be required to ensure airway patency. The person may be admitted to a critical care unit and intravenous antibiotic therapy is initiated. Ceftriaxone may be prescribed. Dexamethasone, a systemic corticosteroid, is also given to suppress the inflammatory response and rapidly reduce swelling of the epiglottis.

Nursing care for the person with acute epiglottitis focuses on monitoring and maintaining airway patency. Monitor oxygen saturation continuously. Observe closely for signs of airway obstruction, including nasal flaring, restlessness, stridor, use of accessory muscles and decreased oxygen saturation measurements. If the person is not intubated, supplies for emergency intubation should be kept within the unit for easy access. Epiglottitis can be frightening for both the person and the nurse as the risk of the airway being compromised is present. Maintaining a calm, reassuring manner is an essential nursing role to reduce patient anxiety.

Laryngitis

Laryngitis, inflammation of the larynx, is a common disorder that may occur alone or in conjunction with other upper respiratory infections such as the common cold. It is frequently associated with a viral URTI such as influenza. It may also occur with bronchitis, pneumonia or other respiratory infections. Excessive use of the voice, sudden changes in temperature or exposure to dust, irritating fumes, smoke or other pollutants can also cause acute or chronic laryngitis. It is more common in the winter and in colder climates.

In laryngitis, the mucous membrane lining the larynx becomes inflamed; the vocal cords also may become oedematous. The primary symptom of laryngitis is a change in the voice. Hoarseness or *aphonia*, complete loss of the voice, may occur. The throat is often sore and scratchy, and a dry, harsh cough may be present.

There is no specific treatment for viral laryngitis. Any identified precipitating factors such as overuse of the voice and exposure to irritants should be eliminated. Management includes resting the voice and abstinence from tobacco and alcohol, which are chemical irritants. Treatment may also include inhaling steam or spraying the throat with antiseptic solutions. Identifying and eliminating irritants are helpful to prevent future attacks.

Impaired verbal communication is a key nursing priority for people with laryngitis. The meaning of messages is conveyed not only by the words used but also by the tone and loudness of voice. Instruct to rest the voice as much as possible. Encourage speaking in short sentences or using alternate methods of communication, such as writing. Resting the voice hastens recovery and decreases throat discomfort. Advise the person to use soothing throat lozenges, sprays or other comfort measures such as gargling with a warm antiseptic solution. Help identify potential irritants, such as fumes, cigarette smoke, chemicals or cold temperature, to prevent future bouts of laryngitis.

THE PERSON WITH PERTUSSIS

Pertussis, or *whooping cough*, is a highly contagious acute upper respiratory infection caused by the bacterium *Bordetella pertussis*. Although it is thought by many to be a childhood disease that has been virtually eliminated through immunisation of infants, up to 45% of people affected by pertussis are adolescents and adults.

Pathophysiology

B. pertussis is a Gram-negative rod that is spread by respiratory droplets. The bacteria attach to ciliated epithelial cells of the nasopharynx, multiplying and invading respiratory tissues. The damage and effects of pertussis are not due to the infection itself but to toxins produced by the bacteria. These toxins damage the mucosa and paralyse the cilia. As a result, clearance of respiratory secretions is impaired, increasing the risk of secondary infection such as pneumonia. The toxins also prompt an inflammatory response and inhibit immune defences.

Although immunisation does not appear to confer lifetime immunity, the disease tends to be milder in adolescents, adults and people who have been immunised. These infected individuals can, however, transmit the disease to other susceptible people, including unimmunised or under-immunised infants, elderly people and immunocompromised patients (Wilkinson et al., 2021).

Young infants have the highest risk of complications of the disease, such as death, pneumonia and neurological complications. Neurological complications are thought to result from hypoxia due to prolonged paroxysms of coughing. Complications in adolescents and adults may occur as a result of increased intrathoracic pressure during prolonged coughing spells. These may include pneumothorax, weight loss, inguinal hernia, rib fracture associated with consistent coughing and *cough syncope* (fainting due to hypoxia) (Wilkinson et al., 2021).

Manifestations

Classic pertussis follows a predictable pattern, with typical URTI symptoms (coryza, sneezing, low-grade fever and mild cough) beginning 7–10 days after exposure. After 1–2 weeks, the cough becomes more frequent, occurring in paroxysms or bursts of rapid coughs, often ending with an audible whoop caused by rapid inspiration. This whoop is less common in adolescents and adults, often delaying diagnosis. Vomiting may follow episodes of coughing (Guiso, 2021). Coughing paroxysms vary in frequency from several per hour to 5–10 per day, interfering with eating and sleep. This stage of the disease, called the *paroxysmal stage*, usually lasts no more than 6 weeks, after which coughing becomes less severe and gradually resolves over a period of up to 3 months.

In adolescents and adults, pertussis is suspected when an upper respiratory infection produces a cough that persists longer than 7 days, is accompanied by vomiting and is worse at night.

INTERPROFESSIONAL CARE

Active immunisation with pertussis vaccine is the primary preventive strategy for pertussis. Acellular pertussis vaccines that are effective but produce fewer adverse reactions than traditional whole-cell vaccines are available and preferred for immunisation.

The diagnosis of pertussis is established by culture of nasopharyngeal secretions. However, nasopharyngeal secretions may remain positive for the organism for only about 3 weeks after the onset of symptoms, so blood tests for antibodies to the organism may be necessary to confirm the diagnosis. Lymphocytosis (elevated lymphocyte count) may be present.

Azithromycin and clarithromycin are the antibiotics of choice to eradicate *B. pertussis* infection. In individuals where macrolide antibiotics are contraindicated, trimethoprim-sulfamethoxazole may be used (Wipperman, Ofei-Dodoo & Nilsen, 2022). Hospitalisation rarely is required for adults, although children and infants with severe disease often are hospitalised to prevent complications such as neurological effects of hypoxia and malnutrition. Respiratory isolation is instituted for 5 days after antibiotic therapy is started. Prophylactic antibiotics may be given to household and close contacts of the infected person depending on age, health, and immunisation status.

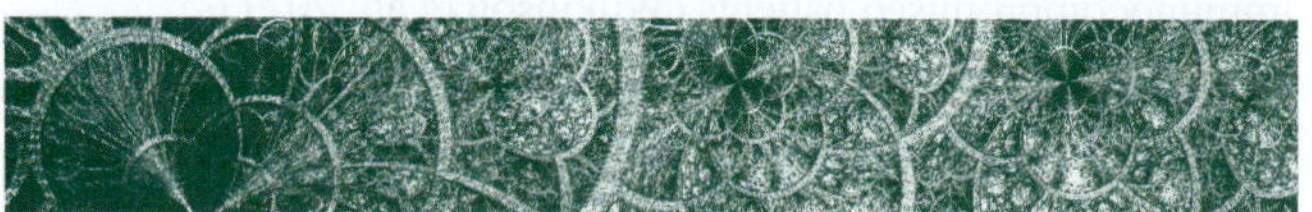

Nursing care

Nurses are instrumental in promoting effective immunisation of all infants and young children against pertussis. Australia's National Immunisation Program recently has started to recommend that parents, grandparents and carers of infants under 6 months of age should receive a single pertussis vaccine (dTpa) booster at least 2 weeks before beginning close contact with the infant (Department of Health and Aged Care, 2022b; Seale et al., 2021). Education is a key nursing role related to immunisation, as significant incorrect and inappropriate information exists about potential long-term adverse consequences of vaccination programs.

Recommend nasopharyngeal culture for people complaining of persistent cough, especially when the cough is accompanied by vomiting or is significantly worse at night, or if other members of the household or close contacts have a similar illness.

CONSIDERATION FOR PRACTICE

Pertussis is a reportable communicable disease. All probable and confirmed cases must be reported to the local health department.

Education is a primary nursing role related to pertussis. Adults usually remain in the community for treatment. Educate the patient and family about respiratory isolation measures to be used until the disease is no longer communicable. Discuss ways to control respiratory secretions and the importance of disposing of tissues and secretions personally to prevent exposure of others. Stress the importance of prophylactic treatment for all household and close contacts. Discuss measures to maintain fluid and nutrient intake and use of a cough suppressant at night to promote rest. Encourage increased fluid intake to promote expectoration of respiratory secretions. Educate the patient and family about the prescribed antibiotic, including its potential adverse effects and measures to reduce them, such as taking the prescribed antibiotic erythromycin with meals to prevent gastric irritation. Contact the state or territory health department for follow up of contacts and compliance with prescribed treatment.

CONSIDERATION FOR PRACTICE

The National Immunisation Program requires the diphtheria, tetanus and acellular pertussis immunisation to be administered at 2, 4 and 6 months of age, with a booster to be administered at 4 years, and also between 10 and 15 years (Department of Health and Aged Care, 2022b).

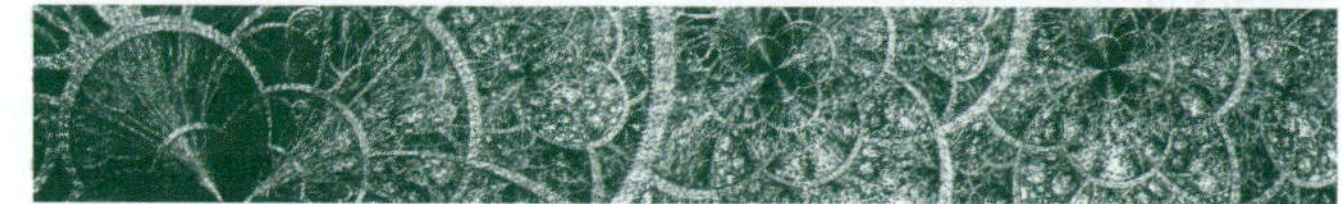

Upper respiratory trauma or obstruction

Obstruction of the upper airway due to trauma (fracture of the nasal septum or the larynx), bleeding (e.g. epistaxis) or a tumour is not only frightening for the person but also may interfere with the ability to breathe.

THE PERSON WITH EPISTAXIS

The nose has a rich blood supply, receiving major arterial vessels from both the internal and external carotid artery systems. **Epistaxis**, or nosebleed, may be precipitated by a number of factors. Trauma (picking the nose or blunt trauma) can cause epistaxis, as can drying of nasal mucous membranes, infection, substance abuse (e.g. cocaine), arteriosclerosis or hypertension. Epistaxis may also indicate a bleeding disorder related to acute leukaemia, thrombocytopenia, aplastic anaemia or severe liver disease. Additionally, treatment with an anticoagulant or antiplatelet drug may cause an increased risk of the vessels in the nose bleeding. In adults, men more frequently have nosebleeds than women.

Pathophysiology and manifestations

Ninety per cent of all nosebleeds arise in the anterior nasal septum from Kiesselbach's area, a rich vascular plexus. Because of their location, these vessels are susceptible to trauma from nose picking, drying and infection. Posterior epistaxis more often develops secondarily to systemic disorders such as blood dyscrasias, hypertension or diabetes. In posterior epistaxis, bleeding is from the terminal branches of the sphenopalatine and internal maxillary arteries. Posterior epistaxis tends to be more severe and occurs more frequently in the older adult.

Anterior nosebleeds usually produce obvious bleeding from the nares, as well as bleeding into the posterior nasal and oral pharynx. Bleeding from a posterior nosebleed may be less obvious, with most of the blood draining into the posterior nasopharynx and swallowed by the person. Nausea and vomiting may occur due to swallowed blood.

INTERPROFESSIONAL CARE

The goal of treatment for epistaxis is to identify and control the source of bleeding.

Anterior bleeding can usually be managed by simple first-aid measures, such as applying pressure (pinching the nose towards the septum) for 5 to 10 minutes and applying ice packs to the nose and forehead to cause vasoconstriction. The person is placed in a sitting position to decrease blood flow to the head and reduce venous pressure. Leaning forward reduces drainage of blood backward into the nasopharynx and decreases swallowing of blood. The person is instructed to spit out the blood to help estimate the amount of bleeding and to prevent nausea and vomiting as a result of swallowed blood.

If applying pressure does not control the bleeding, medications, nasal packing or surgery may be necessary.

Medications

Topical vasoconstrictors such as cocaine (0.5%), phenylephrine (Neo-Synephrine) (1:1,000) or adrenaline (1:1,000) may be used to control anterior bleeding. These medications may be applied by nasal spray or on a cotton swab held against the bleeding site. Chemical cauterisation of the bleeding vessel may be done using agents such as silver nitrate. A topical anaesthetic such as lignocaine or cocaine may be used prior to nasal packing. If posterior nasal packing is required, prophylactic antibiotic therapy is initiated to prevent sinusitis or possible toxic shock syndrome. Toxic shock syndrome (TSS) is caused by *Streptococcus pyogenes* or *Staphylococcus aureus*. TSS can be life threatening; if suspected, the patient should present to a hospital as soon as possible. Signs and symptoms include rapid onset of fever above 38°C, low blood pressure and non-specific flu-like symptoms.

Nasal packing

If bleeding cannot be controlled with pressure and local medications, a nasal tampon (a soft balloon filled with air) may be used to apply direct pressure to the bleeding vessel or the nasal cavity may be packed with 2.5–5 cm petroleum gauze as indicated by the patient's comfort level and width of the nares. For an anterior pack, approximately 1–1.5 m of packing may be placed carefully and systematically along the floor of the nasal cavity and then into the vault of the nose. This is often available prepacked, impregnated with triamcinoline and an antibiotic cream. Anterior nasal packs are usually left in place for 24 to 72 hours. If epistaxis is caused by a bleeding disorder, the packing may be left in place for 4 to 5 days while the disorder is treated.

Posterior nosebleeds are more difficult to control, requiring both anterior and posterior packing (see Figure 34.2). Posterior packs are usually left in place for 2 to 5 days. A loose anterior nasal pack may also be inserted. Posterior nasal packing is very uncomfortable and can cause respiratory and cardiovascular complications. Hypoxaemia is common; supplementary oxygen is administered. Endotracheal intubation may be necessary to maintain adequate ventilation and gas exchange. If indicated, narcotic analgesics are prescribed to manage the discomfort. Hypertension, arrhythmias and even acute myocardial infarction may occur in people with severe cardiovascular disease. Toxic shock syndrome is another potential complication of posterior nasal packing. The pack may occlude the eustachian tube and sinus openings, resulting in ear discomfort, possible otitis media or sinusitis. Oral and nasal dryness can be minimised by use of a high-humidity face tent. Nursing care of the person with nasal packing is outlined in the accompanying box.

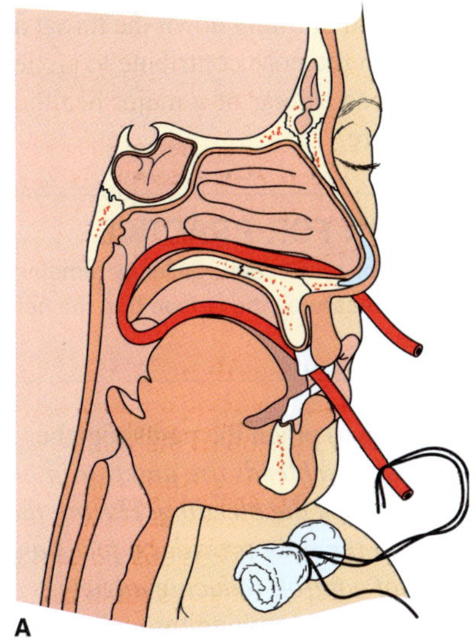

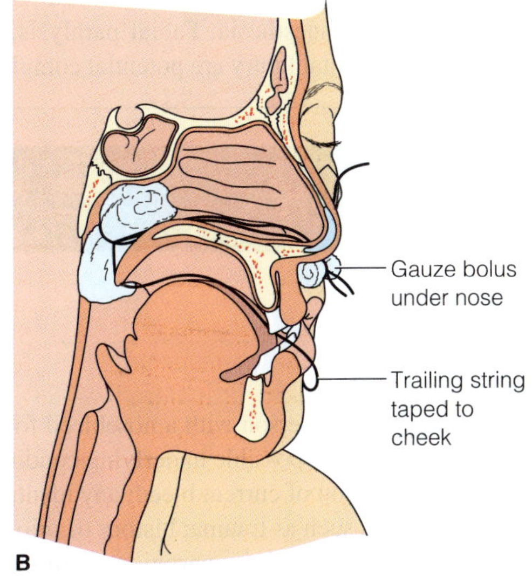

FIGURE 34.2 ***Posterior nasal packing. A, A rubber catheter is inserted through the nose and out the mouth and attached to the packing. B, The catheter is withdrawn through the nose to position the packing in the posterior nasopharynx. Ties exiting through the nose and mouth are used to stabilise the packing in position and remove it when it is no longer needed***

NURSING CARE OF THE PERSON with nasal packing

- Continuously monitor oxygen saturation. Administer supplementary oxygen as ordered. *Posterior nasal packing can cause hypoxaemia. Supplemental oxygen is given to maintain tissue oxygenation.*
- Frequently monitor vital signs and respiratory rate or pattern. *Posterior nasal packing increases the risk of respiratory and cardiovascular complications. Tachycardia and tachypnoea may be early signs of cardiac or respiratory compromise.*
- Inspect the mouth and oropharynx. Notify the doctor if the packing is seen in the oropharynx. *Misplacement of nasal packing can obstruct the upper airway.*
- Elevate the head of the bed. *Elevating the head of the bed facilitates ventilation.*
- Encourage deep, slow breathing through the mouth. Provide psychological support, reassurance and teaching. *Inability to breathe through the nose causes anxiety and fear.*
- Check for blood at the back of the throat and frequent swallowing. *Visible blood or frequent swallowing could indicate posterior bleeding.*
- Report haematemesis. *Bleeding from the posterior portion of the nose often drains down the nasopharynx and is swallowed. Haematemesis may indicate continued bleeding.*
- Apply cold compresses to nose. *An ice or cold compress decreases pain and promotes vasoconstriction, decreasing bleeding and swelling.*
- Provide for rest. *Rest reduces the metabolic demands and oxygen consumption.*
- Ensure adequate oral fluid intake. *Fluid intake helps maintain fluid balance and decreases dryness of oral mucous membranes because of mouth breathing.*
- Provide frequent oral hygiene. Use a bedside humidifier. *These measures reduce drying of oral mucous membranes and promote comfort.*

An indwelling catheter or inflatable nasal balloon may be used as an alternative to posterior nasal packing for effective tamponade without the risk of TSS. The catheter or nasal balloon is inserted through the nose into the nasopharynx, inflated and left in place for 2 to 3 days.

Surgery

Chemical or surgical cautery procedures may be used to sclerose involved vessels in the anterior aspect of the nose. The resulting scab must be left undisturbed until the mucosa has healed, or further bleeding may occur.

Surgical procedures to control bleeding are often preferred to posterior nasal packing for posterior bleeding. The bleeding vessel may be cauterised using an endoscopic approach. In some cases, surgery is required to occlude the internal maxillary artery by ligation (tying off) or embolisation. These procedures may be done under either conscious sedation and local anaesthesia or general anaesthesia. Facial paralysis, paraesthesia, facial pain and dental injury are potential complications.

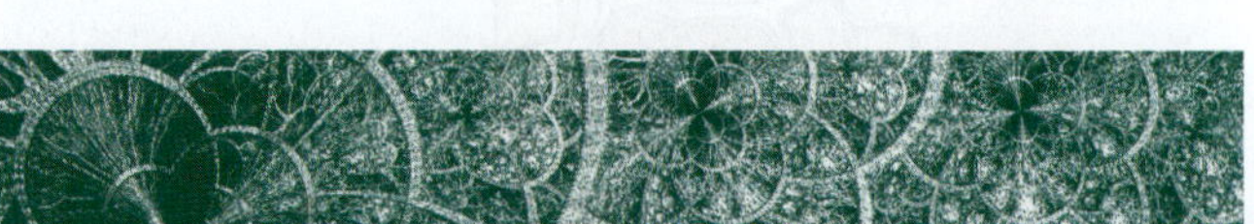

Nursing care

Assessment

Nursing assessment of the person with a nosebleed focuses on the immediate problem and possible underlying conditions.

- *Health history*: duration of current bleed; any identified precipitating factors such as trauma; history of prior nosebleeds; current medications; chronic conditions such as hypertension or bleeding disorders.
- *Physical examination*: estimated amount of bleeding; presence of blood in oropharynx; vital signs; evidence of facial or nasal trauma.
- *Diagnostic tests*: haemoglobin, haematocrit and FBC as indicated; oxygen saturation; tests of organ function such as liver function tests (bilirubin, AST, ALT, LDH) or kidney function tests (serum creatinine and urea).

Nursing diagnoses and interventions

Nosebleeds can be frightening, particularly when they occur without preceding trauma. Nurses provide care for people with epistaxis in outpatient and emergency settings and may care for hospitalised people with nasal packing. Support, reassurance and education are important nursing roles related to epistaxis. Priority nursing concerns include assisting with possible anxiety and monitoring to reduce the potential risk of aspiration.

Anxiety

The amount of blood lost in a nosebleed can be frightening. The sensation of blood draining down the throat and the inability to breathe through the nose contribute to anxiety. Spontaneous epistaxis may lead to fear of a major health problem such as high blood pressure.

CONSIDERATION FOR PRACTICE

Maintain an attitude of calm reassurance. By remaining calm and confident, the nurse reassures the person that the nosebleed is not a life-threatening event.

- Instruct the person to pinch the nares together at the bridge of the nose. *Most nosebleeds are anterior in origin; direct pressure usually stops the bleeding. Having the person place pressure on the nose provides a focus and helps restore a sense of control, reducing anxiety.*
- Encourage slow, deep breathing through the mouth. *Controlled mouth breathing maintains lung ventilation and reduces anxiety.*
- Provide a basin and tissues; encourage the person to expectorate blood, not swallow it. *These measures give the*

person greater control and reduce the fear of choking on blood.

- Apply ice or a cold compress to the nose. *Cold causes vasoconstriction, reducing bleeding*.

> **CONSIDERATION FOR PRACTICE**
> **Assess the person with nasal packing frequently for adequate oxygenation. Maintain supplemental oxygen as ordered. Cerebral hypoxia produces a sense of apprehension and fear.**

Risk of aspiration

Anxiety and blood draining into the nasopharynx increase the risk of aspiration of blood into the trachea. When nasal packing is in place, the person is unable to breathe through the nose, increasing the risk of aspiration when food or fluids are consumed.

> **CONSIDERATION FOR PRACTICE**
> **Position upright with head forward. Provide an appropriate receptacle for expectorating blood. These measures minimise the amount of blood draining down the nasopharynx and swallowed, reducing the risk of aspiration and minimising nausea from swallowed blood. Vomiting of swallowed blood can increase the risk of aspiration.**

> **CONSIDERATION FOR PRACTICE**
> **Position the person with nasal packing with the head elevated and on the side, when asleep. This position reduces the risk of aspiration of oral secretions.**

Community-based care

Following an episode of epistaxis, teaching for home care focuses on measures to prevent further bleeding. Include the following teaching topics:

- Avoid strenuous exercise for several days or weeks, depending on the severity of the nosebleed and its treatment.
- Do not blow the nose or engage in activities such as heavy lifting or bending that could increase pressure and dislodge the crust; sneeze with the mouth open to avoid increasing pressure in nasal vessels.
- For an anterior nosebleed, use petroleum jelly or a water-soluble lubricant to lubricate nasal mucosa and reduce the risk of spontaneous bleeding.
- Use a humidifier or vaporiser to minimise dryness of the mucous membranes.
- Do not forcefully blow the nose or pick the nose.
- For spontaneous nosebleed, seek medical evaluation for any possible underlying problem, such as hypertension or a bleeding disorder.

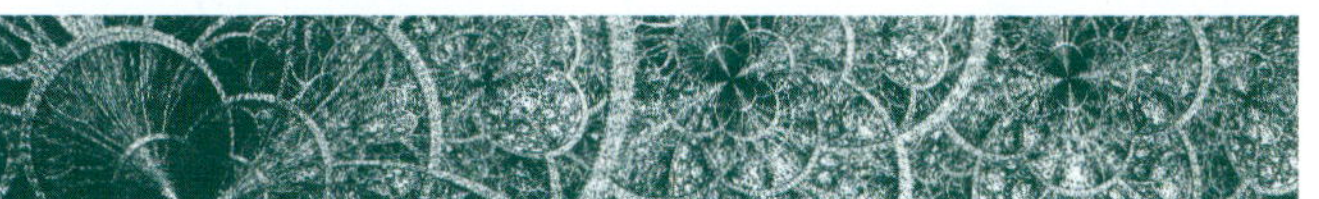

THE PERSON WITH NASAL TRAUMA OR SURGERY

The nose is the most commonly broken bone of the face. A nasal fracture (broken nose) usually is caused by a sports injury or trauma related to violence or motor vehicle crashes. The nasal septum normally divides the nose into two equal parts. Deviation of the septum can result from nasal trauma. Soft tissue trauma commonly accompanies nasal fracture.

Pathophysiology and manifestations

One or both sides of the nose may be broken. A *unilateral fracture* involves only one side of the nose. It causes little displacement or cosmetic deformity. It is usually not serious, but septal deviation and swelling can obstruct the airway. *Bilateral fractures* are more common, with depression or displacement of both nasal bones to one side. The nose appears flattened or deviated with an S or C configuration. *Complex fractures* may also involve the septum, ascending processes of the maxilla and frontal bones of the face. Pain is associated with all types of fractures of the face.

Soft tissue trauma commonly accompanies nasal fracture. Mucous membrane tears cause epistaxis. Soft tissue haematomas (black eye) are also frequent. Swelling develops rapidly following the injury and may obscure the fracture. Bony crepitus may be felt on gentle palpation. Septal haematoma may develop, increasing the risk of infection. The manifestations of nasal fracture are listed in the accompanying box.

Complications

Potential complications of nasal fracture include septal haematoma, abscess formation, septal perforation or deviation, and cerebrospinal fluid (CSF) leakage. Septal haematoma can lead to complete and bilateral nasal obstruction. If undrained, the presence of a haematoma increases the risk of staphylococcal abscess, which can lead to necrosis of septal cartilage and *saddle nose deformity*.

Septal deviation causes varying degrees of nasal obstruction. The septal cartilage bulges or deviates to one side, partially or totally obstructing the nares. Mild deviation is generally asymptomatic. Partial obstruction of air flow through one side may cause noisy breathing while awake and snoring during sleep. Major deviations can cause pain because of sinus obstruction or infection. They may also cause nosebleeds due to dryness of the nasal mucosa. Occasionally, the defect is severe enough to cause cosmetic deformity. Perforations are usually not serious and do not usually require repair unless obstruction or external deformity occurs.

> MANIFESTATIONS **Nasal fracture**
> - Epistaxis
> - Deformity or displacement to one side
> - Crepitus
> - Periorbital oedema and ecchymosis
> - Nasal bridge instability
> - Pain

Fractures of other facial bones may accompany a broken nose, particularly when facial trauma is severe. Fractures in the nasoethmoidal or frontal region can disrupt the dura, causing CSF leakage or rhinorrhoea. CSF rhinorrhoea is suspected if watery nasal drainage tests positive for glucose.

INTERPROFESSIONAL CARE

The main treatment goals for nasal fractures are to maintain a patent airway, prevention of a potential deformity and pain management. Respirations are closely monitored.

Diagnosis

Head and facial x-rays are done to identify the fracture and assess for other facial fractures. The intranasal cavity is examined using a nasal speculum to rule out septal haematoma. If a CSF leak is suspected, a CT scan is done. A radiopaque substance or fluorescein dye may be instilled into the intrathecal or lumbar subarachnoid space to identify the site of leakage.

Treatments

Ideally, the fracture is reduced early, before significant oedema develops. Nasal fractures heal rapidly. Simple reduction may be done in the emergency department with local anaesthesia. An external splint may be applied for 7 to 10 days to maintain proper alignment as healing occurs. The splint is padded to prevent skin breakdown. Ice may be gently applied to the face and nose to control oedema and bleeding. Nasal packing may be used to control epistaxis.

Surgery

Complex nasal fractures, nasal septal deviation or persistent CSF leakage may require surgical repair or realignment of nasal bones. Rhinoplasty with concurrent septoplasty is the most common procedure used to repair nasal fracture or a deviated nasal septum.

Rhinoplasty is surgical reconstruction of the nose. It is done to relieve airway obstruction and repair visible deformity of the nose following fracture. If oedema is excessive after a nasal fracture or associated injury, surgery is delayed for 7 to 10 days to allow swelling to subside. Using an intranasal incision, the nasal skin is lifted and the framework of the nose reshaped by removing, rearranging or augmenting bone or cartilage. The skin is then repositioned over the reconstructed frame. Prosthetic implants may help reshape the nose. Either local or general anaesthesia may be used; hospitalisation is often unnecessary. Following surgery, nasal packing is left in place for up to 72 hours to minimise bleeding and provide tissue support. A temporary plastic splint moulded to the shape of the nose is removed in 3 to 5 days. The splint protects the reshaped nose and helps to control swelling. Most swelling and bruising subside within 10 to 14 days and normal sensation returns within several months following surgery. Rhinoplasty generally has few complications (Heiman et al., (2022).

Either a septoplasty or a submucosal resection may be done under local anaesthesia to correct a deviated septum. *Septoplasty* involves incising one side of the septum, elevating the mucous membrane and removing or straightening the deviated portion of septal cartilage. In a *submucosal resection*, bone and cartilage are removed. In both procedures, packing is applied to both sides of the nose to prevent bleeding and to keep the septal mucosa in the midline position.

Small defects in the cribriform plate, fovea ethmoidalis or sphenoid sinus associated with persistent CSF leakage may require endoscopic repair. Either a tissue graft or fibrin glue may be used to repair the defect. The graft or glue is held in place with absorbable packing. Large defects may require craniotomy for repair.

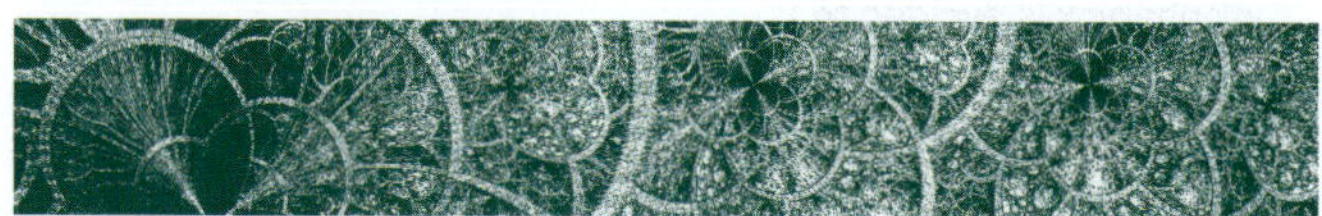

Nursing care

Health promotion

Teach all people—children and adolescents, in particular—about the importance of wearing appropriate protective equipment during exercise or sports. Reinforce the compulsory use of seat belts and air bags in vehicles to reduce the risk of facial injury in motor vehicle crashes.

Assessment

Focused nursing assessment for the person with a suspected nasal fracture includes:

- *Health history*: nature and circumstances of the injury; pain; ability to breathe through the nose.
- *Physical examination*: evident trauma, swelling, ecchymosis or deformity of the nose; vital signs, respiratory rate and ease; gently palpate nose and facial bones for crepitus; inspect oropharynx for drainage; test nasal discharge for glucose.

Nursing diagnoses and interventions

Nursing care for the person with nasal fracture focuses on controlling pain, bleeding and swelling. Airway management is a priority. Most nasal fractures are managed on an outpatient basis and education is a vital nursing function in preparing patients.

Risk of airway compromise

Immediately following nasal trauma and fracture, the airway is at risk of obstruction by bleeding and oedema. Deformity resulting from inappropriate fracture position during healing also can impair nasal airway clearance. This is a consideration when inserting nasogastric tubes or suctioning people with septal deviation.

> **CONSIDERATION FOR PRACTICE**
>
> **Monitor airway patency. Oedema and bleeding may obstruct the airway, causing signs of respiratory distress such as tachypnoea, dyspnoea, shortness of breath, tachycardia and use of accessory muscles.**

- Monitor cough effectiveness and ability to clear airway secretions. *Pain, oedema and nasal bleeding may impair the ability to cough effectively.*
- Maintain adequate hydration. Assess mucous membranes and skin turgor for evidence of dehydration. *Decreased oral fluid intake may lead to dehydration and thick, viscous secretions that are more difficult to expectorate.*

> **CONSIDERATION FOR PRACTICE**
> Have patent suction equipment available. Airway patency is a priority; oropharyngeal suctioning may be necessary to remove secretions and maintain a clear airway. Suctioning of the nasopharynx is avoided to prevent additional tissue trauma.

- Assess patency of both nares before inserting a nasogastric tube or feeding tube. If airflow is obstructed through one side, insert the tube through the unobstructed nare. Carefully monitor respiratory status following tube insertion. *The nasogastric tube is inserted through the unobstructed nare to avoid mucosal trauma; however, a large gastric tube may interfere with nasal breathing, necessitating close monitoring.*

Risk of infection

The person with a nasal fracture is at increased risk of infection. The nasal mucosa is a natural barrier to infection, and trauma increases the risk of invasion by pathogens. Septal haematoma can lead to abscess formation and staphylococcal infection. A cerebrospinal fluid leak indicates disruption of the dura, increasing the risk of ascending infection and meningitis.

> **CONSIDERATION FOR PRACTICE**
> Test watery, clear fluid dripping from the ear or nose for glucose. CSF will test positive for glucose on a glucose test strip.

- Avoid suctioning if possible. *Suction catheters could introduce microorganisms and cause additional trauma to tissues.*
- Monitor vital signs every 4 hours. *A rise in temperature may indicate infection.*
- Administer antibiotics as ordered. *Antibiotics may be prescribed to prevent abscess formation and, if CSF leakage is present, to prevent meningitis.*
- Assess the patient for signs of infection: increased swelling, pain and redness.

Community-based care

Provide the following teaching when preparing the person with a nasal fracture for home care:

- Elevate the head of the bed and apply ice or cold packs to the nose for 20 minutes four times a day to reduce swelling.
- Swelling usually subsides in several days; bruising may persist for several weeks.
- It is difficult to determine the final cosmetic outcome until swelling has subsided.
- If indicated, discuss the potential benefits of rhinoplasty for fracture reduction or correction of this malformation.

If CSF leakage is present, also include the following instructions:

- Rest in bed with the head of the bed elevated to 30 to 45 degrees.
- Restrict fluid intake as ordered and take the prescribed diuretic to reduce intracranial pressure and CSF leakage.
- Distribute allowed fluids throughout the day.
- List the name, purpose, effects and precautions for any prescribed medication.
- Avoid straining, blowing the nose, sneezing or vigorous coughing until allowed by the doctor.
- Immediately report manifestations of infection, including stiff neck, headache and fever, to the doctor.

Following rhinoplasty or septoplasty, provide the following instructions:

- Apply ice packs to the nose to relieve discomfort and reduce swelling.
- Elevate the head of the bed to decrease local oedema.
- Do not blow the nose for 48 hours after the packing is removed to prevent bleeding.
- Vigorous coughing or straining, such as during the Valsalva manoeuvre if the patient is constipated, may cause bleeding and should be avoided.
- Clean teeth and mouth frequently and increase fluid intake to decrease oral dryness due to mouth breathing.
- Bruising around the eyes and nose will last for several days.

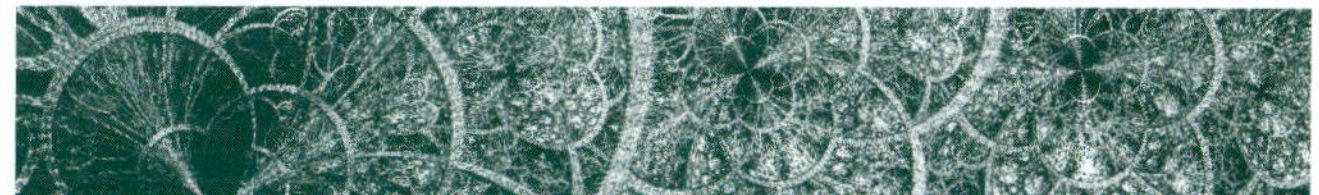

THE PERSON WITH LARYNGEAL OBSTRUCTION OR TRAUMA

The larynx is the narrowest portion of the upper airway. As such, it is at risk of obstruction. Laryngeal obstruction is a life-threatening emergency. Blows to the neck or traumatic injuries may damage the larynx, interfering with its patency and function.

Pathophysiology and manifestations

The larynx may be partially or fully obstructed by aspirated food or foreign objects or by laryngospasm or oedema due to inflammation, injury or anaphylaxis. Anything that occludes the larynx can obstruct the airway. The most common cause of obstruction in adults is ingested meat that lodges in the airway. Risk factors for food aspiration include ingesting large boluses of food and chewing them insufficiently, consuming excess alcohol and wearing dentures. A foreign body in the larynx causes pain, laryngospasm, dyspnoea and inspiratory stridor. Aspirated foreign bodies may pass through the larynx into the trachea and lungs, causing pneumonitis.

Laryngospasm occurs due to repeated or traumatic intubation attempts, chemical irritation or hypocalcaemia. An acute type I hypersensitivity response may cause anaphylaxis with release of inflammatory mediators, leading to angioedema of upper airways and severe laryngeal oedema. This is a life-threatening situation.

The most common manifestations of laryngeal obstruction are coughing, choking, gagging, obvious difficulty breathing with use of accessory muscles and inspiratory stridor. As the airway is obstructed, signs of asphyxia rapidly become apparent. Respirations are laboured and noisy with wheezing and stridor. Cyanosis may develop. Respiratory arrest and possible death may result without prompt treatment.

Trauma to the larynx can occur in motor vehicle crashes or assaults (e.g. blows to the neck or attempted strangulation). The larynx also may be traumatised during endotracheal intubation or tracheotomy. Trauma may fracture thyroid and/or cricoid cartilage, resulting in loss of airway patency. Soft tissue injuries can cause swelling that further impairs the airway. Manifestations of laryngeal trauma may include subcutaneous emphysema or crepitus, voice changes, dysphagia and pain with swallowing, inspiratory stridor, haemoptysis and cough.

INTERPROFESSIONAL CARE

The treatment goal is to maintain an open airway. If airway obstruction is partial and the person is able to cough and move air in and out of the lungs, radiological and laryngoscopic examination may be done to locate the foreign body. An endotracheal tube may be inserted to maintain airflow through the larynx in spasm or an oedematous larynx. For anaphylaxis, adrenaline may be administered to reduce laryngeal oedema and relieve obstruction.

A CT scan is used to identify laryngeal fractures; however, emergency treatment may be required prior to diagnosis to ensure airway patency and preserve life. Soft tissue injuries may be managed conservatively with a bedside humidifier, intravenous fluids, antibiotics and corticosteroids to reduce oedema. More severe injuries require endotracheal intubation or immediate tracheostomy. Nursing care related to caring for the person with a tracheostomy is presented later in this chapter. See the chapter 'Nursing care of people with gas exchange disorders' for more information about endotracheal intubation and nursing care for the intubated person.

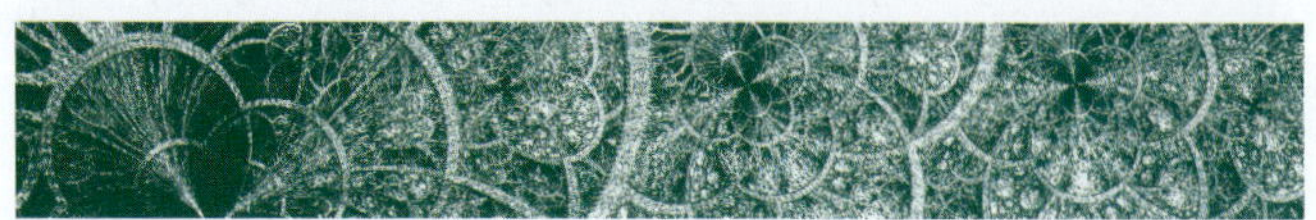

Nursing care

CONSIDERATION FOR PRACTICE

The priority of nursing care in laryngeal obstruction or trauma is restoring a patent airway to prevent cerebral anoxia and death. Laryngeal obstruction and trauma are medical emergencies requiring immediate intervention.

Closely monitor people at risk of laryngeal obstruction (e.g. following neck trauma, newly extubated people and people receiving medications with a high risk of anaphylaxis, such as intravenous antibiotics or radiological dyes) for manifestations of obstruction or anaphylaxis, including dyspnoea, nasal flaring, tachypnoea, anxiety, wheezing and stridor. Suction the airway as needed; small aspirated foreign bodies may be removed by suctioning to maintain a patent airway. If obstruction is complete, initiate a cardiopulmonary arrest procedure until the obstruction is relieved or the emergency response team arrives. Prepare to assist with emergency intubation or tracheotomy as required. Provide emotional support, reassurance and teaching for the person (if conscious) and family to reduce anxiety.

Community-based care

Health promotion and teaching for home care focus on preventing laryngeal obstruction and early intervention techniques. Everyone should be aware of the risk factors for adult aspiration. Caution people who wear dentures to take small bites, chewing each bite carefully before swallowing. Discuss the relationship between excess alcohol intake and food aspiration. Participate in promoting training of the general public in CPR and the appropriate manoeuvres such as back, chest or abdominal thrusts. The more people who are adequately trained in emergency procedures, the more likely it is that emergency procedures will be initiated in a timely manner. Individuals with a known risk of anaphylaxis, such as people with a previous anaphylactic response and those with allergies such as an allergy to bee venom, should wear a MedicAlert® tag and carry an anaphylaxis kit to allow early intervention to prevent severe laryngeal oedema and spasm.

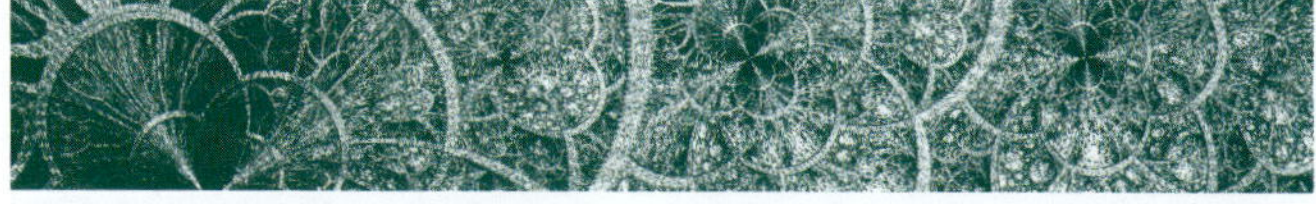

THE PERSON WITH OBSTRUCTIVE SLEEP APNOEA (OSA)

Obstructive **sleep apnoea**, intermittent absence of airflow through the mouth and nose during sleep, is a serious and potentially life-threatening disorder. It affects at least 2% of middle-aged women and 4% of middle-aged men. Sleep apnoea is a leading cause of excessive daytime sleepiness and may contribute to other problems such as poor work performance and motor vehicle crashes (Riha, 2021). Recent studies have linked sleep apnoea with an increased risk of hypertension, ischaemic heart disease and exacerbation of heart failure.

Types of sleep apnoea include obstructive, central and complex, or mixed sleep, apnoea. In *obstructive sleep apnoea*, the more common type, the respiratory drive remains intact but airflow ceases due to occlusion of the oropharyngeal airway. During sleep, the pharyngeal dilator muscle relaxes within the oropharyngeal airway. However, in obstructive sleep apnoea, these structures narrow and collapse, causing an obstruction. The risk of obstructive sleep apnoea increases with age and lifestyle factors such as smoking and obesity. Apnoea in obstructive sleep apnoea is defined as cessation of airflow for a 10-second period. Reduced airflow during sleep is defined as hypopnoea.

Central sleep apnoea is a rare neurological disorder that involves transient impairment of the neurological drive to respiratory muscles, typically for intermittent cycles of 10 to 30 seconds or more. Central sleep apnoea is often due to an impairment of the autonomic nervous system in the brain.

Complex, or *mixed, sleep apnoea* is a combination of obstructive sleep apnoea and central sleep apnoea.

Risk factors

Risk factors for sleep apnoea include:

- male gender (Bullock & Hales, 2019)
- excessive weight/morbid obesity
- advancing age
- large neck circumference (Bullock & Hales, 2019)
- enlarged tonsils or tongue
- gastro-oesophageal reflux
- allergies
- ongoing sinus issues
- a family history of sleep apnoea
- hypertension
- deviated septum
- use of alcohol and other CNS depressants.

Pathophysiology

During sleep, skeletal muscle tone decreases (except the diaphragm). The most significant decrease occurs during rapid eye movement (REM) sleep. Loss of normal pharyngeal dilator muscle tone permits the pharynx to collapse during inspiration as pressure within the airways becomes negative in relation to atmospheric pressure. The tongue is also pulled against the posterior pharyngeal wall by gravity during sleep, causing further obstruction. Obesity or skeletal or soft tissue changes that decrease inspiratory tone, such as a relatively large tongue in a relatively small oropharynx, contribute to the problem. Airflow obstruction causes the oxygen saturation, PO_2 and pH to fall and the PCO_2 to rise. This progressive asphyxia causes brief arousal from sleep, which restores airway patency and airflow. Sleep can be severely fragmented because these episodes may occur hundreds of times each night.

Manifestations

Narrowed upper airways produce loud snoring during sleep, often years before obstructive sleep apnoea occurs. Excessive daytime sleepiness, headache, irritability and restless sleep also are common manifestations. See the 'Manifestations' box.

Complications

Recurrent episodes of apnoea and arousal during sleep can have secondary physiological effects. Sleep fragmentation and loss of slow-wave sleep are thought to contribute to neurological and behavioural problems such as excessive daytime sleepiness, impaired intellect, memory loss and personality changes. Recurrent nocturnal asphyxia and negative intrathoracic pressure due to airway obstruction increase the workload of the heart. People with coronary heart disease may develop myocardial ischaemia and angina. Arrhythmias such as significant bradycardia and dangerous tachyarrhythmias may develop. Left ventricular function may be impaired and heart failure may occur. Systemic blood pressure remains high during sleep and may contribute to systemic hypertension. Pulmonary hypertension may also develop. Sudden cardiac death is believed to be a potentially fatal complication of obstructive sleep apnoea.

Obstructive sleep apnoea is a common condition in people who are morbidly obese. When these individuals undergo any surgery, sleep apnoea places them at significant risk of postoperative respiratory complications. Obesity not only interferes with chest movement and ventilation, but also increases metabolic demands and carbon monoxide production. Anaesthetic and analgesics used during surgery and in the postoperative period can lead to hypoxaemia due to muscle relaxation and depression of the respiratory drive. Individuals with OSA also experience an increased risk of pneumonia (Bullock & Hales, 2019).

Obesity hypoventilation syndrome can affect some obese and morbidly obese patients in association with obstructive sleep apnoea. This syndrome arises from a multifaceted interaction that occurs between diminished respiratory drive and sleep-disordered breathing. Patients with obesity hypoventilation syndrome have obstructive sleep apnoea characterised by interrupted sleep, snoring, periods of apnoeic episodes and excessive diurnal sleepiness (Bullock & Hales, 2019).

MANIFESTATIONS Obstructive sleep apnoea

- Loud, cyclical snoring
- Periods of apnoea lasting 15 to 120 seconds during sleep
- Gasping or choking during sleep
- Restlessness, thrashing during sleep
- Daytime fatigue and sleepiness
- Morning headache
- Personality changes, depression
- Intellectual impairment
- Impotence
- Hypertension

INTERPROFESSIONAL CARE

The goal of care for OSA is to restore airflow and prevent the adverse effects of the disorder. Sustained weight loss may assist in reducing and sometimes curing obstructive sleep apnoea.

Diagnosis

The diagnosis of OSA is based on *polysomnography*, an overnight sleep study. Several variables are recorded during the study, including:

- electroencephalogram and measurements of ocular activity and muscle tone
- recordings of ventilatory activity and airflow
- continuous arterial oxygen saturation readings
- heart rate.

Transcutaneous arterial PCO_2 readings also may be monitored during the study. Because sleep studies are time consuming and expensive, overnight monitoring of oxygen saturation by pulse oximetry may be used to confirm the diagnosis of sleep apnoea when symptoms indicate a high probability of the disorder. Nursing implications for pulmonary function studies and pulse oximetry are presented in the chapter 'A person-centred approach to assessing the respiratory system'. See the chapter 'A person-centred approach to assessing the nervous system' for more information about electroencephalography.

Treatments

Mild to moderate obstructive sleep apnoea may be treated by weight reduction, alcohol abstinence, improving nasal patency and avoiding the supine position for sleep. Although weight reduction may cure the disorder, maintaining optimal weight is often difficult. Oral appliances designed to keep the mandible and tongue forward also may be prescribed.

Nasal continuous positive airway pressure (CPAP) is the treatment of choice for obstructive sleep apnoea. Positive pressure generated by an air compressor and administered through a tight-fitting nasal mask (see Figure 34.3) splints the pharyngeal airway, preventing collapse and obstruction. With proper training, this device is well tolerated and improves quality of life. Nasal airways can become dry and irritated with CPAP, so an in-line humidifier or a room humidifier may be utilised. A newer device, the bilateral BiPAP ventilator, delivers higher pressures during inhalation and lower pressures during expiration, providing less resistance to exhaling.

Surgery

Tonsillectomy and adenoidectomy may relieve upper airway obstruction in some people. Excision of obstructive tissue from the soft palate, uvula and posterior lateral pharyngeal wall may be accomplished by *uvulopalatopharyngoplasty (UPPP)*. Although only about 50% of these surgeries are successful in treating sleep apnoea, UPPP is useful in selected cases. In severe cases, tracheostomy may also be performed to bypass the area of obstruction.

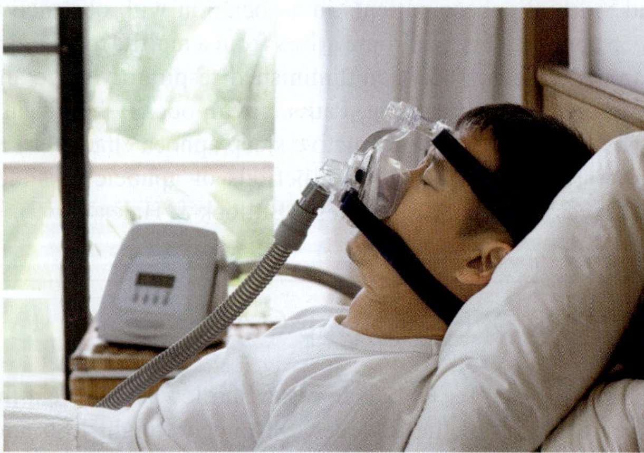

FIGURE 34.3 ***A person using a nasal mask and CPAP to treat sleep apnoea***

Source: sakphuket/123RF.

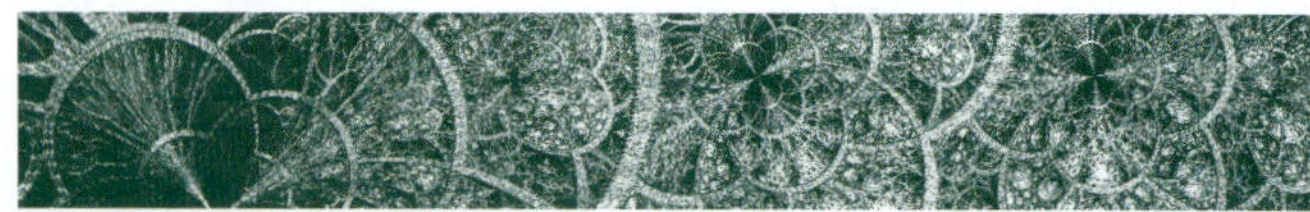

Nursing care

Obstructive sleep apnoea usually is treated in the home. Nursing care focuses on educating the person and family about equipment use and strategies to decrease contributing factors such as obesity and alcohol intake. The following nursing diagnoses are appropriate for individuals with sleep apnoea:

- *Disturbed sleep pattern* related to repeated apnoeic episodes manifested by continual interruptions to the sleep cycle.
- *Fatigue* related to interrupted sleep patterns manifested by tiredness and lack of attention.
- *Ineffective breathing pattern* related to obstruction of upper airway during sleep manifested by alterations in the normal sleep and breathing cycle.
- *Impaired gas exchange* related to altered lung ventilation during obstructive episodes manifested by changes in blood chemistry when assessed.
- *Risk of injury* related to daytime somnolence and altered judgment manifested by increasing number of accidents due to inattention.
- *Risk of sexual dysfunction* related to impotence resulting from sleep apnoea manifested by inability to achieve or maintain an erection.

Community-based care

Effective sleep apnoea management depends on the person's understanding and willingness to participate in care. Provide teaching about the following topics:

- relationship between obesity and sleep apnoea
- plans, resources and referrals as needed for weight loss (e.g. programs such as Weight Watchers to provide additional support)
- relationship of alcohol and sedatives to sleep apnoea; referral to an alcohol treatment program or Alcoholics Anonymous as indicated
- how to use CPAP if ordered
- maintenance of the device including cleaning and servicing
- the importance of using CPAP continuously at night
- measures to reduce airway dryness, including supplemental humidity and an adequate fluid intake to maintain moist mucous membranes.

If a support group for people with sleep apnoea syndrome is available in the local area, a referral can be made for the patient and their family to attend.

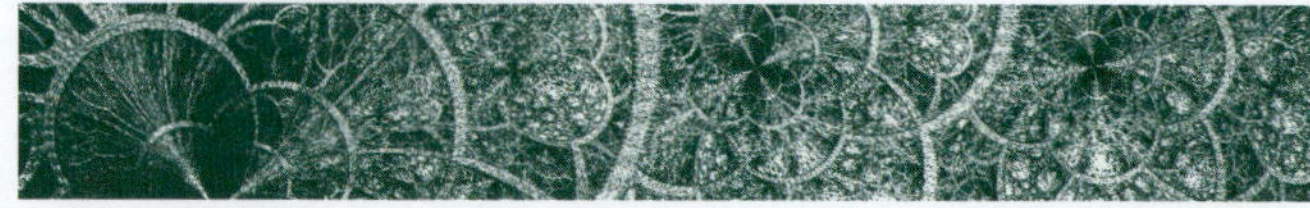

Upper respiratory tumours

Although tumours of the upper respiratory tract are relatively uncommon, they have the potential to impair the upper airways and interfere with breathing and ventilation of the lungs. Of the upper respiratory tract structures, the larynx is affected by abnormal growths most often.

THE PERSON WITH NASAL POLYPS

Nasal polyps are benign grape-like growths of the mucous membrane lining the nose. These benign tumours can interfere with air movement through nasal passages or obstruct sinus openings, leading to sinusitis. They usually affect people who have chronic allergic rhinitis or asthma.

Pathophysiology and manifestations

Chronic irritation and swelling of the mucous membranes from allergic rhinitis may cause slow polyp formation. Polyps form in areas of dependent mucous membrane, presenting as pale, oedematous masses covered with mucous membrane. They are usually bilateral and have a stem-like base, making them fairly movable. Polyps can continue to enlarge, eventually becoming larger than a grape. Polyps may be asymptomatic, although large polyps may cause nasal obstruction, rhinorrhoea and loss of sense of smell. Manifestations of sinusitis can develop as a complication related to nasal polyps. The voice may have a nasal tone.

INTERPROFESSIONAL CARE

When polyps occur in conjunction with an acute upper respiratory infection, they may regress spontaneously with resolution of the infection. When symptomatic, polyps may be managed with topical corticosteroid nasal sprays or low-dose oral corticosteroids to shrink the oedematous polyps and manage allergic symptoms. However, polyps continue to enlarge when corticosteroid therapy is discontinued and therefore surgery is sometimes required.

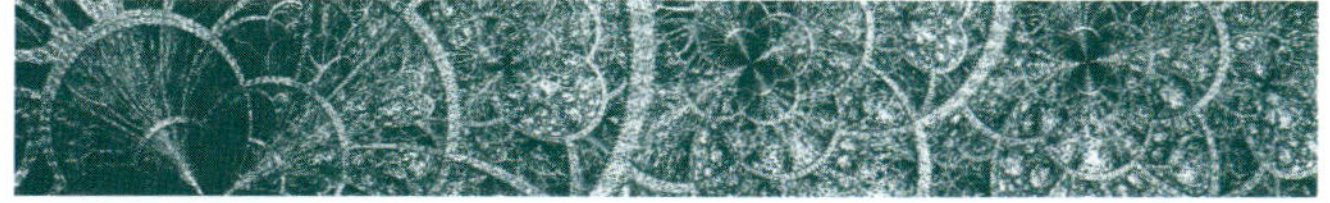

Nursing care

Teaching about home care following polypectomy is the primary nursing responsibility for the person with nasal polyps. Provide postoperative care instructions and discuss measures to reduce the risk of bleeding:

- Apply ice or cold compresses to the nose to decrease swelling, promote comfort and prevent bleeding.
- Avoid blowing the nose for 24 to 48 hours after nasal packing is removed.
- Avoid straining to defecate, vigorous coughing and strenuous exercise.

Discuss manifestations of possible bleeding, such as frequent swallowing or visible blood at the back of the throat. Swallowed blood may cause nausea and vomiting. Encourage the person to rest for 2–3 days after surgery to reduce the risk of bleeding and dislodgement of clots. Instruct to increase fluid intake and clean mouth frequently to reduce oral dryness associated with mouth breathing while nasal packing is in place.

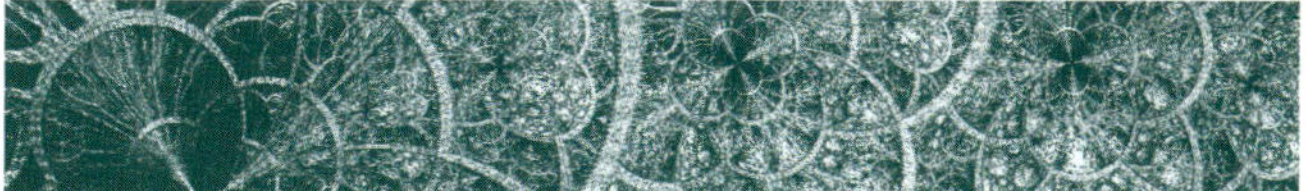

THE PERSON WITH A LARYNGEAL TUMOUR

Laryngeal tumours may be either benign or malignant. Benign tumours of the larynx include papillomas, nodules and polyps. People who chronically shout, project or vocalise in an abnormally high or low tone, abusing the voice, are at risk of developing benign laryngeal tumours. In adults, vocal cord nodules are often referred to as 'singer's nodules'; public speakers may also develop them. Voice abuse also contributes to the development of vocal cord polyps, as do cigarette smoking and chronic irritation from industrial pollutants. Malignant tumours of the larynx, although uncommon, can have devastating effects if diagnosis and treatment are delayed.

Risk factors

Men are affected by laryngeal cancer more than three times as often as women. Cancer of the larynx usually develops between ages 50 and 70. Tobacco use is the main risk factor for laryngeal cancer: the risk of developing laryngeal cancer is significantly greater in smokers (cigarette, pipe or cigar) than in non-smokers. A person who smokes one pack a day is 20 times more at risk of laryngeal cancer than a non-smoker (Dai et al., 2022). Alcohol consumption is a significant co-factor in increasing the risk. Other risk factors include poor nutrition, human papillomavirus infection, exposure to asbestos and other occupational pollutants. Race is also considered a risk factor, with Aboriginal and Torres Strait Islander Australians and Māori New Zealanders experiencing higher rates of laryngeal cancer (Australian Institute of Health and Welfare, 2021).

Pathophysiology and manifestations

Papillomas are small, wart-like growths believed to be viral in origin. Polyps and nodules may develop on the vocal cords of the larynx as a result of voice abuse (see Figure 34.4). Nodules occur as paired lesions on the free edges of the vocal cords. Hoarseness and a breathy voice quality are manifestations of benign vocal cord tumours.

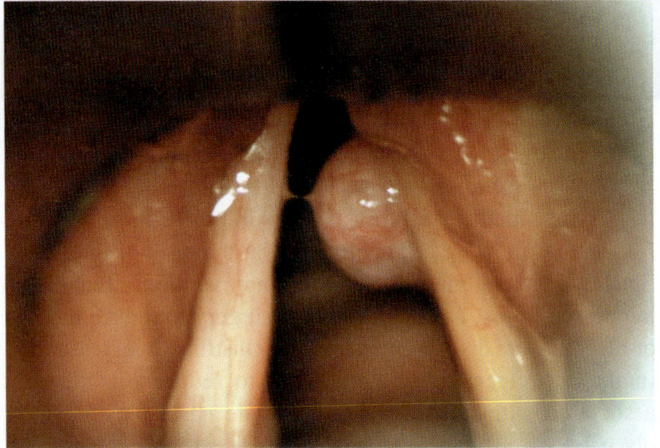

FIGURE 34.4 *Laryngoscopy showing a polyp on the left vocal cord*

Source: CC, ISM/Science Photo Library.

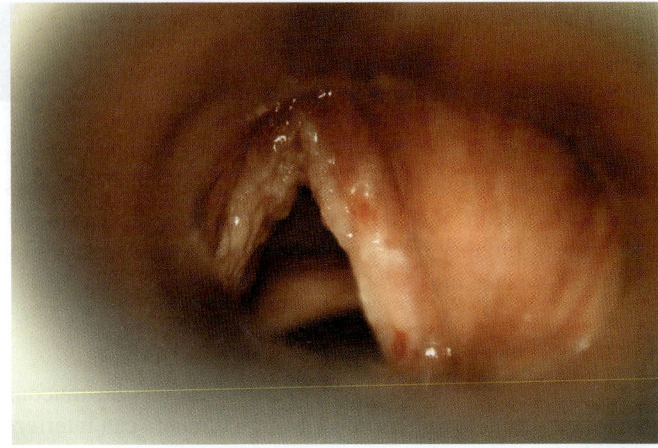

FIGURE 34.5 *Cancer of the larynx and epiglottis*

Source: CC, ISM/Science Photo Library.

Laryngeal cancer

Squamous cell carcinoma is the most common malignancy of the larynx. Changes in the laryngeal mucosa occur over time as it is subjected to noxious irritants such as cigarette smoke. White, patchy, precancerous lesions known as *leucoplakia* appear. Red, velvety patches, called *erythroplakia*, are thought to represent a later stage of carcinoma development. The initial cancerous lesion, carcinoma in situ (CIS), is superficial. Malignant cells replace the lining layer, but do not invade into deeper tissues. Untreated, most CIS lesions develop into squamous cell cancer (Cancer Council Australia, 2022).

Laryngeal cancer spreads both by direct invasion of surrounding tissues and by metastasis. It may metastasise to the lungs; however, metastases from other cancers to the larynx are rare.

Laryngeal cancer may develop in any of the three areas of the larynx: the glottis, the supraglottis and the subglottis. Manifestations vary according to the site of the lesion.

Lesions of the true vocal cords or glottis account for nearly 60% of all laryngeal cancers. Fortunately, these cancers tend to be well differentiated and slow growing. Metastasis occurs late in the course of the disease because of a limited lymphatic supply. The usual symptom of glottic cancer is hoarseness or a change in the voice because the tumour prevents complete closure of the vocal cords during speech.

Approximately 35% of laryngeal cancers develop in the supraglottic area, which includes the epiglottis, aryepiglottic folds, arytenoid muscles and cartilage, and false vocal cords (see Figure 34.5). Lymphatic supply to this region of the larynx is rich; tumours often invade locally and metastasise early. Symptoms often do not develop until the tumour is relatively large, delaying diagnosis. Manifestations of supraglottic cancer include painful swallowing, sore throat or a feeling of a lump in the throat. Later manifestations include dyspnoea, foul breath and pain that radiates to the ear.

Subglottic tumours (below the vocal cords) are the least common, accounting for the remaining 5% of laryngeal tumours. They often are asymptomatic until the enlarging tumour obstructs the airway. Common manifestations of laryngeal cancer are listed in the accompanying box.

MANIFESTATIONS Laryngeal cancer

- Hoarseness
- Change in the voice
- Painful swallowing
- Dyspnoea
- Foul breath
- Palpable lump in neck
- Earache

INTERPROFESSIONAL CARE

Benign laryngeal tumours may resolve with correction of the underlying problem, such as voice training with a speech therapist or smoking cessation. Treatment of laryngeal malignancy varies with the extent of the cancer. Early diagnosis and treatment are important to support successful outcomes, with a single, local treatment modality and/or radiation or surgery (Koroulakis & Agarwal, 2022).

Diagnosis

- *Direct* or *indirect laryngoscopy* is used for initial evaluation when laryngeal cancer is suspected. A fibre-optic laryngoscope is used for direct laryngoscopy; mirrors are used to visualise the larynx in indirect laryngoscopy.
- *Biopsy* is obtained from suspicious lesions to examine the cells. Biopsy is usually obtained under general anaesthesia or conscious sedation. Tissue may be obtained via endoscopy or by fine-needle aspiration of the mass.
- *Imaging studies* such as CT scan, MRI and chest x-ray are obtained to evaluate the size of the mass, possible extension into deeper tissues, involvement of lymph nodes and possible metastasis to the lungs. A barium swallow may be done to evaluate the effects of the tumour on swallowing. A positron emission tomography (PET) scan also may be done (possibly in conjunction with CT) to detect tumour metastasis.

Treatments

An inhaled steroid spray may be used for vocal cord polyps. In some cases, surgical excision of benign nodules or polyps is required. This usually is performed via laryngoscopy, using microforceps or a laser. A biopsy of the tumour is done to rule out malignancy.

Laryngeal cancer treatment is determined by *staging* the cancer. Information such as tumour size and location (T), number of involved lymph nodes (N) and presence or absence of metastases (M) is combined to assign a stage, designated by Roman numerals I to IV. The staging also takes into consideration whether the laryngeal cancer is supra-, peri- or subglottic.

RADIATION THERAPY Radiation therapy is often the treatment of choice for early laryngeal cancer. Radiation disrupts the DNA of the cell, causing it to die. External radiation commonly is used; brachytherapy, implants of iridium seeds placed into hollow plastic needles that are inserted directly into or near the tumour site during surgery to deliver radiation, is less frequently used for laryngeal or hypopharyngeal cancer. Radiation therapy is extremely effective for treating glottic cancer, with cure rates equal to those achieved by surgery. Radiation therapy preserves the voice, although the tone or timbre of the voice may be affected.

Radiation therapy may be used in combination with chemotherapy (*chemoradiotherapy*) to treat more advanced laryngeal cancers. In some institutions, and depending on the stage of cancer, chemoradiotherapy may be used in place of laryngectomy (Wang et al., 2022). Radiation therapy also may be used in conjunction with surgery to destroy any remaining cancerous cells or as a palliative treatment for advanced tumours. See the chapter 'Nursing care of people with cancer' for more information about radiation therapy and its nursing implications.

CHEMOTHERAPY Chemotherapy is used in combination with radiation therapy as the primary treatment for some laryngeal cancers. It also is used to treat distant metastasis and for palliation when the tumour is unresectable. See the chapter 'Nursing care of people with cancer' for the nursing implications for chemotherapy.

Surgery

The type of surgery used to treat laryngeal cancer is based on site, size and invasiveness of the tumour into the larynx and surrounding tissues. The goals of surgery are to remove the malignancy, maintain airway patency and achieve optimal cosmetic appearance.

Carcinoma in situ, vocal cord polyps and early vocal cord cancers may be removed by laser during a laryngoscopy procedure. The cure rate for early tumours using this method is excellent. This surgery may be performed on an outpatient basis. The degree of trauma to the vocal cords varies, depending on the size of the lesion. The voice is preserved, but total voice rest with whispering only may be ordered for a week or more following surgery. In some cases, a temporary tracheostomy may be done at the time of surgery to ensure that swelling does not interfere with airway patency. Once the tracheostomy tube is removed and the opening is closed, the person can eat, speak and breathe normally.

Laryngectomy, removal of the larynx, may be necessary. A partial laryngectomy (hemilaryngectomy, vertical partial laryngectomy) may be used for tumours localised to a portion of the larynx with limited extension beyond the larynx. In a partial laryngectomy, 50% or more of the larynx is removed. The voice generally is well preserved, although it may be changed by the surgery. A tracheostomy tube may be inserted for early postoperative airway management. It is usually removed in 5 to 7 days as postoperative swelling subsides and the stoma is allowed to close. Normal speaking, breathing and swallowing are restored. If the epiglottis has been removed, careful monitoring for aspiration is necessary. Enteral tube feedings or parenteral nutrition may be required for several weeks after surgery. Swallowing techniques to prevent aspiration are taught.

A *total laryngectomy* is required for cancers that extend beyond the vocal cords. The entire larynx is removed, along with the epiglottis, thyroid cartilage, several tracheal rings and the hyoid bone. Because the trachea and the oesophagus are permanently separated by this surgery (see Figure 34.6), there is no risk of aspiration during swallowing. Normal speech is lost and a permanent tracheostomy is created. The tracheostomy tube inserted during surgery may be left in place for several weeks and then removed, leaving a natural stoma, or it may be left in place permanently. See the accompanying box for nursing care of the person undergoing a total laryngectomy. Procedure 34.1 outlines tracheostomy care.

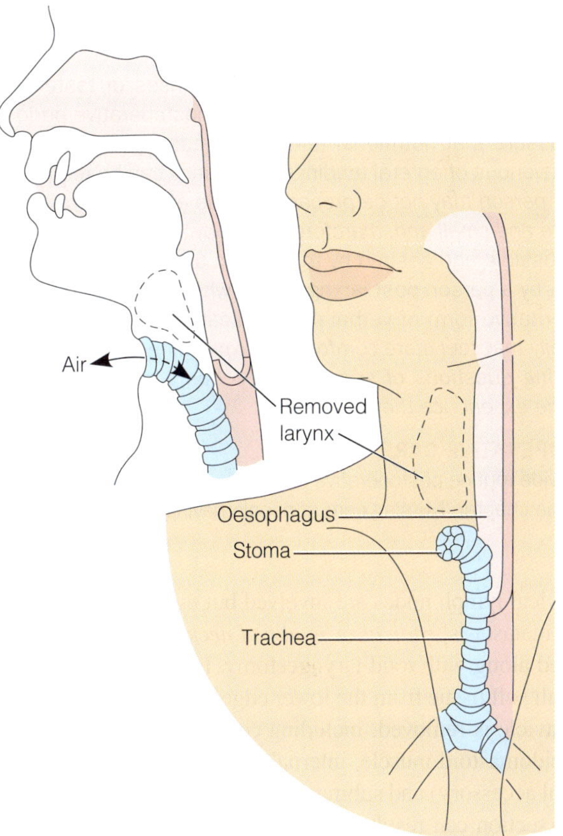

FIGURE 34.6 ***Following a total laryngectomy, the person has a permanent tracheostomy. No connection between the trachea and oesophagus remains***

NURSING CARE OF THE PERSON having a total laryngectomy

PREOPERATIVE CARE

- Provide routine preoperative care and teaching as explained in the chapter 'Nursing care of people having surgery'.
- Assess knowledge and understanding of the diagnosis and proposed surgery. Clarify information and reinforce previous teaching as needed. *A clear understanding by the person and family of the purpose, anticipated benefits and consequences of total laryngectomy prior to surgery is vital to promote postoperative recovery.*
- Assess anxiety levels of the person and family related to the diagnosis and proposed surgery. *High levels of anxiety interfere with learning and the ability to cooperate in care. Interventions to reduce anxiety may be required prior to teaching and providing preoperative instructions.*
- Without increasing fear, emphasise that total laryngectomy results in a loss of speech and that the person will breathe through a permanent stoma in the neck. *Although person and family members may verbalise an understanding of the loss of speech following surgery, they may believe that verbal communication will still be possible through the stoma.*
- Establish a means of communicating postoperatively, using an alphabet board, eye or hand signals, or other strategies. *Learning techniques for communicating preoperatively decreases the person's and family's postoperative anxiety. Long-term speech rehabilitation measures, such as the tracheoesophageal puncture, are not appropriate for use in the immediate postoperative period.*
- Point out that surgery will affect the senses of taste and smell, and hence eating, in the initial postoperative period. Reassure that nutritional and fluid needs will be met with intravenous or enteral feedings until eating can be resumed. *The person may not be prepared for the effect of surgery on taste and smell and, therefore, the enjoyment of food.*
- If possible and desired by the person and family, arrange a visit by a person post laryngectomy who effectively uses an alternative form of verbal communication. *The person and family may feel more comfortable expressing their fears and asking questions of someone who has gone through the same experience they are facing.*

POSTOPERATIVE CARE

- Provide routine postoperative care and monitoring as explained in the chapter 'Nursing care of people having surgery'.
- Frequently monitor airway patency and respiratory status, including respiratory rate and pattern, lung sounds and oxygen saturation. *Excessive or retained respiratory secretions can impair gas exchange, increase the work of breathing and lead to complications such as pneumonia.*
- Encourage deep breathing and coughing. *Deep breathing helps ensure adequate ventilation of lower airways; coughing helps to move secretions out of airways.*
- Elevate the head of the bed. *The upright position promotes effective ventilation of the lungs and reduces oedema and swelling of the neck.*
- Maintain humidification of inspired gases. *With a tracheostomy, humidification of inspired air in the upper airways is lost. Humidified air helps maintain moist mucous membranes and secretions, promoting secretion removal by coughing or suctioning.*
- Maintain an adequate fluid intake (intravenously, enterally and orally when allowed). *Adequate hydration keeps secretions liquid and mucous membranes moist.*
- Suction via tracheostomy using sterile technique as needed. *Surgery, impaired nutrition and the effects of radiation therapy may cause fatigue and a weak cough effort. Suctioning may be necessary to clear secretions and maintain airway patency.*
- Provide tracheostomy care as needed (see Procedure 34.1). *Periodic cleaning of the tracheostomy tube is necessary to remove accumulated secretions and maintain airway patency.*
- Teach to protect the stoma from particulate matter in the air with gauze square or other stoma protector. *Permanent tracheostomy results in loss of the protective mechanisms of the upper airway that prevent foreign material from entering the lungs.*
- Instruct to support the head when moving in bed. *Additional head support reduces the strain on tissues in the operative area.*
- Place the call bell within easy reach at all times; answer the call bell promptly. *The person who is unable to speak needs reassurance that help is within reach at all times.*
- Encourage family members to remain present when possible. *Supportive family presence helps reassure the person that they will not be left alone or helpless.*
- Spend as much time as possible with the person. When leaving the room, specify the time when you will return. *These measures help establish trust and relieve anxiety.*

If cervical lymph nodes are involved but there is no evidence of distal metastasis, *radical* or *modified neck dissection* may be performed along with total laryngectomy. In a radical neck dissection, all soft tissue from the lower edge of the mandible down to the clavicle is removed, including cervical lymph nodes, the sternocleidomastoid muscle, internal jugular vein, cranial nerve XI (spinal accessory) and submaxillary salivary gland. Extensive tissue dissection can result in significant deformity. Skin grafts or flaps may be used to close the wound. Bellovac drains are placed in the wound to prevent haematoma and extensive oedema formation. After surgery, the person may have difficulty lifting and turning the head because of muscle loss. Resection of the spinal accessory nerve causes shoulder drop on the affected side. In a modified neck dissection, neck contents are removed, with the exception of the sternocleidomastoid muscle, internal jugular vein and spinal accessory nerve.

A gastrostomy also may be performed to maintain nutrition in the person with laryngeal or hypopharyngeal cancer. See the chapter 'Nursing care of people with upper gastrointestinal disorders' for more information about caring for the person with a gastrostomy tube.

Speech rehabilitation

Various techniques may be used to restore speech after total laryngectomy. *Tracheoesophageal puncture (TEP)* is the usual method used to restore speech. A small fistula is created between the posterior tracheal wall and the anterior oesophagus. A small, one-way shunt valve is fitted into the fistula (see Figure 34.7).

PROCEDURE 34.1 Providing tracheostomy care

GATHER SUPPLIES

- Dressing pack
- Sterile suction catheter and glove kit
- Sterile disposable replacement inner cannula, if appropriate
- Cleaning solutions (e.g. sterile normal saline)
- Sterile 4 × 4 gauze dressings (not cotton filled) or pre-cut dressing
- Sterile cotton-tipped applicators
- Single-use tracheostomy tube holder or cotton twill ties
- Scissors
- Clean exam gloves

BEFORE THE PROCEDURE

Provide for privacy. Explain the procedure. Provide for a means of communication (e.g. eye blinking or raising a finger to indicate distress). If the person's condition permits, provide a pencil and paper for questions. Place in semi-Fowler's or Fowler's position to facilitate lung ventilation. Assess lung sounds; suction the tracheostomy using sterile technique as needed.

DURING THE PROCEDURE

- Use standard precautions.
- Wearing a clean disposable glove, remove the tracheostomy dressing. Dispose of the glove and dressing.
- Open sterile supplies and add additional materials (dressing, cleaning solution etc). Don gloves.
- Clean area using aseptic technique.
- If the tracheostomy tube has an inner cannula that can be removed for disposal or cleaning, remove the tube and set it aside for disposal or clean with solution. Cleanse the flange of the outer cannula. Clean reusable inner cannulas using a small brush, pipe cleaners or cotton-tipped applicators.
- Rinse the inner cannula thoroughly in normal saline. Tap it gently against the inner aspect of the sterile bowl to remove excess liquid.
- Suction the outer cannula using sterile technique.
- Replace the inner cannula into the tracheostomy tube.
- Replace the dressing, using either a commercially prepared tracheostomy dressing or an opened gauze 4 × 4 refolded into a V shape (see the accompanying figure). Do not cut the dressing or use a cotton-filled dressing to prevent aspiration of foreign material into the respiratory tract.
- Apply a clean tracheostomy holder or clean ties.
- Once the clean ties are secured, remove the old ties.

AFTER THE PROCEDURE

Assess breathing and tolerance of the procedure. Dispose of supplies and used solutions. Wash hands. Chart the procedure and any observations made during the procedure such as amount, colour and consistency of sputum and appearance of the incision.

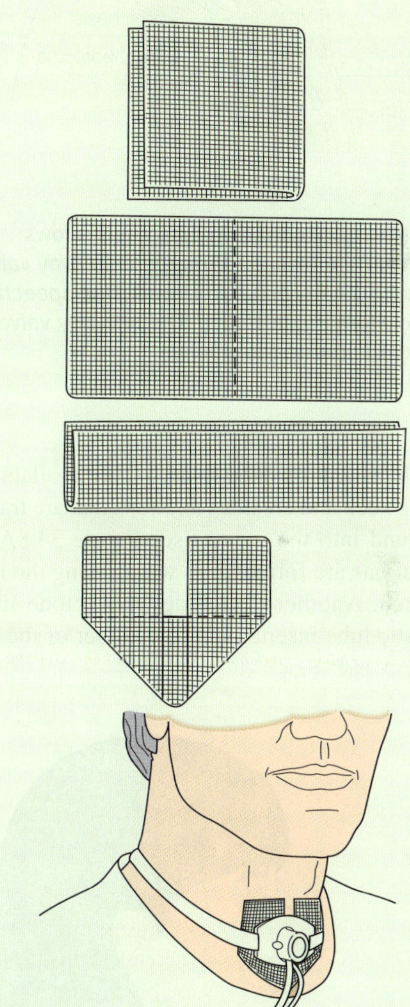

Steps for folding a gauze 4 × 4 into a tracheostomy dressing

Occluding the tracheostomy stoma with a finger forces exhaled air through the valve into the oesophagus and hypopharynx, creating vibration and sound. The muscles of speech are used to form words. The one-way valve prevents aspiration from the oesophagus into the trachea. An external tracheostoma valve may be used to avoid using the hand to occlude the stoma. This device covers the entire tracheal stoma and closes during exhalation, forcing air directly into the voice prosthesis. Not all post-laryngectomy people are candidates for this device because its use requires motivation and manual dexterity.

Oesophageal speech uses swallowed air to create sound and form words as it is expelled in a controlled belch. The pharyngoesophageal segment vibrates with the belch, creating sound. Muscles of the mouth and tongue are used to control the sound and to form words. This form of speech takes practice and fluent speech may not be restored.

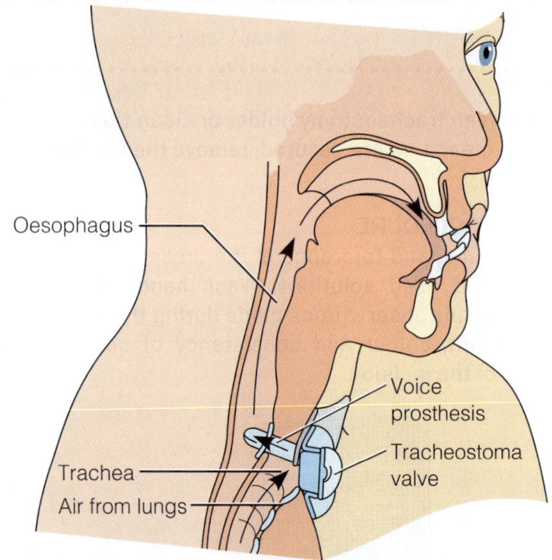

FIGURE 34.7 ***The tracheoesophageal prosthesis allows diversion of air from the trachea through a one-way valve into the oesophagus and oropharynx, producing speech when the tracheostomy stoma is occluded. The one-way valve prevents food from entering the trachea***

Several speech generators (electrolarynx) are available. One type is held to the neck and creates vibrations that are transmitted to the neck and into the mouth (see Figure 34.8A). The transmitted vibrations are formed into words using the normal muscles of speech. Another device delivers a tone into the mouth via a plastic tube inserted into the corner of the mouth (see Figure 34.8B). The lips, tongue and mouth muscles are used to form the sound into words.

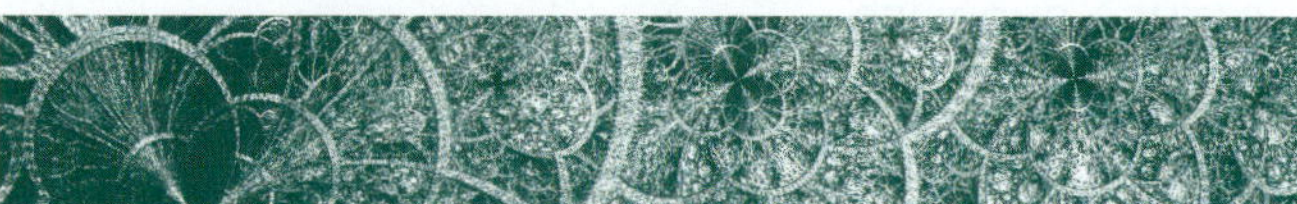

Nursing care

Nurses can be instrumental in early identification and treatment of laryngeal disorders by emphasising the need for the person with any new symptoms, such as chronic hoarseness, to seek treatment.

Health promotion

Health promotion activities to prevent laryngeal cancer focus on preventing smoking by children, adolescents and young adults, and promoting smoking cessation in people who do smoke. Activities to promote abstinence or moderate alcohol use also are beneficial in reducing a significant risk factor for laryngeal cancer.

Assessment

Nurses can be instrumental in identifying early signs of laryngeal cancer, facilitating early diagnosis and treatment.

- *Health history*: current changes, signs and symptoms, including voice change, difficulty swallowing, throat pain; risk factors such as voice abuse, family history of cancer, occupational exposures; smoking history, use of alcohol and amount consumed.
- *Physical examination*: voice character; general appearance and apparent state of health; swallowing ability; visible or palpable mass in neck.

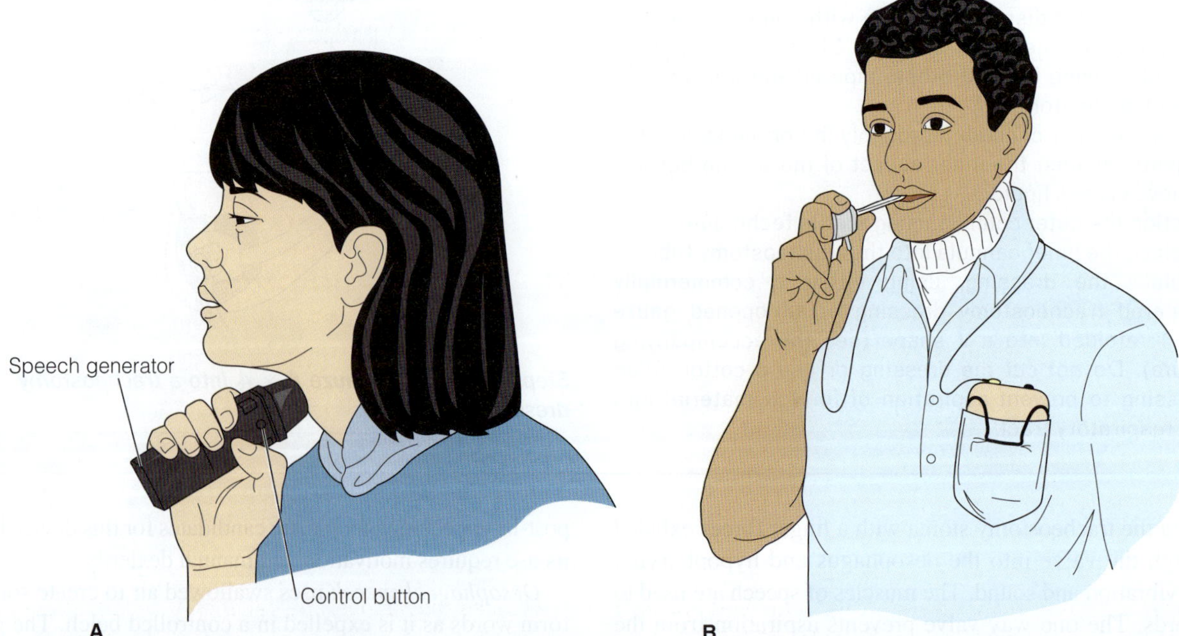

FIGURE 34.8 ***Speech generators. A, The person holds the vibrating tip of the speech generator against the throat, using the mouth to form words. B, A plastic handpiece of the generator is held in the corner of the mouth. The audible tone produced by the generator is formed into words***

Nursing diagnoses and interventions

Nursing care for the person with a benign tumour of the larynx focuses on maintaining a patent airway and teaching about the disorder and strategies to prevent its recurrence. The person with laryngeal cancer has multiple nursing care needs. The risk of impaired verbal communication is significant. Dysphagia may interfere with swallowing and nutrition. Nutrition may also be impaired by radiation, chemotherapy and surgery. The diagnosis of cancer is frightening for most people, no matter what the potential for cure is with treatment. See the accompanying nursing care plan for additional nursing diagnoses and interventions.

CONSIDERATION FOR PRACTICE

During the immediate postoperative period, closely monitor for signs of airway obstruction, such as laboured breathing or inspiratory stridor. The larynx is the narrowest portion of the upper airways. Tissue oedema following surgery can further restrict the airway, interfering with lung ventilation and gas exchange.

Risk of impaired airway clearance

Following resection of a benign or malignant vocal cord nodule, local tissue oedema may interfere with airway patency.

NURSING CARE PLAN A person with total laryngectomy

David Tom is a 61-year-old accountant who is divorced and has two adult children. He has smoked two packets of cigarettes daily since high school and usually has three or four rum and cokes each evening. After several months of persistent sore throat and hoarseness, Mr Tom was diagnosed with cancer of the larynx. He has been admitted to the surgical care unit from the critical care unit 2 days post total laryngectomy.

ASSESSMENT

Mr Tom's vital signs are stable: BP 146/84, P 92 and regular, R 18, T 36.7°C axillary. A tracheostomy tube is sutured in place and he is receiving humidified oxygen at 28% per tracheostomy collar. Pulse oximetry is 94%. He is receiving continuous tube feeding per nasogastric feeding tube. Two Bellovac wound drains are present in the right neck area. A moderate amount of oedema is noted in the right facial and submandibular area. Mr Tom is ambulatory within the room.

DIAGNOSES

- *Risk of airway compromise* related to postoperative oedema manifested by difficulty in clearing secretions.
- *Risk of ineffective breathing* related to pain and anxiety manifested by decreased oxygen intake and symptoms of increased pain and anxiety.
- *Disturbed body image* related to total laryngectomy and presence of tracheostomy stoma manifested by the person self-reporting body image issues or reluctance to engage in the community.
- *Impaired verbal communication* related to total laryngectomy manifested by difficulty communicating verbally when required.
- *Pain* related to surgical procedure manifested by increased respiratory rate and pulse and the person self-reporting discomfort.
- *Nutritional imbalance* related to insufficient oral intake manifested by lack of appetite and pain when eating and difficulty swallowing fluids.

PLANNING

- Assess respiratory status, including rate, pattern, lung sounds and cough effectiveness, at least every 4 hours.
- Monitor quantity, colour and odour of secretions.
- Assess vital signs and pain at least every 4 hours. Administer analgesics as ordered.

Expected outcomes

- Maintain clear airways and normal lung sounds.
- Maintain oxygen saturation level greater than 92%.
- Demonstrate interest in providing incision and stoma care.
- Accept information about potential communication strategies.
- Communicate effective pain management.
- Maintain appropriate body weight.
- Maintain a healthy and balanced diet.

IMPLEMENTATION

- Schedule time to sit with Mr Tom and discuss his concerns and feelings intermittently throughout your shift.
- Provide written information as requested.
- Monitor intake, output and daily weight.
- Arrange dietary consultation to determine kilojoule requirements.

EVALUATION

Mr Tom reports in writing that his pain is adequately controlled. His respiratory status is stable with clear breath sounds throughout and an oxygen saturation of 94%. He is afebrile. Mr Tom is tolerating tube feedings well and expresses a desire to begin eating. The dietitian has visited and assisted in planning to begin oral feedings. Intake and output are stable, as is his weight. Mr Tom has been receptive to receiving information about follow-up care and exploration of various modalities of speech.

CRITICAL THINKING IN THE NURSING PROCESS

1. Compare and contrast advantages and disadvantages of various methods to allow speech following total laryngectomy.
2. Develop a plan of care for Mr Tom for the nursing diagnosis of *Disturbed body image*.
3. Discuss nursing interventions to provide wound care for the person with laryngectomy and radical neck dissection.
4. List strategies to optimise ventilation.

REFLECTION ON THE NURSING PROCESS

1. Discuss the various strategies that can be utilised when communicating with Mr Tom and evaluate which patient education strategies may be most useful in this situation.
2. Outline what you have learned from the case study that you will implement in your future practice.

- Apply cold packs to the neck as ordered or indicated. *Cold application constricts local blood vessels and reduces oedema development.*
- Withhold food and fluids until the cough and gag reflexes have returned. *Local anaesthesia used during removal of benign tumours and nodules impairs the cough and gag reflexes, increasing the risk of aspiration.*

Impaired verbal communication

Treatment of laryngeal cancer often alters the quality of the voice, results in short-term restriction of speaking or, in the case of total laryngectomy, causes loss of the voice. The person ultimately determines treatment choices for laryngeal cancer; some choose to forgo laryngectomy to avoid voice loss when the chance for long-term success and cancer cure is minimal.

- Prior to surgery, assess for additional obstacles to communication, develop alternative methods of communication and ensure the patient is familiar with using assistive devices. *Communication may be impaired by hearing loss, illiteracy or weakness associated with the disease process, altering the ability to use alternative communication strategies.*
- Assess the importance of verbal communication to self-concept, occupation and lifestyle. *Many factors influence adaptation to the loss of normal verbal communication. If the ability to speak is central to an occupation (e.g. school teacher, singer) or self-concept (e.g. politician or barrister), adapting to a total laryngectomy may be difficult. For these people, laryngectomy may mean a loss of employment or career.*

> **CONSIDERATION FOR PRACTICE**
>
> **Prior to surgery, introduce non-verbal communication strategies such as pencil and paper, an alphabet board or a white board and marker. Encourage the person to practise using each method and to choose the most acceptable one. Having the person determine a means of communication prior to surgery helps to alleviate anxiety and increases their sense of control.**

- Arrange consultation with a speech therapist about alternative forms of oral communication prior to surgery if possible. *Determining a means of communicating on a continuing basis prior to surgery helps to relieve fear of inability to communicate and may guide the choice of a surgical procedure.*

> **CONSIDERATION FOR PRACTICE**
>
> **After surgery, assess frequently. Place the call bell at hand. The presence of a caring nurse helps to decrease anxiety and promotes communication. Knowing that help is readily available enhances feelings of security and decreases anxiety.**

- Reinforce teaching about alternative communication strategies. *Anxiety or information overload may impair the ability to retain information; reinforcement facilitates learning.*
- Maintain a positive attitude about postoperative communication, but do not promote unrealistic expectations. *Not everyone is able to use all alternative methods of verbal communication after the laryngectomy. Some people remain non-verbal.*
- If desired, arrange a visit by a rehabilitated laryngectomy person who has mastered an alternative form of verbal communication and has a positive attitude about rehabilitation. *Many people and their families find that they are better able to communicate their fears with someone who has gone through the same experience they are facing.*

Impaired swallowing

Disruption of laryngeal structures by the tumour itself or due to radiation or surgery can impair the swallowing mechanism. Additionally, even when a total laryngectomy has been performed and a connection between the oropharynx and trachea no longer exists, swallowing may cause fear of choking.

- Maintain intravenous fluids and enteral feedings or parenteral nutrition until adequate food and fluids can be ingested orally. *It is important to maintain nutritional and fluid balance until normal eating can be resumed.*
- Postoperatively, initiate oral intake with soft foods, not liquids. *Soft foods are easier to handle and swallow initially. As recovery progresses, thickened liquids can be swallowed and, eventually, a normal diet can be resumed.*
- Following total laryngectomy, reassure that choking is not possible because there is no connection between the oesophagus and trachea. *People often fear that swallowing will result in choking and they will be unable to cough effectively.*
- Instruct to initiate a swallow by placing a small amount of food on the back of the tongue, flex the head forward and then think 'swallow'. *Swallowing is no longer an automatic function and needs to be relearned.*

> **CONSIDERATION FOR PRACTICE**
>
> **Provide for privacy during initial attempts at eating. Eating in the presence of others may cause embarrassment until confidence in eating is regained. Privacy also reduces risk of impaired nutrition and distractions, allowing concentration on swallowing.**

Nutritional imbalance related to insufficient oral intake

Large laryngeal tumours often place pressure on the oesophagus and may cause dysphagia (difficulty swallowing) or odynophagia (painful swallowing). In either case, difficulty eating may ultimately impair nutrition. Additionally, cancer often produces a hypermetabolic state, increasing kilojoule requirements. If surgery is performed, difficulty swallowing and a fear of aspiration in the early postoperative period also interfere with eating. Enteral or parenteral feedings are usually needed initially to meet nutritional status. After a total laryngectomy, the senses of taste and smell are disrupted. Although the sense of taste may be partially recovered, people may complain that eating no longer is pleasurable.

- Assess nutritional status using height and weight charts, reported weight loss and anthropometric measurements such as skin folds. *Thorough assessment of nutritional status is important in planning to meet current and anticipated kilojoule needs.*

CONSIDERATION FOR PRACTICE
Monitor food and fluid intake and urinary output. Pain or fatigue, rather than a sensation of fullness, may prompt the decision to stop eating, resulting in inadequate intake. Additional education and support may be indicated.

- Evaluate current and preferred eating habits and foods, as well as understanding of nutrition. *This evaluation provides additional information about nutrition as well as a basis for future planning.*
- Refer to a dietitian for further evaluation, planning and education. *A professional can identify nutritional needs and help plan a diet that will meet them.*
- Encourage experimentation with foods of different textures and temperatures. *Very cold foods, or foods of a soft texture, may be easier to swallow.*

CONSIDERATION FOR PRACTICE
Weigh daily. Daily weight is an accurate measure of both fluid balance and nutritional status.

- Encourage frequent, small meals rather than three large meals per day. *Frequent, small quantities of food improve overall intake when dysphagia, odynophagia or fatigue interfere with nutrition.*
- Recommend liquid supplements, such as Ensure, when kilojoule needs are not being met. Provide information about where to obtain nutritional supplements. *Liquid dietary supplements provide balanced nutrition as well as additional kilojoules and are an effective way of increasing intake. They are available without prescription in major supermarkets.*
- Provide mouth care before meals and supplemental feedings. Provide a topical anaesthetic such as viscous lignocaine before eating for stomatitis or oesophagitis related to radiation or chemotherapy. *The tumour or its treatment may cause bad breath or a foul taste in the mouth, which suppresses appetite. Inflamed mucosa may make eating uncomfortable. A topical anaesthetic may relieve this discomfort and thus promote food intake.*
- Provide an anti-emetic 30 minutes before eating as needed to relieve nausea. *Nausea interferes with food intake. An anti-emetic can relieve nausea and make eating possible.*
- Suggest enteral (tube) feedings via nasogastric or gastrostomy tube if the person is unable to consume enough food to maintain weight and nutritional status. *Both cancer and surgery increase kilojoule needs. Supplemental enteral feedings may be necessary to prevent catabolism and to promote healing and recovery.*

CONSIDERATION FOR PRACTICE
Following laryngectomy, place in semi-Fowler's or Fowler's position. Elevating the head of the bed facilitates swallowing of oral secretions and helps prevent regurgitation of tube feedings.

- Instruct to perform mouth rinses before initiating feeding postoperatively. *Rinsing helps clean the mouth and also provides practice in using tongue and cheek muscles to control fluid in the mouth.*
- Refer to a physical or speech therapist for swallowing rehabilitation following laryngectomy. *Because surgery changes the relationship of the trachea, oesophagus and oropharynx, swallowing needs to be relearned before eating.*
- Reinforce swallowing instructions. *Reinforcement promotes learning.*

Anticipatory grieving

The person with laryngeal cancer faces not only the diagnosis of cancer, which is often perceived as a death sentence, but also the prospect of mutilating surgery. If laryngectomy is necessary, the person grieves the loss of both a body part and an important function, speech, which is a vital aspect of social interaction and often necessary for their career. It also enables people to express their needs when they cannot meet them alone. The loss of speech, therefore, is a major loss. In addition, the tracheal stoma changes the manner in which the person breathes. If radical neck dissection is required, loss of neck musculature and function also alters body image and self-concept.

- Provide opportunities for expressing feelings of grief, anger or fear about the diagnosis of cancer, the impending surgery and the anticipated loss of speech. Refer to a psychologist as required. *The person with laryngeal cancer needs the opportunity (and may need permission) to grieve anticipated losses. A cancer diagnosis may precipitate grieving for unfulfilled plans and expectations, even though a cure may be anticipated. Laryngectomy causes a major change in body image, with loss of a vital body part and creation of a stoma. The person also grieves the loss of speech. This loss can have a significant impact on occupation and social interaction.*
- Help the person and family discuss the potential impact of the loss on family structure and function. *Discussion helps family members understand each other's feelings and support one another.*
- Refer for psychological or spiritual counselling as appropriate. *Counselling and spiritual guidance can help the person and family deal with the diagnosis and proposed treatment and help prevent a sense of defeat and hopelessness.*

CONSIDERATION FOR PRACTICE
Provide a calm, empathetic and supportive environment with adequate privacy and emotional support for the person and family members as they work through the grieving process. It is important for the person and family to know that their feelings of loss are real and accepted by caregivers and that there is no timeframe placed on the grieving process as it is very individual.

TRANSLATION TO PRACTICE **Evidence-based practice: quality of life after total laryngectomy**

A study by Perry, Casey and Cotton (2015) assessing psychosocial and functional issues following a laryngectomy surveyed 86 people from New South Wales and Victoria, measuring various functional and quality-of-life indicators.

The results demonstrated significant declines in quality of life and social relationship indicators. The individuals also had higher levels of depression and anxiety than normative samples. A strong relationship was demonstrated between the psychological wellbeing scores and important functional measures of speech and swallowing.

IMPLICATIONS FOR NURSING

Psychosocial health is an important part of rehabilitation following a laryngectomy. Follow up with experienced mental health practitioners and methods to support psychosocial health should be pivotal following surgery. Nurses and other healthcare professionals such as speech pathologists need to work together to maximise speech and swallowing function to not only assist individuals with critical safety issues, but also to support and maximise a person's psychosocial wellbeing following laryngectomy and well beyond discharge.

CRITICAL THINKING IN PERSON-CENTRED CARE

1. In this study, there was a strong relationship between swallowing and speech function and the person's psychological wellbeing. As the nurse caring for a person who has had a laryngectomy, what can you do prior to discharge to assist with swallowing and speech function?
2. There were no data comparing male and female outcomes as the number of females in the cohort was too small. Would you expect there to be any difference in quality of life or psychological wellbeing scores between men and women laryngectomees? Explain.
3. How will the findings of this study impact on the care that you give to the person having a laryngectomy or partial laryngectomy?

- Help identify additional resources, such as coping strategies that have been successfully used in the past to deal with crises. *This exercise helps the person and family identify strengths they can use to deal with the present situation.*

Community-based care

Teaching for the person with a benign laryngeal tumour emphasises management of contributing factors. Stress the importance of not yelling or screaming. Refer people, particularly singers, to a speech therapist for voice training. Emphasise the need to keep the voice within its normal range to reduce vocal cord stress. Encourage smoking cessation, particularly if the person is also a singer. Discuss the relationship of industrial pollutants to laryngeal tumours and help explore ways of reducing pollutant exposure.

Teaching the person and family about laryngeal cancer, treatment options and home care related to those treatments is an important nursing responsibility. Include the following topics when teaching:

- Clarification of treatment options, including risks and benefits.
- Importance of early intervention to reduce the risk of local spread and metastases.
- If a total laryngectomy is proposed, options for communication after surgery, including the pros and cons of each:
  a. The tracheoesophageal puncture device requires some manual dexterity to manipulate.
  b. Only about 30% of people are able to master oesophageal speech.
  c. A trial of the speech generator prior to surgery may reduce frustration in learning to use it postoperatively.
- Care related to radiation therapy, including skin and mouth care, management of secretions (see the chapter 'Nursing care of people with cancer' for more information about radiation therapy and its effects).
- Strategies and resources for smoking cessation and alcohol abstinence.
- Ways to achieve and maintain optimal nutrition.
- Tracheostomy stoma care and preventing respiratory infection. Provide opportunities to practise and re-demonstrate techniques. Clean technique (rather than sterile) is used; the tracheostomy tube may not be needed once the stoma is fully healed. Discuss these additional measures:
  a. Using a humidifier or vaporiser to add humidity to inspired air.
  b. Increasing fluid intake to maintain mucosal moisture and loosen secretions.
  c. Shielding the stoma with a stoma guard, such as a gauze square on a tie around the neck, to prevent particulate matter from entering the lower respiratory tract.
  d. Promptly removing secretions from skin surrounding the stoma to prevent irritation and skin breakdown.
  e. Water sports are contraindicated with a permanent tracheostomy; there is no restriction on other activities, although lifting may be more difficult because of inability to hold the breath (the Valsalva manoeuvre).
  f. Showering and bathing (without submerging the neck or head) are allowed; protect the stoma with a cupped hand or washcloth.
- Manifestations of potential complications of laryngectomy to be reported to the doctor, including loss of hearing or facial expression due to auditory or facial nerve injury or shoulder drop due to damage to the spinal accessory nerve.

The person and family need emotional and motivational support through this trying time. Refer to local support groups. If the person and family are having difficulty adjusting to the diagnosis of cancer and the effects of treatment, provide referral to counselling.

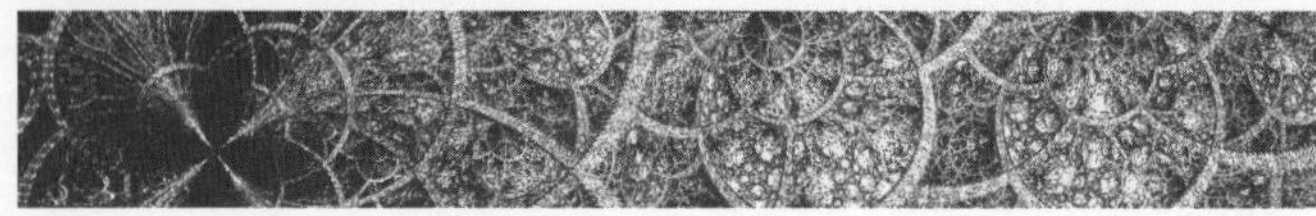

CHAPTER HIGHLIGHTS

- Upper respiratory infections (the common cold) are caused by a multitude of different viruses. Most are mild, self-limiting infections, appropriate for self-care; some viruses, however, such as RSV, can cause serious lower respiratory illness in the very young or very old.
- COVID-19 is a novel coronavirus that it is a new virus not previously seen in humans.
- Three different strains of influenza virus are identified; type A causes most outbreaks of influenza. Because this disease increases the risk of pneumonia in older adults, people with chronic diseases and people who are immunocompromised, annual immunisation is important for these populations and their caregivers.
- Influenza is differentiated from URTI primarily by the presence of systemic manifestations, the duration and degree of fever, and the presence of persistent cough.
- Pharyngitis (sore throat) may be either viral or bacterial in origin; manifestations are similar. People with persistent or severe symptoms that include fever, enlarged lymph nodes and myalgias should be evaluated to rule out streptococcal pharyngitis, which can have significant complications such as rheumatic fever or post-streptococcal glomerulonephritis.
- The incidence of pertussis, a highly contagious reportable disease, is increasing due to waning immunity and improved identification of the infection in adults. In adults, it is often recognised by prolonged and persistent coughing spells. Pertussis is treated in community settings with antibiotic therapy.
- Epistaxis (nosebleed) and nasal fracture are relatively common and pose a risk only when airway clearance is impaired. Emergency care for epistaxis includes pinching the nares or bridge of the nose, sitting upright and leaning forward and applying ice to the nose. When nasal packing is required to control bleeding, close monitoring of respiratory status (respiratory rate and effort, oxygen saturation) is critical.
- Persistent voice hoarseness is the primary manifestation of laryngeal cancer. When identified and treated early, the rate of cure for laryngeal cancer is high. Some laryngeal tumours, however, have few manifestations until advanced. They may be treated by radiation therapy, chemotherapy or surgery (laryngectomy and neck dissection).
- Following total laryngectomy, a permanent tracheostomy is created and the upper trachea and oesophagus are separated, preventing aspiration when feedings are resumed. A tracheoesophageal puncture may be created to allow verbal communication following total laryngectomy.

CONCEPT CHECK

1 A person with hypertension asks the nurse what he can do to relieve the symptoms of an acute URTI. The nurse recommends that he:
1 ask his doctor for an antibiotic prescription
2 use an over-the-counter decongestant such as pseudoephedrine to relieve symptoms
3 take 1,000 mg of vitamin C and zinc tablets on a regular basis
4 use an over-the-counter nasal spray for no more than 3 days to relieve congestion

2 Which of the following health promotion activities planned by a nurse working with a group of community-dwelling senior citizens would be most likely to prevent influenza and pneumonia?
1 Indoor exercise programs during winter months.
2 Influenza vaccine clinics at the senior centre.
3 Teaching effective handwashing.
4 Advising seniors to avoid crowds.

3 In teaching a person with bacterial sinusitis about home care, the nurse stresses the importance of:
1 completing the antibiotic prescription as ordered
2 sleeping with the head of the bed elevated to 45 degrees
3 using a humidifier to promote sinus drainage
4 maintaining a liberal fluid intake to help liquefy secretions

4 Which of the following nursing interventions for the person with posterior nasal packing is of highest priority?
1 Elevate the head of the bed.
2 Apply cold compresses to the nose.
3 Maintain oxygen therapy.
4 Provide frequent oral hygiene.

5 A person in the emergency department following facial trauma complains that his nose 'just keeps dripping'. The drainage appears like watery blood. The most appropriate nursing action would be to:
1 provide a box of tissues
2 reassure the person that this is expected with a nasal fracture
3 suction the nasopharynx
4 obtain a specimen for glucose testing

6 Expected findings in a person with obstructive sleep apnoea would include (select all that apply):
1 confusion and signs of dementia
2 enlarged tongue
3 complaints of daytime sleepiness
4 decreased oxygen saturation levels while awake
5 elevated blood pressure
6 complaints of morning headache

7 The nurse in a doctor's office notes that a person's voice is hoarse, a change from previous visits. The most appropriate question to ask the person would be:
1 'How long has your voice been hoarse?'
2 'Do you smoke?'
3 'Do you have a sore throat?'
4 'Would you like a prescription for throat lozenges?'

8 The nurse evaluates his teaching as effective when a person with stage I laryngeal cancer states:
1 'I'm glad I don't have to worry about treating this cancer now because it is so early.'
2 'I hate to think about eventually losing the ability to speak, but I'd rather treat it aggressively than lose my life to cancer.'
3 'I'm glad this was diagnosed early, when it can be treated with radiation, so I won't lose my voice.'
4 'Thank goodness this type of cancer usually doesn't spread anywhere else.'

9 **Place the following nursing interventions for a person who has undergone total laryngectomy and radical neck dissection in order of priority.**

1 Arrange consultation with speech therapist.
2 Provide small, frequent meals.
3 Encourage to express feelings regarding loss of voice.
4 Suction via tracheostomy as needed.
5 Instruct to support head when moving.

10 **When providing tracheostomy care, the nurse:**

1 cuts the dressing using sterile scissors
2 secures clean ties before removing soiled ones
3 uses clean technique to cleanse the outer cannula
4 cleanses the incision with an iodine-based antiseptic

BIBLIOGRAPHY

Australian Institute of Health and Welfare (2021). *Australian cancer incidence and mortality (ACIM) books: Laryngeal cancer*. Canberra: AIHW.

Branche, A. R., Saiman, L., Walsh, E. E. et al. (2022). Incidence of respiratory syncytial virus infection among hospitalized adults, 2017–2020. *Clinical Infectious Diseases*, *74*(6), 1004–1011.

Bullock, S. & Hales, M. (2019). *Principles of pathophysiology* (2nd ed.). Sydney: Pearson.

Cancer Council Australia (2022). *Throat cancer*. Retrieved from https://www.cancer.org.au

Dai, X., Gil, G. F., Reitsma, M. B. et al. (2022). Health effects associated with smoking: A burden of proof study. *Nature Medicine*, *28*, 2045–2055. https://doi.org/10.1038/s41591-022-01978-x

Dekker, M., Jongerden, I., de Bruijne, M., Jelsma, J., Vandenbroucke-Grauls, C. & van Mansfeld, R. (2022). Strategies to improve the implementation of infection control link nurse programmes in acute-care hospitals. *Journal of Hospital Infection*, *128*, 54–63. https://doi.org/10.1016/j.jhin.2022.07.005

Department of Health and Aged Care (2022a). *Australian influenza surveillance report*. Retrieved from https://www.health.gov.au/

Department of Health and Aged Care (2022b). *The Australian immunisation handbook*. Retrieved from https://www.health.gov.au/

Guiso, N. (2021). What is whooping cough and how can we protect ourselves? *Frontiers*. Retrieved from https://kids.frontiersin.org/

Heiman, A. J., Nair, L., Kanth, A., Baltodano, P., Patel, A. & Ricci, J. A. (2022). Defining regional variation in nasal anatomy to guide ethnic rhinoplasty: A systematic review. *Journal of Plastic, Reconstructive & Aesthetic Surgery*, *75*(8), 2784–2795. doi: 10.1016/j.bjps.2022.04.058

Holford, P., Carr, A. C., Jovic, T. H. et al. (2020). Vitamin C—An adjunctive therapy for respiratory infection, sepsis and COVID-19. *Nutrients*, *12*(20), 3760. doi: 10.3390/nu12123760

Karron, R. A. (2021). Preventing respiratory syncytial virus (RSV) in children. *Science*, *372*(6543), 686–687.

Koroulakis, A. & Agarwal, M. (2022). *Laryngeal cancer*. StatPearls. Treasure Island (FL): StatPearls Publishing. Retrieved from https://www.ncbi.nlm.nih.gov/

Mohammed, H., McMillan, M., Andraweera, P. H., Elliott, S. R. & Marshall, H. S. (2021). A rapid global review of strategies to improve influenza vaccination uptake in Australia. *Human Vaccines & Immunotherapeutics*, *17*(12), 5487–5499.

Nguyen, T. Q., Rollon, R. & Choi, Y. K. (2021). Animal models for influenza research: Strengths and weaknesses. *Viruses*, *13*(6), 1011. doi: 10.3390/v13061011

Ortega, H., Nickle, D. & Carter, L. (2021). Rhinovirus and asthma: Challenges and opportunities. *Reviews in Medical Virology*, *31*(4), e2193. doi: 10.1002/rmv.2193

Perry, A., Casey, E. & Cotton, S. (2015). Quality of life after total laryngectomy: Functioning, psychological well-being and self-efficacy. *International Journal of Language and Communication Disorders*, *50*(4), 467–475.

Riha, R. L. (2021). Defining obstructive sleep apnoea syndrome: A failure of semantic rules. *Breathe*, *17*(3). doi: 10.1183/20734735.0082-2021

Rouf, R., Uddin, S.J., Sarker, D. K. et al. (2020). Antiviral potential of garlic (allium sativum) and its organosulfur compounds: A systematic update of pre-clinical and clinical data. *Trends in Food Science and Technology*, *104*, 219–234. doi: 10.1016/j.tifs.2020.08.006

Seale, H., McFadden, K., Dyda, A., Kaufman, J. & Heywood, A. (2021). The pendulum has swung: How do we ensure a life course approach to immunisation in Australia? *Frontiers in Public Health*, *94*(9). doi: 10.3389/fpubh.2021.801176

Uyeki, T. M. (2020). High-risk groups for influenza complications. *JAMA*, *324*(22), 2334.

Wang, D. Y., Eccles, R., Bell, J. et al. (2021). Management of acute upper respiratory tract infection: The role of early intervention. *Expert Review of Respiratory Medicine*, *15*(12), 1517–1523. doi: 10.1080/17476348.2021.1988569

Wang, W., Huangfu, H., Hou, Y., Feng, Y., Zhang, C., Zhai, S. & Li, M. (2022). Study on the indication of concurrent chemoradiotherapy for locally advanced laryngeal carcinoma. *Lin Chuang er bi yan hou tou Jing wai ke za zhi = Journal of Clinical Otorhinolaryngology, Head, and Neck Surgery*, *36*(9), 721–725.

Wilkinson, K., Righolt, C. H., Elliott, L. J., Fanella, S. & Mahmud, S. M. (2021). Pertussis vaccine effectiveness and duration of protection—A systematic review and meta-analysis. *Vaccine*, *39*(23), 3120–3130.

Wipperman, J., Ofei-Dodoo, S. & Nilsen, K. (2022). Are antibiotics effective in treating children with chronic productive cough? *Evidence-Based Practice*, *25*(4), 32–33.

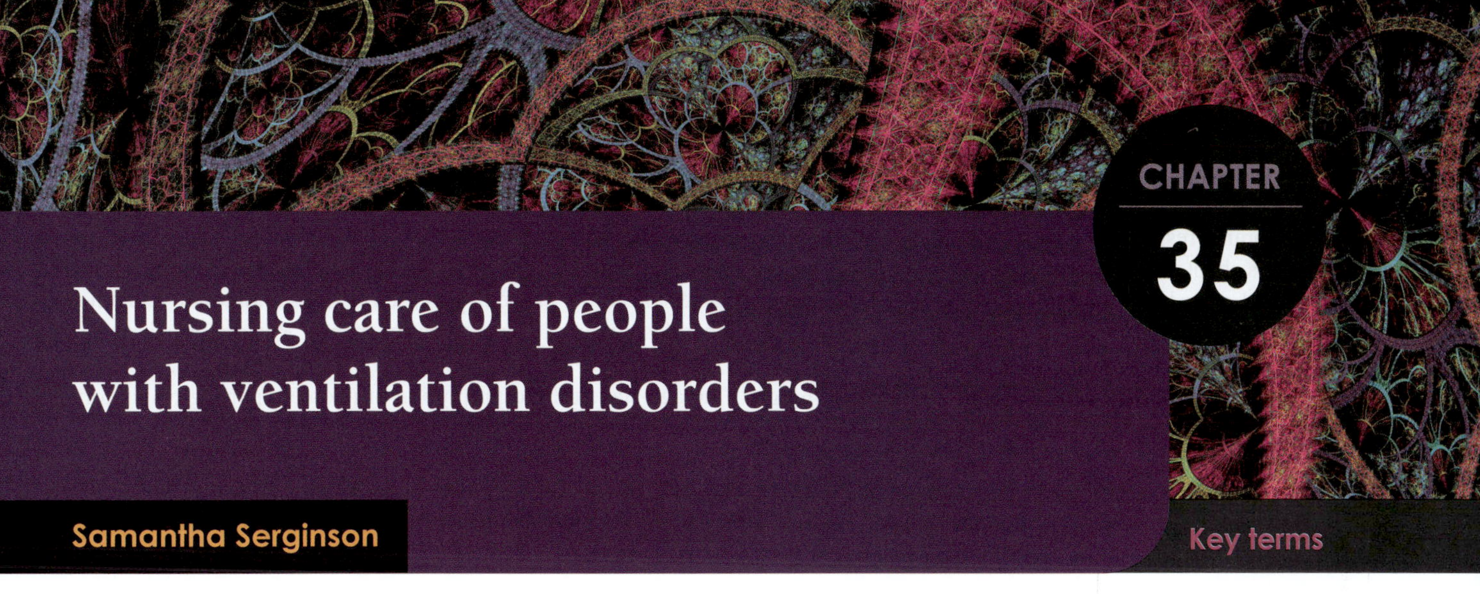

CHAPTER 35

Nursing care of people with ventilation disorders

Samantha Serginson

Key terms

Learning outcomes

- Relate the pathophysiology of lower respiratory tract infections and inflammatory disorders to a person's alteration in oxygenation.
- Discuss the development, consequences and management of a person experiencing selected pleural disorders.
- Explore the pathophysiology, clinical considerations and care of an individual experiencing a thoracic or inhalation injury.
- Review the causes and consequences of lung cancer and responsibilities of caring for individuals requiring surgery or other invasive procedures.

Clinical competencies

- Assess the lower respiratory tract and chest wall disorders on ventilation and gas exchange.
- Use assessment data and knowledge of the effects of lower respiratory tract disorders to identify priority nursing care.
- Use the nursing process and evidence-based nursing research to plan and implement individualised nursing care.
- Develop measures to promote ventilation and gas exchange.
- Plan and provide appropriate teaching for health promotion in vulnerable populations.
- Evaluate the effectiveness of nursing interventions and teaching, revising strategies and teaching plans as needed.
- Coordinate interprofessional care and administer prescribed medications and treatments for people with lower respiratory tract disorders.

Disorders affecting the lower respiratory tract (below the larynx), pleural cavity and chest wall can affect the ability to effectively move air into and out of the lungs (ventilation). The exchange of oxygen and carbon dioxide across the alveolar–capillary membrane (respiration) is also affected. The disorders discussed in this chapter—respiratory infections and inflammation, trauma and disorders of the chest wall or pleural cavity, and neoplasms of the lung—all affect the ability to maintain clear and patent airways and ventilate the lungs. Nursing care for individuals with these disorders focuses on maintaining airway patency, expectoration of sputum and an effective breathing pattern. Disorders that primarily affect gas exchange are discussed in the chapter 'Nursing care of people with gas exchange disorders'.

The lower respiratory tract and chest wall disorders discussed here and in the chapter 'Nursing care of people with gas exchange disorders' both have local and systemic effects. Local effects include cough, excess mucus production, **dyspnoea** (shortness of breath), **haemoptysis** (bloody sputum) and chest pain. Systemic effects may include fever, anorexia and malaise, **cyanosis** (grey/blue skin colour caused by oxygen-poor haemoglobin) and other manifestations of impaired gas exchange. Respiratory disease is very common in both adults and children. Figure 35.1 shows the age-standardised proportion of people reporting respiratory disease for Indigenous and non-Indigenous Australians.

Before continuing, review the anatomy, physiology and assessment of the lower respiratory tract in the chapter 'A person-centred approach to assessing the respiratory system'.

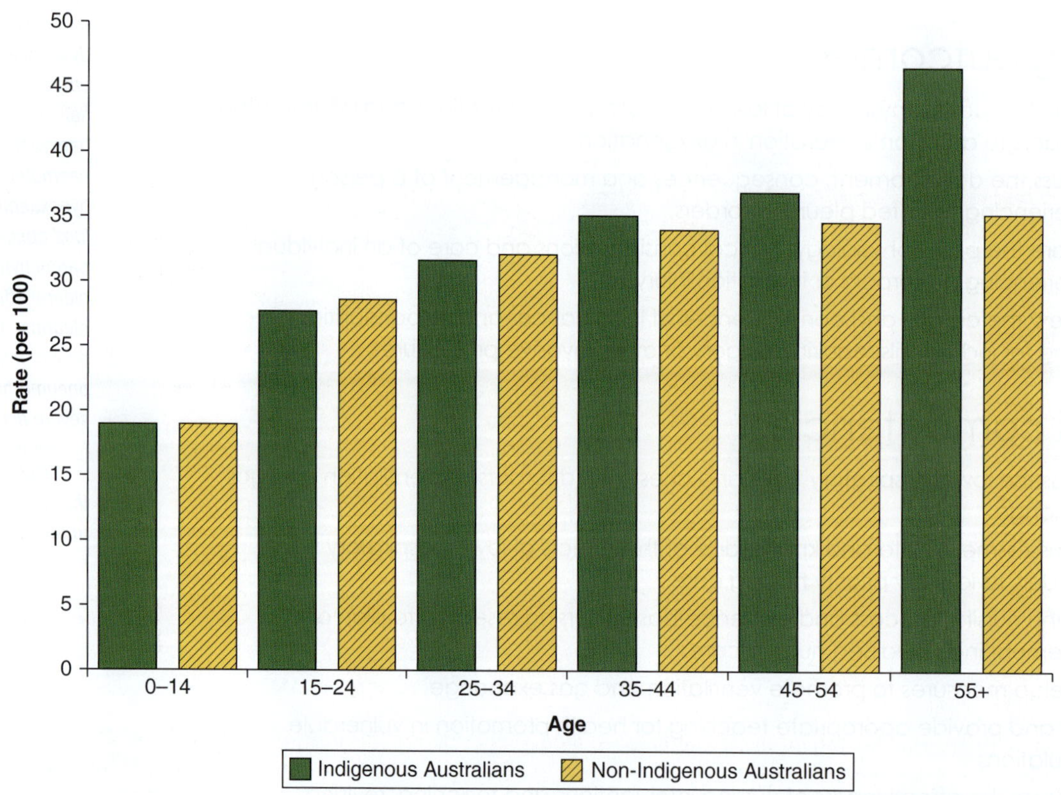

FIGURE 35.1 ***Age-standardised proportion reporting respiratory disease for Indigenous and non-Indigenous Australians (2018–2019)***

Source: Generated using data from Australian Institute of Health and Welfare (AIHW). (2020). *Aboriginal and Torres Strait Islander Health Performance Framework summary report. National Aboriginal and Torres Strait Islander Health Survey 2018–19.* Retrieved from https://indigenoushpf.gov.au/measures/1-04-respiratory-disease/data#DataVisualisation. Licensed under a Creative Commons Attribution 4.0 International licence, https://creativecommons.org/licenses/by/4.0/.

Infections and inflammatory disorders

Infection and inflammation of the lower respiratory tract are common varying in type and severity. The respiratory tree is constantly exposed to the environment as air moves into and out of the lower respiratory tract. In addition, the oropharynx is colonised by large numbers of microorganisms that may be aspirated into the bronchial tree. Both anatomical and physiological defences help maintain the sterility of the lower respiratory tract. When these defences are impaired, the risk of infection increases. Drugs, alcohol or neuromuscular disease may suppress the cough reflex and infections such as the influenza virus can leave the respiratory epithelium vulnerable to bacterial infection. Even in healthy people, microorganisms and other foreign material occasionally enter the bronchial tree and lung parenchyma, bypassing the body's natural defences.

THE PERSON WITH ACUTE BRONCHITIS

Bronchitis, inflammation of the bronchi, may be either an acute or a chronic condition. Acute bronchitis is relatively common in adults. Impaired immune defences, exposure to environmental irritants and cigarette smoking increase the risk of acute bronchitis (Singh, Avula & Zahn, 2022). In otherwise healthy adults, it typically follows a viral upper respiratory tract infection (URTI) as a post-viral infection. Chronic bronchitis is a component of chronic obstructive pulmonary disease (COPD) and is discussed in the chapter 'Nursing care of people with gas exchange disorders'.

FAST FACTS

Chronic obstructive pulmonary disease (COPD) is sometimes referred to by other names:

- COAD—chronic obstructive airways disease
- COLD—chronic obstructive lung disease
- CORD—chronic obstructive respiratory disease
- CAL—chronic airways limitation

The accepted terminology in Australia is COPD: chronic obstructive pulmonary disease.

Pathophysiology and manifestations

Infectious bronchitis can be caused by any pathogen. However, it is most commonly caused by bacteria and viruses that damage the respiratory mucosa. In healthy adults, bacterial bronchitis generally only occurs as a complication of viral infection. Inhalation of toxic gases or chemicals can lead to inflammatory bronchitis (Bullock & Hales, 2019).

The inflammatory response to infection or tissue damage from inhaled substances causes capillary dilation and oedema of the mucosal lining of the bronchi. Inflammatory cells infiltrate the affected mucosa, leading to exudate formation and increased mucus production. Ciliated epithelium is damaged by the inflammatory response and ciliary function is impaired (Papadakis, McPhee & Rabow, 2022), causing build-up of excessive mucus in the airways. The immune response of lymphocytes and tissue macrophages is inhibited by some viruses and mycobacteria, increasing the risk of bacterial infection. Mucosal irritation and increased mucus production initiate the cough reflex. The respiratory tract may become hyperirritable for an extended period of time, leading to paroxysms of coughing and bronchospasm (Bullock & Hales, 2019).

Acute bronchitis is typically characterised by a non-productive cough that becomes productive. The cough often occurs in paroxysms and may be aggravated by cold, dry or dusty air. Pleuritic pain (chest pain related to lung issues), often substernal, is common. Other manifestations include moderate fever and general malaise (Bullock & Hales, 2019).

INTERPROFESSIONAL CARE

The diagnosis of acute bronchitis typically is based on the history, clinical presentation and, when indicated, clinical investigations. A chest x-ray may be ordered to exclude pneumonia because the presenting manifestations can be similar. Other diagnostic testing is rarely indicated. Management focuses on symptom relief and includes rest, increased fluid intake and the use of paracetamol to relieve discomfort, fever and malaise. Bronchodilators may also be beneficial in some circumstances. While antibiotics have been used excessively, it has been found that both antibiotics and corticosteroids are of limited value in the management of an individual with bronchitis as 85–95% of viruses are responsible for causing acute bronchitis in healthy adults. Common viruses include rhinovirus, adenovirus, influenza A and B; however, bacteria are known to cause bronchitis in people with underlying health problems (Dalziel et al., 2022; Glasziou et al., 2022). Other medications may include a codeine-based preparation to ease the coughing paroxysms. However, care must be taken when using medication to suppress the cough reflex, as the infection will have affected the mucociliary escalator and therefore the cough will be the last line of defence in expelling mucus.

In 2020–2021, around 7.5 million (30%) Australians reported having chronic respiratory conditions, of which 5.1 million (20%) had allergic rhinitis, 2.7 million (11%) had asthma and 2.0 million (80%) had chronic sinusitis. It should be noted that this data was drawn during the COVID-19 pandemic and therefore cannot be compared with data from previous years (AIHW, 2022a).

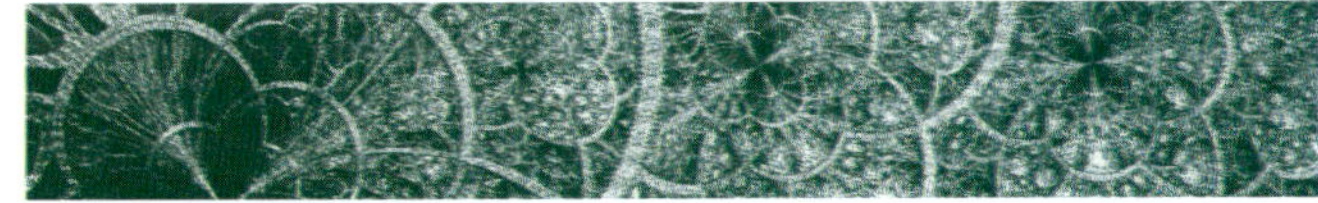

Nursing care

Nursing interventions for people with acute bronchitis are primarily education and should include these teaching topics:

- Increase fluid intake to keep mucus thin and meet increased fluid loss related to fever. Caution should be noted if the person has other comorbidities where fluid balance is measured daily.
- Use over-the-counter (OTC) analgesics and cough preparations containing pseudoephedrine for symptom relief with caution.
- Be aware of the ingredients of each of the preparations so as not to overdose on a drug that may be in several of the combination medications taken such as paracetamol.
- Stress the importance of smoking cessation (as appropriate).

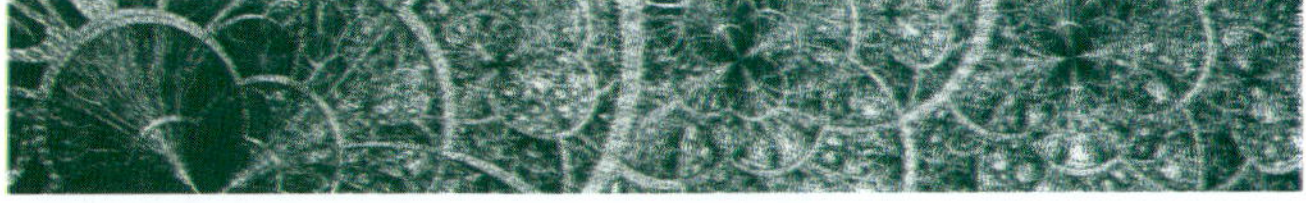

TABLE 35.1 Common organisms causing pneumonia in adults

HOSPITAL ACQUIRED	HEALTHCARE ASSOCIATED	COMMUNITY ACQUIRED	OPPORTUNISTIC
Staphylococcus aureus	*Streptococcus pneumoniae*	*Streptococcus pneumoniae*	*Pneumocystis jiroveci*
Pseudomonas aeruginosa	*Staphylococcus aureus*	*Mycoplasma pneumoniae*	*Mycobacterium tuberculosis*
Klebsiella pneumoniae	*Haemophilus influenzae*	*Haemophilus influenzae*	Cytomegalovirus (CMV)
Legionella spp.	Influenza virus	*Chlamydia pneumoniae*	Atypical mycobacteria
Escherichia coli	*Enterobacter* spp.	*Legionella* spp.	Fungi
		Influenza virus	

THE PERSON WITH PNEUMONIA

Inflammation of the lung **parenchyma** (the respiratory bronchioles and alveoli) is known as **pneumonia**.

Pneumonia may be either infectious or non-infectious. Bacteria, viruses, fungi, protozoa and other microbes can lead to infectious pneumonia. Non-infectious causes include aspiration of gastric contents and inhalation of toxic or irritating gases. Pneumonias are often classified as community acquired, healthcare associated (ventilator associated), nosocomial (hospital acquired) or opportunistic (person is immunosuppressed). Currently, as no universal nomenclature for the classification of pneumonia exists, there is some disparity in the use of these terms. Some authors use the terms 'nosocomial' and 'healthcare associated' interchangeably. Some authors consider exposure to a pathogen from an aged care facility, dialysis unit, long-term ventilation support or outpatient clinic as a type of community-acquired pathogen. However, within this textbook these are considered healthcare associated. They often differ from both hospital-acquired and community-acquired pneumonia, not only in transmission but also in causative pathogens.

Different organisms are implicated in each of these classifications (see Table 35.1). The most common causative organisms for community-acquired pneumonia are the respiratory viruses *Streptococcus pneumoniae* (also called pneumococcus) and *Mycoplasma pneumonia. Haemophilus influenza*, *Legionella* species and *Chlamydia* species are also common community-acquired pneumonia pathogens (AIHW, 2022a). *Staphylococcus aureus* and Gram-negative bacteria such as *Pseudomonas aeruginosa*, *Klebsiella pneumoniae* and enteric bacilli, including *Escherichia coli*, are often implicated as nosocomial causes of pneumonia. Organisms such as *Pneumocystis jiroveci* generally cause infections more often in immunocompromised people (opportunistic infections).

Physiology review

In health, the lower respiratory tract is sterile. Several defence mechanisms help maintain this sterile environment. Infectious particles trapped by the mucous membranes of the nose are removed by sneezing, while those deposited in the nasopharynx usually are swallowed or expectorated. Reflex closure of the epiglottis and the branching bronchial tree present anatomical barriers to entry of microorganisms and other possible contaminants. The cilia and mucus that line the respiratory tract and the cough reflex serve to trap and eliminate foreign matter that enters the lower respiratory tract. Organisms that make it past these barriers are usually rapidly phagocytised in the alveolus by resident macrophages, then attacked by the inflammatory and immune defences of the body. Ageing impairs these immune responses, increasing the risk of pneumonia in the older population.

Pathophysiology

The most common portal of entry for pathogens into the lung is aspiration of oropharyngeal secretions containing microbes. Microorganisms also may be inhaled after having been released when an infected person coughs, sneezes or talks. Finally, bacteria may spread to the lungs through the bloodstream from infection elsewhere in the body. Host defences must be overwhelmed either by the number of organisms or their *virulence* (disease-causing ability) in order for an infection to develop.

FOCUS ON CULTURAL DIVERSITY

- Aboriginal and Torres Strait Islander children are five times more likely than non-Indigenous Australians to die from pneumonia. However, mortality rates in these children have been declining over recent decades and mortality is now rare. This is likely attributed to improved and early diagnosis and management (O'Grady et al., 2018).
- In Victoria, a group evaluating the primary health needs of the local refugee population within its area determined that, although the local refugees were 23% more likely to present to an emergency department and 47% more likely to be admitted for healthcare issues than non-refugee locals, the refugees were no more likely than non-refugees within the area to require admission for pneumonia or influenza (Cheng et al., 2011).

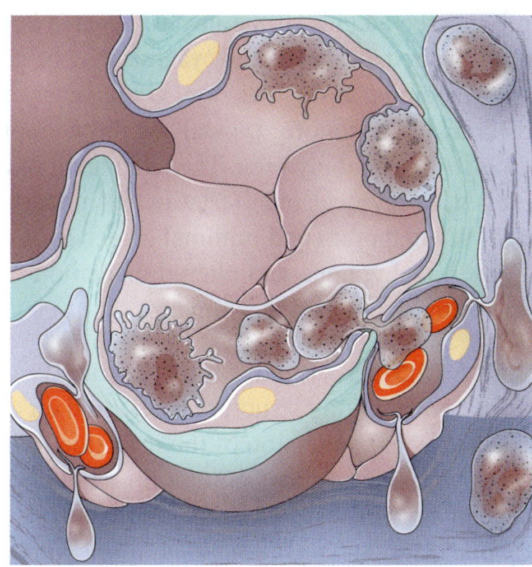

FIGURE 35.2 ***In pneumonia, the inflammatory response causes fluid to accumulate in the alveoli and oedema to form as alveolar capillaries dilate and allow fluid to leak into interstitial tissues***

When the invading microorganisms colonise the alveoli, an inflammatory and immune response is initiated. The body's antigen–antibody response and endotoxins released by some organisms damage bronchial and alveolar mucous membranes, causing inflammation with vascular congestion and oedema. Infectious debris and exudate can fill alveoli, interfering with ventilation and gas exchange (see Figure 35.2). Pneumonia may develop in four distinct patterns: lobar pneumonia, bronchopneumonia, interstitial pneumonia and miliary pneumonia (see Table 35.2). The pathological process, anatomical location and manifestations of pneumonias vary according to the infective organism.

Lifespan considerations

When compared with an adult, the anatomical development and physiological maturation of an infant's respiratory tract increases the child's risk of developing respiratory tract infections. At birth, only 10% of alveoli are present, resulting in a greater surface area to volume ratio. Alveolar multiplication occurs until approximately 8 years of age. Airway lumens in children are smaller and chest wall recoil and underdeveloped respiratory musculature can result in fatigue sooner than in an adult. The breathing zone of a child is lower and therefore heavier particles can travel deeper into the respiratory system.

However, in advancing age, several changes associated with ageing and disease also affect respiratory function and airway clearance. The number of cilia decreases and the cough weakens. Gag and cough reflexes diminish. The older adult is at greater risk of dehydration, leading to thick, viscous mucus that is difficult to expectorate. Immune function declines with ageing. These factors increase the risk of pulmonary infection and reduce the older adult's ability to respond effectively to infectious processes (Bullock & Hales, 2019). Other factors also may increase the risk for and severity of lower respiratory tract infections in the older adult: immobility, smoking history, surgical procedures, use of multiple medications, malnutrition and such diseases as COPD and heart disease.

Acute bacterial pneumonia

Of the bacterial pneumonias, the pathogenesis of pneumococcal (*Streptococcus pneumoniae* pneumonia is best understood (see Figure 35.3). These bacteria reside in the upper respiratory tract of up to 70% of adults. They may be spread by droplet contamination—inhalation of infectious particles in the environment. In many cases, infection results from aspiration of resident bacteria. In the lower respiratory tract, the inflammatory response initiated by these organisms causes alveolar oedema and the formation of exudate. As alveoli and respiratory bronchioles fill with serous exudate, blood cells, fibrin and bacteria, *consolidation* (swelling) of lung tissue occurs. The lower lobes of the lungs are usually affected because of gravity. Consolidation of a large portion of an entire lung lobe is known as *lobar pneumonia*. This is the typical pattern for pneumococcal pneumonia. *Bronchopneumonia* is patchy consolidation involving several lobules. Other bacterial pneumonias often present with the patchy involvement of bronchopneumonia; pneumococcal pneumonia may also follow this pattern

TABLE 35.2 Patterns of lung involvement in pneumonia

PATTERN OF INVOLVEMENT	DESCRIPTION
Lobar pneumonia	Typically involves an entire lobe of a lung. Early in the process, when the immune response is minimal, bacteria spread throughout the affected lobe by rapid accumulation of fluid exudate. As the immune and inflammatory responses develop, RBCs and neutrophils, damaged epithelial cells and fibrin accumulate in the alveoli. Purulent exudate containing neutrophils and macrophages forms. As alveoli and respiratory bronchioles fill with exudate, blood cells, fibrin and bacteria, *consolidation* (solidification) of lung tissue occurs. Finally, the process resolves as enzymes destroy the exudate and residual debris is reabsorbed, phagocytised or coughed out.
Bronchopneumonia	Usually involves dependent portions of lung tissue, characterised by patchy consolidation. Exudate tends to remain primarily in the bronchi and bronchioles, with less oedema and congestion of the alveoli than in lobar pneumonia.
Interstitial pneumonia	The inflammatory process primarily involves the interstitium: the alveolar walls and connective tissue supporting the bronchial tree. Involvement may be patchy or diffuse as lymphocytes, macrophages and plasma cells infiltrate the alveolar septa. While alveoli typically do not contain significant exudates, protein-rich hyaline membranes may line the alveoli, interfering with gas exchange.
Miliary pneumonia	In miliary pneumonia, numerous discrete inflammatory lesions develop as a result of spread of the pathogen to the lungs via the bloodstream. Miliary pneumonia is primarily seen in people who are severely immunocompromised. As a result, the immune response is poor and damage to pleural tissue may be significant.

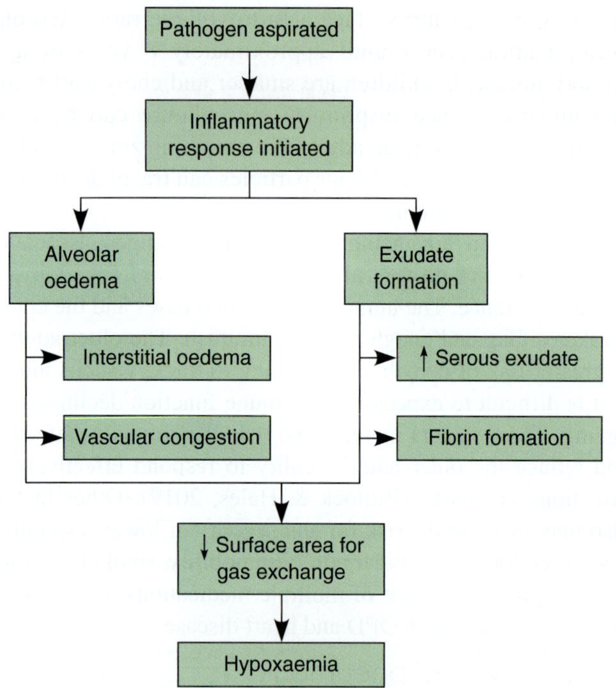

FIGURE 35.3 *The pathogenesis of pneumonia*

(see Figure 35.4). The process resolves when macrophages predominate, digesting and removing inflammatory exudate from the infected lung.

MANIFESTATIONS The presentation of bacterial pneumonia is usually acute, with rapid onset of chills, fever and cough productive of rust-coloured or purulent sputum. Chest aching or *pleuritic pain* (sharp, localised chest pain that increases with breathing and coughing) is common. Limited breath sounds and fine crackles are heard over the affected area of the lung. A pleural friction rub may be audible. If the involved area is large and gas exchange is impaired, dyspnoea and cyanosis may be noted.

A more insidious onset with low-grade fever, cough and scattered crackles is more typical of bronchopneumonia. Dyspnoea is less commonly seen. The older adult or debilitated person may have atypical manifestations of pneumonia, with little cough, scant sputum and minimal evidence of respiratory distress. Fever, tachypnoea and altered mentation or agitation may be the primary presenting symptoms.

COMPLICATIONS Pneumonia typically resolves uneventfully; normal lung structure is restored on completion of the process. Local extension of the infection to involve the pleura (*pleuritis*) is the most common complication. Pneumonia caused by *Staphylococcus aureus*, such as hospital-acquired pneumonia, and some Gram-negative bacteria often cause extensive parenchymal damage with necrosis, lung abscess and empyema or pleural effusion. Progressive destruction of lung tissue and functional impairment is a possible consequence of *Klebsiella* pneumonia.

A *lung abscess* is a local area of necrosis and pus formation within the lung itself. It is relatively uncommon. The manifestations of lung abscess develop slowly and include weight loss, malaise, night sweats, fever and a productive cough. Sputum is foul-smelling and tasting. Rupture of the abscess into a larger airway is evidenced by production of copious amounts of purulent sputum.

Empyema is accumulation of purulent exudate in the pleural cavity. It is identified by chest x-ray or computed tomography (CT) scan. Thoracentesis may be performed or a chest tube inserted to remove purulent exudates. (Nursing care of the person undergoing thoracentesis or with a chest tube is discussed later in this chapter.)

Bacteraemia can spread the infection to other tissues, leading to meningitis, endocarditis or peritonitis, and increasing the risk of mortality.

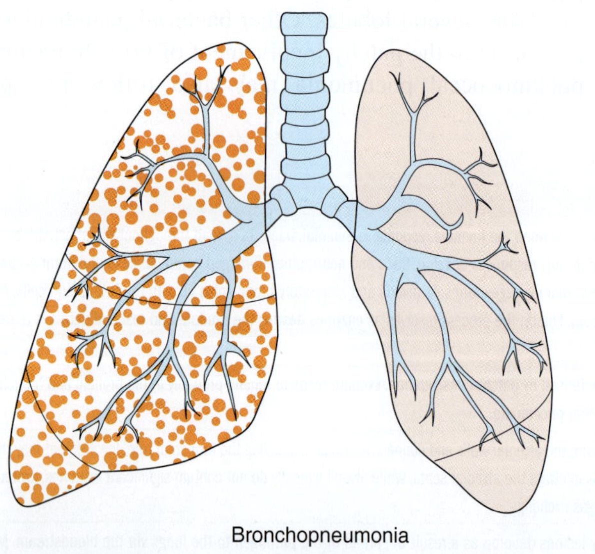

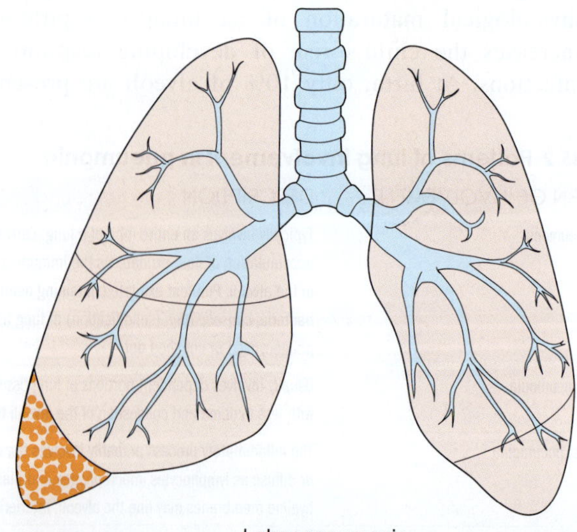

FIGURE 35.4 *Comparison of bronchopneumonia and lobar pneumonia*

Legionnaires' disease

Legionnaires' disease (legionellosis) is a form of atypical bronchopneumonia caused by *Legionella* bacteria. Although there are over 40 strains, not all cause disease in humans. The most common strain is *Legionella pneumophila*. This Gram-negative bacterium is found in warm water or warm damp places. Legionnaires' disease occurs sporadically and in outbreaks, such as that which occurred at an American Legion convention in 1976, when the disease was first recognised. Contaminated water-cooled air-conditioning systems and other water sources have been implicated in its spread (Department of Health and Aged Care, 2022a). See Figure 35.5 for Australian legionellosis statistics.

Smokers, older adults and people with chronic diseases or impaired immune defences are most susceptible to Legionnaires' disease. Symptoms develop gradually, beginning 2 to 10 days after exposure. Dry cough, dyspnoea, general malaise, chills and fever, headache, confusion, anorexia and diarrhoea, myalgias and arthralgias are common manifestations. Consolidation of lung tissue is patchy or lobar.

Viral pneumonia

Viral pneumonia is more common in children (Mosenifar, 2018). However, it is relatively common to have secondary bacterial pneumonia as a direct result of a primary viral infection. Other viruses such as herpes viruses and measles virus also may cause viral pneumonia. As in primary atypical pneumonia, lung involvement in viral pneumonia is limited to the alveolar septum and interstitial spaces.

Viral pneumonia is typically a mild disease that often affects older adults and people with chronic conditions. It usually occurs in community epidemics. Flu-like symptoms of headache, fever, fatigue, malaise and muscle aching are common, along with a dry cough.

See Box 35.1 for examples of emerging zoonotic viral pneumonias.

Aspiration pneumonia

Aspiration of gastric contents into the lungs results in a chemical and bacterial pneumonia known as *aspiration pneumonia*. Major risk factors for aspiration pneumonia include

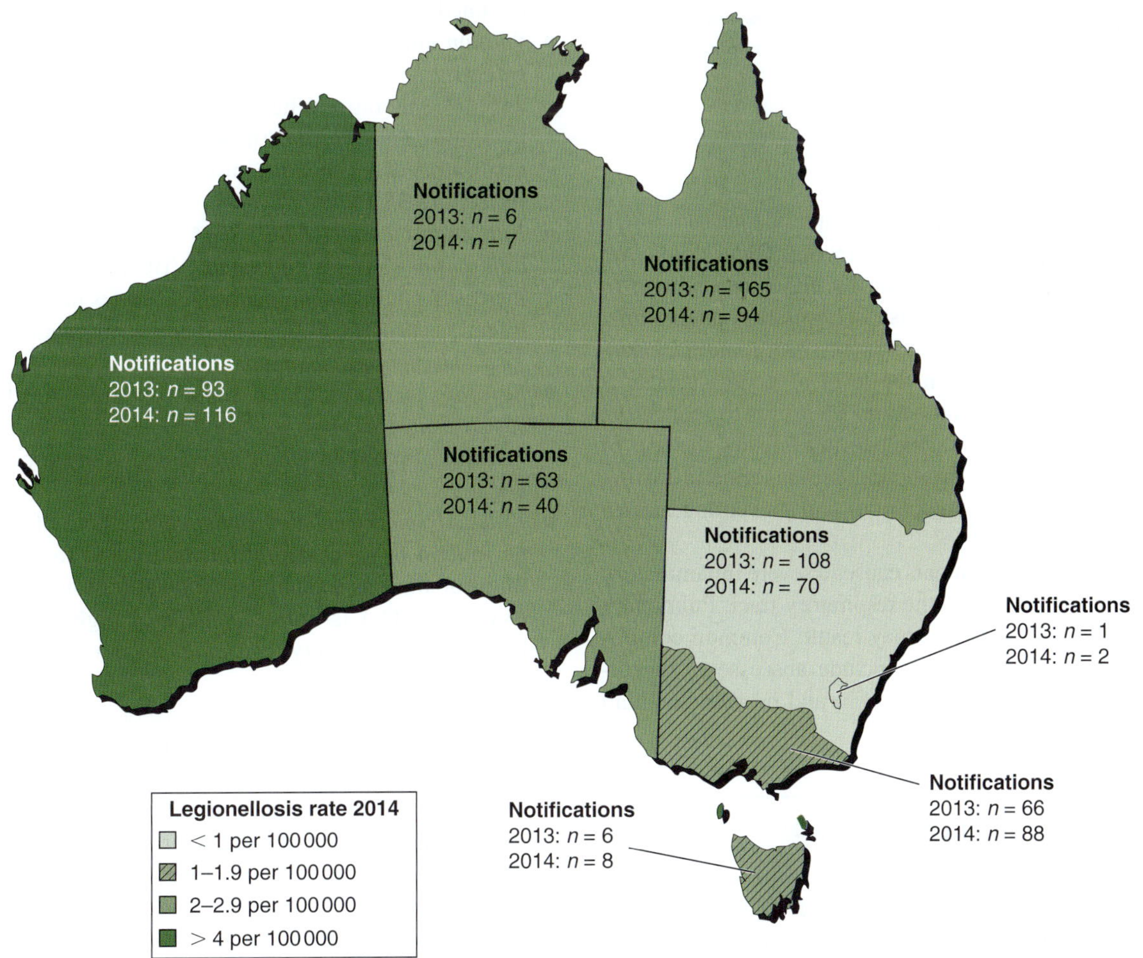

FIGURE 35.5 ***Number of notifications for legionellosis in Australia for 2013 and 2014 (text) and notification rates per 100,000 for 2014 (colour)***

Source: Generated using data from Department of Health (2015). *National Notifiable Diseases Surveillance System. Number of notifications for legionellosis by year, Australia, 1991 to 2015.* Retrieved from https://www9.health.gov.au/cda/source/rpt_4_sel.cfm

BOX 35.1 Emerging zoonotic viral pneumonias

Severe acute respiratory syndrome (SARS) is a lower respiratory tract illness caused by the SARS coronavirus (SARS Co-V). The pathogen is zoonotic (causing disease that can cross the species barrier). First identified in the early 2000s in China, it subsequently spread to four other countries. The World Health Organization (WHO) collaborated with the Global Outbreak Alert and Response Network (GOARN) and local health authorities to provide epidemiological, clinical and logistical support. SARS is an airborne virus with an incubation period of 2–7 days in previously healthy adults (aged 25–70 years). Deaths from SARS are around 3% (WHO, 2022a).

Middle East respiratory syndrome (MERS) is a lower respiratory tract illness caused by the MERS coronavirus (MERS Co-V). It is thought to have originated in Saudi Arabia in 2012. While there are 2,500 cases reported to the WHO, there are currently no reports of MERS cases in Australia (WHO, 2022b).

Typical symptoms of both these viral illnesses include shortness of breath and cough. The person often has a fever and pneumonia is common. Transmission is a most likely droplet. There are currently no vaccines and treatment is supportive, managing the person's signs and symptoms.

emergency surgery or obstetric procedures, depressed cough and gag reflexes, and impaired swallowing. Older adults are at significant risk. Enteral nutrition by either nasogastric or gastric tube also increases the risk of aspiration pneumonia. Vomiting is not always apparent; silent regurgitation of gastric contents may occur when the level of consciousness is decreased, such as during intubation. Measures to reduce the risk of aspiration pneumonia include minimising the use of preoperative medications, promoting pre-anaesthetic fasting (6-hour minimum prior to intubation) and preventing nausea and gastric distension.

The low pH of gastric contents causes a severe inflammatory response when aspirated into the respiratory tract. Pulmonary oedema and respiratory failure may result. Common complications of aspiration pneumonia include abscesses, bronchiectasis (chronic dilation of the bronchi and bronchioles) and gangrene of pulmonary tissue.

INTERPROFESSIONAL CARE

Prevention is a key component in managing pneumonia. Identifying vulnerable populations and instituting preventive strategies (such as adequate vaccination) are measures to reduce the mortality and morbidity associated with pneumonia. With early identification of the infecting organism, appropriate treatment and support of respiratory function, most people recover uneventfully. However, pneumonia remains a serious disease with significant mortality, especially in aged and debilitated populations.

Diagnosis

The history and physical examination, along with diagnostic testing, are used to establish the diagnosis, determine the extent of lung involvement and identify the causative organism. See the chapter 'A person-centred approach to assessing the respiratory system' for more information about the following tests and their nursing implications:

- *A chest x-ray* is obtained to determine the extent and pattern of lung involvement. Fluid infiltrates, consolidated lung tissue and atelectasis (areas of alveolar collapse) appear as densities on the film. The *CT scan* provides a more detailed image of pulmonary tissue and may be used when the chest x-ray is not considered an appropriate diagnostic.
- *Sputum Gram stain* rapidly identifies the infecting organisms as Gram-positive or Gram-negative bacteria. Antibiotic therapy can then be directed at the predominant type of organism until further culture and sensitivity results are obtained.
- *Sputum culture and sensitivity* is ordered to identify the infecting organism and determine the most effective antibiotic therapy. When obtaining sputum for culture, it is important to obtain secretions from the lower respiratory tract, not the mouth and nasal passages (see Procedure 33.1).
- *Full blood count (FBC) with white blood cell (WBC) differential* shows an elevated WBC ($< 10 \times 10^9$/L) with increased circulating immature leucocytes in response to the infectious process. White blood cell changes are minimal in viral and other pneumonias.
- *Serology testing*, blood tests to detect antibodies to respiratory pathogens, may be used to identify the infecting organism when blood and sputum cultures are negative.
- *Pulse oximetry*, a non-invasive method of measuring peripheral oxygen saturation, is ordered to continuously monitor the gas exchange. The saturation of peripheral oxygen (SpO_2) is normally 95% or higher. An SpO_2 of less than 95% may indicate impaired alveolar gas exchange.
- *Arterial blood gases (ABGs)* may be ordered to evaluate gas exchange. Respiratory secretions or pleuritic pain can interfere with alveolar ventilation. Alveolar inflammation can interfere with gas exchange across the alveolar–capillary membrane, especially if exudate or consolidation is present. An arterial oxygen tension (PaO_2) of less than 75 to 80 mmHg indicates impaired gas exchange or alveolar ventilation. See the chapters 'Nursing care of people with altered fluid, electrolyte and acid–base balance' and 'A person-centred approach to assessing the respiratory system' for more information about gas transport, ABGs and normal or expected normal values.

TABLE 35.3 Serotypes in current Australian pneumococcal vaccines

10-VALENT PNEUMOCOCCAL CONJUGATE VACCINE (10VPCV)	13-VALENT PNEUMOCOCCAL CONJUGATE VACCINE (13VPCV)	23-VALENT PNEUMOCOCCAL POLYSACCHARIDE VACCINE (23VPPV)
1, 4, 5, 6B, 7F, 9V, 14, 18C, 19F and 23F	1, 3, 4, 5, 6A, 6B, 7F, 9V, 14, 18C, 19A, 19F and 23F	1, 2, 3, 4, 5, 6B, 7F, 8, 9N, 9V, 10A, 11A, 12F, 14, 15B, 17F, 18C, 19F, 19A, 20, 22F, 23F and 33F

Source: Department of Health and Aged Care (2022b). *The Australian immunisation handbook*. Retrieved from https://immunisationhandbook.health.gov.au/.

- *Fibre-optic bronchoscopy* may be done to obtain a sputum specimen or remove secretions from the bronchial tree (see Figure 33.9). Nursing care related to bronchoscopy is summarised in the 'Diagnostic tests' box in the chapter 'A person-centred approach to assessing the respiratory system'.

Immunisation

Vaccines offer some degree of protection against the most common bacterial and viral pneumonias.

In Australia, a few pneumococcal vaccines are available (see Table 35.3). The critical difference is the number of serotypes contained within the vaccine. Recently the 7-valent pneumococcal vaccine was replaced by a 13-valent one. There is also a pneumococcal vaccine with 10 serotypes and one with 23 serotypes. The individual's medical conditions, age, Indigenous status, overall immunisation status and geographical area can influence the choice of vaccine.

The predominant strain of influenza virus varies from year to year. A new vaccine formulation is prepared yearly, incorporating antigens of the influenza strains predicted to be the most prevalent for the upcoming flu season (typically the winter months). Vulnerable populations for whom yearly vaccine is recommended include individuals with chronic conditions involving lung, heart, diabetes or kidney disease, healthcare workers and residents of long-term care facilities. The vaccine contains egg protein and is not recommended for people who have a severe allergy to eggs or who have previously experienced a severe hypersensitivity response to the vaccine.

Medications

Medications used to treat pneumonia may include antibiotics to eradicate bacterial infection and bronchodilators to reduce bronchospasm and improve ventilation.

Broad-spectrum antibiotic therapy is initially used; then, based on the results of sputum microscopy/culture and sensitivity results, more specific antibiotic therapy may be commenced.

When an inflammatory response to the infection causes bronchospasm and constriction, bronchodilators may be ordered to improve ventilation and reduce hypoxia. Bronchodilators generally belong to one of two main groups: sympathomimetic drugs, such as salbutamol (Ventolin) and anticholinergic drugs, such as ipratropium bromide (Atrovent). The use of these drugs and related nursing implications are discussed in detail in the section on asthma in the chapter 'Nursing care of people with gas exchange disorders'. Figure 35.6 demonstrates the actions of common respiratory drugs.

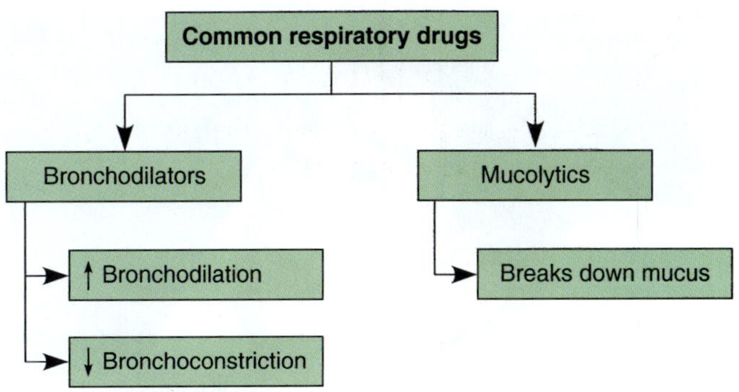

FIGURE 35.6 ***Common drugs used in respiratory disorders***

A mucolytic agent 'breaks up' mucus or reduces its viscosity. Acetylcysteine (Mucomyst) helps to liquefy mucus, making it easier to expectorate. For many people, however, increasing fluid intake is an effective means of liquefying mucus.

Treatments

When mucus secretions are thick and viscous, increasing fluid intake to 2,500 to 3,000 mL per day helps liquefy secretions, making them easier to cough up and expectorate. If the person is unable to maintain an adequate oral intake, intravenous fluids and nutrition may be required.

Incentive spirometry may be used to promote deep breathing, coughing and clearance of respiratory secretions. Endotracheal suctioning may be required if the cough is ineffective. This invasive technique is discussed in the chapter 'Nursing care of people with gas exchange disorders' in Procedure 36.1, describing nursing care for the person undergoing endotracheal suctioning.

OXYGEN THERAPY Oxygen therapy may be indicated for the person who is tachypnoeic or hypoxaemic.

Inflammation of the alveolar–capillary membrane interferes with diffusion of gases across the membrane. Diffusion is affected by several other factors, including the partial pressure of gases on each side of the membrane. Increasing the percentage of inspired oxygen above that of room air (21%) increases the partial pressure of oxygen in the alveoli and enhances its diffusion into the capillaries. Supplemental oxygen improves oxygenation of the blood and tissues in people with pneumonia.

Depending on the degree of hypoxia, oxygen may be administered by either a low-flow or a high-flow system. Low-flow systems include nasal prongs, simple face mask, partial rebreathing mask and non-rebreathing mask (see Figure 35.7). Nasal prongs can deliver 24–45% oxygen concentrations with flow rates of 2 to 4 L/min. The nasal prongs are comfortable and do not interfere with eating or talking. A simple face mask delivers 40–60% oxygen concentrations with flow rates of 5 to 8 L/min. Up to 100% oxygen can be delivered by the non-rebreather mask, the highest concentration possible without

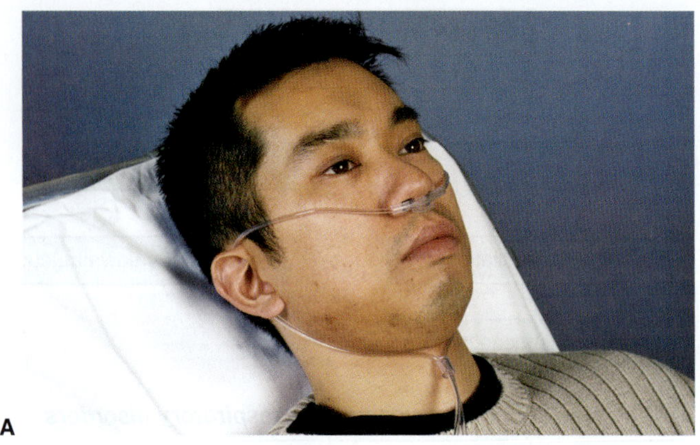
A

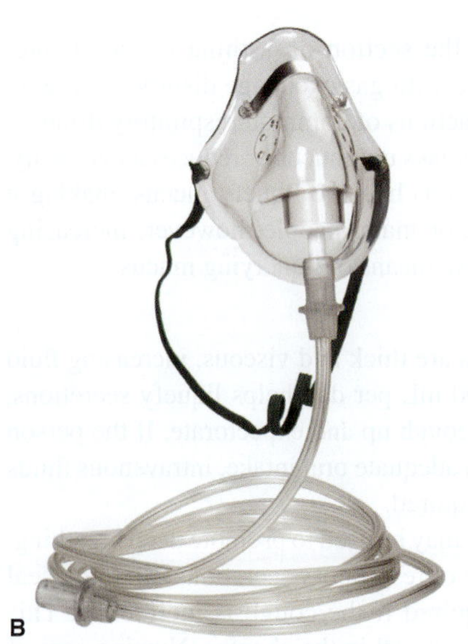
B

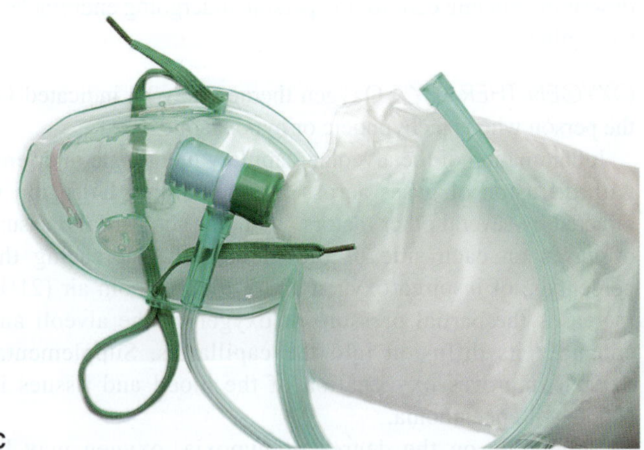
C

FIGURE 35.7 ***Oxygen delivery devices: A, nasal prongs; B, simple face mask; C, non-rebreather mask***

Sources: A, Michal Heron/Pearson Education; B, imagedb.com/Shutterstock; C, 72/Fotolia.

mechanical ventilation. When the amount of oxygen delivered must be precisely regulated, a high-flow system such as a Venturi mask is used (see Figure 35.8). The Venturi mask regulates the ratio of oxygen to room air, allowing precise regulation of the oxygen percentage delivered, from 24% to 50%. Severe hypoxia may necessitate intubation and mechanical ventilation. Endotracheal intubation and methods of mechanical ventilation are discussed in the chapter 'Nursing care of people with gas exchange disorders'.

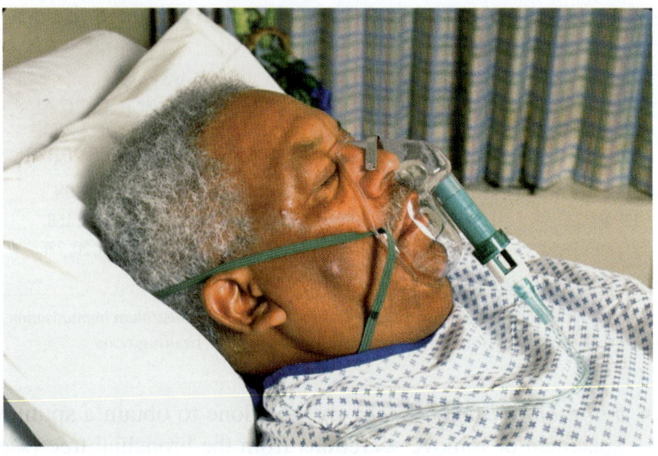

FIGURE 35.8 ***Venturi mask, a high-flow oxygen delivery system***

Source: Michal Heron, Pearson Education/Ph College.

CHEST PHYSIOTHERAPY In recent years, practices in chest physiotherapy, or airway clearance techniques, have changed. A variety of techniques are employed including active cycle of breathing techniques, thoracic expansion exercises, positive expiratory pressure therapy and postural drainage. These techniques must be provided by appropriately trained individuals and may be prescribed to reduce lung consolidation and prevent atelectasis.

Postural drainage uses gravity to facilitate removal of secretions from a particular lung segment. The person is positioned with the segment to be drained superior to or above the trachea or main stem bronchus. Drainage of all lung segments requires a variety of positions (see Figure 35.9); rarely do all segments require drainage. Bronchodilators or nebuliser treatments are administered as ordered prior to postural drainage. It is best to perform postural drainage before meals to avoid nausea and vomiting.

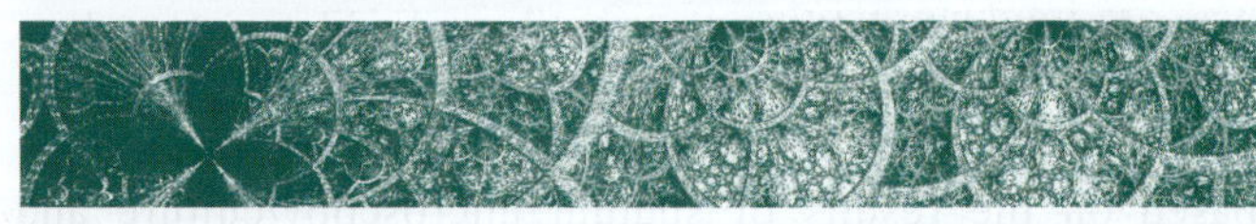

Nursing care

Health promotion

Health promotion activities focus on pneumonia prevention. Make sure individuals in high-risk groups are aware of the benefits of immunisations against influenza and pneumococcal pneumonia. A single dose of the pneumococcus vaccine usually produces immunity to most strains of pneumococcal pneumonia,

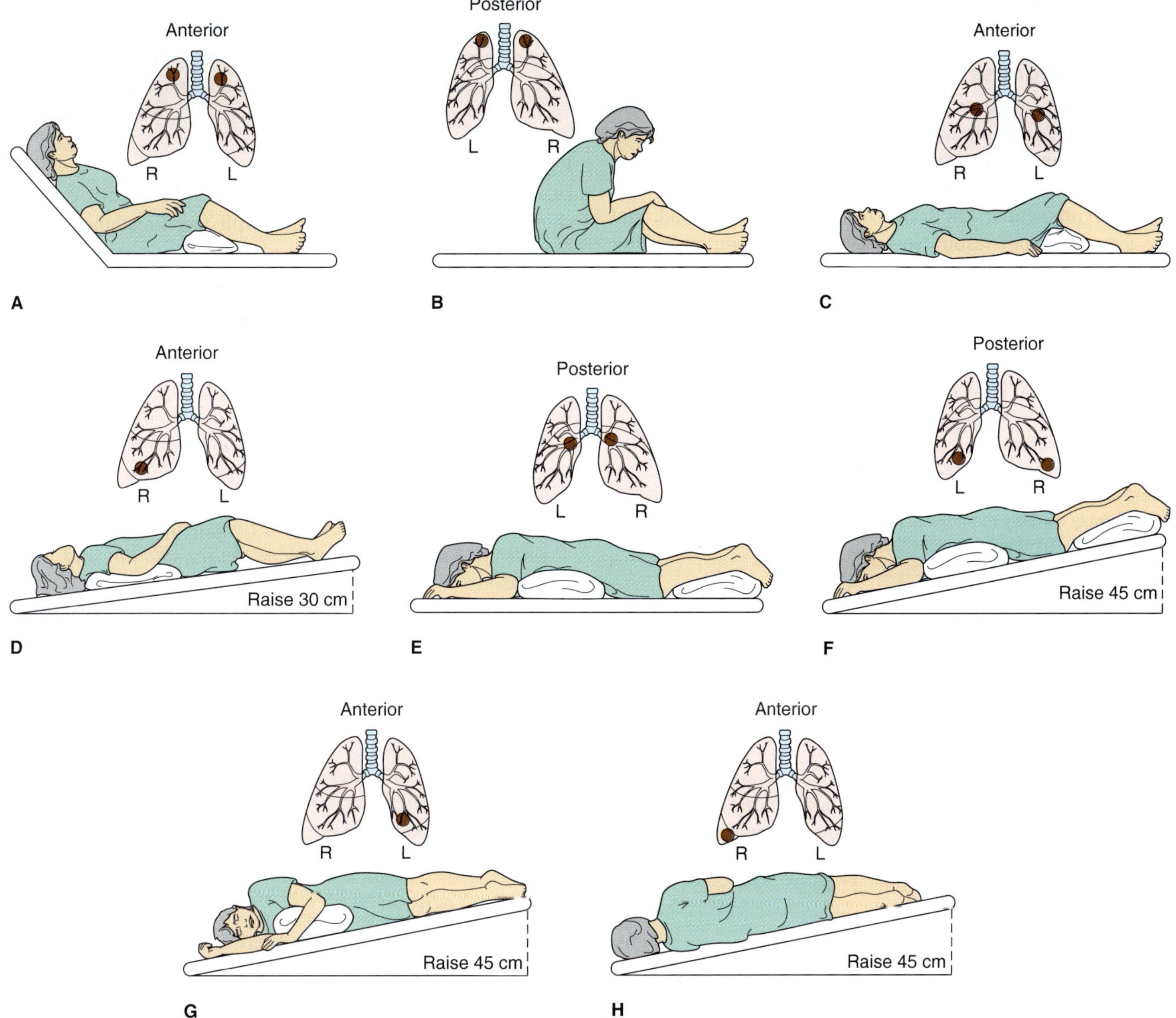

FIGURE 35.9 ***Positions for postural drainage. A, Left and right anterior apical. B, Left and right posterior apical. C, Left and right anterior upper. D, Right middle lobe. E, Left and right superior lower lobes. F, Left and right lower posterior. G, Left lower lateral. H, Right lower lateral***

although repeat doses may be needed for older adults and people who are immunosuppressed. (Pneumococcus vaccine is contraindicated for people receiving immunosuppressive therapy.) Annual influenza vaccine helps prevent pneumonia because pneumonia often occurs as a sequel to influenza.

> **CONSIDERATION FOR PRACTICE**
>
> Inquire about allergic responses to eggs or previous influenza vaccinations prior to administering influenza vaccine. A significant hypersensitivity response may occur in people who are allergic to eggs as the vaccine contains egg protein. Once the vaccine is administered, the patient must stay with the nurse who gave the vaccine for at least 20 minutes in case of a rare allergic reaction.

Assessment

A focused assessment of the person with pneumonia includes the following:

- *Health history*: current symptoms and their duration; presence of shortness of breath, chest pain and its relationship to breathing; cough, productive or non-productive, colour, consistency of sputum; other symptoms; recent upper respiratory or other acute illness; chronic diseases such as diabetes, chronic lung disease or heart disease; current medications; medication allergies.
- *Physical examination*: presentation, apparent distress; level of consciousness; vital signs, including skin colour, temperature; respiratory excursion, use of accessory muscles of respiration; lung sounds.

- *Diagnostic tests*: WBC with differential, sputum Gram stain, culture and sensitivity, chest x-ray or CT scan.

Nursing diagnoses and interventions

People with lower respiratory tract disorders such as pneumonia may have multiple nursing care needs, depending on the severity of the illness. Alveolar ventilation and the process of alveolar respiration can be affected by inflammation and secretions. **Hypoxaemia**, low levels of oxygen in the blood, and tissue hypoxia may result. Nursing care focuses on supporting optimal respiratory function and promoting rest to reduce metabolic and oxygen needs.

CONSIDERATION FOR PRACTICE

Promptly report signs of respiratory distress, including tachypnoea, tachycardia, nasal flaring, use of accessory muscles to breathe adequately, intercostal retractions, cyanosis, increasing restlessness, anxiety or decreased level of consciousness (LOC). These may be early manifestations of respiratory failure and the inability to maintain ventilatory effort.

Ineffective airway clearance

The inflammatory response to infection causes tissue oedema and exudate formation. In the lungs, the inflammatory response can narrow and potentially obstruct bronchial passages and alveoli. Assessment findings supporting this nursing diagnosis include adventitious breath sounds such as crackles (rales) and wheezes; dyspnoea and tachypnoea; coughing; and indicators of hypoxia such as cyanosis, reduced SpO_2 levels, anxiety and apprehension.

- Assess respiratory status, including vital signs, breath sounds, SpO_2 and skin colour, at least every 4 hours. *Early identification of respiratory compromise allows intervention before tissue hypoxia is significant.*
- Assess cough and sputum (amount, colour, consistency and possible odour). *Assessment of the cough and the nature of sputum produced allows evaluation of the effectiveness of respiratory clearance and the response to therapy.*
- Monitor ABG results; report increasing hypoxaemia and other abnormal results to the doctor. *Blood gas changes may be an early indicator of impaired gas exchange due to airway narrowing or obstruction.*
- Place in Fowler's or high-Fowler's position. Encourage frequent position changes and ambulation as allowed. *The upright position promotes lung expansion; position changes and ambulation facilitate the movement of secretions.*
- Assist to cough, deep breathe and use assistive devices. Provide endotracheal suctioning using aseptic technique as required if the person is intubated. *Coughing, deep breathing and suctioning help clear airways.*
- Provide a fluid intake of at least 2,500 to 3,000 mL per day. *A liberal fluid intake helps liquefy secretions, facilitating their clearance. Caution should be exercised based on the individual patient history.*
- Work with the doctor and physiotherapist to provide pulmonary hygiene measures, such as postural drainage, percussion and vibration. *These techniques help mobilise and clear secretions.*
- Administer prescribed medications as ordered and monitor their effects. *If the infecting organism is resistant to the prescribed antibiotic, little improvement may be seen with treatment. Bronchodilators help maintain open airways but may have adverse effects such as anxiety and restlessness.*

Ineffective breathing pattern

Pleural inflammation often accompanies pneumonia, causing sharp localised pain that increases with deep breathing, coughing and movement, which can lead to rapid and shallow breathing, resulting in poor gas exchange. Distal airways and alveoli may not expand optimally with each breath, increasing the risk of atelectasis and decreasing gas exchange. Fatigue from the increased work of breathing is an additional problem in pneumonia. This, too, can lead to decreased lung inflation and an ineffective breathing pattern.

- Provide for rest periods. *Rest reduces metabolic demands, fatigue and the work of breathing, promoting a more effective breathing pattern.*
- Assess for pleuritic discomfort. *Provide analgesics as ordered. Adequate pain relief minimises splinting and promotes adequate ventilation.*
- Provide reassurance during periods of respiratory distress. *Hypoxia and respiratory distress produce high levels of anxiety, which tends to further increase tachypnoea and fatigue and decrease ventilation.*
- Administer oxygen as ordered. *Oxygen therapy increases the alveolar oxygen concentration and facilitates its diffusion across the alveolar–capillary membrane, reducing hypoxia and anxiety.*
- Teach slow abdominal breathing. *This breathing pattern promotes lung expansion and can promote calmness.*

Activity intolerance

Impaired airway clearance and gas exchange interfere with oxygen delivery to body cells and tissues. At the same time, the infectious process and the body's response to it increase metabolic demands on the cells. The net result of this imbalance between oxygen delivery and oxygen demand is a lack of physiological energy to maintain normal daily activities.

- Assess activity tolerance, noting any increase in pulse, respirations, dyspnoea, diaphoresis or cyanosis. *These assessment findings may indicate limited or impaired activity tolerance.*
- Schedule activities, planning for rest periods. *Rest periods minimise fatigue and improve activity tolerance.*
- Provide assistive devices. *Assistive devices facilitate movement and reduce energy demands.*
- Enlist the family's help to minimise stress and anxiety levels. *Stress and anxiety increase metabolic demands and can decrease activity tolerance.*
- Perform active or passive range-of-motion (ROM) exercises. *Exercises help maintain muscle tone and joint mobility and prevent contractures if bed rest is prolonged.*
- Provide emotional support and reassurance that strength and energy will return to normal when the infectious process has resolved and the balance of oxygen supply and demand is restored. *The person may be concerned that*

activity intolerance will continue to be a problem after the acute infection is resolved.

CONSIDERATION FOR PRACTICE

Activity intolerance may be an early sign of cardiorespiratory compromise, particularly in the older adult or person with pre-existing heart disease. New or worsening manifestations of activity intolerance should be reported to the doctor.

Community-based care

Individuals with pneumonia usually are treated in the community, unless their respiratory status is significantly compromised (e.g. altered mental status, tachypnoea, tachycardia, hypotension, hypo- or hyperthermia, and altered blood gases) or if risk factors such as advanced age and/or coexisting heart, kidney or liver disease are present.

Discuss the following topics when preparing the person and family for home care:

- the importance of completing the prescribed medication regimen as ordered
- recommendations for limiting activities and increasing rest
- maintaining adequate fluid intake to keep mucus thin for easier expectoration
- ways to maintain adequate nutritional intake, such as small, frequent, well-balanced meals
- the importance of avoiding smoking or exposure to second-hand smoke to prevent further irritation of the lungs
- manifestations to report to the doctor, such as increasing shortness of breath, difficulty breathing, increased fever, fatigue, headache, sleepiness or confusion.

CONSIDERATION FOR PRACTICE

Beware of any person with cardiac comorbidities who develops a respiratory illness. Individuals with hypertension or cardiac failure may be inadvertently ordered both a sympathomimetic and a beta-blocker concomitantly (e.g. salbutamol and metoprolol). These two classes of drugs are contraindicated—sympathetic agonist and sympathetic antagonist.

The accompanying nursing care plan provides further nursing interventions for people treated in the community.

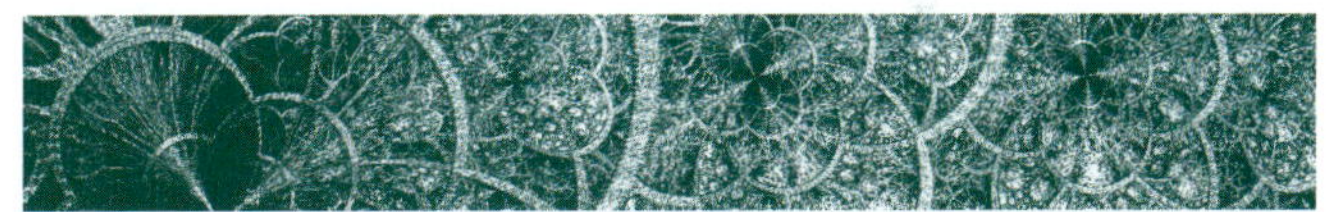

NURSING CARE PLAN A person with pneumonia

Mary O'Neal is a 35-year-old personal assistant and part-time university student. On returning home from class one evening, she begins to experience a chill. She alternates between chills and sweats all night. Staying home from work, she remains in bed most of the next day. Her fever continues and she develops a cough and dull aching chest pain. When the cough becomes productive of rust-coloured sputum the following day, she seeks medical treatment from her family doctor.

ASSESSMENT

Mrs O'Neal is admitted. She denies any previous history of respiratory diseases 'other than the usual colds, flu and such'. She also denies any history of smoking or medication allergies. She says her symptoms began abruptly with the onset of the chills. She describes her chest pain as a dull ache that was initially substernal but now is localised in her lower lateral right chest. The pain increases with deep breathing, coughing and moving. Her cough is increasing in frequency and severity and her sputum appears rusty brown. Her vital signs are BP 116/74, P 104 and regular, R 26, T 38.7°C. Skin warm and flushed, with no evidence of cyanosis. Respirations shallow, unlaboured; respiratory excursion equal. Diminished breath sounds in bases bilaterally, crackles noted in right posterior and lateral base. Faint pleural rub heard at right midaxillary line.

An FBC shows a WBC of 18.4×10^9/L; differential shows increased numbers of neutrophils and immature WBCs (bands). Mrs O'Neal provides a sputum specimen for culture and Gram stain prior to seeing the doctor.

The doctor orders a chest x-ray after examining Mrs O'Neal. Based on her history, examination and chest x-ray, he makes the diagnosis of acute bacterial pneumonia, probably pneumococcal. He prescribes the current antibiotic medication for pneumonia.

DIAGNOSES

- *Ineffective breathing pattern* related to pleuritic chest pain manifested by tachypnoea and shallow breaths.
- *Hyperthermia* related to inflammatory process manifested by febrile temperature.

PLANNING

- Assess knowledge and understanding of pneumonia and its effects.
- Assist to develop a medication schedule that coordinates with normal daily routine.

Expected outcomes

- Maintain normal pulmonary function.
- Describe measures to minimise elevations in body temperature.
- Identify a schedule for taking her medication that will facilitate compliance with the regimen.
- Describe manifestations that should be reported to the doctor.

IMPLEMENTATION

- Teach about the following:
  a. importance of avoiding the use of a cough suppressant except at night to facilitate rest
  b. ways to increase fluid intake to reduce fever and maintain thin mucus for easy expectoration
  c. beneficial effects of rest, especially during the acute phase of her illness
  d. safe use of aspirin and paracetamol to reduce fever
  e. importance of taking all prescribed medication doses as scheduled
  f. common side effects of medications and their management

(continued)

NURSING CARE PLAN A person with pneumonia (continued)

g. early manifestations of a penicillin allergy that necessitate stopping the medication and notifying the doctor

h. signs of complications of pneumonia or worsening pneumonia to report.

EVALUATION

The sputum culture confirms *S. pneumoniae* as the cause of Mrs O'Neal's pneumonia. When she returns for her follow-up appointment, she reports that she began to feel better after 2 days on the penicillin and returned to work the following Monday. Her examination reveals good breath sounds throughout with no adventitious sounds. The follow-up sputum culture is free of pathogens.

CRITICAL THINKING IN THE NURSING PROCESS

1 Do any of the factors identified in the case study increase Mrs O'Neal's risk of acute bacterial pneumonia?

2 Even though Mrs O'Neal has no history of medication allergies, an anaphylactic reaction remains a potential risk. Describe the sequence of events leading to anaphylactic shock, its initial symptoms and immediate nursing interventions.

3 Had Mrs O'Neal required hospitalisation to treat her acute pneumonia, interruption of her usual activities and responsibilities could have led to anxiety. Develop a care plan for this situation, using the nursing diagnosis of *Ineffective role performance* related to hospitalisation.

REFLECTION ON THE NURSING PROCESS

1 Outline what you have learned from this case study that you will apply to your future practice.

2 You developed and undertook an eight-point teaching plan for Mrs O'Neal (see implementation above). Which evaluation data will demonstrate that this comprehensive teaching plan has been understood and will be successful?

CONSIDERATION FOR PRACTICE

Epidemic: when there are more cases in a region than normal.

Pandemic: a worldwide epidemic.

THE PERSON WITH LUNG ABSCESS

A **lung abscess** is a localised area of lung destruction or necrosis and pus formation. The most common cause of lung abscess is aspiration and resulting pneumonia. Risk factors, therefore, are those for aspiration: decreased LOC due to anaesthesia, injury or disease of the central nervous system (CNS), seizure, excessive sedation or alcohol abuse; swallowing disorders; dental caries; and debilitation secondary to cancer or chronic disease. A lung abscess may also occur as a complication of some types of pneumonia, including those due to *S. aureus*, *Klebsiella* and *Legionella*. Many organisms can cause a lung abscess (see Figure 35.10).

Pathophysiology and manifestations

A lung abscess forms after lung tissue becomes consolidated (i.e. after alveoli become filled with fluid, pus and microorganisms). Consolidated tissue may become necrotic. This necrotic process can spread to involve the entire bronchopulmonary segment and progress proximally until it ruptures into a bronchus. With rupture, the contents of the abscess empty into the bronchus, leaving a cavity filled with air and fluid, a process known as

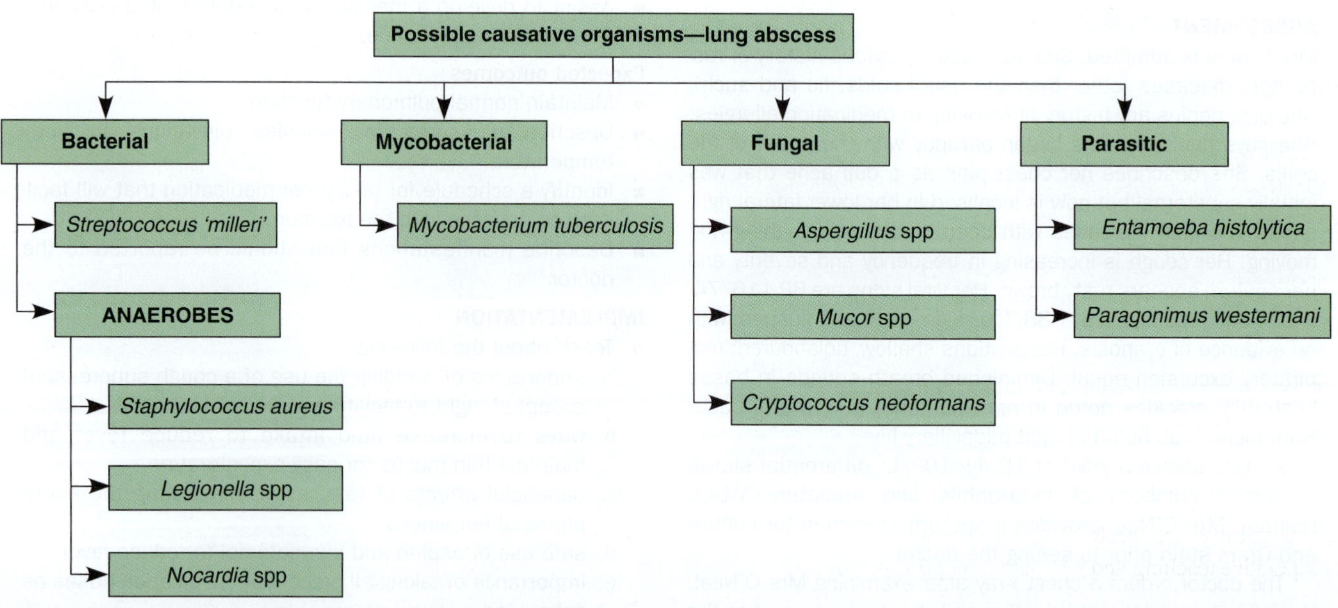

FIGURE 35.10 ***Possible causative organisms—lung abscess***

Source: Generated from information from the Royal College of Pathologists Australasia (RCPA) (2019). *Lung abscess*. Retrieved from https://www.rcpa.edu.au/.

cavitation. If purulent material from the abscess is not expectorated, the infection may spread, leading to diffuse pneumonia or a syndrome similar to acute respiratory distress syndrome.

Manifestations of lung abscess typically develop about 2 weeks after the precipitating event (aspiration, pneumonia and so on). Their onset may be either acute or insidious. Early symptoms are those of pneumonia: productive cough, chills and fever, pleuritic chest pain, malaise and anorexia. The temperature may be significantly elevated, 39.4°C or higher. When the abscess ruptures, the person may expectorate large amounts of foul-smelling, purulent and possibly blood-streaked sputum. Breath sounds are diminished and crackles may be noted in the abscess region. A dull percussion tone is also present.

INTERPROFESSIONAL CARE

The diagnosis of lung abscess usually is based on the history and presentation. The FBC may indicate leucocytosis. A sputum culture may not show the organism involved unless rupture occurs. Chest x-ray shows a thick-walled, solitary cavity with surrounding consolidation, although differentiating lung abscess from consolidation can be difficult until cavitation occurs.

Lung abscess is treated with antibiotic therapy. Postural drainage may be ordered to relieve obstruction and promote drainage. In some cases, bronchoscopy is used to drain the abscess. If the pleural space becomes involved, a chest tube (*tube thoracostomy*) may be used to drain the abscess. See the section on pneumothorax later in this chapter for further discussion of chest tubes.

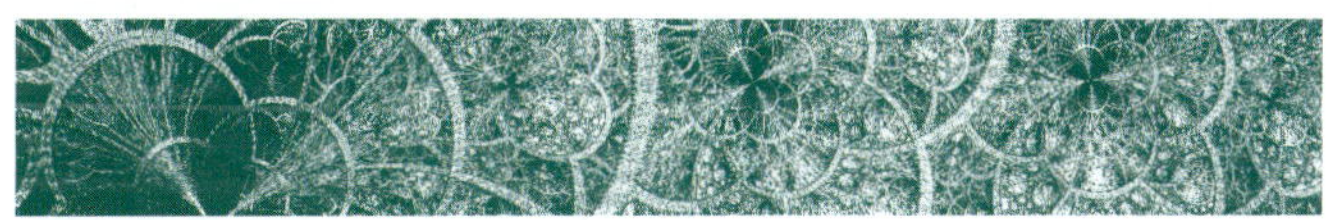

Nursing care

Although most people with lung abscess recover fully with appropriate antibiotic treatment, rupture and drainage of the abscess into a bronchus is a frightening experience. Nursing care needs of the individual relate primarily to maintaining a patent airway and adequate gas exchange.

Health education for the person and family focuses on the importance of completing the prescribed antibiotic therapy. Most lung abscesses are successfully treated with antibiotics; however, treatment may last up to 1 month or more. Emphasise the importance of completing the entire course of therapy to eliminate the infecting organisms. Infection from lung abscess can spread not only to lung and pleural tissue but also systemically, causing sepsis. If postural drainage is ordered, teach the person and family how to perform this procedure. When procedures such as bronchoscopy or thoracostomy are performed to drain the abscess, provide preoperative teaching and instruction on postoperative care.

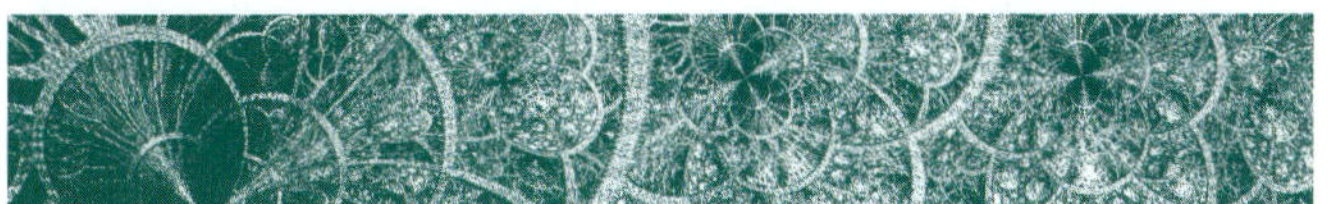

THE PERSON WITH TUBERCULOSIS

Tuberculosis (TB) is a chronic, recurrent infectious disease that usually affects the lungs, although any organ can be affected. The disease caused by *Mycobacterium tuberculosis* is relatively uncommon in Australia.

M. tuberculosis is a relatively slow-growing, slender, rod-shaped, acid-fast organism with a waxy outer capsule, which increases its resistance to destruction. Although the lungs are usually infected, tuberculosis can involve other organs as well. It is transmitted by *droplet nuclei*—airborne droplets produced when an infected person coughs, sneezes speaks or sings. The tiny droplets can remain suspended in the air for several hours. Infection may develop when a susceptible host breathes in air containing droplet nuclei and the contaminated particle eludes the normal defences of the upper respiratory tract to reach the alveoli.

There are two types of TB: (1) *latent*, which is not infectious, so when the person is infected they do not get sick as their immune system is able to fight the infection; and (2) *active*, which is infectious and the person's immune system cannot fight the infection as the bacteria multiply and grow (Healthdirect, 2021).

Incidence and prevalence

In Australia, the incidence of TB has remained low (5.0 and 6.0 per 100,000) for many years. These rates compare favourably with other developed countries; however, no trend of further decrease is noted. Significantly higher rates of TB are seen in specific subgroups: those born overseas and Aboriginal and Torres Strait Islander people (Department of Health and Aged Care, 2022c).

In 2020, TB deaths in Australia occurred in 0.2 cases per 100,000 people (World Data Atlas, 2022). The COVID-19 pandemic had a significant impact on access and delivery of TB diagnostic and treatment services in countries that report high TB incidents and was a financial burden worldwide. During 2019–2020, there was a sharp drop (18%) in TB diagnosis notifications, from 7.1 million in 2019 to 5.8 million in 2020, leading to the need for new reporting methods to be put into place to capture data.

Although TB is both preventable and curable, 1.5 million deaths were recorded in 2020 (WHO, 2021). The emergence of multidrug-resistant (MDR) strains of TB has complicated the treatment and control of this infectious respiratory disease. While MDR-TB continues to be a public health crisis, mechanisms to reduce the development of drug resistance have been implemented to assist with this problem, such as directly observed therapy (DOT) where individuals are observed taking each and every medication (WHO, 2021).

Risk factors

The risk of infection by *M. tuberculosis* is affected by the characteristics of the infectious person, the extent of air contamination, duration of exposure and susceptibility of the host. The number of microbes in the sputum, frequency and force of coughing, and behaviours such as covering the mouth when coughing, affect the production of droplet nuclei. In a small, closed or

Tuberculosis in Australia

Sustainable development goals Australia

FIGURE 35.11 ***Tuberculosis and sustainable development goals in Australia***

Source: World Health Organization (WHO) (2021). *Global tuberculosis report*. Retrieved from https://www.who.int/teams/global-tuberculosis-programme/data.

poorly ventilated space, droplet nuclei become more concentrated, increasing the risk of exposure. Prolonged contact, such as living in the same household, increases the risk. Less-than-optimal immune function—a consistent problem for people in lower socioeconomic groups, injection drug users, the homeless, alcoholics and people with HIV infection—increases the susceptibility of the host.

In 2021, the WHO published its global TB report that provides a comprehensive and current assessment of TB worldwide, including prevention, diagnosis and treatment at global, regional and country levels including Australia (WHO, 2021). The WHO provides interactive visualisations (see Figure 35.11) with current comparative information on TB including:

- number of cases attributed to five risks factors in 2020—HIV, diabetes, undernourishment, smoking and alcohol use disorders
- indicators in the sustainable development goals associated with TB incidence
- end TB strategy milestones.

Pathophysiology

Pulmonary tuberculosis

Minute droplet nuclei containing one to three bacilli that elude upper airway defence systems to enter the lungs implant in an alveolus or respiratory bronchiole, usually in an upper lobe. As the bacteria multiply, they cause a local inflammatory response. The inflammatory response brings neutrophils and macrophages to the site. These phagocytic cells surround and engulf the bacilli, isolating them and preventing their spread. *M. tuberculosis* continues to slowly multiply; some bacilli enter the lymphatic system to stimulate a cellular-mediated immune response. (See the chapter 'Nursing care of people with infections' for a review of immune responses.) Neutrophils and macrophages isolate the bacteria but cannot destroy them. A granulomatous lesion called a *tubercle*, a sealed-off colony of bacilli is formed (Bullock & Hales, 2019). Within the tubercle, infected tissue dies, forming a cheese-like centre, a process called *caseation necrosis*.

If the immune response is adequate, scar tissue develops around the tubercle and the bacilli remain encapsulated. These lesions eventually calcify and are visible on x-ray. The person, although infected by *M. tuberculosis*, does not develop TB, disease. If the immune response is inadequate to contain the bacilli, the disease of TB can develop. Occasionally, the infection can progress, leading to extensive destruction of lung tissue. In *primary tuberculosis*, granulomatous tissue may erode into a bronchus or i blood vessel, allowing the disease to spread throughout the lung or other organs. This severe form of TB is uncommon in adults.

A previously healed TB lesion may be reactivated. *Reactivation tuberculosis* occurs when the immune system is suppressed due to age, disease or use of immunosuppressive drugs. The extent of lung disease can vary from small lesions to extensive cavitation of lung tissue. Tubercles rupture, spreading bacilli into the airways to form satellite lesions and produce tuberculosis pneumonia. Without treatment, massive lung involvement can lead to death or a more chronic process of tubercle formation and cavitation may result (Herchline, 2017). People with chronic disease continue to spread *M. tuberculosis* into the environment, potentially infecting others. 'Pathophysiology illustrated: tuberculosis' illustrates the pathogenesis of TB.

Individuals with HIV are at high risk of developing active TB, due to a primary infection or reactivation. HIV infection suppresses cellular immunity, which is vital to limiting the replication and spread of *M. tuberculosis*.

MANIFESTATIONS AND COMPLICATIONS The initial infection causes few symptoms and typically goes unnoticed until the tuberculin test becomes positive or calcified lesions are seen on a chest x-ray. Manifestations of primary progressive or reactivation TB often develop insidiously and are initially non-specific (see the 'Manifestations' box). Fatigue, weight loss, anorexia, low-grade afternoon fever and night sweats are common. A dry cough develops, which later becomes productive of purulent and/or blood-tinged sputum. It is often at this stage that the person seeks medical attention.

MANIFESTATIONS Pulmonary tuberculosis

- Fatigue
- Weight loss
- Anorexia
- Low-grade afternoon fever and night sweats
- Cough: initially dry, later productive of purulent and/or blood-tinged sputum

NURSING CARE OF THE OLDER ADULT Tuberculosis

Presenting symptoms of tuberculosis in the older adult are often vague, including coughing, weight loss, anorexia, night sweats or periodic fevers. These signs and symptoms should not be dismissed as a normal part of ageing.

Tuberculin skin testing with purified protein derivative (PPD) is required when the diagnosis is considered. A chest x-ray and sputum culture for acid-fast bacilli are obtained if the PPD is positive.

Successful treatment for TB generally requires four drugs for at least 6 months to totally eradicate the organism. Individuals are most often required to take the medication under the direct supervision of a nurse or other healthcare worker to improve adherence to the management regimen and decrease the risk of multidrug-resistant strains forming.

ASSESSING FOR HOME CARE

Community-dwelling older adults are susceptible to tuberculosis as well as those in care facilities.

Assess risk factors for tuberculosis:

- general health and nutritional status, including intake of specific nutrients such as vitamin D (lack of vitamin D is associated with a higher risk of developing active TB)
- presence of a chronic disease such as silicosis, diabetes, alcoholism or HIV infection; past history of a gastrectomy (higher incidence of TB infection has been noted in patients after gastrectomy than in the general population)
- past history of a positive tuberculin test that now has converted to negative
- medications such as corticosteroids or other immunosuppressive drugs.

Assess living and social situation:

- natural light and ventilation in the home
- access to clean water, cooking facilities, supermarkets and other services
- possible exposure to infected people; for example, sharing a household with someone with active TB, crowded living facilities, homelessness, frequent participation in senior activities, volunteer work in residential care facilities or other institutional settings
- access to healthcare.

HEALTH EDUCATION FOR THE PERSON AND FAMILY

Teaching focuses on improving the older adult's ability to self-manage the disease and treatment. Teach about tuberculosis and how it is spread. Emphasise the importance of taking all medications as prescribed and complying with follow-up appointments and testing. Discuss the importance of:

- using disposable tissues to contain respiratory secretions, especially during the first 2 weeks of treatment when the disease may be transmitted to others
- avoiding exposure to crowds or people with infectious diseases
- eating a well-balanced diet with adequate nutrients
- getting adequate rest, sleep and exercise to maintain good general health
- ensuring that housemates or others having frequent contact with the person being tested and receive prophylactic treatment if indicated.
- Teach about possible side effects of the prescribed medications and the importance of reporting these to healthcare providers (see Table 35.4).

TABLE 35.4 Antitubercular medications

DRUG AND DOSAGE	ADVERSE EFFECTS	NURSING IMPLICATIONS
Isoniazid (INH), oral: 300 mg daily or 900 mg 1, 2 or 3 times weekly	Peripheral neuropathy Hepatitis	Administer pyridoxine (vitamin B_6) concurrently. Monitor liver function studies (AST and ALT); avoid other hepatotoxins.
Rifampicin (RMP), oral: 600 mg daily or 2 or 3 times weekly	Hepatitis Flu-like syndrome; fever Colours body fluids—including sweat, urine, saliva, tears and cerebrospinal fluid (CSF)—orange-red	As for INH. Do not miss or skip doses; flu-like syndrome and fever occur when drug is resumed. Contact lenses may become discoloured and should not be worn.
Pyrazinamide (PZA), oral: 1 to 2 g daily; or 2 to 4 g twice weekly	Hyperuricaemia Hepatotoxicity	Monitor uric acid levels. Monitor AST and ALT; avoid other hepatotoxins.
Ethambutol (EMB), oral: 800 mg to 1,600 mg daily; or 2 to 4 g twice weekly	Optic neuritis	Monitor red-green colour discrimination and visual acuity.

Tuberculosis

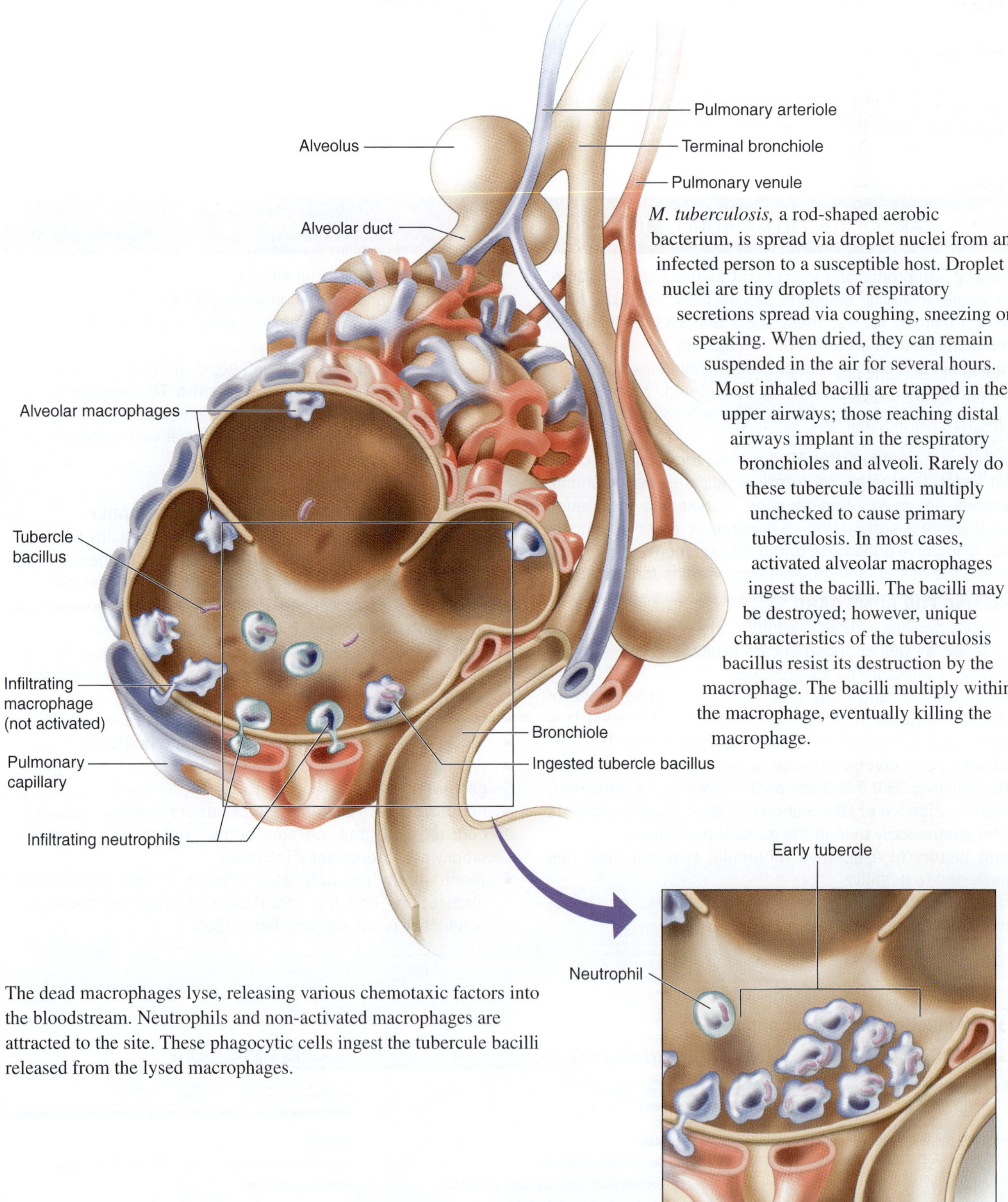

M. tuberculosis, a rod-shaped aerobic bacterium, is spread via droplet nuclei from an infected person to a susceptible host. Droplet nuclei are tiny droplets of respiratory secretions spread via coughing, sneezing or speaking. When dried, they can remain suspended in the air for several hours. Most inhaled bacilli are trapped in the upper airways; those reaching distal airways implant in the respiratory bronchioles and alveoli. Rarely do these tubercule bacilli multiply unchecked to cause primary tuberculosis. In most cases, activated alveolar macrophages ingest the bacilli. The bacilli may be destroyed; however, unique characteristics of the tuberculosis bacillus resist its destruction by the macrophage. The bacilli multiply within the macrophage, eventually killing the macrophage.

The dead macrophages lyse, releasing various chemotaxic factors into the bloodstream. Neutrophils and non-activated macrophages are attracted to the site. These phagocytic cells ingest the tubercule bacilli released from the lysed macrophages.

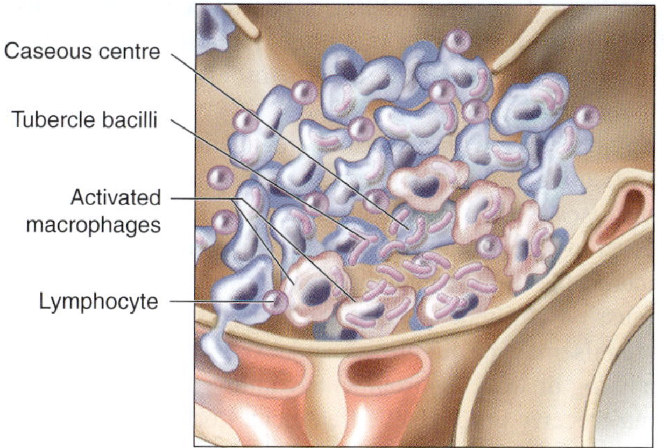

After several weeks, a delayed hypersensitivity response to bacterial antigens destroys many of the macrophages. Concurrently, a cell-mediated immune response activates additional macrophages, which ingest and destroy the bacilli. The lysed macrophages and bacilli are surrounded by a mass of live, activated macrophages and lymphocytes. Scar (granulomatous) tissue forms, encapsulating the primary lesion. Most lesions calcify and are visible on x-ray. These lesions may remain dormant for a year or more (in some cases, many years) before being reactivated to produce secondary or reactivation tuberculosis.

When the immune and macrophage-activating responses are weakened by age or disease (e.g. HIV disease), the tuberculosis bacilli continue to multiply within the lesion. The caseous material at the centre of the lesion liquefies, and the lesion grows.

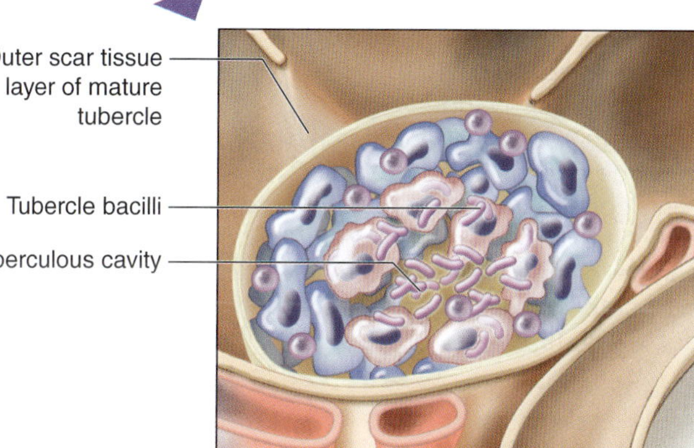

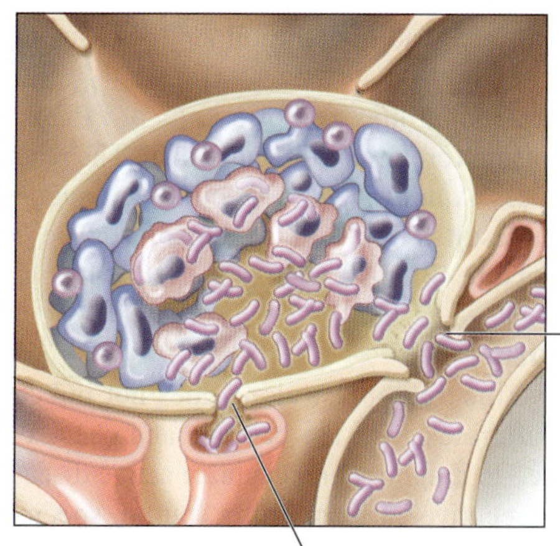

The enlarging lesion damages surrounding bronchial walls and blood vessels. Granulomatous tissue surrounding the lesion can erode into a bronchus, forming an air-filling cavity. Within this cavity, the bacilli multiply, spreading into the airways and the environment via infected sputum. Bacilli also spread via the blood and within macrophages to regional lymph nodes, and from there to many organs and tissues. Resulting extrapulmonary lesions evolve in the same sequence as pulmonary lesions.

Tuberculosis empyema and bronchopleural fistula are the most serious complications of pulmonary tuberculosis. When a tuberculosis lesion ruptures, bacilli may contaminate the pleural space. Rupture may allow air to enter the pleural space from the lung, causing pneumothorax.

Extrapulmonary tuberculosis

When primary disease or reactivation allows live bacilli to enter the bronchi, the disease may spread through the blood and lymph system to other organs. These distant disease metastases may produce an active lesion or may become dormant and reactivate at a later time. Extrapulmonary tuberculosis is especially prevalent in people with HIV.

FAST FACTS

- Immunisation with bacillus Calmette–Guérin (BCG) vaccine is not part of the standard vaccination regimen in Australia. However, individuals with high risk are encouraged to receive it (Department of Health and Aged Care, 2022b).
- High-risk individuals include:
  - Indigenous Australian neonates in high TB incidence regions
  - infants born in Australia to migrant parents
  - children travelling (for an extended period) to countries of high TB prevalence
  - healthcare workers in frequent contact with people with TB.

FAST FACTS

- The organism causing tuberculosis, *M. tuberculosis*, is spread through droplet nuclei that remain suspended in the air for several hours.
- A tubercle is a sealed-off colony of bacilli; if it ruptures, organisms spread, leading to tuberculosis and pneumonia.
- Primary or secondary TB lesions may affect other body systems such as the kidneys, genitalia, bone and brain.

INTERPROFESSIONAL CARE

Tuberculosis was a major public health concern early in the last century, before the development of effective sanitation measures and drug treatment. The development of drug-resistant strains, susceptibility of people with HIV disease and inadequate access to healthcare for high-risk populations contribute to TB continuing to be a significant public health threat. Interprofessional care, therefore, focuses on the following:

- early detection
- accurate diagnosis
- effective disease treatment
- preventing TB spread to others.

With appropriate treatment, individuals become non-infective to others fairly rapidly. Nurses and other healthcare workers are at risk of exposure if the disease has not yet been diagnosed. When a person with TB or suspected TB is hospitalised, maintain respiratory isolation to minimise the risk of infection to other people and the healthcare workers.

Non-adherence with prescribed treatment is a major problem in treating active TB: the person can continue transmitting the disease to others and drug-resistant strains of bacteria can develop when treatment is incomplete. Tuberculosis is a communicable disease and state and territory health authorities must be notified. Contact tracking will commence and individuals may be identified and examined. People who share living or work environments with the person are tested and may receive prophylactic treatment. Local health authorities or services will often continue contact with people who have active TB to facilitate effective containment and infection control.

Screening

The tuberculin test is used to screen for TB infection. A cellular or delayed hypersensitivity response to *M. tuberculosis* develops within 3 to 10 weeks after the infection. Injecting a small amount of *purified protein derivative (PPD)* of tuberculin any time thereafter activates this response, attracting macrophages to the area and causing a pronounced local inflammatory response. The amount of induration surrounding the injection site is used to determine infection (see Figure 35.12).

It is important to remember that a positive response indicates that infection and a cellular (T-cell) response have developed; however, it does not mean that active disease is present or that the person is infectious to others.

Tuberculin testing should only be performed by individuals competent in the administration and assessment of the Mantoux test.

An intradermal injection of 5 units of PPD is administered into the inside forearm of the individual. The reaction is read at 48–72 hours. A negative test is defined as induration < 5 mm. All other results should be considered in the context of the clinical picture (RCPA, 2019).

Diagnosis

A positive tuberculin test alone does not indicate active disease. Sputum tests for the bacillus and chest x-rays are routinely used to diagnose and evaluate active disease. A series of three consecutive early morning sputum specimens are typically examined for bacilli (see Procedure 33.1).

See the 'Diagnostic tests' box in the chapter 'A person-centred approach to assessing the respiratory system' for nursing care related to bronchoscopy.

- *Sputum smear* is microscopically examined for acid-fast bacilli. *M. tuberculosis* resists decolour chemicals after staining. This property is called *acid-fast*. The acid-fast smear provides a rapid indicator of the tubercle bacillus.
- *Sputum culture* positive for *M. tuberculosis* provides the definitive diagnosis. However, *M. tuberculosis* is slow

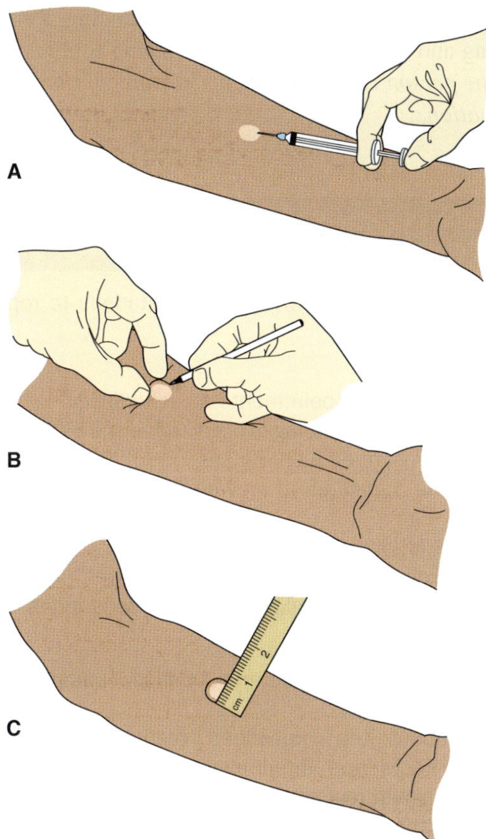

FIGURE 35.12 *A, Intradermal injection for tuberculin testing. B, The injection causes a local inflammatory response (wheal). C, Measurement of induration following tuberculin testing*

growing, requiring 4 to 8 weeks before it can be detected using traditional culture techniques. Automated radiometric culture systems (such as Bactec) allow detection of *M. tuberculosis* in several days.

- Once the organism is detected, *sensitivity testing* is performed to identify appropriate drug therapy.
- *Polymerase chain reaction* (PCR) permits rapid detection of DNA from *M. tuberculosis*.
- *A chest x-ray* is ordered to diagnose and evaluate TB. Typical findings in pulmonary TB include dense lesions in the apical and posterior segments of the upper lobe and possible cavity formation.

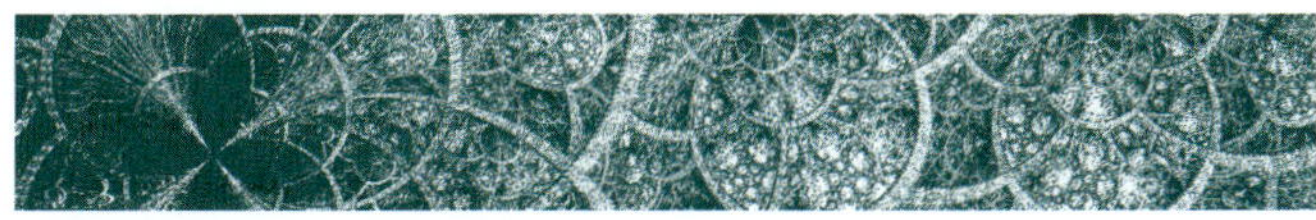

Nursing care

Health promotion

Tuberculosis today presents a greater threat to public health than it does to individuals. Nurses play a key role in maintaining public health. Education and tuberculosis screening are major nursing strategies to prevent TB.

Public health teaching includes increasing awareness of TB as a re-emerging threat. Teach people in all settings how to reduce the spread of TB by covering their mouths when coughing or sneezing and disposing of sputum appropriately. The benefit of screening programs to identify infected (though not necessarily infective) people also needs to be included in public health education.

The best TB prevention is early diagnosis of infections and appropriate treatment to achieve cure. BCG vaccine is recommended for infants born in countries where TB is prevalent.

Assessment

Focused assessment for the person with suspected TB includes the following:

- *Health history*: complaints of fatigue, weight loss, night sweats, difficulty breathing, cough (productive or non-productive), bloody sputum or chest pain; known exposure to TB; most recent tuberculin test and results; living circumstances; alcohol and other recreational drug use.
- *Physical examination*: vital signs, including temperature; general appearance; respiratory rate and lung sounds.
- *Diagnostic tests*: tuberculin test results, presence of acid-fast bacilli in sputum, chest x-ray.

Nursing diagnoses and interventions

Nursing care related to tuberculosis focuses primarily on infection control and compliance with prescribed treatment.

Deficient knowledge

Adequate knowledge and information are necessary to manage the disease and prevent its transmission to others. Educate the person on the importance of prolonged antibiotic therapy and completion of therapy and follow up. Antitubercular agents have side effects, such as increased fatigue, skin rash, nausea, vomiting and anorexia, that the person is required to be aware of so that the impact can be managed to promote compliance.

- Education about TB and the prescribed treatment should include:
  a. nature of the disease and its spread (droplet infection)
  b. purpose of treatment and follow-up procedures (reduces the risk of reoccurrence, risk of bacteria resistance and assists in protecting the community)
  c. measures to prevent spreading the disease to others (using disposable tissues and adopting appropriate coughing and sneezing techniques)
  d. importance of maintaining good general health by eating a well-balanced, high-protein, high-carbohydrate diet; balancing exercise with rest; and avoiding crowds and people with upper respiratory infections
  e. names, doses, purposes and adverse effects of prescribed medications
  f. importance of avoiding alcohol and other substances that may damage the liver while taking chemotherapeutic drugs
  g. fluid intake needs of 2–3 L per day
  h. manifestations to report to the doctor include chest pain, haemoptysis, difficulty breathing; anorexia, nausea or vomiting; yellow tint to skin or sclera; sudden weight gain, swollen feet, ankles, legs or hands; hearing loss, tinnitus or vertigo; change in vision or difficulty discriminating colour.

Tuberculosis is a chronic disease requiring lengthy treatment with antitubercular medications. A good understanding of the disease, its treatment and the potential adverse effects of therapy prepares the person to manage care.

- Document teaching and level of understanding. Reinforce teaching and learning as needed. *Teaching is not complete until the person can demonstrate learning of the information.*

NURSING CARE PLAN A person with tuberculosis

Harry Flanders, aged 53, arrives at a metropolitan public health clinic complaining of aching chest pain that has lasted for the past few days. He says that his sputum also is bloody. He is afraid he might have lung cancer, so he came in to see a doctor.

ASSESSMENT

The public health nurse at the clinic obtains an admission history and physical examination of Mr Flanders. The nurse notes that Mr Flanders is a homeless person who has lived on the streets and in various shelters for the past '10 years or so'. He usually prefers to sleep outdoors, taking refuge in shelters only during very cold or very wet weather. He has a small disability income, but usually scrounges for food or eats with other homeless people at soup kitchens. Mr Flanders states that he has had a cough for a long time, which has become worse recently. It is now productive, especially in the mornings. He also admits that he has recently been waking up drenched with sweat in the middle of the night and is more tired than usual.

Although Mr Flanders' clothes are tattered, he is fairly clean. He answers questions appropriately and intelligently. The nurse does not detect any odour of alcohol on his breath. He is very thin, almost emaciated. Mr Flanders' vital signs are BP 152/86, P 92, R 20 and T 37.8°C.

Suspecting tuberculosis, the nurse obtains a sputum specimen for Gram stain and culture, administers a tuberculin test and sends Mr Flanders for a chest x-ray before he sees the clinic doctor. Although the chest x-ray is inconclusive, the Gram stain is positive for acid-fast bacilli. The diagnosis of probable active pulmonary TB is made. The doctor prescribes isoniazid, 300 mg orally; rifampicin, 600 mg orally; and pyrazinamide, 1,500 mg orally daily for 2 months, to be followed by twice-weekly isoniazid 900 mg orally and rifampicin 600 mg orally. The doctor also orders weekly sputum cultures for the first month.

DIAGNOSES

- *Ineffective health maintenance* related to homelessness.
- *Risk of non-adherence with prescribed treatment* related to lack of understanding and resources manifested by failure to attend clinic for direct observation therapy.
- *Inadequate nutrition* related to increased metabolic needs associated with infection manifested by very low body mass index.
- *Risk of altered sensory perception* related to effects of isoniazid therapy manifested by reports of altered sensory deficits.

PLANNING

- Utilise social work services to facilitate securing accommodation.
- Organise for directly observed medical therapy (DOT) to increase medication compliance and reduce multidrug-resistant TB.
- Identify verbally and in writing manifestations to report to the doctor.

Expected outcomes

- Keep all follow-up appointments as scheduled.
- Verbalise an understanding of his disease and its treatment.
- Follow the prescribed plan of care.
- Demonstrate measures to prevent spread of the organism to others.
- Gain 0.5–1 kg of weight per week.
- Promptly report symptoms of peripheral neuropathy, including numbness, tingling or burning sensations.

IMPLEMENTATION

- Teach about TB and provide an educational pamphlet about the disease.
- Instruct about the prescribed medications, potential adverse effects and the importance of completing the entire prescribed regimen.
- Emphasise the importance of continued follow up.
- Teach and demonstrate sputum and droplet control measures.

EVALUATION

The healthcare team secures Mr Flanders accommodation and community assistance for DOT. He often still sleeps outside when the weather permits but he adheres to the requirement for supervised medication administration because he 'likes the food there'. Always a clean person, Mr Flanders is able to demonstrate appropriate sputum control measures and practises them faithfully. The sputum culture done after 2 months of treatment is negative for tubercle bacilli and his chest x-ray indicates no disease progression.

CRITICAL THINKING IN THE NURSING PROCESS

1. Many homeless people have schizophrenia or other mental diseases. How would you adapt the care plan for a homeless person with schizophrenia with active tuberculosis?
2. The public health nurse was fortunate to have access to an incentive shelter with healthcare workers to supervise medication compliance. Identify available resources in your area for homeless people infected with tuberculosis.
3. Develop a care plan for the nursing diagnosis of *Ineffective airway clearance* related to mucopurulent sputum and weak cough.

REFLECTION ON THE NURSING PROCESS

1. Outline what you have learned from this case study that you will apply to your future practice.
2. In this case study, accommodation was found for Mr Flanders. Consider the situation where an individual chooses not to accept accommodation. Given that tuberculosis is a public health issue, which next steps would be necessary?

Risk of infection

- Place a mask on the person during transport to other parts of the facility for diagnostic or treatment procedures. *Covering the person's nose and mouth during transport minimises air contamination and the risk to visitors and personnel.*
- Inform all personnel having contact with the person of the diagnosis. *This allows personnel to take appropriate precautions.*
- Assist visitors to put on a mask before entering the room. *Providing visitors with appropriate masks or respirators reduces their risk of infection.*
- Teach the person how to limit transmitting the disease to others:
  a. Always cough and expectorate into tissues.
  b. Dispose of tissues properly, placing them in a closed bag.
  c. Wear a mask if you are sneezing or unable to control respiratory secretions.
  d. The disease is not spread by touching inanimate objects, so no special precautions are required for eating utensils, clothing, books or other objects used.

Community-based care

Most people with TB are managed in community settings; few require institutionalisation. In addition to the teaching topics and strategies identified above, discuss the following topics when preparing the person and significant others for home care:

- importance of screening close contacts for infection and possibly prophylactic treatment
- effect, dose and timing for all medications, and potential side effects and their management
- importance of long-term therapy in eradicating the disease
- principles of good nutrition, dietary guidelines for a person with TB and other measures to help maintain good health, such as balancing rest with exercise
- signs and symptoms of complications to report to the doctor or healthcare provider.

Provide referrals as appropriate:

- smoking cessation clinics or support groups
- alcohol treatment facilities, Alcoholics Anonymous, other treatment programs or support groups
- drug treatment facilities, Narcotics Anonymous, other outpatient or inpatient treatment programs or support groups
- community clinics and incentive programs for people with TB
- counselling, support groups and other community resources that provide additional assistance and support.

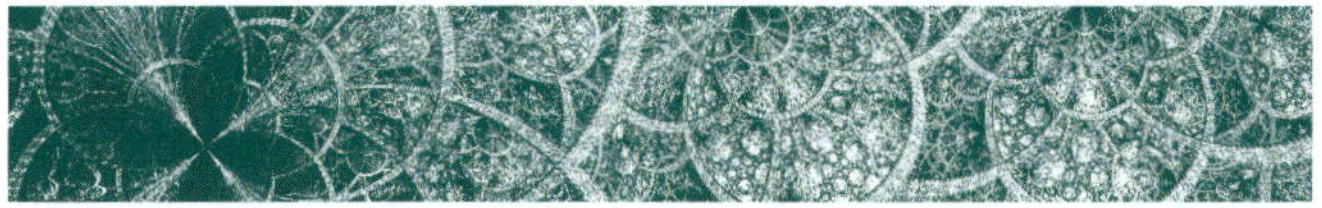

THE PERSON WITH A FUNGAL INFECTION

Fungal spores are endemic and present in the air everyone breathes. Normal respiratory defence mechanisms allow few of these spores to reach the lungs. If they reach the lungs, pulmonary macrophages and neutrophils efficiently remove them in most people. When they do cause infection, it is typically mild and self-limiting. Most fungi are opportunistic and can cause infection only in people who are immunocompromised. For this reason, people with AIDS, kidney failure, leukaemia, burns or chronic diseases, and those receiving corticosteroids or immunosuppressants are particularly susceptible to fungal infections.

The course and manifestations of fungal lung diseases resemble those of tuberculosis. Lung lesions are slow to develop, and symptoms are mild. The fungus can disseminate from the lung to other organs.

Pneumocystis carinii pneumonia

Pneumocystis carinii pneumonia (PCP) is caused by a fungus, recently renamed *Pneumocystis jirovecii*. PCP is common in people with AIDS, and others with significant immunocompromise are at risk of developing an opportunistic pneumonia. Opportunistic infection may develop in people treated with immunosuppressive or cytotoxic drugs for cancer or organ transplant and in people with genetic or acquired immunodeficiency.

Infection with PCP produces patchy involvement throughout the lungs, causing affected alveoli to thicken, become oedematous and fill with foamy, protein-rich fluid. Gas exchange is severely impaired as the disease progresses.

PCP has an abrupt onset with fever, tachypnoea, shortness of breath and a dry, non-productive cough. Respiratory distress can be significant, with intercostal retractions and cyanosis. Table 35.5 compares the manifestations of infectious pneumonias.

Aspergillosis

Aspergillus spores are common in the environment but rarely cause disease, except in immunocompromised people. When they cause infection, *Aspergillus* species invade blood vessels and produce hyphae that branch at acute angles, frequently causing venous or arterial thrombosis. In the lungs, aspergillosis can cause an acute, diffuse, self-limited pneumonitis. The manifestations of pulmonary aspergillosis include dyspnoea, non-productive cough, pleuritic chest pain, chills and fever. If the organism invades a pulmonary blood vessel, haemoptysis or massive pulmonary haemorrhage can occur (Harman, 2018). In individuals with underlying lung disease, balls of *Aspergillus* hyphae may form within cysts or cavities, usually in the upper lobes of the lung. When this occurs, symptoms often are milder and more insidious in onset, with fever, weight loss, night sweats and cough.

INTERPROFESSIONAL CARE

Most fungal lung infections can be diagnosed by microscopic examination of a sputum specimen for the fungus. Blood cultures also may be taken, as well as cultures of cerebrospinal fluid if indicated. A chest x-ray may show typical changes in lung tissue or widening of the mediastinum, depending on the infecting organism.

TABLE 35.5 Manifestations of infectious pneumonias

TYPE	ONSET	RESPIRATORY MANIFESTATIONS	SYSTEMIC MANIFESTATIONS
Pneumococcal or lobar pneumonia	Abrupt	Cough productive of purulent or rust-coloured sputum; pleuritic or aching chest pain; decreased breath sounds and crackles over affected area; possible dyspnoea and cyanosis	Chills and fever
Bronchopneumonia	Gradual	Cough, scattered crackles; minimal dyspnoea and respiratory distress	Low-grade fever
Legionnaires' disease	Gradual	Dry cough; dyspnoea	Chills and fever; general malaise; headache; confusion; anorexia and diarrhoea; myalgias and arthralgias
Primary atypical pneumonia	Gradual	Dry, hacking, non-productive cough	Fever, headache, myalgias and arthralgias predominate
Viral pneumonia	Sudden or gradual	Dry cough	Flu-like symptoms
Pneumocystis pneumonia	Abrupt	Dry cough; tachypnoea and dyspnoea; significant respiratory distress	Fever

A broad-spectrum antifungal agent is commonly prescribed to treat most fungal infections. Some fungal lung diseases and immunocompromised individuals are often treated with intravenous amphotericin B. Surgery (lobectomy) may be indicated for individuals with severe haemoptysis associated with aspergillosis.

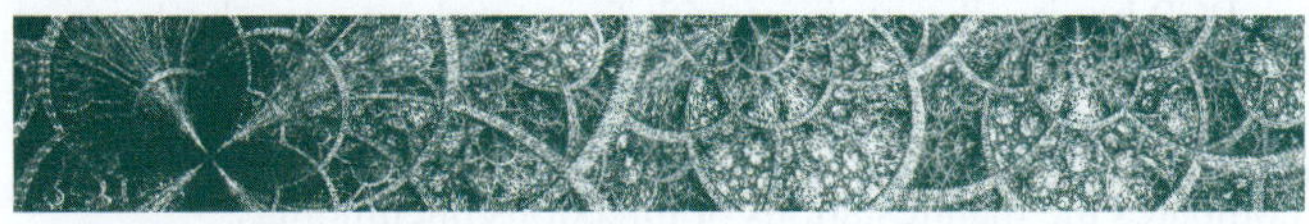

Nursing care

Depending on the disease and their immune status, people with fungal lung infections have different nursing care needs. For most people, nursing care focuses on education. People living in high-prevalence areas or who have specific risk factors such as exposure to bird droppings (e.g. by cleaning chicken coops, pigeon lofts or barns where birds roost), decomposed vegetation, rotting wood or stored grain need to be aware of the risk, common symptoms and measures to reduce the risk. Teach people receiving antifungal drugs about the specific drug, its intended and adverse effects, the duration of therapy and symptoms to report to the doctor. Include teaching about any specific precautions such as drug or food interactions. The person may require treatment with the antibiotic amphotericin B. This medication has many side effects which require management. The initial dose of amphotericin B should be administered slowly. In some instances, a pre-medication, such as an antihistamine and anti-emetic, may be indicated to reduce potential side effects. The person must be monitored carefully during an infusion of amphotericin B for changes in vital signs, hydration, nutrition, weight and urine output and managed as required.

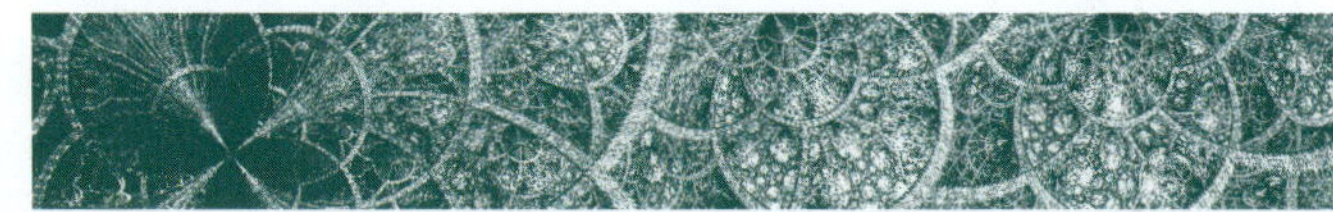

Disorders of the pleura

The *pleura* is a thin membrane with two layers: the visceral pleura, which overlies the lung surface; and parietal pleura, which lines the inner chest wall. A potential space between the pleura layers is the *pleural cavity*, which contains a thin layer of serous fluid. As the thoracic cavity expands during inspiration, the pressure in this space becomes negative to atmospheric and alveolar pressure. The expansible lung is drawn out, and air rushes into the alveoli. When the pleura is inflamed or affected by disease or injury, air or fluid can collect in the pleural cavity, restricting lung expansion, air movement and ventilation.

THE PERSON WITH PLEURITIS

Pleuritis (*pleurisy*), inflammation of the pleura, irritates sensory fibres of the parietal pleura, causing characteristic pain. Pleural inflammation occurs secondarily to another process, such as a viral respiratory illness, pneumonia or rib injury.

The onset of pleuritis is often abrupt. The pain is unilateral and well localised; it is usually sharp or stabbing in nature. Pain may be referred to the neck or the shoulder. Deep breathing, coughing and movement aggravate the pain. Respirations are rapid and shallow, and chest wall movement is limited on the affected side. Breath sounds are diminished, and a pleural friction rub may be heard over the site.

The diagnosis of pleuritis is based on its manifestations. Chest x-ray and ECG may be ordered to rule out other causes of chest pain. Treatment for pleuritis is symptomatic. Analgesics and non-steroidal anti-inflammatory drugs (NSAIDs)—indomethacin (Indocin), in particular—help relieve the pain. Codeine may be ordered, both to alleviate pain and suppress the cough at night to promote regular sleep patterns.

Nursing care for the person with pleuritis is directed towards promoting comfort, including administration of NSAIDs and analgesics. Positioning and splinting the chest while coughing is also helpful.

Teach the individual and family that pleuritis is generally self-limited and of short duration. Discuss symptoms to report to the doctor: high fever, productive cough or shortness of breath. Provide information about prescription and non-prescription NSAIDs and analgesics, including the drug ordered, how to use it and its desired and possible adverse effects.

THE PERSON WITH A PLEURAL EFFUSION

The pleural space typically contains only about 10–20 mL of serous fluid.

Pleural effusion is collection of excess fluid in the pleural space. Pleural effusions result from either systemic or local disease. Systemic disorders that may lead to pleural effusion include heart failure, liver or kidney disease and connective tissue disorders, such as rheumatoid arthritis and systemic lupus erythematosus (SLE). Pneumonia, atelectasis, tuberculosis, lung cancer and trauma are local conditions that may cause pleural effusion.

Pathophysiology and manifestations

Excess pleural fluid may be either *transudate*, formed when capillary pressure is high, or plasma proteins are low, or *exudate*, resulting in increased capillary permeability. Heart failure is the most common precipitating factor in transudate formation; it may also accompany kidney failure, nephrosis, liver failure and malignancy. Exudate, a protein-rich fluid, is seen with inflammatory processes such as infections, systemic inflammation (e.g. rheumatoid arthritis or SLE), pulmonary infarction (leading to tissue necrosis and inflammatory response) and malignancy (Bullock & Hales, 2019). Other pleural fluid collections include *empyema*, pus in the pleural cavity; *haemothorax*, the presence of blood in the cavity; *haemorrhagic pleural effusion*, a mixture of blood and pleural fluid; and *chylothorax*, a collection of lymph in the pleural space. In adults, chylothorax may be iatrogenic resulting from thoracic surgery or placement of a central line in one of the great veins (Adams, 2017).

A large pleural effusion compresses adjacent lung tissue. This causes the characteristic manifestation of dyspnoea. Pain may develop, although, with inflammatory processes, pleuritic pain often is relieved by formation of an effusion, as the fluid reduces friction between inflamed visceral and parietal pleura. Breath sounds are diminished or absent, and a dull percussion tone is heard over the affected area. Chest wall movement may be limited.

INTERPROFESSIONAL CARE

Chest x-ray often provides the first evidence of a pleural effusion. Because fluid typically collects in dependent regions, it is seen at the base of the affected lung on an upright chest x-ray and along the lateral wall when the person is positioned on the affected side. CT scans and ultrasonography also are used to localise and differentiate pleural effusions.

Thoracentesis

If the cause of pleural effusion is not apparent, a thoracentesis is undertaken. **Thoracentesis** is an invasive procedure in which fluid (or occasionally air) is removed from the pleural space with a needle. Aspirated fluid is analysed for appearance, cell counts, protein and glucose content, the presence of enzymes such as LDH and amylase, abnormal cells and culture.

When the pleural effusion is significant and interferes with respirations, thoracentesis is the treatment of choice to remove the fluid (see Figure 35.13). Thoracentesis may be performed at the bedside, in a procedure room or as an outpatient by a trained specialist. Local anaesthesia is used and the procedure can be performed in less than 30 minutes. Percussion, auscultation, radiography or ultrasonography are used to locate the effusion and needle insertion site. The fluid removed is limited to 1,200–1,500 mL at one time to reduce the risk of cardiovascular collapse from the rapid removal of too much fluid. Pneumothorax is a possible complication of thoracentesis if the visceral pleura is punctured or a closed drainage system is not maintained during the procedure. Nursing care for the person undergoing a thoracentesis is outlined in the accompanying box.

Treatments

Because pleural effusion usually occurs secondarily to another disease or disorder, medical management also focuses on treating the underlying condition to prevent further fluid accumulation. An empyema may require repeated drainage as well as high doses of parenteral antibiotics. Occasionally, thoracotomy and surgical excision may be necessary. See the box later in this chapter for nursing care of the person having lung surgery. Recurrent pleural effusions, often due to cancer, may be prevented by instilling an irritant, such as talc, into the pleural space to cause adhesion of the parietal and visceral pleura (*pleurodesis*). Water-seal chest tube drainage is often employed for haemothorax.

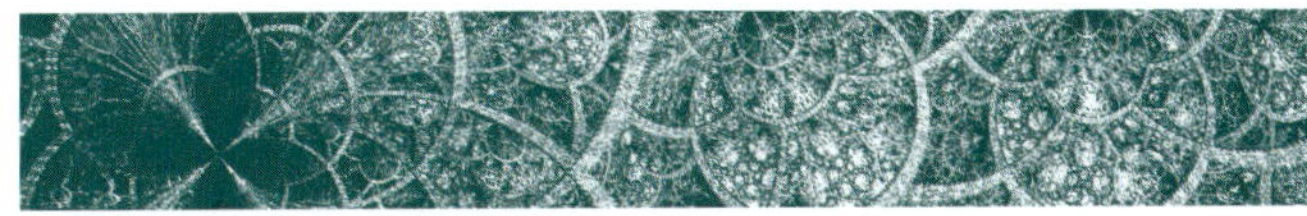

Nursing care

Nursing care for the person with a pleural effusion is directed towards supporting respiratory function and assisting with procedures to evacuate collected fluid. With a large pleural effusion and partial lung collapse, *Impaired gas exchange* and *Activity intolerance* are high-priority nursing problems. *Risk of impaired gas exchange* is a priority problem during the initial period following thoracentesis.

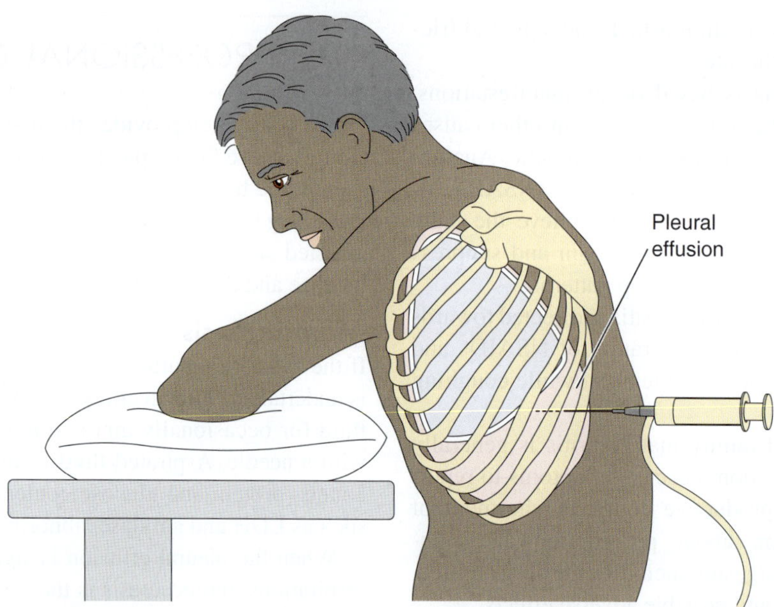

FIGURE 35.13 ***Thoracentesis. With the person seated, a needle is inserted between the ribs into the pleural space to withdraw accumulated fluid***

Teaching for home care focuses on symptoms of recurrent effusion or complications following a thoracentesis to report to the doctor: increasing dyspnoea, cough and haemoptysis. Pleuritic pain may be an early sign of effusion and should also be reported. Further teaching about an underlying condition also may be necessary; for example, the person with heart failure may need education about a salt-restricted diet.

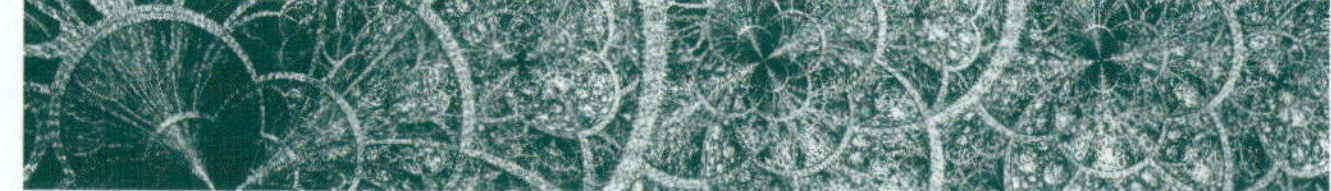

NURSING CARE OF THE PERSON having a thoracentesis

BEFORE THE PROCEDURE

- Verify a signed informed consent for the procedure. *This invasive procedure requires informed consent.*
- Assess knowledge and understanding of the procedure and its purpose; provide additional information as needed. *A fully informed person will be less apprehensive and more able to cooperate during the thoracentesis.*
- Pre-procedure fasting or sedation is not required. *Only local anaesthesia is used in this procedure and the gag and cough reflexes remain intact.*
- Administer a cough suppressant if indicated. *Movement and coughing during the procedure may cause inadvertent damage to the lung or pleura.*
- Obtain a thoracentesis tray, sterile gloves, injectable lignocaine, povidone-iodine, dressing supplies and an extra over-bed table or Mayo stand. *These supplies are used by the doctor performing the procedure.*
- Position the person upright, leaning forward with arms and head supported on an anchored over-bed table. *This position spreads the ribs, enlarging the intercostal space for needle insertion.*
- Inform the person that, although local anaesthesia prevents pain as the needle is inserted, a sensation of pressure may be felt. *A pressure sensation occurs as the needle punctures the parietal pleura to enter the pleural space.*

DURING AND AFTER THE PROCEDURE

- Monitor pulse, colour, oxygen saturation and other signs during thoracentesis. *These are indicators of physiological tolerance to the procedure.*
- Apply a dressing over the puncture site and position on the unaffected side for 1 hour. *This allows the pleural puncture to heal.*
- Label obtained specimen with name, date, time and source; send the specimen to the laboratory for analysis. *Fluid obtained during thoracentesis may be examined for abnormal cells, bacteria and other substances to determine the cause of the pleural effusion.*
- During the first several hours after thoracentesis, frequently assess and document vital signs, oxygen saturation, respiratory status, including respiratory excursion, lung sounds, cough or haemoptysis; and puncture site for bleeding or crepitus. *Frequent assessment is essential to detect possible early complications of thoracentesis, such as pneumothorax.*
- Obtain a chest x-ray. *Chest x-ray is ordered to detect possible pneumothorax.*
- Normal activities generally can be resumed after 1 hour if no evidence of pneumothorax or other complications present. *The puncture wound of thoracentesis heals rapidly.*

THE PERSON WITH PNEUMOTHORAX

Accumulation of air in the pleural space is called **pneumothorax**. Pneumothorax can occur spontaneously, without apparent cause, as a complication of pre-existing lung disease, as a result of blunt or penetrating trauma to the chest, or from an iatrogenic cause (e.g. following thoracentesis).

Pathophysiology

Pressure in the pleural space is normally negative to atmospheric pressure. This negative pressure is vital to the process of breathing. Contraction of the diaphragm and the intercostal muscles enlarges the thoracic space. Negative intrapleural pressure draws the lung outwards, increasing its volume, so air rushes in to fill the expanded lung space.

When either the visceral or the parietal pleura is breached, air enters the pleural space, equalising this pressure. Lung expansion is impaired, and the natural recoil tendency of the lung causes it to collapse to a greater or lesser extent, depending on the size and rapidity of air accumulation. Table 35.6 illustrates the classifications of pneumothorax.

Spontaneous pneumothorax

Spontaneous pneumothorax develops when an air-filled bleb on the lung surface ruptures. A bleb is a small, subpleural, thin-walled air-containing space like a blister. Rupture allows air from the airways to enter the pleural space. Air accumulates until pressures are equalised or until the collapse of the involved lung section seals the leak. Spontaneous pneumothorax may be either *primary* (*simple*) or *secondary* (*complicated*).

Primary pneumothorax affects men who are relatively well, most often smokers, usually tall, slender and between ages 18 and 40 (Daley, 2018). The cause of primary pneumothorax is unknown. Air-filled blebs tend to form in the apices of the lungs. This is considered to be a benign condition, although recurrences are common. Certain activities also increase the risk of spontaneous pneumothorax, such as high-altitude flying and rapid decompression during scuba diving.

Secondary pneumothorax, generally caused by overdistension and rupture of an alveolus, is more serious and potentially life threatening. It develops in people with underlying lung disease, usually COPD. Middle-aged and older adults are primarily affected. Secondary pneumothorax also may be associated with asthma, cystic fibrosis, pulmonary fibrosis, tuberculosis, acute respiratory distress syndrome (ARDS) and other lung diseases. Rarely, a form of secondary pneumothorax called *catamenial pneumothorax* can develop in affected women within 24 to 48 hours of the onset of menstrual flow.

MANIFESTATIONS The manifestations of spontaneous pneumothorax depend on the cause/size of the pneumothorax, extent of lung collapse and any underlying lung disease. Typically, pleuritic chest pain and shortness of breath begin abruptly, often while at rest. The respiratory and heart rates increase as gas exchange is affected. Chest wall movement may be asymmetrical, with less movement on the affected side than the unaffected side. The affected side is hyperresonant to percussion and breath sounds may be diminished or absent. Hypoxaemia may develop, although normal mechanisms that shunt blood flow to the unaffected lung often maintain normal oxygen saturation levels. Hypoxaemia is more pronounced in secondary pneumothorax.

Traumatic pneumothorax

Blunt or penetrating trauma of the chest wall and pleura can cause pneumothorax. Blunt trauma—for example, due to a motor vehicle crash, fall or during cardiopulmonary resuscitation (CPR)—can lead to a *closed pneumothorax*. Fractured ribs penetrating the pleura are the leading cause of pneumothorax due to blunt trauma (Daley, 2018). Fracture of the trachea and a ruptured bronchus or oesophagus also may result from blunt trauma, leading to closed pneumothorax.

Open pneumothorax (*sucking chest wound*) results from penetrating chest trauma such as a stab wound, gunshot wound or impalement injury. With an open pneumothorax, air moves freely between the pleural space and the atmosphere through the wound. Pressure on the affected side equalises with the atmosphere and the lung collapses rapidly. The result is significant hypoventilation.

Iatrogenic pneumothorax may result from puncture or laceration of the visceral pleura during central-line placement, thoracentesis or lung biopsy. During bronchoscopy, bronchi or lung tissue can be disrupted. Alveoli can become overdistended and rupture during anaesthesia, resuscitation procedures or mechanical ventilation.

MANIFESTATIONS With traumatic pneumothorax, manifestations of pain and dyspnoea may be masked or missed due to other injuries. Tachypnoea and tachycardia may be attributed to the primary injury. Focused assessment for evidence of pneumothorax is vital. Chest wall movement on the affected side is diminished and breath sounds are absent. If a penetrating wound is present, air may be heard and felt moving through it with respiratory efforts. Haemothorax frequently accompanies traumatic pneumothorax. The manifestations of iatrogenic pneumothorax are similar to those of spontaneous pneumothorax.

Tension pneumothorax

Tension pneumothorax develops when injury to the chest wall or lungs allows air to enter the pleural space but prevents it from escaping. Pressure within the pleural space becomes positive in relation to atmospheric pressure as air rapidly accumulates with each breath. The lung on the affected side collapses, and pressure on the mediastinum shifts thoracic organs to the unaffected side of the chest, placing pressure on the opposite lung as well. Ventilation is severely compromised and venous return to the heart is impaired. Tension pneumothorax is a medical emergency requiring immediate intervention to preserve respiration and cardiac output.

MANIFESTATIONS In addition to manifestations of pneumothorax, hypotension and distended neck veins are evident as venous return and cardiac output are affected. The trachea is displaced towards the unaffected side due to the mediastinal shift. Signs of shock may be present. See the chapter 'Nursing care of people experiencing trauma and shock' for the manifestations and treatment of shock.

TABLE 35.6 Types of pneumothorax

TYPE	PATHOPHYSIOLOGY	MANIFESTATIONS
A Spontaneous	Rupture of a bleb on the lung surface allows air to enter pleural space from airways. ▪ *Primary pneumothorax* affects previously healthy people. ▪ *Secondary pneumothorax* affects people with pre-existing lung disease (e.g. COPD).	▪ Abrupt onset ▪ Pleuritic chest pain ▪ Dyspnoea, shortness of breath ▪ Tachypnoea, tachycardia ▪ Unequal lung excursion ▪ Decreased breath sounds and hyperresonant percussion tone on affected side
B Traumatic 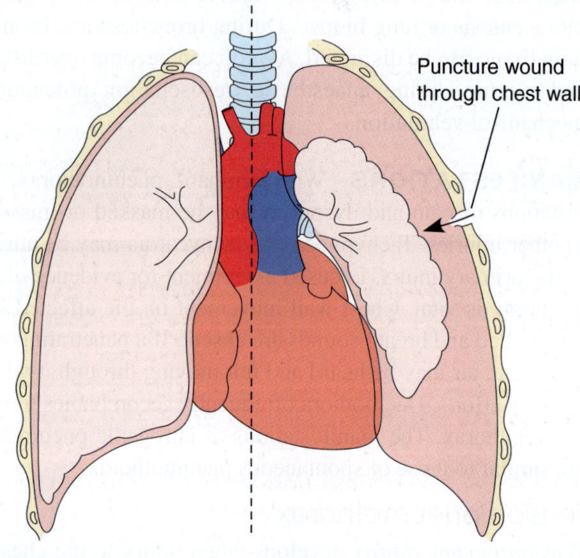	Trauma to the chest wall or pleura disrupts the pleural membrane. ▪ *Open* occurs with penetrating chest trauma that allows air from the environment to enter the pleural space. ▪ *Closed* occurs with blunt trauma that allows air from the lung to enter the pleural space. ▪ *Iatrogenic* involves laceration of visceral pleura during a procedure such as thoracentesis or central-line insertion.	▪ Pain ▪ Dyspnoea ▪ Tachypnoea, tachycardia ▪ Decreased respiratory excursion ▪ Absent breath sounds in affected area ▪ Air movement through an open wound
C Tension 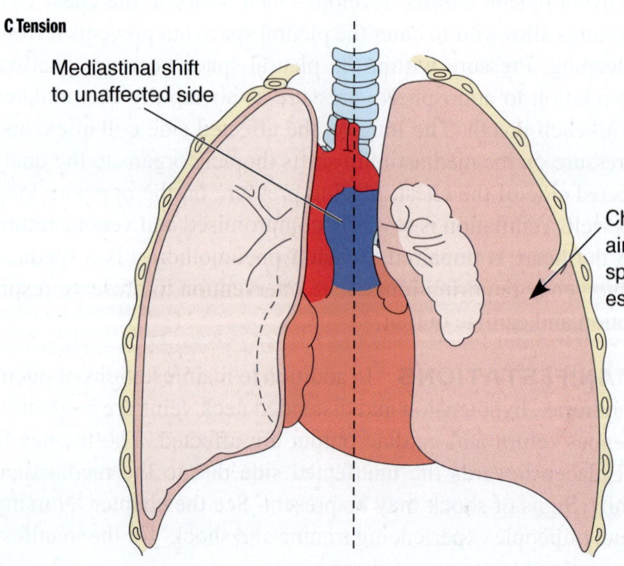	Air enters pleural space through chest wall or from airways but is unable to escape, resulting in rapid accumulation. Lung on affected side collapses. As intrapleural pressure increases, heart, great vessels, trachea and oesophagus shift towards the unaffected side.	▪ Hypotension, shock ▪ Distended neck veins ▪ Severe dyspnoea ▪ Tachypnoea, tachycardia ▪ Decreased respiratory excursion ▪ Absent breath sounds on affected side ▪ Tracheal deviation towards unaffected side

INTERPROFESSIONAL CARE

Treatment for a pneumothorax depends on the severity of the problem. A small, simple pneumothorax may require no treatment other than monitoring with serial x-rays. Air is absorbed from the pleural space, allowing most small pneumothoraces to resolve spontaneously. A large pneumothorax with significant symptoms usually requires treatment with *thoracostomy* or the placement of chest tubes. Surgical intervention may be necessary to prevent recurrent spontaneous pneumothorax.

Diagnosis

Oxygen saturation measurements are obtained to evaluate the effect of pneumothorax on gas exchange. ABGs may be taken to assess gas exchange further.

The chest x-ray is an effective diagnostic tool for pneumothorax. In tension pneumothorax, air is evident on the affected side and mediastinal structures are shifted towards the opposite or unaffected side.

Treatments

CHEST TUBES The treatment of choice for significant pneumothorax is the placement of a closed-chest catheter to allow the lung to re-expand. When a tube is placed in the pleural cavity to remove air or fluid, it must be sealed to prevent air from also entering the tube and, in essence, creating an open pneumothorax.

Chest tubes are sealed with a Heimlich (one-way) valve (see Figure 35.14) or connected to a closed drainage system with a 'water seal'. The valve or water seal prevents air from entering the chest cavity during inspiration and allows air to escape during expiration. Applying a low level of suction to the system helps to re-establish negative pressure in the pleural space, allowing the lung to re-expand. A number of closed-drainage chest tube systems are available. Most are self-contained disposable systems (see Figure 35.15). Drainage from the chest tube is collected in the first collection chamber. This sealed chamber is connected to a water seal chamber, which is connected to the suction control chamber. Nursing care of the person with chest tubes is discussed in the accompanying box.

A large-bore needle or plastic intravenous catheter may be inserted through the chest wall as emergency treatment of a tension pneumothorax. This allows air to escape from the affected side, relieving pressure on mediastinal structures and the opposite lung.

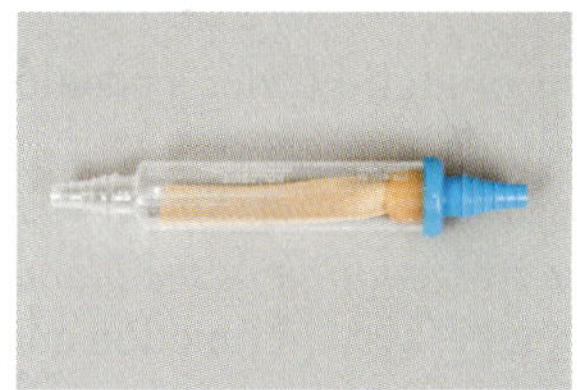

FIGURE 35.14 ***The Heimlich one-way valve allows air to escape from the pleural space, helping to re-establish negative pressure and allowing the lung to re-expand***

Source: George Draper/Pearson Education.

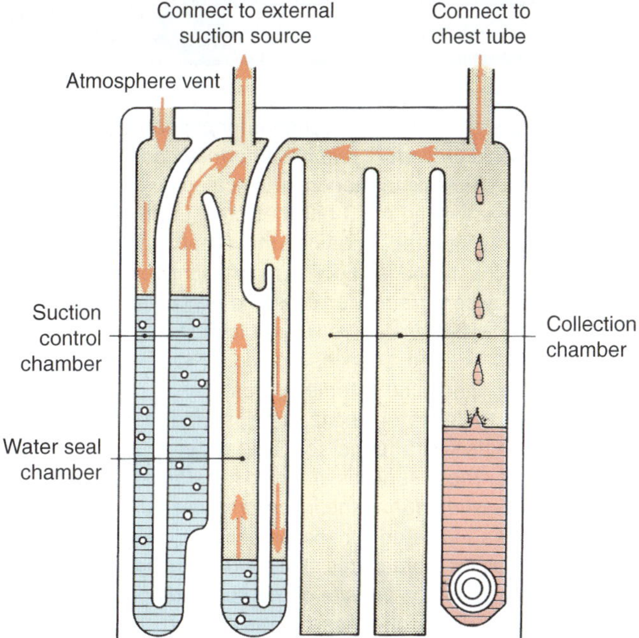

FIGURE 35.15 ***A closed-chest drainage system***

PLEURODESIS Although controversial, *pleurodesis*, or creation of adhesions between the parietal and visceral pleura, may be used to prevent recurrent pneumothorax. This procedure involves instilling a chemical agent such as talc into the pleural space. The subsequent inflammatory response creates scar tissue and adhesions between the pleural layers. This procedure reduces the recurrence rate of recurrent pleurodesis to as low as 2% but can make subsequent surgery more difficult (Daley, 2018).

Surgery

The risk of recurrence of spontaneous pneumothorax increases with each pleurodesis. People at high risk of recurrent pneumothorax may have surgery to reduce the risk of future ruptures. A thoracotomy is done to excise or over-sew blebs (usually at the apices of the lungs) to reduce the risk of complications. The overlying pleura is then roughened or irritated to induce scarring and adhesion to the surface of the lung. In some cases, the parietal pleura may be partially excised. These procedures can be done using video-assisted thoracoscopic surgery (VATS), a minimally invasive surgical technique (Daley, 2018). However, the procedure is conducted under a general anaesthetic.

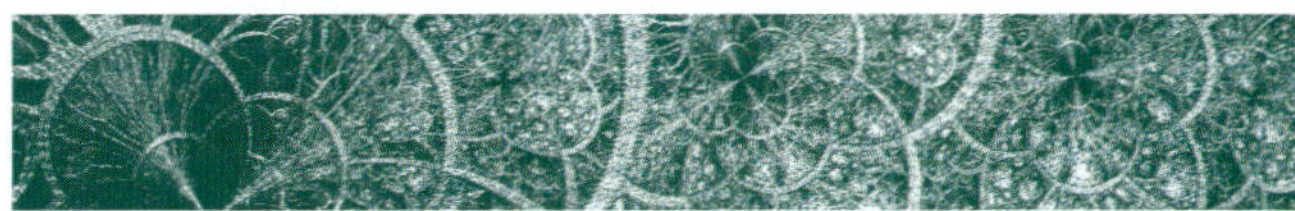

Nursing care

Health promotion

Health promotion activities to prevent spontaneous and traumatic pneumothorax primarily involve health teaching. Initiate and participate in programs to prevent smoking by children and

NURSING CARE OF THE PERSON with chest tubes

BEFORE THE PROCEDURE

- Ensure a signed informed consent for chest tube insertion. *This invasive procedure requires informed consent.*
- Provide additional information as indicated. Explain that local anaesthesia will be used but that pressure may be felt as the trocar is inserted. Reassure that breathing will be easier once the chest tube is in place and the lung re-expands. *The person may be extremely anxious and may need reassurance that this invasive procedure will provide relief.*
- Gather all needed supplies, including thoracostomy tray, injectable lignocaine, sterile gloves, chest tube drainage system, sterile water and a large, sterile, catheter-tipped syringe to use as a funnel for filling water-seal and suction chambers. *These supplies are used to establish a water-seal drainage system during the insertion procedure.*
- Position as indicated for the procedure. *Either an upright position (as for thoracentesis) or a side-lying position may be used, depending on the site of the pneumothorax.*
- Assist with chest tube insertion as needed. The procedure may be performed in a procedure room, in the surgical suite or at the bedside by a trained specialist. *Although chest tube insertion is a relatively simple procedure, nursing assistance is necessary to support the person and rapidly establish a closed drainage system.*
- Local anaesthetic will be given prior to insertion of the tube. *Administer pain relief as required.*

AFTER THE PROCEDURE

- Patient vital signs are assessed as follows: 15 minutely for 1 hour and 1 hourly for 4 hours, then 4 hourly. *Frequent assessment is necessary to monitor respiratory status and the effect of the chest tube.*
- Maintain a closed system. Tape all connections and secure the chest tube to the chest wall. *These measures are essential to prevent inadvertent tube removal or disruption of system integrity.*
- Keep the intercostal catheter's underwater-seal drain system below chest level. *Pleural fluid drains into the collection apparatus by gravity flow.*
- Check tubes frequently for kinks or loops. *These could interfere with drainage and potentially cause a tension pneumothorax.*
- Check the water seal frequently. The water level should fluctuate with respiratory effort. If it does not, the system may not be patent or intact. Periodic air bubbles in the water-seal chamber are normal and indicate that trapped air is being removed from the chest. *Frequent assessment of the system is essential to ensure appropriate functioning.*
- Measure swinging, bubbling and drainage every hour, marking the level on the drainage chamber. Report drainage that is cloudy, in excess of 70 mL per hour or red, warm and free flowing. *Red, free-flowing drainage indicates haemorrhage; cloudiness may indicate an infection.*
- Periodically assess water level in the suction control chamber, adding water as necessary. *Adequate water in the suction control chamber prevents excess suction from being placed on delicate pleural tissue.*
- Assist with frequent position changes and sitting and ambulation as allowed. Chest tubes should not prevent the performance of permitted activities. *Care is needed to prevent inadvertent disconnection or removal of the tubes.*
- When the chest tube is removed, immediately apply a sterile occlusive dressing. *An occlusive dressing prevents air from re-entering the pleural space through the chest wound.*

teenagers. Teach safe behaviours such as always wearing a seat belt in a motor vehicle, driving safely and using precautions to prevent falls when working or spending recreation time in high-altitude environments.

Assessment

The person with pneumothorax may be in acute respiratory distress, necessitating rapid and focused assessment.

- *Health history*: current symptoms and duration; precipitating factors or activities if known; previous episodes of pneumothorax; smoking history; chronic pulmonary diseases such as COPD.
- *Physical assessment*: general appearance and degree of apparent respiratory distress; evidence of chest trauma; vital signs, oxygen saturation, skin colour, LOC; respiratory excursion, percussion tone and breath sounds anterior and posterior chest; neck vein inspection, position of the trachea; peripheral pulses.
- *Diagnostic tests*: chest x-ray, ABGs.

Nursing diagnoses and interventions

Maintaining or restoring adequate alveolar ventilation and gas exchange is the highest priority for the person with a pneumothorax. Chest tubes may interfere with physical mobility, contributing to an increased risk of injury.

Impaired gas exchange

Loss of negative pressure in the pleural cavity and the resulting collapse of lung tissue can cause poor chest expansion and loss of alveolar ventilation. As the pneumothorax is removed or reabsorbed, ventilation and gas exchange improves.

- Assess and document vital signs and respiratory status, including rate, depth, lung sounds and oxygen saturation, at least every 4 hours. *Frequent assessment is essential to monitor the adequacy of respirations and lung expansion.*
- Place in Fowler's or high-Fowler's position. *This position facilitates lung expansion.*
- Administer oxygen as ordered. *Supplemental oxygen is given to improve oxygenation of the blood and tissues.*
- Assess the chest tube, system function and drainage every hour. The system must remain patent and intact to function effectively. Assess swinging, bubbling and draining, replacing the water seal fluid as required.
- Provide rest. *Adequate rest is essential to conserve energy and reduce oxygen demand.*

> **CONSIDERATION FOR PRACTICE**
> **Provide emotional support, particularly during the early stages and chest tube insertion. Dyspnoea and hypoxaemia can cause extreme anxiety and apprehension, impairing the ability to cooperate with procedures.**

Risk of injury

Pain and the presence of chest tubes can reduce the perceived ability to ambulate and provide self-care. Moderate activity is encouraged unless respiratory function is significantly impaired. Caution is taken to maintain the integrity of the chest tube system. If the tube is inadvertently pulled out or system integrity is disrupted, the pneumothorax may increase, or infection may develop.

> **CONSIDERATION FOR PRACTICE**
> **Avoid placing tension on chest tubes during positioning, ambulation and care activities. The chest tubes are minimally secured to the chest wall and can be dislodged if tension is placed on them.**

- Secure a loop of drainage tubing to the gown. *Looping the drainage tubing prevents direct pressure on the chest tube itself.* Be sure not to dislodge the tube when removing the patient's gown.
- When turning to the affected side, ensure that neither the chest tube nor the drainage tubing is kinked or occluded under the person. *This maintains patency of the system.*
- Teach the person how to ambulate with the drainage system, keeping the system lower than the chest. In most cases, suction can be discontinued during ambulation. *Ambulation facilitates lung ventilation and expansion. Drainage systems are portable to allow ambulation while chest tubes are in place. Keeping the drainage system lower than the chest promotes drainage and prevents reflux.*
- Observe insertion site for redness, swelling, pain or drainage. Report any signs of infection, including fever, to the doctor. *Interruption of skin integrity by chest tube insertion increases the risk of infection.*
- If a connection comes loose, reconnect it as soon as possible. *A closed, sealed system is vital to prevent air from entering the pleural space and an open pneumothorax.*

Community-based care

People who have experienced spontaneous pneumothorax require education about their future risks. After a single episode of spontaneous pneumothorax, the risk of recurrence is 15–30%. This risk increases with subsequent episodes (Daley, 2018). Stress the importance of quitting smoking to reduce the risk. Other activities that precipitate recurrent episodes include exposure to high altitudes (such as mountain climbing), flying in unpressurised aircraft and scuba diving (Daley, 2018). The person may be advised to avoid contact sports.

Following a pneumothorax, instruct the person gradually to increase exercise and activity to previous levels. Stress the importance of follow-up care and monitoring. Discuss manifestations to report to the doctor: upper respiratory infections; fever, cough or difficulty breathing; sudden, sharp chest pain; or redness, pain, swelling, tenderness or drainage from the chest tube puncture wound.

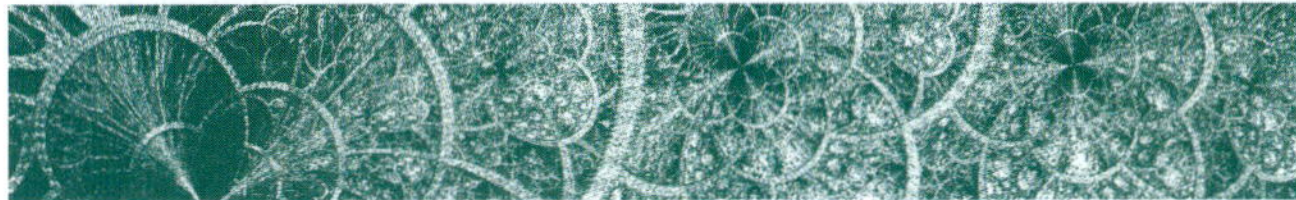

THE PERSON WITH HAEMOTHORAX

Haemothorax, or blood in the pleural space, usually occurs due to chest trauma, surgery or diagnostic procedures. Haemothorax develops in about 30–60% of people with chest trauma, usually due to a laceration of the lung, an intercostal vessel or the internal mammary artery. If a major thoracic vessel is disrupted, haemorrhage can be substantial (Mancini, 2018; Papadakis et al., 2022). Tumours, pulmonary infarction and infections such as tuberculosis also can cause haemothorax. When blood collects in the pleural space, pressure on the affected lung impairs ventilation and gas exchange. With significant haemorrhage, a high risk of shock exists.

Haemothorax causes symptoms similar to those of pneumothorax or pleural effusion. Lung sounds are diminished, and a dull percussion tone is noted over the collected blood, typically at the base of the lung. A chest x-ray is used to confirm the diagnosis of haemothorax.

Thoracentesis or thoracostomy with chest tube drainage removes blood from the pleural space. With significant haemorrhage (e.g. due to trauma or surgery), the blood may be collected for subsequent autotransfusion; this blood should be collected and reinfused within 4 hours. Strict aseptic technique is used in collecting the blood. It is collected through a gross particulate filter into a container primed with anticoagulant and reinfused when the container is full or when transfusion is necessary. Air is removed from the blood container before reinfusion and a filter is used to eliminate debris such as degenerating blood cells, fat particles and fibrin.

Priority nursing care for the person with haemothorax focuses on assessing and maintaining adequate respiratory function and cardiac output. The priority of care depends on the rate and extent of haemothorax. In a large, slow-developing haemothorax, the ventilatory status may be affected significantly. In this instance, *Impaired gas exchange* and *Ineffective breathing patterns* are priority nursing diagnoses. When haemothorax develops rapidly and haemorrhage is significant, additional priority nursing diagnoses include *Decreased cardiac output* and *Risk of deficient fluid volume*.

When preparing the person for home care following a haemothorax, discuss the importance of avoiding smoking and preventing respiratory infection. Include symptoms to report to the doctor. If trauma or infection caused the haemothorax, discuss measures to prevent future trauma and continue treatment for the infection as indicated.

Trauma of the chest or lung

Chest injury is a leading cause of death from trauma. It is commonly associated with motor vehicle crashes, violent crime and falls. Chest injuries can range from mild, such as a simple rib fracture, to severe and fatal. Traumatic injury to the chest may involve the chest wall and underlying thoracic structures, including the lungs, heart, great vessels and oesophagus. Chest and lung injury can result from several different mechanisms: penetrating trauma, such as a stab or gunshot wound; blunt trauma, such as a fall, motor vehicle accident (MVA), vehicle–pedestrian impact or crush injury; or inhalation injuries, such as smoke inhalation or immersion/submersion.

Rapid and continuing primary survey assessing airway, breathing and circulation (ABC) is vital in chest or lung injuries. Chest trauma can disrupt any or all of these functions. Chest injuries that may be life threatening include airway obstruction, tension pneumothorax, open pneumothorax, massive haemothorax and flail chest with pulmonary contusion.

THE PERSON WITH A THORACIC INJURY

Thoracic injuries may be minor and have little effect on respiratory status; for example, a simple rib fracture in a previously healthy person. The risk is more significant when pain or chest wall instability impairs breathing, or the underlying lung tissue is damaged. Thoracic trauma usually is caused by motor vehicle crashes or falls.

Pathophysiology and manifestations

Acceleration–deceleration injury and direct mechanisms of injury (e.g. crush injuries) are the most common mechanisms of thoracic injuries. Acceleration–deceleration injuries are caused by a rapid change in velocity such as in an MVA or fall. The body stops suddenly, but the tissues and organs within the chest cavity continue to move forward until they impact the chest wall. Injuries sustained can be significant, depending on the velocity (speed) of the vehicle or body at the point of impact, the surface with which the body impacts and individual characteristics (e.g. size and bone structure).

Rib fracture

Simple rib fracture, usually involving a single rib, is the most common chest wall injury. Rib fracture generally is tolerated well and heals rapidly in a young, previously healthy person. In an older adult or person with pre-existing lung disease, however, a fractured rib may lead to significant complications, such as pneumonia, atelectasis and, potentially, respiratory failure. Displaced fractured ribs can penetrate the pleura, leading to pneumothorax and possible haemothorax. Fractures of certain ribs are more frequently associated with underlying tissue damage. Intrathoracic vessels may be damaged or torn with fractures of the first and second ribs. Fractures of the seventh to tenth ribs may cause liver or spleen injuries.

Rib fracture causes pain on inspiration and coughing. This leads to voluntary splinting, with rapid, shallow respirations and inhibited coughing. Bruising may be seen over the fracture and crepitus may be palpated with respiratory movement. Breath sounds are diminished, especially in the bases, due to splinting. If pneumothorax develops, chest wall movement on the affected side may be reduced and breath sounds may be absent or significantly diminished. A hyperresonant percussion tone usually is noted. Haemothorax also causes diminished or absent breath sounds, with a dull percussion note on the affected side.

Flail chest

Multiple rib fractures may impair chest wall stability and normal chest wall function. When two or more consecutive ribs are fractured in multiple places, a free-floating segment of the chest wall, or **flail chest**, results. The physiological function of the chest wall is impaired as the flail segment is sucked inwards during inhalation and moves outwards with exhalation. This is known as *paradoxical movement* (see Figure 35.16).

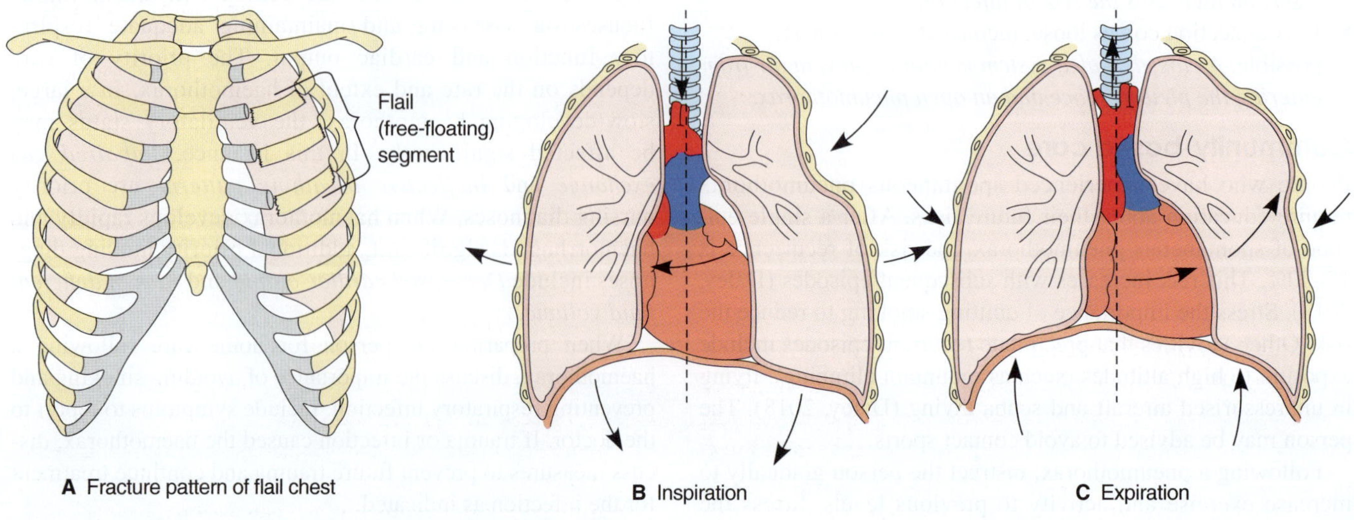

FIGURE 35.16 ***Flail chest with paradoxical movement***

A flail chest can significantly affect ventilation and, consequently, gas exchange. Lung expansion is impaired, and the work of breathing increases. A flail chest is frequently associated with underlying pulmonary contusion, which may lead to respiratory failure.

Flail chest causes dyspnoea and pain, especially on inspiration. Paradoxical chest movement is evident with inspection. Chest expansion is unequal and palpable crepitus is present. Breath sounds are diminished and crackles may be heard on auscultation.

Pulmonary contusion

Pulmonary contusion, or lung tissue injury, is frequently associated with flail chest and other blunt chest trauma. It may occur unilaterally or bilaterally. Pulmonary contusion often results from abrupt chest compression followed by sudden decompression, as can occur with MVA, a significant fall or crush injury. Alveoli and pulmonary arterioles rupture, causing intra-alveolar haemorrhage and interstitial and bronchial oedema. The resulting inflammatory response increases capillary permeability, leading to oedema, which may be localised to the damaged lung tissue or more generalised. Inflammation and oedema impair surfactant production within the alveoli, decreasing compliance. Pulmonary vascular resistance increases, and blood flow decreases. Airway obstruction, atelectasis and impaired gas diffusion result. Associated chest wall injury impairs the ability to clear secretions effectively and the work of breathing is significantly increased.

Manifestations of pulmonary contusion may not be apparent until 12 to 24 hours after the initial injury. Increasing shortness of breath, restlessness, apprehension and chest pain are early signs. Copious sputum, which may be blood tinged, is present. Later manifestations include tachycardia, tachypnoea, dyspnoea and cyanosis. Even with appropriate treatment, pulmonary contusion can lead to acute respiratory distress and potential death.

INTERPROFESSIONAL CARE

Diagnosis

A chest x-ray is used to identify most chest wall injuries. Rib fractures are evident on x-ray. Pulmonary contusion may show as initial patchy opacifications progressing to diffuse opacification or 'white out'. Changes in oxygen saturation and ABGs depend on the degree to which the injury affects ventilation and gas exchange.

Management

Simple rib fractures typically heal uneventfully. Providing adequate analgesia to promote breathing, coughing and movement is the primary intervention. An intercostal nerve block may be used with multiple rib fractures to ensure adequate ventilation. Rib belts, binders and taping to stabilise the rib cage are not recommended because they may interfere with ventilation and lead to atelectasis. Even with a simple rib fracture, older people and individuals with pre-existing lung disease require close monitoring to prevent and detect atelectasis, pneumonia and associated complications.

Intercostal nerve blocks or continuous epidural analgesia may be employed to manage the pain associated with flail chest. For a small flail chest, analgesia combined with supplemental oxygen therapy may be adequate. In some cases, internal or external fixation of the flail segment may be required.

Mechanical ventilation

The preferred treatment for flail chest is intubation and mechanical ventilation. Positive-pressure ventilation supports and stabilises the flail segment and improves ventilation and gas exchange. The work of breathing is decreased and healing improved.

People with pulmonary contusion often are critically ill, requiring intensive care management. Treatment is supportive, directed at maintaining adequate ventilation and alveolar gas exchange. Endotracheal intubation and mechanical ventilation are necessary in most cases. Repeated bronchoscopy may be done to remove secretions and cellular debris, preventing atelectasis. Although adequate hydration is necessary to prevent shock, overhydration can increase the risk of pulmonary oedema developing. Pulmonary arterial pressure monitoring with a Swan–Ganz catheter and frequent ABG measurement is sometimes used to assist in assessing optimal fluid replacement and managing ventilatory support. See the chapter 'Nursing care of people with gas exchange disorders' for nursing care of the person who is intubated and ventilated.

Unilateral pulmonary contusion may present a unique management problem. Mechanical ventilation with positive end-expiratory pressure (PEEP) to maintain open alveoli and adequate gas exchange can damage the unaffected lung. Intubation with a double-lumen endotracheal tube that permits independent lung ventilation may be used.

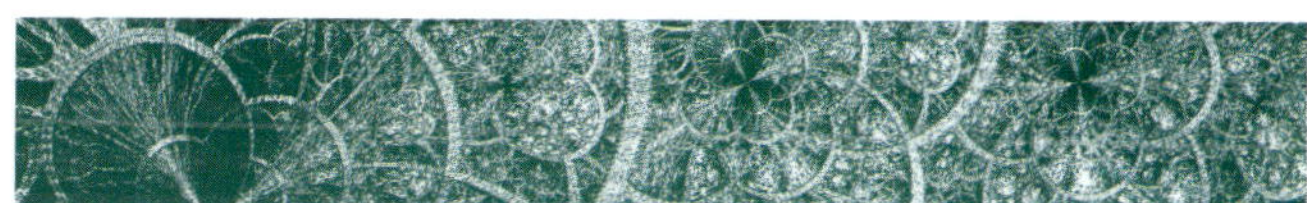

Nursing care

Health promotion

Encourage the use of seat belts, shoulder harnesses and supplemental restraint systems such as airbags to significantly reduce the incidence of thoracic injury associated with motor vehicle crashes. Discuss the importance of appropriate protective equipment and gear for people engaging in potentially hazardous activities such as contact sports or mountain climbing and occupations such as roofing or house painting.

Assessment

The nursing assessment of the person with a thoracic injury may need to be rapid and focused.

- *Health history*: pain, difficulty breathing; circumstances of the injury, including position in the motor vehicle, use of restraints, speed and type of impact; distance of a fall, surface, position and place on impact; history of chronic lung or heart disease; smoking history.
- *Physical examination*: airway, breathing, circulation; LOC; pallor, vital signs; respiratory rate, depth, ease; symmetry of chest movement; lung sounds and percussion tone; the presence of bruising, crepitus or paradoxical chest movement.

Nursing diagnoses and interventions

Chest wall trauma can interfere with adequate chest expansion and alveolar ventilation. Gas exchange is also affected when a pulmonary contusion is present. Priorities for nursing management include controlling pain, ensuring adequate ventilation and promoting gas exchange.

Acute pain

With many thoracic injuries, pain interferes with lung expansion and coughing, leading to complications such as pneumonia and atelectasis. Adequate pain management is a critical component of medical and nursing management for these individuals.

- Frequently assess pain using a standard pain scale and objective data. *Increased respiratory rate, shallow respirations, diminished breath sounds, reluctance to move and cough may indicate inadequate pain control in a thoracic injury.*
- Administer analgesics by patient-controlled analgesia or on a schedule to maintain pain control. *Analgesics are more effective when pain is not allowed to become intense.*

> **CONSIDERATION FOR PRACTICE**
> Assess for possible respiratory depression due to narcotic analgesia. Respiratory depression can further compromise ventilation in the person with thoracic injury.

- Notify the doctor if pain relief is inadequate or excess sedation and respiratory depression occur. An intercostal nerve block may reduce the need for narcotic analgesia. *Assess for bleeding and adequate ventilation following a nerve block.*

Ineffective airway clearance

Aggressive respiratory hygiene may be necessary to maintain open airways and adequate ventilation.

- Assess lung sounds and respiratory rate, depth and effort frequently. Encourage to cough, deep breathe, change position every 1 to 2 hours and use the incentive spirometer. *Frequent assessment and measures to maintain airway patency are vital to prevent complications in the person with thoracic injury.*
- Teach how to splint the affected area with a blanket or pillow when coughing. *Splinting reduces movement and discomfort of the affected area.*
- Suction airway as indicated. Work with respiratory therapy to maintain optimal mechanical ventilation. Secure the endotracheal tube to maintain appropriate position and lung ventilation. *Endotracheal tube security is critical when a double-lumen endotracheal tube is in place because malposition can occlude one main bronchus and prevent ventilation of the affected lung.*
- Elevate the head of the bed. *Elevating the head of the bed facilitates lung expansion and reduces the work of breathing.*

Impaired gas exchange

Impaired gas exchange is of particular concern in pulmonary contusion. Alveolar damage and pulmonary oedema can significantly impair blood oxygenation and carbon dioxide removal.

- Monitor vital signs, colour, oxygen saturation and ABGs. Assess for manifestations such as anxiety or apprehension, restlessness, confusion, lethargy or complaints of headache. *These assessment data alert the nurse and care providers to potential hypoxaemia or hypercapnia due to impaired gas exchange.*
- Maintain oxygen therapy and mechanical ventilation as ordered—hyperoxygenate prior to suctioning. Oxygen and mechanical ventilation support alveolar gas exchange. *Hyperoxygenation prior to suctioning reduces the degree of hypoxaemia that occurs during suctioning.*
- Monitor intake and output, weigh daily and monitor central venous pressure and pulmonary artery pressure as ordered. Maintain any ordered fluid restriction. *Fluid volume status is monitored to reduce the effects of pulmonary oedema on lung tissues.*
- Maintain bed rest or activity restriction as ordered. Space activities to allow periods of uninterrupted rest. *Rest reduces the metabolic rate and oxygen consumption.*

Community-based care

Simple rib fractures and minor chest wall injuries often are managed on an outpatient basis. Include the following topics when teaching for home care:

- pain management and its importance in preventing respiratory complications
- importance of coughing and deep breathing; how to splint the rib cage during coughing
- reasons for not taping or wrapping the chest
- symptoms to report to the doctor: chills and fever, productive cough, purulent or bloody sputum, shortness of breath and increasing chest pain
- avoiding respiratory irritants, such as cigarette smoke and occupational or environmental pollutants.

A significant pulmonary contusion can result in long-term respiratory insufficiency. Discuss activity modifications and occupational changes with the person and family as indicated. Refer to home care services if needed.

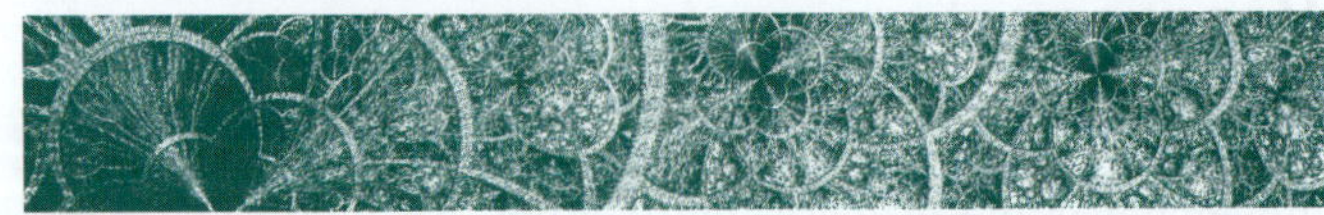

THE PERSON WITH INHALATION INJURY

The lungs' internal environment is normally protected from noxious substances by respiratory defence mechanisms. If these defences are breached, inhaled agents, such as gases, fumes, toxins and water, can cause internal lung trauma.

Pathophysiology and manifestations

Smoke inhalation

Pulmonary injury due to inhalation of hot air, smoke, toxic gases or particulate matter is the leading cause of death in burn injury (Galeiras, 2021). Smoke inhalation can significantly affect normal respiratory function through three different mechanisms:

1. thermal damage to the airways, leading to impaired ventilation
2. carbon monoxide or cyanide poisoning, resulting in tissue hypoxia
3. chemical damage to the lung from noxious gases, which can impair gas exchange.

Smoke inhalation is suspected whenever a burn occurs in a closed space; if there are burns to the face or upper torso or singed nasal hairs; if sputum contains ash-like material; and when manifestations such as dyspnoea, wheezing, or rales develop.

The lower airways of the lungs are typically protected from thermal damage by cooling the inhaled gases in the upper airway and laryngeal spasm. Upper airway obstruction due to tissue oedema and laryngeal spasm can occur quickly, resulting in **asphyxiation**, or oxygen deprivation, without lung damage. Steam inhalation can cause thermal damage to tissues of the lower respiratory tract.

Inhalation of carbon monoxide or cyanide gas poses an immediate threat to life. Carbon monoxide is a colourless, odourless gas produced in a fire. It binds readily with haemoglobin. The affinity of carbon monoxide for haemoglobin is 200 to 250 times stronger than that of oxygen. Haemoglobin bound to carbon monoxide reduces the oxygen-carrying capacity of blood and oxygen delivery to cells of the body. Carbon monoxide poisoning is suspected if the burn occurred in a closed space, if there is evidence of inhalation injury or if dyspnoea develops.

The manifestations of carbon monoxide poisoning depend on the level of carboxyhaemoglobin saturation. When haemoglobin is 10–20% saturated with carbon monoxide, symptoms include headache, dizziness, dyspnoea and nausea. A characteristic cherry-red colour of the skin and mucous membranes may be seen. With increasing levels, confusion, visual disturbances, irritability, hallucinations, hypotension, seizures and coma develop. Permanent neurological deficit can occur in survivors of severe, acute carbon monoxide poisoning.

Many other toxic chemicals may be present in smoke, especially in a house fire or industrial plant fire. Hydrogen cyanide can be lethal when inhaled. Inhalation of toxic chemicals causes bronchospasm and oedema of the airways and alveoli. Acute respiratory distress syndrome may develop within 1 to 2 days. Sloughing of damaged mucosa leads to airway obstruction and atelectasis. Pneumonia is common following smoke inhalation.

Immersion/submersion

Immersion/submersion (previously known as near drowning) is a leading cause of preventable accidental death in Australia. Between July 2016 and June 2017, 291 people died of drowning (Royal Life Saving Society, 2018). In 2014–2015, 566 people were admitted to hospital for an immersion/submersion (AIHW, 2019).

In a small percentage of drowning victims, laryngeal spasm causes asphyxiation, not the aspiration of water. This is known as 'dry drowning'. However, in most cases, asphyxiation and hypoxaemia result from fluid aspiration. Loss of consciousness can occur within 3 to 5 minutes after total immersion. Circulatory impairment, brain injury and brain death can occur within 5 to 10 minutes. Immersion in icy water and the *dive reflex*—a protective mechanism that slows the heartbeat, constricts peripheral vessels and shunts blood to the brain and heart—may prolong survival.

When aspirated, the type of water will directly affect the outcome. Freshwater is hypotonic; when aspirated, it is rapidly absorbed from the alveoli, leading to hypervolaemia and haemodilution. Haemolysis occurs as blood cells are subjected to a hypotonic environment, and serum electrolytes are diluted. Electrolyte imbalances can cause cardiac arrhythmias and death. Haemolysis can lead to acute tubular necrosis and acute kidney failure. Aspiration of freshwater impairs pulmonary surfactant and damages the alveolar–capillary membrane. Respiratory failure can result. Nearly the opposite effects occur with saltwater aspiration. As a hypertonic fluid, saltwater draws fluid into the alveoli, resulting in hypovolaemia. Haemolysis is insignificant and small elevations in serum sodium, and chloride levels rarely cause life-threatening effects. With either type of immersion/submersion episode, inhaled microorganisms and debris can lead to pneumonia. The pathophysiological changes associated with freshwater and saltwater immersion/submersion are illustrated in Figure 35.17.

Manifestations of immersion/submersion may include altered LOC, restlessness and apprehension. The person may complain of headache or chest pain. Other signs include vomiting, possible cyanosis, apnoea, tachypnoea and wheezing. If pulmonary oedema is present, pink froth may be visible in the mouth and nose. Other manifestations include tachycardia, arrhythmias, hypotension, shock and cardiac arrest. Hypothermia may be present.

INTERPROFESSIONAL CARE

With inhalation injuries, the most effective treatment is prevention. A working smoke detector (with functioning batteries) could prevent the majority of deaths from smoke inhalation occurring in the home. The statement, 'A smoke detector was found, but the batteries had been removed' is all too familiar in news reports of fire-related deaths.

The second most important line of defence against death or permanent injury from inhalation injuries is removing the victim from the area of the fire or water and administering effective CPR. In many cases, immediate restoration of effective breathing and circulation is key to preserving life. Hypoxaemia progresses rapidly until breathing is restored; reversal of tissue hypoxia depends on adequate circulation. In both smoke inhalation and immersion/submersion, intubation may be necessary to establish a patent airway. Oxygen is administered as soon as possible. Attempts to drain water from the lungs of the immersion/submersion victim can waste time

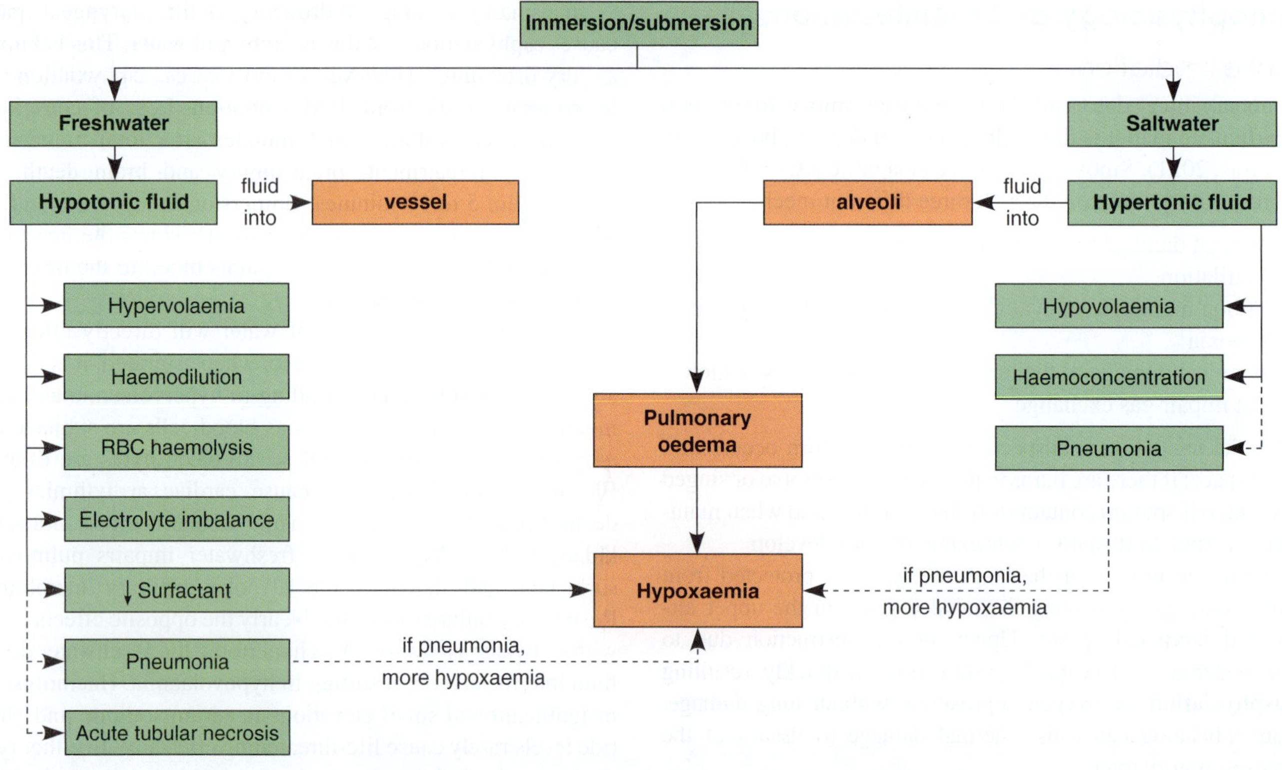

FIGURE 35.17 *The pathogenesis of immersion/submersion: freshwater and saltwater*

and is generally ineffective in restoring alveolar ventilation. External cardiac defibrillation may be necessary to re-establish an effective cardiac rhythm and circulation. When the victim is hypothermic, resuscitation measures are continued until the core body temperature reaches approximately 32°C. The basic rule in hypothermia is that the person is not declared dead until the body has been rewarmed and life signs remain absent.

To prevent drowning, life preservers and flotation vests or jackets should be worn on the body, not stored in the hold of the boat, when people are sailing and involved in any boat activities. These devices are designed to keep the head above water. Even accomplished swimmers should never enter the water alone in unguarded areas. Just as alcohol and driving do not mix, neither do alcohol and boating or other water sports.

Diagnosis

When inhalation injury is known or suspected, the following diagnostic tests may be done:

- *ABGs* are drawn to evaluate gas exchange and the degree of hypoxaemia. Combined respiratory and metabolic acidosis may be apparent. With effective ventilation and supplemental oxygen, acidosis may reverse quickly. With carbon monoxide poisoning, arterial PO_2 may be normal but oxyhaemoglobin saturation is less than normal.
- *Carboxyhaemoglobin levels* are drawn in suspected carbon monoxide poisoning. Normal levels are less than 5% in non-smokers and less than 10% in smokers. Higher levels indicate carbon monoxide poisoning. Levels less than 20% are considered mild poisoning; between 20% and 40% is moderate poisoning; and 40% to 60% is severe poisoning. Levels higher than 60% are generally fatal. *Serum electrolytes* and *osmolality levels* vary in immersion/submersion, depending on the type of water aspirated. In freshwater drowning, serum electrolyte levels and osmolality may be significantly reduced. With saltwater drowning, serum sodium and chloride may be somewhat high, and osmolality is increased because of hypovolaemia.
- *Chest x-ray* is done but may not show changes until 12 or more hours after the insult. Evidence of ARDS may be seen 24 to 48 hours after inhalation injury.
- *Bronchoscopy* may be ordered to inspect damaged lung tissue, particularly with smoke inhalation and possible thermal injury.

Treatments

Treatment of inhalation injury is generally supportive. Endotracheal intubation and mechanical ventilation often are required to maintain the airway and provide adequate alveolar ventilation and oxygenation. All people with inhalation injuries require supplemental oxygen, even when intubation and ventilation are not needed. *Hyperbaric oxygen therapy*, the delivery of 100% oxygen at increased atmospheric pressure, may be used to treat carbon monoxide poisoning. This treatment carries some risks, such as oxygen toxicity and potential trauma to lung tissues, sinuses and ears due to the increased pressure.

Other treatment measures may include bronchodilator therapy to manage bronchospasm. Bronchodilators can be administered by aerosol inhalation or intravenous infusion.

Coughing and suctioning are essential to remove secretions and debris. Chest physiotherapy with percussion and postural drainage may be performed.

Intravenous fluids may be ordered; if significant haemolysis has occurred, packed red blood cells may be given to improve the oxygen-carrying capacity of the blood. Fluid therapy is monitored carefully, using pulmonary artery or central venous pressures to reduce the risk of pulmonary oedema.

With immersion/submersion victims, measures such as inducing hypothermia or barbiturate-induced coma and administering corticosteroids and osmotic diuretics may be employed to help prevent neurological damage.

Careful monitoring for complications such as pneumonia and ARDS is vital throughout treatment. Respiratory status, vital signs and other data are frequently assessed to identify complications and allow early intervention and treatment.

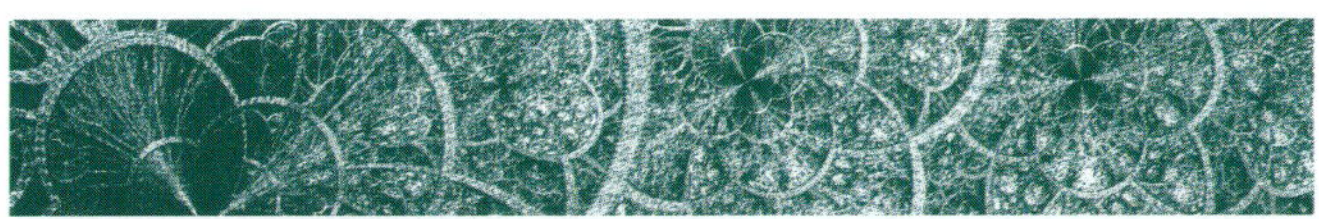

Nursing care

Health promotion

Prevention of inhalation injuries is an important nursing responsibility. Provide education on the value of having a working smoke detector, especially in the sleeping areas of the house. Encourage families to develop an escape plan in case of fire and to use fire drills to rehearse getting out of the house. Provide education on reducing smouldering cigarettes, a leading cause of house fires; help people develop a plan to stop smoking if this is a concern. Teach people to drop and roll should clothing catch fire. (Flames rise, increasing the risk of respiratory injury when upright.)

Learning to swim safely is essential to prevent drowning. Educate individuals never to swim alone when fatigued or immediately following a meal. Remind people that knowing how to swim will not prevent drowning in icy water or large bodies of water, such as lakes, rivers or the ocean. Instruct to always wear flotation devices while boating, water skiing, surfing, windsurfing or when participating in any water recreational activities. Wetsuits help prevent hypothermia during activities in icy water. Advise covering or fencing swimming pools and ponds to prevent inadvertent entry and drowning, and having a safely secured pool with a high fence and a gate with a self-closing latch to reduce the risk of infants entering a pool area unsupervised.

A population well trained in effective, safe CPR provides the best second line of defence against inhalation injury. Rapid restoration of breathing is essential to prevent hypoxia and brain damage. Encourage all people to be trained and regularly update CPR skills. Work with communities to increase the number of qualified people. Refer individuals to the Australian Red Cross, Surf Life Saving, St John's Ambulance or any other accredited CPR training facility.

Assessment

Inhalation injuries may be a medical emergency, necessitating focused and timely nursing assessment.

- *Health history*: circumstances of the injury, including duration of exposure to smoke or time underwater, explosion or fire in a closed area, type and temperature of water immersed in; resuscitation measures used; allergies and current medical problems.
- *Physical examination*: airway, breathing, circulation; LOC; pallor, oxygen saturation level; vital signs; heart and lung sounds; urine output; evidence of burns or soot around nares or mouth.
- *Diagnostic tests*: carboxyhaemoglobin levels, serum electrolytes and osmolality; ABGs; chest x-ray.

Nursing diagnoses and interventions

Nursing care priorities for the person with an inhalation injury are determined by the type of injury or tissue damage. Airway clearance is a major concern in all inhalation injuries, as is impaired gas exchange. Tissue hypoxia also can be a significant problem.

Ineffective airway clearance

Nursing measures to maintain an adequate airway begin with careful and frequent assessment of respiratory status, including rate, depth, effort and breath sounds. Note the amount, colour and consistency of sputum. Assist to cough frequently and suction the intubated person as needed to remove secretions. Elevate the head of the bed to facilitate alveolar ventilation unless otherwise ordered. If the person is intubated, stabilise the endotracheal tube to prevent displacement into a mainstem bronchus, which could lead to ventilation of only one lung. Report changes in the character of secretions that may indicate complications: pink, frothy sputum suggesting pulmonary oedema or purulent sputum suggestive of pneumonia. Administer bronchodilators as ordered. Perform percussion and postural drainage ordered.

Impaired gas exchange

Support gas exchange by administering supplemental oxygen, with or without mechanical ventilation, as required. Frequently assess oxygen saturation, skin colour and mental status. Decreasing level of consciousness may be an early sign of hypoxaemia. Monitor exhaled carbon dioxide, ABGs and pulmonary artery pressures as ordered and indicated. Report changes to the doctor. Maintain oxygen flow rates as ordered. Provide frequent mouth care to reduce the discomfort of dry mucous membranes and prevent tissue breakdown. Work with physiotherapists to maintain effective oxygen delivery with mechanical ventilation. Administer sedation as required. Maintain fluid restriction if ordered.

Ineffective cerebral tissue perfusion

Impaired cerebral tissue perfusion is a priority problem, especially with immersion/submersion. Hypoxia and possible hypervolaemia can lead to cerebral oedema and increased intracranial pressure (IICP), further impairing blood flow. Monitor vital signs and neurological status frequently.

A change in level of consciousness or behaviour is typically the earliest sign of IICP. Changes noted on an intracranial pressure monitor also provide early evidence of IICP. Increasing systolic blood pressure, pulse pressure and slowed heart rate are late signs. Other manifestations may include pupillary changes and decreasing muscle strength. Report changes promptly to the doctor. Elevate the head of the bed and keep the head in a neutral position to promote drainage from the cranial vault. Maintain effective ventilation and oxygenation; hypercapnia and hypoxaemia increase cerebral oedema. Administer sedation, osmotic diuretics or corticosteroids as ordered to reduce cerebral oedema. Maintain fluid restriction and a strict fluid balance record to monitor input and output. Space activities and promote rest to reduce metabolic demands.

Community-based care

Teach individuals who do not require hospitalisation for inhalation injury about symptoms that may indicate a complication and should be reported to the doctor: increasing dyspnoea, cough productive of purulent or pink frothy mucus, confusion or other changes. Manifestations of respiratory damage may not be apparent for 24 to 48 hours following the injury.

Significant hypoxia due to immersion/submersion or carbon monoxide poisoning may cause permanent neurological effects. Work with the family to develop communication techniques and identify remaining strengths. Help the family identify future care needs and means for meeting them, such as community-based care, personal care aides or access to long-term care facilities. Facilitate social services and support group referrals.

Lung cancer

THE PERSON WITH LUNG CANCER

Incidence and risk factors

Lunch cancer continues to be the fifth most diagnosed cancer in Australia. In 2022, an estimated 14,529 (7,707 males and 6,822 females) were diagnosed; a person has a 1 in 20 (5.0%) chance of being diagnosed with lung cancer by the age of 85. Lung cancer was also the most common cancer diagnosis for Indigenous Australians and the second most common cancer diagnosis for each gender. Lung cancer remains the most common cause of cancer death in Australia, with 8,693 deaths in 2021 (AIHW, 2021). See Figure 35.18.

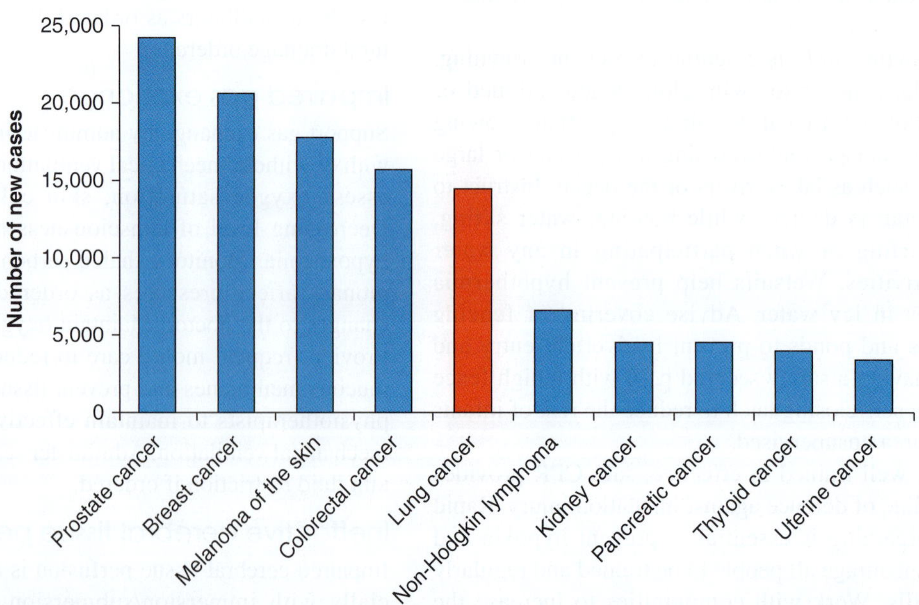

FIGURE 35.18 *Cancer data in Australia*

Source: AIHW (2022b). *Cancer data in Australia.* Retrieved from https://www.aihw.gov.au/reports/cancer/cancer-data-in-australia.

Tobacco use was the risk factor that contributed the most by far to cancer burden (AIHW, 2021). Nearly 90% of lung cancers are caused by tobacco smoking and smokers have 16 times more chance than non-smokers of developing lung cancer. Cigarette smoke, which contains over 40 known chemical carcinogens and cancer promoters, is the most significant cause of lung cancer. Even former smokers who have abstained for several years have a higher risk than non-smokers of developing lung cancer (Greenhalgh, Scollo & Winstanley, 2022).

Pathophysiology

Lung cancer develops as damaged bronchial epithelial cells mutate over time to become neoplastic. The genetic abnormality commonly seen is on chromosome 3, with loss of genetic material. Alterations of suppressor genes are also seen in some types of lung cancer.

The vast majority of primary lung lesions are bronchogenic carcinoma tumours of the airway epithelium. These tumours are further differentiated by cell type: small-cell carcinoma, adenocarcinoma, squamous cell carcinoma and large-cell carcinoma. For clinical purposes, the latter three cell types are frequently classified together as non-small-cell carcinomas. *Small-cell carcinomas*, which account for approximately 18% of lung cancers, proliferate and spread early. These tumours have paraneoplastic properties; producing manifestations at sites that are not directly affected by the tumour. Small-cell lung carcinomas can synthesise bioactive products and hormones such as adrenocorticotropic hormone (ACTH), antidiuretic hormone (ADH), a parathormone-like hormone and gastrin-releasing peptide. *Non-small-cell carcinoma* accounts for about 70% of lung cancers. Each cell type differs in its incidence, presentation and manner of spread.

Table 35.7 outlines the incidence and unique characteristics of each cell type.

TABLE 35.7 Comparison of lung cancer cell types

	CELL TYPE AND PREVALENCE	PRESENTATION AND ASSOCIATED MANIFESTATIONS	SPREAD
	Small-cell (oat-cell) carcinoma: 18% of all lung cancers	Central lesion with hilar mass common, early mediastinal involvement, no cavitation; SIADH, Cushing's syndrome, thrombophlebitis	Aggressive tumour; more than 40% of people have distant metastasis at time of presentation
	Adenocarcinoma: 32% of all lung cancers	Peripheral mass involving bronchi; few local symptoms; hypertrophic pulmonary osteoarthropathy	Early metastasis to CNS, skeleton and adrenal glands
	Squamous cell carcinoma: 29% of all lung cancers	Central lesion located in large bronchi; person presents with cough, dyspnoea, atelectasis and wheezing; hypocalcaemia common	Spreads by local invasion
	Large-cell carcinoma: 9% of all lung cancers	Usually, peripheral lesion that is larger than that associated with adenocarcinoma and tends to cavitate; gynaecomastia, thrombophlebitis	Early metastasis

Regardless of cell type, bronchogenic cancer tends to be aggressive and locally invasive, and have widespread metastatic lesions. Tumours begin as mucosal lesions that grow to form masses obstructing bronchi or invade adjacent lung tissue. All types frequently spread via the lymph system to nodes and other organs such as the brain, bones and liver.

Manifestations

The manifestations of lung cancer are related to the location and spread of the tumour. People may present with symptoms related to the primary tumour, manifestations of metastatic disease or with systemic symptoms. Initial symptoms often are attributed to smoking or chronic bronchitis. Chronic cough is common, as is haemoptysis. Wheezing and shortness of breath occur as a result of airway obstruction. Dull, aching chest pain occurs as the tumour spreads to the mediastinum; pleuritic pain occurs when the pleura is invaded. Hoarseness and/or dysphagia indicate pressure of the tumour on the trachea or oesophagus.

Systemic and paraneoplastic manifestations of lung cancer include weight loss, anorexia, fatigue and weakness; bone pain, tenderness and swelling; clubbing of the fingers and toes; and various endocrine, neuromuscular, cardiovascular and haematological symptoms.

Confusion, impaired gait and balance, headache and personality changes may indicate brain metastasis. Bone metastases cause bone pain, pathological fractures and possible spinal cord compression, as well as thrombocytopenia and anaemia if bone marrow is invaded. When the liver is affected, symptoms of liver dysfunction and biliary obstruction—including jaundice, anorexia and upper right quadrant pain—are evident.

See 'Multisystem effects of lung cancer'.

Complications and course

Superior vena cava syndrome, partial or complete obstruction of the superior vena cava, is a potential complication of lung cancer, particularly the tumour involves the superior mediastinum or the mediastinal lymph nodes. Obstructed venous flow from the head and neck produces the symptoms of superior vena cava syndrome (oedema of the neck and face, headache, dizziness, vision disturbances and syncope) and may develop acutely or more gradually. Veins of the upper chest and neck are dilated; flushing occurs, followed by cyanosis. Cerebral oedema may affect the level of consciousness; laryngeal oedema may impair respiration.

Paraneoplastic syndromes commonly associated with lung cancer include syndrome of inappropriate ADH secretion (SIADH) with fluid retention, hyponatraemia and oedema, Cushing's syndrome (see the chapter 'Nursing care of people with endocrine disorders') related to abnormal ACTH production and hypercalcaemia. Lung tumours may also produce procoagulation factors, increasing the risk of venous thrombosis, pulmonary embolism and thrombotic endocarditis (Bullock & Hales, 2019). In lung cancer, neuromuscular symptoms such as muscle weakness and wasting of the limbs may be the first indication of the disease.

At the time of diagnosis, cancer of the lung may be well advanced, with distant metastasis present in 55% of people and regional lymph node involvement in another 25%. The chance of surviving lung cancer for at least 5 years is 19% (Cancer Council, 2021).

INTERPROFESSIONAL CARE

Because lung cancer typically is advanced when diagnosed and the prognosis generally is poor, prevention of the disease must be a primary goal for all healthcare providers. Reducing cigarette smoking can significantly impact the death rate from lung cancer—a far greater impact than advances in treatment.

Establishing an accurate diagnosis is the first step in treating lung cancer. Treatment decisions are based on the tumour location, type of cancer cell, staging of the tumour and the person's ability to tolerate treatment. Lung cancer is staged by the tumour size, location, degree of invasion of the primary tumour and the presence of metastatic disease. Lung cancer staging is summarised in Table 35.8. Surgery is the treatment of choice for most forms of lung cancer.

Diagnosis

- *Chest x-ray* usually provides the first evidence of lung cancer. It is particularly reliable as a diagnostic tool when compared with a previous chest x-ray. In high-risk populations, the chest x-ray may be used as a screening tool for lung cancer.

TABLE 35.8 Lung cancer staging

	PRIMARY TUMOUR (T STAGE)	REGIONAL LYMPH NODES (N)	DISTANT METASTASIS (M)
Stage 0	T_0—No evidence of primary tumour T_X—Malignant cells in bronchopulmonary secretions, but no tumour visualised		M_X—Presence of distant metastasis cannot be assessed
Stage I	T_1S—Carcinoma in situ T_1—Tumour that is 3 cm in diameter or less, with no evidence of invasion	N_0—No regional lymph node metastasis	M_0—No distant metastasis
Stage II	T_2—Tumour that is greater than 3 cm in diameter or invades visceral pleura or has associated atelectasis or pneumonitis	N_1—Metastasis or direct extension to peribronchial or ipsilateral hilar nodes	
Stage III	T_3—Tumour with direct extension into an adjacent structure or any tumour with associated pleural effusion or atelectasis or pneumonitis of entire lung	N_2—Metastasis to ipsilateral mediastinal or subcarinal nodes	
Stage IV	T_4—Tumour that invades mediastinum or involves the heart, great vessels, trachea, oesophagus, vertebral body or carina; presence of malignant pleural effusion	N_3—Metastasis to contralateral mediastinal, scalene or supraclavicular nodes	M_1—Distant metastasis present

Multisystem effects of lung cancer

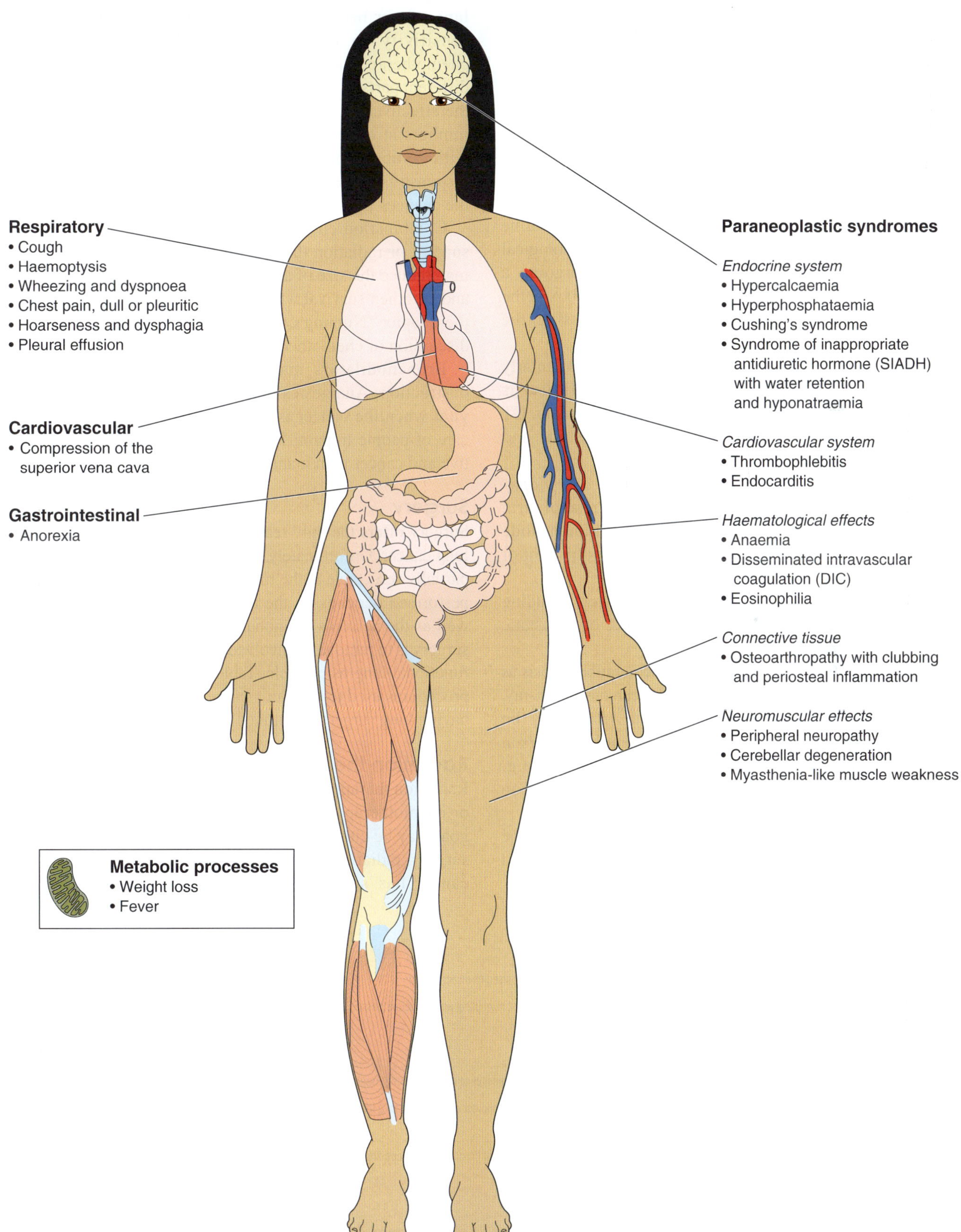

- *Sputum specimen* is sent for *cytological examination* to establish the diagnosis of lung cancer. The sputum sample is collected on arising in the morning. More expensive and invasive examinations may be considered unnecessary if malignant cells are found in the sputum. However, a sputum sample negative for malignant cells does not rule out lung cancer; it may simply indicate that the tumour is not shedding cells into mucus secretions.
- *Bronchoscopy* is frequently done to visualise and obtain tissue for biopsy from the tumour. When a tumour mass or suspicious tissue is identified visually, a cable-activated instrument is used to obtain a biopsy specimen. If the tumour cannot be seen, the airways may be flushed with a saline solution (bronchial washing) to obtain cells for cytological examination. Nursing care of the person undergoing a bronchoscopy is included in the 'Diagnostic tests' box in the chapter 'A person-centred approach to assessing the respiratory system'.
- *CT scan* is used to evaluate and localise tumours, particularly tumours in the lung parenchyma and pleura. It also is completed prior to needle biopsy to localise the tumour. CT scanning can also detect distant tumour metastasis and evaluate tumour response to treatment.
- *Cells or tissue for cytological examination and biopsy* may be obtained by aspirating fluid from a pleural effusion, percutaneous needle biopsy and lymph node biopsy. These procedures may be done in an outpatient or a surgical setting.
- *FBC*, *liver function studies* and *serum electrolytes*, including calcium, are obtained to evaluate for evidence of metastatic disease or paraneoplastic syndromes.
- *Tuberculin test (PPD)* is performed to rule out tuberculosis as the cause of symptoms and abnormalities seen on chest x-ray.
- *Respiratory function tests (RFTs)* and *ABGs* may be performed prior to the initiation of treatment if the person has manifestations of respiratory insufficiency (e.g. dyspnoea, activity intolerance, low oxygen saturation levels).

See the chapter 'A person-centred approach to assessing the respiratory system' for nursing care related to commonly used diagnostic tests for lung cancer.

Medications

Combination chemotherapy (often combined with radiation therapy and/or surgery) is the treatment of choice for small-cell lung cancer because of its rapid growth, dissemination and sensitivity to cytotoxic drugs. Used in combination, chemotherapeutic drugs allow tumour cells to be attacked at different parts of the cell cycle and in different ways, increasing the effectiveness of therapy. Fifty per cent of individuals with tumours at early stages achieve complete tumour remission with combination chemotherapy. When a complete tumour response is achieved in the first few cycles of chemotherapy, the chances for long-term survival are much greater.

Combination chemotherapy is also used as an adjunct to surgery or radiation therapy for other types of lung cancer. It may reduce the size of advanced local tumours prior to surgery and lengthen survival when distant metastases are present. See the chapter 'Nursing care of people with cancer' for further discussion of chemotherapy.

Bronchodilators may be prescribed to reduce airway obstruction. Analgesics and pain management strategies are vital when the cancer is advanced. See the chapter 'Nursing care of people in pain' for more information about postoperative and cancer pain management.

Surgery

Surgery offers the only real chance for a cure in non-small-cell lung cancer. Unfortunately, most tumours are inoperable or only partially resectable at the time of diagnosis. The type of surgery performed depends on the location and size of the tumour, as well as the person's pulmonary and general health. The goal of surgery is to remove all involved tissue while preserving as much functional lung as possible. Table 35.9 outlines various surgical procedures used to treat lung cancer. Nursing care for the person having lung surgery is outlined in the accompanying box.

Radiation therapy

Radiation therapy is used alone or in combination with surgery or chemotherapy for lung cancer (Tan, 2018). The treatment goal may be either cure or symptom relief (palliative). Prior to surgery, radiation therapy is used to 'debulk' tumours. When cancer has spread by direct extension to other thoracic

TABLE 35.9 Types of surgery for lung cancer

PROCEDURE	DESCRIPTION	USED FOR
Laser bronchoscopy	Bronchoscopy-guided laser used to resect tumour	Tumours localised in a main bronchus
Mediastinoscopy	Visualisation of the mediastinum using an endoscope passed through a suprasternal incision	Evaluation and biopsy of a mediastinal tumour and lymph nodes
Thoracotomy	Incision into the chest wall	Access the lung and thoracic cavity for surgery
Wedge resection	Removal of a small section (wedge) of peripheral lung tissue	Small, peripheral lung tumours
Segmental resection	Removal of an individual bronchovascular segment of a lobe	Peripheral lung tumour with no evidence of extension to the chest wall or metastasis
Sleeve resection (bronchoplastic reconstruction)	Resection of a section of a major bronchus with reconstruction of remaining normal bronchus	Small lesion of a major bronchus
Lobectomy	Removal of a single lung lobe	Tumours confined to a single lobe
Pneumonectomy	Removal of an entire lung	Tumour widespread throughout the lung, involving the main bronchus or fixed to the hilum

structures and surgery is not feasible, radiation therapy may be the treatment of choice. It also may relieve manifestations such as cough, haemoptysis, pain due to bone metastasis and dyspnoea from bronchial obstruction. Complications of lung cancer, such as superior vena cava syndrome, may be treated with radiation.

Radiation therapy may be delivered by external beam to the primary tumour site or by intraluminal radiation or brachytherapy. Radiation therapy and related nursing care are discussed further in the chapter 'Nursing care of people with cancer'. Specific nursing measures for the person undergoing radiation therapy for lung cancer are outlined in the 'Nursing care' box.

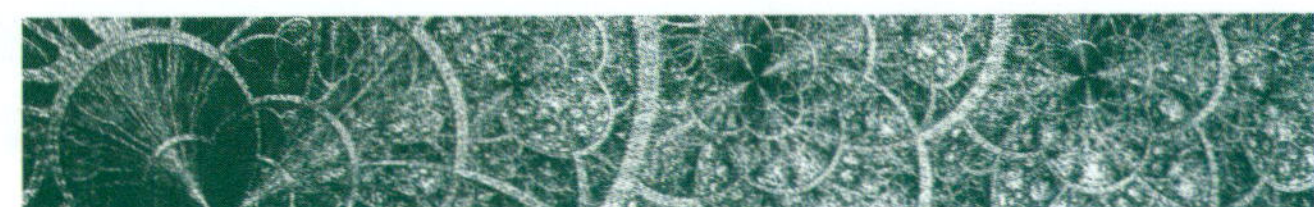

Nursing care

Health promotion

Teach people of all ages, particularly children and teenagers, about the link between cigarette smoking and lung cancer. Not smoking and avoiding exposure to second-hand smoke, is the primary preventive measure for lung cancer. In addition, explain the risk of lung cancer to people with occupational risk factors—exposure to asbestos products, in particular.

NURSING CARE OF THE PERSON **having lung surgery**

PREOPERATIVE CARE

- Provide routine preoperative nursing care as outlined in the chapter 'Nursing care of people having surgery'.
- Note any history of smoking, respiratory and cardiac diseases, and other chronic conditions in the nursing history. *These factors may affect the response to surgery and the risk of postoperative complications.*
- Provide emotional and psychological support for the person and family. *In addition to facing surgery, the individual may be adjusting to a new diagnosis of cancer and the possibility that surgical intervention will be only partially successful.*
- Instruct about postoperative procedures, including respiratory therapy, breathing exercises and coughing techniques. *Allow practice time. Learning will be easier in the preoperative period when pain and analgesia are not affecting mental function.*
- If the person will return from surgery with an endotracheal tube and mechanical ventilation, establish a means of communication using hand or eye signals or a magic slate. *Establishing a means of communication prior to surgery reduces postoperative anxiety at being unable to speak.*
- If the person will return to the critical care unit, introduce the person and family to the unit and any machines, such as ventilators and monitors that will be used. *The knowledge that this is an expected part of surgical recovery reduces the person's and family's postoperative anxiety.*

POSTOPERATIVE CARE

- Assess and provide routine postoperative care as outlined in the chapter 'Nursing care of people having surgery'.
- Assess for adequate pain control and provide analgesics as needed. *Incisional pain commonly causes altered breathing patterns in the person who has undergone lung surgery.*
- Frequently assess respiratory status, including colour, oxygen saturation, respiratory rate and depth, chest expansion, lung sounds, percussion tone and ABGs. *Maintaining adequate ventilation and gas exchange postoperatively is vital to reduce mortality and morbidity. Gas exchange may be impaired by complications of lung surgery, including pneumothorax, atelectasis, bronchospasm, pulmonary embolus, bronchopleural fistula and ARDS.*
- Assist with effective coughing techniques, postural drainage and incentive spirometry. Perform endotracheal suctioning as needed while intubated. *Surgical manipulation and anaesthesia can increase mucus production, leading to airway obstruction. Aggressive respiratory hygiene is important to prevent this complication.*
- Monitor and maintain effective mechanical ventilation. *This is vital to ensure adequate ventilation and gas exchange in the early postoperative period.*
- Maintain patent chest tubes and a closed drainage system. Monitor chest tube output every hour initially and then every 2 to 4 or 8 hours as indicated. Notify the doctor if chest tube output exceeds 70 mL per hour and/or is bright red, warm and free flowing. *Maintaining a patent, intact chest drainage system is vital for re-establishing negative pressure within the chest cavity and re-expansion of the lungs. Increased amounts of warm, free-flowing blood indicate intrathoracic haemorrhage that may necessitate surgical intervention.*
- Assess for signs of infection involving the incision or chest tube site(s). Use strict aseptic technique in caring for incisions and invasive monitoring devices. *The postoperative period poses risks for individuals from incisional infections, empyema in the chest cavity and pneumonia.*
- Assist with turning and encourage the person to ambulate as soon as possible. *Early mobility is important to prevent possible complications, such as pneumonia or pulmonary embolus.*
- Assess and maintain nutritional status. Initiate enteral or parenteral nutrition early if intubation and mechanical ventilation will be required for an extended period. Provide frequent small feedings once extubated. *Maintaining nutritional status promotes wound healing and prevents negative nitrogen balance. Giving frequent small feedings reduces the fatigue associated with eating.*

NURSING CARE OF THE PERSON receiving radiation therapy

Although radiation therapy is well controlled and specifically directed towards the tumour cells, some normal cells are also damaged in the process of treatment. Nursing care and teaching help the person cope with uncomfortable side effects associated with radiation therapy.

NURSING RESPONSIBILITIES

- Monitor for potential complications:
  a. radiation pneumonitis—dyspnoea on exertion, dry cough, fever
  b. pericarditis—chest pain, pericardial friction rub; muffled heart sounds, paradoxical pulse, ECG abnormalities (notify the doctor if symptoms develop)
  c. oesophagitis—pain, sore throat, difficulty swallowing.
- Encourage adequate fluid intake to liquefy respiratory secretions.
- Provide local analgesics and local anaesthetics such as viscous lignocaine as ordered to relieve dysphagia and sore throat.
- Offer small frequent meals of soft, cool foods and liquids to maintain nutritional status.

HEALTH EDUCATION FOR THE PERSON AND FAMILY

- If dyspnoea or pneumonitis develops, teach positioning, pursed-lip techniques and relaxation exercises to facilitate breathing.
- Reassure that pneumonitis is generally a self-limiting process and should resolve when the course of radiotherapy is completed.
- Teach the manifestations of pericarditis, which may develop during treatment or up to 1 year after its completion. Chest pain or pressure, rapid heartbeat and fever may signal pericarditis; increasing fatigue, dyspnoea and light-headedness can indicate a chronic process with pericardial effusion and possible cardiac tamponade.
- Instruct to eliminate hot, spicy or acidic foods from the diet if oesophagitis is a problem. Alcohol and tobacco should also be avoided.
- Adequate rest and nutrition are important to alleviate the symptoms of radiation fatigue, which is common in people receiving radiation therapy for lung cancer. The fatigue is generally temporary.

Assessment

Nursing assessment related to lung cancer focuses on identifying risk factors for the disease, early manifestations of lung cancer and respiratory function in the person undergoing treatment.

- *Health history*: current symptoms, including chronic cough, shortness of breath, blood-tinged sputum; systemic manifestations such as recent weight loss, fatigue, anorexia, bone pain; smoking history; occupational exposure to carcinogens; chronic diseases such as COPD.
- *Physical examination*: general appearance; skin colour, evidence of clubbing; weight and height; vital signs; respiratory rate, depth, excursion; lung sounds to percussion and auscultation.
- *Diagnostic tests*: FBC and coagulation studies, serum electrolytes and osmolality, liver and renal function studies; chest x-ray and CT scan results; ABGs and oxygen saturation levels.

Nursing diagnoses and interventions

The person with lung cancer is facing invasive treatments with undesirable side effects, possibly surgery and typically a poor prognosis for long-term survival. Nursing care needs are diverse, related to respiratory status, cancer itself and possible metastases, and the treatment plan. Priority nursing diagnoses related to respiratory function include *Ineffective breathing patterns* and *Activity intolerance. Pain* and *Anticipatory grieving* also are likely to be high-priority problems. See the accompanying nursing care plan.

NURSING CARE PLAN A person with lung cancer

After coughing up bloody sputum one morning, James Mueller, a 68-year-old retired mill worker, sees his doctor. A chest x-ray shows a suspicious density in the central portion of his right lung. Mr Mueller is admitted to the hospital the following Monday for diagnostic tests.

ASSESSMENT

Mr Mueller is admitted to the oncology unit and the nurse obtains a nursing history. Mr Mueller is married and has three grown children. He worked in a local paper mill for 35 years before retiring at age 62. He describes himself as 'pretty healthy', except for a chronic smoker's cough. He started smoking as a young man in the army. He has a 50-pack-a-year smoking history, having smoked a packet a day for 50 years since age 18. Mr Mueller says he briefly quit smoking following a small heart attack 3 years ago but started again after 4 months. On further questioning, Mr Mueller says his cough has been productive for the past few months, especially in the morning, and that he is more short of breath than usual with activity.

Mr Mueller's examination data include BP 162/86, P 78 and regular, R 20 and T 36.9°C. Colour good, skin warm and dry. Inspiratory and expiratory wheezes noted in right chest but good breath sounds throughout. No other abnormal findings are noted on examination. The doctor orders early-morning sputum specimens for 3 days for cytological examination and schedules a CT scan of the chest the morning after admission.

Mr Mueller's FBC shows mild anaemia, but the remaining routine laboratory tests are essentially normal. Sputum cytology is positive for small-cell bronchogenic cancer. The CT scan shows a central mass approximately 4 cm in diameter with involved mediastinal and subclavicular lymph nodes. A small mass is also noted on the lumbar spine. After conferring with his doctor and an oncologist, Mr Mueller decides to undergo a trial course of chemotherapy.

NURSING CARE PLAN A person with lung cancer (continued)

DIAGNOSES

- *Impaired gas exchange* related to tumour mass and effects of chronic cigarette smoking manifested by increased shortness of breath.
- *Risk of inadequate nutrition* related to effects of chemotherapy manifested by weight loss and/or anorexia.
- *Risk of increased stress and anxiety* related to new diagnosis of lung cancer manifested by behavioural changes, sleep disturbances and/or changes in eating habits.
- *Knowledge deficit* about lung cancer and aids to smoking cessation manifested by continued smoking habits despite significant health challenges.

PLANNING

- Discuss symptoms to report to the doctor: increased dyspnoea or haemoptysis, severe stridor or wheezing and chest pain.
- Discuss measures to relieve nausea associated with chemotherapy, including premedication with a prescribed anti-emetic.
- Discuss possible effects of lung cancer with Mr and Mrs Mueller.
- Encourage Mr and Mrs Mueller to call a family conference to discuss the disease with their children and grandchildren.
- Refer to a local cancer support group.
- Refer to community services for follow up and further teaching.
- Ask the doctor for a prescription for nicotine patches or gum for Mr Mueller.

Expected outcomes

- Maintain a patent airway.
- Maintain current weight.
- Express feelings and concerns about the effect of cancer on the family unit.
- Participate in care.
- Contact appropriate support groups.
- Verbalise an understanding of the disease, its treatment and prognosis.
- Develop a plan to stop smoking.

IMPLEMENTATION

- Evaluate family members' knowledge and understanding of lung cancer, correcting misinformation and teaching as needed.
- Teach coughing, deep breathing and hydration measures to facilitate airway clearance.
- Have a dietitian consult with Mr and Mrs Mueller to develop a diet plan for maintaining ideal weight.
- Have an Australian Lung Foundation volunteer contact the family.
- Work with Mr Mueller to develop a plan to stop smoking.

EVALUATION

Mr Mueller had his first chemotherapy treatment in the hospital and was discharged 4 days after admission. After 3 months of chemotherapy, his tumour shows little regression and a liver scan reveals further metastasis. He and his wife decide to stop chemotherapy, a decision with which the children reluctantly agree. Mr and Mrs Mueller are referred to hospice services. With the help of hospice nurses and volunteers, Mr Mueller is able to remain at home. His pain is managed initially with oral MS Contin, a sustained-release form of morphine sulfate, and later with an intravenous morphine infusion. Mr Mueller dies at home with his family at his side 9 months after his diagnosis of lung cancer.

CRITICAL THINKING IN THE NURSING PROCESS

1. The oncologist prescribed a chemotherapy regimen of cyclophosphamide, doxorubicin and vincristine. Describe how each of these drugs works against cancer cells and discuss the rationale for using this combination.
2. Develop a care plan to deal with the specific side effects of the above treatment regimen.
3. Mr Mueller had small-cell (oat-cell) cancer. How would his presentation and treatment differ if the diagnosis had been non-small-cell adenocarcinoma, stage $T_2N_2M_0$?

REFLECTION ON THE NURSING PROCESS

1. Outline what you have learned from this case study that you will apply to your future practice.
2. Given that Mr Mueller has continued to smoke even after experiencing a myocardial infarction, which communication and education strategies could you use to assist him with success in quitting smoking now he has developed lung cancer?

Ineffective breathing pattern

Breathing patterns and ventilation may be affected by the tumour itself or by treatment of the tumour. Thoracic surgery increases the risk due to the incision and disruption of the muscles of respiration. Maintaining effective lung ventilation is particularly important postoperatively to re-expand remaining lung tissue and prevent surgical complications.

- Assess and document respiratory rate, depth and lung sounds at least every 4 hours; evaluate more frequently in the immediate postoperative period or as indicated by condition. *Early detection of signs of respiratory compromise or adventitious lung sounds is vital for effective intervention.*

> **CONSIDERATION FOR PRACTICE**
>
> **Monitor oxygen saturation and/or blood gas results, reporting changes from normal. Changes in levels of blood oxygen may be early indications of respiratory compromise.**

- Frequently assess and document pain level (using a standard pain scale); provide analgesics as needed. *Pain and attempting to avoid chest movement to prevent additional pain can lead to rapid, shallow respirations and ineffective ventilation.*
- Elevate the head of the bed to 60 degrees. *Elevating the head of the bed reduces pressure on the diaphragm from the abdominal contents and permits optimal lung expansion.*

- Assist to turn, cough and deep breathe, and use incentive spirometry. Help splint the chest with a pillow or blanket when coughing. *These measures promote airway clearance.*
- Suction airway as needed. *Suctioning may be required to remove secretions that the person cannot cough up and expectorate.*

> **CONSIDERATION FOR PRACTICE**
> **Maintain chest tube integrity and patency by ensuring uninterrupted gravity flow. Chest tubes help re-establish negative pressure in the thoracic cavity, allowing the lung to fully re-expand.**

- Provide chest physiotherapy with percussion and postural drainage as needed or ordered. *Percussion and postural drainage help maintain airway patency and effective respirations.*
- If mechanical ventilation is instituted, work with respiratory therapy and use analgesia or sedation as needed to synchronise respirations with the ventilator. *Coordination of the person's respiratory effort with ventilator-delivered breaths is essential for fully effective mechanical ventilation.*
- Provide reassurance and emotional support. *These measures help relieve anxiety and promote an effective breathing pattern.*

Activity intolerance

Both resectional lung surgery and inoperable lung cancer reduce the amount of functional lung tissue and surface area for gas diffusion. This can lead to activity intolerance if the oxygen supply is insufficient to meet the body's oxygen demand.

> **CONSIDERATION FOR PRACTICE**
> **Assess and document physiological responses to activity, including pulse, respiratory rate, dyspnoea and fatigue. These assessments are good indicators of activity tolerance.**

- Plan rest periods between activities and procedures. *Rest periods reduce oxygen demands and fatigue.*
- Assist the person to increase activities gradually in the postoperative period. *Increasing activity levels gradually improves exercise tolerance.*
- Teach measures to conserve energy while performing ADLs, such as sitting while showering and dressing and wearing slip-on shoes. *These energy-conserving measures reduce oxygen demand and allow the person to remain independent as long as possible.*
- Keep frequently used objects within easy reach. *This helps conserve energy.*
- Administer oxygen as prescribed. Teach the person and family about home oxygen use if appropriate. *Supplemental oxygen can help improve activity and exercise tolerance.*
- Encourage maintenance of physical activity to tolerance. *Maintaining activity levels to the degree possible improves physical and emotional wellbeing.*
- Allow family members to assist as needed. *This helps the person conserve energy and allows the family to retain a sense of usefulness.*

Pain

Pain is a priority problem in both the postoperative period and terminal stages of cancer. Poorly managed pain prolongs recovery from surgery. In the person with terminal cancer, chronic and acute pain must be managed effectively to allow for a peaceful death.

- Assess and document pain using a standardised pain scale and objective data. Pain is a subjective experience, best evaluated by the person. *Changes in vital signs, guarded movement or unwillingness to move may indicate unreported pain.*
- Provide analgesics as needed to maintain comfort. *Postoperative recovery and restoration of function are facilitated by adequate pain management.*
- For cancer pain, maintain an around-the-clock medication schedule using narcotic, non-steroidal anti-inflammatory drugs and other medications as ordered. *Addiction is not a concern in terminal cancer; providing adequate pain relief that does not allow 'breakthrough' pain is essential.*
- Provide or assist with comfort measures, such as massage, positioning, distraction and relaxation techniques. *These techniques promote relaxation and enhance pain relief.*
- Assist the person and family to plan and engage in activities that distract from the pain, such as reading, watching television and engaging in social interactions. *Distraction helps the individual focus away from the pain.*
- Spend as much time with the person as possible; allow family members to remain with the person. *The physical presence of the nurse and family provides emotional support for the individual.*

Anticipatory grieving

Because lung cancer is often advanced when diagnosed, the person faces the very real prospect of dying from the disease. Grieving for the anticipated loss of life is a normal response as the person and family begin to adapt to the diagnosis. Nursing care goals are to promote expressing feelings and thoughts about the loss and to help the person and family initiate grief work, make decisions and use appropriate resources and coping mechanisms to deal with the loss.

- Spend time with the person and family. *Time is necessary to develop a trusting, therapeutic relationship.*
- Answer questions honestly; do not deny the probable outcome of the disease. *Honesty reinforces reality and provides a sense of control over decisions to be made.*
- Encourage the person and family to express their feelings, fears and concerns. *Open expression of feelings helps to promote understanding and acceptance.*
- Assist with understanding the grieving process and acceptance of feelings as normal. *Feelings of guilt, anger or depression may cause the person to withdraw from others. Explanation of the grieving process enhances understanding and ability to cope.*

- Help identify strengths and coping measures used effectively in the past. Provide positive reinforcement for effective coping behaviour. *Past effective coping measures can help the person and family deal with the present situation and regain a sense of control.*
- Help the person and family make decisions regarding treatment and care. *This is also important to give them a sense of control.*
- Encourage use of other support systems, such as spiritual and social groups. Refer the individual and family to support groups, social support services and hospice care as indicated. Provide Cancer Council literature and information as appropriate. *These support systems provide emotional support and help the person and family cope with the diagnosis.*
- Discuss advance directives (living wills) and power of attorney for healthcare with the individual and family. *These documents give the person and family a sense of control over the medical care provided if the person can no longer express their own wishes.*

Community-based care

A primary teaching need to prepare the person and family affected by lung cancer for home care is information about the disease itself, expected prognosis and planned treatment strategies. Provide honest information; do not promote false hope. Include the following additional topics in teaching for home care:

- importance of quitting smoking, especially if surgery has been performed. (The person with lung cancer may have difficulty recognising the need to stop smoking. Include information about the effects of nicotine and the tars in cigarette smoke on healing and already compromised lung tissue.)
- planned treatments such as chemotherapy or radiation therapy, including expected effects and usual side effects of each
- strategies to cope with noxious effects of radiation or chemotherapy
- activities and exercises to improve strength and regain function for the individual in the postoperative period
- the need to continue coughing and deep-breathing exercises at home
- symptoms to report to the doctor: fever, increasing or continued shortness of breath, cough, increased or purulent sputum, redness, pain, swelling or incisional drainage
- use of prescribed medications, including desired and potential side effects and interactions with other drugs or foods
- use of analgesics and other pain-relief measures for postoperative or cancer pain
- information about hospice services, community support, local cancer support groups for individuals and caregivers, and Cancer Council services.

Refer the person and family for home health services, including nursing care, assistance with ADLs, respiratory care and respite care as needed.

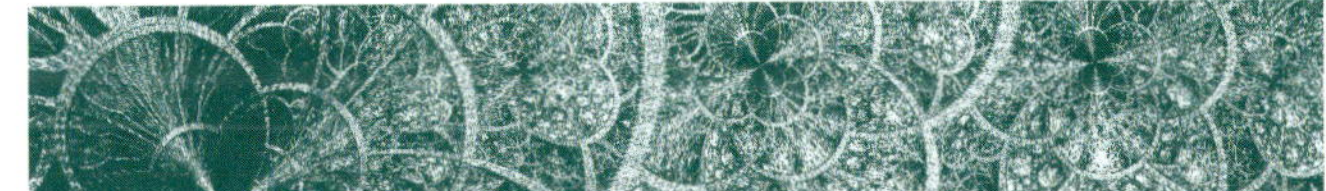

TRANSLATION TO PRACTICE How can communication practices in a multidisciplinary lung cancer care team influence a person's care?

Qualitative research by Rowlands and Callen (2013) was part of a larger mixed-methods study exploring the methods and efficacy of communication within and between the multidisciplinary, hospital-based lung cancer care team. Twenty-two members were interviewed using semi-structured in-depth interviews. A thematic grounded theory approach was used to determine that two key themes were emerging. First, that the characteristics of communication were influenced by roles within the team, where doctors dominated, and second, that current mediums for communication and traditional influences on role delineation impacted communication. It was noted that face-to-face verbal communication was preferred and that existing cancer care guidelines did not address team communication barriers.

IMPLICATIONS FOR NURSING

Specific attention must be placed on introducing and developing communication skills between nurses and other healthcare team members to benefit the management of individuals with lung cancer and all people in need of quality healthcare. Healthcare professionals must work effectively together. When staff work within professional 'silos', the concept of a functioning team fails to exist. Also, when face-to-face communication is preferred, there is a risk that failure to document observations or changes to care can compromise the integrity and completeness of the person's medical record. Further investigation and professional development are required to ensure that failures in communication do not compromise a person's care.

CRITICAL THINKING IN PERSON-CENTRED CARE

1 In this study, the findings indicated that although some literature suggests that multidisciplinary communication is well developed within healthcare, more work is required to ensure that a person's care is not compromised. Which characteristics and interventions should be undertaken to improve a team's communication? Make a table outlining both individual characteristics and team characteristics that will promote improved communication.
2 How will the study findings impact on how you will approach communication with other healthcare colleagues? Which further education requirements would be needed to improve multidisciplinary team communication?

CHAPTER HIGHLIGHTS

- Pneumonia, inflammation of the respiratory bronchioles and alveoli are usually bacterial. Different organisms are typically found in hospital-acquired pneumonia than in community-acquired pneumonia. Nursing care promotes airway clearance, supporting effective gas exchange and promoting rest.
- Infection control measures, including standard, airborne and contact precautions, are vital to prevent the spread of viral severe acute respiratory syndrome.
- Tuberculosis affects many people worldwide; in Australia, the primary affected populations are migrants, people with compromised immunity and people living in crowded or unsanitary conditions.
- The tuberculin test (PPD) detects a cellular immune response to *M. tuberculosis*, indicating infection but not necessarily active disease.
- Effective tuberculosis treatment is a public health concern, requiring therapy and compliance monitoring, contact follow up and assessment for adverse treatment effects.
- Disorders of the pleura, such as pleural effusion and pneumothorax, can affect lung expansion, ventilation and gas exchange when significant.
- Tension pneumothorax develops when air enters the pleural space but cannot escape, collapsing the lung on the affected side and placing pressure on the unaffected lung and mediastinum. Ventilation, gas exchange, venous return and cardiac output can be significantly affected.
- Trauma may affect the chest wall (rib fracture, flail chest), the surface of the lungs (pulmonary contusion) or the airways and alveoli (smoke inhalation and immersion/submersion). Flail chest and pulmonary contusion often occur concurrently; haemothorax also frequently develops with chest trauma. Chest trauma (chest wall or airways) can endanger effective ventilation and gas exchange.
- Lung cancer, the leading cause of cancer deaths, typically is advanced when diagnosed. Surgery, radiation therapy and chemotherapy are used to treat lung cancer, often in combination.

CONCEPT CHECK

1 Admitting orders for a person with acute bacterial pneumonia include an intravenous antibiotic every 8 hours, oxygen per nasal prongs at 5 L/min, continuous pulse oximetry monitoring, bed rest with bathroom privileges and chair at bedside as desired, diet as tolerated, sputum specimen for culture and sensitivity, FBC, urinalysis and electrolytes. Which order should the nurse carry out first?

1 Start the oxygen per nasal prongs.
2 Insert an intravenous catheter and start the prescribed antibiotic.
3 Provide a dinner tray to the person.
4 Obtain the sputum specimen.

2 When assessing a person with bacterial pneumonia, the nurse notes that the person's overall skin tone is somewhat grey and there is a bluish tinge around the person's fingertips. The nurse should (place the following in the correct order of priority):

1 start oxygen
2 assess breath sounds
3 notify the doctor
4 raise the head of the bed
5 obtain oxygen saturation level

3 The nurse evaluating a tuberculin test result 72 hours after it was administered notes an area of induration 9 mm in diameter. What additional information would indicate to the nurse that this is a positive result? The person:

1 resides in a long-term care facility
2 was born in South-East Asia
3 has HIV disease
4 is an injection drug user

4 The nurse teaching a person taking prophylactic daily isoniazid (INH) following tuberculin test conversion includes which of the following in the instructions?

1 This drug turns your urine red-orange. This is harmless.
2 Report numbness and tingling of your extremities to your doctor.
3 You will need to have periodic eye examinations during treatment.
4 Do not use aspirin while taking this drug because abnormal bleeding may occur.

5 Which of the following statements made by a person with a new lung cancer diagnosis indicates that the nurse's teaching has been effective?

1 'Well, since I'm going to die anyway, I may as well go home, put my affairs in order and spend the rest of my time in the easy chair.'
2 'I understand that because cancer has already spread, I will undergo aggressive cancer treatment for the next several years to beat this.'
3 'Even though I can't undo the damage caused by cigarette smoking, I will try to quit to prevent further damage to my lungs.'
4 'Having the "big C" is very scary; I'm just glad it is one of the more curable forms of cancer.'

6 The nurse caring for a person following a lobectomy notes 100 mL of red drainage in the chest drainage container since checking it 30 minutes previously. The nurse should (select all that apply):

1 empty the chest tube drainage system
2 note the finding and re-evaluate drainage in 30 minutes
3 notify the surgeon
4 assess vital signs and level of consciousness
5 apply pressure to the chest tube insertion site

7 The nurse caring for a person having a thoracentesis appropriately assists the person to:

1 sit upright leaning forward during the procedure
2 breathe deeply as the needle is inserted
3 remain on quiet bed rest for 4 hours following the procedure
4 cough as the fluid is withdrawn

8 The nurse teaches a person being discharged from the emergency department with a diagnosis of a fractured rib to:

1 avoid using pain medications to prevent respiratory depression
2 heavily tape the chest wall and promote comfort
3 remain on bed rest for a week to allow the fracture to stabilise
4 use a small pillow to splint the area when coughing

9 Which of the following assessment findings of a person with smoke inhalation does the nurse find of greatest concern?

1 Ash-like material in the sputum
2 Respiratory rate of 36
3 Skin and mucous membranes pink
4 Fine crackles in bilateral bases

10 Which nursing diagnosis does the nurse identify as the highest priority for a person with tension pneumothorax?

1 *Decreased cardiac output*
2 *Ineffective breathing patterns*
3 *Acute pain*
4 *Risk of aspiration*

BIBLIOGRAPHY

Adams, S. (2017). Chylothorax. *Emedicine*. Retrieved from http://emedicine.medscape.com/

Australian Institute of Health and Welfare (AIHW) (2019). *National hospital morbidity database: T75.1 Drowning and nonfatal submersion*. Retrieved from https://www.aihw.gov.au/

Australian Institute of Health and Welfare (AIHW) (2020). *Aboriginal and Torres Strait Islander Health Performance Framework summary report. National Aboriginal and Torres Strait Islander Health Survey 2018–19*. Retrieved from https://www.aihw.gov.au/

Australian Institute of Health and Welfare (AIHW) (2021). *Cancer in Australia*. Retrieved from https://www.aihw.gov.au/

Australian Institute of Health and Welfare (AIHW) (2022a). *Chronic respiratory conditions*. (Cat. no. ACM 24.) Canberra: AIHW.

Australian Institute of Health and Welfare (AIHW) (2022b). *Cancer data in Australia*. Retrieved from https://www.aihw.gov.au/

Bullock, S. & Hales, M. (2019). *Principles of pathophysiology* (2nd ed.). Sydney: Pearson.

Cancer Council (2021). *Lung cancer*. Retrieved from https://www.cancer.org.au/

Cheng, I.-H., Russell, G., Bailes, M. & Block, A. (2011). *An evaluation of the primary healthcare needs of refugees in southeast metropolitan Melbourne. A report by the Southern Academic Primary Care Research Unit to the Refugee Health Research Consortium*. Melbourne: Southern Academic Primary Care Research Unit.

Daley, B. (2018). Pneumothorax. *Emedicine*. Retrieved from http://emedicine.medscape.com/

Dalziel, S. R., Haskell, L., O'Brien, S., Borland, M. L., Plint, A. C., Babl, F. E. & Oakley, E. (2022). Bronchiolitis. *The Lancet*. https://doi.org/10.1016/S0140-6736(22)01016-9

Department of Health (2015). *National Notifiable Diseases Surveillance System. Number of notifications for legionellosis by year, Australia, 1991 to 2015*. Retrieved from https://www9.health.gov.au/

Department of Health and Aged Care (2022a). *Legionellosis*. Retrieved from https://www.health.gov.au/

Department of Health and Aged Care (2022b). *The Australian immunisation handbook*. Retrieved from https://immunisationhandbook.health.gov.au/

Department of Health and Aged Care (2022c). *Tuberculosis CDNA national guidelines for public health units*. Retrieved from https://www.health.gov.au/

Galeiras, R. (2021). Smoke inhalation injury: A narrative review. *Mediastinum*, *5*(16). doi: 10.21037/med-21-7

Glasziou, P., Dartnell, J., Biezen, R., Morgan, M. & Manski-Nankervis, J. A. (2022). Antibiotic stewardship. *Australian Journal of General Practice*, *51*(1/2), 15–20.

Greenhalgh, E. M., Scollo, M. M. & Winstanley, M. H. (2022). *Tobacco in Australia: Facts and issues*. Melbourne: Cancer Council Victoria. Retrieved from www.TobaccoInAustralia.org.au

Harman, E. (2018). Aspergillosis. *Emedicine*. Retrieved from http://emedicine.medscape.com/

Healthdirect (2021). *Tuberculosis*. Retrieved from https://www.healthdirect.gov.au/

Herchline, T. (2017). Tuberculosis. *Emedicine*. Retrieved from http://emedicine.medscape.com/

Mancini, M. (2018). Hemothorax. *Emedicine*. Retrieved from http://emedicine.medscape.com/

Mosenifar, Z. (2018). Viral pneumonia. *Emedicine*. Retrieved from http://emedicine.medscape.com/

O'Grady, K. F., Hall, K. K., Bell, A., Chang, A. B. & Potter, C. (2018). Review of respiratory diseases among Aboriginal and Torres Strait Islander children. *Australian Indigenous Health Bulletin*, *18*(2). Retrieved from http://healthbulletin.org.au/

Papadakis, M., McPhee, S. J. & Rabow, M. W. (2022). *Current medical diagnosis and treatment* (61st ed.). New York: McGraw-Hill Education.

Rowlands, S. & Callen. J. (2013). A qualitative analysis of communication between hospital-based multidisciplinary lung cancer team members. *European Journal of Cancer Care*, *22*(1), 20–31. doi: 10.1111/ecc.12004

Royal College of Pathologists Australasia (RCPA) (2019). *Lung abscess*. Retrieved from https://www.rcpa.edu.au/

Royal Life Saving Society (2018). *Royal Life Saving national drowning report 2017*. Retrieved from https://www.royallifesaving.com.au/

Singh, A., Avula, A. & Zahn, E. (2022). *Acute bronchitis*. Retrieved from https://www.ncbi.nlm.nih.gov/

Tan, W. (2018). Non-small-cell lung cancer. *Medicine*. Retrieved from http://emedicine.medscape.com/

World Data Atlas (2022). *Tuberculosis Australia*. Retrieved from https://knoema.com/

World Health Organization (WHO) (2021). *Global tuberculosis report*. Retrieved from http://www.who.int/

World Health Organization (WHO) (2022a). *Severe acute respiratory syndrome (SARS)*. Retrieved from http://www.who.int/

World Health Organization (WHO) (2022b). *MERS-COV*. Retrieved from http://www.who.int/

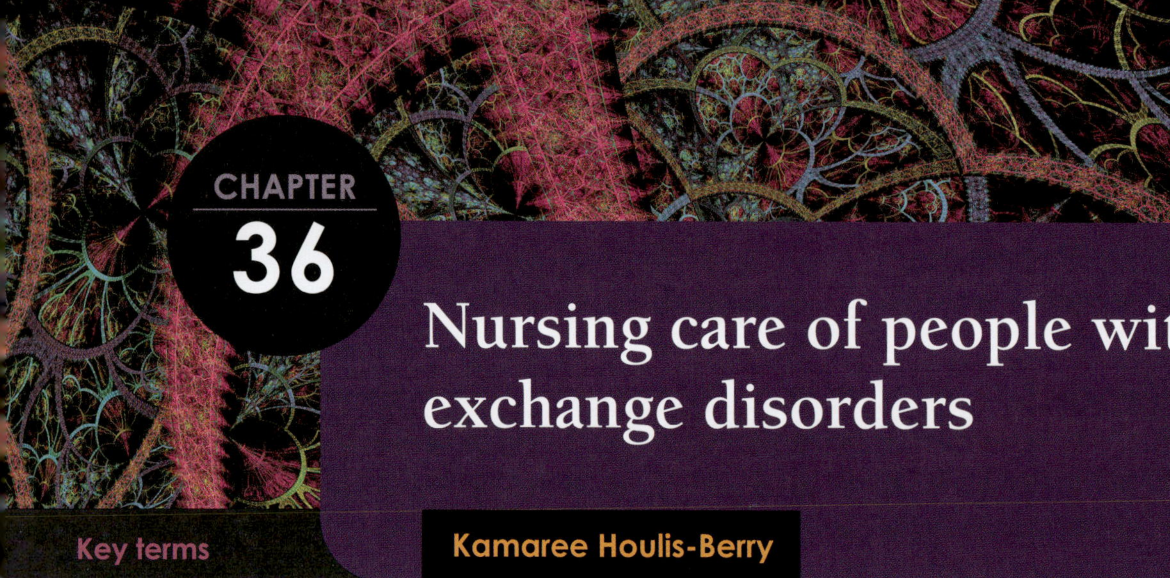

Nursing care of people with gas exchange disorders

Kamaree Houlis-Berry

Key terms

acute respiratory distress syndrome (ARDS) 1346
asthma 1295
atelectasis 1323
bronchiectasis 1323
chronic bronchitis 1308
chronic obstructive pulmonary disease (COPD) 1308
cor pulmonale 1332
cystic fibrosis (CF) 1320
emphysema 1309
pulmonary embolism 1327
pulmonary hypertension 1331
respiratory failure 1333
sarcoidosis 1326
status asthmaticus 1298
weaning 1342

Learning outcomes

- Describe the epidemiology, pathophysiology, manifestations and management of a person with asthma.
- Differentiate between the types, pathophysiology and management of an individual experiencing a chronic obstruction pulmonary disease.
- Compare the progression and potential outcomes for a person with a lung disease such as cystic fibrosis, atelectasis or bronchiectasis.
- Describe the influence on gas exchange for a person experiencing an occupational lung disease or sarcoidosis.
- Differentiate between the types of pulmonary vascular disorders in relation to aetiology, manifestations and management.
- Identify the types, pathophysiology, manifestations and management options for a person with respiratory failure.

Clinical competencies

- Assess functional health status of a person with a disorder affecting ventilation and gas exchange.
- Use data and knowledge of the effects of the disorder and prescribed treatment to identify priority nursing diagnoses and to plan care for a person with a disorder affecting ventilation and gas exchange.
- Use the nursing process and evidence-based nursing research to plan and implement individualised nursing care for individuals, including measures to promote ventilation and gas exchange.
- Plan and provide appropriate teaching for health promotion in vulnerable populations and to prepare individuals and families for community-based care.
- Evaluate the effectiveness of nursing interventions and teaching, revising strategies and teaching plans as needed.
- Coordinate safe interprofessional care and administer prescribed medications and treatments for people with disorders affecting ventilation and gas exchange.

Normal function of the lower respiratory tract depends on several organ systems: the central nervous system, which stimulates and controls breathing; chemoreceptors in the brain, aortic arch and carotid bodies, which monitor the pH and oxygen content of blood; the heart and circulatory system, which provide for blood supply and gas exchange; the musculoskeletal system, which provides an intact thoracic cavity capable of expanding and contracting; and the lungs and bronchial tree, which allow air movement and gas exchange. Impaired function of any of these systems affects ventilation. As a result, tissues may become *hypoxic*, with inadequate oxygen to support metabolic activity.

Although some of the disorders discussed in this chapter can affect ventilation (air movement into and out of the airways and alveoli), all can have significant effects on gas exchange. The mechanisms by which they affect gas exchange differ:

- In reactive airway disease (asthma, thunderstorm asthma), coronavirus (COVID-19) and obstructive disorders, air trapping reduces the amount of oxygen available to drive gas exchange.
- Interstitial lung disorders affect the ability of the lungs to expand and the work of breathing—again, reducing alveolar oxygenation and gas exchange.
- Pulmonary vascular disorders affect blood flow to the lungs or a portion of the lungs, reducing gas exchange through their effects on perfusion of the lungs.
- Respiratory failure is the ultimate consequence of impaired gas exchange; the lungs cannot adequately oxygenate the blood or eliminate sufficient carbon dioxide.

With a few exceptions, the disorders discussed in this chapter are relatively common, chronic lung diseases.

Disorders of other body systems, such as neurological disorders (e.g. head injury, spinal cord trauma or disorders, multiple sclerosis and myasthenia gravis) can also affect gas exchange through their effects on the central or peripheral nervous systems. These disorders and their effects on the respiratory system are discussed in subsequent chapters of this text.

Ageing affects pulmonary ventilation and gas exchange as well. The number of alveoli decrease and emphysematous changes reduce the surface area for gas exchange. Alveoli become less elastic, causing increased air trapping and dead space. For older adults who remain active, these changes have minimal effect on exercise tolerance and activities of daily living (ADLs). When combined with lung disease, however, age-related pulmonary changes increase the person's risk of developing respiratory failure.

The National Aboriginal and Torres Strait Islander health survey (ABS, 2019) showed that chronic lower respiratory diseases ranked third overall as the leading cause of death for both males and females.

FAST FACTS

- Approximately 7 million Australians live with a chronic respiratory condition.
- Approximately 11% of Australians have asthma (12% females and 9.4% males).
- Over 9.7 million Australians have acquired COVID-19.
- Approximately 1.5% have a chronic obstructive pulmonary disease (COPD).
- For those who have chronic obstructive pulmonary disease (COPD), 91.3% suffer from another condition.
- Chronic lower respiratory disease is one of the leading causes of death in Australia.

Sources: Australian Bureau of Statistics (ABS), (2021, 2022a); Australian Institute of Health and Welfare (AIHW) (2020b); Department of Health and Aged Care (2022a).

Reactive airway disease

In reactive airway disease, the airways narrow in response to a stimulus. Airway narrowing limits airflow both into and out of the alveoli. Limited airflow increases the work of breathing and the residual volume of the lungs as air is trapped behind narrowed airways. Inspired air mixes with an abnormally large volume of residual air, effectively reducing the amount of oxygen available in the alveoli. Decreased alveolar ventilation further reduces oxygen available for exchange.

THE PERSON WITH ASTHMA

Asthma is a chronic inflammatory disorder of the airways characterised by recurrent episodes of wheezing, breathlessness, chest tightness and coughing. Inflammation causes increased responsiveness of the airways to multiple stimuli. The widespread airflow obstruction that occurs during acute episodes usually reverses either spontaneously or with treatment. While most episodes or asthma 'attacks' are relatively brief, some individuals with asthma may experience longer episodes with some degree of airway impairment daily. In rare cases, an acute episode of asthma is so severe that respiratory failure and death result.

Prevalence and risk factors

In Australia, approximately 11% of the population had asthma in 2017–2018. Rates are decreasing in children and young adults but have remained stable in adults 35 years and older (AIHW, 2019a). Australia has one of the highest prevalence rates of asthma in the world, with 1 in 10 people affected. Females were more likely than males to have asthma (12.0% compared to 9.4%), with the rate of asthma similar in boys and girls aged 0–14 years (9.5% and 7.9%). In 2020, 417 people died of asthma (143 males and 274 females). Asthma hospitalisation rates were 158 per 100,000 population. The rate for children aged 0–14 was 363 per 100,000, which was markedly higher than those aged 15 years and over (106 per 100,000). Asthma remains a significant problem and burden on healthcare resources (see Figure 36.1) (AIHW, 2019b, 2020a; Asthma Australia, 2021; National Asthma Council Australia (NACA), 2021).

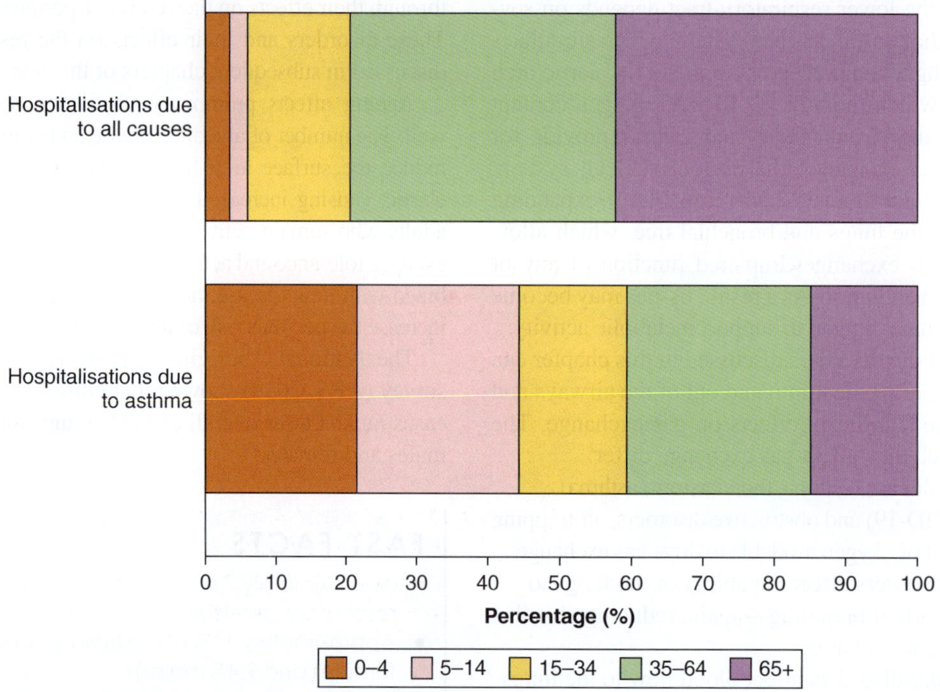

FIGURE 36.1 ***Comparison of hospitalisations due to all causes versus asthma by age group***

Source: Australian Institute of Health and Welfare, AIHW analysis of the AIHW National Hospital Morbidity Database. http://www.aihw.qov.au. Licensed under a Creative Commons BY 4.0 (CC-BY 4.0) licence, https://creativecommons.org/licenses/by/4.0/.

A number of risk factors can be identified for asthma, although many people develop the disease in the absence of known risk factors. Allergies play a strong role in childhood asthma but a lesser role in adults. There is a strong genetic component to the disease, although a specific pattern of inheritance has not been identified. More than 50 different genes have been identified as being involved in a variety of processes contributing to the development of asthma (Weiss, 2021). Environmental factors, including dust mites, animal and fungal allergens, pollution and occupational exposure to industrial compounds, may contribute. Respiratory viruses, such as rhinovirus, influenza and COVID-19, and other contributory factors including exercise (particularly in cold air) and emotional stress can precipitate asthma attacks (NACA, 2022a).

Physiology review

Airways within the lungs contain criss-crossing strips of smooth muscle that control their diameter. This muscle is innervated by the autonomic nervous system. Parasympathetic (cholinergic) stimulation leads to bronchoconstriction or narrowing of the airways. Sympathetic stimulation through β_2-adrenergic receptors causes bronchodilation or expansion of the airways (Martini, Nath & Bartholomew, 2018) and slight bronchoconstriction normally predominates. However, when increased airflow is necessary (e.g. during exercise), the parasympathetic system is inhibited and stimulation of the sympathetic system causes bronchodilation. Inflammatory mediators (such as histamine) released during an antigen–antibody response act directly on bronchial smooth muscle to produce bronchoconstriction.

FAST FACTS

- One in 4 people aged over 15 with asthma have a written action plan.
- Data show that females over 15 years of age are 2.3 times more likely than males to be admitted to hospital for asthma.
- Respiratory tract infections are frequently identified as an exacerbating factor in admission to hospital.

Sources: Data extracted from AIHW (2019a, 2019b); NACA (2022a).

Pathophysiology

In asthma, the airways are in a persistent state of inflammation. During symptom-free periods, airway inflammation in asthma is subacute or quiet. Even during these periods, however, inflammatory cells such as eosinophils, neutrophils and lymphocytes may be found in airway tissues, and oedema may be present. An acute inflammatory response, during which resident inflammatory cells interact with inflammatory mediators, cytokines and additional infiltrating inflammatory cells, may be triggered by a variety of factors (Bullock & Hales, 2019). Common triggers for an acute asthma attack include exposure to allergens, respiratory tract infection, exercise, inhaled irritants and emotional upsets.

Attack triggers

Childhood asthma (which may continue into adulthood) is most often linked to inhalation of allergens such as pollen, animal dander (shed skin flakes) or household dust. Individuals with allergic asthma often have a history of other allergies. Environmental pollutants, such as tobacco smoke and irritant

FOCUS ON CULTURAL DIVERSITY Prevalence of asthma in certain populations

- Asthma prevalence is higher in Aboriginal and Torres Strait Islander people in every age group, as shown in the table below:

AGE IN YEARS	ABORIGINAL AND TORRES STRAIT ISLANDER AUSTRALIANS	NON-INDIGENOUS AUSTRALIANS
0-14	11.5	9.7
15-24	13.8	10.2
25-34	15.0	10.6
35-44	17.0	11.2
45-54	20.8	12.4
> 55	25.7	11.1

- The proportion of people with asthma in remote areas (9%) is around half that of people living in non-remote areas (17%).
- Prevalence of asthma is lower in people living in Australia who were born overseas, as shown in the following table:

COUNTRY OF BIRTH	RELATIVE PERCENTAGE OF POPULATION
Australia	12.8%
Overseas	6.0%

Sources: Data extracted from ABS (2019). *National Aboriginal and Torres Strait Islander health survey.* Retrieved from https://www.abs.gov.au; ABS (2022b). *Australian health survey*. Retrieved from https://www.abs.gov.au.

gases (e.g. sulfur dioxide, nitrogen dioxide and ozone), can provoke asthma. Exposure to second-hand smoke as a child is associated with a higher risk and increased severity of asthma. Agents found in the workplace, such as noxious fumes and gases, chemicals and dusts, may cause occupational asthma.

Respiratory infections—viral, in particular—are a common internal stimulus for an asthmatic attack. Exercise-induced asthma attacks are also relatively common. Loss of heat or water from the bronchial surface may contribute to exercise-induced asthma. Exercising in cold, dry air increases the risk of an asthma attack in susceptible people.

Emotional stress is a significant aetiological factor for attacks in almost half of people with asthma. Common pharmacological triggers include aspirin and other non-steroidal anti-inflammatory drugs, sulfites (used as preservatives in wine, beer, fresh fruits and salad) and beta-blockers.

See Box 36.1 for triggers of asthma.

BOX 36.1 Triggers of asthma

- **Environmental allergens (often small glycoproteins; e.g. dust mites, animal dander, pollen, fungi)**
- **Cigarette smoking**
- **Pollution**
- **Irritants (fumes from volatile compounds; e.g. cleaning agents, glues, paints)**
- **Respiratory tract infections**
- **Medications (aspirin, non-steroidal anti-inflammatory drugs, beta-blockers)**
- **Physical factors (exercise, changes in temperature)**
- **Gastro-oesophageal reflux**
- **Emotional stress**
- **Occupational exposure to organic compounds**
- **Food additives**

Responses

When a trigger such as inhalation of an allergen or irritant occurs, an acute or *early response* develops in the hyperreactive airways predisposed to bronchospasm. Sensitised mast cells in the bronchial mucosa release inflammatory mediators such as histamine, prostaglandins and leukotrienes. Resident and infiltrating inflammatory cells also produce inflammatory mediators such as cytokines, bradykinin and growth factors. These mediators stimulate parasympathetic receptors and bronchial smooth muscle to produce bronchoconstriction. They also increase capillary permeability, which allows plasma to escape and leads to mucosal oedema. Mucus production is stimulated; excess mucus collects in the narrowed airways (Bullock & Hales, 2019).

The attack is prolonged by the *late phase response*, which develops 4 to 12 hours after exposure to the trigger. Inflammatory cells such as basophils and eosinophils are activated, which damage airway epithelium, produce mucosal oedema, impair mucociliary clearance and produce or prolong bronchoconstriction. The degree of hyperreactivity depends on the extent of inflammation. Together, bronchoconstriction, oedema and inflammation, and mucus secretion narrow the airway. Airway resistance increases, limiting airflow and increasing the work of breathing (see Figure 36.2).

Limited expiratory airflow traps air distal to the spastic, narrowed airways. Trapped air mixes with inspired air in the alveoli, reducing its oxygen tension and gas exchange across the alveolar–capillary membrane. Distended alveoli compress alveolar capillaries, reducing blood flow and further affecting gas exchange. As a result, hypoxaemia develops. Hypoxaemia and increased lung volume due to trapping stimulate the respiratory rate. Hyperventilation causes the $PaCO_2$ to fall, leading to respiratory alkalosis. (See the chapter 'Nursing care of people with altered fluid, electrolyte and acid–base balance' for more information about acid–base imbalances.)

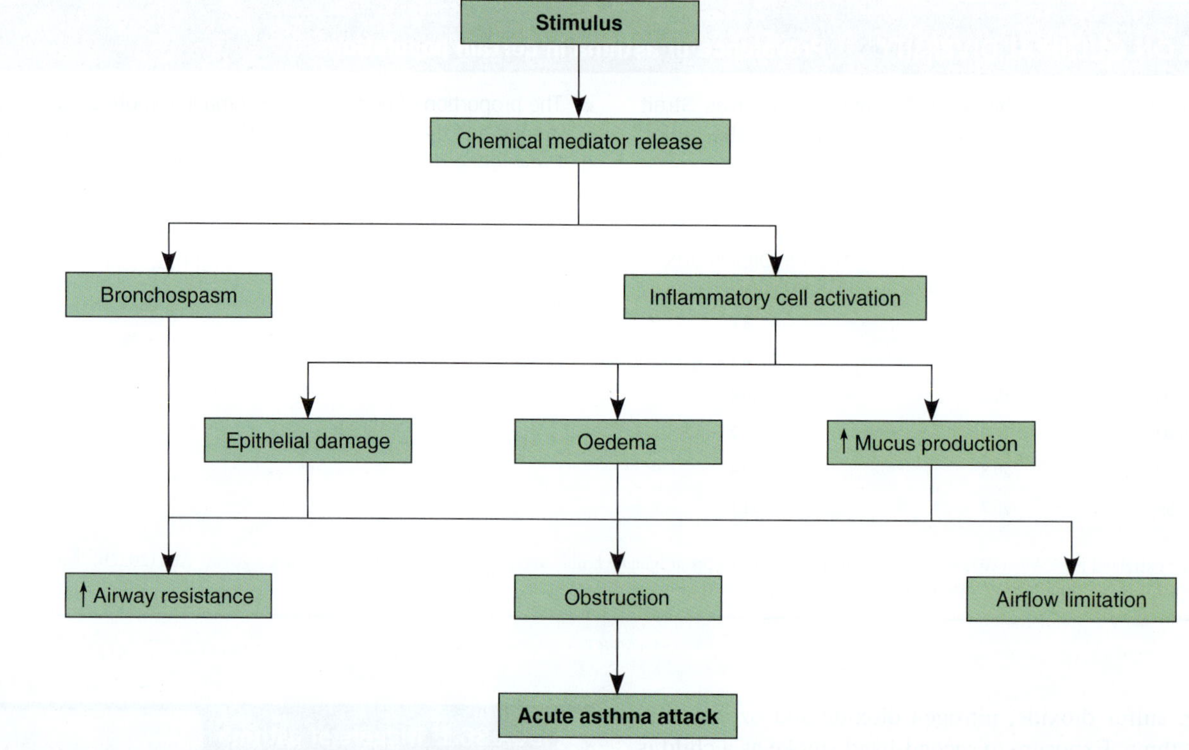

FIGURE 36.2 *Pathogenesis of an acute episode of asthma*

To summarise, in an acute asthma attack inflammatory mediators are released from sensitised airways followed by activation of inflammatory cells. These events lead to bronchoconstriction, airway oedema and impaired mucociliary clearance. Airway narrowing limits airflow and increases the work of breathing; trapped air mixes with inhaled air, impairing gas exchange.

Manifestations and complications

An asthma attack is characterised by a subjective sensation of chest tightness, cough, dyspnoea and wheezing (see the 'Manifestations' box). The onset of symptoms may be either abrupt or insidious, and an attack may subside rapidly or persist for hours or days. A sense of chest constriction and non-productive cough are common early manifestations of an attack. During an attack, tachycardia, tachypnoea and prolonged expiration are common. Diffuse wheezing is heard on auscultation. With more severe attacks, use of the accessory muscles of respiration, intercostal retractions, loud wheezing and distant breath sounds may be noted. Fatigue, anxiety, apprehension and severe dyspnoea that allows speaking only one or two words between breaths may occur with persistent severe episodes. The onset of respiratory failure is marked by inaudible breath sounds with reduced wheezing and an ineffective cough. Without careful assessment, this apparent relief of symptoms can be misinterpreted as an improvement.

The frequency of attacks and severity of symptoms vary greatly from person to person. Although some people have infrequent, mild episodes, others have nearly continuous manifestations of cough, dyspnoea on exertion and wheezing, with periodic severe exacerbations. **Status asthmaticus** is severe, prolonged asthma that does not respond to routine treatment. Without aggressive therapy, status asthmaticus can lead to respiratory failure with hypoxaemia, hypercapnia and acidosis. Endotracheal intubation, mechanical ventilation and aggressive drug treatment may be necessary to sustain life.

MANIFESTATIONS Acute asthma

- Dyspnoea
- Tachypnoea
- Tachycardia
- Chest tightness
- Wheezing
- Cough
- Anxiety
- Poor mental health

In addition to acute respiratory failure, other complications associated with acute asthma include dehydration, respiratory infection, atelectasis, pneumothorax and cor pulmonale.

Cough-variant asthma

A common symptom of asthma is a cough which is usually non-productive and non-paroxysmal (Gao et al., 2020). Cough can be initiated by either upper airway irritants (e.g. post-nasal drip or gastro-oesophageal reflux disease) or by inflammation or constriction of the lower airways. Most commonly, cough associated with asthma is accompanied by classic asthma symptoms such as chest constriction, dyspnoea and wheezing. Individuals with *cough-variant asthma*, however, have persistent cough without wheezing or dyspnoea, often delaying diagnosis. These individuals do have significant airway inflammation and demonstrate the pathophysiological features of asthma.

INTERPROFESSIONAL CARE

The diagnosis of asthma is based primarily on the history and manifestations. Treatment goals are twofold. Daily management focuses on controlling symptoms and preventing acute attacks. During an acute attack, therapy is directed towards restoring airway patency and alveolar ventilation.

Diagnosis

Diagnostic tests are used to determine the degree of airway involvement during and between acute episodes, and to identify causative factors such as allergens. See the chapter 'A person-centred approach to assessing the respiratory system' for more information about and the nursing care related to these diagnostic tests.

- *Respiratory function tests (RFTs)* are used to evaluate the degree of airway obstruction. Respiratory function testing done before and after use of an aerosolised bronchodilator helps determine the reversibility of airway obstruction. The residual volume of the lungs may be increased and the vital capacity decreased or normal even during periods of remission. The forced expiratory volume and peak expiratory flow rate are the most valuable respiratory function studies to evaluate the severity of an asthma attack and the effectiveness of treatment measures.
- *Challenge*, or *bronchial*, *provocation testing* uses an inhaled substance such as methacholine or histamine with RFTs to confirm the diagnosis of asthma by detecting airway hyperresponsiveness.
- *Arterial blood gases (ABGs)* are drawn during an acute attack to evaluate oxygenation, CO_2 elimination and acid–base status. ABGs initially show hypoxaemia with a low PaO_2 and mild respiratory alkalosis with an elevated pH and low $PaCO_2$ due to tachypnoea. Severe airflow obstruction causes significant hypoxaemia and respiratory acidosis (pH < 7.35 and $PaCO_2 > 42$ mmHg), indicative of respiratory failure and the need for mechanical ventilation. See the chapter 'Nursing care of people with altered fluid, electrolyte and acid–base balance' for more information about arterial blood gases and their interpretation.
- *Skin testing* may be done to identify specific allergens if an allergic trigger is suspected for asthma attacks.

Disease monitoring

Peak expiratory flow rate (PEFR) is used on a day-to-day basis to evaluate the severity of bronchial hyperresponsiveness. Small, inexpensive meters to measure PEFR are available. Readings taken at varying times of day over several weeks are used to establish the person's personal best or normal PEFR. This value is then used to evaluate the severity of airway obstruction. Some people with asthma may benefit from regular peak flow monitoring, which enables not only the individual but also asthma healthcare professionals to monitor and recognise exacerbations early (NACA, 2022a).

Preventive measures

Asthma attacks often can be prevented by avoiding allergens and environmental triggers. Modifying the home environment by controlling dust, removing carpets, covering mattresses and pillows to reduce dust mite populations and installing air-filtering systems may be useful. Pets may need to be removed from the household. Eliminating all tobacco smoke in the home is vital. Wearing a mask that retains humidity and warm air while exercising in cold weather may help prevent attacks of exercise-induced asthma. Early treatment of respiratory infections is vital to prevent asthma exacerbations. National guidelines recommend that all individuals with asthma have a written asthma action plan. Despite the recommendation being in place for over 20 years, the majority of people with asthma in Australia do not have a plan. Healthcare professionals should work towards ensuring that all individuals in their care have a written asthma action plan.

Asthma first aid

Friends and family should be aware of how to manage an individual who is having an asthma attack. The NACA provides information on selecting and adjusting medications for adults and adolescents as well as asthma first aid charts for children under 12 and people 12+ years. These charts clearly identify steps to assist an individual who is having an asthma attack (see Figures 36.3 and 36.4).

Medications

Medications are used to prevent and control asthma symptoms, reduce the frequency and severity of exacerbations, and reverse airway obstruction. Drugs used for long-term control of asthma are taken daily to maintain control of the disease. The primary drugs in this group are anti-inflammatory agents, long-acting bronchodilators and leukotriene receptor antagonists. Quick-relief medications provide prompt relief of bronchoconstriction and airflow obstruction with associated wheezing, cough and chest tightness. Short-acting adrenergic stimulants (rapid-acting bronchodilators), anticholinergic drugs and methylxanthines fall into this category.

The NACA's (2022a) asthma handbook provides information related to COVID-19 and asthma and recommends a five-step approach for managing asthma (see Figure 36.5) including individual assessments, written action plan, regular medications for daily maintenance and good symptom control, and specialist treatment if additional interventions and/or medications are required. Many of the drugs used for continued asthma management and relief of an acute attack can be administered by a metered-dose inhaler (MDI), dry powder inhaler (DPI) or nebuliser. The advantages of administering medications locally by inhalation include rapid onset and reduced systemic effects of the drugs. In an MDI, a chemical propellant is used to deliver the medication when the canister is depressed. In contrast, DPI contains no propellant. Instead, the medication is released by inhaling rapidly through the mouthpiece.

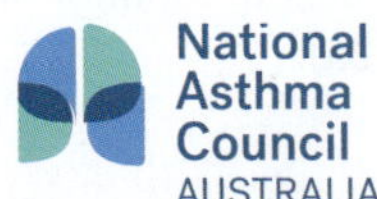

FIRST AID FOR ASTHMA

CHILDREN UNDER 12

USE BLUE/GREY PUFFER (E.G. ASMOL, VENTOLIN, ZEMPREON)

Use child's own reliever puffer, if possible. If not, use blue/grey puffer from first aid kit or borrow one.

1 **Sit the child comfortably upright.**
Stay calm and reassure them.

2 **Give 4 puffs of blue/grey puffer**
How to do this:
Add 1 puff into spacer – child takes 4 breaths in and out of spacer.
Repeat until 4 puffs have been given.
See instructions below: **How to use a blue/grey puffer with spacer**

3 **Wait 4 minutes.** Stay with child – watch carefully and reassure them. Call 000 for an ambulance **at any time** if you need to. Say that a child is having an asthma attack.

4 **After 4 minutes.**

Worse or no better?
If getting worse or severe breathing problem, **call 000** for ambulance NOW.
Keep giving 4 puffs every 4 minutes until ambulance arrives.
(Give 4 separate puffs, 4 breaths with each puff.)

Still hard to breathe?
If the child still cannot breathe normally, **give 4 more puffs.**
If still cannot breathe normally within a few minutes, **call 000.**
Keep giving 4 puffs every 4 minutes until ambulance arrives.
(Give 4 separate puffs, 4 breaths with each puff.)

Breathing normally?
If the child feels better and is breathing normally, get them to a doctor for a check-up.

Signs of an asthma attack in a child (any of these): Sudden shortness of breath, cough, chest tightness or wheezing.

Not sure it's asthma?
If child stays conscious and main problem seems to be breathing use **blue/grey puffer.** It is unlikely to harm them, even if not asthma.
CALL AMBULANCE (000)

Severe allergic reactions/ anaphylaxis
If child is allergic to foods, insect stings or medicines **AND** has sudden breathing problems (e.g. cough, wheeze, hoarse voice): Give adrenaline injection first. Use their own autoinjector (e.g. EpiPen, Anapen) if available. Do this even if no other signs of allergic reaction. **Then** give blue/grey puffer by following the 4 steps shown here.
CALL AMBULANCE (000)

If someone is unconscious, start life support. Scan code for ANZCOR Basic Life Support Flowchart

If you need an interpreter, call 131 450

HOW TO USE A BLUE/GREY PUFFER WITH SPACER

WITHOUT MASK (older children)
- Remove puffer cap and shake puffer.
- Insert puffer upright into spacer.
- Put mouthpiece of spacer between child's teeth and seal lips around it.
- Press once firmly on puffer to release 1 puff into spacer.
- Get child to take 4 breaths in and out of spacer.
- Repeat, 1 puff at a time till 4 puffs taken.
- Replace cap on puffer.

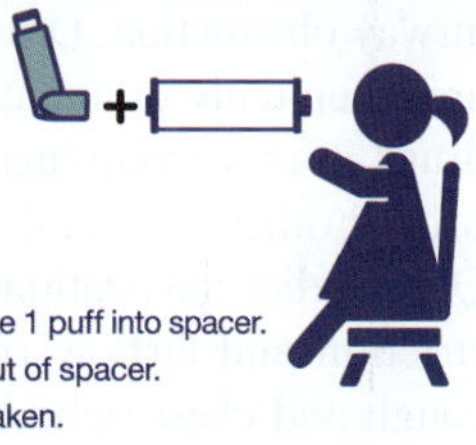

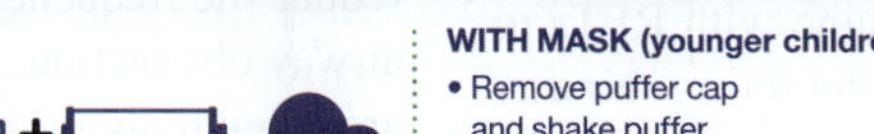

WITH MASK (younger children)
- Remove puffer cap and shake puffer.
- Insert puffer upright into spacer.
- Attach mask to spacer.
- Hold mask firmly over child's nose and mouth.
- Press once firmly on puffer to release 1 puff into spacer.
- Get child to take 4 breaths in and out of spacer.
- Repeat, 1 puff at a time, till 4 puffs taken.
- Replace cap on puffer.

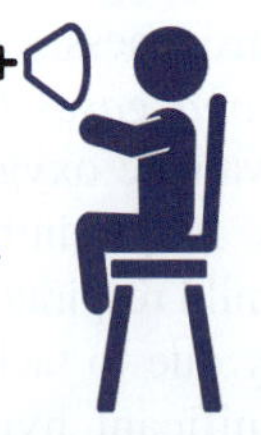

! No spacer?
Use a plastic drink bottle or rolled-up paper
Go to nationalasthma.org.au or scan code

! No blue/grey asthma puffer is available and the person's own asthma reliever inhaler is not blue/grey?
Go to nationalasthma.org.au or scan code

Allergic Reactions

SIGNS OF ALLERGIC REACTION: Can include swelling of lips/face/eyes, tingling mouth, hives/welts, (abdominal pain/ vomiting if insect allergy)

WATCH FOR ANY OF THESE SIGNS OF ANAPHYLAXIS (severe reaction): Difficult/noisy breathing, swelling of tongue, swelling or tightness in throat, wheeze, persistent cough, difficulty talking, hoarse voice, persistent dizziness or collapse, pale and floppy (young children)

ALWAYS GIVE ADRENALINE INJECTOR FIRST, and then asthma reliever puffer if someone with known asthma and allergy to food, insects or medication has SUDDEN BREATHING DIFFICULTY (including wheeze, persistent cough or hoarse voice), even if there are no skin symptoms.

When to call 000 for an ambulance
- Child is drowsy
- Child looks blue around lips
- Child with breathing problem has allergies to foods, insect stings, or medicines
- Breathing problem is severe
- Child is not getting better
- You are not sure what to do

FIGURE 36.3 *First aid for asthma for children under 12*

Source: NACA (2022b). *First aid for asthma: Children under 12*. Retrieved from https://www.nationalasthma.org.au/. Reproduced with permission of National Asthma Council Australia, 2023. National Asthma Council guidelines are reviewed annually; please visit https://www.nationalasthma.org.au/ for current guidelines.

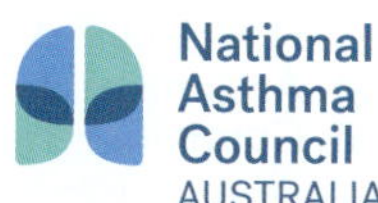

FIRST AID FOR ASTHMA

AGES 12+

USE BLUE/GREY PUFFER (E.G. ASMOL, VENTOLIN, ZEMPREON)

Use person's own reliever inhaler, if possible. If not, use blue/grey puffer from first aid kit or borrow one.

1 **Sit the person comfortably upright.**
Stay calm and reassure them.

2 **Give 4 puffs of blue/grey puffer**
How to do this:
Add 1 puff into spacer – person takes 4 breaths in and out of spacer.
Repeat until 4 puffs have been given.
See instructions below: **How to use a blue/grey puffer with spacer**

3 **Wait 4 minutes.** Stay with person – watch carefully and reassure them. Call 000 for an ambulance **at any time** if you need to. Say that someone is having an asthma attack.

4 **After 4 minutes.**

Worse or no better?
If getting worse or severe breathing problem, **call 000** for ambulance **NOW**.
Keep giving 4 puffs every 4 minutes until ambulance arrives.
(Give 4 separate puffs, 4 breaths with each puff.)

Still hard to breathe?
If the person still cannot breathe normally, **give 4 more puffs.**
If still cannot breathe normally within a few minutes, **call 000.**
Keep giving 4 puffs every 4 minutes until ambulance arrives.
(Give 4 separate puffs, 4 breaths with each puff.)

Breathing normally?
If the person feels better and is breathing normally, get them to a doctor for a check-up.

Signs that someone is having an asthma attack (any of these): Sudden shortness of breath, can't talk normally, cough, chest tightness or wheezing.

Not sure it's asthma?
If a person stays conscious and their main problem seems to be breathing, use blue/grey reliever puffer and call ambulance on 000. This medicine is unlikely to harm them even if they do not have asthma.

Severe allergic reactions/ anaphylaxis If someone is allergic to foods, insect stings or medicines **AND** they have sudden breathing problems (e.g. cough, wheeze, hoarse voice):
Give adrenaline **first**.
Use their own autoinjector (e.g. EpiPen, Anapen) if available. Do this even if there are no other signs of an allergic reaction – see below.
Then give asthma reliever puffer by following the 4 steps shown here.
CALL AMBULANCE (000)

If someone is unconscious, start life support. Scan code for ANZCOR Basic Life Support Flowchart

If you need an interpreter, call 131 450

HOW TO USE A BLUE/GREY PUFFER WITH SPACER

- Remove puffer cap and shake puffer.
- Insert puffer upright into spacer.
- Put mouthpiece of spacer between person's teeth and seal lips around it.
- Press once firmly on puffer to release one puff into spacer.
- Get them to take 4 breaths in and out of spacer.
- Repeat, 1 puff at a time, until 4 puffs taken.
- Replace cap on puffer.

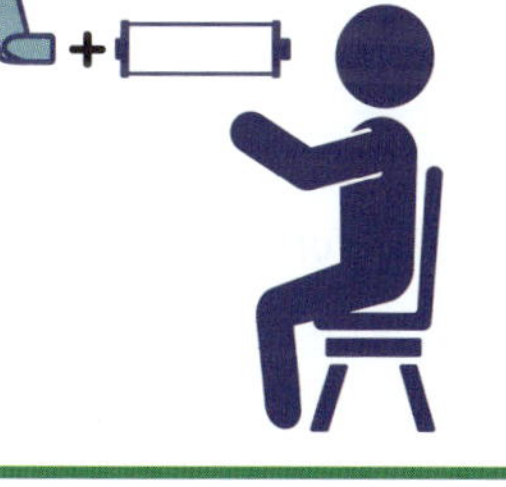

! No spacer?
Use a plastic drink bottle or rolled-up paper
Go to nationalasthma.org.au or scan code

! No blue/grey asthma puffer is available and the person's own asthma reliever inhaler is not blue/grey?
Go to nationalasthma.org.au or scan code

Allergic Reactions

SIGNS OF ALLERGIC REACTION: Can include swelling of lips/face/eyes, tingling mouth, hives/welts, (abdominal pain/ vomiting if insect allergy)

WATCH FOR ANY OF THESE SIGNS OF ANAPHYLAXIS (severe reaction): Difficult/noisy breathing, swelling of tongue, swelling or tightness in throat, wheeze, persistent cough, difficulty talking, hoarse voice, persistent dizziness or collapse, pale and floppy (young children)

ALWAYS GIVE ADRENALINE INJECTOR FIRST, and then asthma reliever puffer if someone with known asthma and allergy to food, insects or medication has SUDDEN BREATHING DIFFICULTY (including wheeze, persistent cough or hoarse voice), even if there are no skin symptoms.

When to call 000 for an ambulance

- Person is drowsy
- Person looks blue around lips
- Person with breathing problem has allergies to foods, insect stings, or medicines
- Breathing problem is severe
- Person is not getting better
- You are not sure what to do

 More information: www.nationalasthma.org.au

FIGURE 36.4 *First aid for asthma for those aged 12+*

Source: NACA (2022c). *First aid for asthma: Ages 12+*. Retrieved from https://www.nationalasthma.org.au/. Reproduced with permission of National Asthma Council Australia, 2023. National Asthma Council guidelines are reviewed annually; please visit https://www.nationalasthma.org.au/ for current guidelines.

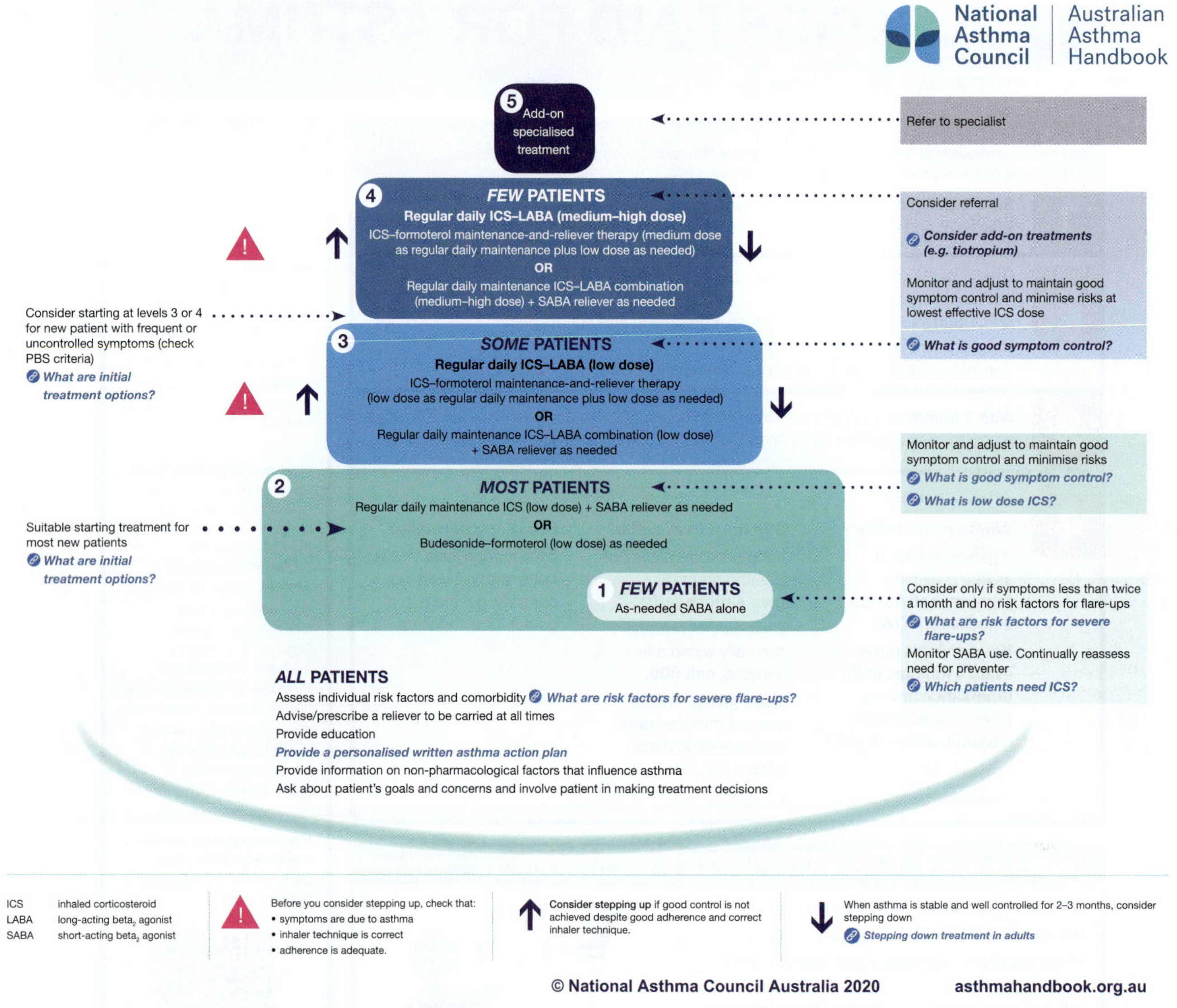

FIGURE 36.5 *Selecting and adjusting medication for adults and adolescents*

Source: Adapted from NACA (2022a). *Australian asthma handbook* (V2.2). Retrieved from https://www.asthmahandbook.org.au. Reproduced with permission of National Asthma Council Australia, 2023. National Asthma Council guidelines are reviewed annually; please visit https://www.nationalasthma.org.au/ for current guidelines.

Nursing implications for medications used to treat asthma are outlined in the 'Medication administration' box.

BRONCHODILATORS Most asthmatics need bronchodilator therapy to control their symptoms (see Table 36.1). Inhalation of nebulised medication is the preferred means of administration. The primary bronchodilators used include adrenergic stimulants and anticholinergic agents. These drugs often are administered in combination with an anti-inflammatory agent.

Adrenergic stimulants (β_2-agonists) affect receptors on smooth muscle cells of the respiratory tract, causing smooth muscle relaxation and bronchodilation. Long-acting adrenergic stimulants (inhaled salmeterol) and oral sustained-release salbutamol are used in conjunction with anti-inflammatory drugs to control symptoms but are not appropriate to treat an acute episode of asthma. Inhaled short-acting beta-adrenergic agonists (salbutamol and terbutaline), administered by MDI or DPI, are the treatment of choice for quick relief. They act within minutes, but their duration generally is short, lasting only 4–6 hours. Tachycardia and muscle tremors, common side effects of adrenergic agonists, are minimal with inhalation therapy.

Anticholinergic medications prevent bronchoconstriction by blocking parasympathetic input to bronchial smooth muscle. Ipratropium bromide, an anticholinergic drug administered by MDI, is useful when asthma symptoms are poorly controlled by adrenergic stimulants alone. Anticholinergic drugs act more slowly than adrenergic stimulants, requiring up to 60–90 minutes to achieve maximal effect.

ANTI-INFLAMMATORY AGENTS Corticosteroids and two non-steroidal anti-inflammatory agents, cromolyn sodium and nedocromil, are used to suppress airway inflammation and reduce asthma symptoms.

MEDICATION ADMINISTRATION Asthma

ADRENERGIC STIMULANTS

Adrenergic stimulants affect sympathetic receptors in the respiratory tract. Administered by MDI or dry powder inhalers, these drugs are the treatment of choice for acute bronchial asthma. Nearly all of the drugs in this class (adrenaline and isoprenaline being the exceptions) selectively activate β_2-receptors at the doses typically used to treat asthma. β_2-receptor activation results in smooth muscle relaxation and bronchodilation. Salmeterol and eformoterol are highly selective to β_2-receptors, resulting in fewer adverse effects. However, they have been shown to increase the risk of serious asthma exacerbations and death by masking the symptoms of worsening inflammation. Salmeterol (or eformoterol) should be used with concomitant corticosteroid therapy to prevent rapid deterioration from serious bronchospasm (MIMS, 2018a).

Oral forms of adrenergic agonists may be used for prophylaxis but are not effective in treating an acute attack because of their slow onset. When administered orally or parenterally, their effect on sympathetic nervous system receptors can produce undesirable side effects, such as nervousness, irritability, tachycardia and cardiac arrhythmias.

Nursing responsibilities

- Use with caution in individuals with hypertension, cardiovascular disease or arrhythmias, hyperthyroidism or diabetes.
- When given to a person who is hypoxaemic and acidotic, these drugs may cause potentially dangerous cardiac stimulation.
- Observe for desired effect of reduced dyspnoea and wheezing. CNS stimulation (anxiety, irritability and insomnia) and tremors are common side effects.

Health education for the person and family

- Follow the first aid for asthma charts (see Figures 36.3 and 36.4).
- Use the prescribed inhaler or nebuliser as directed.
- Use the bronchodilator first to open airways to enhance the effectiveness of the second medication.
- Rinse mouth after using inhalers to reduce systemic absorption of the medication.
- Keep a log to track bronchodilator use. If the drug becomes less effective or if higher doses are needed, contact a doctor.
- Report palpitations, irregular pulse and other side effects to the doctor.

ANTICHOLINERGICS

Anticholinergics are potent bronchodilators, blocking muscarinic receptors of the parasympathetic nervous system. Activation of muscarinic receptors produces smooth muscle contraction and bronchoconstriction; blockade of these receptors facilitates smooth muscle relaxation and bronchodilation. Atropine is used infrequently because of its tendency to dry secretions of the mucous membranes and other side effects. Ipratropium and tiotropium bromide are available as inhalers and have fewer side effects than atropine.

Nursing responsibilities

- Assess for possible contraindications to the drug, including hypersensitivity, glaucoma, prostatic hypertrophy or bladder-neck obstruction.
- Assess for desired and/or adverse effects: improving or worsening symptoms; nausea, vomiting, abdominal cramping; anxiety; dizziness; headache.
- Provide ice chips or sips of clear fluid to relieve dry mouth.

Health education for the person and family

- Take the drugs as prescribed.
- If the drug becomes less effective over time, notify the doctor; an adjustment in dosage may be needed.

CORTICOSTEROIDS

The anti-inflammatory effect of corticosteroids helps both prevent and treat acute episodes. Corticosteroids are used to reduce the frequency and severity of asthma attacks and allow reduced dosages of other drugs. The beneficial effects of corticosteroids for asthma result from their ability to decrease the synthesis and release of inflammatory mediators (such as histamine and leukotrienes), reduce inflammatory cell activation and infiltration and decrease airway oedema. Corticosteroids also increase the number and receptivity of β_2-receptors. The cushingoid side effects of corticosteroids, always a major concern with their use, are minimised when they are inhaled (Blakey et al., 2021). Note that the combination product salmeterol/fluticasone is associated with an increased risk of serious asthma exacerbations and death. It is a second-line drug, recommended for use only when asthma is inadequately controlled using other preparations (MIMS, 2018b).

Nursing responsibilities

- Administer inhaler doses after bronchodilators to facilitate transit of the medication to distal airways.
- Assess for common side effects: sore throat; hoarseness; and oropharyngeal or laryngeal *Candida albicans* infection.
- Administer antifungal medications or gargles as ordered.

Health education for the person and family

- Rinse the mouth after using the inhaler and maintain good oral hygiene to reduce the risk of fungal infections.
- These medications should not be used to alleviate the symptoms of an acute attack.
- Several weeks of continued therapy may be required before a beneficial effect is noticed.
- Notify the doctor if you develop weight gain, fluid retention, muscle weakness, redistribution of fat or mood changes.

MAST CELL STABILISERS

Cromolyn sodium and nedocromil sodium inhibit inflammatory cells in the airway, blocking early and late responses to inhaled antigens. Both drugs also prevent bronchoconstriction in response to inhaling cold air. These drugs act primarily by stabilising the cytoplasmic membrane of mast cells, preventing the cells from releasing inflammatory mediators such as histamine. These drugs are used only for preventing asthma attacks, not to treat an acute attack. They are administered by metered-dose inhaler and have a wide margin of safety. Individuals using nedocromil may complain of an unpleasant taste (Minutello & Gupta, 2022; Wang et al., 2019).

(continued)

MEDICATION ADMINISTRATION **Asthma (continued)**

Nursing responsibilities

Evaluate for potential adverse effects of wheezing and bronchoconstriction.

Health education for the person and family

- Gargling or sipping water can decrease the throat irritation associated with nebuliser treatment.
- Use appropriate technique. Inhale deeply with head tipped back to open airways, hold breath and then exhale. Repeat until all the drug dose has been inhaled.
- These drugs are used only to prevent asthma attacks; they are not effective in treating an acute attack.
- Several weeks may be required before a beneficial effect is noted.

LEUKOTRIENE RECEPTOR ANTAGONISTS

Leukotriene receptor antagonists interfere with the inflammatory process in the airways by suppressing the effects of leukotrienes, a group of inflammatory mediators. Leukotrienes are powerful bronchoconstrictors and vasodilators; blocking their synthesis or binding to their receptors improves airflow, decreases symptoms and reduces the need for short-acting bronchodilators. They are used for maintenance therapy in adults and children over the age of 12 as an alternative to inhaled corticosteroid therapy. They are not used to treat an acute attack.

Nursing responsibilities

- Administer orally either before or after meals depending on which medication has been prescribed (montelukast or zafirlukast) (Choi & Azmat, 2022).
- These drugs are generally well tolerated. However, they may inhibit some liver enzymes, affecting the metabolism of warfarin and possibly terfenadine and theophylline.
- Monitor liver enzymes (these drugs may be hepatotoxic), prothrombin times and theophylline blood levels.

Health education for the person and family

- Take the drugs as prescribed.
- Notify the doctor if a change in colour of stools or urine is noted or if jaundice or any other adverse side effects develop.

METHYLXANTHINES

The methylxanthines are central nervous system (CNS) stimulants chemically related to caffeine. These drugs produce bronchodilation through relaxation of bronchial smooth muscle. As CNS stimulants, they produce adverse effects such as nervousness, insomnia and tremors. When administered in large doses, convulsions may result.

Once the drugs of choice for preventing and treating asthma attacks, methylxanthines are now used primarily to prevent nocturnal asthma. Theophylline has a narrow margin of safety and high potential for toxicity. Because the metabolism and excretion of theophylline vary significantly from person to person—affected by such factors as age, smoking, genetic factors, alcoholism and other chronic diseases—monitoring of serum levels is vital.

Nursing responsibilities

- The therapeutic blood level for theophylline is 10 to 20 mg/L.
- Monitor for manifestations of toxicity. Anorexia, nausea, vomiting, restlessness, insomnia, cardiac arrhythmias and seizures are early manifestations. Other manifestations include epigastric pain, haematemesis, diarrhoea, headache, irritability, muscle twitching, palpitations, tachycardia, flushing and circulatory failure.
- Administer with meals or a full glass of water or milk to minimise gastric irritation.
- Monitor effect closely when administering concurrently with medications such as barbiturates, anticonvulsants, thyroid hormone, beta-blockers, bronchodilators and others.

Health education for the person and family

- Oral methylxanthines are ineffective to treat an acute asthma attack; do not delay other treatment by using these drugs.
- Check with the doctor before taking any over-the-counter (OTC) medications or other prescription drugs while on theophylline.
- Do not smoke while using this drug.
- Report adverse effects to the doctor.

CONSIDERATION FOR PRACTICE

The treatment of chronic health conditions becomes complicated in women of childbearing age. Women are advised to update their asthma action plan and continue with preventive medications during pregnancy. Before administering *any* medication, the pregnancy category should be assessed (see the table below).

Pregnancy category for common medications used in asthma

DRUG	CATEGORY	DRUG	CATEGORY
acetylcysteine	B2	methylprednisolone (IV)	A
beclomethasone	B3	montelukast	B1
budesonide	A	nedocromil	B1
ciclesonide	B3	omalizumab	B1
dexamethasone	A	prednisolone	A
dornase alfa	B1	prednisone	A
eformoterol	B3	salbutamol (MDI)	A
fluticasone	B3	salmeterol	B3
hydrocortisone	A	sodium cromoglycate	A
ipratropium bromide	B1	terbutaline	A
isoprenaline	A	zafirlukast	B1

Sources: Therapeutic Goods Administration (2022). *Updates to the prescribing medicines in pregnancy database*. Retrieved from https://www.tga.gov.au/updates-prescribing-medicines-pregnancy-database; extract from information in MIMS (2018c). *Full product information—Various drugs*. Retrieved from https://www.mimsonline.com.au.

TABLE 36.1 Asthma medications and delivery devices

GENERIC NAME	COMMON TRADE NAMES	DEVICE OR PRESENTATION	ROUTE OF DELIVERY	CLASS
Relievers				
Salbutamol	Airomir Asmol Butamol Epaq Ventolin	Autohaler MDI Nebulising solution Syrup Injection *(often for obstetric purposes)*	Inhaled Oral Subcut injection IMI IV	SAßa
Terbutaline	Bricanyl	Turbuhaler Elixir Solution for injection	Inhaled Oral Subcut injection	
Preventers				
Ciclesonide	Alvesco	MDI	Inhaled	ICS
Fluticasone propionate	Flixotide Seretide	Accuhaler MDI	Inhaled	ICS
Budesonide	Pulmicort Symbicort	Turbuhaler Nebulising suspension	Inhaled	ICS
Beclomethasone dipropionate	Qvar	MDI Autohaler	Inhaled	OCS
Sodium cromoglycate	Intal Forte	Nebulising solution	Inhaled	Mast cell stabiliser
Nedocromil sodium	Tilade	MDI	Inhaled	Mast cell stabiliser
Montelukast	Singulair	Tablet	Oral	LTRA
Symptom controllers				
Eformoterol fumarate dehydrate	Oxis Foradile	Turbuhaler	Inhaled	LAßa
Salmeterol xinafoate	Serevent	Accuhaler	Inhaled	LAßa
Combination medications				
Fluticasone and salmeterol	Seretide	Accuhaler MDI	Inhaled	LAßa + ICS
Beclomethasone and eformoterol Budesonide and eformoterol	Symbicort	Turbuhaler	Inhaled	LAßa + ICS

ICS = inhaled corticosteroids; LAβa = long-acting, selective beta$_2$-adrenoreceptor agonist; MDI = metered-dose inhaler; SAβa = short-acting beta agonist; LTRA = leukotriene receptor antagonist.

Corticosteroids block the late response to inhaled allergens and reduce bronchial hyperresponsiveness. The preferred route of administration is by MDI or DPI to minimise systemic absorption and reduce the adverse effects of prolonged steroid use (cushingoid effects). For a severe acute attack, corticosteroids may be given systemically to alleviate symptoms and induce remission.

Cromolyn sodium and nedocromil are used to prevent acute episodes of asthma. They reduce airway hyperreactivity and inhibit the release of mediator substances. These drugs are used for long-term control of asthma, not quick relief. They have a wide margin of safety and few side effects.

LEUKOTRIENE ANTAGONISTS Leukotriene modifiers, montelukast and zafirlukast, are oral medications that reduce the inflammatory response in asthma. They appear to improve lung function, diminish symptoms and reduce the need for short-acting bronchodilators. These drugs affect the metabolism and excretion of other medications such as warfarin and theophylline and may cause liver toxicity.

METHYLXANTHINE Theophylline is an old drug of the methylxanthine class, which is used less commonly nowadays because of its frequent adverse effects. Many other drugs available have more efficiency and fewer adverse effects attributed to their use. Theophylline should never be used as a first-line drug for the treatment of asthma, but is occasionally used as adjunctive treatment. It relaxes bronchial smooth muscle, inhibits the release of chemical mediators of the inflammatory response and increases diaphragmatic contractility. Theophylline has significantly more adverse effects associated with its use (NACA, 2022a).

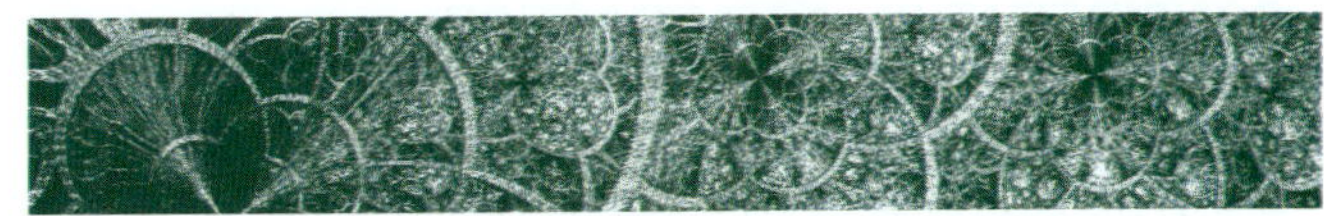

Nursing care

Nurses encounter individuals with asthma both in the acute care setting during an acute exacerbation and as outpatients or in homes. The priority nursing care needs differ with each individual presentation, severity and setting.

Health promotion

Although specific measures to prevent asthma have not yet been identified, the link between parental smoking and childhood asthma is strong. Discuss this link with young people and families with children if relevant. Encourage all individuals to avoid ever starting smoking and, if they already do smoke, to quit. Provide referrals to smoking cessation clinics, help groups or a care provider for nicotine patches as needed to facilitate quitting.

Assessment

Assessment of the person experiencing an acute asthma attack must be very focused and timely.

- *Health history*: current symptoms, including chest tightness, dyspnoea; duration of current attack; measures used to relieve symptoms and their effect; identification of precipitating factors for the attack; frequency of attacks; current medications; known allergies.
- *Physical examination*: apparent level of distress; colour; vital signs; respiratory rate and excursion, breath sounds throughout lung fields; apical pulse.
- *Diagnostic tests*: forced expiratory volume, peak expiratory flow rate; arterial blood gases.

Nursing diagnoses and interventions

An acute asthma attack causes fear as breathing becomes increasingly difficult and hypoxaemia develops. Anxiety in turn tends to increase the severity and manifestations of the attack. Priority nursing care needs during an acute attack focus on improving airway clearance and reducing fear and anxiety. Teaching about prevention of future attacks and home management must be postponed until adequate ventilation is restored.

Ineffective airway clearance

Bronchospasm and bronchoconstriction, increased mucus secretion and airway oedema narrow the airways and impair airflow during an acute attack of asthma. Both inspiratory and expiratory volumes are affected, decreasing the oxygen available at the alveolus for the process of respiration. Narrowed air passages increase the work of breathing, increasing the metabolic rate and tissue demand for oxygen.

- Monitor skin colour and temperature and level of consciousness (LOC). *Cyanosis, cool clammy skin and changes in LOC (agitation, lethargy or confusion) indicate worsening hypoxia.*

> **CONSIDERATION FOR PRACTICE**
> **Assess respiratory status at least every 1 to 2 hours. Observe respiratory rate and depth, chest movement or excursion, breath sounds and peak expiratory flow rate. Respiratory status can change rapidly during an acute asthma attack and its treatment. Decreasing PEFRs indicate worsening airflow restriction. Slowed, shallow respirations with significantly diminished breath sounds and decreased wheezing may indicate exhaustion and impending respiratory failure. Immediate intervention is necessary.**

- Assess ABG results and pulse oximetry readings; notify the doctor of abnormal values or changes in status. *These values provide information about gas exchange and the adequacy of alveolar ventilation. A fall in SpO_2 levels is an early indicator of impaired gas exchange.*

> **CONSIDERATION FOR PRACTICE**
> **Assess cough effort and sputum for colour, consistency and amount. Ineffective cough may also signal impending respiratory failure.**

- Place in Fowler's, high-Fowler's or orthopnoeic (with head and arms supported on the over-bed table) position to facilitate breathing and lung expansion. *These positions reduce the work of breathing and increase lung expansion, especially of basilar areas.*
- Administer oxygen as ordered. If a mask is used, monitor closely for feelings of claustrophobia or suffocation. *Supplemental oxygen reduces hypoxaemia. Although the mask is a very effective oxygen delivery system, it may increase anxiety.*
- Administer nebuliser treatments and provide humidification as ordered. *Nebuliser treatments are used to administer bronchodilators and other medications; humidity helps loosen secretions.*
- Initiate or assist with chest physiotherapy, including percussion and postural drainage. *Percussion and postural drainage facilitate the movement of secretions and airway clearance.*
- Increase fluid intake. *Increasing fluids helps reduce the viscosity of the secretions.*
- Provide endotracheal suctioning as needed. *Endotracheal suctioning may be necessary to remove secretions and improve ventilation if the person is unable to clear secretions by coughing.*

Ineffective breathing pattern

The physiological changes in lung ventilation that occur during an acute asthma attack impair both lung expansion and emptying. Anxiety caused by hypoxia and dyspnoea compounds the problem by increasing the respiratory rate. Collaborative and nursing interventions can help restore a more normal breathing pattern and adequate lung ventilation.

- Monitor vital signs and laboratory results. *Tachypnoea, tachycardia, an elevated blood pressure and increasing hypoxaemia and hypercapnia are signs of compromised respiratory status.*

> **CONSIDERATION FOR PRACTICE**
> **Frequently assess respiratory rate, pattern and breath sounds. Note manifestations of ineffective breathing, including rapid rate, shallow respirations, nasal flaring, use of accessory muscles, intercostal retractions and diminished or absent breath sounds. Early identification of ineffective respirations allows timely initiation of interventions.**

- Assist with ADLs as needed. *This conserves energy and reduces fatigue.*
- Provide rest periods between scheduled activities and treatments. *Scheduled rest is important to prevent fatigue and reduce oxygen demands.*
- Teach and assist to use techniques to control breathing pattern:
  a. pursed-lip breathing
  b. abdominal breathing
  c. relaxation techniques, including visualisation and meditation.

  Pursed-lip breathing helps keep airways open by maintaining positive pressure and abdominal breathing improves lung expansion. Relaxation techniques reduce anxiety and its effect on the respiratory rate.
- Administer medications, including bronchodilators and anti-inflammatory drugs, as ordered. Monitor for desired and possible adverse effects. *Medications are used to improve airway status and facilitate breathing.*

Anxiety

Acute exacerbations of asthma can produce significant anxiety. Fear of being unable to breathe and feelings of suffocation associated with acute asthma are significant. Financial or other concerns may cause the person to want to avoid hospitalisation. Increasingly frequent and severe episodes may cause fear for the future. Hypoxia contributes to anxiety as well, stimulating the sympathetic nervous system and the fight-or-flight response.

- Assess level of anxiety. *Interventions for severe anxiety or panic differ from those for mild or moderate anxiety.*
- Assist to identify coping skills that have been successful in the past. *Successful coping helps the person to regain control of the situation, reducing anxiety.*
- Listen actively to concerns; do not deny or negate the fear of dying or of being unable to breathe. *Active listening promotes trust and helps the person express concerns.*
- Include the person in care planning and decisions as appropriate, without making excessive demands. *Participating in decision making increases the person's sense of control. Because high levels of anxiety interfere with the ability to make decisions, it is important to avoid placing demands on the person that may further increase the level of anxiety.*
- Reduce excessive environmental stimuli and maintain a calm demeanour. *This promotes rest.*

> **CONSIDERATION FOR PRACTICE**
> **Provide physical and emotional support. Remain with the person during episodes of severe anxiety; schedule time every 1 to 2 hours to be with the mildly or moderately anxious person. Answer call lights promptly. The severely anxious person may fear being alone or believe that they will die if someone is not on hand. Knowing that the nurse is readily available and will return quickly reduces anxiety.**

> **CONSIDERATION FOR PRACTICE**
> **Provide clear, concise directions and explanations about procedures. Avoid presenting more information than the person is able to assimilate. Anxiety interferes with the ability to learn. Explanations may need to be repeated frequently.**

- Allow supportive family members to remain with the person. *Significant others provide additional support and can help reduce anxiety.*
- Assist to use relaxation techniques, such as guided imagery, muscle relaxation and meditation. *These techniques help restore psychological balance and reduce sympathetic stimulation and responses.*

Ineffective therapeutic regimen management

Once acute asthma is under control and effective respirations have been re-established, it is important to help the person identify contributing factors to the attack. This helps the person prevent future episodes.

- Assess level of understanding about asthma and the prescribed treatment regimen. Provide additional information and teaching as indicated. *Assessment helps to identify and clarify misperceptions and difficulties with disease management.*
- Discuss the person's perception of the illness and its effect on their lifestyle. *Open discussion can help identify conflicts between lifestyle and the treatment regimen.*
- Assist the person and significant others to identify problems or difficulties integrating the treatment regimen into their lifestyle. *Asthma and its management may necessitate lifestyle modifications to prevent acute exacerbations. This can significantly impact on family members—for example, eliminating cigarette smoking or pets from the household, removing carpets or daily damp dusting to remove dust mites.*
- Assess knowledge and understanding of prescribed medications and use of OTC preparations. *This is important to determine misperceptions or possible misuse of medications.*
- Provide verbal and written instructions. *Written instructions reinforce teaching and allow future reference.*

> **CONSIDERATION FOR PRACTICE**
> **Assist to identify factors that contributed to the acute episode. Identifying contributing factors increases the person's awareness of the disease and of strategies to prevent future exacerbations.**

- Refer to counselling, support groups or self-help organisations. *These can help the person and family adapt to living with asthma and the treatment regimen.*

Community-based care

Asthma is a chronic disease that is best managed by the person with assistance from medical personnel. Teaching for home care focuses on promoting the highest level of wellness and preventing and managing acute episodes and exacerbations of the disease. Topics to include in teaching are as follows:

- Suggestions for lifestyle changes to avoid specific triggers for asthma attacks—for example:
  - Warm up slowly before exercising in cold weather; wear a special mask or scarf to retain air warmth and humidity while exercising.
  - Substitute indoor exercises during cold, dry weather.
  - Reduce the risk of respiratory infections (e.g. adequate rest, good nutrition and stress management to maintain immune function, yearly influenza vaccines and immunisation against pneumococcal pneumonia and COVID-19).
  - Use techniques to reduce or manage physical and psychological stress.
- Using peak expiratory flow rate (PEFR) meter to monitor airway status; how to manage the disease based on results.
- Using prescribed medications, including:
  - name, frequency, dose and desired effect
  - potential adverse effects and their management, including effects to report to the doctor
  - potential interactions with other drugs (including OTC herbal preparations) or foods
  - if tolerance is a potential risk, how to identify it and steps to take.

Provide referrals to local or regional resources for further teaching and support as needed. Consider the need for community-based services, home respiratory care services and others as needed.

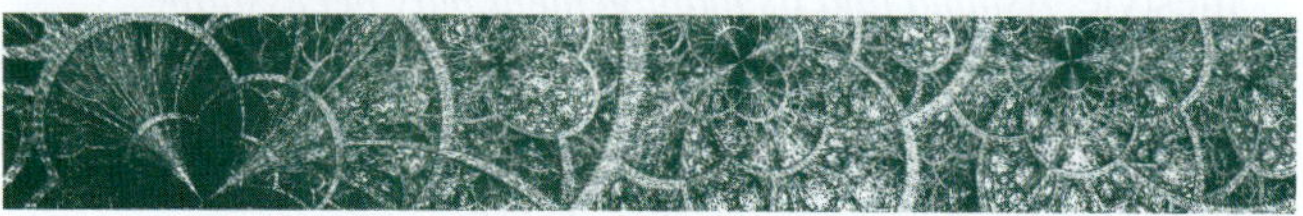

CHRONIC OBSTRUCTIVE PULMONARY DISEASE

Individuals with chronic airflow obstruction due to chronic bronchitis and/or emphysema are said to have **chronic obstructive pulmonary disease (COPD)**.

Incidence and risk factors

COPD is one of the most prevalent chronic conditions in Australia and 9 out of 10 (91.3%) people with COPD also suffer from another condition. In 2020–2021, 375,800 (1.5%) people across all ages had COPD, with 7,102 deaths recorded, making it the fifth leading cause of death in Australia. COPD mortality rates are also higher for Indigenous Australians. Between 2014 and 2018, 835 Aboriginal and Torres Strait Islander people aged over 45 died from COPD, a mortality rate of 114 per 100,000 population (ABS, 2022a; AIHW, 2020b).

Obstructive lung disease typically affects middle-aged and older adults. Cigarette smoking is clearly implicated as the primary cause of COPD. It is estimated that over 70% of deaths in people with COPD are attributed to smoking (Greenhalgh, Scollo & Winstanley, 2022). Cigarette smoke and the irritants it contains impair ciliary movement, inhibit the function of alveolar macrophages and cause mucus-secreting glands to hypertrophy. Smoke also produces emphysema or airway destruction and constricts smooth muscle, increasing airway resistance. Other contributing factors include air pollution, occupational exposure to noxious dusts and gases, airway infection and familial and genetic factors.

FAST FACTS

- In 2020–2021 in Australia, COPD was the fifth leading cause of death (4.5%).
- The financial burden was estimated to be over $980 million.
- The World Health Organization (WHO) predicts that by 2030, COPD will become the third leading cause of death worldwide.

Sources: ABS (2022a); AIHW (2020b); Cousins et al. (2020).

Pathophysiology

COPD is characterised by slowly progressive obstruction of the airways. The disease is one of periodic exacerbations, often related to respiratory infection, with increased symptoms of dyspnoea and sputum production. Unlike acute processes in which lung tissues recover, airways and lung parenchyma do not return to normal following an exacerbation; instead, they demonstrate progressive destructive changes.

Although one or the other may predominate, COPD typically includes components of both chronic bronchitis and emphysema, two distinctly different processes. Small airways disease, narrowing of small bronchioles, is also part of the COPD complex. Through different mechanisms, these processes cause airways to narrow, resistance to airflow to increase and expiration to become slow or difficult (see Figure 36.6). The result is a mismatch between alveolar ventilation and blood flow or perfusion, leading to impaired gas exchange.

Chronic bronchitis

Chronic bronchitis is a disorder of excessive bronchial mucus secretion. It is characterised by a productive cough lasting 3 or more months in 2 consecutive years. Cigarette smoke is the main factor implicated in the development of chronic bronchitis.

Inhaled irritants lead to a chronic inflammatory process with vasodilation, congestion and oedema of the bronchial mucosa. Goblet cells increase in size and number, and mucous glands enlarge. Thick, tenacious mucus is produced in increased amounts. Changes in bronchial squamous cells impair the ability to clear mucus. Narrowed airways and excess secretions obstruct airflow; expiration is affected first, then inspiration. Because ciliary function is impaired, normal defence mechanisms are unable to clear the mucus and any inhaled pathogens (Bullock & Hales, 2019).

Recurrent infection is common in chronic bronchitis. An imbalance between ventilation and perfusion leads to hypoxaemia, hypercapnia and pulmonary hypertension. Pulmonary hypertension often leads to right-sided heart failure.

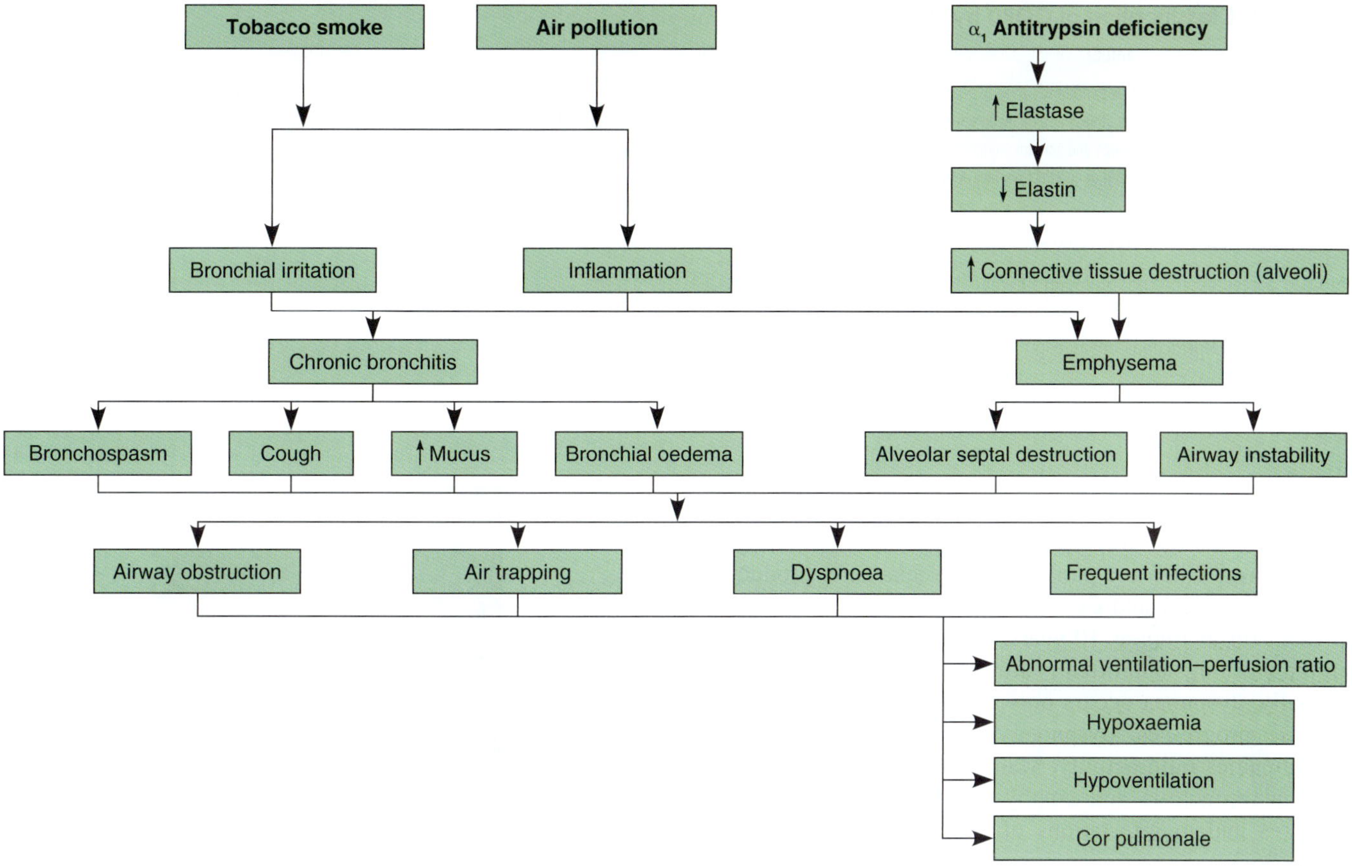

Tobacco smoke
Air pollution
α_1 Antitrypsin deficiency
↑ Elastase
↓ Elastin
Bronchial irritation
Inflammation
↑ Connective tissue destruction (alveoli)
Chronic bronchitis
Emphysema
Bronchospasm
Cough
↑ Mucus
Bronchial oedema
Alveolar septal destruction
Airway instability
Airway obstruction
Air trapping
Dyspnoea
Frequent infections
Abnormal ventilation–perfusion ratio
Hypoxaemia
Hypoventilation
Cor pulmonale

FIGURE 36.6 ***Pathogenesis of chronic obstructive pulmonary disease***

Emphysema

Emphysema is characterised by destruction of the walls of the alveoli, with resulting enlargement of abnormal air spaces. As in chronic bronchitis, cigarette smoking is strongly implicated as a causative factor in most cases of emphysema. Deficiency of a_1-antitrypsin, an enzyme that normally inhibits the activity of proteolytic enzymes and tissue destruction in the lungs, contributes to the development of emphysema, especially when combined with exposure to cigarette smoke.

Inflammatory cells that collect in distal airway tissues appear to lead to destruction of elastic fibres in the respiratory bronchioles and alveolar ducts. Alveolar wall destruction causes alveoli and air spaces to enlarge, with loss of corresponding portions of the pulmonary capillary bed. As a result, the surface area for alveolar–capillary diffusion is reduced, affecting gas exchange. Elastic recoil is lost, reducing the volume of air that is passively expired. The loss of support tissue also affects airways, increasing the risk of expiratory collapse and further air trapping. Anatomically, either respiratory bronchioles or alveoli may be the primary tissue involved.

To summarise, COPD is a progressive, non-reversible process of airway narrowing and loss of supporting tissue. Three separate processes typically are involved:

1. chronic bronchitis with persistent airway oedema, excessive mucus production and impaired airway clearance
2. emphysema with loss of interstitial membranes and airway support tissue, resulting in airway collapse and loss of alveolar surface area for gas exchange
3. small airways disease with bronchoconstriction.

The result of these processes and their combined effects is increased work of breathing, impaired expiration with air trapping and impaired gas exchange.

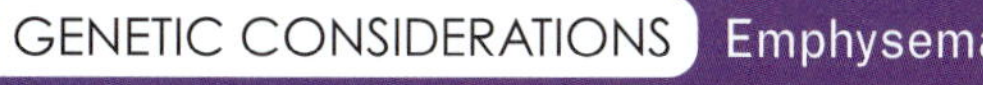

Severe α_1-antitrypsin (alpha-1 antitrypsin or ATT) deficiency, present in about 1% of people with COPD, is a proven risk factor for COPD. Normal alpha-1 antitrypsin levels are associated with the common M allele. Two other alleles, the S allele and the Z allele, lead to reduced alpha-1 antitrypsin levels. Different concentrations of alpha-1 antitrypsin can be produced, depending on the inherited phenotype (observable characteristic or trait). It is estimated there are 30,000 people in Australia and New Zealand with alpha-1 antitrypsin deficiency (AATD). However, fewer than 10% of these people have been diagnosed (Lung Foundation Australia, 2020).

Manifestations

The clinical presentation of COPD varies from simple chronic bronchitis without disability to chronic respiratory failure and severe disability. Table 36.2 outlines the classifications of COPD severity.

TABLE 36.2 Classification of COPD by severity

	MILD	MODERATE	SEVERE
Typical symptoms	Few symptoms Breathlessness on moderate exertion Cough and sputum production Little or no effect on daily activities	Breathlessness walking on level ground Increasing limitation of daily activities Recurrent chest infections Exacerbations requiring oral corticosteroids and/or antibiotics	Dyspnoea on minimal exertion Daily activities severely curtailed Exacerbations of increasing frequency and severity
Typical lung function	$FEV_1 \approx 60-80\%$ predicted	$FEV_1 \approx 40-59\%$ predicted	$FEV_1 < 40\%$ predicted

FEV_1 = forced expiratory volume in 1 second.

Source: Lung Foundation Australia (2021). *The COPD-X: Plan: Australian and New Zealand guidelines for the management of chronic obstructive pulmonary disease* (V2.65). Retrieved from https://copdx.org.au/copd-x-plan/.

Manifestations are typically absent or minor early in the disease. When the person finally seeks care, productive cough, dyspnoea and exercise intolerance often have been present for as long as 10 years. The cough typically occurs in the mornings and often is attributed to 'smoker's cough'. Initially, dyspnoea occurs only on extreme exertion; as the disease progresses, dyspnoea becomes more severe and accompanies mild activity. Manifestations characteristic of chronic bronchitis and emphysema develop. The clinical features and manifestations of COPD are summarised in Table 36.3.

Manifestations of chronic bronchitis are a productive cough with copious amounts of thick, tenacious sputum, cyanosis and evidence of right-sided heart failure, including distended neck veins, oedema, liver engorgement and an enlarged heart. Adventitious lung sounds, including loud rhonchi and possible wheezes, are prominent on auscultation.

Emphysema is insidious in onset. Dyspnoea is the initial symptom occurring only with exertion, dyspnoea may progress to become severe even at rest. Cough is minimal or absent. Air trapping and hyperinflation increase the anterior–posterior chest diameter, causing *barrel chest*. The person often is thin, tachypnoeic, uses accessory muscles of respiration and often assumes a position of sitting and leaning forward (see Figure 36.7). The expiratory phase of the respiratory cycle is prolonged. On auscultation, breath sounds are diminished and the percussion tone is hyperresonant.

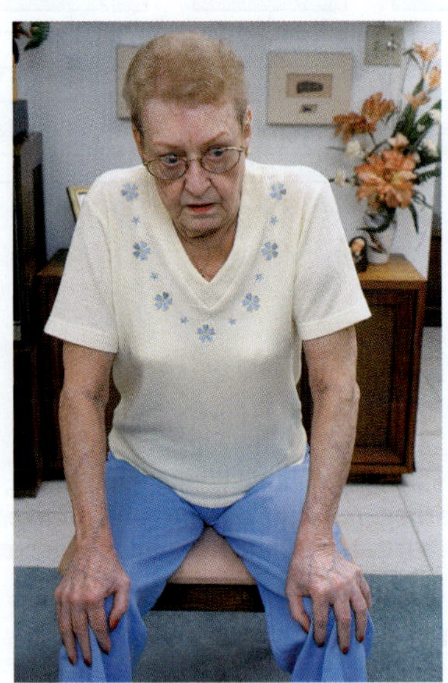

FIGURE 36.7 ***Typical appearance of a person with emphysema. Note the person's anxious expression and assumption of the tripod position, leaning forward with the hands on the knees***

Source: Courtesy of Michal Heron/Pearson Education/PH College.

INTERPROFESSIONAL CARE

Although COPD is preventable and treatable, it cannot be cured. Smoking abstinence is the only certain way to prevent COPD and to slow its progression. To a certain extent, airway

TABLE 36.3 Clinical features and manifestations of COPD

	FEATURE	CHRONIC BRONCHITIS	EMPHYSEMA
History	Onset	After age 35; recurrent respiratory infections	After age 50; insidious progressive dyspnoea
	Smoking	Usual	Usual
	Cough	Persistent, productive of copious mucopurulent sputum	Absent or mild with scant clear sputum, if any
Physical examination	Appearance	Often obese; oedematous and cyanotic; distended neck veins and other symptoms of right-sided heart failure	Usually thin and cachectic; barrel chest; prominent accessory muscles of respiration
	Chest	Adventitious sounds with wheezing and rhonchi; normal percussion note	Distant or diminished breath sounds; hyper-resonant percussion note
Other features	Blood gases	Hypercapnia and hypoxaemia; respiratory acidosis	Normal or mild hypoxaemia; normal pH
	Pulmonary function studies	Normal or decreased total lung capacity; moderately increased residual volume	Increased total lung capacity; markedly increased residual volume
	Pulmonary hypertension	May be severe	Only when advanced

obstruction can be reversed and disability minimised early in the disease. Treatment generally focuses on relieving symptoms, minimising obstruction and slowing disability.

Diagnosis

In clinical practice, diagnosis is usually based on:

- symptoms of exertional breathlessness, cough and sputum
- a history of smoking or exposure to other noxious agents
- FEV1/FVC < 0.7 post-bronchodilator.

Diagnostic tests are used to help establish the diagnosis of COPD and identify the predominant component, emphysema or chronic bronchitis (Lung Foundation Australia, 2021). These procedures are also used to assess respiratory status and monitor treatment effectiveness (see the chapter 'A person-centred approach to assessing the respiratory system' for diagnostic procedures and related nursing care).

- *Respiratory function testing* is performed to establish the diagnosis and evaluate the extent and progress of COPD (see Box 33.1). Results are based on calculated norms for each person by age, height, sex and weight as well as all current medications on the requisition. In COPD, total lung capacity and residual volume typically are increased. The forced expiratory volume (FEV_1) and forced vital capacity (FVC) are decreased due to narrowed airways and resistance to airflow (see Figure 36.8).
- *Ventilation–perfusion scanning* may be performed to determine the extent of ventilation–perfusion mismatch—that is, the extent to which lung tissue is ventilated but not perfused (dead space) or perfused but inadequately ventilated (physiological shunting) (see Figure 36.9). A radioisotope is injected or inhaled to illustrate areas of shunting and absent capillaries.

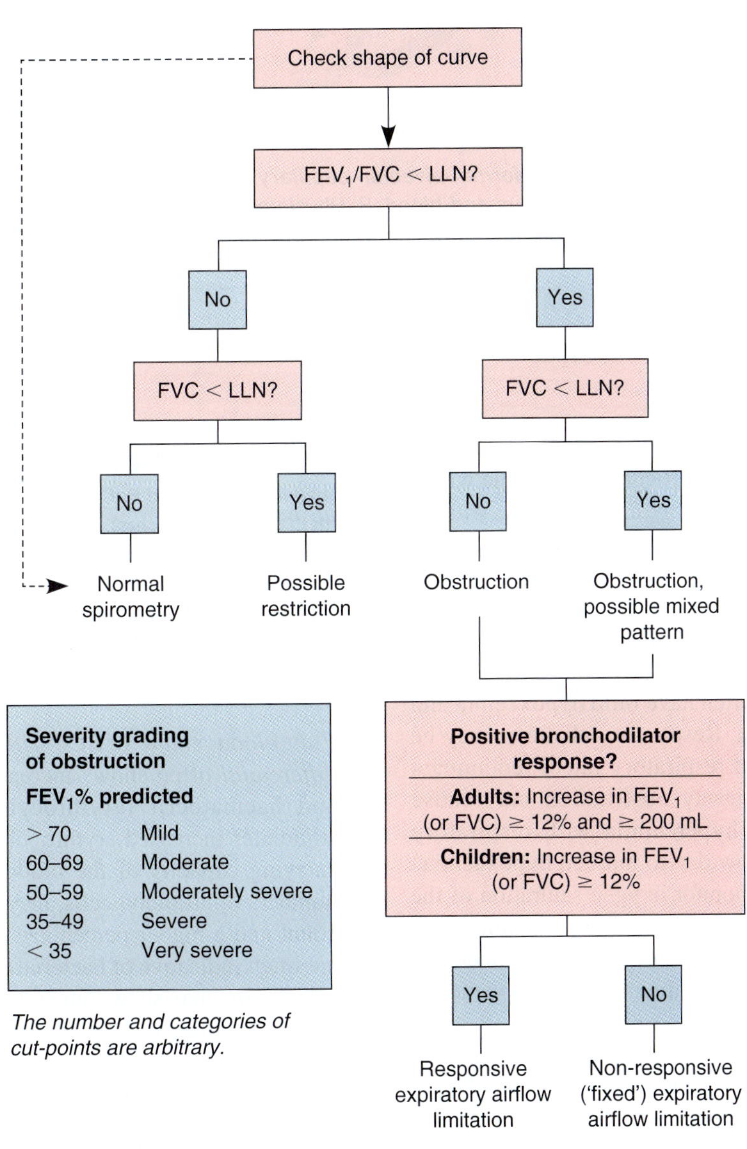

FIGURE 36.8 ***Guideline for spirometry interpretation***

FEV_1 = forced expiratory volume; FVC = forced vital capacity; LLN = lower limit of normal.

Source: NACA (2020). *Spirometry quick reference guide.* Melbourne: National Asthma Council Australia. Reproduced with permission of National Asthma Council Australia, 2023. National Asthma Council guidelines are reviewed annually; please visit https://www.nationalasthma.org.au/ for current guidelines.

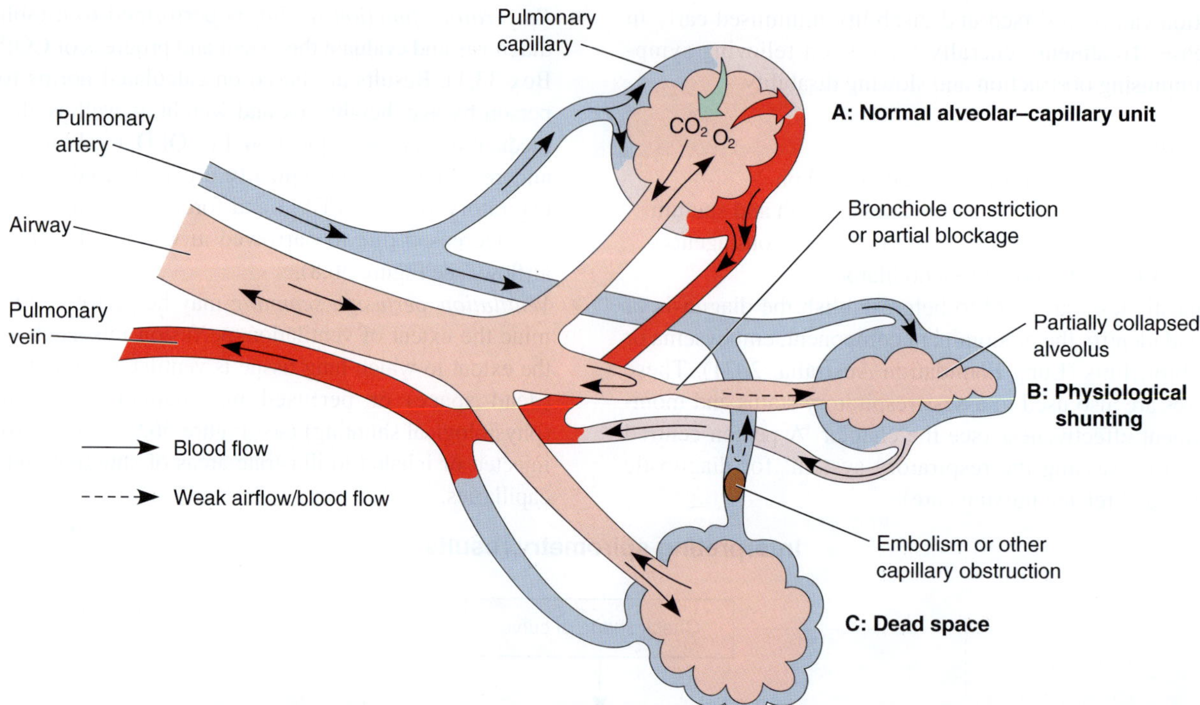

FIGURE 36.9 ***Ventilation–perfusion relationships. A, Normal alveolar–capillary unit with an ideal match of ventilation and blood flow. Maximal gas exchange occurs between alveolus and blood. B, Physiological shunting: a unit with adequate perfusion but inadequate ventilation. C, Dead space: a unit with adequate ventilation but inadequate perfusion. In the latter two cases, gas exchange is impaired***

- *Serum α_1-antitrypsin (alpha-1 antitrypsin) levels* may be drawn to screen for deficiency, particularly in people with a family history of obstructive airway disease, those with an early onset, women and non-smokers. Normal adult serum alpha-1 antitrypsin levels range from 90 to 200 mg/dL. Fasting is not required prior to this test.
- ABGs are drawn to evaluate gas exchange, particularly during acute exacerbations of COPD. Individuals with predominant emphysema often have mild hypoxaemia and normal or low CO_2 tension. Respiratory alkalosis may be present due to an increased respiratory rate. Predominant chronic bronchitis and airway obstruction may cause marked hypoxaemia and hypercapnia with respiratory acidosis. SpO_2 levels are low due to marked hypoxaemia.
- *Pulse oximetry* is used to monitor oxygen saturation of the blood. Marked airway obstruction and hypoxaemia often cause oxygen saturation levels $< 95\%$. Pulse oximetry is continuously monitored to assess the need for supplemental oxygen.
- *Exhaled* CO_2 (*capnogram* or $ETCO_2$) may be measured to evaluate alveolar ventilation. The normal $ETCO_2$ reading is 35 to 45 mmHg; it is elevated when ventilation is inadequate and decreased when pulmonary perfusion is impaired. $ETCO_2$ monitoring can reduce the frequency of ABG determinations.

CONSIDERATION FOR PRACTICE

Hypercapnia (elevated $PaCO_2$ levels) is often chronic in individuals with COPD (CO_2 retainers). In these individuals, administering excessive oxygen flows can actually reduce respiratory rate which results in increased $PaCO_2$, potentially leading to somnolence and acute respiratory failure. While oxygen is the drug of choice for treating individuals with COPD, close monitoring is necessary during oxygen therapy.

- *Full blood count (FBC) with white blood cell (WBC) differential* often shows increased red blood cells (RBCs) and haematocrit (erythrocytosis) as chronic hypoxia stimulates increased erythropoiesis to improve the oxygen-carrying capacity of the blood. *Polycythaemia*, increased numbers of all blood cells, may be evident. Increased WBC count and a higher percentage of immature WBCs (bands) are often indicative of bacterial infection.
- *Chest x-ray* may show longer lung fields and flattening of the diaphragm due to hyperinflation and evidence of pulmonary infection if present. The anterior–posterior (AP) diameter is wider (see Figure 36.10).

Quitting smoking

Smoking cessation can not only prevent COPD from developing but can also improve lung function once the disease has been

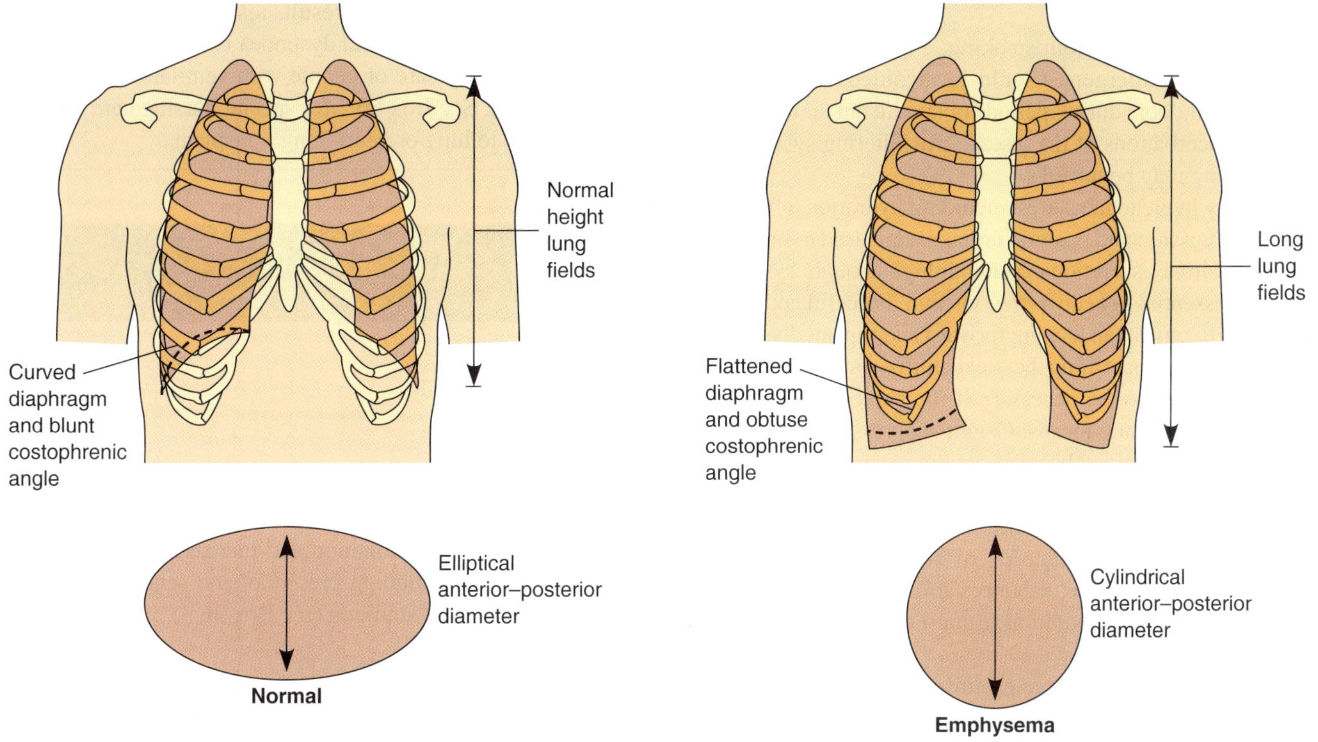

FIGURE 36.10 *Anatomical changes related to emphysema*

diagnosed. FEV_1 improves and survival is prolonged, largely due to lower rates of lung cancer and heart disease. Sustained quitting is difficult; however, various methods may assist people.

- Nicotine replacement therapy can increase the rate of quitting by up to 70%.
- Partial nicotine agonists such as varenicline can increase the rate of quitting by up to 50%.
- The non-nicotine oral therapy bupropion can improve the rate of quitting more than a placebo but less successfully than varenicline.
- Group counselling can improve quitting success above minimal support.
- Brief motivational advice from healthcare professionals has a success rate of 3–6%.

Interventions such as hypnotherapy, acupuncture, naltrexone, aversive smoking, biomedical feedback, novel and emerging nicotine and tobacco products (e.g. e-cigarettes, heated tobacco products (HTPs), vaping), physical activity, the Alan Carr method or the consumption of St John's wort (*Hypericum perforatum*) herb extract do not demonstrate sufficient good-quality empirical evidence to support their success (Royal Australian College of General Practitioners, 2021; WHO, 2022).

Medications

Immunisation against pneumococcal pneumonia and influenza is recommended yearly to reduce the risk of respiratory infections. If the infection is considered to be bacterial, a broad-spectrum antibiotic is prescribed. Antibiotics should be administered in times of exacerbation. However, prophylactic antibiotics, although they have a statistically significant reduction in number of sick days experienced, do not have a place in routine medication regimens as the risk of increasing antibiotic resistance is too great (Lung Foundation Australia, 2021).

Short- and long-acting bronchodilators improve airflow and reduce air trapping in COPD, resulting in improved dyspnoea and exercise tolerance. Bronchodilators may be given by MDI, DPI, nebuliser or orally. Oral administration may promote adherence but is associated with much higher rates of adverse effects. A spacer may facilitate effective use of an MDI. Ipratropium bromide, an anticholinergic agent administered by MDI, is frequently prescribed. It has a longer duration of action than the short-acting β_2-adrenergic stimulant bronchodilators and few side effects. Salmeterol, a longer-acting β_2-agonist, may be used in combination therapy. Bronchodilators are discussed in further detail in the section on asthma and their nursing implications are outlined in the 'Medication administration: asthma' box earlier in this chapter.

Corticosteroid therapy may be used when asthma is a major component of COPD. It also improves symptoms and exercise tolerance and may reduce the severity of exacerbations and the need for hospitalisation. Oral corticosteroids, such as prednisone, are used initially. If a beneficial response occurs, the amount is reduced to the lowest effective dose. Every-other-day dosing or administration by inhaler is preferred to minimise steroid side effects, such as cushingoid effects and an increased risk of osteoporosis and vertebral fractures.

Alpha-1 antitrypsin replacement therapy is not common practice in Australia.

Treatments

In addition to refraining from smoking, exposure to other airway irritants and allergens should be avoided. The person should remain indoors during periods of significant air pollution to prevent exacerbations of the disease. Air-filtering systems or air conditioning may be useful.

Respiratory hygiene measures, including hydration, effective coughing, percussion and postural drainage, are used to improve clearance of airway secretions. Maintaining adequate systemic hydration is essential to keep secretions thin. Forceful coughing is often less effective than leaning forward and repeatedly 'huffing', with relaxed breathing between huffs. Percussion and postural drainage may be necessary if the person is unable to clear secretions by usual means. Cough suppressants and sedatives generally are avoided because they may cause retention of secretions.

Unless disabling cardiac disease is present, there is strong evidence supporting the benefits of regular exercise as it improves exercise tolerance, enhances ability to perform ADLs and prevents further deterioration (Lung Foundation Australia, 2021).

A program of regular aerobic exercise designed to gradually increase exercise tolerance is recommended. Activities that strengthen the muscles used for breathing and ADLs, including Tai Chi, swimming and golf, also are beneficial.

Breathing exercises are used to slow the respiratory rate and relieve accessory muscle fatigue. Pursed-lip breathing slows the respiratory rate and helps maintain open airways during exhalation by keeping positive pressure in the airways. Abdominal breathing relieves the work of accessory muscles of respiration.

OXYGEN Long-term oxygen therapy is used for severe and progressive hypoxaemia. It improves exercise tolerance, mental functioning and quality of life in advanced COPD. It also reduces the rate of hospitalisation and increases length of survival. Oxygen may be used intermittently, at night or continuously. For severely hypoxaemic individuals, the greatest benefit is seen with continuous oxygen. Home oxygen may be supplied as liquid oxygen, compressed gas cylinders or oxygen concentrators.

An acute exacerbation of COPD may necessitate oxygenation and inspiratory positive-pressure assistance with a face mask or intubation and mechanical ventilation. Oxygen administered without intubation and mechanical ventilation requires caution: administering oxygen to individuals with chronic elevated CO_2 levels in the blood can actually increase the $PaCO_2$, leading to increased somnolence and even respiratory failure. Close monitoring of LOC and ABGs during oxygen therapy is vital.

Surgery

When medical therapy is no longer effective, lung transplantation may be an option; however, it has been shown to have limited survival benefit (Lung Foundation Australia, 2020). Lung reduction surgery is an experimental surgical intervention for advanced diffuse emphysema and lung hyperinflation. The procedure reduces the overall volume of the lung, reshapes it and improves elastic recoil. As a result, respiratory function and exercise tolerance improve and dyspnoea is reduced (see box in the chapter 'Nursing care of people with ventilation disorders' for nursing care). See Box 36.2 for special nursing care considerations related to lung or heart–lung transplant.

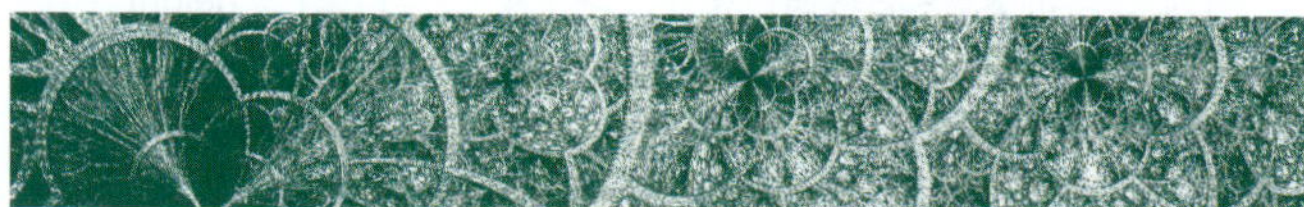

Nursing care

Health promotion

Not smoking—never starting or quitting—is the best preventive measure for COPD. Even in individuals with COPD, smoking cessation improves lung function and increases survival. Educate all individuals, including preschool and school-aged children, about the risks of smoking (see Box 36.3).

Assessment

Focused assessment for the person with COPD includes:

- *Health history*: current symptoms, including cough, sputum production, dyspnoea, activity tolerance; frequency of respiratory infections and most recent episode; previous diagnosis of emphysema, chronic bronchitis or asthma; current medications; smoking history (in pack years—packets per day times number of years smoked), history of exposure to second-hand smoke, occupational or other pollutants.
- *Physical examination*: general appearance, weight for height, mental status; vital signs, including temperature; skin colour and temperature; anterioposterior and lateral chest diameter, use of accessory muscles, nasal flaring or pursed-lip breathing; respiratory excursion and diaphragmatic excursion; percussion tone; breath sounds throughout; neck veins, apical pulse and heart sounds, peripheral pulses, oedema.
- *Diagnostic tests*: FVC and FEV_1, ABGs, haematocrit.

Nursing diagnoses and interventions

Individuals with COPD, whether hospitalised or in the community, have multiple nursing care needs. Because of the obstructive nature of the disease, airway clearance is a high priority. Nutritional deficit is common, particularly when emphysema is predominant. Because this chronic disease affects all functional health patterns, psychosocial issues are also of concern in planning nursing care. In addition to the nursing diagnoses presented here, see the accompanying nursing care plan.

Ineffective airway clearance

Both chronic bronchitis and emphysema affect the ability to maintain open airways. In chronic bronchitis, copious amounts of thick, tenacious mucus are produced. Ciliary action is impaired, making it difficult to clear mucus from the airways.

BOX 36.2 Nursing considerations related to lung transplant

While immediate postoperative care for individuals undergoing lung or heart–lung transplant is provided by specially trained interprofessional teams in transplant centres, increased survival following transplant means that these individuals are more commonly seen in community-based settings, non-transplant units and on general nursing care wards. An understanding of common post-transplant complications and care needs of the person following transplant facilitates appropriate nursing care.

Common post-transplant complications

In the early post-transplant period, the most common complications relate to the surgical procedure itself or to rejection of the transplanted organ(s).

- *Rejection.* Acute organ rejection can occur at any time following the transplant. An acute change in FEV_1 and FVC on home spirometry is often the first indication of acute rejection. Other manifestations of rejection include fever, dyspnoea and an elevated WBC count. Because these manifestations are similar to those of infection, the person is instructed to contact their doctor or transplant coordinator for further investigation. Acute rejection is treated with increased corticosteroids and adjustment of the immunosuppressive regimen (see the chapter 'Nursing care of people with altered immunity'). Chronic rejection is less amenable to therapy, ultimately necessitating retransplant.
- *Infection.* Prevention of infection is vital in a person following lung transplantation. Individuals are encouraged to reduce their risk of infection by avoiding contact with people who have an infectious disease (e.g. upper respiratory tract infection (URTI), shingles, diseases of childhood). The transplant recipient may not have typical manifestations of infection due to immunosuppression. Any vague symptoms with or without fever or leucocytosis are investigated. Recurrent viral infections such as cytomegalovirus have been associated with chronic rejection; hence, they are aggressively treated with antiviral therapy. Treatment of other infections is targeted to the infectious organism.

Nursing considerations for the person following transplant

Reverse isolation procedures are not necessary unless the neutrophil count is very low ($< 500/mm^3$). Use good hand-washing and standard precautions at all times and aseptic technique for dressing changes, IV starts, site care and other invasive procedures (such as urinary catheterisation). Do not allow caregivers or visitors with URTI to have contact with the person; a mask may be provided for short visits if contact is unavoidable. Skin surveillance and care is vital following transplant. Intact skin reduces the risk of infection; however, corticosteroid therapy increases the risk of skin tears and breakdown.

The effect of all medications on immunosuppressive therapy and the transplanted organ(s) should be carefully investigated prior to administration. Some antibiotics and other drugs can affect blood levels of immunosuppressants.

Particular attention must be paid to respiratory hygiene. Denervation of the transplanted lung eliminates the usual cough stimuli (Whitson, 2022). Regularly scheduled coughing and deep breathing, and the use of vibration, percussion and postural drainage, are important to prevent accumulation of secretions (Cavallaro Goodman & Fuller, 2020).

BOX 36.3 Cigarette smoking and tobacco use

The use of tobacco reaches back to early civilisations when it was used in religious ceremonies and as an offering of friendship. At one time tobacco was thought to have medicinal qualities effective against all common diseases. Widespread use of tobacco in the male population of the industrialised world began during World War I.

Tobacco is now recognised as the leading cause of preventable illness in the world. Diseases directly related to tobacco use are responsible for the deaths of more than 20,500 Australians every year (ABS, 2021). In spite of this knowledge, aggressive marketing of the product continues and its worldwide use is increasing, especially in developing countries.

The link between tobacco use and lung cancer was reported as early as 1912. Today, 90% of lung cancer in men and 65% in women is considered to be caused by smoking tobacco (Greenhalgh et al., 2022). The WHO reported that tobacco smoke contributes to the death of 8 million people a year worldwide (WHO, 2022).

Cigarette smoke contains over 4,000 chemicals, including nicotine (WHO, 2022). Nicotine is a highly addictive psychoactive substance that is relatively cheap and readily available. It produces euphoria, which acts as a positive reinforcer for continued use.

Tar is the particulate matter in cigarette smoke that is responsible for most of its carcinogenic and pathological effects on the lungs. Smoke also paralyses the cilia, reducing their ability to remove the tar. The risk of cancer and other lung diseases is dose related, affected by the age at which smoking began, the number of cigarettes smoked per day and the number of years smoked. Smoking cessation reduces the risks associated with tobacco use. For some, such as those at risk of coronary heart disease, quitting smoking yields rapid benefits. For others, the degree of risk reduction is less immediate, but still significant.

Nurses need to do more than simply advise individuals to quit smoking and talk about the risks of smoking, including e-cigarettes and vaping. Nurses can take an active role in smoking cessation. Identify smoking habits, related illnesses and previous efforts to quit. Work with the person to identify barriers and obstacles to quitting. Educate about the addictive nature of nicotine and explain the manifestations of nicotine withdrawal (anxiety, irritability, headache and disturbed sleep). Develop a plan that specifies a target date to quit and includes ways to deal with obstacles to quitting, withdrawal symptoms and the temptation to resume smoking. Offer self-help material at an appropriate reading level. Refer to a counsellor, doctor, self-help group or smoking cessation clinic. If a

(continued)

BOX 36.3 Cigarette smoking and tobacco use (continued)

relapse occurs, accept it as a normal part of rehabilitation from any addictive substance. Continue to provide support and encouragement, helping the person to avoid further relapses.

Nurses can be especially effective in primary prevention of smoking and the diseases associated with it as nurses can target all demographics with programs to prevent smoking. In addition, nurses need to become active in reducing minors' access to tobacco and associated products.

Nursing diagnoses that may be appropriate related to smoking include the following:

- *Ineffective maintenance of health* related to tobacco use evidenced by cough, haemoptysis, or shortness of breath.
- *Decisional conflict related* to tobacco use evidenced by inability to determine a 'quit smoking date'.
- *Ineffective denial related* to substance abuse and dependence evidenced by statements discounting health concerns related to tobacco smoking.

The loss of supporting tissue caused by emphysema increases the risk of airway collapse. In both cases, air is trapped distally and less oxygen is available to the alveoli for diffusion. Normal respiratory defence mechanisms are impaired and mucus-plugged airways provide an ideal environment for bacterial growth. Respiratory infection further impairs airway clearance and is often the cause of an acute exacerbation.

- Assess respiratory status every 1–2 hours or as indicated. Assess rate and pattern; cough and secretions (colour, amount, consistency and odour); and breath sounds, both normal and adventitious. *Frequent assessment is vital to monitor current status and response to treatment. Adventitious sounds should decrease with effective intervention. Diminished or absent breath sounds may indicate increasing airway obstruction and possible atelectasis.*

CONSIDERATION FOR PRACTICE

Promptly report changes in SpO_2, skin colour or mental status. A drop in SpO_2, increasing cyanosis or altered LOC indicate hypoxaemia, which may be related to airway obstruction.

- Monitor ABG results. *Increasing hypoxaemia, hypercapnia and respiratory acidosis may indicate increasing airway obstruction.*
- Weigh daily, monitor intake and output, and assess mucous membranes and skin turgor. *Dehydration causes respiratory secretions to become thicker, more tenacious and difficult to expectorate; fluid overload can further compromise respiratory status.*

NURSING CARE PLAN A person with COPD

Anna Mercurio is an 83-year-old widow who lives with her two adult sons. During the past 15 years, Mrs Mercurio has become increasingly short of breath while gardening and walking, two favourite activities. She also has developed a chronic cough that is particularly bad in the mornings. Ten years ago her family doctor told her that she had emphysema. She is admitted to the hospital with possible pneumonia and acute exacerbation of COPD.

ASSESSMENT

Mrs Mercurio was admitted to the medical unit. In the nursing history, the nurse notes that she denies ever smoking, but says that her husband and two sons have been smokers 'for practically their whole lives'. She says she lived an active life before developing lung disease, but her breathing difficulties and cough have progressed so that she now must rest after just a few minutes of housework or other activity. Her cough is productive of moderate to large amounts of sputum, particularly in the mornings. She developed increasing shortness of breath and sputum 2 days ago; this morning, she could not complete her morning activities without resting, so she contacted her doctor.

On physical examination, Mrs Mercurio demonstrated the following: skin very warm and dry, colour dusky. Pauses frequently while speaking to breathe. Respiratory rate 36, fairly shallow; coughs frequently, producing large amounts of thick, tenacious green sputum. Other vital signs: P 115 and irregular, BP 186/60, T 39°C. Appears very thin; weight 43.6 kg, height 160 cm. Anteroposterior and lateral chest diameter increased; moderate kyphosis noted. Chest hyperresonant to percussion. Auscultation reveals distant breath sounds with scattered wheezes and rhonchi throughout lung fields. Chest x-ray shows flattening of diaphragm, long lung fields, slight cardiac enlargement, prominent vascular and bronchial markings, and patchy infiltrates. Initial laboratory work reveals moderate erythrocytosis, leucocytosis and low serum albumin. Arterial blood gas results: pH 7.19; PaO_2 54 mmHg; $PaCO_2$ 59 mmHg; HCO_3^- 30 mg/dL and SpO_2 88%. Admitting orders include sputum specimen for culture; intravenous penicillin G, 2 million units every 4 hours; salbutamol/ipratropium inhaler, two puffs every 6 hours; salmeterol/fluticasone dry powder inhaler, twice a day; bed rest with bathroom privileges; oxygen per nasal prongs at 2 L/min continuously; and regular diet.

NURSING CARE PLAN A person with COPD (continued)

DIAGNOSES

- *Ineffective airway clearance* related to pneumonia and COPD evidenced by increased shortness of breath and respiration rate.
- *Impaired gas exchange* related to acute and chronic lung disease evidenced by low SpO_2.
- *Risk of impaired ventilation* related to loss of hypoxaemic respiratory drive and respiratory muscle fatigue evidenced by decreasing respiration rate and SpO_2.
- *Impaired home maintenance* related to activity intolerance evidenced by inability to undertake activities of daily living.

PLANNING

- Closely monitor response to oxygen therapy, including skin colour, SpO_2, sputum consistency and respiratory drive.
- Assess respiratory status and LOC every 1–2 hours until stable, then at least every 4 hours.
- Contact respiratory therapy for percussion and postural drainage following inhaler treatments.
- Meet with Mrs Mercurio and her sons to develop a post-discharge care plan.
- Refer to home health department for nursing follow up.
- Refer to social services for possible assistance with home maintenance.

Expected outcomes

- Expectorate secretions effectively.
- Return to level of respiratory function prior to acute exacerbation.
- Demonstrate improved ABG and SpO_2 values.
- Maintain spontaneous respirations without excess fatigue.
- Verbalise willingness to allow sons or a housekeeper to assist with daily household tasks.

IMPLEMENTATION

- Increase fluid intake to at least 2,500 mL per day and provide bedside humidifier.
- Elevate head of bed to at least 30 degrees at all times.
- Teach 'huff' coughing technique.
- Administer medications as ordered, providing ipratropium inhaler before beclomethasone inhaler. Provide mouth care after inhalers.
- Provide for uninterrupted rest periods following treatments and procedures.

EVALUATION

After the first day in the hospital Mrs Mercurio's condition begins to improve slowly. On discharge 6 days later she is able to provide self-care with less fatigue and dyspnoea. She is using oxygen at night only, admitting that it is only for security. Although a few scattered wheezes and rhonchi are still present in her lungs, her sputum is thinner, white and easily expectorated. She will continue taking oral penicillin V for an additional 10 days at home. She will also continue using the inhalers as prescribed. Although her sons admit they will probably never be able to quit smoking, they have agreed to smoke only in the garage or outside. A community health nurse will initially evaluate Mrs Mercurio's progress three times weekly. Arrangements have been made for a housekeeper to come twice a week for cleaning and laundry. Mrs Mercurio is glad to be returning home and grateful for the arrangements that have been made.

CRITICAL THINKING IN THE NURSING PROCESS

1. Mrs Mercurio has never been a smoker but has had long-term exposure to second-hand smoke. How does second-hand smoke contribute to lung diseases in adults and children?
2. The nursing care plan included the nursing diagnosis *Risk of impaired ventilation* related to loss of hypoxaemic respiratory drive and respiratory muscle fatigue. Identify the normal physiological events that stimulate breathing and describe how these differ for the person with chronic hypoxaemia and hypercapnia.
3. The person with an acute exacerbation of COPD is at risk of respiratory failure. Which changes in Mrs Mercurio's assessment findings could indicate this complication?
4. Develop a nursing care plan for Mrs Mercurio for the nursing diagnosis *Deficient diversional activities* related to inability to continue preferred activities.

REFLECTION ON THE NURSING PROCESS

1. Outline what you have learned from this case study that you will take into your future practice.
2. In individuals experiencing acute exacerbations, extreme shortness of breath can result in an inability to speak in sentences of more than a couple of words. How might this impact on communication and the ability to collect an adequate detailed health history? How should you prioritise the information required at that point in time? Which techniques would you use to facilitate adequate communication without further compromising a person's oxygenation?

- Encourage a fluid intake of at least 2,000–2,500 mL per day unless contraindicated. *Adequate fluid intake helps keep mucus secretions thin.*
- Place in Fowler's, high-Fowler's or orthopnoeic position; encourage movement and activity to tolerance. *Upright positions improve ventilation and reduce the work of breathing. Activity helps mobilise secretions and prevent them from pooling.*
- Assist with coughing and deep breathing at least every 2 hours while awake. Position seated upright, leaning forward during coughing. *The upright position promotes chest expansion, increasing the effectiveness of coughing and reducing the work involved.*
- Provide tissues and a paper bag to dispose of expectorated sputum. *This important infection control measure reduces the spread of respiratory organisms to other people.*
- Refer to a respiratory therapist and assist with or perform percussion and postural drainage as needed. *Percussion helps loosen secretions in airways; postural drainage facilitates movement of these secretions out of the respiratory tract.*
- Provide rest periods between treatments and procedures. *The person with COPD fatigues easily; adequate rest is important to conserve energy and reduce fatigue.*

TRANSLATION TO PRACTICE Evidence-based practice: self-management programs in people with COPD in Australia

Programs such as a Tasmanian controlled study demonstrated that a community nurse can facilitate improved quality of life and early healthcare utilisation to reduce the risk of exacerbation in people with COPD; a randomised controlled trial with COPD patients recruited from The Prince Charles Hospital, Brisbane, was designed to integrate an innovative mobile health program (including telehealth) within a clinical COPD care service and lived experiences of COPD patients in rural Australia. Results demonstrated an increase in quality of life, adherence to interventions and the opportunity to improve community patient care using innovative healthcare approaches (Ding et al., 2019; Glenister, Haines & Disler, 2019; Wood-Baker et al., 2012).

IMPLICATIONS FOR NURSING

Years of life lost, readmission for exacerbation and reduced quality of life are serious social and financial costs of COPD. Programs that directly facilitate better outcomes in any of these factors should be considered beneficial in the management of individuals with COPD. It would be reasonable to consider that financial gains from reducing exacerbation and improving a person's quality of life would easily offset costs of such a program. Among other things, this study reaffirmed the fact that nursing support via various methods appears to be an important factor in the risk of readmission for exacerbation.

CRITICAL THINKING IN PERSON-CENTRED CARE

1 Identify factors that may be important in such programs. Consider the practicalities of offering such programs including necessary content, volume, type of support and logistical issues, such as provision of support for individuals in rural and remote regions.
2 Which factors would be important to measure in order to determine an improvement in a person with COPD?
3 People with COPD generally have comorbidities. What implications would cardiac, renal or hepatic disease have on an individual with COPD?

- Administer expectorant and bronchodilator medications as ordered. Correlate timing with respiratory treatments. *Using expectorants and bronchodilators prior to coughing, percussion and postural drainage increases their effectiveness in clearing airways.*

CONSIDERATION FOR PRACTICE

Provide endotracheal, oral or nasopharyngeal suctioning as necessary. Suctioning may be necessary to stimulate cough and help clear secretions.

- Provide supplemental oxygen as ordered. *Supplemental oxygen helps maintain adequate blood and tissue oxygenation.*

CONSIDERATION FOR PRACTICE

Prepare for intubation and mechanical ventilation if respiratory status deteriorates (increasing hypoxaemia and hypercapnia, decreased LOC, cyanosis or worsening airway obstruction). Respiratory failure is a possible complication of an acute exacerbation of COPD and requires immediate intervention to preserve life.

Inadequate nutrition

With advanced COPD, minimal activity, including eating, can cause fatigue and dyspnoea. The person may be unable to consume a full meal without resting. At the same time, the increased work of breathing increases metabolic demands and more kilojoules are required. The person may appear cachectic (thin and wasted). Poor nutritional status further impairs immune function and increases the risk of a complicating infection.

- Assess nutritional status, including diet history, weight for height (use reference tables of desired weights) and anthropometric (skinfold) measurements. *It is important to differentiate nutritional status from body type rather than assume a nutritional impairment.*
- Observe and document food intake, including types, amounts and kilojoule intake. *This information can provide direction for supplementation, if needed.*
- Monitor laboratory values, including serum albumin and electrolyte levels. *These values provide information about the adequacy of nutritional intake, including protein.*
- Consult with a dietitian to plan meals and nutritional supplements that meet kilojoule needs. More concentrated sources of high-energy foods may be required to maintain kilojoule intake without excess fatigue. *A diet high in proteins and fats without excess carbohydrates is recommended to minimise CO_2 production during metabolism. (Carbohydrates are metabolised to form CO_2 and water.)*
- Provide frequent, small feedings with between-meal supplements. *Frequent, small meals help maintain intake and reduce fatigue associated with eating.*
- Place seated or in high-Fowler's position for meals. *An upright position promotes lung expansion and reduces dyspnoea.*
- Assist to choose preferred foods from the menu; encourage family members to bring food from home if allowed. *Providing preferred foods encourages eating.*
- Keep snacks at the bedside. *Snacks provide additional kilojoule intake.*
- Provide mouth care prior to meals. *This helps enhance the appetite.*
- If unable to maintain oral intake, consult with the doctor about enteral or parenteral feedings. *Maintenance of kilojoule and nutrient intake is vital to prevent catabolism.*

Compromised family coping

Chronic illness affects the entire family structure. Roles and relationships change; additional demands are placed on the family. Family members may blame the person for causing the illness and may have distorted perceptions about it, even denying its existence. They may refuse to assist or participate in care. The person may develop an attitude of helplessness or dependence, or may demonstrate anger, hostility or aggression.

- Assess interactions between individuals and their family. *Assessment helps identify desired and potential destructive behaviours.*
- Assess the effect of the illness on the family. *Assessment of family interactions, roles and relationships assists in planning appropriate interventions.*
- Help the person and family identify strengths for coping with the situation. *Identifying personal and family strengths helps the family regain a sense of control.*
- Provide information and teaching about COPD. *Education helps the family gain an understanding of the individual's condition and needs.*
- Encourage expression of feelings. *Avoid judging feelings expressed by family members as 'good' or 'bad', 'right' or 'wrong'. It is important that the nurse remain objective to maintain the therapeutic relationship.*
- Help family members recognise behaviours and attitudes that may hinder effective treatment, such as continuing to smoke in the house. *Family members may be unaware of the effect of their behaviour on the person's ability to change habits and cope with a disabling disease.*
- Encourage family members to participate in care. *This helps develop skills for use at home.*
- Initiate a care conference involving the person, family and healthcare team members from a variety of disciplines. *A wide range of perspectives and areas of expertise aids in problem solving and facilitates communication.*
- If dysfunctional family relationships interfere with measures to enhance coping, advocate for the person, reaffirming his or her right to make decisions. *Dysfunctional family relationships are not likely to change simply because of illness. The nurse can better meet the person's needs by accepting their limitations in dealing with family members.*
- Refer the person and family to support groups and respiratory rehabilitation programs, as available. *Support groups and structured rehabilitation programs enhance coping abilities.*
- Arrange a social services consultation. *This can help the person and their family identify care and support service needs.*
- Refer community agencies or home services such as Meals on Wheels as appropriate. *Agencies or community services can provide additional support beyond the family's means or capability.*

Conflict: smoking

Smoking is more than a habit; it is an addiction. The person who must quit is facing a significant loss, not only of nicotine but also of a lifestyle. Although the person may fully comprehend the consequences of continuing to smoke, the decision to give up a part of their life is not easy. This fear may be expressed in such concerns as 'I'll gain weight' or 'What will I do with my hands?' In addition to providing practical information, a plan and assistance with nicotine withdrawal, the nurse must support the person's decision-making process to comply with an order to stop smoking.

- Assess knowledge and understanding of the choices involved and possible consequences of each. *The decision to quit smoking ultimately belongs to the individual. They need a full understanding of the consequences of quitting or continuing to smoke.*
- Acknowledge concerns, values and beliefs; listen non-judgmentally. *The nurse needs to avoid imposing their own values and beliefs about smoking on the person.*
- Spend time with the person, encouraging expression of feelings. *This demonstrates acceptance of the person and their right to make the decision.*
- Help plan a course of action for quitting smoking and adapt it as necessary. *When the person develops the plan, they have more ownership in it and interest in making it work.*
- Demonstrate respect for decisions and the right to choose. *Respect supports self-esteem and the ability to cope.*
- Provide referral to a counsellor or other professional as needed. *Counsellors or other people trained to assist with smoking cessation can help with decision making.*

Community-based care

As with any chronic disease, the person and family will have primary responsibility for disease management. Teaching is vital to promote optimal health and slow disease progression. Teaching for home care focuses on effective coughing and breathing techniques (see Box 36.4), preventing exacerbations and managing prescribed therapies.

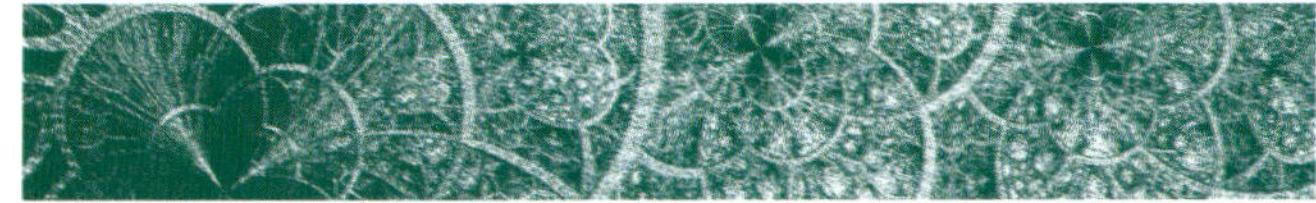

BOX 36.4 Person-centred teaching: effective coughing and breathing techniques

Pursed-lip and diaphragmatic breathing techniques help minimise air trapping and fatigue. Pursed-lip breathing helps maintain open airways by maintaining positive pressures longer during exhalation. Teach the person to:

1. Inhale through the nose with the mouth closed.
2. Exhale slowly through pursed lips, as though whistling or blowing out a candle, making exhalation twice as long as inhalation.

Diaphragmatic or abdominal breathing helps conserve energy by using the larger and more efficient muscles of respiration. Teach the person to:

1. Place one hand on the abdomen, the other on the chest.
2. Inhale, concentrating on pushing the abdominal hand outwards while the chest hand remains still.
3. Exhale slowly, while the abdominal hand moves inwards and the chest hand remains still.

(continued)

BOX 36.4 Person-centred teaching: effective coughing and breathing techniques (continued)

Repeat these exercises as often as necessary until the techniques become incorporated into normal breathing.

Several different coughing techniques may be useful. For controlled cough technique, teach the person to:

1. Following prescribed bronchodilator treatment, inhale deeply and hold breath briefly.
2. Cough twice, the first time to loosen mucus, the second to expel secretions.
3. Inhale by sniffing to prevent mucus from moving back into deep airways.
4. Rest. Avoid prolonged coughing to prevent fatigue and hypoxaemia.

For 'huff' coughing, teach the person to:

1. Inhale deeply while leaning forwards.
2. Exhale sharply with a 'huff' sound to help keep airways open while mobilising secretions.

In addition, include the following topics when teaching for home care:

- maintaining adequate fluid intake (at least 2 L of fluid daily)
- avoiding respiratory irritants, including cigarette smoke, both primary and secondary, other smoke sources, dust, aerosol sprays, air pollution and very cold, dry air
- preventing exposure to infection, especially upper respiratory infections
- importance of pneumococcal vaccine and annual influenza immunisation
- prescribed exercise program, maintaining ADLs and balancing rest and exercise
- maintaining nutrient intake (e.g. eating small frequent meals and using nutritional supplements to provide adequate kilojoules)
- ways of reducing sodium intake if prescribed
- identifying early signs of an infection or exacerbation and the importance of seeking medical attention for the following: fever, increased sputum production, purulent (green or yellow) sputum, upper respiratory infection, increased shortness of breath or difficulty breathing, decreased activity tolerance or appetite, increased need for oxygen
- prescribed medications, including purpose, proper use and expected effects
- avoiding use of OTC medications unless approved by the doctor
- other prescribed therapies, such as use of home oxygen, percussion, postural drainage and nebuliser treatments
- use, cleaning and maintenance of any required special equipment
- importance of wearing an identification band and carrying a list of medications at all times in case of an emergency.

Provide referrals to home care services such as home health, assistance with ADLs as needed, home maintenance services, respiratory therapy and home oxygen services, and other agencies such as Meals on Wheels as indicated.

Other selected lung diseases affecting the airway

THE PERSON WITH CYSTIC FIBROSIS

Cystic fibrosis (CF) is an autosomal recessive disorder that affects epithelial cells of the respiratory, gastrointestinal and reproductive tracts and leads to abnormal exocrine gland secretions. Although it can affect many organ systems, CF is particularly damaging to the lungs, leading to COPD in childhood and early adulthood. Respiratory manifestations of CF are the usual cause of morbidity and death from this disease. The gastrointestinal tract also is affected significantly; exocrine pancreatic insufficiency is characteristic of CF. Abnormally high sweat electrolytes also occur in CF.

Incidence and prevalence

In 2020, 3,538 people were recorded as having CF; of these, 1,965 (55.5%) were adults (18+ years), with 12.8% of people aged 40 years and over. Diagnosis was via newborn screening (53.2%), 33.6% had clinical symptoms or signs at the time of diagnosis, 7.6% had a family history of CF and 2.0% had a diagnosis confirmed by prenatal screening. There were 18 deaths recorded from CF in Australia (Australian Cystic Fibrosis Data Registry (ACFDR) & Monash University, 2020).

Pathophysiology

The CFTR protein is involved in membrane transport of chloride and sodium in cells lining the ducts of exocrine glands (sweat glands, pancreas, liver and reproductive systems). The genetic abnormality of CF leads to a lack or abnormality of this protein, with resulting abnormal electrolyte transport across epithelial cell membranes (see the 'Genetic considerations' box). Defective chloride transport causes more water and sodium reabsorption than normal. Secretions in affected organs become thick and viscous, obstructing glands and ducts. This obstruction causes dilation of secretory glands and damage to exocrine tissue (Bullock & Hales, 2019). The hallmark pathophysiological effects of CF include:

- excess mucus production in the respiratory tract with impaired ability to clear secretions and progressive COPD
- pancreatic enzyme deficiency and impaired digestion
- abnormal elevation of sodium and chloride concentrations in sweat.

In the lungs, viscous mucus plugs small airways and impairs mucociliary clearance, leading to atelectasis, infection, bronchiectasis and dilation of distal airways. Lower respiratory infections with *Staphylococcus aureus* and *Pseudomonas*, *Haemophilus*

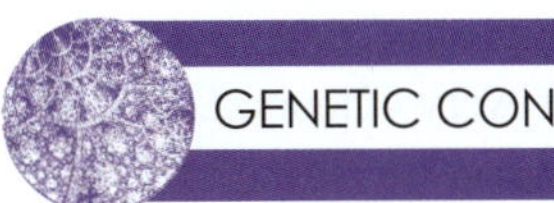

GENETIC CONSIDERATIONS Cystic fibrosis

The gene responsible for cystic fibrosis is at a single locus on the long arm of chromosome 7. This gene codes for a protein known as the *cystic fibrosis transmembrane conductance regulator (CFTR)*. More than 1,000 mutations of this gene have been identified. The most common mutation in Australia, identified as F508del, accounts for about 49% of cystic fibrosis (ACFDR & Monash University, 2020). Cystic fibrosis is an autosomal recessive disorder: it is not transmitted as a sex-linked trait and the normal gene is dominant. People with one abnormal gene do not have the disorder but can transmit this abnormal gene to their offspring. When a child inherits an abnormal gene from both parents, the disorder is seen. Genetic screening of family members can detect 70–75% of carriers of the CF gene. Screening for the CF gene is not recommended for the general population.

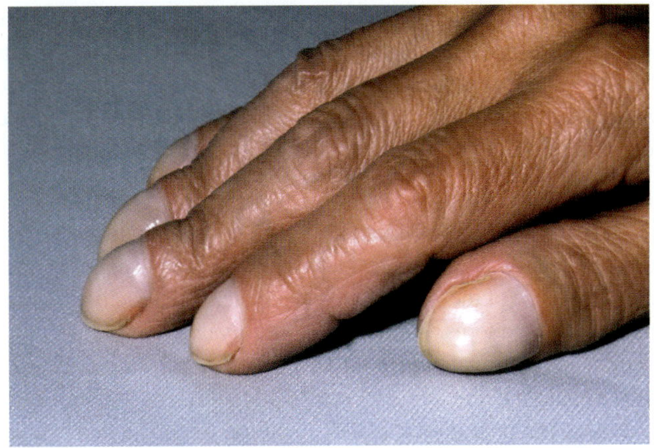

FIGURE 36.11 ***Clubbing of fingers caused by chronic hypoxaemia***

Source: Mediscan/Alamy Stock Photo.

influenza and *Escherichia coli* are common (ACFDR & Monash University, 2020). A multidrug-resistant bacteria *Burkholderia cepacia* (previously *Pseudomonas cepacia*) is clinically significant as it may also hamper the potential for lung transplantation. Acute and chronic damage to lung parenchyma causes tissue loss and extensive scarring and fibrosis. The upper lobes are involved to a greater extent than the lower lobes. Severe airway obstruction and chronic hypoxaemia lead to pulmonary hypertension, right ventricular hypertrophy and eventual cor pulmonale. Death usually results from a combination of cardiovascular changes and respiratory failure.

Pancreatic insufficiency is a frequent component of CF. It can range from slight pancreatic dysfunction to complete absence of function due to obstruction of pancreatic ducts with thick mucus and degenerative and fibrotic changes. Pancreatic insufficiency and impaired enzyme secretion lead to impaired digestion and absorption of proteins, carbohydrates and fats.

Around 24% of individuals with CF over 12 years of age develop diabetes mellitus. More than 40% of individuals experience osteoporosis or osteopenia. Gastric oesophageal reflux and liver disease are also potential complication of the disease (ACFDR & Monash University, 2020). Because the genetic defect also affects cells of the reproductive tract, males with CF usually are sterile. Although females may have difficulty conceiving, pregnancies are usually carried to term. Depending on a women's pre-pregnancy health, pregnancy can be tolerated well despite at least a moderate decrease in lung function (Jain et al., 2022).

Manifestations

Manifestations of CF in a young adult include a history of chronic lung disease. Recurrent pneumonia, exercise intolerance and chronic cough are typical. Other pulmonary manifestations include *clubbing* of the fingers and toes (see Figure 36.11), increased anteroposterior chest diameter (barrel chest), hyperresonant percussion tone and basilar crackles on auscultation. Distended neck veins, ascites and peripheral oedema accompany right-sided heart failure. Abdominal pain and *steatorrhoea* (excess fat in the stools, causing frequent, bulky, foul-smelling stool) commonly result from associated pancreatic insufficiency. Growth and development are often retarded, resulting in small stature. Initial research showed COVID-19 resulted in serious consequences for some people with CF, although overall it appeared to have been less severe than originally thought (McClenaghan et al., 2020).

INTERPROFESSIONAL CARE

The treatment plan for cystic fibrosis is multidisciplinary, with the goals of preventing or treating respiratory complications and maintaining adequate nutrition. Psychosocial care is vital, as is genetic and occupational counselling.

Diagnosis

Although evidence of lung disease and pancreatic insufficiency suggests CF, analysis of Cl^- concentration in sweat is used to confirm the diagnosis. In CF, the Cl^- concentration is > 70 mEq/L. Pilocarpine (a parasympathomimetic agent) and a small electric current are used to increase sweat production on the forearm. Absorbent paper or gauze is used to collect the sweat for analysis.

ABGs and SpO_2 levels show hypoxaemia. Pulmonary function studies reveal reduced airflow, reduced forced vital capacity (see Box 33.1) and reduced total lung capacity. Alveolar–capillary diffusion also is typically reduced.

Medications

Immunisation against respiratory infections is vital to promote optimal health. Yearly influenza vaccine is recommended, along with measles and pertussis boosters as needed. COVID-19 vaccines and booster doses are recommended for people with CF, depending on age and risk factors.

Bronchodilator inhalers may be used to control airway constriction. Acute pulmonary infections are treated with appropriate antibiotic therapy as determined by sputum culture and sensitivity tests. A prolonged treatment course or multiple antibiotics may be required to eradicate pulmonary infections. Antibiotics may be administered by several routes, including inhalation, to achieve the desired concentration in large airways (Sharma, 2020).

Dornase alfa, recombinant human DNase, breaks down the excess DNA in the sputum of individuals with CF, decreasing its viscosity and making it easier to clear. Dornase alfa, administered by aerosol, reduces the frequency of hospitalisations and the need for antibiotics for some individuals.

Treatments

Chest physiotherapy with percussion and postural drainage is used to promote airway clearance. Newer airway clearance techniques include the use of the 'huff' cough technique with specified breathing cycles or patterns. In one technique, a valved mask or mouthpiece is used to maintain positive expiratory pressure (PEP) for approximately 20 breaths, followed by three to five 'huff' coughs. This cycle is repeated for a total of 20 minutes. The autogenic drainage technique, a form of biofeedback, involves controlled breathing at specific lung volumes and patterns to facilitate the movement of mucus into larger airways, where it can be cleared with the 'huff' cough. A flutter valve device, which looks like a fat pipe, contains a steel ball within an inner cone. The weight of the ball provides intermittent PEP, which vibrates airway walls to loosen secretions.

Oxygen therapy may be required for hypoxaemia. A liberal fluid intake helps reduce the viscosity of mucus secretions. A diet high in protein, fat and kilojoules may be necessary to maintain weight. Vitamins and minerals are supplemented to counteract excess losses in the sweat and stools. Enteral or parenteral nutrition may be required during acute exacerbations of the disease.

Surgery

Lung transplantation currently offers the only definitive treatment for CF. Lung transplantation lengthens lifespan and improves quality of life. Single-lung, double-lung and heart–lung transplants have been successfully completed. Because the donor lungs do not have the CF gene, they do not develop the pathophysiological changes of CF. Although the other defects characteristic of CF remain, they can be managed with pharmacological therapy.

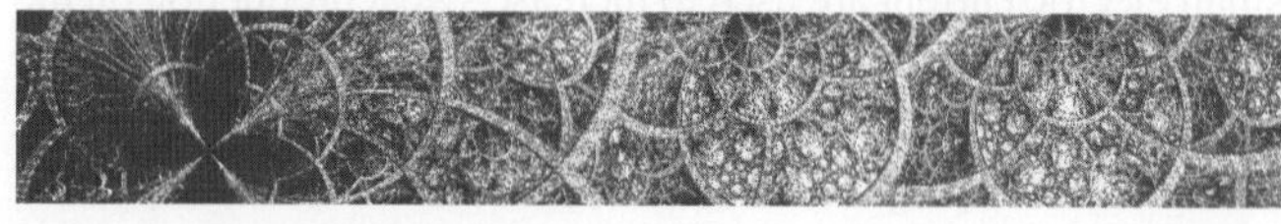

Nursing care

Nursing care for the person with cystic fibrosis is much the same as that for any chronic obstructive lung disease. Promoting airway clearance is the priority of nursing care. The genetic component of the disease and the person's age are important considerations. Adults with CF are just entering their productive years and face a lifespan that is likely to be shortened significantly. Females who do conceive face the prospect of transmitting the defective gene to their offspring.

Nursing diagnoses and interventions

Ineffective airway clearance

Bronchial hygiene measures, including vibration, percussion and postural drainage, are the mainstay of treatment for a person with CF.

- Assess respiratory status, including vital signs, breath sounds, SpO_2 and skin colour, at least every 4 hours. *Early identification of respiratory compromise allows intervention before tissue hypoxia is significant.*
- Assess cough and sputum (amount, colour, consistency and possible odour). *Assessment of the cough and nature of sputum produced allows evaluation of the effectiveness of respiratory clearance and the response to therapy.*
- Monitor ABG results; report increasing hypoxaemia and other abnormal results to the doctor. *Blood gas changes may be an early indicator of impaired gas exchange due to airway obstruction.*
- Place in Fowler's or high-Fowler's position. Encourage frequent position changes and ambulation as allowed. *The upright position promotes lung expansion; position changes and ambulation facilitate the movement of secretions.*
- Assist to cough, deep breathe and use assistive devices. *Coughing and deep breathing help clear airways.*
- Provide a fluid intake of at least 2,500–3,000 mL per day. *A liberal fluid intake helps liquefy secretions, facilitating their clearance.*
- Work with the doctor and respiratory therapist to provide pulmonary hygiene measures, such as postural drainage, percussion and vibration. *These techniques help mobilise and clear secretions.*
- Administer prescribed medications as ordered and monitor their effects. If the infecting organism is resistant to the prescribed antibiotic, little improvement may be seen with treatment. *Bronchodilators help maintain open airways but may have adverse effects such as anxiety and restlessness.*

Anticipatory grieving

The person with CF and family members face the knowledge that their lifespan is likely to be short.

- Spend time with the person and family. *Time is necessary to develop a trusting, therapeutic relationship.*
- Answer questions honestly; do not deny the probable outcome of the disease. *Honesty reinforces reality and provides a sense of control over decisions to be made.*
- Encourage the person and family to express their feelings, fears and concerns. *Open expression of feelings helps to promote understanding and acceptance.*
- Assist with understanding the grieving process and acceptance of feelings as normal. *Feelings of guilt, anger or depression may cause the person to withdraw from others. Explanation of the grieving process enhances understanding and ability to cope.*
- Help the individual and their family make decisions regarding treatment and care. *This also is important to give them a sense of control.*
- Encourage use of other support systems, such as spiritual and social groups. Refer the person and their family to support groups, social support services and hospice care as indicated. *These support systems provide emotional support and help the person and family cope with the diagnosis.*
- Discuss advance directives (living wills) and power of attorney for healthcare with the person and their family. *These documents give the person and their family a sense of control over the medical care provided if the person is no longer able to express their own wishes.*

Community-based care

Education of the person and family affected by CF is essential to maintaining optimal health. The adult whose disease was diagnosed in infancy or childhood has grown up with the disease and often has a much greater knowledge level than many caregivers. However, when the initial diagnosis is made as an adolescent or young adult, teaching needs are significant. Include the following topics when teaching for home care:

- respiratory care techniques, including percussion, postural drainage and controlled cough techniques
- specific breathing and coughing exercises and procedures
- the importance of avoiding respiratory irritants, such as cigarette smoke, air pollution and occupational dusts and gases
- measures to prevent respiratory infection, such as maintaining immunisations and optimal general health and avoiding exposure to large crowds and infected people.

Refer to a dietitian for planning and teaching to maintain adequate nutrition and minimise gastrointestinal symptoms. Referral to community agencies and support groups such as Cystic Fibrosis Australia is also helpful.

Discuss the genetic transmission of cystic fibrosis and refer for counselling and possible genetic testing. Help the individual and their family sort through the impact of the disease on future pregnancies and generations. Remember that the possibility of CF may present an ethical dilemma regarding future pregnancies. Provide support as needed.

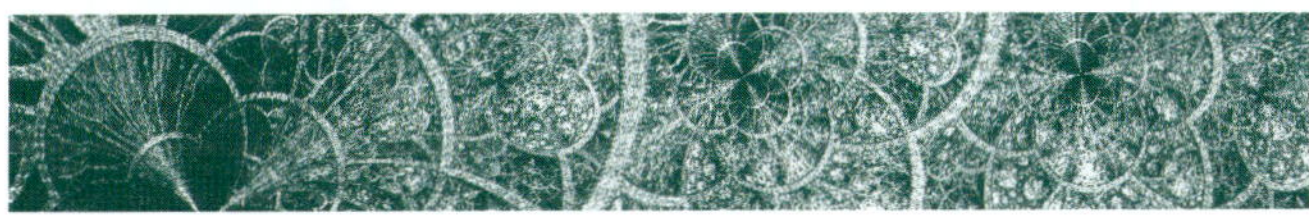

THE PERSON WITH ATELECTASIS

Atelectasis is not a disease but a condition associated with many respiratory disorders. It is a reversible state of partial or total lung collapse of the small airways leading to impaired gas exchange of CO_2 and O_2 (Grott, Chauhan & Dunlap, 2022). It may be acute or chronic. The most common cause of atelectasis is obstruction of the bronchus ventilating a segment of lung tissue. The affected segment may be small or an entire lobe. Atelectasis is common in patients who recently had a general anaesthetic, with incidents as high as 90%. Other causes include compression of the lung by pneumothorax, pleural effusion or tumour; or loss of pulmonary surfactant and inability to maintain open alveoli.

The manifestations of atelectasis depend on its size. Diminished breath sounds over the affected area may be the only sign of a small atelectasis. If a large lung segment is affected, manifestations may include tachycardia, tachypnoea, dyspnoea, cyanosis and other signs of hypoxaemia. Chest expansion may be reduced and breath sounds absent on the affected side. Fever and other manifestations of infection may be present.

Chest x-ray shows an area of airless lung. Computed tomography (CT) scan may help determine the cause of atelectasis. Arterial blood gas may identify arterial hypoxaemia and respiratory alkalosis (Grott et al., 2022).

The primary therapy for atelectasis is prevention. Individuals with COPD, smokers undergoing surgery and people on prolonged bed rest or mechanical ventilation should have vigorous chest physiotherapy to maintain open airways as they are at high risk of atelectasis. Frequently assess respiratory status, including rate, breath sounds and spirometry readings, for early detection and treatment.

When atelectasis develops, treatment focuses on the underlying cause. Vigorous coughing and chest therapy may relieve obstruction by a mucus plug. Bronchoscopy may be necessary to remove the obstruction. Antibiotic therapy is ordered to treat infectious causes.

Nursing care to prevent and treat atelectasis is directed towards airway clearance. Position the person with atelectasis on the unaffected side to promote gravity drainage of the affected segment. Encourage frequent position changes, ambulation, coughing and deep breathing. Unless contraindicated, encourage fluids to help liquefy secretions. Teach the person at high risk of developing atelectasis about respiratory care measures, fluid intake and preventing respiratory infections.

THE PERSON WITH BRONCHIECTASIS

Bronchiectasis is characterised by permanent abnormal dilation of one or more large bronchi and destruction of bronchial walls. Infection often is present. The destructive process of bronchiectasis is initiated by inflammation, usually due to recurrent airway infections. About half of all cases of bronchiectasis are related to cystic fibrosis. Other causes include infections, such as severe pneumonia, tuberculosis or fungal infections; lung abscess; exposure to toxic gases; abnormal lung or immunological defences; and localised airway obstruction due to a foreign body or tumour. Inflammation and airway obstruction are common to all of these processes. Bronchial walls become weakened and dilated as a result, leading to pooling of secretions and further infection and inflammation.

A chronic cough productive of large amounts of mucopurulent sputum is characteristic. Other manifestations of bronchiectasis include haemoptysis, recurrent pneumonia, wheezing and shortness of breath, malnutrition, right-sided heart failure and cor pulmonale.

Collaborative care for bronchiectasis focuses on maintaining optimal pulmonary function and preventing progression of the disorder. The diagnosis is typically based on the history and physical examination. Chest x-ray and CT scan may be ordered to help confirm the diagnosis and determine the extent of lung damage.

Currently there is no cure for bronchiectasis; therefore, early treatment is important to help improve quality of life, manage symptoms and maintain normal lung function (AIHW, 2020c). Antibiotics are prescribed at the first indication of infection and may also be used prophylactically. Inhaled bronchodilators may be ordered. Chest physiotherapy is a vital component of continuing care for bronchiectasis. Percussion and postural drainage help mobilise secretions. Oxygen may be prescribed. Bronchoscopy may be used to clear retained secretions or obstruction, or to evaluate haemoptysis. If lung destruction is localised and unresponsive to conservative management, surgical lung resection may be necessary.

Clinical practice guidelines in Australia and New Zealand recommend early diagnosis and coordination of multidisciplinary care needs (AIHW, 2020c). Nursing care of the person with bronchiectasis is similar to that for individuals with other obstructive lung diseases. Airway clearance is a primary problem, as is ineffective breathing pattern. Other applicable nursing diagnoses may include *Impaired gas exchange*, *Inadequate nutrition* and *Self-care deficit.*

Interstitial pulmonary disorders

Many lung diseases damage the interstitial or connective tissue of the lung. Occupational lung diseases and sarcoidosis are interstitial lung diseases. Toxic drugs and radiation also cause interstitial damage. Table 36.4 identifies common causes of interstitial lung disorders. These disorders may be acute or insidious. Their rate of progression varies from person to person, as does the degree of disability they produce. Statistics are difficult to locate. However, in Australia, it is estimated that occupational exposure contributes to 29% of lung cancers in males and 5.3% in females (Safe Work Australia, 2021).

THE PERSON WITH AN OCCUPATIONAL LUNG DISEASE

Occupational lung diseases are a diverse group of disorders directly related to inhalation of noxious substances in the work environment. In 2019, Australia established the National Occupational Respiratory Disease Registry (NORDR) to record the nature and extent of these diseases and capture incident data to support targeted intervention and prevention strategies (Department of Health and Aged Care, 2022b). There are two main classifications of occupational lung diseases:

1. *Pneumoconiosis*: chronic fibrotic lung diseases caused by inhalation of inorganic dusts and particulate matter.
2. *Hypersensitivity pneumonitis*: allergic pulmonary diseases caused by exposure to inhaled organic dusts.

Physiology review

Lung tissue contains elastin and collagen fibres. Elastin fibres are easily stretched, facilitating lung expansion. Collagen fibres, in contrast, resist stretching. This increases the work of breathing. Both elastin and collagen affect lung compliance or the ease with which the lungs are inflated (Jumat et al., 2021). Other factors affecting compliance include the water content of lung tissue and surface tension.

Pathophysiology and manifestations

When a noxious substance is inhaled, the response to that substance depends on:

- the size of particulates
- its nature (organic or inorganic)
- where it deposits in the respiratory tract
- the susceptibility of the individual.

Relatively large particles, larger than 6 μm, are too big to reach lower airways and often are deposited in the nose. Smaller particles can be carried with inspired air into the alveoli. Normal lung defences, including alveolar macrophages, lymph channels and the mucociliary escalator, attempt to remove particulate matter from the alveoli. Cigarette smoking, alcohol ingestion or hypersensitivity reactions can impair these defences.

The inhaled substance damages alveolar epithelium, leading to an inflammatory process of the alveoli and interstitial tissue of the lung. The inflammatory response produces further damage and abnormal fibrotic (scar) tissue replaces the elastin fibres of normal lung tissue. As a result, the lungs become stiff and non-compliant. Lung volumes decrease, the work of breathing increases and alveolar–capillary diffusion is impaired, leading to hypoxaemia.

Asbestosis

Inhalation of asbestos fibres is a common cause of occupational lung disease. *Asbestosis* is a diffuse interstitial fibrotic disease involving the terminal airways, alveoli and pleurae. Exposure to

TABLE 36.4 Selected causes of interstitial lung disorders

CAUSE	EXAMPLES
Inorganic dusts	Silica (silicosis), asbestos (asbestosis), coal (coal worker's pneumoconiosis), talc (talcosis)
Organic dusts	Cotton (byssinosis), sugar cane (bagassosis), mouldy hay (farmer's lung)
Drugs	Antineoplastic agents, antibiotics, gold salts, phenytoin
Radiation	External radiation or inhaled radioactive materials
Infections	Widespread tuberculosis or fungal infections, viral or *Pneumocystis carinii* pneumonia
Poisons and noxious gases	Paraquat, nitrogen dioxide, chlorine, ammonia, sulfur dioxide
Systemic diseases	Uraemia, pulmonary oedema
Unknown causes	Sarcoidosis, idiopathic pulmonary fibrosis, connective tissue disorders

asbestos fibres occurs during mining, milling, manufacturing and application of asbestos products. Although symptoms may not become apparent until 20 years after exposure, they tend to progress, even when further exposure has been halted. Asbestosis is also associated with an increased risk of bronchogenic carcinoma, especially in cigarette smokers. Mesothelioma, a rare cancer of the pleural membrane, is also associated with asbestos exposure. The period between asbestos exposure and tumour development in mesothelioma is long, ranging from 20 to 30 years. People exposed to asbestos prior to the imposition of strict environmental controls may only now be developing manifestations of this disease.

The manifestations of asbestosis include exertional dyspnoea, exercise intolerance and inspiratory crackles. Diffuse, small, irregular or linear opacities appear on chest x-ray, primarily in the lower lobes. As the disease progresses, respiratory failure and marked hypoxaemia may develop.

Silicosis

Inhalation of silica dust by hard-rock miners, foundry workers, sandblasters, pottery makers and granite cutters can lead to *silicosis*, a nodular pulmonary fibrosis (Jedynak, 2020). In silicosis, macrophages are destroyed as they engulf silica particles, releasing substances that damage lung tissue and lead to fibrosis and scarring.

Simple silicosis is asymptomatic with no demonstrable respiratory impairment. Complicated silicosis, in contrast, is characterised by large conglomerate densities in the upper lungs. These individuals may be severely dyspnoeic and have a productive cough. Respiratory function testing shows both restrictive and obstructive changes. The increasing size of conglomerate masses can lead to severe disability, cor pulmonale and death. In 2019, there were around 350 cases in Australia. Given that over 500,000 Australians are exposed silica in the workplace annually, silicosis has the potential for huge socioeconomic impact (Austin, James & Tessier, 2021).

Coal worker's pneumoconiosis

Ingestion of coal dust by alveolar macrophages causes 'coal macules' to form, leading to *coal worker's pneumoconiosis (CWP)*, or *black lung disease*. Coal macules appear on chest x-ray as diffuse, small opacities primarily affecting the upper lungs.

In the US, 37,965 cases of CWP were reported from 1968 to 2015; in China between 2003 and 2016, 21,719 cases were diagnosed. Australia has had only one person diagnosed with CWP since 2015 (Karatela, Caruana & Paul, 2022; Wong, 2019).

Simple CWP generally is asymptomatic. A small percentage of individuals (1–2%) develop progressive massive fibrosis, which destroys the pulmonary vascular bed and airways of the upper lungs. This progressive form of the disease causes symptoms similar to those of complicated silicosis. There is no known cure to date.

Hypersensitivity pneumonitis

Workers exposed to organic dusts and gases may develop *hypersensitivity pneumonitis*, an allergic pulmonary disease affecting the airways and alveoli. Byssinosis, resulting from cotton dust exposure; bagassosis, due to exposure to mouldy sugar cane fibre; farmer's lung and bird-fancier's lung are examples of hypersensitivity pneumonitis.

Either acute or subacute illness can occur. Acute illness occurs 4–8 hours after exposure and is heralded by sudden onset of malaise, chills and fever, dyspnoea, cough and nausea. The subacute syndrome is characterised by an insidious onset of chronic cough, progressive dyspnoea, anorexia and weight loss. Diffuse fibrosis occurs after repeated exposure to the organic material, leading to respiratory insufficiency.

INTERPROFESSIONAL CARE

Prevention is a key strategy for all occupational lung diseases. Containing dust and wearing personal protective devices that limit the amount of inhaled particles are essential for people who work in industries with known risks.

Investigations

Chest x-ray, pulmonary function studies, bronchoscopy and possibly lung biopsy are used to establish the diagnosis of pneumoconiosis. Characteristic patterns are seen for each disorder on x-ray. Pulmonary function testing shows restrictive impairment of lung ventilation, with reduced vital capacity and reduced total lung capacity. The diffusing capacity of the lungs is also decreased. Blood gas analysis reveals hypoxaemia, especially with exercise. Bronchoscopy may be performed to obtain tissue for biopsy. Specialised lung scans may be used to determine the extent of fibrosis.

Management

Eliminating further exposure to the offending agent is an important part of disease management. There is no specific therapy. Anti-inflammatory drugs, such as corticosteroids, may reduce the inflammatory response and slow the progression of the disease. Preventing exposure to other damaging substances such as cigarette smoke and pollution is vital. Pneumococcal vaccine and annual influenza immunisations are recommended to reduce the risk of lower respiratory infections. COVID-19 vaccines may also be recommended by the GP. Other care is supportive, similar to that for COPD.

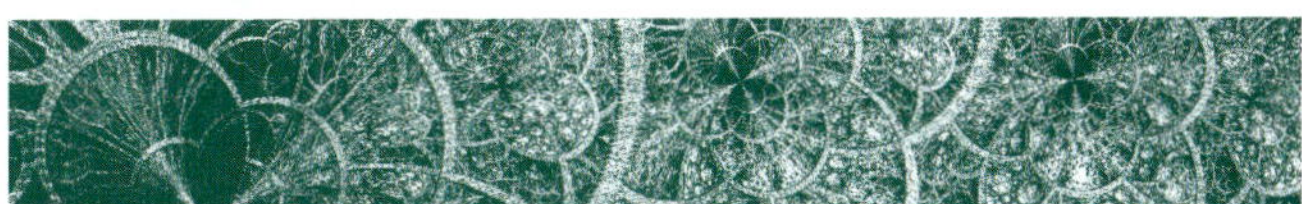

Nursing care

Health promotion

Teaching about the dangers of occupational lung diseases and ways to reduce their risks needs to begin early, before the disease develops. Nurses in industrial and public health settings can begin by recognising potential dangers and teaching workers about measures to reduce dust in their work area and the use of personal protective devices such as masks. Nurses working with affected families have an excellent opportunity to begin educating children about the risks associated with the occupation.

Nursing diagnoses and interventions

Nursing care for the person with occupational lung diseases is similar to that for those with COPD. Activity intolerance is a high-priority problem for many individuals. Severe dyspnoea can significantly interfere with ADLs. Nursing measures to reduce energy expenditures and provide for rest are essential. Caregiver role strain, either actual or potential, must be considered when the person with severe disability is being cared for at home.

For both the individual and their family, coping may be compromised. Many of these diseases develop after 20–30 years of exposure to the hazardous material. Individuals who entered the industry following high school may develop evidence of disease in their forties and face the possibility of changing their occupation or developing significant disability. The resulting role strain affects all members of the family.

Other nursing diagnoses to consider for the person with an occupational lung disease are:

- *Ineffective oxygenation* related to restrictive lung disease evidenced by low SpO_2.
- *Situational low self-esteem* related to effects of ill health, evidenced by reduced ability to maintain self-care.

Community-based care

The affected person and their family need teaching in preparation for home care, including:

- prevention of further lung damage—for example, avoiding cigarette smoke and heavy air pollution
- recommendations for pneumococcal and annual influenza immunisations; yearly tuberculin testing for individuals with silicosis
- respiratory hygiene measures, such as liberal fluid intake, coughing and deep-breathing exercises
- use and care of oxygen therapy equipment if required
- use and effects of any prescribed or recommended OTC medications.

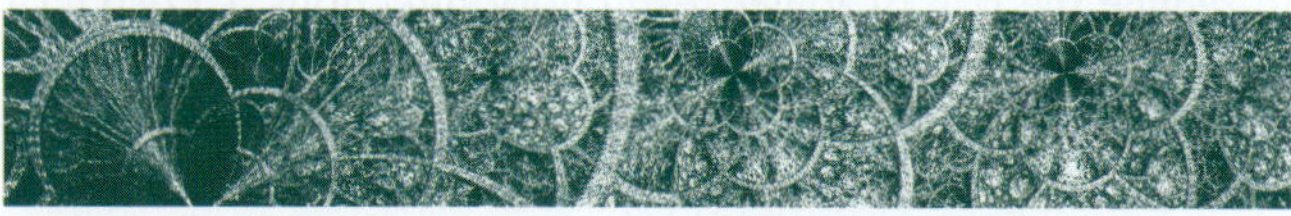

THE PERSON WITH SARCOIDOSIS

Sarcoidosis is a chronic multisystem disease characterised by an exaggerated cellular immune response in involved tissues. This abnormal immune response leads to granuloma formation in the lungs, lymph nodes, liver, eyes, skin and other organs. Its cause is unknown and it is neither a malignant nor an autoimmune disease (Kamangar, 2022). It primarily affects adults between the ages of 20 and 40 and is seen in 20–40 per 100,000 population in Australia (Lung Foundation Australia, 2019). Although the disease occurs worldwide, incidences are low as it is sometimes misdiagnosed as tuberculosis (Kamangar, 2022).

In sarcoidosis, multiple granulomas form; these lesions may resolve spontaneously or proceed to fibrosis. The lungs are affected in most individuals with sarcoidosis. Pulmonary haemorrhage and cardiac and respiratory failure from pulmonary fibrosis are the leading causes of death from sarcoidosis.

The manifestations of sarcoidosis vary depending on the organ system affected. It may be asymptomatic, diagnosed by characteristic findings on routine chest x-ray. Symptoms may be insidious, with anorexia, fatigue, weight loss, fever, dyspnoea, arthralgias and myalgias. Skin lesions, uveitis, lymphadenopathy, hepatomegaly or other manifestations may also develop.

Leucopenia, eosinophilia and an elevated erythrocyte sedimentation rate (ESR) typically are noted in sarcoidosis. The chest x-ray helps to determine the extent of pulmonary involvement. Biopsy of a granulomatous lesion may be required to confirm the diagnosis. Pulmonary function tests reveal decreased compliance and impaired diffusing capacity.

Sarcoidosis often resolves spontaneously; therefore, treatment is indicated only when symptoms are severe or disabling. Corticosteroid therapy is prescribed to suppress the inflammatory process when indicated. Relapse frequently occurs when corticosteroids are discontinued. Other anti-inflammatory or immune-modifier medications may also be used.

Nursing care for individuals with sarcoidosis is directed by involved organ systems and related manifestations. Respiratory care is supportive and includes avoiding respiratory irritants and maintaining adequate ventilation. Refer for smoking cessation assistance as needed.

Educate individuals about the disease and symptoms to report to a healthcare provider, including shortness of breath, tearing and eye inflammation, chest pain or irregular pulse, skin lesions and swollen and painful joints. Also educate about infection control strategies and provide advice regarding relevant vaccinations, such as influenza and COVID-19 (Crawford & Ruth-Sahd, 2021). If corticosteroid therapy is prescribed, teach the importance of taking the drug as prescribed and not stopping it abruptly. Include information about managing the side effects of corticosteroids by limiting sodium and increasing potassium in the diet, taking the medication with food or milk to minimise gastric irritation and identifying early signs of infection.

Pulmonary vascular disorders

The cardiovascular and respiratory systems are closely interrelated. As blood flows through the capillary network of the pulmonary vascular system, oxygen diffuses into it and CO_2 diffuses out. An effective match of alveolar ventilation and capillary perfusion is essential to maintain this process and, ultimately, tissue oxygenation and function of all organ systems. Both vascular and alveolar changes can alter gas exchange. Arteriosclerotic changes in pulmonary vasculature reduce blood flow to the alveolus. Nearly all lower respiratory system disorders potentially can affect ventilation. Many also have a secondary effect on lung perfusion, because breakdown or fibrosis of alveolar walls destroys the capillary network as well. This section focuses on primary disorders of the pulmonary vascular system.

THE PERSON WITH PULMONARY EMBOLISM

A **pulmonary embolism** (or *thromboembolism*) is obstruction of blood flow in part of the pulmonary vascular system by an embolus. *Thromboemboli*, or blood clots, that develop in the venous system (deep venous thrombosis, or DVT) or right side of the heart are the most frequent cause of pulmonary embolism. Other sources of emboli include tumours that have invaded venous circulation, fat or bone marrow entering the circulation due to fracture or other trauma, amniotic fluid released into the circulation during childbirth and intravenous injection of air or other foreign substances.

Pulmonary embolism (PE) is a medical emergency. Most people who die from PE will generally die within the first few hours (Ouellette, 2020). In many cases, DVT has not been recognised or treated; often embolisation also goes undetected. Prevention is the most effective treatment strategy for PE.

Incidence and risk factors

More than 17,000 Australians are diagnosed with an embolism every year. It is estimated to be one of the leading preventable causes of death in hospitals, costing the healthcare system over $1.7 billion annually (Australian Commission on Safety and Quality in Health Care, 2020). PE is considered an adverse outcome of poor health and chronic diseases, leading to disproportional high rates of hospitalisation among Indigenous Australians. Although many substances can become emboli, thrombus arising from the deep veins of the legs is the leading cause of PE. The risk factors for a pulmonary embolus are those for DVT: stasis of venous blood flow, vessel wall damage and altered blood coagulation.

Prolonged immobility; trauma, including hip and femur fractures; surgery (orthopaedic, pelvic and gynaecological surgery, in particular); myocardial infarction and heart failure; obesity; acute medical illness (e.g. AIDS, congestive heart failure (CHF)); drug abuse; hereditary factors; and advanced age. Women who use oral contraceptives or oestrogen therapy are at risk, as are women during pregnancy and childbirth. See the chapter 'Nursing care of people with vascular and lymphatic disorders' for more information about DVT.

Physiology review

The right heart receives deoxygenated blood from the systemic venous circulation. The entire output of the right ventricle enters the pulmonary circulation via the pulmonary artery. This artery branches into successively smaller arteries, arterioles and capillaries of the pulmonary vascular system. Each alveolus of the lungs is surrounded by a meshwork of capillaries. Oxygen and CO_2 readily diffuse across the alveolar–capillary membrane, driven by a concentration gradient. The partial pressure of oxygen in the alveolus is greater than in the capillary; therefore, it diffuses into the blood. CO_2 diffuses from the capillaries into the alveoli, driven by the higher pressure of dissolved CO_2 in venous blood.

A match between blood flow through the pulmonary vascular system (perfusion) and lung ventilation is necessary for effective *respiration* (gas exchange). Local factors regulate ventilation and perfusion to maintain this match. A low alveolar PO_2 constricts alveolar capillaries, directing blood flow to better-ventilated areas of the lung. High alveolar PCO_2 levels cause local bronchodilation, increasing airflow and eliminating excess CO_2.

Pathophysiology

There are respiratory and haemodynamic consequences related to PE (Ouellette, 2020). Thrombi affecting only the deep veins of the calf rarely embolise to the pulmonary circulation. However, thrombi often propagate proximally to the popliteal and ileofemoral veins. From there, they may break loose to become an embolus. As vessels of the venous system become progressively larger, the embolus moves freely until it enters the pulmonary arterial system, with its progressively smaller vessels leading to the pulmonary capillary beds (see Figure 36.12).

The impact of a pulmonary embolus depends on the extent to which pulmonary blood flow is obstructed, the size of the embolus, its nature and secondary effects of the obstruction. The effects can range widely:

- Occlusion of a large pulmonary artery with sudden death. Gas exchange is significantly reduced or prevented, and cardiac output falls dramatically as blood fails to move through the pulmonary vascular system and return to the left heart.
- Lung tissue infarction due to occlusion of a significant portion of pulmonary blood flow. Fewer than 10% of pulmonary emboli result in pulmonary infarction.
- Obstruction of a small segment of the pulmonary circulation with no permanent lung injury.
- Chronic or recurrent, possibly multiple, small emboli with recurring symptoms.

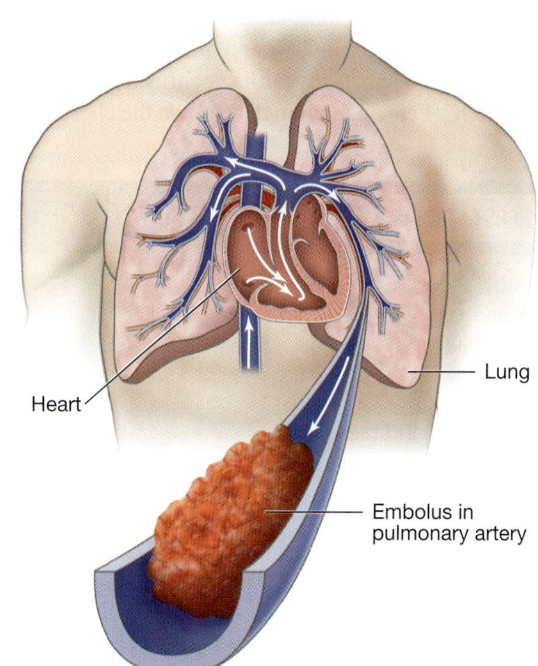

FIGURE 36.12 ***A thromboembolism lodged in a pulmonary vessel***

Obstruction of pulmonary blood flow by an embolus affects both perfusion and ventilation. Neurohumoral reflexes triggered by obstruction cause vasoconstriction, increasing pulmonary vascular resistance. In severe cases, this can lead to pulmonary hypertension and right ventricular heart failure. Systemically, hypotension and a drop in cardiac output may develop. Bronchoconstriction occurs in the affected area of lung. Dead space (areas of the lung that are ventilated but not perfused) increases. Alveolar surfactant decreases, increasing the risk of atelectasis.

If infarction does not occur, the thrombolytic system (see the chapter 'Nursing care of people with coronary heart disease') ultimately dissolves the clot and pulmonary function returns to normal. Infarcted tissue becomes scarred and fibrotic.

Fat emboli are the most common non-thrombotic pulmonary emboli. A fat embolism usually occurs after fracture of long bone (typically the femur) releases bone marrow fat into the circulation. Adipose tissue or liver trauma may also lead to fat emboli.

Manifestations

The manifestations of PE depend on its size and location. Small emboli may be asymptomatic. Manifestations usually develop abruptly, over a period of minutes. The most common symptoms are dyspnoea and pleuritic chest pain. Anxiety, a sense of impending doom and cough are also common (see the 'Manifestations' box). Diaphoresis and haemoptysis may develop. Massive pulmonary embolus can cause syncope and cyanosis. On examination, tachycardia and tachypnoea are noted. Crackles may be heard on auscultation of the chest and a cardiac gallop (S_3 and possibly S_4) may be noted. A low-grade fever may develop. It is difficult to differentiate PE from myocardial infarction or pneumonia by manifestations (Ouellette, 2020).

Characteristic manifestations of fat emboli include sudden onset of cardiopulmonary and neurological symptoms: dyspnoea, tachypnoea, tachycardia, confusion, delirium and decreased LOC. Petechiae often develop on the chest and arms.

MANIFESTATIONS Pulmonary embolism

COMMON

- Dyspnoea
- Chest pain
- Anxiety
- Cough
- Tachycardia and tachypnoea
- Crackles (rales)
- Low-grade fever

LESS COMMON

- Diaphoresis
- Haemoptysis
- Syncope
- Cyanosis
- S_3 and/or S_4 gallop

INTERPROFESSIONAL CARE

Because deep venous thrombosis may not be identified until PE occurs, prevention is the primary goal in treating PE.

Early ambulation is an effective means of preventing venous stasis and reducing the incidence of PE. External pneumatic compression of the legs is also effective for individuals undergoing neurosurgery, urological surgery or major surgery of the hip or knee or when anticoagulant therapy is contraindicated. Other preventive measures include elevating the legs and active and passive leg exercises.

When PE occurs, treatment is supportive. Oxygen therapy is initiated and analgesics may be ordered to relieve severe pleuritic pain and anxiety. Pulmonary artery and wedge pressures are monitored with a balloon (Swan–Ganz) catheter. Vena cave filters may be inserted if indicated. Cardiac outputs also may be assessed. Cardiac rhythm is monitored to detect arrhythmias.

Diagnosis

The studies performed to identify DVT differ from those used to diagnose a PE. See the chapter 'Nursing care of people with vascular and lymphatic disorders' for diagnostic studies for venous thrombosis.

- *Plasma d-dimer levels* detect inflammation. A d-dimer is a fragment of fibrin formed during lysis of a blood clot; elevated blood levels indicate thrombus formation and lysis (e.g. DVT and PE).
- *Chest CT with contrast* is the principal test used to diagnose PE. Chest CT effectively shows large, central PE; newer-generation scanners also can detect peripheral emboli.
- *Lung scans*, including perfusion and ventilation scans, may be used. In a perfusion lung scan, radio-tagged albumin is injected intravenously and distributed in the lungs by the pulmonary blood flow. The lungs are then scanned for distribution of the isotope. An area of lung in which the isotope is undetectable is suggestive of occluded blood flow and PE. For a ventilation scan, a radio-tagged gas is inhaled and the lungs are scanned for gas distribution. Combined perfusion and ventilation scans allow identification of areas of the lungs that are ventilated but not perfused, a characteristic of PE.
- *Pulmonary angiography* is the definitive test for PE when other, less invasive tests are inconclusive. It is possible to detect very small emboli with angiography. A contrast medium injected into the pulmonary arteries illustrates the pulmonary vascular system on x-ray.
- *Chest x-ray* often shows pulmonary infiltration and occasionally pleural effusion.
- *Electrocardiogram (ECG)* is ordered to rule out acute myocardial infarction as the cause of symptoms. ECG findings commonly associated with PE include tachycardia and non-specific T-wave changes.
- *ABGs* usually show hypoxaemia (PaO_2 less than 80 mmHg) and often respiratory alkalosis ($pH > 7.45$, $PaCO_2 < 38$ mmHg) due to tachypnoea and hyperventilation.

- *$ETCO_2$* may be measured to evaluate alveolar perfusion. The normal $ETCO_2$ reading is 35 to 45 mmHg; it is decreased when pulmonary perfusion is impaired.
- *Coagulation studies* are ordered to monitor the response to therapy. The *activated partial thromboplastin time (aPTT* or *PTT*) is used to assess the intrinsic clotting pathway and the response to heparin therapy. Desired levels with anticoagulant therapy are 1.5 to 2 times the control value. The risk of recurrent thromboembolism is high at lower levels; the risk of bleeding increases at higher levels. The *International Normalized Ratio (INR)* is used to assess the extrinsic clotting system and oral anticoagulation with warfarin (Coumadin). The goal of anticoagulant therapy is to achieve a therapeutic range of 2.0 to 3.0.

Medications

Anticoagulant therapy is the standard treatment to prevent pulmonary emboli. It is often instituted in high-risk individuals who have no evidence of PE to prevent possible devastating effects. In the person with DVT or a pulmonary embolus, anticoagulants are administered to prevent further clotting and embolisation. See the chapter 'Nursing care of people with vascular and lymphatic disorders' for more information about anticoagulant therapy to prevent and treat DVT. See the 'Medication administration' box on anticoagulant therapy in the chapter 'Nursing care of people with vascular and lymphatic disorders' for the nursing implications for such therapy.

For PE, heparin therapy is initiated with an intravenous bolus of 5,000 to 10,000 units of heparin, followed by continuous infusion at the rate of 1,000 to 1,500 units per hour. The aPTT or PTT is monitored frequently until stabilised. Heparin therapy is typically continued for about 5 days or until oral anticoagulant therapy has become fully effective.

Oral anticoagulant therapy with warfarin sodium is initiated at the same time as heparin. Warfarin alters the synthesis of vitamin-K-dependent clotting factors and requires 5 to 7 days to be fully effective. Anticoagulant therapy is continued for 2 to 3 months when few risk factors for thromboemboli exist; long-term therapy is used when chronic disorders that increase the risk of thromboemboli are present.

Bleeding is a risk associated with anticoagulant therapy. Although major haemorrhage is uncommon, it occurs in approximately 5% of individuals receiving intravenous heparin. Cardiac, hepatic and renal disease increase the risk of significant bleeding in people aged over 60 years. Protamine, a protein that combines with heparin to inactivate it, is used to stop its anticoagulant effect if major bleeding occurs. Vitamin K is given to treat bleeding associated with warfarin therapy.

Thrombolytic therapy may be used to treat massive pulmonary embolus and hypotension. Streptokinase, urokinase or tissue plasminogen activator (tPA) are used to *lyse* (disintegrate) the embolus, restore pulmonary blood flow and reduce pulmonary artery and right heart pressures. Although thrombolytic therapy may not reduce mortality associated with pulmonary embolus, it may reduce the incidence of pulmonary hypertension, which develops 3–5 years after an embolism. Thrombolysis significantly increases the risk of bleeding, particularly cerebral bleeding. Contraindications to thrombolysis include intracranial disease, recent stroke, active bleeding or a bleeding disorder, pregnancy, severe hypertension and recent surgery or trauma. Because of the increased risk of haemorrhage, invasive procedures are avoided after thrombolysis. See the chapter 'Nursing care of people with coronary heart disease' for further discussion of thrombolytic therapy and its nursing implications.

Surgery

When anticoagulant therapy fails to prevent recurrent emboli or is contraindicated, an umbrella-like filter may be inserted into the inferior vena cava to trap large emboli while allowing continued blood flow. The filter usually is inserted percutaneously, via either the femoral or the jugular vein. A surgical embolectomy may also be considered in patients with massive PE where fibrinolysis is contraindicated or who continue to be unstable post fibrinolysis (Ouellette, 2020).

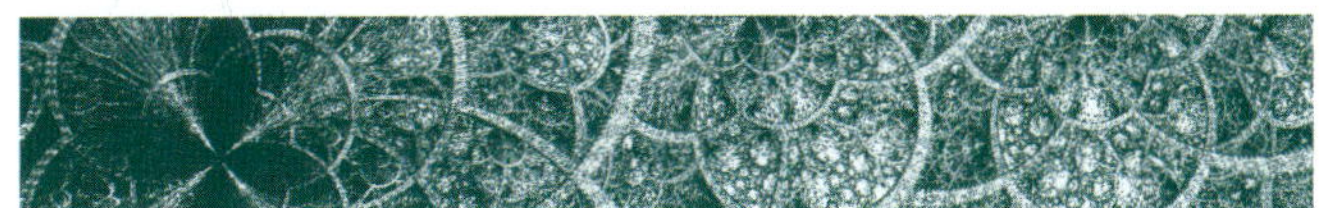

Nursing care

Health promotion

Nurses are pivotal in preventing PE. Encouraging individuals to ambulate after surgery or illness, applying compression stockings or pneumatic compression devices, teaching and encouraging leg exercises, discouraging the use of pillows under the knees—all of these measures help prevent DVT and subsequent PE.

Teach individuals to reduce the risks associated with long periods of immobility, stopping every 1–2 hours during long automobile trips for a brief stretch and walk, getting up every hour or so and doing leg exercises while seated during long flights and avoiding crossing the legs to prevent venous stasis and pooling. Regular exercise such as walking also reduces the risk of DVT. Instruct individuals who stand for long periods to use well-fitted elastic stockings, being careful to avoid hose that bind around the knee or thigh.

Assessment

Because pulmonary embolus can be a medical emergency, assessment may be very focused. In other instances, when emboli are small and not life threatening, a more extensive nursing assessment may be done.

- *Health history*: chest pain, dyspnoea, other symptoms, including onset, severity, precipitating factors; history of recent surgery, venous thrombosis or other risk factor such as childbirth or malignancy; current medications.
- *Physical examination*: level of consciousness, presence of respirations and pulse; colour, skin temperature and moisture; vital signs, including apical pulse and temperature; breath sounds and heart sounds; SpO_2 level; neck vein distension, peripheral oedema.

- *Diagnostic tests*: plasma d-dimer levels, coagulation studies; chest x-ray and other imaging studies; SpO_2 and ABGs; ECG.

Nursing diagnoses and interventions

A large pulmonary embolus can cause a significant mismatch between pulmonary ventilation and circulation. Impaired gas exchange is a priority problem and focus for interventions. Cardiac output may be significantly affected by obstructed pulmonary blood flow. Thrombolytic and anticoagulant therapy affect the clotting process, increasing the risk of bleeding. Anxiety accompanies PE almost universally.

Impaired gas exchange

PE results in areas of the lung that are ventilated but not perfused; they receive no capillary blood flow. If the embolus is large and a major segment of the lung is not perfused, gas exchange is significantly affected. Nursing interventions are directed towards compensating for impaired gas exchange.

- Frequently assess respiratory status, including rate, depth, effort, lung sounds and SpO_2. *Impaired ventilation will further compromise gas exchange and worsen hypoxaemia. Oxygen saturation can be monitored continuously and non-invasively to evaluate gas exchange.*

> **CONSIDERATION FOR PRACTICE**
> **Monitor and record LOC, mental status and skin colour. Hypoxaemia often causes confusion and agitation; hypercapnia may reduce LOC. Cyanosis indicates significant hypoxaemia.**

- Place in Fowler's or high-Fowler's position, with the lower extremities dependent. *This position facilitates maximal lung expansion and reduces venous return to the right side of the heart, lowering pressures in the pulmonary vascular system.*

> **CONSIDERATION FOR PRACTICE**
> **Start oxygen per nasal prongs or mask. Obtain a doctor's order if one has not been written. Supplemental oxygen increases alveolar and arterial oxygenation. Oxygen is a drug and must be prescribed by the doctor. However, it may be initiated by the nurse in an emergency to prevent tissue hypoxia.**

- Monitor ABG results, reporting abnormal findings as indicated. An arterial line may be inserted for monitoring arterial pressure and arterial blood sampling. *ABGs are used to assess gas exchange and tissue oxygenation.*
- Maintain bed rest. *Bed rest reduces metabolic demands and tissue needs for oxygen.*

Decreased cardiac output

The impact of a large pulmonary embolus on haemodynamic status can be significant. Pressures in the pulmonary vascular system and right heart increase; blood return to the left heart and cardiac output may significantly decrease. Nursing interventions focus on preserving an adequate blood pressure and organ function until cardiopulmonary status stabilises. A central line for haemodynamic monitoring may be instituted. (See the chapter 'Nursing care of people with cardiac disorders' for nursing care related to haemodynamic monitoring.)

- Auscultate heart sounds every 2–4 hours, reporting any abnormalities. *Sounds such as an S_3 or S_4 gallop may indicate cardiac compromise.*

> **CONSIDERATION FOR PRACTICE**
> **Assess and record vital signs and cardiopulmonary status every 15–30 minutes initially, then every 2–4 hours as condition stabilises. Frequent assessment facilitates timely interventions to maintain cardiovascular status and preserve organ function.**

> **CONSIDERATION FOR PRACTICE**
> **Record intake and output hourly. Decreased urinary output often is an early indicator of decreased cardiac output. Maintaining renal perfusion is vital to preserve renal function and prevent acute renal failure.**

- Assess skin colour and temperature. *These assessments monitor tissue perfusion.*
- Monitor cardiac rhythm. *A drop in cardiac output and other haemodynamic alterations resulting from PE can precipitate arrhythmias. Arrhythmias, in turn, can further impair cardiac output.*
- Administer vasopressors and other medications as ordered. Carefully monitor the response to prescribed medications. *Drugs may be prescribed to maintain adequate arterial pressure and tissue perfusion. Potent drugs such as vasopressors require careful monitoring for desired and adverse effects.*
- Monitor pulmonary artery pressures, neck vein distension and peripheral oedema. Report findings as indicated. *Right-sided heart failure is a potential complication of PE because of increased pulmonary artery pressures.*
- Maintain intravenous and arterial access sites as well as central lines. *The person may be in an unstable and critical condition, potentially needing immediate interventions to maintain life.*
- Instruct to report chest pain or other symptoms. *Decreased cardiac output and an increased workload due to pulmonary hypertension may cause anginal pain.*

> **CONSIDERATION FOR PRACTICE**
> **Provide frequent skin care. Impaired tissue perfusion and oxygenation increase the risk of skin and tissue breakdown.**

Ineffective protection

Thrombolytics and anticoagulant therapy impair normal clotting mechanisms, increasing the risk of bleeding and haemorrhage. This risk is particularly acute during the first 24–48 hours following thrombolytic drug administration.

- Assess frequently for overt and covert signs of bleeding: bleeding gums; haematuria; obvious or occult blood in stool or vomitus; incisional bleeding, bleeding or bruising of injection sites or with minor trauma; joint pain or immobility; abdominal or flank pain.

Careful monitoring is necessary to identify early signs of abnormal bleeding and prevent potential haemorrhage.

- Report coagulation study results outside the desired range for anticoagulant therapy. *Levels less than the target range may indicate an increased risk of further clot development and pulmonary emboli; levels above the target range indicate an increased risk of bleeding.*

CONSIDERATION FOR PRACTICE

Promptly report changes in neurological status. Although cerebral bleeding is not evident externally, changes in LOC and other neurological signs suggest it and should be reported immediately.

- Keep protamine sulfate available for heparin therapy and vitamin K available for warfarin therapy. *Bleeding or haemorrhage due to excess anticoagulant may require antidote administration to rapidly reverse anticoagulant effects.*
- Assess medication regimen for possible drug interactions that could potentiate or inhibit anticoagulant effects. *Drug interactions can increase the risk of haemorrhage or further embolus formation.*
- Avoid invasive procedures, injections and venipunctures when possible, particularly during and following thrombolytic therapy. *Invasive procedures increase the risk of tissue trauma and bleeding.*
- Maintain firm pressure on injection and venipuncture sites. Maintain pressure for 30 minutes following arterial puncture. *Firm pressure reduces the risk of bleeding into the tissues.*
- Maintain adequate fluid intake. Administer stool softeners as ordered. *These measures help prevent constipation and straining, which may precipitate bleeding of haemorrhoids.*

CONSIDERATION FOR PRACTICE

Use an infusion device to administer heparin infusion. Using an infusion pump or device helps prevent administration of excess medication.

Anxiety

PE is a physiological and psychological threat to safety and integrity. It is a major physiological stressor, eliciting a strong neuroendocrine stress response. The feeling of suffocation and inability to catch one's breath that accompanies a pulmonary embolus is also a strong psychological stressor. Fear and anxiety are common responses.

- Assess anxiety level. *Appropriate interventions are determined by the level of anxiety.*

CONSIDERATION FOR PRACTICE

Provide reassurance and emotional support, listening to fears. Do not negate the fear of dying, but reassure that treatment usually restores effective respiratory function. The fear of death is very real and must not be discounted; however, it is important to provide reassurance to alleviate excess anxiety.

- Remain with the person as much as possible. *The presence of a caring nurse helps reduce fear.*
- Explain procedures and treatments, using short, simple sentences. *Providing clearly understood, simple instructions reduces fear of the unknown.*
- Reduce environmental stimuli and use a calm, reassuring manner. *These measures help reduce anxiety (for both the nurse and the individual).*
- Allow supportive family members to remain with the person as much as possible. *Calm, supportive family members provide further reassurance.*
- Administer morphine sulfate as ordered. *Morphine is given to reduce pain and anxiety.*

Community-based care

Discuss the following topics when preparing the person with PE and family members for home care:

- use of prescribed anticoagulant, including drug interactions, scheduled laboratory testing and manifestations of bleeding to report to the primary care provider
- using a soft toothbrush and electric razor to reduce the risk of bleeding
- avoiding aspirin (unless prescribed) and other OTC medications unless approved by the doctor
- importance of wearing a MedicAlert® tag for anticoagulant use
- health-promotion measures to reduce the risk of recurrent PE
- symptoms of recurrent PE, such as sudden chest pain, shortness of breath and, possibly, bloody sputum.

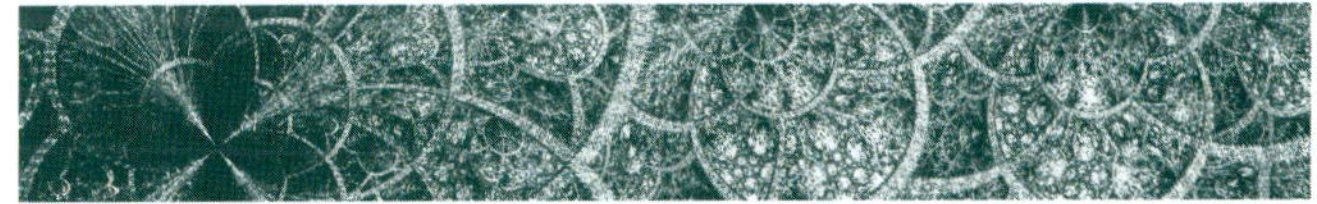

THE PERSON WITH PULMONARY HYPERTENSION

The pulmonary vascular system is normally a high-flow, low-pressure, low-resistance system that can accommodate large increases in blood flow when necessary (e.g. during exercise). The normal mean arterial pressure in the pulmonary system is 12–15 mmHg (25–28 systolic/8 diastolic). **Pulmonary hypertension** is abnormal elevation of the pulmonary arterial pressure. In Australia, approximately 3–10 people per million have idiopathic pulmonary hypertension. A family history is present in 10–12% of cases (PHA Australia, 2022).

Pathophysiology

Pulmonary hypertension can develop as a primary disorder, but usually occurs secondarily to another condition. In both instances, changes in the pulmonary artery lead to abnormal growth and remodelling of pulmonary vessels. Smooth muscle cells and fibroblasts proliferate, leading to abnormal vasoconstriction and fibrosis of pulmonary vessels. Once initiated, pulmonary vascular changes are progressive and non-reversible. Vasoconstrictive substances such as endothelin 1 and thromboxane A_2 are produced in excess, while the production of vasodilating substances such as nitric oxide is reduced. This further contributes to vasoconstriction and increased pulmonary artery pressures. Thromboxane A_2 also stimulates platelet aggregation, promoting clot formation in pulmonary vessels. Inflammation may contribute to progression of the disease. Vasoconstriction and increased pressures in the pulmonary system increase the workload of the right ventricle, ultimately leading to right ventricular failure (Oudiz, 2022; Schwab, 2022).

Primary pulmonary hypertension

Primary pulmonary hypertension is an uncommon disorder without identified cause. It occurs in both familial and sporadic patterns. In the familial form, a gene transmitted in an autosomal dominant pattern affects a protein receptor in the walls of pulmonary arteries, leading to abnormal vessel growth and remodelling. Primary pulmonary hypertension mainly affects women in their thirties or forties.

Secondary pulmonary hypertension

Secondary pulmonary hypertension is more common than primary. HIV infection and collagen diseases (e.g. scleroderma and lupus) may lead to secondary pulmonary hypertension. However, its usual cause is the reduced size of the pulmonary vascular bed, which may be due to vasoconstriction or widespread vessel destruction or obstruction. Hypoxaemia is a potent pulmonary vasoconstrictor and common initiating factor in pulmonary hypertension. Chronic lung diseases, sleep apnoea and hypoventilation due to obesity or neuromuscular disease can lead to hypoxaemia. Alveolar wall destruction associated with emphysema leads to loss of pulmonary capillaries. Large or multiple pulmonary emboli may cause vessel obstruction. Left ventricular failure or mitral stenosis also can lead to elevated pulmonary pressures. Once initiated, pulmonary hypertension becomes self-sustaining, as pulmonary vessels undergo changes that further narrow the pulmonary bed.

Manifestations

The manifestations of pulmonary hypertension are progressive dyspnoea, fatigue, angina and syncope with exertion. In secondary pulmonary hypertension, the signs and symptoms often are masked by those of the underlying disease. Dull, retrosternal chest pain may occur in addition to the manifestations of the primary disease. Primary pulmonary hypertension is a progressive disorder that generally causes a steady decline to death within 3 to 4 years.

Complications

Cor pulmonale is a condition of right ventricular hypertrophy and failure resulting from long-standing pulmonary hypertension. Chronic obstructive pulmonary disease is the most common cause of cor pulmonale.

The manifestations of cor pulmonale are those of the underlying pulmonary disorder and right-sided heart failure. Chronic productive cough, progressive dyspnoea and wheezing are common. With right-sided heart failure, peripheral oedema and distended neck veins are seen. Skin is warm, moist and cyanotic because of increased numbers of RBCs and hypoxaemia.

INTERPROFESSIONAL CARE

An FBC commonly shows *polycythaemia*, increased numbers of red blood cells. ABGs and SpO_2 measurements reveal hypoxaemia. A chest x-ray shows right heart enlargement and dilation of central pulmonary arteries. Typical ECG changes are those of right ventricular hypertrophy. An echocardiogram may be done to identify cardiac changes occurring either as a cause or a result of pulmonary hypertension. Doppler ultrasonography is a non-invasive means of estimating pulmonary artery pressure, but cardiac catheterisation may be required for definitive diagnosis. See the chapter 'A person-centred approach to assessing the cardiovascular and lymphatic systems' for nursing care of the person undergoing cardiac catheterisation.

Treatment for pulmonary hypertension focuses on slowing the course of the disease, preventing thrombus formation and reducing pulmonary vasoconstriction. Oxygen is administered to reduce hypoxaemia and improve activity tolerance. If polycythaemia is present, venesection is performed to reduce the viscosity of the blood.

Medications including calcium channel blockers nifedipine or diltiazem may be given to reduce pulmonary vascular resistance and improve cardiac output. Short-acting direct vasodilators such as intravenous epoprostenol or oral bosentan may be used for individuals who do not respond to calcium channel blockers. An oral anticoagulant (warfarin) is given to prevent clotting. Sildenafil, a smooth muscle relaxant, is given to reduce the blood pressure in the pulmonary arteries and increase in cardiac output (Oudiz, 2022; Schwab, 2022).

Bilateral lung or heart–lung transplant is the most effective long-term treatment for primary pulmonary hypertension.

When cor pulmonale is present, salt and water restrictions as well as diuretic therapy are added to the above regimen to manage the right-sided heart failure.

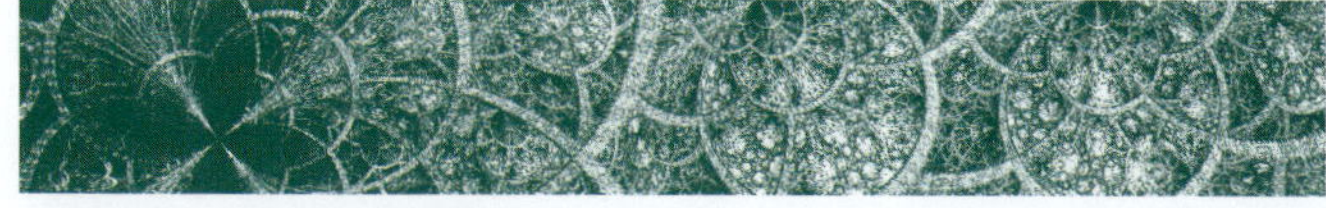

Nursing care

Nursing care for the person with pulmonary hypertension or cor pulmonale is largely supportive. The focus is on the underlying lung disease. Impaired gas exchange due to contraction of the pulmonary vascular system is a significant problem that causes many secondary problems, such as activity intolerance, anxiety and fatigue. Nursing interventions for impaired gas exchange are directed towards maintaining adequate alveolar ventilation, oxygenation and perfusion. The following measures may be included:

- monitoring breath sounds, respiratory rate, skin colour and use of accessory muscles
- positioning for optimal lung expansion
- coughing, deep breathing and chest physiotherapy
- administering prescribed vasodilators.

It is important to assess fatigue and dyspnoea with activities and to plan frequent rest periods. Assist with self-care as needed to conserve energy.

With primary pulmonary hypertension, *Anticipatory grieving* and *Hopelessness* are additional potential nursing diagnoses. When cor pulmonale is present, *Decreased cardiac output*, *Excess fluid volume* and *Ineffective individual coping* must be considered.

Community-based care

Most care for these chronic conditions is provided in the home and community settings. Teaching is directed both at the underlying lung disease, if present, and the resulting hypertensive process. Refer to the section on COPD for teaching related to this disease, the most frequent underlying cause of cor pulmonale. In addition, provide teaching about the following topics for the person and their family:

- disease process, its management and the prognosis
- manifestations or changes in condition to report to the doctor, such as a change in activity tolerance, increased oedema and signs of respiratory infection or exacerbation, and COVID-19
- importance of planned rest periods between activities and measures to conserve energy, such as using a shower chair
- importance of not smoking due to its irritant and vasoconstrictive effects
- prescribed medications, including their use and effects.

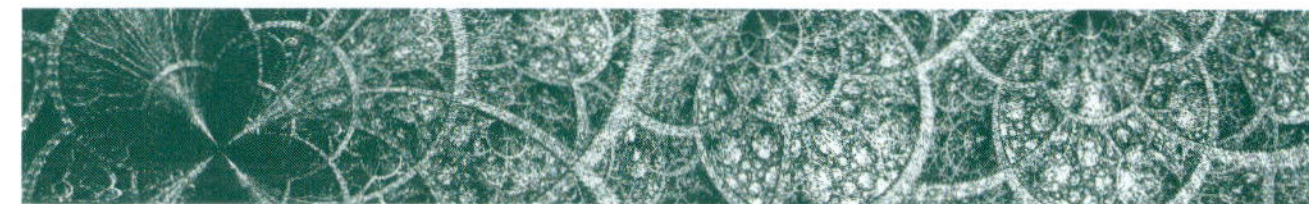

Respiratory failure

Many of the conditions discussed in this chapter and in the chapter 'Nursing care of people with ventilation disorders', from pneumonia to ARDS, can lead to respiratory failure. In **respiratory failure**, the lungs are unable to oxygenate the blood and remove CO_2 adequately to meet the body's needs, even at rest.

THE PERSON WITH ACUTE RESPIRATORY FAILURE

Respiratory failure is not a disease but a consequence of severe respiratory dysfunction. It is often defined by ABG values. An arterial oxygen level (PaO_2) of less than 50–60 mmHg and an arterial carbon dioxide level ($PaCO_2$) of greater than 45 mmHg are generally accepted as indicators of respiratory failure. However, individuals with advanced COPD may be alert and functional with blood gas values that would indicate respiratory failure in someone whose respiratory function was previously normal. In people with COPD, respiratory failure is indicated by an acute drop in blood oxygen levels along with increased CO_2 levels.

Respiratory failure can result from inadequate alveolar ventilation (hypoventilation), impaired gas exchange or a significant ventilation–perfusion mismatch. COPD is the most common cause of respiratory failure. Other lung diseases, chest injury, inhalation trauma, neuromuscular disorders and cardiac conditions can also lead to respiratory failure. Selected causes of acute respiratory failure are identified in Table 36.5.

Pathophysiology

Respiratory failure may be characterised by primary hypoxaemia or a combination of hypoxaemia and hypercapnia (see Figure 36.13). In hypoxaemic respiratory failure, PaO_2 is significantly reduced, whereas $PaCO_2$ remains normal or is low due to stimulation of the respiratory centre and tachypnoea. Impaired diffusion across the alveolar–capillary membrane and a ventilation–perfusion mismatch can cause a drop in arterial oxygen levels that is more rapid than the rise in CO_2. Metabolic acidosis results from tissue hypoxia. The increased work of breathing can eventually lead to respiratory muscle fatigue and hypoventilation.

Hypoventilation, or reduced movement of air into and out of the lung, causes CO_2 retention. With significant hypoventilation, the CO_2 level in the blood rises rapidly, leading to

TABLE 36.5 Selected causes of respiratory failure

TYPE OF DYSFUNCTION	EXAMPLES
Impaired ventilation	
• Airway obstruction	Laryngospasm, foreign body aspiration, airway oedema
• Respiratory disease	Asthma, COPD
• Neurological causes	Spinal cord injury, poliomyelitis, Guillain-Barré syndrome, drug overdose, stroke
• Chest wall injury	Flail chest, pneumothorax
Impaired diffusion	
• Alveolar disorders	Pneumonia, pneumonitis, COPD
• Pulmonary oedema	Heart failure, ARDS, immersion/submersion
• **Ventilation-perfusion mismatch**	PE

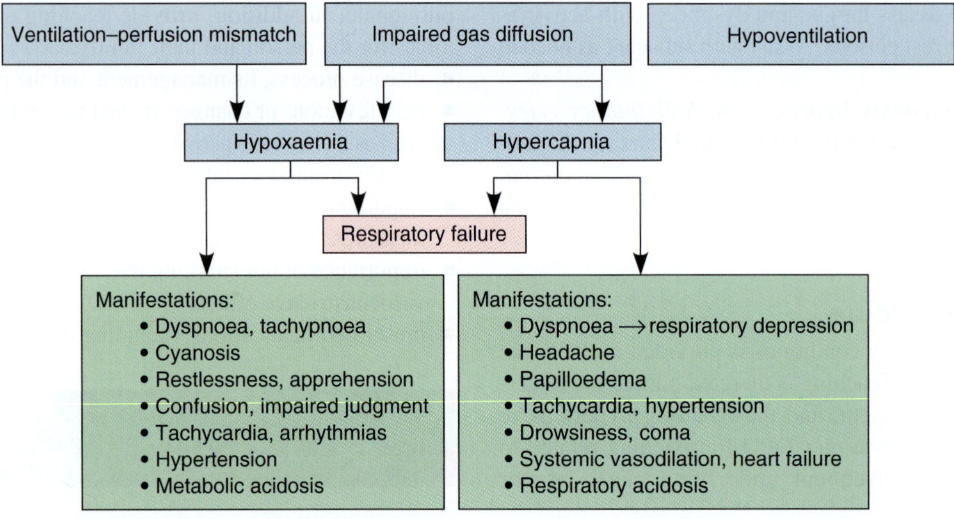

FIGURE 36.13 ***Causes and manifestations of respiratory failure***

respiratory acidosis. Hypoxaemia develops more slowly and responds readily to administration of oxygen unless gas exchange also is impaired.

In summary, hypoxaemia without a corresponding rise in CO_2 levels indicates a failure of oxygenation; hypoxaemia with hypercapnia is the result of lung hypoventilation.

See 'Pathophysiology illustrated'.

Manifestations and course

The manifestations of respiratory failure are caused by hypoxaemia and hypercapnia, as well as the underlying disease process. Hypoxaemia causes dyspnoea and neurological symptoms such as restlessness, apprehension, impaired judgment and motor impairment. Tachycardia and hypertension develop as the cardiac output increases in an effort to bring more oxygen to the tissues. Cyanosis is present. As hypoxaemia progresses, arrhythmias, hypotension and decreased cardiac output may develop.

Increased CO_2 levels depress CNS function and cause vasodilation. Dyspnoea and headache are early signs. Other manifestations include peripheral and conjunctival vasodilation, papilloedema, neuromuscular irritability and decreased LOC. As hypercapnia worsens, the respiratory centre may be depressed, reducing dyspnoea and slowing respirations. Increased CO_2 and hydrogen ion concentrations no longer stimulate the respiratory centre; hypoxaemia provides the primary active breathing stimulus. Administering oxygen without ventilatory support may further reduce the drive to breathe, leading to respiratory arrest.

The prognosis for acute respiratory failure varies, depending on the underlying disease process. Respiratory failure resulting from uncomplicated drug overdose generally resolves quickly without long-term effects. When respiratory failure results from underlying lung disease, the course may be prolonged and the outcome less favourable.

INTERPROFESSIONAL CARE

Treatment of respiratory failure focuses on correcting the underlying cause or disease, supporting ventilation and correcting hypoxaemia and hypercapnia. Care related to disorders that can precipitate respiratory failure is discussed in the sections specific to each disorder.

Diagnosis

Exhaled CO_2 and ABGs are used to diagnose and monitor treatment of respiratory failure.

- *$ETCO_2$* is used to evaluate alveolar ventilation. The normal $ETCO_2$ is 35–45 mmHg; it is elevated when ventilation is inadequate and decreased when pulmonary perfusion is impaired.
- *ABGs* also are used to evaluate alveolar ventilation and gas exchange. With hypoxaemic respiratory failure, the $PaCO_2$ may be normal, 38–42 mmHg, or even low due to tachypnoea. A pH of less than 7.35 and low bicarbonate levels indicate metabolic acidosis, typical of hypoxaemic respiratory failure.

In respiratory failure due to hypoventilation, the $PaCO_2$ is elevated, usually greater than 50 mmHg. The pH is low due to respiratory acidosis. Acidosis develops rapidly in hypoxaemia and hypercapnia because of increased acid production (metabolic) and decreased acid elimination (respiratory).

Medications

Drugs used in treating respiratory failure depend on the underlying cause of the failure and the need for intubation and mechanical ventilation.

Beta-adrenergic (sympathomimetic) or anticholinergic medications may be administered by inhalation to promote bronchodilation. If mechanical ventilation is required, the drugs may be given by nebuliser attached to the ventilator. See the 'Medication administration: asthma' box and the asthma section of this chapter for more information about bronchodilators and their nursing

MEDICATION ADMINISTRATION Neuromuscular blockers

NON-DEPOLARISING NEUROMUSCULAR BLOCKERS

Non-depolarising neuromuscular blockers competitively block the action of acetylcholine (ACh) at skeletal muscle receptors, preventing muscle depolarisation and contraction. Complete muscle paralysis is achieved within minutes. Facial muscles are affected first, followed by muscles of the limbs, neck and trunk. The muscles of respiration (the diaphragm and intercostal muscles) are least sensitive to the effects of neuromuscular blockers and are paralysed last. When the drug is discontinued or an antagonist is given, muscles recover in reverse order; respiratory function is recovered first.

Nursing responsibilities

- Prior to administering, assess endotracheal tube placement and ensure effective mechanical ventilator function. The risk of hypoxaemia and organ damage is significant if respiratory muscles are paralysed without adequate ventilatory support in place.
- Administer the drug by slow intravenous injection and/or intravenous infusion as prescribed.
- Keep an acetylcholinesterase (AChE) inhibitor such as neostigmine available at the bedside to rapidly reverse neuromuscular effects if needed.
- Administer morphine sulfate, diazepam, midazolam or other anti-anxiety agent or sedative as ordered. Neuromuscular blockers provide no sedation or pain relief; muscle paralysis in a conscious person produces extreme anxiety.
- Instil artificial tears every 2–4 hours.
- Suction oral cavity as needed to remove saliva.
- Ensure ventilator alarms are always on and appropriate for the person especially when administering neuromuscular blockers. Should the tubing become disconnected or plugged, the person is unable to breathe independently. Begin manual intermittent positive pressure ventilation with an air viva bag or bag/valve system and/or call for assistance.
- Treat the person as though awake and alert. Although unable to respond, mental function is unaffected.

Health education for the person and family

- Reassure that the ability to move and communicate will return when the drug is discontinued.
- Teach the family about the effects of the drug and the reason for its use. Explain that the person can hear and understand what is going on.

implications. Corticosteroids, administered by inhalation or intravenously, may be ordered to reduce airway oedema. Antibiotics are given to treat any underlying infection.

Sedation and analgesia often are required during mechanical ventilation to decrease pain and anxiety. Benzodiazepines such as diazepam, lorazepam or midazolam may be used for sedation and to inhibit the respiratory drive. Intravenous morphine or fentanyl provides analgesia and also inhibits the respiratory drive, allowing more effective mechanical ventilation. Occasionally, the person's respiratory drive competes with the ventilator despite sedation, decreasing its effectiveness and increasing the work of breathing. A neuromuscular blocking agent may be necessary to induce paralysis and suppress the ability to breathe. Nursing implications of neuromuscular blockers are described in the 'Medication administration' box.

Oxygen therapy

Oxygen is administered to reverse hypoxaemia in acute respiratory failure. In general, the goal is to achieve an SpO_2 of 90% or greater without oxygen toxicity. A PaO_2 of about 60 mmHg usually is adequate to meet the oxygen needs of body tissues. Higher levels do not significantly increase SpO_2 and may lead to hypoventilation in individuals with chronic hypercapnia. As little as 1–3 L of oxygen per nasal prongs or 28% oxygen per Venturi mask may correct hypoxaemia in advanced COPD. Oxygen concentrations of 40–60% may be required when diffusion is impaired (e.g. pneumonia or ARDS). High concentrations are used only for short periods to avoid oxygen toxicity. Both the oxygen concentration and duration of therapy contribute to oxygen toxicity. Continued high oxygen concentrations impair the synthesis of surfactant, reducing lung compliance (ease of inflation). ARDS or absorption atelectasis may develop.

When respiratory failure is caused by hypoventilation or usual oxygen delivery systems do not correct hypoxaemia, a tight-fitting mask to maintain *continuous positive airway pressure (CPAP)* may be used. CPAP increases lung volume, opening previously closed alveoli, improving ventilation of under-ventilated alveoli and ventilation–perfusion relationships.

Airway management

If the upper airway is obstructed or positive-pressure mechanical ventilation is necessary to correct hypoxaemia and hypercapnia, an endotracheal tube that extends from the mouth or nose into the trachea is inserted (see Figure 36.14). To maintain positive-pressure ventilation, the tube is cuffed with an air-filled balloon just above the end of the tube. When the cuff is inflated it obstructs the upper airway, preventing air from escaping back

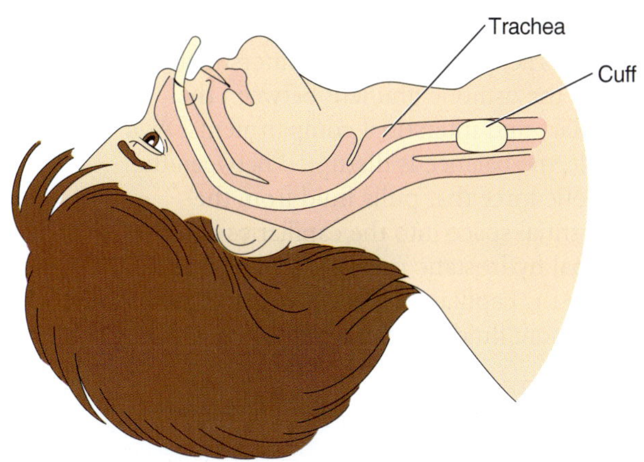

FIGURE 36.14 *Nasal endotracheal (nasotracheal) intubation*

Acute respiratory distress syndrome

Acute respiratory distress syndrome (ARDS) is a severe form of acute respiratory failure that occurs in response to pulmonary or systemic insults. ARDS is characterised by non-cardiogenic pulmonary oedema caused by inflammatory damage to alveolar and capillary walls. Many disorders such as COVID-19 may precipitate ARDS, although sepsis is the most common.

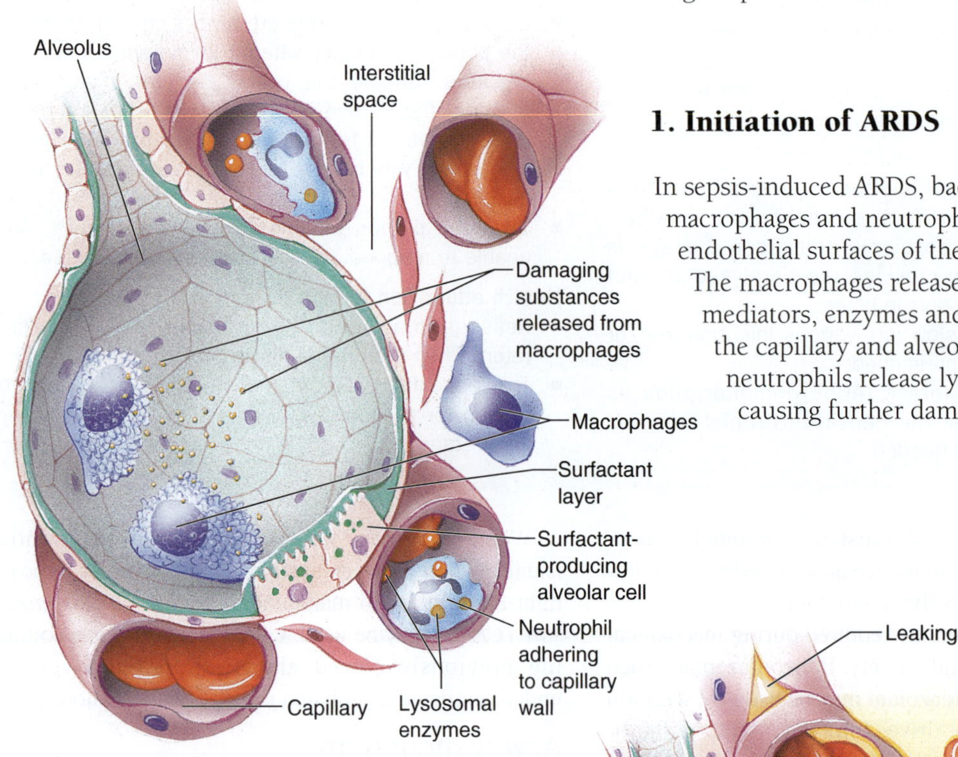

1. Initiation of ARDS

In sepsis-induced ARDS, bacterial toxins cause macrophages and neutrophils to adhere to endothelial surfaces of the alveoli and capillaries. The macrophages release oxidants, inflammatory mediators, enzymes and peptides that damage the capillary and alveolar walls. In response, neutrophils release lysosomal enzymes, causing further damage.

2. Onset of pulmonary oedema

The damaged capillary and alveolar walls become more permeable, allowing plasma, proteins and erythrocytes to enter the interstitial space. As interstitial oedema increases, pressure in the interstitial space rises and fluid leaks into alveoli. Plasma proteins accumulating in the interstitial space lower the osmotic gradient between the capillary and interstitial compartments. As a result, the balance is disrupted between the osmotic force that pulls fluid from the interstitial space into the capillaries and the normal hydrostatic pressure that pushes fluid out of the capillaries. This imbalance causes even more fluid to enter alveoli.

4. End-stage ARDS

Fibrin and cell debris from necrotic cells combine to form hyaline membranes, which line the interior of the alveoli and further reduce alveolar compliance and gas exchange. Because CO_2 cannot diffuse across hyaline membranes, $PaCO_2$ levels now begin to rise while PaO_2 levels continue to fall. Rising $PaCO_2$ levels can lead to respiratory acidosis. Without respiratory support, respiratory failure will develop. Even with aggressive treatment, almost 50% of people with ARDS die.

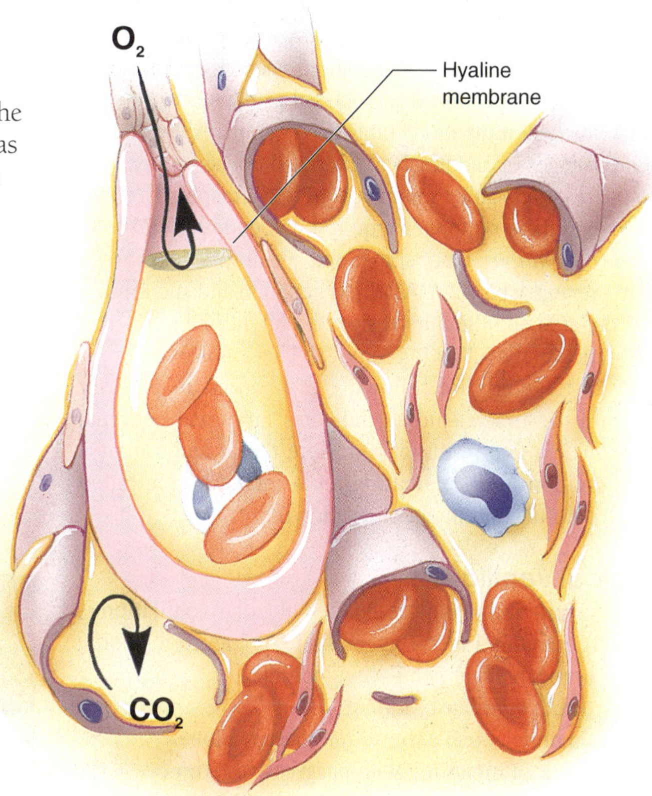

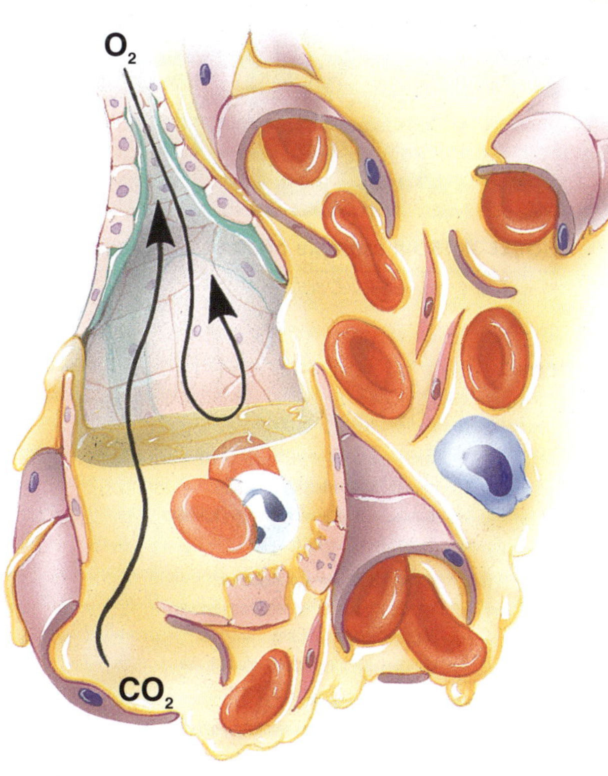

3. Alveolar collapse

Protein-rich fluid accumulates in the alveoli, inactivating surfactant and damaging type II alveolar cells that produce surfactant. (Surfactant is important in maintaining alveolar compliance—the ability of tissue to stretch or distend.) As active surfactant is lost, the alveoli stiffen and collapse, leading to atelectasis, which increases breathing effort.

Decreased alveolar compliance, atelectasis and fluid-filled alveoli interfere with gas exchange across the alveolar-capillary membrane. Blood oxygen (PaO_2) levels fall. Because CO_2 diffuses more readily than oxygen, however, blood carbon dioxide ($PaCO_2$) levels also fall initially as tachypnoea causes more CO_2 to be expired.

into the nose or mouth. Excess pressure from the cuff can cause tissue ischaemia and necrosis of the trachea. To minimise this risk, high-volume, low-pressure ('floppy') cuffs are used. Tubes with low-pressure cuffs may be left in place for 3–4 weeks.

A tracheostomy may be performed if long-term ventilatory support is required. Although a tracheostomy is more comfortable and easier to secure in place, complications such as cuff necrosis and increased risk of infection are associated with tracheostomy as well as endotracheal intubation. Table 36.6 compares the advantages, disadvantages of endotracheal tubes and tracheostomy.

When the person is able to maintain effective respirations and ventilatory support is no longer required, the endotracheal tube is removed (*extubation*). Gag, cough and swallow reflexes must be intact to prevent aspiration. After oxygenation and suctioning, the cuff is deflated and the tube removed. Humidified oxygen is provided immediately following removal. Close observation for respiratory distress is vital following extubation. Inspiratory stridor within the first 24 hours indicates laryngeal oedema, which may necessitate re-intubation. Sore throat and a hoarse voice are common after extubation. Oral intake is reinitiated slowly, with careful assessment of swallowing.

Mechanical ventilation

Mechanical ventilation is indicated when alveolar ventilation is inadequate to maintain blood oxygen and CO_2 levels. Specific indications for mechanical ventilation include:

- apnoea or acute ventilatory failure
- hypoxaemia unresponsive to oxygen therapy alone
- increased work of breathing with progressive fatigue.

One of the most common indicators for ventilatory support is respiratory muscle fatigue or its potential. Drug overdose, neural disorders, chest wall injury and airway problems such as severe asthma or COPD can lead to acute ventilatory failure. Disorders that affect alveolar–capillary diffusion, such as pulmonary contusion, pneumonia and ARDS, may necessitate mechanical ventilation to attain adequate oxygenation. Positive-pressure ventilation increases lung volume, helps redistribute fluid from the alveolar to the interstitial space and helps reduce the oxygen demand caused by increased work of breathing.

TYPES OF VENTILATORS Two broad general classifications of mechanical ventilators are available. Negative-pressure ventilators create negative (subatmospheric) pressure externally to draw the chest outwards and air into the lungs, mimicking spontaneous breathing. The iron lung and cuirass ventilator are examples of negative-pressure ventilators. Negative-pressure ventilators are rarely used nowadays.

Positive-pressure ventilators are used more often especially in treating acute respiratory failure (see Figure 36.15). These ventilators push air into the lungs, rather than drawing it in like negative-pressure ventilators. Either invasive ventilation using an endotracheal tube or tracheostomy or non-invasive positive-pressure ventilation may be used. Increasingly, non-invasive techniques, which use a nasal or face mask, nasal plugs or an oral mouthpiece, are being used with various levels of success (Byrd, 2018; Soo Hoo, 2020).

Non-invasive ventilation (NIV) provides ventilator support using a tight-fitting face mask, thus avoiding intubation. Its primary use is to support individuals with obstructive sleep apnoea, neuromuscular disease or impending respiratory failure (e.g. advanced COPD). NIV also may be used for individuals in

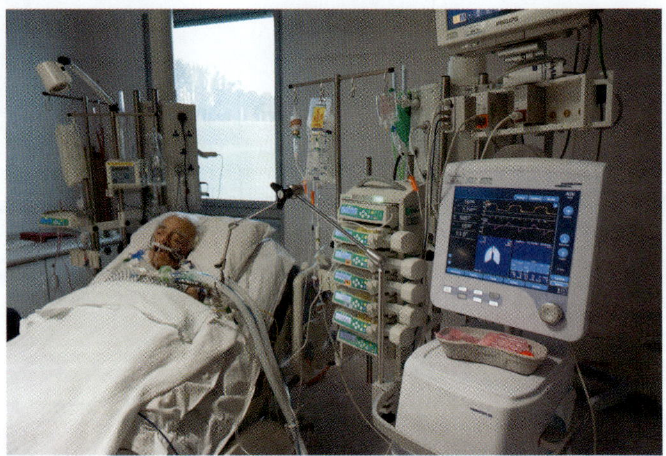

FIGURE 36.15 ***An example of a positive-pressure ventilator***

Source: Yon Marsh/Alamy Stock Photo.

TABLE 36.6 A comparison of endotracheal tubes and tracheostomy

	ADVANTAGES	DISADVANTAGES
Oral endotracheal tube	Easily inserted Larger-size tube can be used Easier to facilitate breathing and suctioning	Can be displaced or obstructed by biting or trismus Injury risk to lips, teeth, soft tissue Increased risk of lower respiratory infection Tracheo-oesophageal fistula
Nasal endotracheal tube	Well tolerated Easily secured and stabilised Facilitates patient communication	Risk of obstruction or displacement Smaller tube impeding secretion removal Pressure necrosis of nares Increased lower respiratory infection risk
Tracheostomy	Enables speech and oral hygiene Easily secured and stabilised Avoids upper airway complications	Requires surgical incision Increased risk of lower respiratory infection, site haemorrhage and infection Tracheal infarction and stenosis

respiratory failure who refuse intubation. The degree of success varies, primarily limited by the person's intolerance due to the physical and psychological discomfort of wearing a mask when dyspnoeic (Soo Hoo, 2020). NIV tends to be more successful in individuals without significant underlying lung disease (e.g. respiratory failure related to neuromuscular disease).

Several variables are used to trigger, cycle and limit airflow with positive-pressure ventilators. The *trigger* prompts the ventilator to deliver a breath. The individual's inspiratory effort triggers ventilator-assisted breaths. *Ventilator-controlled breaths* usually are triggered by a preset time interval (e.g. a breath is delivered every 5 seconds for a rate of 12 breaths per minute). The *ventilator cycle*, or duration of inspiration, can be limited by volume, pressure, flow or time. *Volume-cycled ventilators* deliver air until a preset volume is delivered. *Pressure-cycled ventilators* cycle off when a preset pressure is achieved within the airways. *Flow-cycled ventilators* are cycled by a preset inspiratory flow rate, and *time-cycled ventilators* deliver air for a set time interval. Airflow delivered by the ventilator also can be limited by factors such as airway pressure (e.g. a volume-cycled ventilator can be set to immediately stop inspiratory flow if airway pressure exceeds a preset value).

MODES OF VENTILATION A number of different *modes* or patterns of ventilation may be used with positive-pressure ventilators. The mode determines whether a breath is initiated by the person or the ventilator and the pattern of airway support provided by the ventilator. CPAP, bi-level airway pressure support, assist-control mode ventilation, synchronised intermittent mandatory ventilation, positive end-expiratory pressure, pressure support ventilation and pressure-control ventilation are common modes of ventilation in use today (see Table 36.7).

Continuous positive airway pressure applies positive pressure to the airways of a person who is spontaneously breathing. CPAP may be used with either endotracheal intubation or a tight-fitting face mask. All breathing is spontaneous (triggered by the person) and pressure controlled. CPAP is used to help maintain open airways and alveoli, decreasing the work of breathing. *Bi-level ventilators (BiPAP)* provide inspiratory positive airway pressure as well as airway support during expiration. Bi-level ventilation is primarily used at night with a tight-fitting mask (nasal, facial or oral). Three modes of ventilation can be used with BiPAP: spontaneous breathing (S); timed mode (T), in which pressure-supported breaths are delivered at a predetermined rate; and spontaneous/timed (S/T), in which the ventilator switches to timed mode if spontaneous breathing falls below a preset rate (Soo Hoo, 2020).

Assist-control mode ventilation (ACMV or AC) is frequently used to initiate mechanical ventilation and when the person is at risk of respiratory arrest (e.g. overdose or head injury). Assisted breaths are triggered by inspiratory effort; however, if the respiratory rate falls below a preset number (e.g. 14 per minute), ventilator-controlled breaths are delivered. All breaths, assisted and controlled, are delivered at a specific tidal volume or pressure and inspiratory flow rate.

Synchronised intermittent mandatory ventilation (SIMV) allows the person to breathe spontaneously, without ventilator assistance, between delivered ventilator breaths. Mandatory or ventilator-controlled breaths are delivered at a preset rate, volume and/or pressure, coordinated with the individual's inspiratory efforts. New evidence appearing suggests that respiratory muscles may not be able to rest between mandatory breaths and, therefore, this mode may result in fatigue which actually prolongs the need for ventilation (Byrd, 2018; Soo Hoo, 2020).

Positive end-expiratory pressure (PEEP) requires intubation and can be applied to any of the previously described ventilator modes. With PEEP, a positive pressure is maintained in the airways during exhalation and between breaths. Keeping alveoli open between breaths improves ventilation–perfusion relationships and diffusion across the alveolar–capillary membrane. This reduces hypoxaemia and allows use of lower percentages of inspired oxygen. PEEP is particularly useful for treating ARDS.

In *pressure support ventilation (PSV)*, ventilator-assisted breaths are delivered when the person initiates an inspiratory effort. The cycle is flow limited; inspiration is terminated when inspiratory airflow falls below a preset rate. This mode decreases the work of breathing. It can be used in combination with SIMV when the respiratory drive is depressed. Ventilator support can be gradually withdrawn during weaning.

Pressure-control ventilation (PCV), in contrast, controls pressure within the airways to reduce the risk of airway trauma (e.g. following thoracic surgery). Ventilation is time triggered and time cycled, but pressure is limited. The ventilator maintains a preset airway pressure throughout inspiration. Because all breaths are controlled by the ventilator, heavy sedation may be required to prevent competition between inspiratory effort and ventilator control.

Pressure-regulated volume control (PRVC) is a newer mode. It enables the desired tidal volume to be preset and permits the ventilator to deliver a pressure-limited (controlled) breath. Some benefits include automatic breath-to-breath adjusting according to the individual's lung compliance, resulting in the lowest peak inspiratory pressure needed to achieve a preset tidal volume.

VENTILATOR SETTINGS In addition to choosing the mode of ventilation, other parameters are set to meet individual's needs when positive-pressure ventilation is used (see Table 36.8).

For most adults, the rate is initially set between 12 and 15 breaths per minute. With ACMV or SIMV, the person's respiratory rate often is higher than the ventilator setting due to spontaneous breathing. Exhaled carbon dioxide ($ETCO_2$) or the $PaCO_2$ may be used to determine the rate. A $PaCO_2$ of less than 38 mmHg indicates hyperventilation and respiratory

TABLE 36.7 Modes of positive-pressure ventilator operation

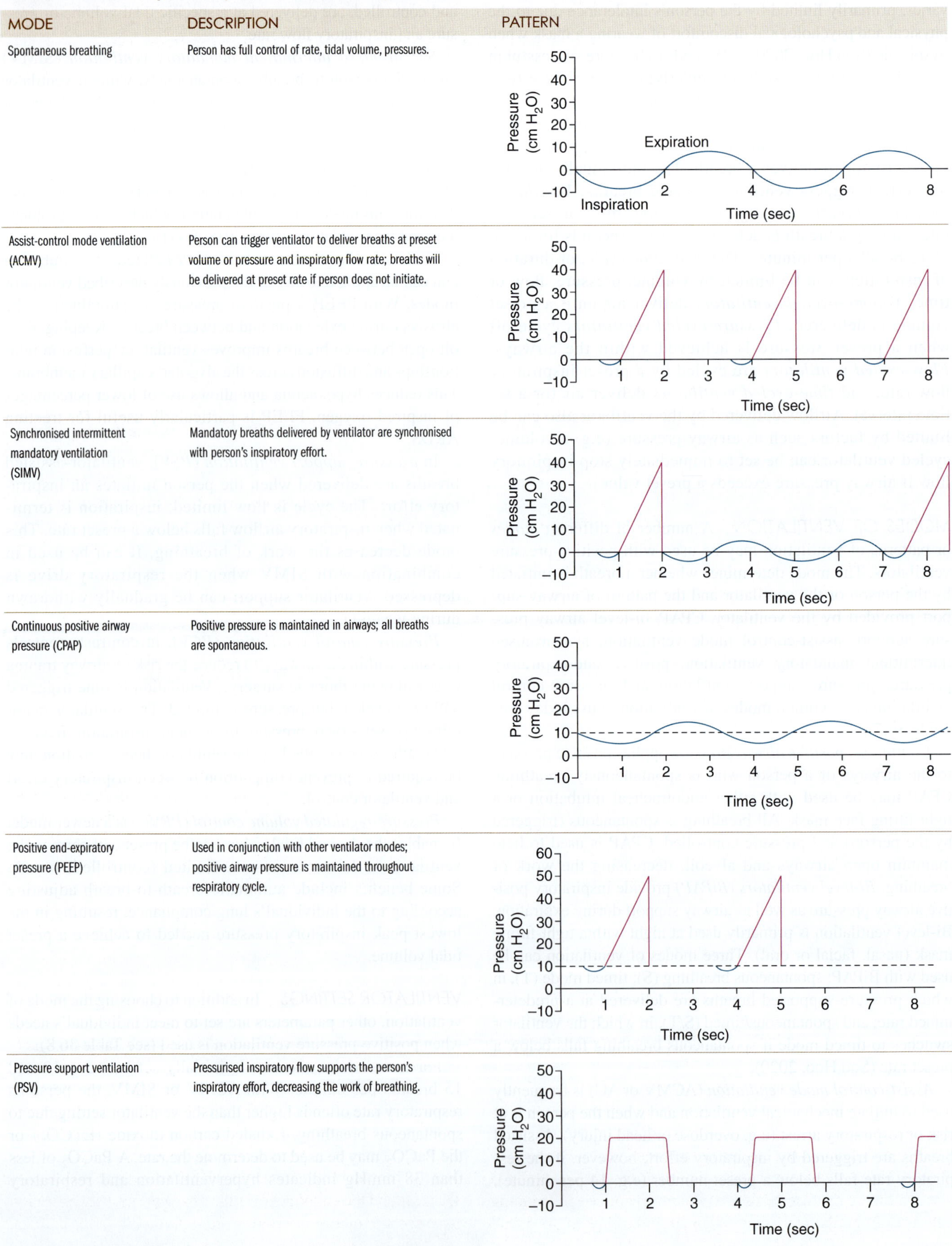

MODE	DESCRIPTION	PATTERN
Spontaneous breathing	Person has full control of rate, tidal volume, pressures.	
Assist-control mode ventilation (ACMV)	Person can trigger ventilator to deliver breaths at preset volume or pressure and inspiratory flow rate; breaths will be delivered at preset rate if person does not initiate.	
Synchronised intermittent mandatory ventilation (SIMV)	Mandatory breaths delivered by ventilator are synchronised with person's inspiratory effort.	
Continuous positive airway pressure (CPAP)	Positive pressure is maintained in airways; all breaths are spontaneous.	
Positive end-expiratory pressure (PEEP)	Used in conjunction with other ventilator modes; positive airway pressure is maintained throughout respiratory cycle.	
Pressure support ventilation (PSV)	Pressurised inspiratory flow supports the person's inspiratory effort, decreasing the work of breathing.	

TABLE 36.8 Ventilator settings

PARAMETER	DESCRIPTION
Rate (*f*)	Number of ventilator-delivered breaths per minute: usually 10-15 in adults using ACMV; may be lower in SIMV
Tidal volume (*VT*)	Amount of gas delivered with each ventilator breath: usually 8-10 mL/kg of body weight
Oxygen concentration (FiO_2)	Percentage of oxygen delivered with ventilator breaths; can be set between 21% (room air) and 100%
I:E ratio	Duration of inspiration to expiration: usually 1:2 to 1:1.5
Flow rate	Speed at which air is delivered
Sensitivity	Effort required to initiate a ventilator-assisted breath
Pressure limit	Maximal pressure within airways that will terminate a ventilator breath

alkalosis; the set rate is reduced. A $PaCO_2$ above 42 mmHg or an $ETCO_2$ greater than 45 mmHg indicates hypoventilation and a need to increase the rate.

The tidal volume setting controls the amount of gas delivered with each ventilator breath. Depending on various factors, an average normal adult tidal volume at rest may range between 5 and 10 mL/kg of body weight. The tidal volume delivered by mechanical ventilation is slightly higher to compensate for tubing dead space. Higher tidal volumes can cause lung tissue trauma.

The percentage of oxygen delivered with ventilator breaths is adjusted to maintain the SpO_2 and PaO_2 within acceptable ranges. Because prolonged delivery of high oxygen concentrations increases the risk of oxygen toxicity and pulmonary fibrosis, the FiO_2 is set at the lowest possible level for adequate tissue oxygenation. For most individuals, the goal is to maintain SpO_2 level of greater than 90%. Lower SpO_2 levels may be appropriate for individuals with longstanding COPD.

COMPLICATIONS Although endotracheal intubation and mechanical ventilation can be lifesaving in respiratory failure, they are not without risk. Improper endotracheal tube placement or advancement of the tube into a mainstem bronchus can result in ventilation of one lung only. The inflated lung becomes over-distended and traumatised and the uninflated lung develops atelectasis. In non-invasive ventilation, associated complications include gastric dilation, aspiration, facial skin necrosis, drying of the eyes and mucous membranes, stress and claustrophobia (Soo Hoo, 2020).

Healthcare-associated pneumonia Infection is a significant risk associated with intubation and mechanical ventilation. Normal upper respiratory tract defence mechanisms are bypassed, with loss of air humidification and trapping of pathogens. Oral secretions and gastric contents can enter the respiratory tree through the open epiglottis. Frequent, meticulous oral hygiene, upright positioning with the head of the bed elevated > 30 degrees, gastric ulcer prophylaxis, minimised ventilator time, removal of condensate from circuits and frequent and thorough hand hygiene from the healthcare professionals are vital interventions in reducing the risk of ventilator-associated pneumonia (Aitken, Marshall & Chaboyer, 2019). Often the cough reflex is inhibited or impaired by the underlying disease process and the continued presence of the endotracheal tube. Secretions often become thick and tenacious, increasing the risk of atelectasis.

Barotrauma *Barotrauma* (also called *volutrauma*) is lung injury due to alveolar over-distension. Both the volume of delivered gas and the pressures under which it is delivered can contribute to barotraumas. As a result, over-distended alveoli rupture, allowing air to escape into the pulmonary interstitial spaces and the mediastinum, pleural space and other tissues. Subcutaneous emphysema, pneumothorax and pneumomediastinum are possible results of barotrauma.

Subcutaneous emphysema, or air in the subcutaneous tissue, causes tissue swelling of the chest, neck and face. A 'crackling' or air-bubble-popping sensation is felt on palpation of subcutaneous emphysema. Swelling may be massive. Once the cause is corrected, the air is gradually reabsorbed.

Pneumothorax is identified by signs of unequal chest expansion, a sudden loss or significant decrease in breath sounds on the affected side and a hyperresonant percussion tone. Rapid chest tube insertion is necessary to prevent tension pneumothorax and cardiovascular compromise.

Pneumomediastinum is the presence of air in the mediastinum, the space between the lungs that contains the heart, great vessels, trachea and oesophagus. Air in the mediastinal space can interfere with the function of all of these organs and lead to such complications as pneumopericardium (air in the pericardial sac). Pneumomediastinum may have few manifestations, but the chest x-ray shows widening of the mediastinal space.

Cardiovascular effects Positive-pressure ventilation increases intrathoracic pressure, which can interfere with venous return to the heart and ventricular filling. As a result, cardiac output falls. Use of PEEP increases the effects of mechanical ventilation on cardiac output. The decreased cardiac output can affect liver and kidney function secondarily.

Gastrointestinal effects Gastrointestinal complications are commonly associated with prolonged mechanical ventilation. Stress ulcers (erosive gastritis) may develop, leading to painless gastrointestinal haemorrhage. Histamine H_2-receptor blockers are often used to prevent stress ulcers. Air leaks around the endotracheal tube can cause gastric distension; a nasogastric tube is inserted to prevent vomiting. Sedation and other medications used during mechanical ventilation can slow intestinal motility, leading to constipation.

WEANING The process of removing ventilator support and re-establishing spontaneous, independent respirations is called **weaning**. Weaning begins only after the underlying process causing respiratory failure has been corrected or stabilised. The process and time required for weaning depend on factors such as pre-existing lung condition, duration of mechanical ventilation and the person's general condition, both physical and psychological. In all cases, the vital signs, respiratory rate, extent of dyspnoea, blood gases and clinical status are used to evaluate weaning and its progress. More rapid weaning protocols are common in people with no underlying pulmonary condition who have only been ventilated for a short period of time. In this situation, care must be taken to avoid failed extubation (Aitken et al., 2019).

Following a brief period of mechanical ventilation, a T-piece or CPAP may be used for weaning. In T-piece weaning, the ventilator is removed for brief periods during which oxygen is delivered using a T-piece (see Figure 36.16). The duration of periods off the ventilator is gradually increased until the person can maintain adequate independent respirations for several hours. Vital signs, SpO_2, $ETCO_2$ and PaO_2 are carefully monitored during the process. The person is placed back on the ventilator at previous settings if signs of respiratory distress develop. When mechanical ventilation is no longer needed, the endotracheal tube is removed. CPAP weaning follows a similar process, with trials of spontaneous breathing supported by the ventilator in CPAP mode.

SIMV and PSV are used for weaning when the duration of mechanical ventilation has been longer and reconditioning of respiratory muscles is needed. When SIMV is used, the number of mandatory ventilator-assisted breaths is gradually decreased as ABGs, $ETCO_2$ and the respiratory rate are monitored.

Weaning is the primary use for pressure-support ventilation. Initially, PSV is set slightly below the peak inspiratory pressures required during volume-cycled ventilation. Pressure support levels are gradually decreased, often in a cyclical pattern of periods of minimal support alternating with higher support to recondition respiratory muscles. Various weaning protocols exist; however, some parameters used identify an individual's readiness for extubation including a respiratory rate of less than 25 breaths per minute, a tidal volume of greater than 5 mL/kg and a PaO_2 of greater than 80 mmHg (Byrd, 2018; Soo Hoo, 2020).

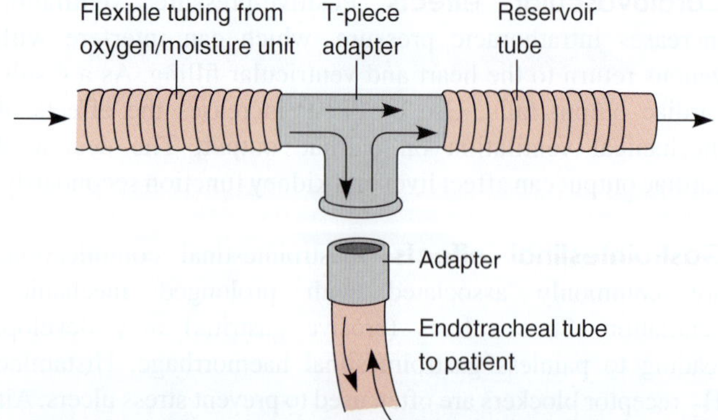

FIGURE 36.16 ***A T-piece for weaning from mechanical ventilation***

Terminal weaning When an illness is terminal or irreversible with a poor prognosis, terminal weaning may be requested by the person or their family. *Terminal weaning* is the gradual withdrawal of mechanical ventilation when survival without assisted ventilation is not expected. Unlike weaning when recovery is expected, which usually occurs in a critical care unit, the person is moved to a quiet critical care or hospice room or even home prior to initiating terminal weaning. Family members are encouraged to remain with the person throughout the process. If possible, decisions about sedation and analgesia prior to and during weaning are made with the person, as are decisions about hydration and nutritional support following weaning. Ventilator support is gradually withdrawn using the same modes described earlier (SIMV, PSV). Analgesia and sedation are given to promote comfort during weaning.

Nutrition and fluids Attention also must be paid to fluid and electrolyte status and adequate nutrition. Mechanical ventilation promotes sodium and water retention due to its effects on cardiac output. Renal perfusion is decreased, stimulating the renin–angiotensin–aldosterone system to retain sodium and water. A Swan–Ganz catheter is often inserted to monitor pulmonary artery pressures and cardiac output. An arterial line allows repeated blood gas analysis and continuous arterial pressure monitoring. Serum electrolytes are drawn frequently and intake, output and daily weight are carefully monitored.

Enteral or parenteral nutrition are provided during mechanical ventilation because the endotracheal tube prohibits eating. A nasogastric, gastrostomy or jejunostomy feeding tube is placed for enteral nutrition. A jejunostomy tube may be used to reduce the risk of regurgitation and aspiration.

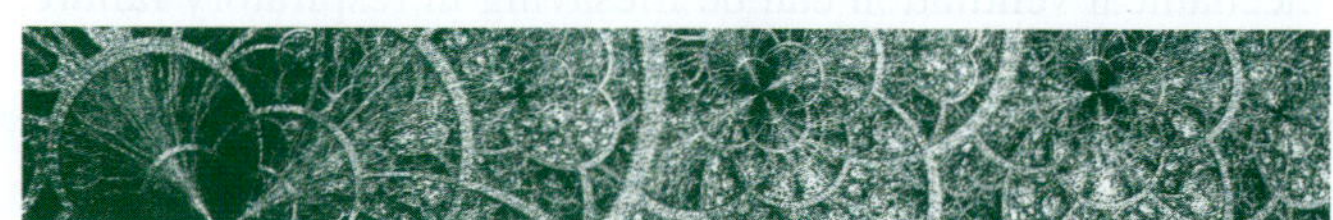

Nursing care

Health promotion

Education is a primary strategy to prevent respiratory failure. Teach all individuals and the public about the risks of smoking, water safety, the value of a working smoke detector and measures to prevent smoke inhalation in a fire. Discuss the importance of immunisations (pneumococcal, annual influenza, COVID-19) for people who are at high risk, including those over age 65 and people with chronic diseases. Teach individuals with spinal cord injury or neuromuscular disease to use effective breathing and coughing techniques to maintain airway patency. Work with individuals addicted to narcotic drugs to attain and maintain drug-free status. Teach individuals with COPD about measures to reduce their risk of respiratory infection and symptoms to report to the doctor.

Assessment

Focused assessment data related to respiratory failure include the following:

- *Health history*: current manifestations, their duration and identified precipitating factors (may need to be obtained from family members if mental status is affected); history of previous episodes; chronic diseases such as COPD, occupational lung disease; current medications.
- *Physical examination*: LOC, mental status; vital signs; colour and SpO_2; respiratory assessment, including rate and depth, use of accessory muscles, respiratory excursion, auscultation; cardiovascular assessment, including heart rate and sounds, neck vein distension, peripheral pulses, evidence of clubbing.
- *Diagnostic tests*: ABGs, chest x-ray, pulmonary artery pressure and wedge pressure readings, cardiac output.

Nursing diagnoses and interventions

Individuals in respiratory failure are often unstable and critically ill. They require both intensive medical care and intensive nursing care. Priority nursing needs relate to maintaining ventilation and a patent airway. Perhaps less obvious, but no less critical, nursing care needs to relate to preventing injury and managing anxiety.

Impaired spontaneous ventilation

In acute respiratory failure, fatigue from the work of breathing may impair the ability to maintain adequate ventilation. This is a concern both prior to initiation of mechanical ventilation and during the weaning process.

- Assess and document respiratory rate, vital signs and SpO_2 every 15–30 minutes. *Close monitoring is vital to detect early signs of increasing respiratory distress and inability to sustain adequate breathing.*

> **CONSIDERATION FOR PRACTICE**
>
> **Promptly report signs of respiratory distress, including tachypnoea, tachycardia, nasal flaring, use of accessory muscles, intercostal retractions, cyanosis, increasing restlessness, anxiety or decreased LOC. These may be early manifestations of respiratory failure and inability to maintain ventilatory effort.**

- Promptly report worsening ABGs and SpO_2 levels. *Close assessment of these values allows timely intervention as needed.*
- Administer oxygen as ordered, monitoring response. Observe closely for respiratory depression, especially in the person with COPD. *Oxygen administration reduces the hypoxic respiratory drive. Chronically high $PaCO_2$ levels depress the respiratory centre; hypoxaemia may provide the only respiratory drive.*
- Place in Fowler's or high-Fowler's position. *Sitting positions decrease pressure on the diaphragm and chest, improving lung ventilation and decreasing the work of breathing.*
- Minimise activities and energy expenditures by assisting with ADLs, spacing procedures and activities, and by allowing uninterrupted rest periods. *Rest is vital to reduce oxygen and energy demands.*

> **CONSIDERATION FOR PRACTICE**
>
> **Avoid sedatives and respiratory depressant drugs. These medications can further depress the respiratory drive, worsening respiratory failure.**

- Prepare for endotracheal intubation and mechanical ventilation:
  a. Obtain an intubation tray with a selection of sterile endotracheal tubes and laryngoscope with a variety of adult blades.
  b. Check laryngoscope bulb; replace battery or bulb as needed.
  c. Set up for endotracheal suction, bringing suction equipment and gloves to the bedside.
  d. Set up the ventilator.
  e. Notify radiology that a portable chest x-ray will be needed on completion of intubation to verify correct placement of the endotracheal tube.

  Intubation and mechanical ventilation may be required to maintain ventilation and gas exchange.
- Explain the procedure and its purpose to the person and their family, providing reassurance that this is a temporary measure to reduce the work of breathing and allow rest. Inform the person and their significant others that talking is not possible while the endotracheal tube is in place and establish a means of communication. *Thorough explanation is important to relieve anxiety.*

Ineffective airway clearance

Ineffective airway clearance may either cause respiratory failure or occur as a result of interventions. Impaired ventilation frequently leads to acute respiratory failure, particularly in a person with COPD or asthma. Chest trauma also can impair airway patency as a result of pulmonary contusion and ineffective cough. Although intubation and mechanical ventilation can be lifesaving measures, they also increase the risk of respiratory infection and ineffective secretion management.

- Suction as needed to maintain a patent airway. Indicators for suctioning include crackles and rhonchi on auscultation, frequent coughing or setting off of the high-pressure alarm, and increasing restlessness or anxiety. Procedure 36.1 outlines endotracheal suctioning. *Although individuals with a tracheostomy can usually cough up secretions, the length and diameter of endotracheal tubes make this extremely difficult. Even with humidification, secretions often become thick and tenacious, further inhibiting their removal.*

> **CONSIDERATION FOR PRACTICE**
>
> **Frequently assess respiratory rate, chest movement, lung sounds, SpO_2, $ETCO_2$ and ABGs. Intubation and mechanical ventilation do not ensure adequate oxygenation and ventilation. Displacement of the endotracheal tube or obstruction by respiratory secretions impairs ventilation.**

PROCEDURE 36.1 Endotracheal suctioning

GATHER SUPPLIES

- Suction unit with connecting tubing and connector at the bedside
- If an in-line suction catheter is not present:
  a. sterile suction catheter (a simple formula for sizing) is: if ETT < 6 mm (Fr $=$ ETT size (mm) $\times 2$) if ETT ≥ 6 mm (Fr $=$ ETT size (mm) $- 2 \times 2$)
  b. a solution (e.g. water) to clean suction tubing following intervention
- Personal protective devices as indicated: goggles, mask, gown

BEFORE THE PROCEDURE

Explain the procedure and why it is being done. Tell the person that although suctioning is not painful, it is uncomfortable. While suction is being applied, breathing is difficult but these periods last only 10 seconds. Stress that suctioning allows removal of secretions, stimulates coughing and helps clear secretions. Establish a means of communicating; for example, tell the person to raise a finger or rapidly blink if unable to tolerate suctioning.

DURING THE PROCEDURE

1 Use standard precautions.

2 Prepare the suction unit by turning it on and regulating it to no more than −80 to −120 mmHg.

3 Open sterile saline bottle and pour approximately 50 mL of saline into the opened sterile container.

With an in-line catheter

- Wearing exam gloves, attach the catheter to the suction tubing.
- Adjust the oxygen (FiO_2) to 100%; allow three breaths.
- Manipulating the catheter through the plastic shield (to maintain its sterility), insert the catheter without applying suction until resistance is met; apply suction while slowly withdrawing the catheter with a twirling motion.
- Suction for no longer than 10 seconds (count the seconds or watch the clock—the time passes more quickly than you think. Holding your own breath during this time also gives you an indication of how quickly the technique needs to be completed), then allow to rest for three to five breaths. Repeat the procedure as needed for a total of no more than three times.
- Remove suction tubing from the catheter, clear the tubing, turn off suction and remove and discard gloves.

As an open suction technique

- Open suction catheter. Ensure that there is water to clean the catheter between attempts.
- With a non-touch technique, attach catheter to suction tubing, keeping dominant hand clean; remove the outside package with the non-dominant hand and take the sterile catheter with the dominant hand.
- Use the non-dominant hand to adjust oxygen (FIO_2) to 100%; allow three breaths.
- Using the non-dominant hand, disconnect ventilator tubing from the endotracheal tube. Manipulating the suction catheter with the dominant hand and the suction control valve with the non-dominant hand, insert the catheter, without applying suction, until resistance is met. Then, apply suction intermittently while slowly withdrawing the catheter, using a twirling motion.
- Suction for no longer than 10 seconds. Reconnect the ventilator and allow the person to rest for three to five breaths; clear suction tubing as per protocol.
- Repeat the preceding two steps as needed for a total of three times.
- Reconnect ventilator tubing to the endotracheal tube.
- Clear suction tubing, turn off suction and remove the catheter, discarding it with the gloves.

4 Provide three additional breaths at 100% oxygen and then readjust to the previous ordered level.

5 Note colour, quantity, consistency and odour of sputum.

6 Assess lung sounds and tolerance of the procedure.

7 Wash hands.

AFTER THE PROCEDURE

Document results of suctioning procedure, along with the character of the sputum and the person's tolerance of the procedure. Report changes in sputum character, such as purulence or an odour that may indicate infection.

- Obtain sputum for culture if it appears purulent or is odorous. *Culture is necessary to identify pathogens and guide antibiotic therapy.*
- Perform percussion, vibration and postural drainage as required. *These techniques help loosen secretions and move them into larger airways for removal by coughing or suctioning.*

CONSIDERATION FOR PRACTICE

Evaluate endotracheal tube cuff pressure by measurement (no more than 20–25 mmHg of pressure). The minimum effective cuff pressure to maintain alveolar ventilation is used to reduce the risk of tracheal ischaemia and necrosis.

- Firmly secure endotracheal or tracheostomy tube. Provide adequate slack on ventilator tubing to prevent tension on the tube when turning, positioning or transferring to chair or stretcher. *These measures are important to ensure proper airway placement and prevent its inadvertent removal.*
- Assess fluid balance and maintain adequate hydration. *Adequate hydration helps liquefy secretions.*

Risk of injury

Many factors increase the risk of injury in acute respiratory failure. Hypoxaemia and hypercapnia affect the level of consciousness and may impair mental status. Endotracheal intubation and mechanical ventilation carry risks of tracheal damage and trauma to the lungs. Neuromuscular blockade, if used, presents a significant risk of injury as the person is unable to breathe spontaneously, communicate and move.

- Assess frequently, noting the following:
  a. LOC, orientation and awareness
  b. condition of mucosa of mouth and nose
  c. respiratory: lung sounds, chest excursion and ventilator pressures
  d. cardiovascular: vital signs, skin colour, capillary refill and peripheral pulses
  e. gastrointestinal: bowel sounds; test gastric secretions and faeces for occult blood
  f. genitourinary: urine output, daily weight
  g. skin and extremities.

  Complications associated with respiratory failure and mechanical ventilation can affect many body systems. Frequent assessment allows early detection and intervention.
- Report condition changes such as increasing air leak around the cuff and decreased breath sounds or chest movement. *These may be manifestations of a complication of intubation and ventilation, such as tracheal necrosis, displacement of the endotracheal tube into the right mainstem bronchus, pneumothorax or atelectasis.*

CONSIDERATION FOR PRACTICE

Do not bypass or turn off any ventilator alarms. A person who is intubated is unable to communicate verbally and cannot call for help. If neuromuscular blockers are used, the person is also unable to breathe without ventilator support.

- Turn and reposition frequently, taking care to stabilise endotracheal tube during movement. *Repositioning helps maintain tissue perfusion and prevent skin and tissue breakdown.*
- Keep skin and bed linen clean, dry and wrinkle-free. Protect pressure areas with padding, egg crate or heel and elbow protectors. *The person may not be able to perceive and report pain and move voluntarily to reduce pressure, necessitating excellent skin care.*
- Perform passive range-of-motion exercises every 4–8 hours. *These exercises maintain joint flexibility and help prevent contractures associated with long-term immobility.*
- Keep side rails up and use soft restraints as needed. *These safety measures are important to prevent falls, inadvertent disconnection of the ventilator or dislodging of the endotracheal tube.*
- Administer histamine H_2-blockers as ordered. *Stress gastritis and possible gastrointestinal haemorrhage are common, preventable complications of mechanical ventilation.*

Anxiety

Critical illness creates anxiety for any person. In acute respiratory failure, this anxiety is compounded by the presence of an endotracheal tube or tracheostomy, mechanical ventilator, numerous monitors and equipment, and, potentially, neuromuscular blockade and paralysis of voluntary muscles. Fear of continued dependence on the mechanical ventilator and inability to return to a normal life may compound this anxiety.

CONSIDERATION FOR PRACTICE

Frequently monitor anxiety level. High levels of anxiety increase oxygen use and often interfere with the ability to work with the respirator. This can increase hypoxaemia and further increase anxiety; intervention is necessary to break this cycle.

See the 'Translation to practice' box for information about assessing and managing anxiety in individuals who are intubated.

- Remain with the person as much as possible. *The frequent and continuing presence of a caregiver provides reassurance that help is readily available.*
- Explain all monitors, procedures, unusual sounds and machinery. *Understanding of the environment and various sounds and alarms reduces anxiety.*
- Provide a simple means of communication, such as a slate, picture board or alphabet board. Reassure that endotracheal tube removal restores the ability to speak. *The inability to speak and call out for help is frightening for the person. Providing an alternate means of communication helps reduce anxiety.*
- Encourage frequent family visits, especially if the time of visitations is being limited. Encourage family participation in care. *Family visits help reduce anxiety and feelings of abandonment. Allowing family members to participate in care helps reduce their anxiety as well.*
- Explain to the family that the person can hear and understand. Emphasise the importance of talking to the person, not over or about the person. *The family may not understand that the person may be mentally alert although unable to respond. Talking to the person about everyday things reduces the person's sense of isolation and fear.*
- Provide distraction with radio or television if available. *Distraction helps reduce the focus on machines and unusual sounds of monitors and alarms.*
- Attend to physical needs promptly and completely. *This provides reassurance that needs will be met even though the person is unable to ask for assistance.*
- Reassure that intubation and mechanical ventilation are temporary measures to allow the lungs to rest and heal. Reinforce that the person will be able to breathe independently again. *The person may fear continued dependence on mechanical ventilation.*

CONSIDERATION FOR PRACTICE

Provide sedation and anxiolytic medications as needed, especially when neuromuscular blockade is used. Although neuromuscular blockade paralyses voluntary muscles, the level of consciousness is unimpaired.

TRANSLATION TO PRACTICE Evidence-based practice for the person who is intubated

Individuals who are intubated cannot communicate verbally. A number of worldwide studies of critically ill people who were intubated have identified that while effective patient and staff communication has contributed to patients having positive memories, communication difficulties and psychoemotional distress (involving fear and anger) were noted. These difficulties were a positive predictor for psychological distress, with a significant percentage of patients displaying emotional and behavioural problems, including symptoms consistent with post-traumatic stress disorder. It was found that a multidisciplinary approach supporting alternative communication methods, including use of technology, pictures and non-verbal gestures, has been used to further enhance patient communication (Freeman-Sanderson, Morris & Elkins, 2019; Khalaila et al., 2011; Schwartzstein & Campbell, 2022).

IMPLICATIONS FOR NURSING

People who are intubated and receiving mechanical ventilation are critically ill. Stress can contribute to physical deterioration; therefore, identifying and attempting to remove stressors can have a positive effect on a person's recovery. Research in this area reinforces the need to ensure that methods to reduce frustration and fear related to communication difficulties from endotracheal intubation should continue.

CRITICAL THINKING IN PERSON-CENTRED CARE

1 Why is a person who is mechanically ventilated unable to communicate verbally?
2 What tools are available to assist the nurse in facilitating improved communication skills with people who are unable to communicate verbally?
3 Is there any way that a person who is undergoing neuromuscular blockade and mechanical ventilation can communicate with the nurse? Which factors need to be considered in this circumstance?
4 How can a nurse be sure that the information the person is trying to express is the same information that is being received by the nurse?

Community-based care

Prior to hospital discharge, teach the person and their family about the following topics:

- factors that precipitated respiratory failure and measures to prevent it in the future (e.g. the impact of respiratory irritants on compromised lungs)
- measures to prevent future episodes, such as remaining indoors with an air filter or air conditioning when pollution levels are high, obtaining influenza and pneumonia immunisations, and avoiding exposure to cigarette smoke
- effective coughing and pulmonary hygiene measures such as percussion, vibration and postural drainage.

Acute respiratory failure resulting from an acute insult such as pneumonia or near-drowning often resolves with few long-term sequelae. When respiratory failure results from an underlying disease such as COPD, the prognosis is less optimistic. Individuals with end-stage COPD may have repeated episodes of respiratory failure, with a gradual loss of respiratory function and reserve. These individuals may choose terminal weaning rather than a future of increasing disability. Discuss what to expect during the terminal weaning process with the person and their family. Discuss use of sedation prior to and during the weaning process. Explain that medications are used to reduce respiratory distress and dyspnoea during weaning. Assure the person and family that nursing support is continuously available during the weaning process and that family and other supporters such as clergy are allowed to remain with the person.

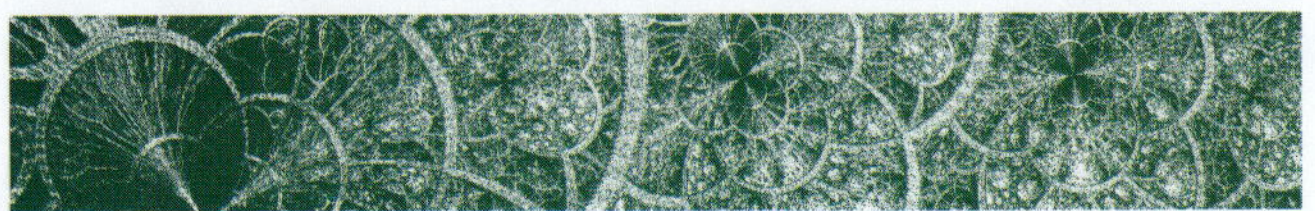

THE PERSON WITH ACUTE RESPIRATORY DISTRESS SYNDROME

Acute respiratory distress syndrome (ARDS) is characterised by non-cardiac pulmonary oedema and progressive refractory hypoxaemia. First identified in 1967, ARDS has been known by various names, such as shock lung and adult hyaline membrane disease. It is widely recognised as a severe form of acute respiratory failure.

Although the exact cause of ARDS is unclear, it is known that ARDS does not occur as a primary process but may follow a number of diverse conditions producing direct or indirect lung injury (see Table 36.9). Individuals who develop ARDS as a complication of an acute lung injury or condition are more likely to fully recover than individuals with chronic conditions.

Pathophysiology

The underlying pathology in ARDS is acute lung injury resulting from an unregulated systemic inflammatory response to acute injury or inflammation. Inflammatory cellular responses and biochemical mediators damage the alveolar–capillary membrane.

TABLE 36.9 Conditions associated with the development of ARDS

CONDITIONS	EXAMPLES
Shock	Haemorrhagic shock, septic shock
Inhalation injuries	Aspiration of gastric contents, smoke and toxic gases, immersion/submersion, oxygen toxicity
Infections	Gram-negative sepsis, viral pneumonias, *Pneumocystis carinii* pneumonia
Drug overdose	Heroin, methadone, aspirin
Trauma	Burns, head injury, lung contusion, fat emboli
Other	COVID-19, disseminated intravascular coagulation, pancreatitis, uraemia, amniotic fluid and air emboli, multiple transfusions, open heart surgery with cardiopulmonary bypass

This damage develops rapidly, often within 90 minutes of the systemic inflammatory response and within 24 hours of the initial insult. Damaged capillary membranes allow plasma and blood cells to escape into the interstitial space. Increased interstitial pressure and damage to the alveolar membrane allow fluid to enter the alveoli. Within the alveolus, the fluid dilutes and inactivates surfactant. Surfactant-producing cells are damaged by the inflammatory process, leading to a deficit of surfactant, increased alveolar surface tension and alveolar collapse with atelectasis. The lungs become less compliant and gas exchange is impaired. As the syndrome progresses, hyaline membranes form, further reducing gas exchange and compliance. Finally, fibrotic changes occur in the lungs. Intra-alveolar septa thicken and alveolar surface area for gas exchange is reduced. Hypoxaemia becomes refractory or resistant to improvement with supplemental oxygen and the $PaCO_2$ rises as diffusion is further impaired. Figure 36.17 illustrates the pathogenesis of ARDS.

As ARDS progresses, tissue hypoxia becomes significant and metabolic acidosis develops. Carbon dioxide exchange is impaired as well as oxygen exchange, leading to combined respiratory and metabolic acidosis. Sepsis and multiple-organ-system dysfunction of the kidneys, liver, gastrointestinal tract, CNS and cardiovascular system are the leading causes of death in ARDS. If the process is halted before this occurs, the long-term prognosis for recovery is good.

Manifestations

Initial manifestations of ARDS typically develop within hours or up to 7 days after the initial insult. Dyspnoea, tachypnoea and anxiety are early manifestations. Progressive respiratory distress develops, with increasing respiratory rate, intercostal retractions and use of accessory muscles of respiration, and low SpO_2 despite being delivered 100% oxygen. Cyanosis develops that may not improve with oxygen administration. Breath sounds are initially clear, but crackles (rales) and rhonchi develop later. As respiratory failure progresses, mental status changes such as agitation, confusion and lethargy occur (Diamond et al., 2022).

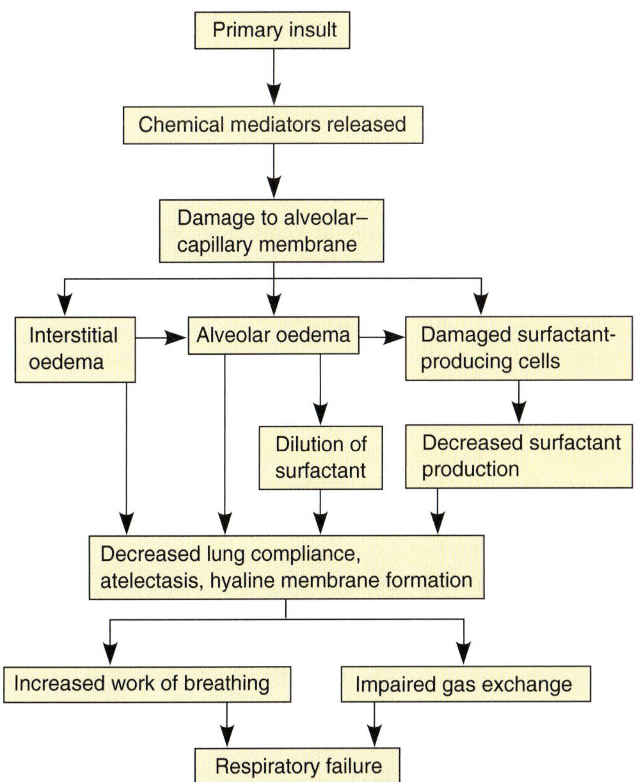

FIGURE 36.17 *The pathogenesis of ARDS*

INTERPROFESSIONAL CARE

ARDS management is directed towards identifying and treating its underlying cause and providing aggressive respiratory support and supportive care.

- *ABGs* initially show hypoxaemia with a PaO_2 of less than 60 mmHg and respiratory alkalosis due to tachypnoea.
- *Chest x-ray* changes may not be evident for as long as 24 hours after the onset of ARDS. Diffuse infiltrates are seen initially, progressing to a 'white out' pattern. Chest CT scan provides a better illustration of the pattern of alveolar consolidation and atelectasis in ARDS.
- *Pulmonary function testing* shows decreased lung compliance with reduced vital capacity, minute volume and functional vital capacity (see Box 33.1).
- *Pulmonary artery pressure monitoring* shows normal pressures in ARDS, helping distinguish ARDS from cardiogenic pulmonary oedema.
- Increase oxygen delivery, decrease oxygen consumption and avoid further injury (Diamond et al., 2022).

Medications

Although there is no definitive drug therapy for ARDS, a number of medications may be used. Inhaled nitric oxide reduces intrapulmonary shunting and improves oxygenation by dilating blood vessels in better ventilated areas of the lungs. Surfactant therapy may be prescribed. Surfactant is a complex mixture of phospholipids, neutral lipids and proteins that forms a thin layer atop a thin layer of water on the inner surface of the alveolus, reducing the surface tension within the alveoli. Surface tension tends to pull the walls of the alveoli together, increasing the likelihood of collapse during exhalation. Surfactant, by reducing surface tension, helps maintain open alveoli, decreasing the work of breathing, improving compliance and gas exchange, and preventing atelectasis.

Diagnosis

Refractory hypoxaemia (hypoxaemia that does not improve with oxygen administration) is the hallmark of ARDS.

Interventions to block the inflammatory response are under investigation, such as using non-steroidal anti-inflammatory agents and corticosteroids. Corticosteroids may be used late in the course of ARDS to improve oxygenation and lung mechanics when fibrotic changes occur.

Mechanical ventilation

The mainstay of ARDS management is endotracheal intubation and mechanical ventilation. With ARDS, it is rarely possible to maintain adequate tissue oxygenation with oxygen therapy alone.

With mechanical ventilation, the FiO_2 is set at the lowest possible level to maintain a PaO_2 higher than 60 mmHg and SpO_2 of approximately 90%. When the PaO_2 cannot be maintained with less than 50% inspired oxygen, there is a risk that oxygen toxicity will accentuate ARDS. Often it is necessary to add CPAP, BiPAP or PEEP to mechanical ventilation settings to maintain blood and tissue oxygenation. Maintaining open airways and alveoli enhances gas diffusion and reduces ventilation–perfusion mismatch. PEEP decreases cardiac output and increases the risk of barotrauma, necessitating close monitoring. Either assist-control or SIMV may be used along with PEEP or CPAP in treating ARDS.

It is important to remember that mechanical ventilation does not cure ARDS; it simply supports respiratory function while the underlying problem is being identified and treated.

Treatments

Atelectasis frequently occurs in dependent lung regions in ARDS. Prone positioning in conjunction with mechanical ventilation reduces the pressure of surrounding tissue on dependent regions and improves oxygenation (Johnson et al., 2022).

Other management strategies include careful fluid replacement, attention to nutrition, treatment of any infection and correction of the underlying condition. A Swan–Ganz line may be placed to monitor pulmonary artery pressures and cardiac output. Fluid replacement is carefully tailored to these measurements to avoid fluid imbalances, which may worsen hypoxia and ARDS. Enteral or parenteral feeding is necessary to maintain nutritional status and prevent tissue catabolism. Infections are treated with intravenous antibiotic therapy tailored to the causative organism. Low-molecular-weight heparin may be ordered to prevent thrombophlebitis and possible pulmonary embolus or disseminated intravascular coagulation, a possible complication of ARDS.

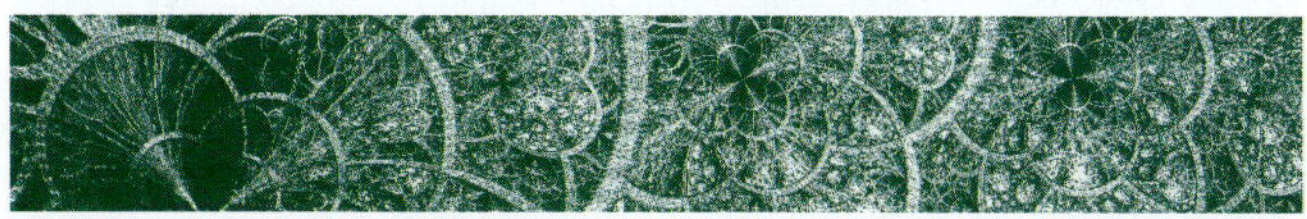

Nursing care

The nursing care needs of the person with ARDS are very similar to those of any individual with acute respiratory failure. Maintaining adequate ventilation and respirations is of highest priority, along with preventing injury and managing anxiety. See the section on acute respiratory failure for nursing care related to these diagnoses. Additional high-priority nursing care concerns for the person with ARDS are related to the effects of PEEP on cardiac output and potential problems of weaning ventilatory support. See the accompanying nursing care plan for additional nursing interventions for the person with ARDS.

Nursing diagnoses and interventions

Decreased cardiac output

With positive-pressure ventilation, increased intrathoracic pressure decreases cardiac output. When PEEP is applied, intrathoracic pressure increases further; this can significantly decrease venous return, ventricular filling, stroke volume and cardiac output. Manifestations of decreased cardiac output include hypotension and compensatory tachycardia as the heart attempts to maintain cardiac output despite decreased stroke volume. In the person who is already hypoxic because of ARDS, this drop in cardiac output can increase tissue damage. Urine output falls and arrhythmias may develop.

- Monitor and record vital signs, including apical pulse, at least every hour; more frequently immediately following initiation of mechanical ventilation or the addition of PEEP. *Frequent assessment is vital to detect early signs of decreased cardiac output.*
- Assess level of consciousness at least every 4 hours. *Altered LOC, confusion and restlessness are early signs of cerebral hypoxia due to decreased cardiac output.*
- Monitor pulmonary artery pressures, central venous pressure and cardiac output readings every 1 to 4 hours. *Changes in these measurements may indicate worsening cardiac status.*
- Assess heart and lung sounds frequently. *Increasing crackles or abnormal heart sounds may indicate heart failure.*
- Weigh daily at the same time. *Accurate daily weights are the best indicator of fluid volume status.*
- Frequently provide good skin care, keeping skin clean and dry and protecting pressure points. *Tissue hypoxia increases the risk of skin breakdown, which in turn increases the risk of infection and sepsis.*
- Maintain intravenous fluids as ordered. *Intravenous fluids are given to maintain vascular volume and prevent dehydration.*
- Administer analgesics, sedatives and neuromuscular blockers as needed. *These medications may be prescribed to decrease cardiac workload.*

Dysfunctional ventilatory weaning response

The person with dysfunctional ventilatory weaning response has difficulty adjusting to reduced mechanical ventilator support, prolonging the weaning process. Airway congestion, inadequate rest or nutrition, pain, anxiety and a non-supportive environment are factors that can contribute to difficulty weaning. With ARDS, the pathological processes of the disease and its effects on gas exchange may be responsible for a prolonged or ineffective weaning process.

Assessment findings indicative of dysfunctional weaning include:

- dyspnoea, apprehension or agitation
- decreasing SpO_2 level
- cyanosis or pallor, diaphoresis
- increased blood pressure, pulse and respiratory rate
- diminished or adventitious breath sounds, use of accessory muscles
- decreased LOC
- deteriorating ABG values
- shallow, gasping breaths or paradoxical abdominal breathing.

NURSING CARE PLAN A person with ARDS

Peggy Adamson is a 36-year-old (75 kg) admitted to the hospital following an immersion/submersion at the local lake. On admission to the emergency department, she is alert and oriented, having been rescued and resuscitated within 2 minutes of the accident. Rescuers report that she seemed to have aspirated 'a lot' of water as she was water-skiing when the accident occurred. She is admitted to the critical care unit for observation. Oxygen is started per nasal prongs at 6 L/min, intravenous fluids are administered to correct electrolyte imbalances and 40 mg of frusemide is given intravenously for hypervolaemia.

ASSESSMENT

Throughout her stay, Ms Adamson has remained alert and oriented with stable vital signs. Her respiratory rate has been 20–24 per minute, with scattered crackles, SpO_2 around 94%, and a PaO_2 of 75–80 mmHg on 6 L/min of oxygen. Her pulse has been 96–100 and regular. On her initial assessment, the nurse notes that she seems apprehensive and anxious. Although her blood pressure is 116/74, unchanged from previous levels, her heart rate is up to 106 and respiratory rate is 28 per minute. Her lungs have scattered crackles but good breath sounds throughout, unchanged from previous assessments. Her SpO_2 has dropped to 84%, her oxygen is increased to 8 L/min. ABG results show PaO_2 65 mmHg; respiratory alkalosis, pH 7.48; and $PaCO_2$ 32 mmHg.

Portable chest x-rays were ordered. The doctor orders a non-rebreather mask at 8 L/min and repeat ABGs in 1 hour. The chest x-ray reveals scattered infiltrates and a normal heart size.

Ms Adamson's SpO_2 continues to fall and subsequent blood gases show a PaO_2 of 55 mmHg. The attending doctor diagnoses probable ARDS. She is intubated via endotracheal tube and is commenced on mechanical ventilation.

DIAGNOSES

- *Impaired gas exchange* related to effects of immersion/submersion evidenced by increased respiration rate and decreasing SpO_2.
- *Anxiety* related to hypoxaemia evidenced by decreasing oxygen saturations.
- *Risk of decreased cardiac output* related to mechanical ventilation evidenced by decreasing blood pressure and increasing heart rate.
- *Risk of injury* related to endotracheal intubation evidenced by haemoptysis.

PLANNING

- Obtain all necessary supplies and radiology in preparation for intubation and mechanical ventilation.
- Explain the purpose and procedure of intubation.
- Provide an opportunity to express fears related to intubation and mechanical ventilation; answer questions and provide reassurance.
- Discuss communication strategies while intubated; obtain a magic slate.

Expected outcomes

- Breathe effectively with the mechanical ventilator.
- Demonstrate improved SpO_2, $ETCO_2$ and ABG values.
- Express fears related to intubation and mechanical ventilation.
- Demonstrate reduced anxiety levels (relaxed facial expression, ability to rest).
- Maintain adequate cardiac output and tissue perfusion.
- Tolerate endotracheal intubation and mechanical ventilation without evidence of infection or barotrauma.

IMPLEMENTATION

- Administer analgesics and/or sedatives as ordered.
- Monitor SpO_2 and $ETCO_2$ levels every 30–60 minutes initially after mechanical ventilation is commenced; report changes to the doctor.
- Obtain ABGs as ordered or indicated; monitor and report results.
- Suction via endotracheal tube as needed to maintain clear airways.
- Provide periods of uninterrupted rest.
- Monitor vital signs every 1–2 hours.
- Assess skin colour, capillary refill and the presence of oedema every 4 hours.
- Monitor urine output hourly; report output of less than 30 mL per hour.
- Assess lung sounds and chest excursion every 1–2 hours.

EVALUATION

Ms Adamson is intubated and placed on a volume-cycled ventilator at 50% FiO_2 and a tidal volume of 730 mL in the assist-control mode at 16 breaths per minute. She has difficulty working with the ventilator initially, so morphine and midazolam are ordered to reduce her anxiety. Her SpO_2, $ETCO_2$ and ABG results do not begin to improve until 5 mmHg of PEEP is added to ventilator settings. After 3 days of mechanical ventilation with PEEP and aggressive fluid and diuretic therapy, Ms Adamson begins to improve. She is placed on SIMV and, over the course of another 3 days, is gradually weaned off the ventilator to a face mask with CPAP. She eventually recovers fully, with minimal apparent long-term effects.

CRITICAL THINKING IN THE NURSING PROCESS

1. Endotracheal intubation and mechanical ventilation were effective in supporting Ms Adamson's respiratory status as she recovered from ARDS. Discuss a possible sequence of events had it not been possible to wean her from the ventilator.
2. How might the presentation and management of an acute episode of respiratory failure due to ARDS differ from respiratory failure related to COPD?
3. What measures can nurses take to prevent the development of ARDS?
4. Develop a nursing care plan for Ms Adamson for the nursing diagnosis *Powerlessness* related to endotracheal intubation and mechanical ventilation.

REFLECTING ON THE NURSING PROCESS

1. Outline what you have learned from this case study that you will apply to your future practice.
2. Communication from the nurse to the individual and their significant others is important. Given Ms Adamson's diagnosis of ARDS, what information and education should be communicated to both Ms Adamson and her significant others? Create a different list for both.

Nursing interventions for dysfunctional weaning include the following:

- Observe the person closely following changes in ventilator settings and during T-piece trials. *Vital signs—heart and respiratory rates, in particular—can provide early signs of hypoxaemia and poor tolerance of the weaning process.*

CONSIDERATION FOR PRACTICE

Frequently monitor SpO_2, $ETCO_2$ and ABGs following changes in ventilator settings. These values are used to assess the adequacy of ventilation and gas exchange during the weaning process.

- Place in Fowler's or high-Fowler's position. *Fowler's position facilitates lung expansion and reduces the work of breathing.*
- Fully explain all weaning procedures, along with expected changes in breathing. *Adequate explanations help reduce anxiety and improve the ability to cooperate.*
- Remain with the person during initial periods following changes of ventilator settings or T-piece trials. *This provides reassurance and allows close monitoring of the response.*
- Limit procedures and activities during weaning periods. *Reducing energy expenditures and cardiac work facilitates the weaning process.*
- Provide diversion, such as television or radio. *Diversion helps distract the focus from breathing.*
- Begin weaning procedures in the morning, when the person is well rested and alert; weaning may be discontinued overnight to provide rest. *The work of breathing increases during the weaning process; adequate rest is important.*
- Avoid administering drugs that may depress respirations during the weaning process (except as ordered at night to facilitate rest when ventilator support is provided). *Sedatives or analgesics that depress respirations can impair the weaning process.*
- Keep oxygen at the bedside following weaning and extubation. *Supplemental oxygen may be necessary to maintain adequate blood and tissue oxygenation.*

CONSIDERATION FOR PRACTICE

Frequently assess respiratory status following weaning and extubation. Keep an intubation kit readily available following extubation; be prepared for emergency re-intubation.

- Provide pulmonary hygiene with percussion and postural drainage. *Maintaining patent airways and adequate alveolar ventilation is vital during the weaning process.*

Community-based care

When preparing the person who has recovered from ARDS and the family for home care, discuss the following topics:

- ARDS did not result from something they did or did not do, but developed as a consequence of serious illness. Provide factual information about ARDS.
- Maximal respiratory function following ARDS is usually achieved within 6 months; respiratory function may remain significantly impaired. This may necessitate changes in occupation, lifestyle and family roles.
- Avoiding smoking and exposure to second-hand smoke and environmental pollutants is vital to prevent further lung damage.
- Obtain immunisation for pneumococcal pneumonia and annual influenza immunisations to prevent further episodes of serious respiratory disease.

Provide referrals to community health and respiratory care services as indicated, as well as for occupational therapy and counselling as needed.

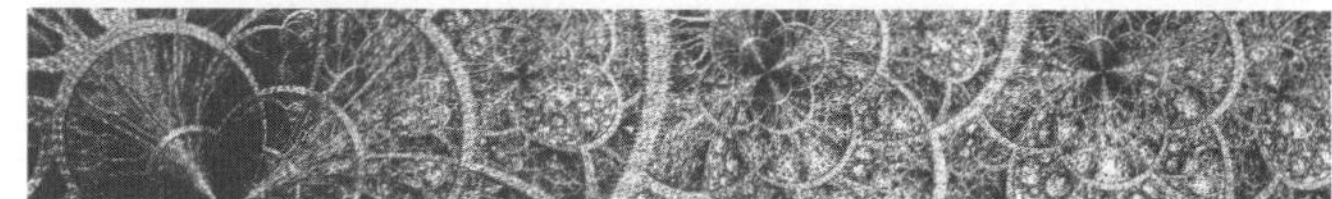

CHAPTER HIGHLIGHTS

- **Obstructive disorders of the lower respiratory system, including asthma, COVID-19, COPD and cystic fibrosis, impair airflow into and out of the lungs, often affecting outflow of air to a greater extent than inflow. As a result, air trapped in the alveoli increases the residual volume of the lungs and reduces functional residual capacity. Alveolar ventilation is reduced as well. The net result is less available oxygen in the alveoli and impaired gas exchange.**
- **In many instances, acute episodes of asthma can be avoided through the use of inhaled steroids to reduce airway inflammation, inhaled long-acting bronchodilators and frequent self-monitoring of expiratory flow rate. Nursing care focuses on teaching for self-management and providing care during acute episodes of airway constriction.**
- **COPD is a long-term process of progressive lung dysfunction. COPD involves two different disease processes: chronic bronchitis, characterised by airway oedema; and excessive mucus production and emphysema, characterised by destruction of supporting tissue with enlargement of respiratory bronchioles and alveolar spaces and loss of surface area for gas exchange.**
- **Smoking and exposure to tobacco smoke is the single greatest risk factor for COPD. A small percentage of cases result from an inherited deficiency of α_1-antitripsin, an enzyme that inhibits lung tissue destruction. Although smoking cessation does not reverse COPD, it does slow the progress of the disease.**
- **Cystic fibrosis, inherited as an autosomal recessive disorder, causes thick, viscous secretions in affected organs, primarily the lungs, pancreas, sweat glands and reproductive tract. In the lungs, small airway clearance is impaired, leading to atelectasis, bronchiectasis, infection and dilation of distal airways with air trapping and impaired gas exchange. Chest physiotherapy and early treatment of respiratory infections are key components of disease management. Ultimately, lung or heart–lung transplant may be required.**
- **Occupational lung diseases, pneumoconiosis and hypersensitivity pneumonitis damage interstitial tissues of the lungs, leading to fibrosis and scarring that causes the lungs to become stiff and**

non-compliant. Lung volumes decrease, the work of breathing increases and gas diffusion is impaired. Most occupational lung diseases are progressive and non-reversible. Interprofessional care is similar to that provided for individuals with COPD.

- Pulmonary vascular disorders affect blood flow through the pulmonary vascular system and gas exchange. PE, obstruction of pulmonary blood flow, is a potentially critical condition usually resulting from deep venous thrombosis. Sudden onset of chest pain and dyspnoea with changes in haemodynamic status are possible manifestations of PE. Prevention through early ambulation, lower extremity exercises and sequential compression devices is the most effective treatment for PE.
- In primary and secondary forms of pulmonary hypertension, constriction of pulmonary vessels and remodelling of the pulmonary vascular bed increase pressure in the pulmonary system and right heart, ultimately leading to right-sided heart failure (cor pulmonale).
- Treatment focuses on slowing disease progression through oxygen therapy, administration of vasodilators and anticoagulants, and supporting function.
- Hypoventilation, impaired gas exchange and significant ventilation–perfusion mismatch (e.g. PE) can lead to respiratory failure. Hypoventilation leads to hypoxaemia and hypercapnia, whereas in impaired gas exchange or ventilation–perfusion mismatch, hypoxaemia predominates.
- The manifestations of respiratory failure relate directly to the effects of hypoxaemia (dyspnoea, restlessness, apprehension, impaired judgment, motor impairment, tachycardia, hyper- or hypotension, and cyanosis) and hypercapnia (dyspnoea, headache, peripheral and conjunctival vasodilation, papilloedema, neuromuscular irritability and decreased LOC).
- Respiratory support often is required, using positive-pressure ventilators. Variables of mechanical ventilation include the mode or cycle of ventilation, the flow rate and amount, pressures delivered and the oxygen concentration. Either invasive or non-invasive techniques may be used.
- Complications of mechanical ventilation include lung and mucous membrane trauma and infection, reduced cardiac output, gastric dilation, impaired communication and stress.
- ARDS is non-cardiac pulmonary oedema caused by a diffuse inflammatory response with increased pulmonary capillary permeability leading to interstitial and alveolar oedema and impaired gas exchange. As the process continues, lung compliance decreases, increasing the work of breathing, and atelectasis and consolidation of lung tissue develop. Respiratory failure with refractory hypoxaemia results.
- Mechanical ventilation and measures to support physiological function are the primary treatments for ARDS. The mortality rate, however, remains high at about 50%.

CONCEPT CHECK

1 All of the following nursing diagnoses are appropriate for a person with an acute asthma attack. Which is of highest priority?

1 *Anxiety* related to difficulty breathing
2 *Ineffective airway clearance* related to bronchoconstriction and increased mucus production
3 *Ineffective breathing pattern* related to anxiety
4 *Ineffective health maintenance* related to lack of knowledge about attack triggers and appropriate use of medications

2 The nurse caring for a person with asthma notices that the individual's respirations have slowed and he is no longer coughing. Breath sounds are diminished throughout his lung fields and absent in the bases. The nurse should:

1 notify the doctor
2 allow the person to rest undisturbed
3 obtain a chest x-ray
4 ask family members to leave

3 When teaching use of an MDI, the nurse's instruction should be:

1 take quick shallow breaths in rapid succession while holding the canister down
2 use the inhaler containing the anti-inflammatory drug first, then the bronchodilator
3 use the anti-inflammatory drug as needed to treat acute episodes of wheezing
4 rinse the mouth after using the inhaler to reduce systemic absorption of the drug

4 Which of the following would be an expected assessment finding in a person admitted with COPD?

1 AP chest diameter equal to or greater than lateral chest diameter
2 mental confusion and lethargy
3 3+ pitting oedema of ankles and lower legs
4 SpO_2 readings of 85% or less

5 An appropriate goal for a person admitted with an acute exacerbation of COPD would be:

1 will verbalise self-care measures to regain lost lung function
2 arterial blood gases will be within normal limits by discharge
3 will maintain SpO_2 (saturation or peripheral oxygen) of 90% or higher
4 will identify strategies to help reduce number of cigarettes smoked per day

6 Which of the following statements best represents a nurse's understanding of use of supplemental oxygen in individuals with COPD?

1 The individual should not smoke because oxygen supports combustion.
2 Oxygen is used only at night for individuals with COPD.
3 Oxygen is never used for individuals with COPD because they may become dependent on it.
4 The person needs to be closely monitored for signs of respiratory depression.

7 The community health nurse working with a person who has cystic fibrosis specifically directs the home care aide to report which of the following? (Select all that apply.)

1 thick, tenacious milky white sputum
2 fever
3 bulky, fatty stools
4 difficulty clearing mucus secretions
5 increasing shortness of breath and fatigue

8 A person in skeletal traction suddenly develops right-sided chest pain and shortness of breath. The nurse should:

1 check for Homans' sign
2 start oxygen per nasal prongs
3 administer the prescribed analgesic
4 elevate the head of the bed to 45 degrees

9 **The nurse caring for a person with COPD recognises which of the following as an early sign of possible respiratory failure?**
1 restlessness and tachypnoea
2 deep coma
3 hypotension and tachycardia
4 decreased urine output

10 **The nurse caring for a person undergoing mechanical ventilation for acute respiratory failure plans and implements which of the following measures to help maintain effective alveolar ventilation?**
1 keeps the person in supine position
2 increases the tidal volume on the ventilator
3 maintains ordered oxygen concentration
4 performs endotracheal suctioning as indicated

BIBLIOGRAPHY

Aitken, L., Marshall, A. & Chaboyer, W. (2019). *ACCCN's critical care nursing* (4th ed.). Chatswood, NSW: Elsevier.

Asthma Australia (2021). *Asthma statistics and facts.* Retrieved from https://asthma.org.au/

Austin, E. K., James, C. & Tessier, J. (2021). Early detection methods for silicosis in Australia and internationally: A review of the literature. *International Journal of Environmental Research and Public Health, 18*(15). https://doi.org/10.3390/ijerph18158123

Australian Bureau of Statistics (ABS) (2019). *National Aboriginal and Torres Strait Islander health survey.* Retrieved from www.abs.gov.au/

Australian Bureau of Statistics (ABS) (2021). *Causes of death, Australia.* Retrieved from www.abs.gov.au/

Australian Bureau of Statistics (ABS) (2022a). *Health conditions prevalence.* Retrieved from www.abs.gov.au/

Australian Bureau of Statistics (ABS) (2022b). *Australian health survey.* Retrieved from www.abs.gov.au/

Australian Commission on Safety and Quality in Health Care (2020). *Venous Thromboembolism Prevention Clinical Care Standard.* Sydney: ACSQHC.

Australian Cystic Fibrosis Data Registry (ACFDR) & Monash University (2020). *Australian Cystic Fibrosis Data Registry annual report, 2020.* Retrieved from https://www.cysticfibrosis.org.au/

Australian Institute of Health and Welfare (AIHW) (2019a). *Monitoring asthma in Australia.* Retrieved from https://www.aihw.gov.au/

Australian Institute of Health and Welfare (AIHW) (2019b). *National asthma indicators.* Retrieved from https://www.aihw.gov.au/

Australian Institute of Health and Welfare (AIHW) (2020a). *Asthma.* Retrieved from https://www.aihw.gov.au/

Australian Institute of Health and Welfare (AIHW) (2020b). *COPD.* Retrieved from https://www.aihw.gov.au/

Australian Institute of Health and Welfare (AIHW) (2020c). *Bronchiectasis.* Retrieved from https://www.aihw.gov.au/

Blakey, J., Chung, L. P., McDonald, V. M. et al. (2021). Oral corticosteroids stewardship for asthma in adults and adolescents: A position paper from the Thoracic Society of Australia and New Zealand. *Respirology, 26*(12), 1112–1130. https://doi.org/10.1111/resp.14147

Bullock, S. & Hales, M. (2019). *Principles of pathophysiology* (2nd ed.). Sydney: Pearson.

Byrd, R. (2018). Mechanical ventilation. *Emedicine.* Retrieved from http://emedicine.medscape.com/

Cavallaro Goodman, C. & Fuller, K. S. (2020). *Pathology: Implications for the physical therapist* (5th ed.). New York: Elsevier.

Choi, J. & Azmat, C. E. (2022). *Leukotriene receptor antagonists.* Retrieved from https://www.ncbi.nlm.nih.gov/

Cousins, J. L., Wood-Baker, R., Wark, P. A. B. et al. (2020). Management of acute COPD exacerbations in Australia: Do we follow the guidelines? *ERJ Open Research, 6.* doi: 10.1183/23120541.00270-2019

Crawford, A. & Ruth-Sahd, L. (2021). Sarcoidosis: What nurses need to know. *Nursing, 51*(12), 20–26. doi: 10.1097/01.NURSE.0000800084.63457.b6

Department of Health and Aged Care (2022a). *Coronavirus (COVID-19) case numbers and statistics.* Retrieved from https://www.health.gov.au

Department of Health and Aged Care (2022b). *National Occupational Respiratory Disease Registry.* Retrieved from https://www.health.gov.au

Diamond, M., Peniston, H. L., Sanghavi, D. & Mahapatra, S. (2022). *Acute respiratory distress syndrome.* Retrieved from https://www.ncbi.nlm.nih.gov/

Ding, H., Karunanithi, M., Ireland, D. et al. (2019). Evaluation of an innovative mobile health programme for the self-management of chronic obstructive pulmonary disease (MH-COPD): Protocol of a randomised controlled trial. *BMJ Open, 9*(4). doi: 10.1136/bmjopen-2018-025381

Freeman-Sanderson, A., Morris, K. & Elkins, M. (2019). Characteristics of patient communication and prevalence of communication difficulty in the intensive care unit: An observational study. *Australian Critical Care, 32*(5), 373–377. https://doi.org/10.1016/j.aucc.2018.09.002

Gao, J., Wu, F., Wu, S. & Yang, X. (2020). Inflammatory subtypes in classic asthma and cough variant asthma. *Journal of Inflammation Research, 13,* 1167–1173. doi: 10.2147/JIR.S269795

Glenister, K., Haines, H. & Disler, R. (2019). Benefits of the 'village': A qualitative exploration of the patient experience of COPD in rural Australia. *BMJ Open,* 9(10). doi: 0.1136/bmjopen-2019-030953

Greenhalgh, E. M., Scollo, M. M. & Winstanley, M. H. (2022). *Tobacco in Australia: Facts and issues.* Melbourne: Cancer Council Victoria. Retrieved from www.TobaccoInAustralia.org.au

Grott, K., Chauhan, S. & Dunlap, J. D. (2022). *Atelectasis.* Retrieved from https://www.ncbi.nlm.nih.gov/

Jain, R., Kazerski, T. M., Zuckerwise, L. C. et al. (2022). Pregnancy in cystic fibrosis: Review of the literature and expert recommendations. *Journal of Cystic Fibrosis, 21*(3), 397–395. https://doi.org/10.1016/j.jcf.2021.07.019

Jedynak, A. R. (2020). Silicosis and coal worker's pneumoconiosis imaging. *Emedicine.* Retrieved from http://emedicine.medscape.com/

Johnson, C., Giordano, N. A., Patel, L. et al. (2022). Pressure injury outcomes of a prone positioning protocol in patients with COVID and ARDS. *American Journal of Critical Care, 31*(1), 34–41. https://doi.org/10.4037/ajcc2022242

Jumat, M. I., Hayati, F., Rahim, S. S. S. A. et al. (2021). Occupational lung disease: A narrative review of lung conditions from the workplace. *Annals of Medicine and Surgery, 64.* https://doi.org/10.1016/j.amsu.2021.102245

Kamangar, N. (2022). Sarcoidosis. *Emedicine.* Retrieved from http://emedicine.medscape.com/

Karatela, S., Caruana, S. & Paul, G. (2022). Prevalence of respiratory disease in the population of Queensland communities in proximity to coal mines and coal mining activities. *International Journal of Community Medicine and Public Health, 9*(7), 3014–3022. https://dx.doi.org/10.18203/2394-6040.ijcmph20221776

Khalaila, R., Zbidat, W., Anwar, K., Bayya, A., Linton, D. & Sviri, S. (2011). Communication difficulties and psychoemotional distress in patients receiving mechanical ventilation. *American Journal of Critical Care, 20*(6), 470–479.

Lung Foundation Australia (2019). *Sarcoidosis.* Retrieved from https://lungfoundation.com.au/

Lung Foundation Australia (2020). *Alpha-1 antitrypsin deficiency.* Retrieved from https://lungfoundation.com.au/

Lung Foundation Australia (2021). *The COPD-X: plan: Australian and New Zealand guidelines for the management of chronic obstructive pulmonary disease* (V2.65). Retrieved from https://copdx.org.au/copd-x-plan/

Martini, F., Nath, J. & Bartholomew, E. (2018). *Fundamentals of anatomy & physiology* (11th ed.). Harlow, Essex: Pearson.

McClenaghan, E., Cosgriff, R., Brownlee, K. et al. (2020). *Journal of Cystic Fibrosis, 19,* 868–871. https://doi.org/10.1016/j.jcf.2020.10.003

MIMS (2018a). *Foradile.* Retrieved from https://www.mimsonline.com.au

MIMS (2018b). *Seretide.* Retrieved from https://www.mimsonline.com.au

MIMS (2018c). *Full product information—Various drugs.* Retrieved from https://www.mimsonline.com.au

Minutello, K. & Gupta, V. (2022). *Cromolyn sodium.* Retrieved from https://www.ncbi.nlm.nih.gov/

National Asthma Council Australia (NACA) (2020). *Spirometry quick reference guide.* Retrieved from https://www.nationalasthma.org.au/

National Asthma Council Australia (NACA) (2021). *Asthma deaths remain stubbornly high in Australia.* Retrieved from https://www.nationalasthma.org.au/

National Asthma Council Australia (NACA) (2022a). *Australian asthma handbook* (V2.2). Retrieved from https://www.nationalasthma.org.au/

National Asthma Council Australia (NACA) (2022b). *First aid for asthma: Children under 12.* Retrieved from https://www.nationalasthma.org.au/

National Asthma Council Australia (NACA) (2022c). *First aid for asthma: Ages 12+.*

Oudiz, R. (2022). Idiopathic pulmonary arterial hypertension. *Emedicine*. Retrieved from http://emedicine.medscape.com/

Ouellette, D. (2020). Pulmonary embolism. *Emedicine*. Retrieved from http://emedicine.medscape.com/

Pulmonary Hypertension Association (PHA) Australia (2022). *What is pulmonary hypertension?* Retrieved from http://www.phaaustralia.com/

Royal Australian College of General Practitioners (2021). *Supporting smoking cessation: A guide for health professionals*. Retrieved from https://www.racgp.org.au/

Safe Work Australia (2021). *Occupational lung diseases*. Retrieved from https://www.safeworkaustralia.gov.au/

Schwab, K. (2022). Pulmonary arterial hypertension. *Emedicine*. Retrieved from http://emedicine.medscape.com/

Schwartzstein, R. M. & Campbell, M. L. (2022). Dyspnea and mechanical ventilation: The emperor has no clothes. *American Journal of Respiratory and Critical Care Medicine, 205*(8). https://doi.org/10.1164/rccm.202201-0078ED

Sharma, G. (2020). Cystic fibrosis. *Emedicine*. Retrieved from http://emedicine.medscape.com/

Soo Hoo, G. (2020). Noninvasive ventilation. *Emedicine*. Retrieved from http://emedicine.medscape.com/

Therapeutic Goods Administration (2022). *Updates to the prescribing medicines in pregnancy database*. Retrieved from https://www.tga.gov.au/

Wang, R. S., Croteau-Chonka, D. C., Silvermann, E. K. et al. (2019). Pharmacogenomics and placebo response in a randomized clinical trial in asthma. *Clinical Pharmacology & Therapeutics, 106*(6), 1261–1267. https://doi.org/10.1002/cpt.1646

Weiss, S. T. (2021). Genetics of asthma. *Emedicine*. Retrieved from http://emedicine.medscape.com/

Whitson, B. (2022). Lung transplantation. *Emedicine*. Retrieved from http://emedicine.medscape.com/

Wong, F. J. (2019). Coal worker's pneumoconiosis (black lung disease). *Emedicine*. Retrieved from https://emedicine.medscape.com/

Wood-Baker, R., Reid, D., Robinson, A. & Walters, E. (2012). Clinical trial of community nurse mentoring to improve self-management in patients with chronic obstructive pulmonary disease. *International Journal of COPD*, 7. doi: 10.2147/COPD.S32220

World Health Organization (WHO) (2022). *Tobacco*. Retrieved from http://www.who.int/

UNIT 9 BUILDING CLINICAL COMPETENCE

Responses to altered respiratory function

Clinical scenario

You have been assigned to work with the following individuals on a respiratory unit. Significant data obtained during report are as follows:

- Jack Holt, a 65-year-old male, has bacterial pneumonia. Vital signs are T 38.3°C, P 94, R 30, BP 146/88. He is complaining of chest pain with breathing and has a productive cough of rusty-coloured sputum. His SpO_2 is 90% in room air.
- Maggie Sawyer, an 82-year-old female, is being discharged today following treatment for a DVT. She has congestive obstructive pulmonary disease. Suddenly she complains of difficulty breathing, chest pain, coughing, restlessness and a feeling that she is going to die.
- James Mohr, a 25-year-old male, sustained head, neck and chest injuries, and has a tracheostomy, from a motor vehicle crash. His vital signs were stable at the last assessment. He begins coughing and puts on his call light.
- Amy Campbell, a 30-year-old female, is being treated after having a severe asthma attack. Her current vital signs are T 37.2°C, P 64, R 26, BP 124/84. She has inspiratory and expiratory wheezing. Her SpO_2 is 94% on 4 L/min O_2 via nasal prongs.

Critical-thinking questions

1 In what order would you visit these individuals after report?
1. ______________________________
2. ______________________________
3. ______________________________
4. ______________________________

2 Which top two priorities would you choose for each of the individuals presented above? Can you explain, if asked, the rationale for your choices?

	Priority #1	Priority #2
Jack Holt		
Maggie Sawyer		
James Mohr		
Amy Campbell		

3 The older adult is prone to respiratory problems due to which age-related changes in the respiratory system? (Select all that apply.)
1. loss of skeletal muscle strength in the thorax
2. increased elastic recoil of lungs during expiration
3. alveoli that are less elastic and more fibrotic
4. decreased residual volume of lung
5. decreased effectiveness of coughing

4 Bacterial pneumonia is spread by droplets. When using standard precautions, which equipment is necessary to prevent its spread?
1. Wear a gown when providing hygiene care for the person.
2. Wear a gown and gloves when touching the person.
3. Wear a mask and gloves when suctioning the person.
4. Wear a cap to keep hair from touching the individual.

5 For the individual receiving percussion and vibration with postural drainage for left lower lobe pneumonia, which position most facilitates removal of secretions?
1. semi-Fowler's position with arms elevated
2. right Sims' position with head in Trendelenberg
3. high-Fowler's position leaning on a bedside tray
4. left Sims' position with head flat

6 On discharge, the nurse teaches Mrs Sawyer ways to prevent PE. Which instruction is appropriate?
1. Use pillows under the knees when in bed.
2. Apply knee-high elastic stockings when ambulating.
3. Exercise the legs vigorously to encourage blood flow.
4. Stop every 1–2 hours to stretch legs when travelling.

7 Mr Mohr will be discharged with a tracheostomy. What should the nurse teach him about tracheostomies?
1. The tracheostomy will not interfere with lifting when returning to work.
2. Water-skiing is allowed, but swimming in a pool or lake is not allowed.
3. Showering is allowed as long as the tracheostomy is covered with a washcloth.
4. A small amount of alcohol is allowed but smoking is not allowed.

8 When admitted to the emergency department, which laboratory studies would you expect to obtain on a person with an inhalation injury?
1. ABGs, carboxyhaemoglobin levels, electrolytes
2. sputum cultures and sensitivity, serology testing, sputum Gram stain
3. methaemoglobin levels, venous blood gases, WBC count
4. FBC count, SpO_2, sputum specimen

9 ABGs are ordered on a person with acute respiratory distress. The results are: pH 7.22; PaO_2 50 mmHg; $PaCO_2$ 58 mmHg; HCO_3^- 29 mEq/L. How would a nurse interpret these results?
1. respiratory acidosis
2. respiratory alkalosis
3. metabolic acidosis
4. metabolic alkalosis

10 Corticosteroids are ordered to decrease the inflammatory process of asthma. Which comment indicates the person understands how to take corticosteroids?
1. 'Corticosteroids have very few side effects to worry about.'
2. 'I understand that I cannot stop taking the medication abruptly.'
3. 'I can stop taking the corticosteroids as soon as I feel better.'
4. 'I can take an over-the-counter medication if I develop a cold.'

11 Which are early manifestations of pulmonary tuberculosis?
1. tachypnoea, tachycardia, activity intolerance
2. bradypnoea, foul-smelling sputum, weight gain
3. blood-tinged sputum, high-grade fever, fatigue
4. low-grade fever, night sweats, dry cough

Case study

Gladys Hamer, an 83-year-old female, presents in the emergency department complaining of shortness of breath and fever. Her vital signs are T 39.1°C, P 115 and irregular, R 35 and shallow, BP 168/66. Her height is 160 cm and weight is 43.5 kg. On assessment, her skin is very dry and warm. Her colour is dusky. Scattered wheezes and rhonchi are heard throughout all lung fields. Her chest is hyperresonant to percussion. A pulse oximeter is applied and SpO_2 is 88%. Mrs Hamer has a past medical history of emphysema for 10 years, complaints of shortness of breath on exertion and has a chronic cough productive of thick, greyish sputum. Her spouse died 5 years ago and she has lived with her two adult sons since then.

Blood is drawn for ABGs and results are pH 7.19; PaO_2 54 mmHg, $PaCO_2$ 55 mmHg; HCO_3^- 30 mEq/L indicating respiratory acidosis. Based on her current assessment, ABG results and past medical history, a medical diagnosis of COPD is determined.

When planning nursing care for Mrs Hamer, the nursing diagnosis of *Impaired gas exchange* related to acute and chronic lung disease is appropriate for implementing nursing interventions.

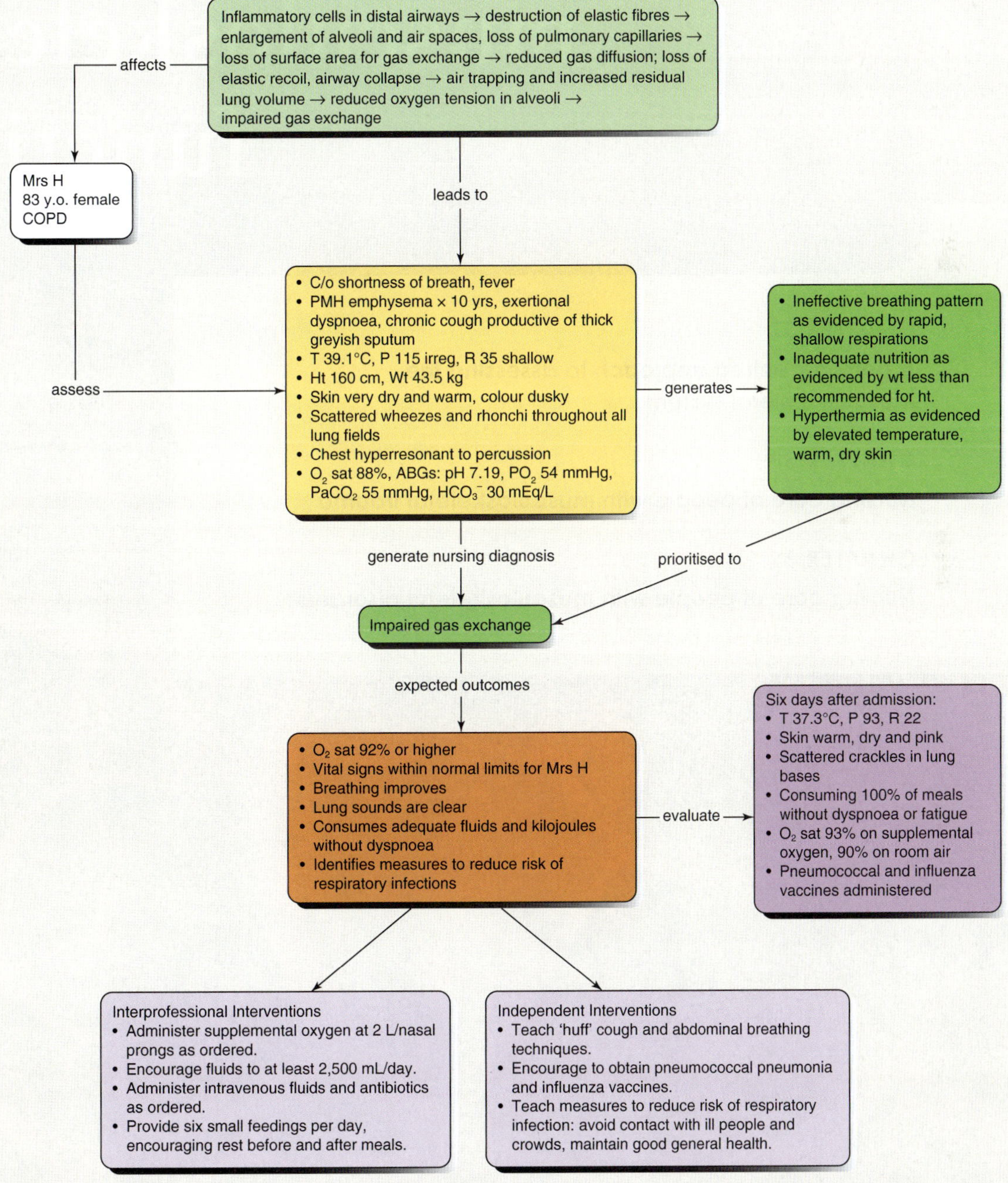

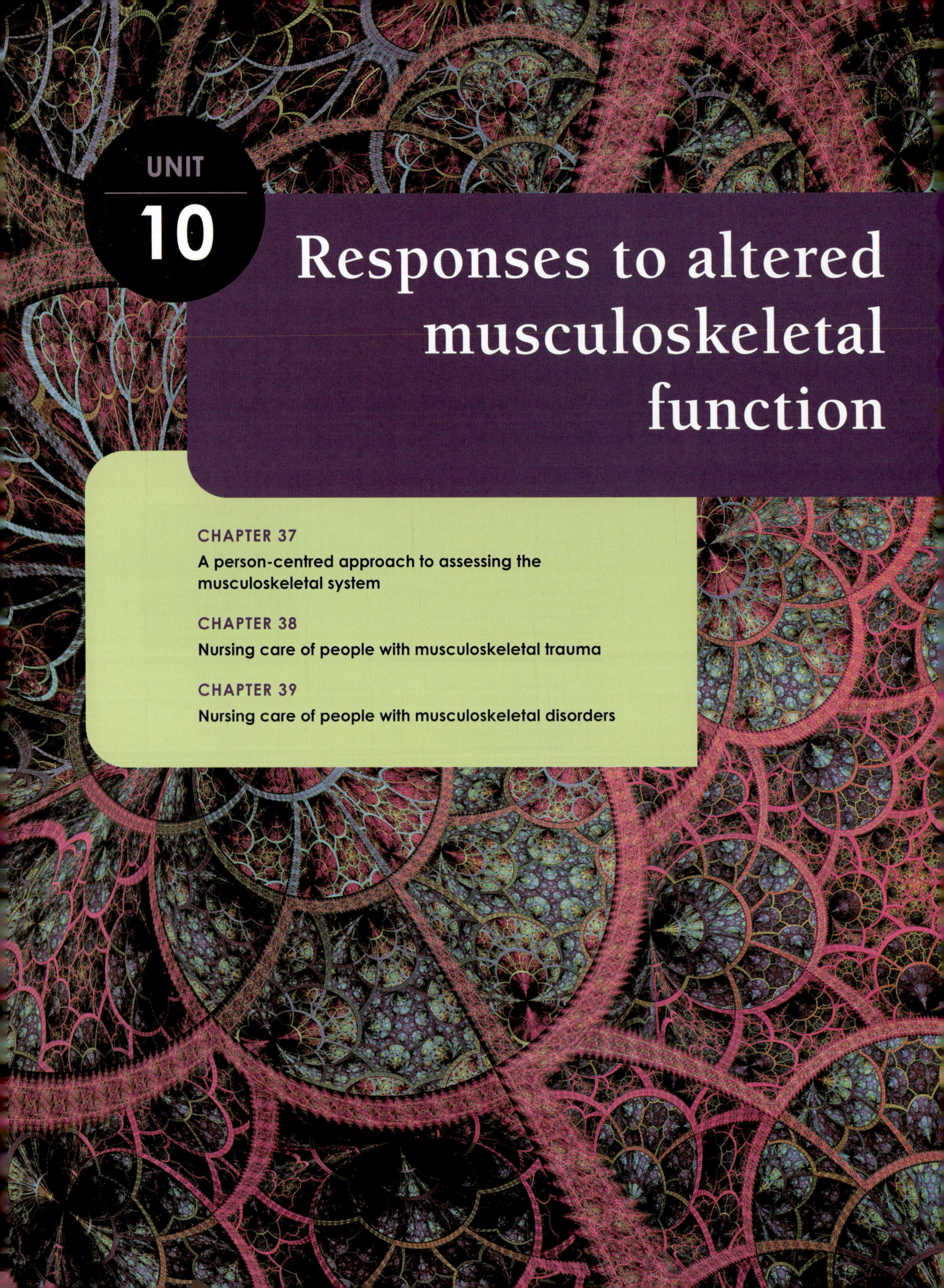

UNIT 10

Responses to altered musculoskeletal function

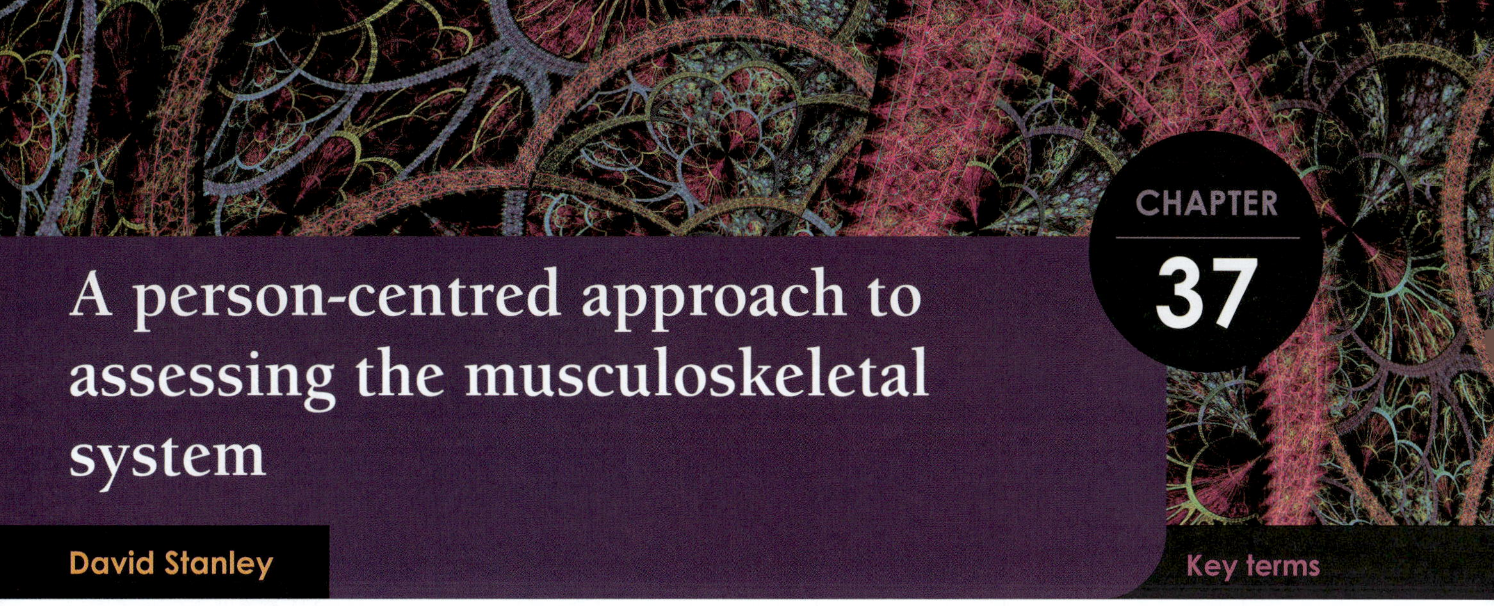

CHAPTER 37

A person-centred approach to assessing the musculoskeletal system

David Stanley

Key terms

bursitis 1372
crepitation 1370
haematopoiesis 1358
kyphosis 1370
lordosis 1370
ossification 1360
scoliosis 1370
synovitis 1373
tendonitis 1372

Learning outcomes

- Describe the anatomy, physiology and functions of the musculoskeletal system.
- Explain the normal movements facilitated by synovial joints.
- Identify specific topics for consideration during a health history interview of the person with health problems involving the musculoskeletal system.
- Describe normal variations in a musculoskeletal assessment for the older adult.
- Identify manifestations of impairment of the musculoskeletal system.

Clinical competencies

- Conduct and document a health history for people who have or are at risk of alterations in the musculoskeletal system.
- Conduct and document a physical assessment of musculoskeletal structures and functions.
- Monitor the results of diagnostic tests and report abnormal findings.

Equipment needed

- Tape measure
- Goniometer (an instrument for the precise measurement of angles)

The tissues and structures of the musculoskeletal system perform many functions, including support, protection and movement. The musculoskeletal system has two subsystems that include the bones and joints of the skeleton, and the skeletal muscles. These two main subsystems work together to allow the body to perform both gross and simple movements, such as closing a door, and fine, complex movements, such as repairing a watch.

Anatomy, physiology and functions of the musculoskeletal system

The musculoskeletal system is composed of bones of the skeletal system; ligaments, tendons and muscles of the muscular system; and joints. The bones serve as the framework for the body and for the attachment of muscles, tendons and ligaments. Innervated by the nervous system, contraction and relaxation of muscles permit movement at joints.

The skeleton

Bones form the body's structure and provide support for soft tissues. They also protect vital organs from injury and serve to move body parts by providing points of attachment for muscles. Bones also store minerals and serve as a site for **haematopoiesis** (blood cell formation).

The human skeleton is made up of 206 bones (see Figure 37.1). Bones of the skeletal system are divided into the axial skeleton and the appendicular skeleton. The axial skeleton includes the bones of the skull, ribs, sternum and vertebral column. The appendicular skeleton consists of all the bones of the upper and lower limbs, shoulder girdles and pelvic girdle.

Bone structure

Bone cells include osteoblasts (cells that form bone), osteocytes (cells that maintain bone matrix) and osteoclasts (cells that resorb bone). Bone matrix is the extracellular element of bone tissue; it consists of collagen fibres, minerals (primarily calcium and phosphate), proteins, carbohydrates and ground substance. Ground substance is a gelatinous material that facilitates diffusion of nutrients, wastes and gases between the blood vessels and bone tissue. Bones are covered with periosteum, a double-layered connective tissue. The outer layer of the periosteum contains blood vessels and nerves; the inner layer is anchored to the bone.

Bones consist of a rigid connective tissue called osseous tissue of which there are two types: compact bone is smooth and dense; spongy bone contains spaces between meshworks of bone. Both types contain the same elements and are found in almost all bones of the body.

The basic structural unit of compact bone is the Haversian system (also called an osteon). The Haversian system consists of a central canal, called the Haversian canal; concentric layers of bone matrix, called lamellae; spaces between the lamellae, called lacunae; osteocytes within the lacunae; and small channels, called canaliculi (see Figure 37.2).

Spongy bone has no Haversian systems. Instead, the lamellae are arranged in concentric layers called trabeculae that branch and join to form meshworks. The spongy sections of long bones and flat bones contain tissue for haematopoiesis. In the adult, these sections, called red marrow cavities, are present in the spongy centre of flat bones (especially the sternum) and in only two long bones: the humerus and the head of the femur. This red marrow is active in haematopoiesis in adults.

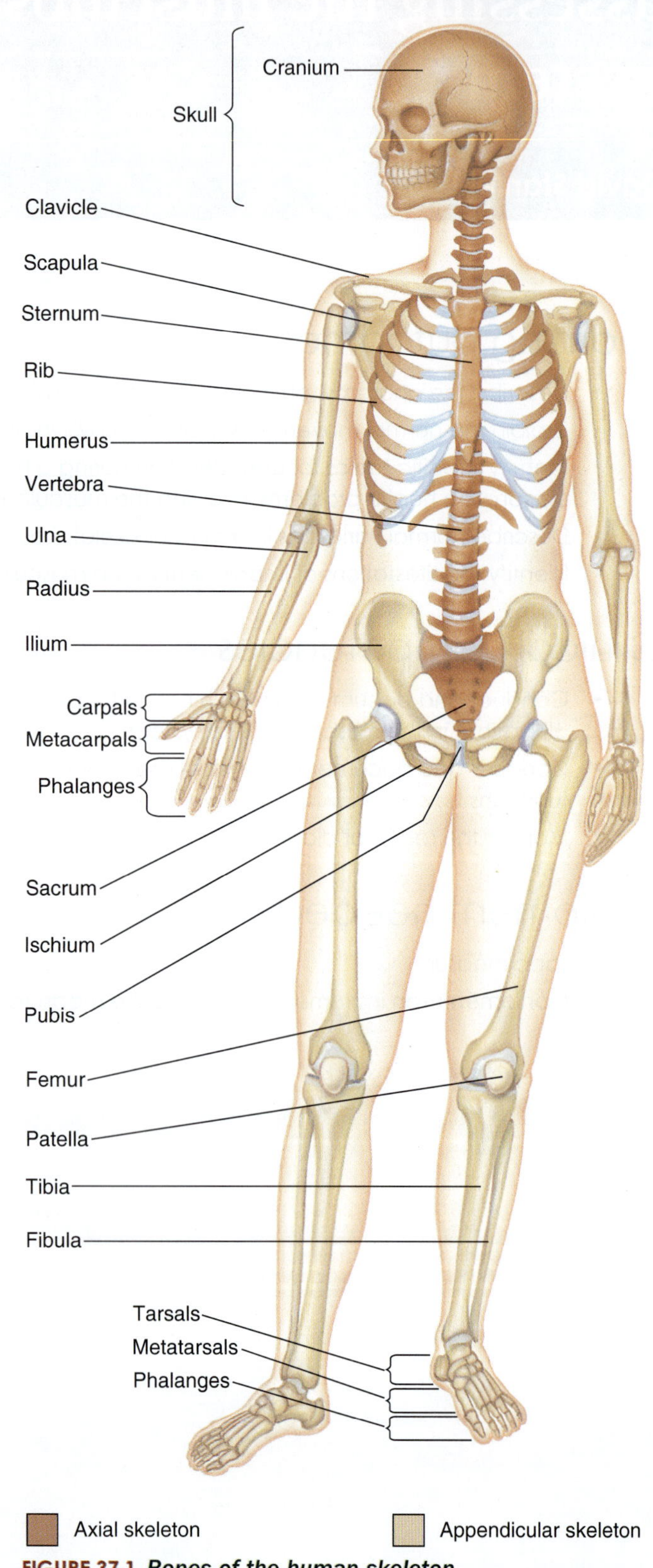

FIGURE 37.1 *Bones of the human skeleton*

Bone shapes

Bones are classified by shape (see Figure 37.3).

- *Long bones* are longer than they are wide. They have a midportion or shaft, called a diaphysis, and two broad ends, called epiphyses (see Figure 37.4). The diaphysis is compact bone and contains the marrow cavity, which is lined with endosteum. Each epiphysis is spongy bone covered by a thin layer of compact bone.

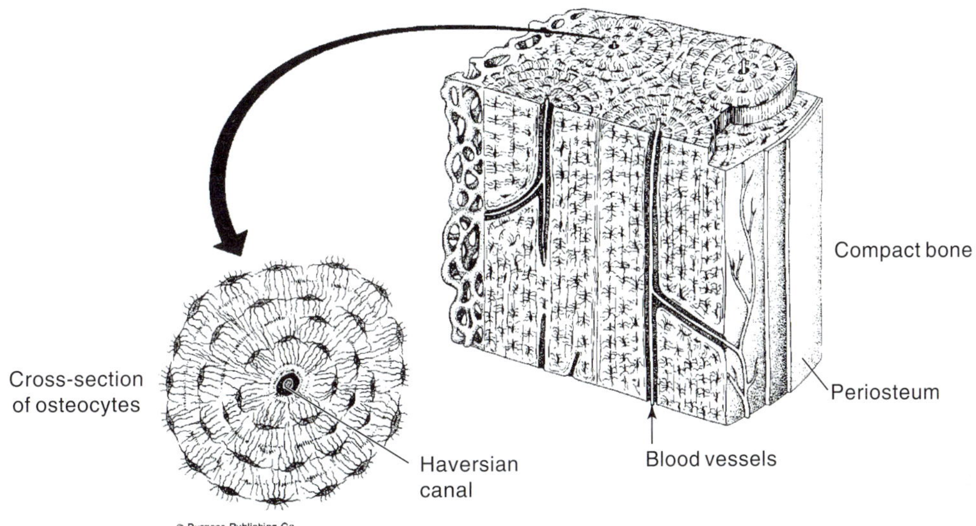

FIGURE 37.2 *The microscopic structure (Haversian system) of compact bone*

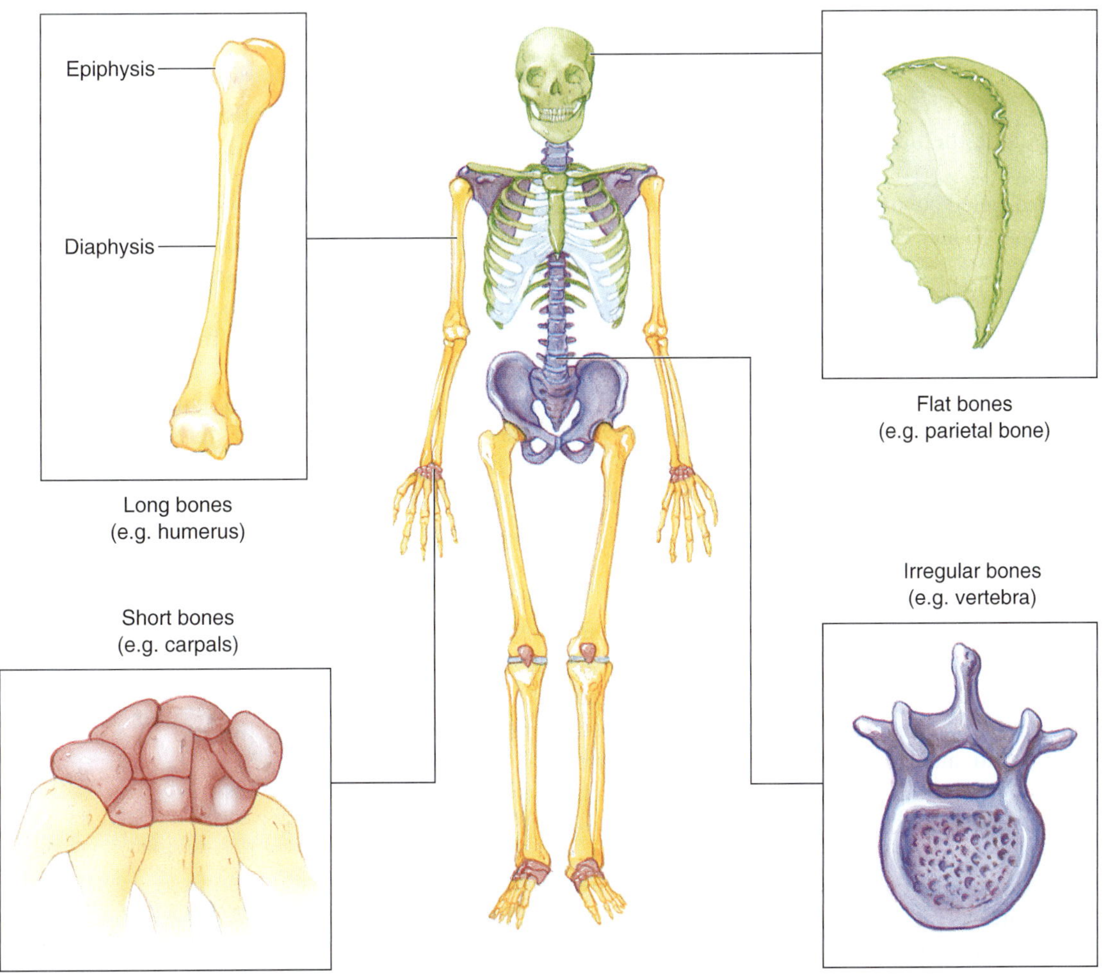

FIGURE 37.3 *Classification of bones according to shape*

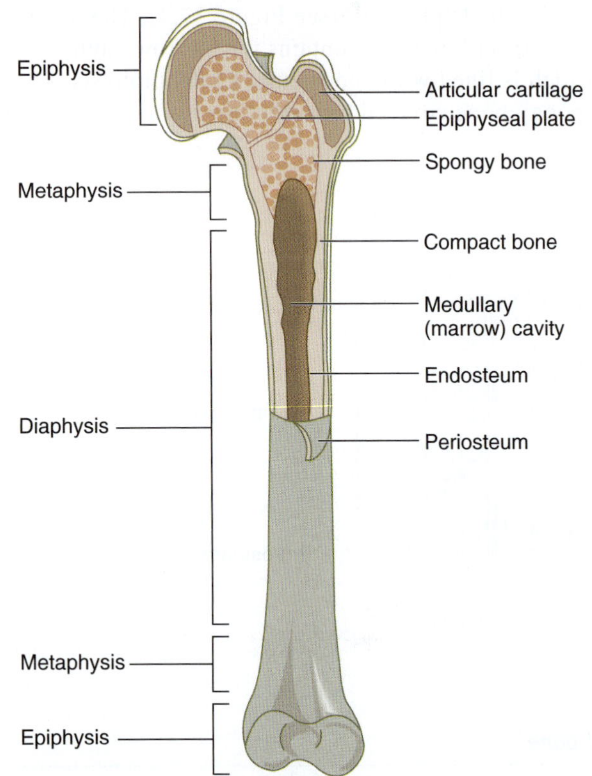

FIGURE 37.4 *Parts of a long bone*

Long bones include the bones of the arms, legs, fingers and toes.

- *Short bones*, also called cuboid bones, are spongy bone covered by compact bone. They include the bones of the wrist and ankle.
- *Flat bones* are thin and flat and most are curved. Their disc-like structure consists of a layer of spongy bone between two thin layers of compact bone. Flat bones include most bones of the skull, the sternum and the ribs.
- *Irregular bones* are of various shapes and sizes and, like flat bones, are plates of compact bone with spongy bone between. Irregular bones include the vertebrae, the scapulae and the bones of the pelvic girdle.

Bone remodelling in adults

Although the bones of adults do not normally increase in length and size, constant remodelling of bones, as well as repair of damaged bone tissue, occurs throughout life. In the bone remodelling process, bone resorption and bone deposit occur at all periosteal and endosteal surfaces. Hormones and forces that put stress on the bones regulate this process, which involves a combined action of the osteocytes, osteoclasts and osteoblasts. Bones that are in use, and are therefore subjected to stress, increase their osteoblastic activity to increase **ossification** (the development of bone). Bones that are inactive undergo increased osteoclast activity and bone resorption.

The hormonal stimulus for bone remodelling is controlled by a negative feedback mechanism that regulates blood calcium levels. This stimulus involves the interaction of parathyroid hormone (PTH) from the parathyroid glands and calcitonin from the thyroid gland. When blood levels of calcium decrease, PTH is released; PTH then stimulates osteoclast activity and bone resorption so that calcium is released from the bone matrix. As a result, blood levels of calcium rise and the stimulus for PTH release ends. Rising blood calcium levels stimulate the secretion of calcitonin, inhibit bone resorption and cause the deposit of calcium salts in the bone matrix. Thus, bones are necessary to regulate blood calcium levels.

Calcium ions are necessary for the transmission of nerve impulses, the release of neurotransmitters, muscle contraction, blood clotting, glandular secretion and cell division. Of the body's 1,200 to 1,400 g of calcium, over 99% is present as bone minerals.

Bone remodelling is also regulated by the response of bones to gravitational pull and to mechanical stress from the pull of muscles. Although the exact mechanism is not fully understood, it is known that bones that undergo increased stress are heavier and larger. This finding supports Wolff's law, which states that bone develops and remodels itself to resist the stresses placed on it.

The process of bone repair following a fracture is discussed in the chapter 'Nursing care of people with musculoskeletal trauma'.

Muscles

The three types of muscle tissue in the body are skeletal muscle, smooth muscle and cardiac muscle (see Table 37.1). This discussion focuses on skeletal muscle, the only muscle that allows musculoskeletal function. Skeletal muscles attach to and cover the bones of the skeleton. Skeletal muscles promote body movement, help maintain posture and produce body heat. They may be moved by conscious, voluntary control or by reflex activity. The body has approximately 600 skeletal muscles (see Figure 37.5).

Skeletal muscles are thick bundles of parallel multinucleated contractile cells called fibres. Each single muscle fibre is itself a bundle of smaller structures called myofibrils. The myofibrils have alternating light and dark bands that give skeletal muscle its striated (striped) appearance under an electron microscope. Myofibrils are strands of smaller repeating units called sarcomeres, which consist of thick filaments of myosin and thin filaments of actin, proteins that contribute to muscle contraction.

TABLE 37.1 Types of body muscle

TYPE	DESCRIPTION	EXAMPLES
Skeletal	Striated, voluntary muscle (can consciously move) can contract rapidly and vigorously, and is adaptable	Biceps, triceps, deltoid, gluteus maximus
Smooth	Non-striated, involuntary muscle (cannot consciously move)	Muscles in the walls of the bladder, stomach and bronchi
Cardiac	Striated, involuntary muscle	Heart muscle

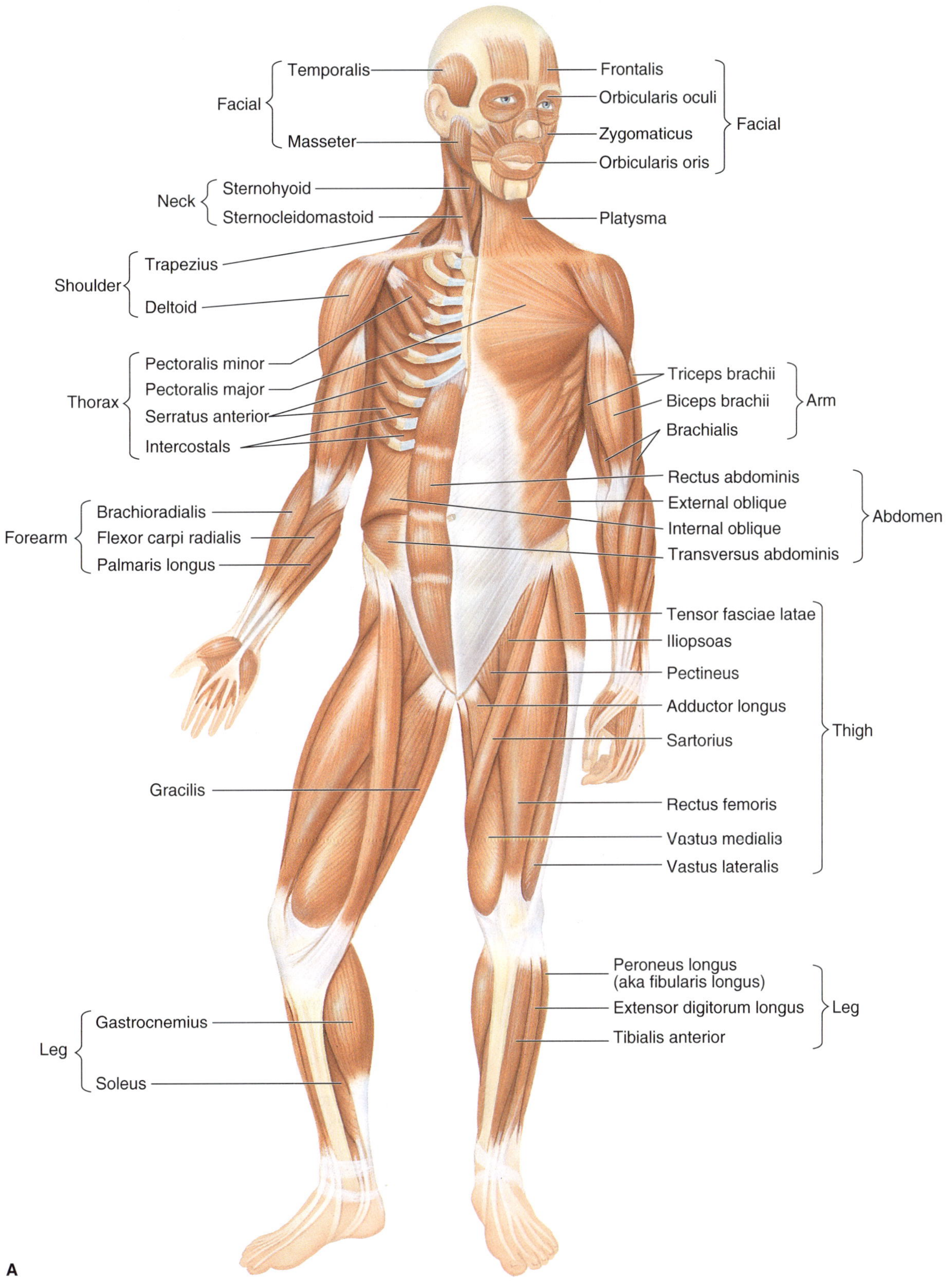

FIGURE 37.5 ***A, Muscles of the anterior body***

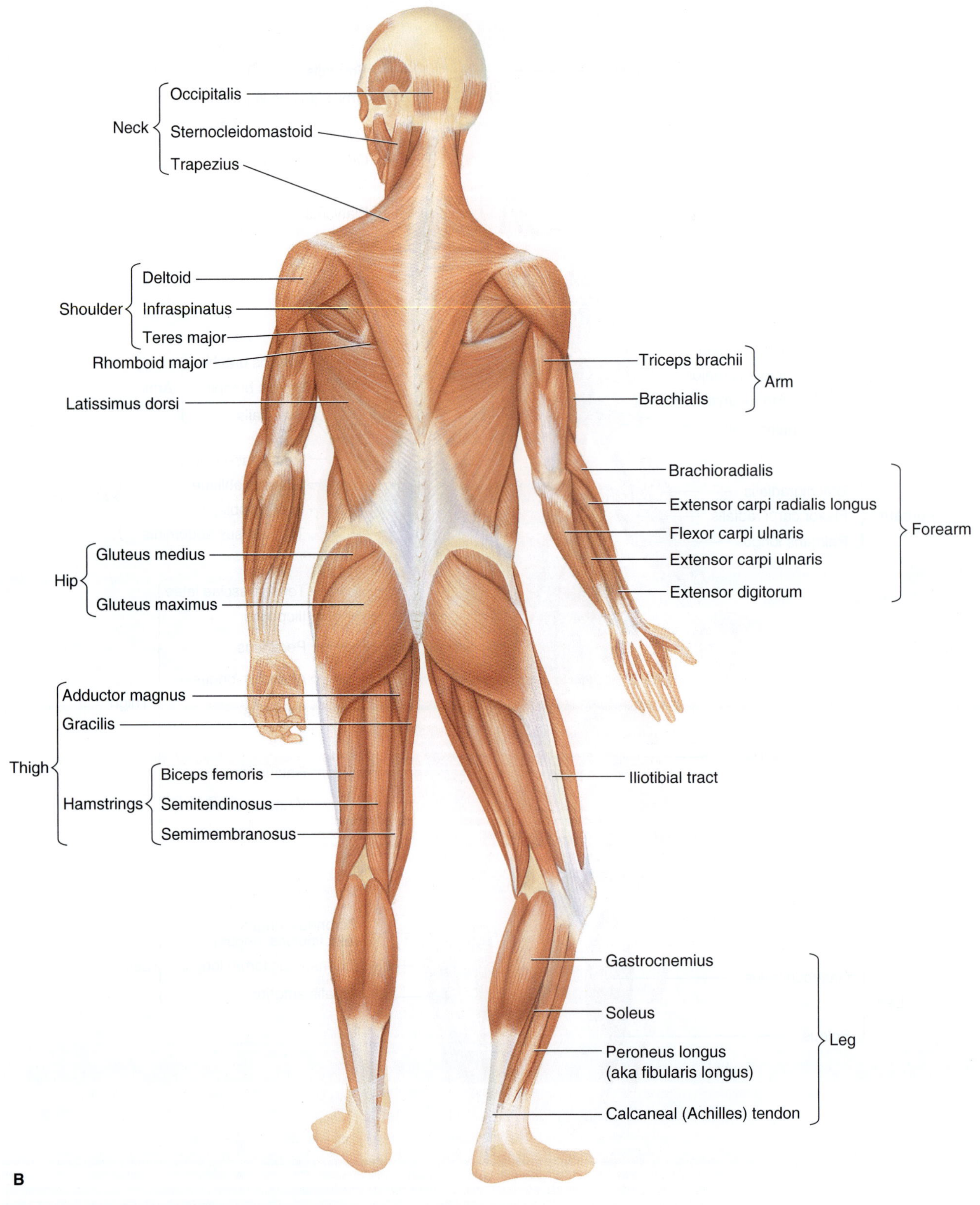

FIGURE 37.5 *B, Muscles of the posterior body*

Skeletal muscle cells have typical functional properties:

- *Excitability*: the ability to receive and respond to a stimulus. The stimulus is usually a neurotransmitter released by a neuron and the response is the generation and transmission of an action potential along the plasma membrane of the muscle cell.
- *Contractibility*: the ability to respond to a stimulus by forcibly shortening.
- *Extensibility*: the ability to respond to a stimulus by extending and relaxing; muscle fibres shorten when they contract and extend when they relax.
- *Elasticity*: the ability to resume its resting length after it has shortened or lengthened.

Skeletal muscle movement is triggered when motor neurons release acetylcholine, a neurotransmitter that crosses the neuromuscular junction and alters the permeability of the muscle fibre. Sodium ions enter the fibre, producing an action potential that causes muscle contraction. The more fibres that contract, the stronger the contraction of the entire muscle.

Prolonged strenuous activity causes continuous nerve impulses and eventually results in a build-up of lactic acid and reduced energy in the muscle, or muscle fatigue. However, continuous nerve impulses are also responsible for maintaining muscle tone. Lack of use results in muscle atrophy, whereas regular exercise increases the size and strength of muscles.

Joints, ligaments and tendons

Joints, or articulations, are regions where two or more bones meet. Joints hold the bones of the skeleton together while allowing the body to move. Joints may be classified by function as synarthroses, amphiarthroses or diarthroses. Table 37.2 describes each of these types. Joints are also classified by structure as fibrous, cartilaginous or synovial.

Fibrous joints

Fibrous joints permit little or no movement because the articulating bones are joined either by short connective tissue fibres that bind the bones together, as with the sutures of the skull, or by short cords of fibrous tissue called ligaments, which permit slight articulation but give no true movement.

TABLE 37.2 Functional classification of joints

TYPE	DESCRIPTION	EXAMPLES
Synarthrosis	Immovable joint	Skull sutures Epiphyseal plates Joint between first rib and manubrium of sternum
Amphiarthrosis	Slightly movable joint	Vertebral joints Joint of the pubic symphysis
Diarthrosis	Freely movable joint	Joints of the limbs Shoulder/hip joints

Cartilaginous joints

Some cartilaginous joints, such as the sternocostal joints of the rib cage, are composed of hyaline cartilage growths that fuse together the articulating bone ends. These joints are immobile. In other cartilaginous joints, such as the intervertebral discs, the hyaline cartilage fuses to an intervening plate of flexible fibrocartilage. This structural feature accounts for the flexibility of the vertebral column.

Synovial joints

Bones in synovial joints are enclosed by a cavity that is filled with synovial fluid, a filtrate of blood plasma (see Figure 37.6). Synovial joints are freely movable, allowing many kinds of movements, as listed and described in Table 37.3. Synovial joints are found at all articulations of the limbs.

They have several characteristics:

- The articular surfaces are covered with articular cartilage.
- The joint cavity is enclosed by a tough, fibrous, double-layered articular capsule; internally, the cavity is lined with a synovial membrane that covers all surfaces not covered by the articular cartilage.
- Synovial fluid fills the free spaces of the joint capsule, enhancing the smooth movement of the articulating bones.

Bursae are small sacs of synovial fluid that cushion and protect bony areas that are at high risk of friction, such as the knee and the shoulder. Tendon sheaths are a form of bursae, but they are wrapped around tendons in high-friction areas.

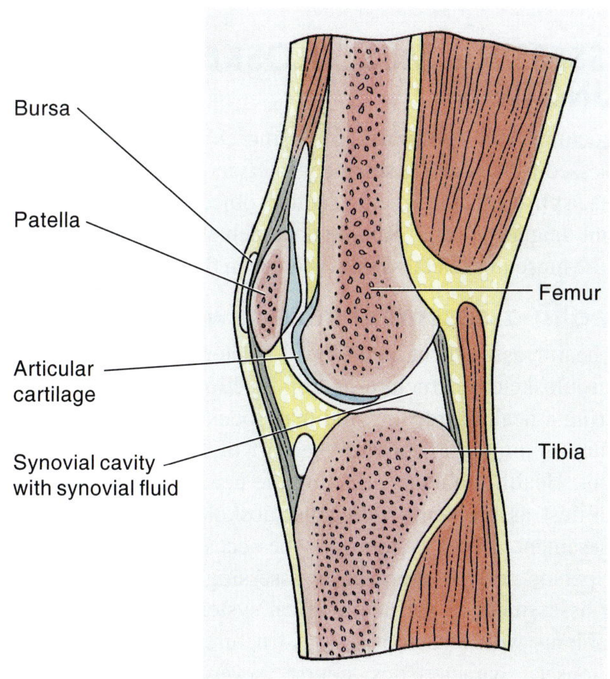

FIGURE 37.6 ***Structure of a synovial joint (knee)***

Source: DK Images.

TABLE 37.3 Movements allowed by synovial joints

TYPE	DESCRIPTION
Abduction	Move limb away from body midline
Adduction	Move limb towards body midline
Extension	Straighten limbs at joint
Flexion	Bend limbs at joint
Dorsiflexion	Bend ankle to bring top of foot towards shin
Plantar flexion	Straighten ankle to point toes down
Pronation	Turn forearm to place palm down
Supination	Turn forearm to place palm up
Eversion	Turn out
Inversion	Turn in
Circumduction	Move in circle
Internal rotation	Move inwards on a central axis
External rotation	Move outwards on a central axis
Protraction	Move forwards and parallel to ground
Retraction	Move backwards and parallel to ground

The fibrous capsules that surround synovial joints are supported by ligaments, dense bands of connective tissue that connect bones to bones. Ligaments limit or enhance movement, provide joint stability and enhance joint strength. Tendons are fibrous connective tissue bands that connect muscles to the periosteum of bones and enable the bones to move when skeletal muscles contract. When muscles contract, increased pressure causes the tendon to pull, push or rotate the bone to which it is connected.

ASSESSING MUSCULOSKELETAL FUNCTION

Structures and functions of the musculoskeletal system are assessed by a health assessment interview to collect subjective data, a physical assessment to collect objective data and findings from diagnostic tests. Sample documentation of an assessment of the musculoskeletal system is given in the accompanying box.

Health assessment interview

A health assessment interview to determine problems with musculoskeletal structure and/or function may be conducted during a health screening and may focus on a chief complaint (such as joint pain) or may be part of a total health assessment. Health problems affecting the neurological system may manifest as problems with musculoskeletal function, and an assessment of both systems may be necessary. (See the chapter 'A person-centred approach to assessing the nervous system' for assessment of the neurological system.) If the person has problems with musculoskeletal structure or function, analyse its onset, characteristics, course, severity, precipitating and relieving factors, and any associated symptoms, noting the timing and circumstances. For example, ask the person:

- Describe the pain you have had in your elbow. Does the pain increase with movement? Have you noticed any redness or swelling?

SAMPLE DOCUMENTATION

Assessment of the musculoskeletal system

7/4/2023 NURS 0900 hrs	58-year-old Caucasian male (preferred pronoun 'he') employed as a roofer, comes to the orthopaedic clinic for evaluation of chronic knee pain. The person states, 'The pain in my knees is worse when I get up in the morning and when I carry something heavy at work.' Posture erect, gait even without obvious limp. Bones of lower extremities appear equal in size and shape bilaterally. No swelling noted, bulge test negative for fluid around knee. Crepitus heard in both knees during flexion and extension. Range of motion (ROM) in both knees slightly decreased. No obvious decrease in muscle mass. The person states that his knee pain during ROM is a 3 on a 1 to 10 scale. Referred to clinic physician for further evaluation, including x-rays of both knees. R Coleman (REX COLEMAN, RN)

- Did you injure your ankle before you began to experience difficulty walking?
- Is your pain worse in the morning or does it get worse throughout the day?

The primary manifestations of altered function of the musculoskeletal system are pain and limited mobility. Specific descriptors of the pain, its location and its nature are important. Other significant information includes associated manifestations, such as fever, fatigue, changes in weight or skin colour, rash and/or swelling. Also collect information about the person's lifestyle: type of employment, ability to carry out activities of daily living (ADLs) and provide self-care, exercise or participation in sports, use of alcohol or drugs, and nutrition. Explore past injuries and measures to self-treat pain (such as over-the-counter (OTC) medications, prescribed medications, application of heat or cold, splinting, wrapping or rest).

Interview questions categorised by functional health patterns are listed in the 'Functional health pattern interview' box.

Physical assessment

Physical assessment of the musculoskeletal system may be performed either as part of a total assessment or alone for a person with specific musculoskeletal problems. The techniques used to assess the musculoskeletal system are inspection, palpation and measurement of muscle mass and range of motion (ROM). The person should be comfortably dressed in clothing that lets you see the movement of all joints clearly. The person may be standing, sitting or lying down; the sequence of the examination should be such that the person does not have frequent position changes. An assessment of an older adult, person in pain or person who is tired may take extra time. Normal age-related findings for the older adult are summarised in Table 37.4.

FUNCTIONAL HEALTH PATTERN INTERVIEW Musculoskeletal system

FUNCTIONAL HEALTH PATTERN	INTERVIEW QUESTIONS AND LEADING STATEMENTS
Health perception–Health management	▪ Have you ever had any muscle or bone diseases or injuries? If so, describe them.
	▪ Describe any surgery, physical therapy, heat or other treatments you have received for problems with your muscles or bones.
	▪ List any medications, such as muscle relaxants or prescribed or over-the-counter (OTC) medications and ointments you use for musculoskeletal problems.
	▪ Do you take any herbal or nutritional supplements for musculoskeletal problems (e.g. calcium tablets)? If so, what and how often?
Nutritional–Metabolic	▪ Describe your dietary intake in a typical 24-hour period. Does your diet include milk, cheese, cottage cheese and vegetables? If so, how often?
	▪ Do you take vitamins and/or additional calcium supplements? If so, what type and how often?
	▪ Have you had a recent weight gain or loss? What do you see as your ideal weight?
	▪ Have you had any redness or swelling in your joints?
Elimination	▪ Does your musculoskeletal problem make it difficult for you to get to the bathroom?
Activity–Exercise	▪ Describe your usual activities for a 24-hour period.
	▪ Describe any musculoskeletal problems (such as limited movement, weakness, stiffness, pain) that limit your activities of daily living (ADLs), such as driving, gardening, dressing, bathing, walking, climbing stairs, cooking or cleaning.
	▪ Has there been a change in your usual ability to move around? Describe.
	▪ Do you regularly exercise or take part in strenuous activities such as heavy lifting? Describe. If you have to lift heavy objects at work, do you use any type of special equipment? Describe.
	▪ Do you use any assistive devices (such as a cane or walker) to help move around?
Sleep–Rest	▪ Does having this problem with your musculoskeletal system interfere with your ability to rest and sleep? If so, how, and what do you do?
Cognitive–Perceptual	▪ Describe any muscle, bone or joint pain that you have. What relieves it or makes it worse?
	▪ Describe any changes in the colour, temperature or sensations in your extremities.
	▪ Describe any muscle weakness you are experiencing.
	▪ Do you have stiffness in your joints when you wake up? Does it get better with movement?
	▪ Do you ever have muscle cramps?
Self-perception–Self-concept	▪ How does having this condition make you feel about yourself?
Role–Relationships	▪ How has having this condition affected your personal/intimate relationships with others?
	▪ Has having this condition interfered with your ability to work? Explain.
	▪ Has anyone in your family had problems with bone, joint or muscle disease? Explain.
Sexuality–Reproductive	▪ Has this condition interfered with your usual sexual activity?
Coping–Stress– Tolerance	▪ Has having this condition created stress for you?
	▪ Have you experienced any kind of stress that makes the condition worse? Explain.
	▪ Describe what you do when you feel stressed.
Value–Belief	▪ Describe how specific relationships or activities help you cope with this problem.
	▪ Describe specific cultural beliefs or practices that affect how you care for and feel about this problem.
	▪ Are there any specific treatments that you would not use to treat this problem?

TABLE 37.4 Age-related changes in the musculoskeletal system

AGE-RELATED CHANGE	SIGNIFICANCE
Bones and joints: • ↓ bone mass and minerals. • ↓ calcium reabsorption, a slow resorption of the interior of long bones and slower production of new bone on the outside surface of bones. • Vertebrae shorten and intervertebral discs thin, and kyphosis often occurs. • Cartilage on bone surfaces in joints deteriorates and bone spurs may occur.	Decreased bone mass as well as decreased calcium absorption contributes to bones that are often thinner and weaker, with an increased risk of fractures with trauma. As the spinal column shortens, height decreases. Loss of joint cartilage and formation of bone spurs makes movement more painful and may even limit mobility. Especially common in older adults.
Muscles: • Muscle fibres atrophy and fibrous tissue slowly replaces muscle tissue. • ↓ muscle mass and strength. • ↓ muscle movements, especially in the arms and legs. • Range of motion decreases. • Tendons shrink and harden. • Muscle cramping is common.	Regular exercise is very important in decreasing the loss associated with ageing in terms of maintaining muscle mass, strength and agility.

Prior to the examination, collect all equipment and explain the techniques to decrease the person's anxiety. The sequence for a musculoskeletal examination follows:

1. Begin the examination with an assessment of gait and posture. Observe how the person walks, sits and/or moves about in bed.
2. Inspect and palpate the bones for any obvious deformity or changes in size or shape. Palpation also will elicit tenderness or pain.
3. Measure the extremities for length and circumference. Before taking measurements, make sure the person is lying in a comfortable position. Remember to compare limbs bilaterally.
4. Assess muscle mass by first inspecting for obvious increase or decrease in size. Assess and document muscle strength on a scale of 0 to 5 (see Table 37.5). Box 37.1 provides instructions for testing the strength of various muscles.
5. Assess joints for swelling, pain, redness, warmth, crepitus and ROM. Only assess the ROM of every joint if the person has a specific musculoskeletal problem; however, assessing one or more joints is a common part of nursing care. Use a goniometer for precise measurements of joint ROM (see Figure 37.7). This device has a pointer joined to a protractor at 0 degrees. The two arms are placed along articulating bones and the angle of joint movement is recorded in degrees.

TABLE 37.5 Muscle grading scale

GRADE	ASSESSMENT DESCRIPTION
0	(No visible) contraction; paralysis
1	Can feel contraction of muscle but there is no movement of limb
2	Passive ROM
3	Full ROM against gravity
4	Full ROM against some resistance
5	Full ROM against full resistance

BOX 37.1 Guidelines for assessing muscle strength

In adults, muscles are usually strong and equally strong bilaterally. However, neuromuscular diseases, disuse, metabolic disorders or infections can cause muscle weakness. Muscle strength is expected to be greater in the dominant arm and leg. In most instances (and especially when moving digits and extremities), the nurse provides resistance by pushing in the opposite direction.

The muscles listed below are routinely tested. Instructions for the person are also provided.

MUSCLE	INSTRUCTIONS FOR THE PERSON
Ocular muscles and lids	Close eyes tightly.
Finger muscles	Shake hands. Make a fist. Spread fingers.
Facial muscles	Blow out cheeks. Stick out tongue.
Hip muscles	Raise straight leg while supine.
Neck muscles	Bend head forwards and backwards.
Gluteal and leg muscles	Alternately cross legs while sitting.
Deltoid muscles	Hold arms up.
Biceps muscle	Bend the arm.
Quadriceps muscle	Straighten leg.
Triceps muscle	Straighten the arm.
Wrist muscles	Bend hand forwards and backwards.
Ankle and foot muscles	Bend foot up and down.

Diagnostic tests

The results of diagnostic tests of musculoskeletal structure and function are used to support the diagnosis of a specific injury or disease, to provide information to identify or modify the appropriate medications or therapy used to treat the disease, and to help nurses monitor the person's responses

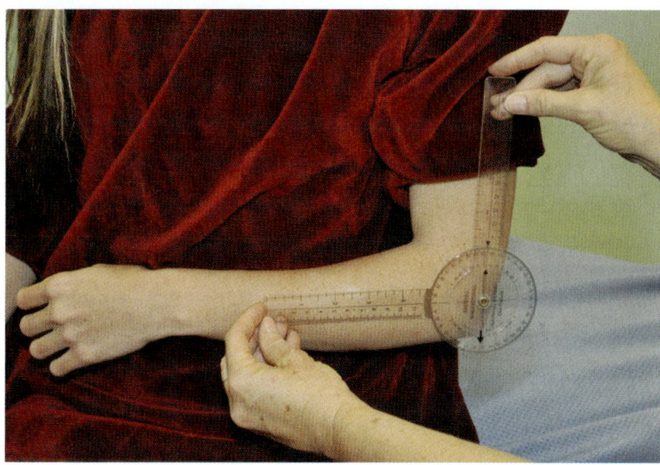

FIGURE 37.7 *Using a goniometer to measure joint ROM*

to treatment and nursing care interventions. Diagnostic tests to assess the structures and functions of the musculoskeletal system are described in the 'Diagnostic tests' box and summarised in the following bulleted list. More information is included in the discussion of specific injuries or diseases in the chapters 'Nursing care of people with musculoskeletal trauma' and 'Nursing care of people with musculoskeletal disorders'.

- Blood tests are used to monitor levels of alkaline phosphatase, calcium, uric acid and creatine kinase, which are commonly increased in bone and joint diseases and muscle trauma (see Table 37.6).
- Radiological examinations, including x-rays, CT scans, MRIs and bone scans, are done to identify and evaluate bone density and structure in conditions such as arthritis, intervertebral disc disease, musculoskeletal trauma, muscle tears, osteomyelitis and bone tumours.
- Bone density examinations (dual energy x-ray absorptiometry (DEXA), quantitative ultrasound (QUS) and bone mineral density (BMD)) are done to evaluate bone mineral density and evaluate the degree of osteoporosis.
- An arthroscopy uses a fibre-optic endoscope to examine the joint interior, to diagnose diseases and to perform surgery. An arthrocentesis is done to withdraw fluid from a joint by needle aspiration.
- Both an electromyogram (EMG) and a somatosensory evoked potential (SSEP) are tests of the electrical activity of skeletal muscle.

Regardless of the type of diagnostic test, the nurse is responsible for explaining the procedure and any special preparation needed, for assessing for medication use that may affect the outcome of the tests, for supporting the person during the examination as necessary, for documenting the procedures as appropriate, and for monitoring the results of the tests.

TABLE 37.6 Blood tests with purposes specific to the musculoskeletal system

NAME OF TEST	PURPOSE	NORMAL VALUE
Alkaline phosphatase (ALP)	To identify bone diseases. Increased in bone cancer, Paget's disease, healing fractures, rheumatoid arthritis and osteoporosis	Neonate: 50–300 U/L Growing child: 70–350 U/L Adult, non-pregnant: 25–100 U/L Higher levels are seen in the third trimester of pregnancy and in individuals over 50 years of age
Calcium (Ca)	To monitor calcium levels and detect calcium imbalances. Decreased with lack of calcium and vitamin D intake and malabsorption from the gastrointestinal tract. Increased in bone cancer and multiple fractures	4.5–5.5 mEq/L or 9–11 mg/dL (serum) Total calcium: 2.10–2.60 mmol/L Corrected calcium: 2.15–2.60 mmol/L Ionised calcium: 1.16–1.30 mmol/L
Phosphorus (P), phosphate (PO_4)	To assess phosphorus levels. Increased with bone tumours and healing fractures	1.7–2.6 mEq/L or 2.5–4.5 mg/dL Adult: 0.8–1.5 mmol/L Levels are slightly higher in children
Rheumatoid factor (RF)	To diagnose rheumatoid arthritis (RA) (positive for RA at > 1:80 titre). Also increased in lupus erythematosus and scleroderma	< 1:20 titre < 30 IU/L
Uric acid	To diagnose and monitor the treatment of gout. Panic level considered > 12 mg/dL	Male: 3.5–8.0 mg/dL Female: 2.8–6.8 mg/dL
Human leucocyte antigen (HLA)	To diagnose diseases such as juvenile rheumatoid arthritis or ankylosing spondylitis	Match or no match; no normal values
Creatine kinase (CK)	To diagnose muscle trauma or disease. Increased in muscular dystrophy and traumatic injuries (specifically, CPK-MM isoenzyme)	Neonate: 70–380 U/L Adult female: 30–180 U/L Adult male: 60–220 U/L

DIAGNOSTIC TESTS The musculoskeletal system

NAME OF TEST Blood chemistry **PURPOSE AND DESCRIPTION** See Table 37.6.	**RELATED NURSING CARE** No special preparation is needed.
NAME OF TEST X-ray **PURPOSE AND DESCRIPTION** X-rays are done to identify and evaluate bone density and structure. Injection of contrast medium with an accompanying x-ray may be done to visualise joint structures, intervertebral discs and wounds deep in muscle.	**RELATED NURSING CARE** No special preparation needed for standard x-rays. If contrast medium is used, assess for allergy to shellfish, iodine or contrast medium used in previous tests. If allergy is present, test will not be performed.
NAME OF TEST Computed tomography (CT) scan **PURPOSE AND DESCRIPTION** Provides a three-dimensional picture used to evaluate musculoskeletal trauma and bony abnormalities.	**RELATED NURSING CARE** No special preparation is needed.
NAME OF TEST Magnetic resonance imaging (MRI) **PURPOSE AND DESCRIPTION** Used in diagnosis and evaluation of avascular necrosis, osteomyelitis, tumours, disc abnormalities and tears in ligament or cartilage. Uses radiowaves and magnetic fields; gadolinium may be injected to increase visualisation of bony or muscular structures.	**RELATED NURSING CARE** Assess for metallic implants or metal on clothing. (Metallic implants, such as clips on aneurysms, pacemakers or shrapnel, will prohibit having an MRI.)
NAME OF TEST Bone scan **PURPOSE AND DESCRIPTION** Degree of uptake of a radioisotope (based on blood supply to bone) is measured with a Geiger counter and recorded on paper. Uptake is increased in osteomyelitis, osteoporosis, cancers of the bone and in some fractures. Uptake is decreased in avascular necrosis.	**RELATED NURSING CARE** No special preparation is needed; tell the person to increase oral fluids after the test to aid in excretion of the radioisotope.
NAME OF TEST Bone density (BD) ■ Dual energy x-ray absorptiometry (DEXA) ■ Quantitative ultrasound (QUS) ■ Bone mineral density (BMD) ■ Bone absorptiometry **PURPOSE AND DESCRIPTION** Bone density examinations are done to evaluate bone mineral density and to evaluate degree of osteoporosis. DEXA can calculate the size and thickness of bone and detect even a 1% loss of bone mass.	Osteoporosis is diagnosed if the peak bone mass level is below > 2.5 standard deviations. **Normal value:** 1 standard deviation below peak bone mass. **RELATED NURSING CARE** No special preparation is needed. Assess for previous fractures, which may increase bone density.
NAME OF TEST Arthroscopy **PURPOSE AND DESCRIPTION** An endoscopic examination of the interior surfaces of a joint, used to perform surgery and diagnose diseases of the patella, meniscus and synovial and extrasynovial membranes. In addition, fluid may be drained from the joint and tissue removed for biopsy. A fibre-optic endoscope is inserted into the joint, with either local or general anaesthesia.	**RELATED NURSING CARE** If general anaesthesia is used, the person is nil by mouth at least 6–8 hours prior to surgery. Following the procedure, assess for bleeding and swelling, apply ice to the area if prescribed and teach the person to avoid excessive use of the joint for 2 to 3 days.

DIAGNOSTIC TESTS **The musculoskeletal system (continued)**

NAME OF TEST Arthrocentesis

PURPOSE AND DESCRIPTION Done to obtain synovial fluid from a joint for diagnosis (such as infections) or to remove excess fluid. A needle is inserted through the joint capsule and fluid is aspirated.

RELATED NURSING CARE No special preparation is needed. Apply compression dressing and assess for bleeding and leakage of fluid following the procedure.

NAME OF TEST Electromyogram (EMG)

PURPOSE AND DESCRIPTION Measures the electrical activity of skeletal muscles at rest and during contraction; useful in diagnosing neuromuscular diseases. Needle electrodes are inserted into skeletal muscle (as on the legs) and electrical activity can be heard, viewed on an oscilloscope and recorded on graph paper. Normally, there is no electrical activity at rest.

RELATED NURSING CARE Tell the person not to drink fluids containing caffeine or to smoke for 3 hours before the test and not to take medications such as muscle relaxants, anticholinergics or cholinergics.

NAME OF TEST Somatosensory evoked potential (SSEP)

PURPOSE AND DESCRIPTION Measures nerve conduction along pathways to evaluate evoked potential of muscle contractions. Used to identify dysfunction of lower motor neurons as well as muscle disease. Transcutaneous or percutaneous electrodes are applied to the skin and provide recordings.

RELATED NURSING CARE No special preparation is needed.

Genetic considerations

When conducting a health assessment interview and a physical assessment, it is important for the nurse to consider genetic influences on health. During the health assessment interview, ask about family members with health problems affecting musculoskeletal structure or function including a family history of arthritis, abnormally long bones, muscular dystrophy and motor neurone disease. During the physical assessment, assess for any manifestations that might indicate a genetic disorder (see the 'Genetic considerations' box). If data are found to indicate genetic risk factors or alterations, ask about genetic testing and refer for appropriate genetic counselling and evaluation. The chapter 'Genetic implications of adult health nursing' provides further information about genetics in medical–surgical nursing (Norris, 2018).

GENETIC CONSIDERATIONS **Musculoskeletal disorders**

- Myotonic dystrophy is an inherited disorder in which the muscles become weak, have a decreased ability to relax and eventually waste away. Other effects are mental deficiency, hair loss and cataracts. Although rare, the disease does increase in severity with each successive generation.
- Marfan syndrome, an autosomal dominant disorder of connective tissue, affects the bones, lungs, eyes, heart and blood vessels. It is characterised by abnormally long extremities and is believed to have affected Abraham Lincoln. The aspect of the disease that is most life threatening is the effect on the cardiovascular system. With advances in the diagnosis, evaluation and management of the organ abnormalities associated with Marfan syndrome, the life expectancy for a person with the disease has nearly doubled in the past 25 years. Today, individuals with Marfan syndrome can expect to have a life expectancy comparable to that of the general population (Marfan Association Victoria, 2022).
- Ellis–van Creveld syndrome is a rare genetic disorder characterised by a variety of physical alterations, including short-limb dwarfism, additional fingers or toes, malformed wrists, cardiac abnormalities and partial tooth eruption.
- Duchenne muscular dystrophy, an X-linked disorder, primarily affects males. It is one of the most common muscular dystrophies and is characterised by rapid muscle degeneration early in life.
- Motor neurone disease is a neurological disease that affects the motor neurons in the spinal cord and brain, eventually resulting in paralysis and death.
- Other musculoskeletal diseases believed to have a genetic component include rheumatoid arthritis, osteoarthritis, gout, muscular dystrophy, ankylosing spondylitis, lupus erythematosus and scleroderma.

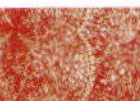

MUSCULOSKELETAL ASSESSMENTS

Technique/normal findings	Abnormal findings
Gait and body posture	
Inspect body posture and gait. *Body posture should be upright; gait should be smooth and steady.*	■ Joint stiffness, pain, deformities and muscle weakness can cause changes in gait and posture.
Inspect the spine for curvature. Ask the person to stand and bend back slowly as far as possible, bend slowly to the right and then to the left as far as possible, turn slowly to the right and left in a circular motion, and bend forwards slowly and try to touch fingers to toes. *When viewed from the back, the cervical and lumbar spine are concave, the thoracic spine is convex and the spine is straight.*	■ With herniated lumbar discs, the lumbar curve flattens and spinal mobility is decreased. ■ An increased lumbar curve, called **lordosis**, may be seen in obesity or pregnancy. ■ A lateral, S-shaped curvature of the spine is called **scoliosis**. Functional scoliosis usually is a compensatory response to painful paravertebral muscles, herniated discs or discrepancy in leg length. It disappears with forward flexion. Structural scoliosis is often congenital and tends to appear during adolescence. It is accentuated with forward bending. ■ **Kyphosis** is an exaggerated thoracic curvature of the spine common in older adults.
Joints	
Inspect the joints for deformity, swelling and redness. *There should be no visible deformity, swelling or redness of joints.*	■ Diseases of the joints may be manifested by such deformities as tissue loss, tissue overgrowth or contractures or irreversible shortenings of muscles and tendons. ■ Disease in a joint may cause obvious bulging. ■ Redness, swelling and pain are evidence of an inflammation or infection in the joint.
Palpate the joints for tenderness, warmth, crepitation, consistency and muscle mass. *Joints should be non-tender and consistent bilaterally and without visible or palpable excess warmth, crepitation or masses.*	■ Inflammation and injury cause joint pain. ■ Arthritis, bursitis, tendonitis and osteomyelitis (infection of a bone) result in painful, hot joints. ■ **Crepitation** (a grating sound) is present in a joint when the articulating surfaces have lost their cartilage, such as in arthritis.
Range-of-motion	
Assess joint ROM by asking the person to perform activities specific to each joint, as described below. *All bilateral joints should move through full range of motion.*	■ Clicking or popping noises, decreased ROM, pain and swelling may indicate temporomandibular joint syndrome or, in rare cases, osteoarthritis.
Temporomandibular joint: 'Open your mouth wide and then close your mouth.' (As the person opens and closes the mouth, palpate the temporomandibular joints with your index and middle fingers, as shown in Figure 37.8.)	

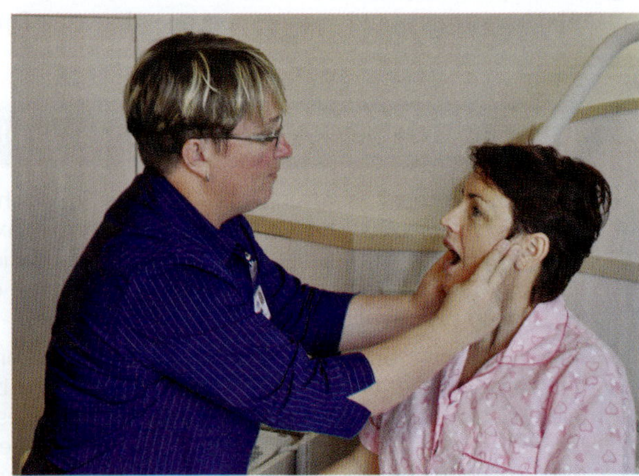

FIGURE 37.8 *Palpating the temporomandibular joints*

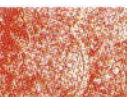

MUSCULOSKELETAL ASSESSMENTS (continued)

Technique/normal findings	Abnormal findings
Cervical spine: 45-degree flexion: 'Touch your chin to your chest.' 55-degree extension: 'Look at the ceiling.' 40-degree lateral bending: 'Try to touch your right ear to your right shoulder.' Repeat with the left side. 70-degree rotation: 'Try to touch your chin to each shoulder.'	■ Neck pain and limited extension with lateral bending are seen with herniated cervical discs and in cervical spondylosis. ■ An immobile neck with head and neck thrust forwards is seen with ankylosing spondylitis.
Lumbar spine: 75 to 90-degree flexion: 'Touch your toes with your fingers' (see Figure 37.9A). 30-degree extension: 'Bend backwards slowly.' 35-degree lateral bending: 'Bend right and left' (see Figure 37.9B). 30-degree rotation: 'Twist your shoulders right and left' (see Figure 37.9C).	■ Decreased movement or pain with movement may indicate an abnormal spinal curvature, arthritis, herniated disc or spasm of paravertebral muscles.

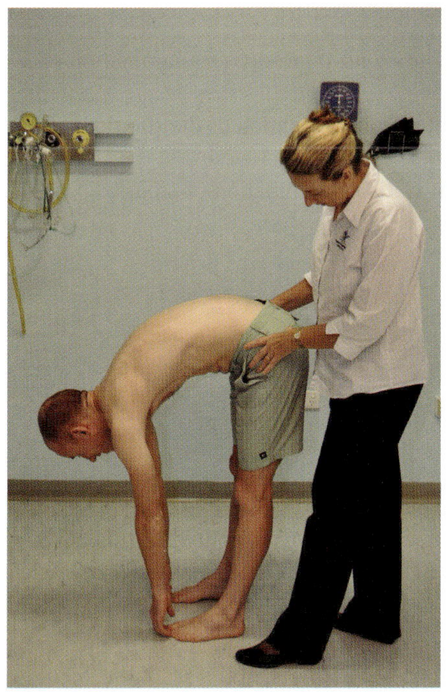

A

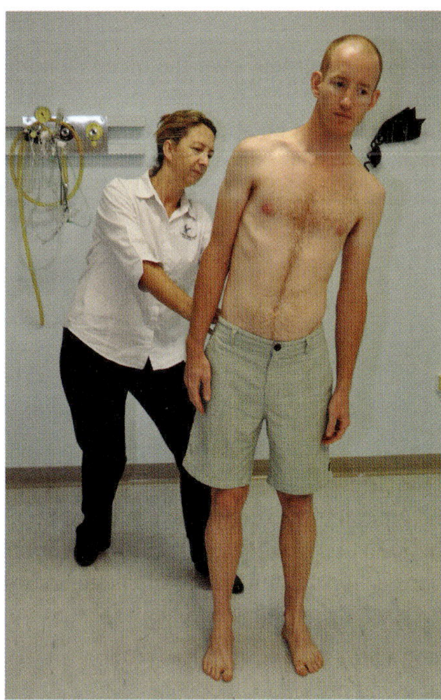

B

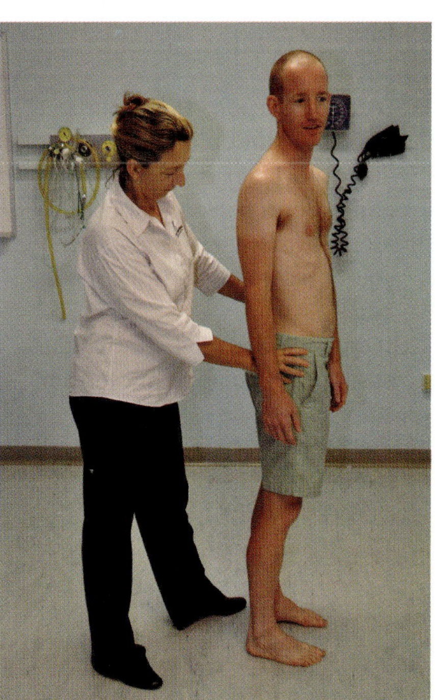

C

FIGURE 37.9 *A, Forward flexion of spine. B, Lateral flexion of spine. C, Rotation of spine*

(continued)

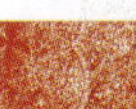

MUSCULOSKELETAL ASSESSMENTS (continued)

Technique/normal findings	Abnormal findings
Fingers: Flexion: 'Make a fist.' Extension: 'Open your hand.' Abduction: 'Spread your fingers.' Adduction: 'Close your fingers.'	■ Flexion and extension of fingers are decreased in arthritis. ■ Heberden's nodes and Bouchard's nodes are hard, non-tender nodules on the dorsolateral parts of the distal and proximal interphalangeal joints, respectively. They are common in osteoarthritis. ■ Stiff, painful, swollen finger joints are seen in acute rheumatoid arthritis. ■ Boutonnière and swan-neck deformities are seen in chronic rheumatoid arthritis. ■ Swollen finger joints with a white chalky discharge may be seen in chronic gout.
Wrists: 90-degree flexion: 'Bend wrist down.' 70-degree extension: 'Bend wrist up.' 55-degree ulnar deviation: 'Bend wrist towards little finger.' 20-degree radial deviation: 'Bend wrist towards thumb.'	■ Bilateral chronic swelling in the wrist is seen in arthritis.
Elbows: 160-degree flexion: 'Touch your hands to your shoulders.' 180-degree extension: 'Straighten your elbows.' 90-degree supination: 'Bend your elbows 90 degrees and turn hands palm up.' 90-degree pronation: 'Bend your elbows 90 degrees and turn fists down.'	■ Swollen, tender, inflamed elbows are apparent in gouty arthritis and rheumatoid arthritis. ■ Pain and tenderness at the lateral epicondyle occur in tennis elbow.
Shoulders: 180-degree flexion: 'Hold your arms straight up and out.' 50-degree hyperextension: 'Put your straight arm behind your back.' 90-degree internal rotation: 'Put your forearm behind your lower back.' 180-degree abduction: 'Raise your straight arm up and out to your side.' 50-degree adduction: 'Put your straight arm across your chest.'	■ Pain and tenderness over the biceps tendon occurs with **tendonitis** (inflammation of a tendon). ■ The arm cannot be abducted fully when the supraspinatus tendon of the shoulder is ruptured. ■ Pain and limited abduction is also seen with **bursitis** (inflammation of a bursa) and calcium deposits in this area.
Toes: 90-degree flexion: 'Walk on your toes.'	■ The great toe is excessively abducted in hallux valgus. ■ The joint above the great toe is swollen, inflamed and painful in gouty arthritis. ■ There is hyperextension of the metatarsophalangeal joint and flexion of the proximal interphalangeal joint with hammer toes.
Ankles: 20-degree dorsiflexion: 'Point your foot to the ceiling.' 45-degree plantar flexion: 'Point your foot to the floor.' 30-degree inversion: 'Walk on the outside of your feet.' 20-degree eversion: 'Walk on the inside of your feet.'	■ Contractures of the Achilles tendon may occur in people with rheumatoid arthritis or following prolonged bed rest.

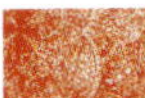

MUSCULOSKELETAL ASSESSMENTS (continued)

Technique/normal findings	Abnormal findings
Knees: 130-degree flexion: 'Do a deep knee bend.' 180-degree extension: 'Sit down and hold your legs straight out in front of you.'	■ Swelling over the suprapatellar pouch is seen with inflammation and fluid in the articular capsule of the knee. **Synovitis** is inflammation of the synovial membrane lining the articular capsule of a joint. It is common with knee trauma. ■ Swelling over the patella is seen in bursitis.
Hips: (The person is lying down.) 120-degree flexion: 'Bring bent knee up to your chest.' 30-degree hyperextension: 'Lie on your abdomen and lift up one leg at a time.' 45-degree abduction: 'Hold your leg straight and move it out to the side.' 40-degree internal rotation: 'Bend your knee and swing it towards your other leg.' 45-degree external rotation: 'Bend your knee and swing it out to the side.'	■ Movement of the hip is limited and/or painful in arthritis.
Special assessments Perform Phalen's test. Ask the person to hold the wrist in acute flexion for 60 seconds (see Figure 37.10). *There should be no tingling, numbness or pain.*	■ Numbness and burning in the fingers during Phalen's test may indicate carpal tunnel syndrome. 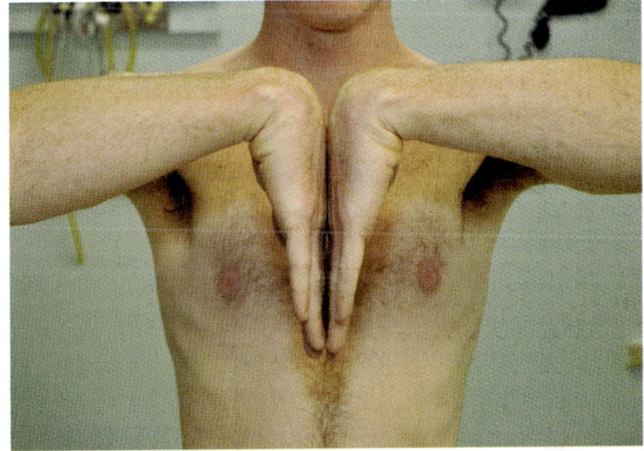 **FIGURE 37.10** ***Phalen's test***
Check for small amounts of fluid on the knee by conducting the bulge test. Milk upwards on the medial side of the knee and then tap the lateral side of the patella (see Figure 37.11). *No bulge of fluid should appear on the medial side of the knee.*	■ A fluid bulge indicates increased fluid in the knee joint rather than soft tissue swelling. 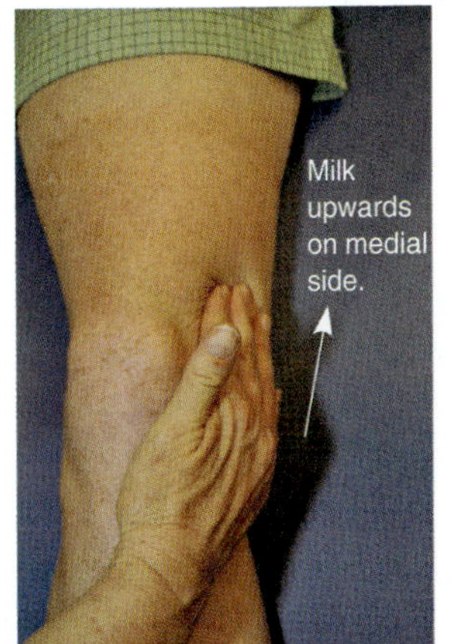 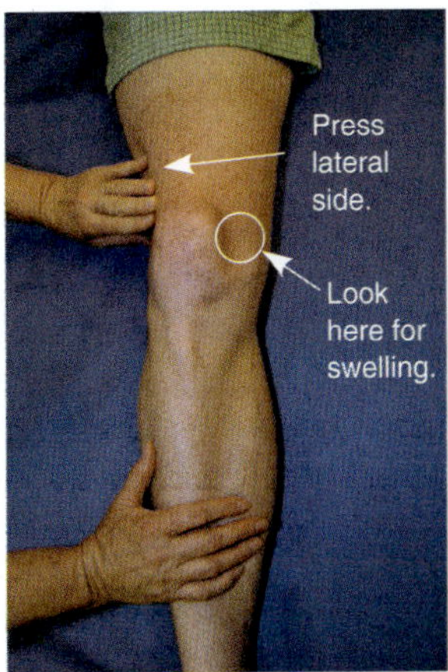 **FIGURE 37.11** ***Checking for the bulge sign***

(continued)

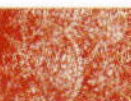

MUSCULOSKELETAL ASSESSMENTS (continued)

Technique/normal findings	Abnormal findings
Conduct the ballottement test to detect large amounts of fluid in the knee. Apply downward pressure on the knee with one hand while pushing the patella backwards against the femur with the other hand (see Figure 37.12). *There should be no movement of the patella. The patella should rest firmly over the femur.*	■ Increased fluid will cause a tapping sound as the patella displaces the fluid and hits the femur.
Perform McMurray's test. While reclining, ask the person to turn the flexed knee towards the centre of the body. Stabilise the knee with one hand and apply pressure on the lower leg with the other hand (see Figure 37.13). *There should be no pain or clicking.*	■ Pain, locking (inability to fully extend the knee) or a popping sound may indicate an injury to a meniscus, a disc of cartilaginous tissue in the knee.
Perform the Thomas test. Ask the person to lie down and extend one leg while bringing the knee of the opposite leg to the chest (see Figure 37.14). *The extended leg should not rise off the table.*	■ A hip flexion contracture will cause the extended leg to rise off the table.

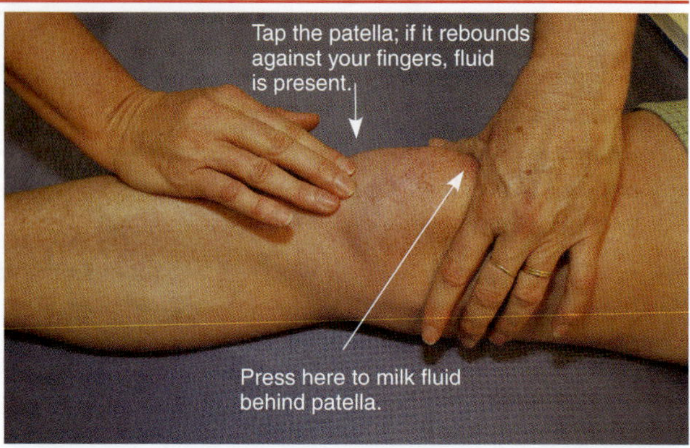

FIGURE 37.12 *Checking for ballottement*

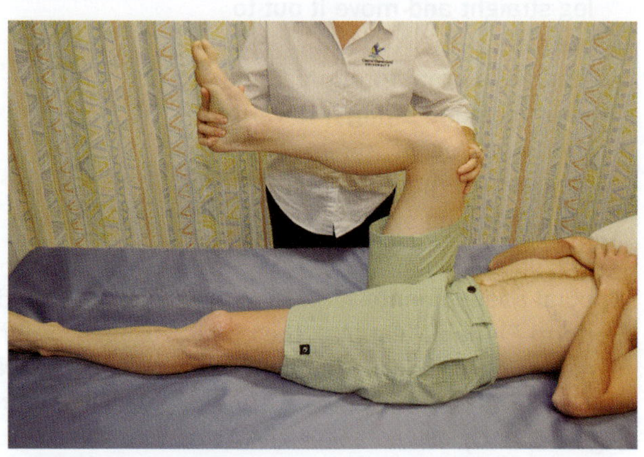

FIGURE 37.13 *McMurray's test*

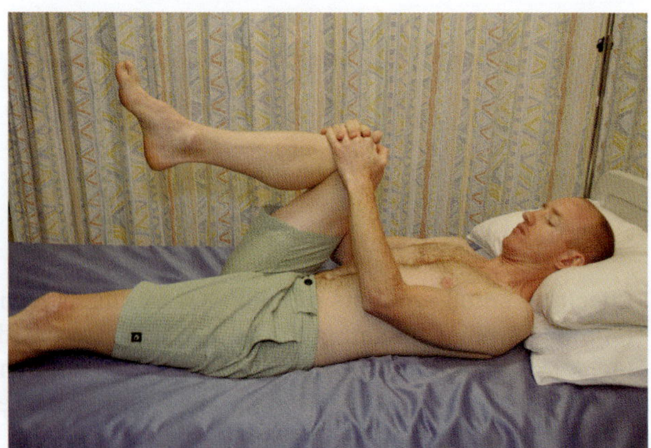

FIGURE 37.14 *Thomas test for hip contracture*

CONCEPT CHECK

1 If a person has an epiphyseal fracture, what is the classification of bone involved?
1 irregular
2 flat
3 long
4 short

2 Select the word describing the movement of an extremity away from the midline of the body:
1 abduction
2 adduction
3 extension
4 flexion

3 A person you are caring for asks you, 'Why is my blood being examined for uric acid?' Which of the following describes the most accurate response?
1 'A uric acid test is done to see if your gout medication is effective.'
2 'A uric acid test is done to diagnose rheumatoid arthritis.'
3 'Do you have a family history of muscle or bone disease?'
4 'Tell me how you got that big bruise on your hip.'

4 State the age at which a female would be most likely to have a bone density examination?
1 as a teenager
2 in her twenties
3 in her forties
4 in her sixties

5 With ageing, bone mass and calcium absorption decrease. State a feature that increases a person's risk as a result.
1 obesity
2 weakness
3 fractures
4 deformity

6 State which of the following instructions is used to assess facial muscle strength.
1 'Close your eyes tightly.'
2 'Stick out your tongue.'
3 'Bend your head forwards.'
4 'Open your eyes wide.'

7 Which term best describes the word used to document a grating sound when a joint is moved?
1 crackles
2 arthritis
3 synovitis
4 crepitation

8 While conducting the ballottement test, you note the patella rebounds against your fingers. Suggest what this finding indicates.
1 deformity of the elbow
2 infection of the metatarsals
3 fluid in the knee joint
4 crepitus in the hip joint

9 During the physical assessment of a young adult, you note a lateral, S-shaped curve of the spine. State the name of this condition.
1 lordosis
2 scoliosis
3 kyphosis
4 musclosis

10 Select the two most common manifestations of musculoskeletal disorders.
1 pain and limited mobility
2 swelling and exaggerated reflexes
3 cyanosis and decreased pulses
4 pallor and decreased ROM

BIBLIOGRAPHY

Marfan Association Victoria (2022). *What is Marfan syndrome?* Retrieved from https://marfan.org/

Norris, T. L. (2018). *Porth's pathophysiology: Concepts of altered health states* (10th ed.). Philadelphia: Lippincott Williams & Wilkins.

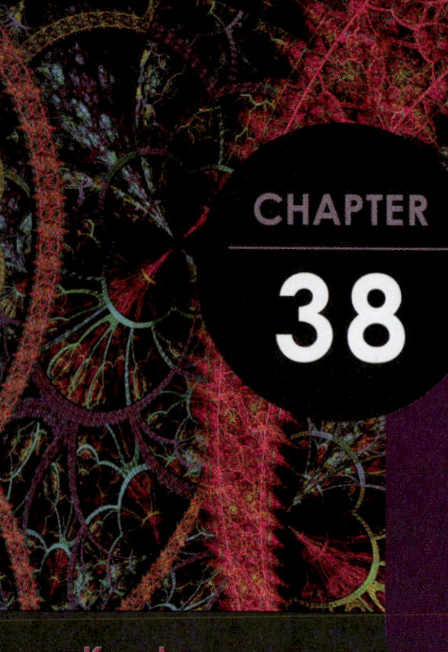

CHAPTER 38

Nursing care of people with musculoskeletal trauma

David Stanley

Key terms

Learning outcomes

- Compare and contrast the causes, risk factors, pathophysiology, manifestations, interprofessional care and nursing care of contusions, strains, sprains, joint dislocations and fractures.
- Describe the stages of bone healing.
- Explain the pathophysiology, manifestations and related treatment for complications of bone fractures: compartment syndrome, fat embolism syndrome, deep venous thrombosis, infection, delayed union and non-union, and reflex sympathetic dystrophy.
- Discuss the purposes and related nursing interventions for casts, traction and stump care.
- Explain the causes, levels, types and potential complications (infection, delayed healing, chronic stump pain, phantom pain and contractures) of an amputation.
- Describe the pathophysiology, interprofessional care and nursing care for repetitive use injuries: carpal tunnel syndrome, bursitis and epicondylitis.

Clinical competencies

- Assess functional health status of people with musculoskeletal injuries and monitor, document and report abnormal manifestations.
- Plan and implement nursing care for people with skeletal pin sites based on relevant, contemporary evidence.
- Determine priority nursing diagnoses, based on assessed data, to select and implement individualised nursing interventions for people with musculoskeletal injuries.
- Provide skilled cast care, traction care and stump care based on relevant, contemporary evidence.
- Integrate interprofessional practices into the care of people with musculoskeletal trauma.
- Provide teaching appropriate for prevention and self-care of traumatic injuries of the musculoskeletal system.
- Revise the plan of care as needed to provide effective interventions to promote, maintain or restore functional health status to people with traumatic injuries of the musculoskeletal system.

Musculoskeletal trauma is an injury to muscle, bone or soft tissue that results from excessive external force. The external force transmits more kinetic energy than the tissue can absorb and injury results. The severity of the trauma depends not only on the amount of force but also on the location of the impact, because different parts of the body can withstand different amounts of force. A wide variety of external forces can cause trauma and the force involved can vary in severity (e.g. a step off the curb, a fall, being tackled in a football game and a motor vehicle crash). See the chapter 'Nursing care of people experiencing trauma and shock' for a detailed discussion of the results of different forces and types of injury from trauma.

Traumatic musculoskeletal injuries include blunt tissue trauma, alterations in tendons and ligaments, and fractures of bones. Various forces that cause musculoskeletal trauma are typical for a specific environment, activity or age group. For example, motorcycle accidents resulting in fractures of the distal tibia, midshaft femur and radius are common in young men. Sports injuries, resulting from either overuse or acute trauma, are seen more often in adolescents and young adults. Falls are the most common cause of injury in people aged 65 or older, with fractures of the vertebrae, proximal humerus and hip seen most often (Norris, 2018). Regardless of the cause, the injury may require rehabilitation and temporary or permanent changes in lifestyle.

Musculoskeletal trauma can result in mild or severe injuries. A person may experience a soft tissue injury, a fracture and/or a complete amputation. In addition, trauma to one part of the musculoskeletal system often produces dysfunction in adjacent structures. For example, a fracture of the femur prevents the adjacent muscles from abducting and adducting. Nursing care helps minimise the effects of trauma, prevents complications and hastens restoration of function. This chapter discusses fractures, amputations, soft tissue injuries, dislocations and repetitive use injuries.

Traumatic injuries of the muscles, ligaments and joints

THE PERSON WITH A CONTUSION, STRAIN OR SPRAIN

Contusions, strains and sprains are among the most commonly reported injuries. They account for about 50% of work-related injuries, with lower back injuries being the most commonly reported occupational injury. However, many sprains and strains are not work related and often are not reported. The lower back and cervical region of the spine are the most common sites for muscle strains; the ankle is the most commonly sprained joint, usually caused by forced inversion of the foot (e.g. during sporting activity).

Pathophysiology and manifestations

A contusion, the least serious form of musculoskeletal injury, is bleeding into soft tissue that results from a blunt force, such as a kick or striking a body part against a hard object. The skin remains intact, but small blood vessels rupture and blood is released into soft tissues. A contusion with a large amount of bleeding is referred to as a *haematoma*. The manifestations of a contusion include swelling and discolouration of the skin. The blood in the soft tissue initially results in a purple-blue colour commonly referred to as a *bruise*. As the blood begins to reabsorb, the area involved becomes brown and then yellow until it disappears.

A **strain** is a stretching injury to a muscle or a muscle–tendon unit caused by mechanical overloading. A muscle that is forced to extend past its elasticity will become strained. Lifting heavy objects without bending the knees or a sudden acceleration–deceleration, as in a motor vehicle crash, can cause strains. The most common sites for a muscle strain are the lower back and cervical regions of the spine. The manifestations include pain, limited motion, muscle spasms, swelling and possible muscle weakness. Severe strains that partially or completely tear the muscle or tendon are painful and disabling.

A **sprain** is a stretch and/or tear of one or more ligaments surrounding a joint. Forces going in opposite directions cause the ligament to overstretch and/or tear, either partially or completely. Although any joint may be involved, sprains of the ankle and knee are most common. Manifestations include loss of the ability to move or use the joint, a feeling of a 'pop' or tear, discolouration, pain and rapid swelling. Motion increases the joint pain. The intensity of the manifestations depends on the severity of the sprain. A comparison of sprains and strains is presented in Box 38.1.

BOX 38.1 Comparison of sprains and strains

Sprain
- Defined as an injury to a ligament that results from a twisting motion.
- Can cause joint instability.
- Pain, oedema and swelling are present.
- Motion increases the joint pain.

Strain
- Defined as a microscopic tear in the muscle.
- Sharp or dull pain is present.
- Pain increases with isometric contraction of the muscle.
- Swelling and local tenderness are present.

INTERPROFESSIONAL CARE

The goal of the initial stage of treating soft tissue trauma is to reduce swelling and pain. People should follow a regimen of rest, ice, compression and elevation (RICE) for the first 24 to 48 hours (see Table 38.1 for RICE therapy). Severe sprains may require surgical repair. Ankle sprains may be immobilised with an air cast, with no limitations on weight bearing. A knee injury often requires a knee immobiliser, such as a knee brace (e.g. Zimmer brace). If an upper extremity is injured, a sling is

TABLE 38.1 RICE therapy for musculoskeletal injuries

ACTION	HEALTH EDUCATION FOR THE PERSON AND FAMILY
Rest	• Decrease regular activities of daily living and exercise as needed. • If advised by your healthcare provider, do not put weight on the injured area for 48 hours. • Crutches may help if you cannot put weight on an ankle or knee. • If you use a cane or crutch for an ankle injury, use it on the uninjured side so you can lean away from and relieve weight on the injured ankle.
Ice	• Apply an ice pack to the injured area for 20 minutes at a time, four to eight times a day. • An ice bag, cold pack, plastic bag filled with ice or a bag of frozen peas may be used. • Do not apply the ice pack for longer than 20 minutes to avoid cold injury and frostbite.
Compression	• Compression often helps reduce swelling. The kind you use will depend on the recommendation of your healthcare provider. • Examples of compression bandages include special boots, air casts and splints.
Elevation	• Keep the injured extremity elevated on a pillow above heart level, to help reduce swelling and pain.

provided. Physical therapy may be recommended for rehabilitation. Time required for healing depends on the severity and location of the injury; for example, a mild ankle sprain will require less time than a severe sprain or a fracture, which will require a longer time to return to full activities (National Institute of Arthritis and Musculoskeletal and Skin Diseases, 2022).

When soft tissue trauma is suspected, x-rays are taken to rule out fractures or confirm soft tissue injury; magnetic resonance imaging (MRI) may be done if further assessment is necessary. Medications used to treat soft tissue trauma include non-steroidal anti-inflammatory drugs (NSAIDs) and analgesics.

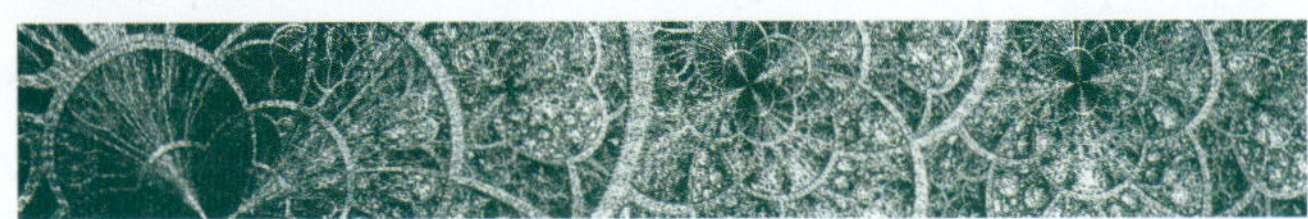

Nursing care

The nursing care of each person is individualised. A strain or sprain may not be as devastating to a person with a desk job as it would be to a professional athlete; therefore, the nurse should determine what the injury means to the particular person.

Nursing diagnoses and interventions

Nursing diagnoses focus on providing information about self-care to decrease pain and return physical mobility to pre-injury levels.

Acute pain

The pain that results from soft tissue trauma is due primarily to the injury to the muscle or ligament and secondarily to bleeding and oedema at the injury site.

- Teach the person to use RICE (rest, ice, compression, elevation) therapy to care for the injury. *The interventions included in RICE therapy allow the injured muscle, ligament or tendon to heal (rest), cause vasoconstriction and reduce pain (ice), decrease oedema formation and pain (compression), and promote venous return to decrease oedema and pain (elevation).*

Impaired physical mobility

Pain causes the person to avoid using or bearing weight on the injured extremity. Always observe the person's use of assistive devices; if the device is inappropriate, the person can face a greater risk of falling. Also consider that the device may be appropriate but the person may not be using it correctly or safely. As a person ages, muscle mass in the upper extremities declines. As a result, the older person with a sprained ankle may not be able to use crutches because crutches require that the person distribute body weight along the upper extremities. Older people may therefore find a walker more useful.

- Teach the correct use of crutches, walkers, canes or slings if prescribed. *Use of the correct technique increases safety and encourages use of these devices.*
- Encourage follow-up care. *Severe sprains may require further evaluation to determine if surgical intervention is indicated.*

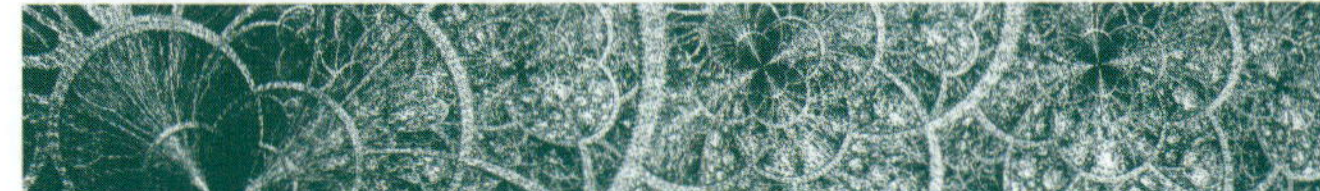

THE PERSON WITH A JOINT DISLOCATION

A **dislocation** is an injury of a joint in which the ends of bones are forced from their normal position. Dislocations usually follow trauma such as a fall or blow, with the bone ends displaced or separated from their normal position in the joint capsule. They commonly are seen in people who take part in contact sports such as football or from falls during activities such as skiing. Although dislocations may occur in any joint, they occur most frequently in the shoulder and acromioclavicular joints. Dislocations may also result from a disease such as rheumatoid arthritis. A **subluxation** is a partial dislocation in which the bone ends are still partially in contact with each other. It is common in young children.

Pathophysiology

Dislocations may be congenital, traumatic or pathological. Congenital dislocations are present at birth and are seen in the hip and knee. Traumatic dislocations result from falls, blows or rotational injuries. Pathological dislocations result from disease of the joint, including infection, rheumatoid arthritis, paralysis and neuromuscular diseases.

Manifestations

The manifestations of a dislocation include pain, deformity and limited motion.

INTERPROFESSIONAL CARE

Care of the person with a dislocation focuses on relieving pain, correcting the dislocation and preventing complications. The dislocation is diagnosed by physical examination and x-rays. The joint is most often reduced (bone ends realigned) by means of manual traction.

Treatment of a shoulder joint dislocation depends on the severity of the dislocation. Reduction of shoulder dislocations may be undertaken in the emergency department or on occasions in the operating theatre. Immobilisation is no longer recommended and only the most severe dislocations are surgically reduced. A dislocated hip requires immediate reduction in the emergency room under sedation to prevent necrosis of the femoral head and injury to the sciatic and femoral nerves. After reduction, the person is placed on bed rest. In some cases, traction is needed for several weeks. If a hip dislocation is accompanied by a fracture, the person will undergo surgery to increase mobility, decrease complications and rapidly stabilise the joint.

Children, generally between the ages of 1 and 4 years, often have common injuries such as a pulled elbow (subluxation). This is a result of the radius slipping out of its normal position at the elbow joint. It is usually caused by a sudden yank or pull on the child's lower arm or wrist. The child presents as distressed and is unable to use the arm, with the elbow in the extension and the forearm in the pronation position. This can be reduced, after diagnosis, with manipulation of the elbow (Perth Children's Hospital, 2021).

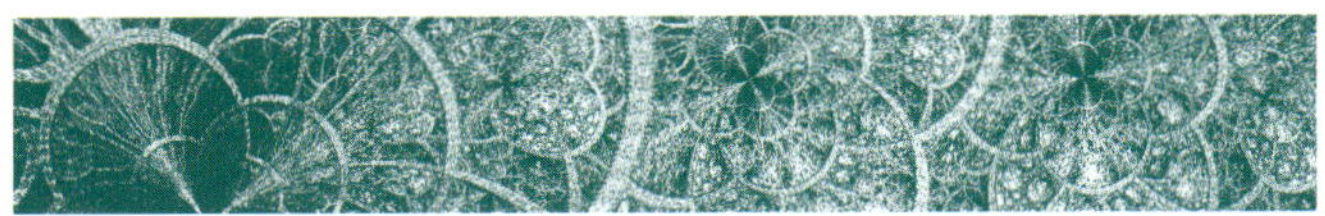

Nursing care

Nursing care of the person with a dislocation or subluxation is individualised to the cause of injury, the type of dislocation and the age of the person. It is important to teach people to seek immediate medical attention, to splint the joint to prevent further damage and to put ice on the injured joint (Mayo Clinic, 2022). Assessment of the affected limb is required to observe for changes in movement, sensation, colour, warmth and increased pain. These changes need to be reported and documented.

Nursing diagnoses and interventions

Nursing diagnoses focus on relieving pain and preventing complications.

Risk of injury

The person with a dislocation requires frequent assessments to ensure that neurovascular compromise does not develop.

- Monitor neurovascular status by assessing the '5 Ps': pain, pulses, pallor, paralysis and paraesthesia. *Neurovascular compromise is indicated by increased pain, decreased or absent pulses, pale skin, inability to move a body part or extremity, and changes in sensation (such as 'pins and needles' sensations or loss of sense of sharp/dull touch).*
- Maintain immobilisation after reduction. *Immobilisation prevents the joint from dislocating again.*

Community-based care

Joint dislocations often tend to be recurring injuries for people actively participating in contact sports and other vigorous physical activities. Prolonged immobilisation (for several weeks after the injury) and aggressive rehabilitation following the initial dislocation can reduce the risk of recurrent dislocation. The following topics should be addressed in preparing the person for community-based care:

- importance of complying with the prescribed length of immobilisation
- skin care and ways to prevent skin-to-skin contact, particularly in the axillary area
- prescribed rehabilitation exercises that will strengthen muscles and other supportive structures in the shoulder, decreasing the risk of future dislocations
- alternatives to activities that precipitate recurrent dislocations
- instructions or referrals to physical therapy if needed for further teaching about using assistive devices
- referrals to physical and occupational therapy and community-based services as needed.

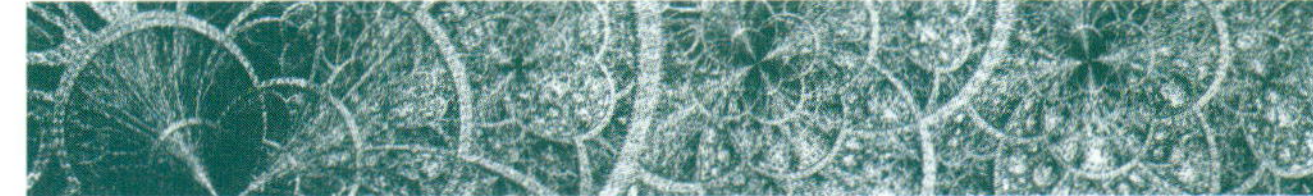

Traumatic injuries of bones

THE PERSON WITH A FRACTURE

A **fracture** is any break in the continuity of a bone. Fractures vary in severity depending on the location and the type of fracture. Although fractures occur in all age groups, they are more common in people who have sustained trauma and in older people.

Pathophysiology

Any of the 206 bones in the body can be fractured. A fracture occurs when the bone is subjected to more kinetic energy than it can absorb. Fractures may result from a direct blow, a crushing force (compression), a sudden twisting motion (torsion), a severe muscle contraction or disease that has weakened the bone (called a *stress* or *pathological fracture*). Two basic mechanisms produce fractures: direct force and indirect force. With direct force, the kinetic energy is applied at or near the site of the fracture. The bone cannot withstand the force. With indirect force, the kinetic energy is transmitted from the point of impact to a site where the bone is weaker. The fracture occurs at the weaker point.

Fractures in adults are classified in the following ways:

- If the skin is intact, the fracture is considered a *closed (simple) fracture*. If the skin integrity is interrupted, the fracture is considered an *open (compound) fracture* (see Figure 38.1). An open fracture allows bacteria to enter the injured area and increases the risk of complications.
- The fracture line may be *oblique* (at an angle to the bone) or *spiral* (curved around the bone). An *avulsed* fracture occurs when the fracture pulls bone and other tissues away from the point of attachment. It may also be described as *comminuted* (the bone breaks into many pieces), *compressed* (the bone is crushed), *impacted* (the broken bone ends are forced into each other) or *depressed* (the broken bone is forced inwards) (see Figure 38.2).
- *Complete fractures* involve the entire width of the bone, whereas incomplete fractures involve only a part of the width of the bone.
- A *stable* (non-displaced) *fracture* is one in which the bones maintain their anatomical alignment. An *unstable* (displaced) *fracture* occurs when the bones move out of correct anatomical alignment. If a fracture is displaced, immediate interventions are required to prevent further damage to soft tissue, muscle and bone.

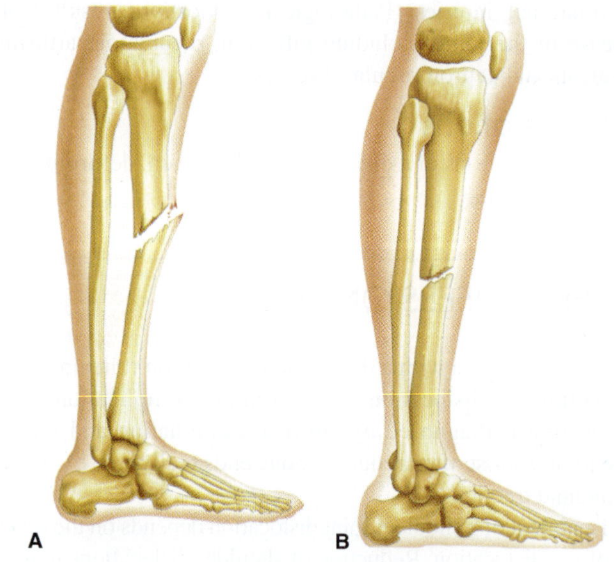

FIGURE 38.1 *A, An open fracture. B, A closed fracture*

Fractures may also be classified by point of reference on the bone, such as midshaft, middle third and distal third. The point of reference may also be specific, such as intra-articular or diaphyseal.

Fracture healing

Regardless of classification or type, fracture healing progresses over three phases: the inflammatory phase, the reparative phase and the remodelling phase (see 'Pathophysiology illustrated'). The bleeding and inflammation that develop at

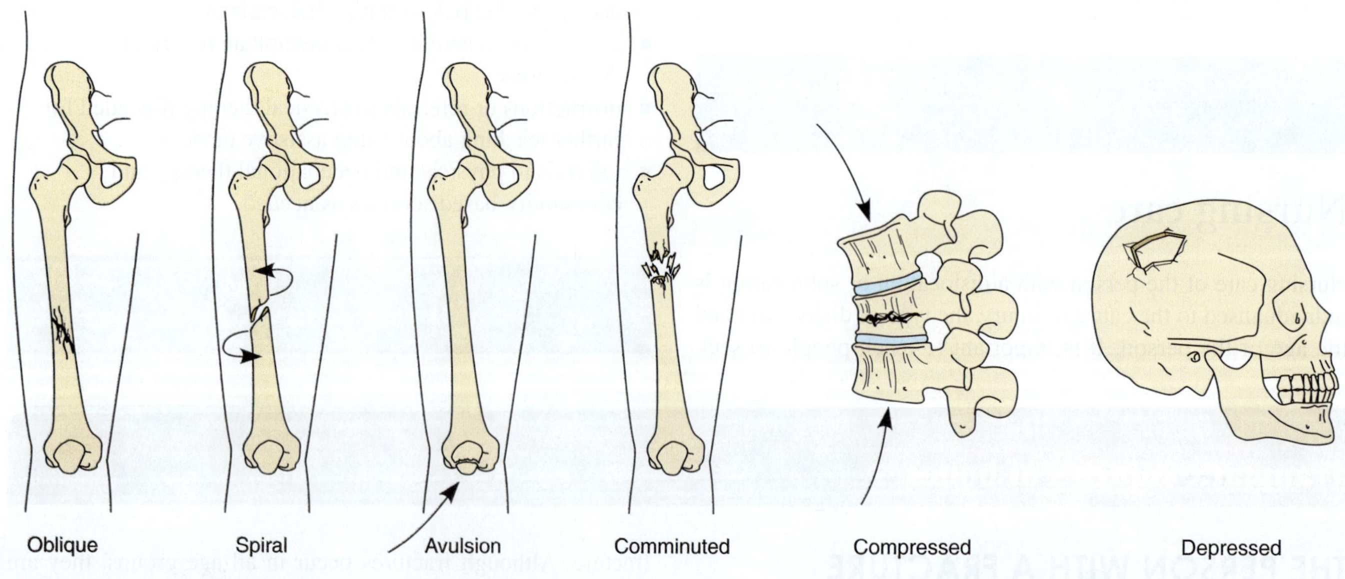

FIGURE 38.2 *Types of fractures*

the site of the fracture initiate the inflammatory phase. A haematoma forms between the fractured bone ends and around the bone surfaces. The osteocytes at the bone ends die as the haematoma clots, obstructing blood flow and depriving them of oxygen and nutrients. Necrosis of the cells heightens the inflammatory response, which in turn leads to vasodilation and oedema. In addition, fibroblasts, lymphocytes, macrophages and even osteoblasts from the bone migrate to the fracture site. Fibroblasts form a fibrin meshwork and promote the growth of granulation tissue and capillary buds. The lymphocytes and macrophages wall off the area, localising and containing the inflammation. The capillary buds invade the fracture site and supply a source of nutrients to promote the formation of collagen. The collagen allows calcium to be deposited.

Once calcium is deposited, a callus begins to form. In this reparative phase, osteoblasts promote the formation of new bone and osteoclasts destroy dead bone and assist in the synthesis of new bone. Collagen formation and calcium deposition continue. During the remodelling phase, excess callus is removed and new bone is laid down along the fracture line. Eventually, the fracture site is calcified and the bone is reunited.

The age, physical condition of the person and the type of fracture sustained influence the healing of fractures. Other factors influence bone healing either positively or negatively and may be grouped according to their local or systemic influence (see Box 38.2). Healing time varies with each individual. An uncomplicated fracture of the arm or foot can heal in 6 to 8 weeks. A fractured vertebra will take at least 12 weeks to heal. Healing of a fractured hip may take from 12 to 16 weeks.

Manifestations

Fractures are often accompanied by soft tissue injuries that involve muscles, arteries, veins, nerves or skin. The degree of soft tissue involvement depends on the amount of energy or force transmitted to the area. Fracture manifestations and their causes are outlined in the 'Manifestations' box.

Complications

Complications of musculoskeletal trauma are associated with pressure from oedema and haemorrhage, development of fat emboli, deep venous thrombosis, infection, loss of skeletal integrity or involvement of nerve fibres. Bone fragments may also result in further injury or complications.

Compartment syndrome

A compartment is a space enclosed by a fibrous membrane, or fascia. The fascia lines the compartment within the limbs and is non-expandable. Compartments within the limbs may enclose and support bones, nerves and blood vessels. **Compartment syndrome** occurs when excess pressure in a limited space constricts the structures within a compartment, reducing circulation to muscles and nerves. Acute compartment syndrome may result from haemorrhage and oedema within the compartment following a fracture or from a crush injury, or from external compression of the limb by a cast that is too tight. Increased pressure within the confined space of the compartment results in entrapment of nerves, blood vessels and muscles (Hoffman, 2020).

BOX 38.2 Factors influencing bone healing

Positive factors

Local:

- Immobilisation
- Timely correction of displacement
- Application of ice
- Electrical stimulation

Systemic:

- Adequate amounts of growth hormone, vitamin D and calcium
- Adequate blood supply
- Absence of infection or diseases
- Younger age
- Moderate activity level prior to injury

Negative factors

Local:

- Delay in correction of displacement
- Open fracture (increases risk of infection)
- Presence of foreign body at fracture site

Systemic:

- Immunocompromised status
- Decreased circulation (as in diabetes or peripheral vascular disease)
- Malnutrition
- Osteoporosis
- Advanced age

MANIFESTATIONS Fracture

MANIFESTATION	CAUSE
Deformity	Abnormal position of bones secondary to fracture and muscles pulling on fractured bone
Swelling	Oedema from localisation of serous fluid and bleeding
Pain/tenderness	Muscle spasm, direct tissue trauma, nerve pressure, movement of fractured bone
Numbness	Nerve damage or nerve entrapment
Guarding	Pain
Crepitus	Grating of bones or entrance of air in an open fracture. *Note*: do not manipulate the extremity to elicit crepitus; doing so may cause additional damage and pain.
Hypovolaemic shock	Blood loss or associated injuries
Muscle spasms	Muscle contraction near the fracture
Ecchymosis	Extravasation of blood into the subcutaneous tissue

Bone healing

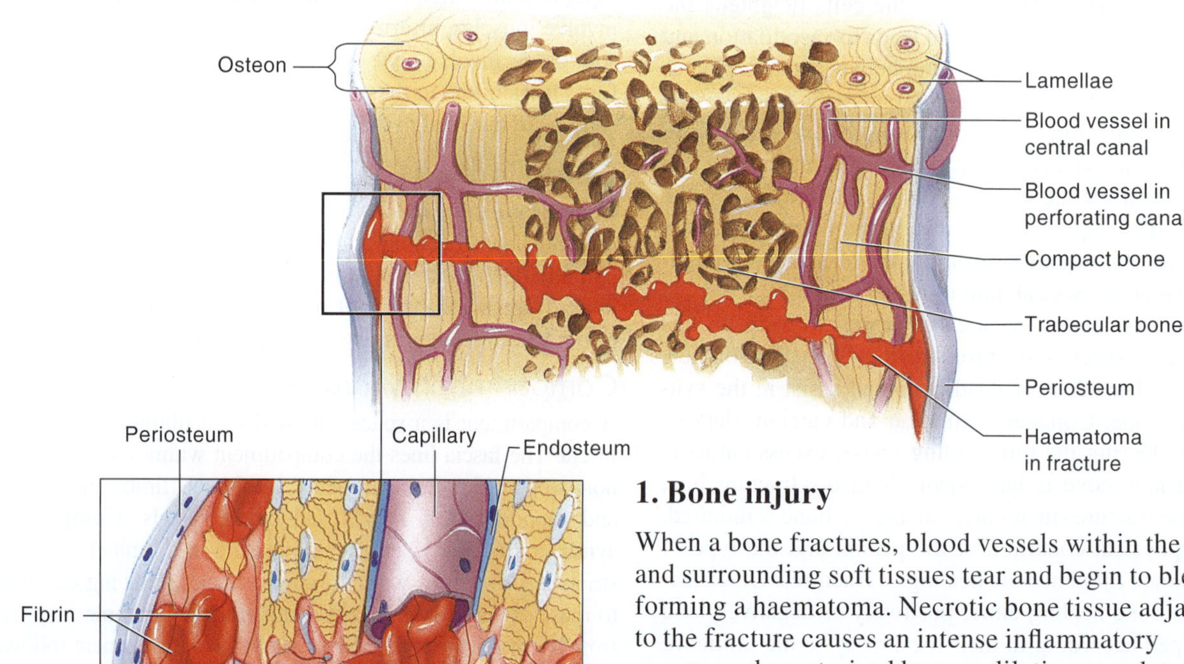

1. Bone injury

When a bone fractures, blood vessels within the bone and surrounding soft tissues tear and begin to bleed, forming a haematoma. Necrotic bone tissue adjacent to the fracture causes an intense inflammatory response characterised by vasodilation, exudate formation and white cell migration to the fracture site.

2. Fibrocartilaginous callus formation

Clotting factors within the haematoma form a fibrin meshwork. Within 48 hours, fibroblasts and new capillaries growing into the fracture form granulation tissue that gradually replaces the haematoma. Phagocytes begin to remove cell debris.

Osteoblasts, bone-forming cells, proliferate and migrate into the fracture site, forming a fibrocartilaginous callus. The osteoblasts build a web of collagen fibres from both sides of the fracture site that eventually unites to connect bone fragments, thus splinting the bone. Chondroblasts lay down patches of cartilage that provide a base for bone growth.

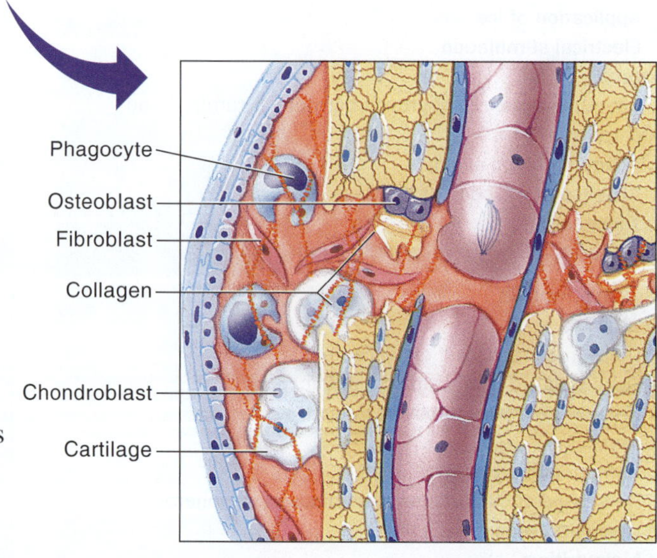

4. Bone remodelling

Osteoblasts continue to form new woven bone, which is in turn organised into the lamellar structures of compact bone. Osteoclasts resorb excess callus as it is replaced by mature bone.

As the bone heals and is subjected to the mechanical stress of everyday use, osteoblasts and osteoclasts respond by remodelling the repair site along the lines of force. This ensures that the repaired section of bone eventually resembles the structure of the uninjured part.

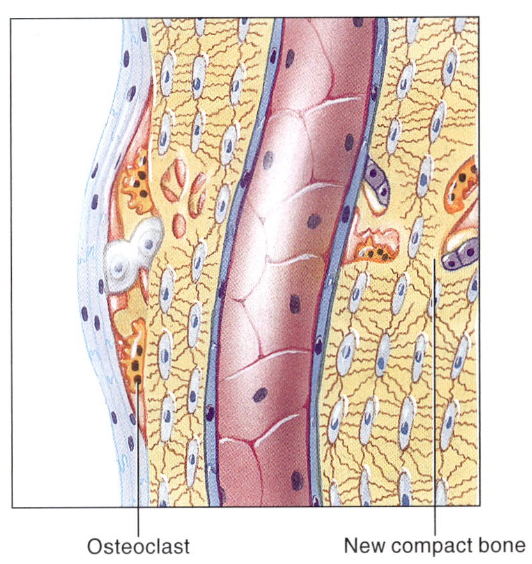

3. Bony callus formation

Osteoblasts continue to proliferate and synthesise collagen fibres and bone matrix, which are gradually mineralised with calcium and mineral salts to form a spongy mass of woven bone. The trabeculae of woven bone bridge the fracture. Osteoclasts migrate to the repair site and begin removing excess bone in the callus. Bony callus formation usually continues for 2 to 3 months.

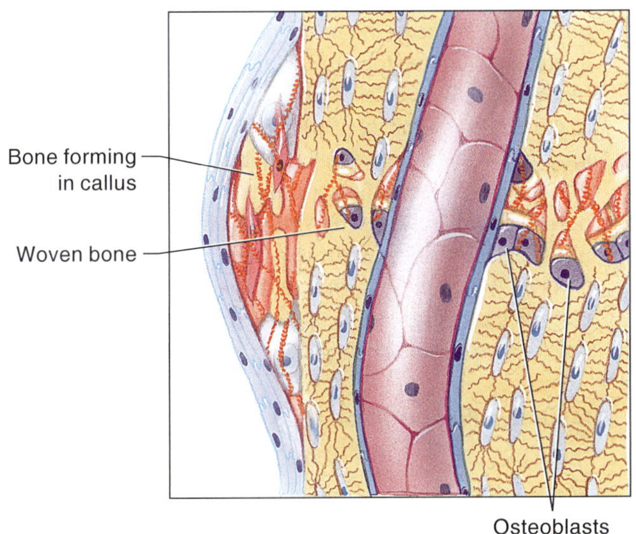

Entrapment of blood vessels limits tissue perfusion, beginning a cycle of events that may result in the loss of the limb. Inadequate oxygen supply causes cellular acidosis, which intensifies as cellular energy requirements are met through anaerobic metabolism. The capillaries inside the compartment dilate in an attempt to increase the supply of blood and oxygen. Additional blood and oxygen are not available and plasma proteins leak out into the interstitial tissues. The interstitial tissue then pulls fluid in to balance the protein load. As a result, oedema within the compartment increases. The oedema causes further compression of the vascular network and the cycle continues. Uninterrupted, this cycle threatens the person's limb and increases the risk of sepsis. Compartment syndrome usually develops within the first 48 hours of injury, when oedema is at its peak. Manifestations of compartment syndrome are listed in the 'Manifestations' box. It is important to note that arterial pulses may remain normal, even when pressure within the compartment is high enough to significantly impair tissue perfusion.

If compartment syndrome develops, interventions to alleviate pressure will be implemented; these may include removal of a tightly fitting cast. If the pressure is internal, a *fasciotomy*, a surgical intervention in which muscle fascia is cut to relieve pressure within the compartment, may be necessary. After a fasciotomy, the incision is left open and passive ROM exercises are performed on the extremity.

Volkmann's contracture, a common complication of elbow fractures, can result from unresolved compartment syndrome. Arterial blood flow decreases, leading to ischaemia, degeneration and contracture of the muscle. Arm mobility is impaired and the person is unable to completely extend the arm.

Fat embolism syndrome

Fat emboli occur when fat globules lodge in the pulmonary vascular bed or peripheral circulation. **Fat embolism syndrome (FES)** is characterised by neurological dysfunction, pulmonary insufficiency and a petechial rash on the chest, axilla and upper arms. Long bone fractures and other major trauma are the principal risk factors for fat emboli; hip replacement surgery also poses a risk of FES.

When a bone is fractured, pressure within the bone marrow rises and exceeds capillary pressure; as a result, fat globules leave the bone marrow and enter the bloodstream. Another contributing factor may be the stress-induced release of catecholamine, which causes the rapid mobilisation of fatty acids. Once the fat globules are released, they combine with platelets and travel to the brain, lungs, kidneys and other organs, occluding small blood vessels and causing tissue ischaemia.

Manifestations usually develop within a few hours to a week after injury. The manifestations result from the occlusion of the blood supply and the presence of fatty acids. Altered cerebral blood flow causes confusion and changes in level of consciousness. Pulmonary circulation may be disrupted and free fatty acids damage the alveolar–capillary membrane. Pulmonary oedema, impaired surfactant production and atelectasis can result in significant respiratory insufficiency and manifestations of acute respiratory distress syndrome (see the chapter 'Nursing care of people with gas exchange disorders'). Fat droplets activate the clotting cascade, causing thrombocytopenia. Petechiae (pin-sized purplish areas from bleeding under the skin) appearing on the skin, buccal membranes and conjunctival sacs are thought to result from either microvascular clotting or the accompanying thrombocytopenia.

Early stabilisation of long bone fractures is preventive for FES. Prompt identification and treatment of the syndrome are necessary to maintain adequate pulmonary function. In severe cases, the person may require intubation and mechanical ventilation to prevent hypoxaemia. Fluid balance is closely monitored. Corticosteroids may be administered to decrease the inflammatory response of lung tissues, stabilise lipid membranes and reduce bronchospasm (Norris, 2018).

Deep venous thrombosis

A *deep venous thrombosis (DVT)* is a blood clot that forms along the intimal lining of a large vein. Three precursors linked to DVT formation are: (1) venous stasis or decreased blood flow, (2) injury to blood vessel walls, and (3) altered blood coagulation (see Table 38.2). Any or all of these precursors can cause a DVT to form. Damage to the lining of the vein causes the platelets to aggregate or clump together, forming the thrombus. Fibrin, white blood cells (WBCs) and red blood cells (RBCs) begin to cling to the thrombus and a tail forms. This tail or the entire thrombus may dislodge and move to the brain, lungs or heart. Five per cent of DVTs dislodge and enter the pulmonary circulation to form a pulmonary embolus. If the thrombus remains in the vein, venous insufficiency may result from scarring and valve damage.

If a DVT is present, there may be swelling, leg pain, tenderness or cramping. Homans' sign (also called dorsiflexion sign test) is a procedure or physical examination that may be used to

MANIFESTATIONS Compartment syndrome

EARLY MANIFESTATIONS

- Pain
- Normal or decreased peripheral pulse

LATER MANIFESTATIONS

- Cyanosis
- Tingling, loss of sensation (paraesthesias)
- Weakness (paresis)
- Severe pain, especially when the extremity is passively flexed
- Eventual renal failure (due to release of myoglobin into the bloodstream; myoglobin molecule is too large for effective filtration and excretion by kidney, and renal failure results)

TABLE 38.2 Precursors of deep venous thrombosis

PRECURSOR	IMPLICATIONS FOR FRACTURES
Decreased blood flow	Common in people with a fracture who are immobilised and less active. Bed rest alone can decrease venous flow by 50%.
Injury to blood vessel wall	May occur as a direct result of the force that caused the fracture or from surgical manipulation.
Altered blood coagulation	May result from active blood loss. The body's attempt to maintain homeostasis leads to increased production of platelets and clotting factor.

test for DVT. To perform this test, have the person actively extend their knee. Then raise the person's straight leg to 10 degrees and passively dorsiflex the foot and squeeze the calf with the other hand. Deep calf pain and tenderness may indicate the presence of a DVT. While clinical evaluation alone cannot be relied on for patient management, when carefully performed it remains useful in determining the need for additional testing for DVT. Not all people experience the manifestations above. For this reason diagnostic tests, such as a venogram or Doppler ultrasound of lower extremities, may be required. A venogram requires intravenous administration of dye in the radiology department, whereas a Doppler ultrasound study is non-invasive and can be performed at the person's bedside. Doppler ultrasonography uses sound waves to form an image on a computer screen.

The best treatment for DVT is prevention. Early immobilisation of the fracture and early ambulation of the person are imperative. The extremity should be elevated above the level of the heart. Frequent assessments of the injured extremity may lead to early recognition of DVT and prevent the formation of pulmonary embolus. Prophylactic anticoagulant administration is beneficial. Anti-embolism stockings and compression boots increase venous return and prevent stasis of blood. Constrictive clothing should be avoided.

The diagnosis of DVT requires rapid intervention. Fibrinolytic agents, which dissolve the clot, may be administered. Heparin may be administered intravenously or subcutaneously, to prevent more clots from forming. Prophylactic warfarin, rivaroxaban or low-molecular-weight heparin (e.g. enoxaparin (Clexane)) may also be administered to prevent DVT (Tiziani, 2017). Monotherapy with rivaroxaban or apixaban is the preferred option for most adults with acute venous thromboembolism, with the initial duration of anticoagulation usually planned for 3 months (Stevens, Tran & Gibbs, 2019).

A vena cava filter may be placed to prevent the existing clot from entering the pulmonary circulation and forming a pulmonary embolus. In extreme cases in which anticoagulation therapy is contraindicated, a thrombectomy (surgical removal of the clot) may be necessary. See the chapter 'Nursing care of people with vascular and lymphatic disorders' for further discussion of DVT.

Infection

Infection is more likely to occur in an open fracture than a closed fracture, but any complication that decreases blood supply increases the risk of infection. Infection may result from contamination at the time of injury or during surgery. *Pseudomonas*, *Staphylococcus* or *Clostridium* organisms may invade the wound or bone. *Clostridium* infection is particularly serious because it may lead to severe gas gangrene and cellulitis, but any infection may delay healing and result in osteomyelitis—infection within the bone that can lead to tissue death and necrosis. (See the chapter 'Nursing care of people with musculoskeletal disorders' for a discussion of osteomyelitis.)

Delayed union and non-union

Delayed union is the prolonged healing of bones beyond the usual period. Many factors may inhibit bone healing, including poor nutrition, inadequate immobilisation, prolonged reduction time, infection, necrosis, age, immunosuppression and severe bone trauma resulting in multiple fragments. Delayed union is diagnosed by means of serial x-ray studies. It is important to note that x-ray findings may lag 1 to 2 weeks behind the healing process; for example, a person may be completely healed by week 13, but this fact may not be apparent on the x-ray until week 14.

Delayed union may lead to **non-union**, which can cause persistent pain and movement at the fracture site. Non-union may require surgical interventions, such as internal fixation and bone grafting. If infection is present, the bones are surgically debrided. Electrical stimulation of the fracture site may be as effective as bone grafting.

Reflex sympathetic dystrophy

Reflex sympathetic dystrophy may occur after musculoskeletal or nerve trauma. This term refers to a group of post-traumatic conditions involving persistent pain, hyperaesthesias, swelling, changes in skin colour and texture, changes in temperature and decreased motion. Diagnosis is made by the person's history and physical examination. X-rays may demonstrate spotty osteoporosis and bone scans may reveal increased uptake of radionuclide. Treatment with a sympathetic nervous system blocking agent often alleviates the manifestations.

INTERPROFESSIONAL CARE

A fracture requires treatment to stabilise the fractured bone(s), maintain bone immobilisation, prevent complications and restore function. The diagnosis of a fracture is primarily based on physical assessments and x-rays.

Emergency care

Emergency care of the person with a fracture includes immobilising the fracture, maintaining tissue perfusion and preventing infection. In the case of serious trauma, normal body alignment must be maintained and may involve cervical immobilisation. Once the person is in a secure location, they are assessed for instability or deformity of the bone. If any deformity or instability is detected, the extremity is rapidly immobilised. Open wounds are covered with sterile dressings and bleeding may be controlled with a pressure dressing. The extremities are assessed for the presence of pulses, movement and sensation. The joints above and below the deformity are immobilised. Pulses, movement and sensation are re-evaluated after splinting.

The fracture is splinted to maintain normal anatomical alignment and prevent the fracture from dislocating. Splinting relieves pain and prevents further damage to the arteries, nerves and bones. Splinting can be accomplished with air splints. If equipment is not available, the limb may be secured to the body. For example, an arm may be secured to the torso with a sling or one leg may be strapped to the other leg.

Diagnosis

Diagnosis of a fracture begins with the history and initial assessment and usually is confirmed by radiographical tests. X-rays and bone scans are used to identify fractures (see Figure 38.3). Blood chemistry studies, full blood count (FBC), group and hold and coagulation studies may be used to assess blood

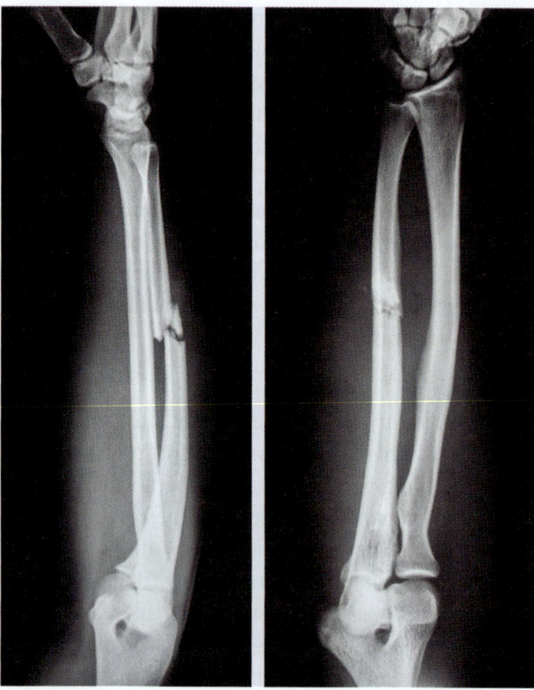

FIGURE 38.3 *X-ray of an oblique fracture of the ulna*

Source: Puwadol Jaturawutthichai/Alamy Stock Photo.

loss, renal function, muscle breakdown and the risk of excessive bleeding or clotting. Diagnostic tests are described in the chapter 'A person-centred approach to assessing the musculoskeletal system'.

Medications

Most people with a fracture require pharmacological interventions. The priority intervention focuses on relieving pain. In the case of multiple fractures or fractures of large bones, narcotics are administered initially. As healing progresses, the person begins to take oral medication for pain. Pain management for the person with a fracture is described in Box 38.3.

Stool softeners may be administered to decrease the risk of constipation secondary to narcotics and immobility. People who have sustained trauma are often placed on anti-ulcer medications or antacids. NSAIDs may be prescribed to decrease inflammation. Antibiotics may be administered prophylactically, particularly to people with open or complex fractures. Anticoagulants may be prescribed to prevent DVT.

Treatments

Fracture treatment may involve a closed reduction and the application of a cast, or may include one or more of the following: traction, casts, surgery and electrical bone stimulation.

TRACTION Muscle spasms usually accompany fractures and may pull bones out of alignment. Traction is the application of a straightening or pulling force to return the fractured bones to or maintain them in normal anatomical position. Weights are applied to maintain the necessary force (see Figure 38.4). Traction is not used often in orthopaedic management due to the advancement of orthopaedic implant technologies and operative techniques. It may be used in the short term for the individual awaiting operative fixation.

BOX 38.3 Pain management in the person with a fracture

The person who has had musculoskeletal trauma experiences pain from many different causes:

- the interruption in the continuity of the bone itself
- damage to ligaments and tendons
- swelling of tissues around the trauma site
- muscle spasms
- tissue anoxia from swelling inside a cast, splint or the muscle fascia sheath
- haematoma formation
- pressure over bony prominences from casts or splints.

The pain is often severe and may be described as sharp, aching or burning. Carefully assess any complaint of pain; pain may be an indication of a serious complication, such as compartment syndrome, decreased tissue perfusion and neurovascular impairment, or pressure ulcers. Do not administer analgesics until the location, character and duration of pain have been carefully assessed. After the cause of the pain has been identified, the following nursing interventions may be implemented:

1. Administer prescribed analgesics, which may include NSAIDs and narcotic analgesics. For serious fractures or following orthopaedic surgery, patient-controlled analgesia (PCA) or epidural methods of providing pain relief may be used. If medications are used on an as-needed basis, tell the person to request the medication before the pain is severe; alternatively, offer the medications at regular intervals for the first 24 to 48 hours. Reassure the person that addiction does not result from taking medications to relieve fracture or surgical pain. Most people require only oral analgesics by the third or fourth day after orthopaedic surgery.
2. Elevate the involved extremity and apply cold (if prescribed) to help decrease swelling.
3. Monitor and drain the accumulated fluids in any drainage devices to ensure patency and to decrease the possibility of haematoma formation.
4. Encourage the person to wiggle fingers or toes on an extremity in a cast or traction to improve venous return and decrease oedema.
5. Assist the person to change positions to relieve pressure and use pillows to provide support.
6. Teach the person alternative methods of pain management, such as relaxation and guided imagery.
7. Notify the doctor of unrelieved pain, which may indicate a serious complication such as compartment syndrome or neurovascular impairment.

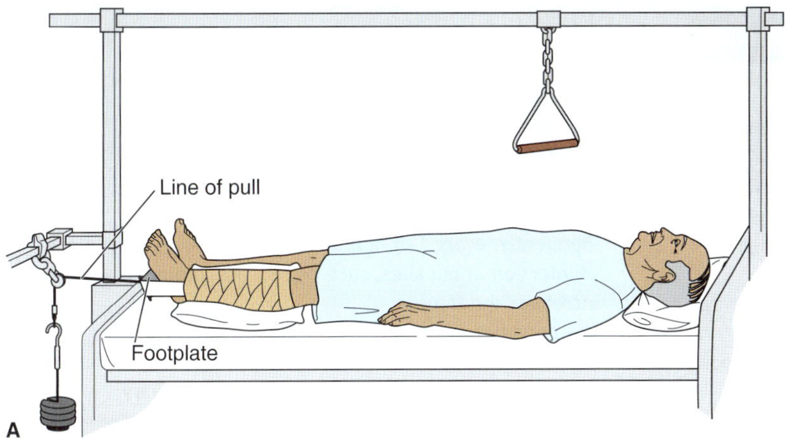

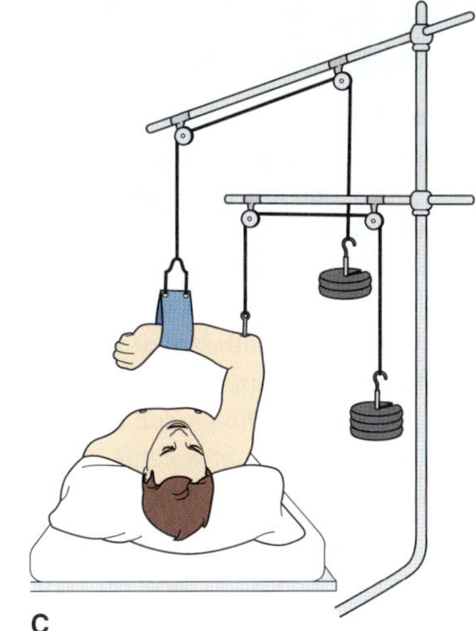

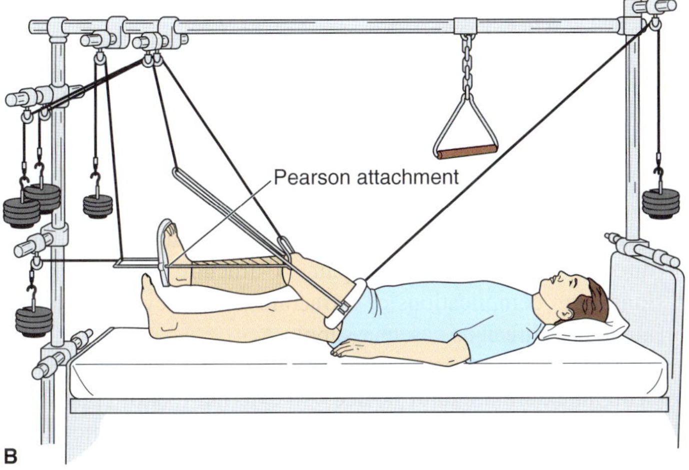

FIGURE 38.4 *Traction is the application of a pulling force to maintain bone alignment during fracture healing. Different fractures require different types of traction. A, Skin traction (also called straight traction), such as Buck's traction shown here, is often used for hip fractures. B, Balanced suspension traction is commonly used for fractures of the femur. C, Skeletal traction, in which the pulling force is applied directly to the bone, may be used to treat fractures of the humerus*

Types of traction are as follows:

- In *manual traction*, the hand directly applies the pulling force.
- *Skin traction* (also called straight traction) is used to control muscle spasms and to immobilise a part of the body before surgery, with traction exerting its grabbing and pulling force through the person's skin. The most common type of skin traction is Buck's traction, in which traction tape or a foam boot is applied to the lower portion of a person's leg and a free-hanging weight is attached to the taped or booted area (see Figure 38.4A). Buck's traction is used to immobilise the leg before surgery to repair a fracture of the proximal femur. The advantage of skin traction is the relative ease of use and ability to maintain comfort. The disadvantage is that the weight required to maintain normal body alignment or fracture alignment cannot exceed the tolerance of the skin—about 13.2 kg per extremity. It is important to ensure that the weights remain hanging freely; they should never rest on the bed or the floor. The nurse may have to reposition the person or the weights if this occurs.
- *Balanced suspension traction* involves more than one force of pull. Several forces work in unison to raise and support the person's injured extremity off the bed and pull it in a straight line away from the body (see Figure 38.4B). The advantage of this type of traction is that it increases mobility without threatening joint continuity. The disadvantage is that the increased use of multiple weights makes the person more likely to slide down in the bed.
- *Skeletal traction* is the application of a pulling force through placement of pins into the bone (see Figure 38.4C). The person may receive a local, spinal or general anaesthetic, and the pins are inserted into the bone. This type of traction must be applied under sterile conditions because of the increased risk of infection. One or more pulling forces may be applied with skeletal traction. The advantage of this type of traction is that more weight can be used to maintain the proper anatomical alignment if necessary. The disadvantages include increased anxiety, increased risk of infection and increased discomfort. The weights used for skeletal traction are not removed by the nurse.

Nursing interventions for people in traction are described in Box 38.4.

CASTS A cast is a rigid device applied to immobilise the injured bones and promote healing. The cast immobilises the joints above and below the fractured bone so that the bone will

BOX 38.4 Nursing interventions for people in traction

- In skeletal traction, never remove the weights.
- In skin traction, remove weights only when intermittent skin traction has been ordered to alleviate muscle spasm.
- For traction to be successful, countertraction is necessary. In most instances, the countertraction is the person's weight. Therefore, do not wedge the person's foot or place it flush with the footboard of the bed.
- Maintain the line of pull:
  a. Centre the person on the bed.
  b. Ensure that weights hang freely and do not touch the floor.
- Ensure that nothing is lying on or obstructing the ropes. Do not allow the knots at the end of the rope to come into contact with the pulley.
- If a problem is detected, assist in repositioning. The area of the fracture must be stabilised when the person is repositioned.
- In skin traction:
  a. Frequently (every 1–4 hours) assess skin for evidence of pressure, shearing or pending breakdown.
  b. Protect pressure sites with padding and protective dressings as indicated.
- In skeletal traction:
  a. Frequent skin assessments should include pin care per policy.
  b. Frequently (every 1–4 hours), observe for and report signs of infection at pin sites, such as redness, drainage and increased tenderness.
  c. The person may require more frequent analgesic administration.
- Perform neurovascular assessments frequently (every 1–4 hours).
- Assess for common complications of immobility, including formation of pressure ulcers, constipation, formation of renal calculi, deep venous thrombosis, pneumonia, paralytic ileus and loss of appetite.
- Teach the person and family about the type and purpose of the traction.

not move during healing. A fracture is first reduced manually (by hand) and a cast is then applied. Casts are applied on people who have relatively stable fractures.

The cast, which may be composed of plaster or fibreglass, is applied over a thin cushion of padding and moulded to the normal contour of the body. The cast must be allowed to dry before any pressure is applied to it; simply palpating a wet cast with the fingertips will leave dents that may cause pressure ulcers. A plaster cast may require up to 48 hours to dry, whereas a fibreglass cast dries in less than 1 hour. The type of cast applied is determined by the location of the fracture (see Figure 38.5). Nursing care of the person with a cast is discussed in the accompanying box. During follow-up appointments, the doctor may x-ray the bone to assess alignment and healing and possibly remove the cast for skin assessment.

SURGERY Surgery is indicated for a fracture that requires direct visualisation and repair, a fracture with common long-term complications or a fracture that is severely comminuted and threatens vascular supply.

The simplest form of surgery is done by external fixation with an external fixator device. An external fixator consists of a frame connected to pins that are inserted perpendicular to the long axis of the bone (see Figure 38.6). The number of pins inserted varies with the type and site of the fracture, but in all cases the same number of pins are inserted above and below the fracture line. The pins require care similar to that of skeletal traction pins. The person is monitored for infection, and frequent neurovascular assessment is performed. The fixator increases independence while maintaining immobilisation.

NURSING CARE OF THE PERSON with a cast

NURSING INTERVENTIONS

- Perform frequent (every 1–4 hours) neurovascular assessments.
- Once dry, palpate the cast for 'hot spots' that may indicate the presence of underlying infection.
- Report any drainage promptly.

HEALTH EDUCATION FOR THE PERSON AND FAMILY

- Do not place any objects in or under the cast.
- If the cast is made of plaster, keep it dry, and have it removed if it becomes excessively wet.
- If the cast is made of fibreglass, dry it with a blow dryer on the cool setting if it becomes wet. Be aware that some padding is not waterproof and therefore will need to be checked prior to the person showering or swimming.
- Assess the injured extremity for coolness, changes in colour, increased pain, increased swelling and/or loss of sensation.
- Use a blow dryer on the cool setting to relieve itching by blowing cool air into the cast.
- If a sling is used, it should distribute the weight of the cast evenly on the support around the neck. Do not roll the sling; this can impair circulation to the neck.
- If crutches are used, arrange for a physiotherapist to teach correct crutch walking technique.
- When the cast is removed, an oscillating cast remover will be used. A guard prevents the cast remover from penetrating past the depth of the cast, so it will not cut the person. It is noisy and the person will feel vibration.

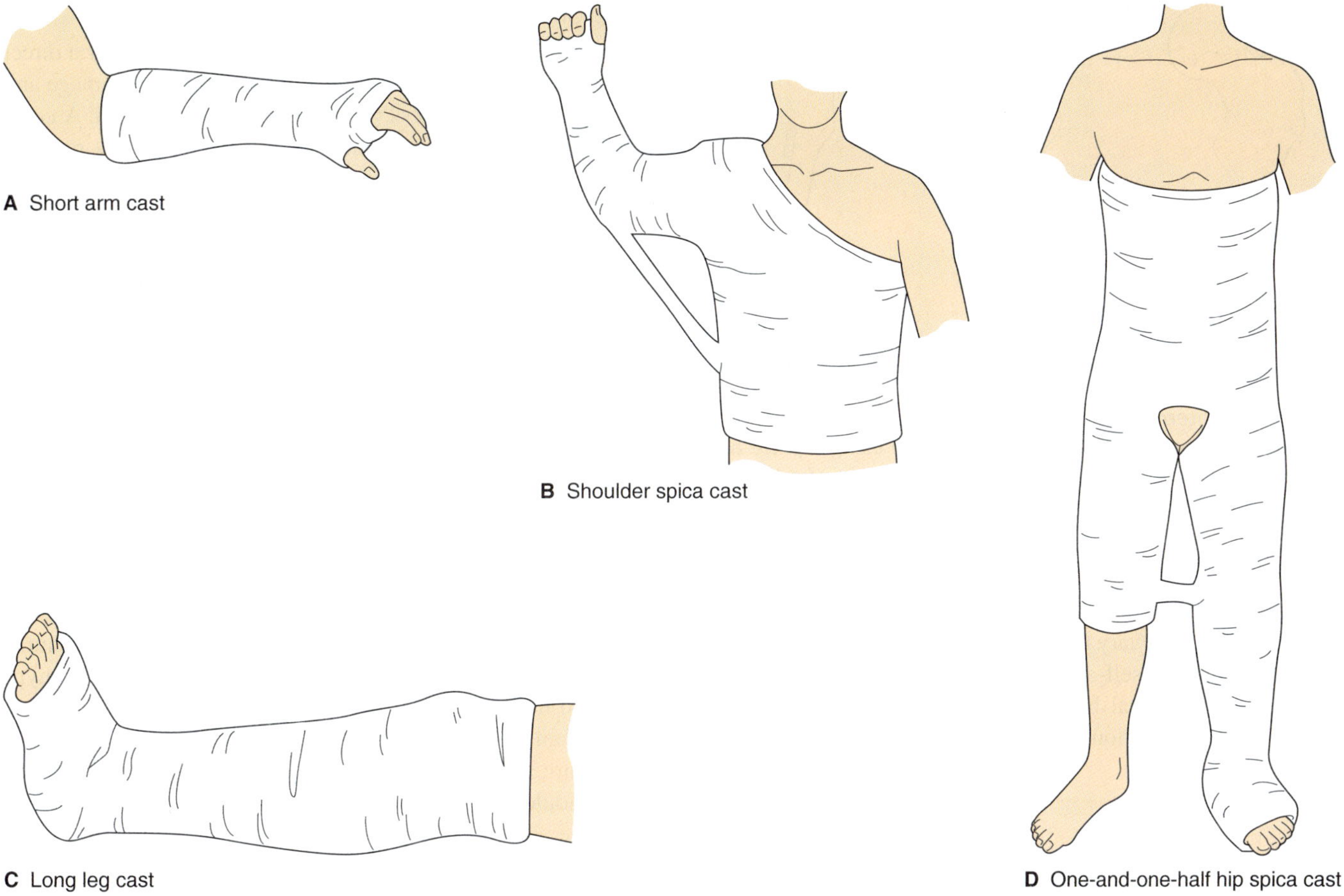

A Short arm cast

B Shoulder spica cast

C Long leg cast

D One-and-one-half hip spica cast

FIGURE 38.5 ***Examples of types of casts used to immobilise fractures***

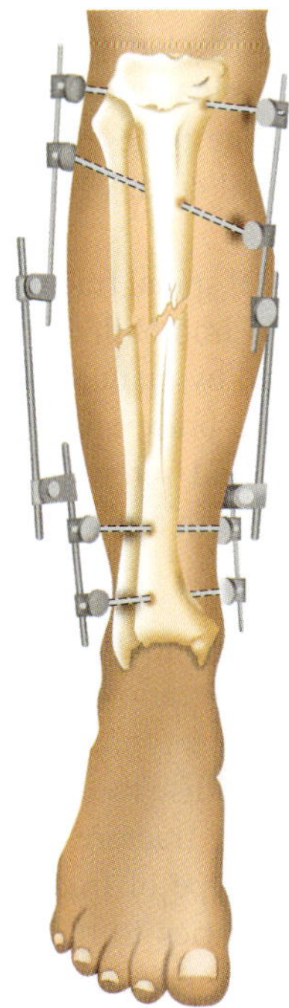

FIGURE 38.6 ***In external fixation, pins are placed through the bone above and below the fracture site to immobilise the bone. External fixation rods hold the pins in place***

Internal fixation can be accomplished through a surgical procedure called an *open reduction and internal fixation (ORIF)*. In this procedure, the fracture is reduced (placed in correct anatomical alignment) and nails, screws, plates or pins are inserted to hold the bones in place (see Figure 38.7). Open fractures of the arms and legs are most commonly repaired in this way. Hip fractures in older people are almost always repaired with ORIF to prevent complications and to allow early rehabilitation. Interventions for postoperative nursing care are presented in Box 38.5.

ELECTRICAL BONE STIMULATION Electrical bone stimulation is the application of an electrical current at the fracture site. It is a painless method of treating fractures that are not healing appropriately. The electrical stress increases the migration of osteoblasts and osteoclasts to the fracture site. Mineral deposition increases, promoting bone healing. Electrical bone stimulation can be accomplished invasively or non-invasively. In invasive stimulation, the surgeon inserts a cathode and a lead wire at the fracture site. The lead wire is attached to an internal or external generator, which delivers electricity through the lead wire to the cathode 24 hours a day. In non-invasive inductive stimulation, a treatment coil encircles the cast or skin directly over the fracture site. The coil is attached to an external generator that runs on batteries. The electricity goes

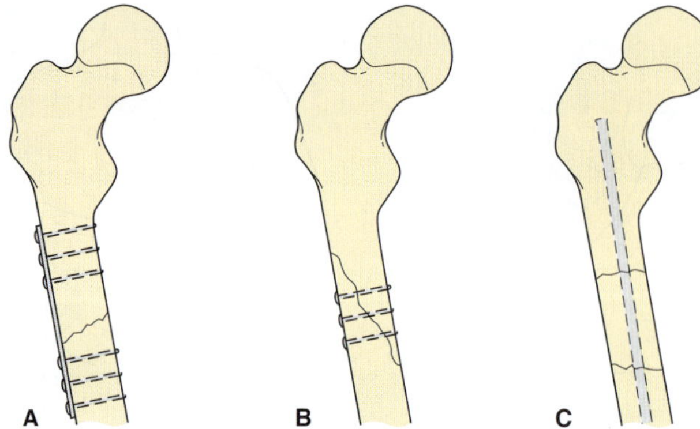

FIGURE 38.7 ***Internal fixation hardware is entirely within the body. A, Fixation of a short oblique fracture using a plate and screws above and below the fracture. B, Fixation of a long oblique fracture using screws through the fracture site. C, Fixation of a segmental fracture using a medullary nail***

through the skin to the fracture site. The time period for external stimulation can vary from 3 to 10 hours per day. The person may be taught to self-administer the non-invasive electrical stimulation. Electrical bone stimulation is contraindicated in the presence of infection and for upper extremities if the person has a pacemaker.

Fractures of specific bones or bony areas

Causes, manifestations, complications, treatment and selected nursing interventions are described for the following fractures: skull, face, spine, clavicle, humerus, elbow, radius/ulna, wrist/hand, ribs, pelvis, femur, hip, tibia/fibula and ankle/foot.

BOX 38.5 Nursing interventions for people with internal fixation

- Expect the person to have sutures and at least one drain (the type depends on the surgeon's choice).
- Perform neurovascular assessments frequently.
- Assess the following:
  a. wounds for drainage
  b. drainage device for the removal of serosanguineous fluid
  c. bowel sounds
  d. lung sounds
  e. lower limbs for DVT.
- Administer medications, such as analgesics and antibiotics, per doctor's orders.
- In hip fractures, place an abductor pillow between the legs to prevent dislocation of the hip joint.
- Arrange for physical and occupational therapy, as ordered.
- Assist with weight-bearing program, if ordered.
- Encourage early mobilisation, coughing and deep breathing, as appropriate, to help prevent complications.

Fracture of the skull

The skull may be fractured as a result of either a fall or a direct blow. The person must be assessed for neurological damage and any loss of consciousness (LOC) must be documented. A complete neurological assessment is conducted: pupillary reaction to light; movement and strength of all extremities; complaints of nausea and vomiting; LOC and orientation to person, place and time are noted. A displaced skull fracture, which is referred to as depressed, may press on the brain and cause neurological damage. Brain injuries related to skull fractures are discussed in the chapter 'Nursing care of people with intracranial disorders'.

Fracture of the face

Fracture of the facial bones may result from a direct blow. The person presents with haematomas, pain, oedema and bony deformity. Non-displaced fractures are monitored to ensure the airway is not compromised. The person is observed for any neurological deficits. Severely displaced or multiple facial fractures are treated with ORIF with wires or plates.

Nursing care focuses on maintaining the airway by helping the person clear secretions from the oropharynx. The nurse monitors the person's breathing for increased effort or tachypnoea and notifies the doctor immediately if these findings are noted. Pain is treated with analgesics and body image disturbances are addressed. If the person asks to see their face, the nurse should plan to stay with the person and answer questions while the person looks in a mirror.

Fracture of the spine

The spine can be injured in many ways, including sports injuries, falls and motor vehicle accidents. The spine can be fractured in the cervical, thoracic, lumbar or sacral area. The most severe complication of spine fracture is injury to the spinal cord (discussed in the chapter 'Nursing care of people with cerebrovascular and spinal cord disorders'). A fracture to the vertebrae may cause the bones to become displaced and apply pressure on the spinal cord, which may in turn result in permanent paralysis.

A non-displaced cervical spinal fracture may be treated with a cervical collar or a halo immobilising brace. The displaced cervical fracture is reduced by manual or skeletal traction and, eventually, application of a brace and/or surgical stabilisation of the bones with plates and screws. Immobilisation after a spinal fracture may last as long as 6 months.

Fracture of the clavicle

A fracture of the clavicle commonly results from a direct blow or a fall. The most common location is midclavicular. A person with a midclavicular fracture typically assumes a protective slumping position to immobilise the arm and prevent shoulder movement. A less common fracture occurs along the distal third of the clavicle. This type of fracture may be associated with ligament damage. Injuries to the clavicle may be associated with skull or cervical fractures. The fractured bone, if displaced, may lacerate the subclavian vessels and result in haemorrhage. The fractured bone may also puncture the lung, resulting in a pneumothorax. Malunion may occur at the fracture site and result in asymmetry of the clavicles. Injury to the brachial plexus may result in numbness and decreased movement of the arm on the affected side.

A deformity may be observed or palpated along the clavicle. Treatment focuses on immobilising the fractured bone in normal anatomical position by applying a clavicular strap, or a surgical repair may be necessary.

Fracture of the humerus

The exact location of the fracture, the presence of displacement and the results of the neurovascular examination determine the severity of a fracture of the humerus and the appropriate interventions. Treatment focuses on immobilising the fractured bone in normal anatomical position. Common complications of humeral fracture include nerve and ligament damage, frozen or stiff joints, and malunion. Early interventions may prevent permanent damage.

Fractures of the proximal humerus are common in older adults. A simple non-displaced fracture of the proximal humerus (near the humeral head) with a normal neurovascular assessment can be safely treated with immobilisation. A more complicated displaced fracture of the proximal humerus with bone fragmentation requires surgical intervention. The more severe the fracture and damage to soft tissue, the more likely it is that the range of motion (ROM) of the shoulder will be impaired. Rehabilitative measures focus on increasing ROM.

The humerus may also fracture along the shaft, usually as a direct result of trauma. If the humeral shaft fracture is simple and non-displaced, a hanging arm cast is applied. This cast maintains alignment of the fracture by using the pulling force of gravity; therefore, the person must be instructed not to rest the cast on anything to alleviate the weight. If the person is on bed rest, a hanging arm cast is not applied because the arm would not be able to hang freely. Instead, the fracture is immobilised with external skeletal traction. This traction places the injured arm in an upright position over the face and weights are hung off the distal portion of the humerus (see Figure 38.4C). Nursing interventions for people with fractures of the humerus are presented in Box 38.6.

BOX 38.6 Nursing interventions for people with fractures of the humerus

- Perform neurovascular assessments frequently (every 1–4 hours).
- Administer prescribed medications to alleviate pain.
- Encourage exercises for people with a hanging cast:
  a. finger exercises: move each finger of the affected arm through complete range of motion
  b. pendulum shoulder exercises: dangle the affected arm at the side and move it forwards and backwards about 30 degrees in each direction.
- If the person is discharged, instruct the person and family in cast care and sling application, neurovascular assessments, exercises, prescribed pain medications and manifestations of complications.
- If the person is admitted to the hospital, provide preoperative teaching.

Fracture of the elbow

The most common location of an elbow fracture is the distal humerus. Elbow fractures usually result from a fall or a direct blow to the elbow. The person guards the injured extremity, holding the arm rigidly in a flexed position or an extended position. Because the radius, ulna or humerus may be involved in the elbow fracture, all three bones must be visualised by x-ray.

Complications of an elbow fracture include nerve or artery damage and haemarthrosis, a collection of blood in the elbow joint. The most serious complication of an elbow fracture is Volkmann's contracture, which results from arterial occlusion and muscle ischaemia. The person complains of forearm pain, impaired sensation and loss of motor function. Rapid interventions are aimed at relieving pressure on the brachial artery and nerve and preventing muscle atrophy.

Non-displaced elbow fractures are treated by immobilising the fracture with a posterior splint or cast. The displaced fracture is first reduced and then immobilised. Nursing interventions focus on alleviating pain, maintaining immobilisation and educating people in neurovascular assessments.

Fracture of the radius and/or ulna

Fractures of the radius and ulna may occur as a result of either indirect injury, such as twisting or pulling on the arm, or direct injury, such as that resulting from a fall. The usual treatment of radius fractures depends on the location. The proximal radial head may be fractured from a fall on an outstretched hand. Blood commonly collects in the elbow joint and must be aspirated. If the fracture is non-displaced, a sling is applied. If the fracture is displaced, surgical intervention is required. After surgical repair of a displaced fracture, the arm is splinted with a posterior plaster splint. The person avoids movement for the first week and then initiates movement gradually.

When both bones are broken, the fracture is usually displaced. The person complains of pain and inability to turn up the palm of the hand. A non-displaced fracture is casted for about 6 weeks and either a shorter cast or a brace is then applied for 6 more weeks. If the fracture is displaced, surgical intervention is performed. The doctor reduces the fracture and may insert pins or screws to keep the bones in alignment. After the surgery, a cast is applied and the person is encouraged to exercise the fingers.

Complications after a radius and/or ulnar fracture include compartment syndrome, delayed healing and decreased wrist and finger movement. After surgery, the person also has an increased risk of infection. Nursing interventions focus on alleviating pain, maintaining immobilisation and educating people in neurovascular assessments, the importance of elevation and the need to inform the doctor of changes in sensation or an increase in pain.

Fractures in the wrist and hand

Wrist fractures often result from a fall onto an outstretched hand or onto the back of the hand. A common type of wrist fracture is *Colles' fracture*, in which the distal radius fractures after a fall onto an outstretched hand. The person with a wrist fracture presents with a bony deformity, pain, numbness, weakness and decreased ROM of the fingers. The capillary refill and sensation of the hand must be assessed.

The hand is composed of many bones. Most commonly, the metacarpals and phalanges are involved in a hand fracture. The injuring mechanism in a hand fracture varies from striking an object with a closed fist to closing a hand in a door. The person presents with complaints of pain, oedema and decreased ROM.

Comparative x-rays may be obtained to compare left and right wrists and hands. Complications of wrist and hand fractures are compartment syndrome, nerve damage, ligament damage and delayed union. A wrist fracture is commonly treated with closed reduction, cast application and elevation of the injured extremity. A hand fracture is splinted and elevated.

Nursing interventions focus on alleviating pain and educating the person in neurovascular assessments, the importance of elevation and how to exercise the fingers to prevent stiffness. If the dominant hand is injured, the person will require assistance in performing activities of daily living (ADLs).

Fracture of the ribs

Rib fractures commonly result from blunt chest trauma. The location of the fracture and involvement of underlying organs determine the severity of the injury. Fractures of the first through to third ribs may result in injury to the subclavian artery or vein. Fractures of the lower ribs may result in spleen and liver injuries.

The person presents with a history of recent chest trauma. Typically, the person complains of pain along the lateral portion of the rib. Palpation of the rib reveals a bony deformity and increases pain. Deep inspiration also increases pain. The skin over the fracture site may be ecchymotic (bruised).

A complication of rib fractures is a flail chest, which results from the fracture of two or more adjacent ribs in two or more places and the formation of a free-floating segment that moves in the opposite direction to the rib cage. The bony instability impairs respirations. Treatment is aimed at stabilising the flail segment and supporting respirations. Other complications of rib fractures include pneumothorax and/or haemothorax. The fractured rib may pierce and injure the lung. The lower ribs may pierce the liver or spleen, resulting in intra-abdominal bleeding. Pneumonia may also develop from ineffective clearing of respiratory secretions.

A simple rib fracture is treated with pain medication and instructions for coughing, deep breathing and splinting. The person is also instructed to return to the emergency room if shortness of breath develops. Nursing interventions focus on alleviating pain and teaching the person about splinting. Because deep inspiration increases pain, people frequently avoid it. The person may be instructed to splint the injured rib with the hand or a pillow, and to take deep breaths and cough to decrease the chance of developing pneumonia and/or atelectasis. Incentive spirometry is encouraged.

Fracture of the pelvis

Pelvic fractures are often caused by trauma, such as a fall or a motor vehicle crash. The person with a pelvic fracture presents with pain in the back or hip area. A single fracture in the pelvis is treated conservatively with bed rest on a firm mattress. Log rolling increases the person's comfort. A pelvic fracture with two fracture sites is considered unstable and treated with surgery. An external fixator may be applied to stabilise the pelvis. In the person who is not stable for surgery, a pelvic sling may be used. The pelvic sling stabilises the pelvis and allows the person to move in bed with less pain. Common complications include hypovolaemia, spinal injury, bladder injury, urethral injury, kidney damage and gastrointestinal trauma.

Nursing care focuses on alleviating discomfort, maintaining immobilisation and preparing the person for surgery if necessary. The nurse monitors the person for increased heart rate, decreased blood pressure and decreasing haemoglobin levels. These findings may indicate impending hypovolaemia due to bleeding into the pelvis. Any blood in the urine should be reported to the doctor; this may indicate kidney, bladder or urethral damage.

Fracture of the shaft of the femur

A large amount of force, such as from motor vehicle crashes, falls or acts of violence, is required to fracture the shaft of the femur. People with femoral shaft fractures often have associated multiple traumas. A fracture of the femoral shaft is manifested by an oedematous, deformed, painful thigh. The person is unable to move the hip or knee. Initial assessment focuses on the circulation and sensation present in the affected extremity. Pedal pulses and capillary refill in the affected extremity are compared to the unaffected extremity. Complications of a femoral shaft fracture include hypovolaemia due to blood loss (which may be as great as 1.0 to 1.5 L), fat embolism, dislocation of the hip or knee, muscle atrophy and ligament damage.

Treatment of fractures of the shaft of the femur initially includes skeletal traction to separate the bony fragments and reduce and immobilise the fracture. Depending on the location and severity of the fracture, traction may be followed by either external or internal fixation. Strength in the affected extremity is maintained through gluteal and quadricep exercises. ROM exercises for unaffected extremities are critical in preparation for ambulation. Although full weight bearing is usually restricted until x-rays demonstrate bone union, the person may be allowed to carry out non-weight-bearing activities with an assistive device.

The nurse assesses pulses in the extremity and compares them bilaterally. Sensation is evaluated by asking whether the person can feel touch and discriminate sharp from dull objects. Nursing interventions include providing pain medication, providing reassurance and decreasing anxiety, and assisting with exercises of the lower legs, feet and toes.

Fracture of the hip

A hip fracture refers to a fracture of the femur at the head, neck or trochanteric regions (see Figure 38.8). Hip fractures are classified as intracapsular or extracapsular. *Intracapsular fractures* involve the head or neck of the femur; *extracapsular fractures* involve the trochanteric region. The majority of hip fractures involve the neck or trochanteric regions. The femoral head and neck lie within the joint capsule and are not covered in periosteum; thus, they do not have a large blood supply. Fractures at this location usually fragment, further decreasing blood supply and increasing the risk of non-union and avascular necrosis. The trochanteric region is covered in periosteum and therefore has more blood supply than the head or neck.

Hip fractures are a common clinical issue in the older adult in both Australia and New Zealand. In Australia, an estimated 19,000 people over the age of 50 are hospitalised with a hip fracture each year (Australian Commission on Safety and Quality in Health Care (ACSQHC), 2016). In both countries, hip fractures are more prevalent in women than in men due to osteoporosis. There is a general increase in mortality for patients with hip fracture, with a higher mortality rate in men than in women. Institutionalisation combined with comorbidities was associated with a higher mortality (Guzon-Illescas et al., 2019).

In 2015–2016, the hospitalisation rate for new hip fractures rose substantially with age. When the influence of age was adjusted for, new hip fractures were 1.7 times higher for women than for men and 5% higher for Indigenous Australians than for other Australians (Australian Institute of Health and Welfare (AIHW), 2022).

Hip fractures cause a decrease in mobility and independence. Factors contributing to falls include problems with gait and balance, neurological and musculoskeletal impairments, dementia, psychoactive medications and visual impairments. Modifiable risk factors include lower body weakness, problems with walking and balance, and taking four or more medications or any psychoactive medications.

Hip fractures occur in older adults as a result of decreased bone mass and the increased tendency to fall. Whether the femur breaks spontaneously and causes the fall, or whether the fall causes the fracture, is not always clear; regardless of the cause of the fracture, rapid interventions are required to prevent bone necrosis. Assessment findings commonly associated with a hip fracture are pain, inability to walk and shortening and external rotation of the affected lower extremity. Rarely, the fracture dislocates posteriorly; if that occurs, the extremity may internally rotate. However, some people with a hip fracture have only vague pain in the buttocks, knees, thighs, groin or back, and their ability to walk is unaffected. If the fracture is not visible on x-ray, a bone scan or MRI may be done to confirm the presence of the fracture.

A hip fracture may be treated with traction to decrease muscle spasms, followed by surgery (however, this is being used less often) (AIHW, 2022) or surgery may be performed immediately or within the first 24 hours. The goal of surgery is to reduce and stabilise the fracture, thereby increasing mobility, decreasing pain and preventing complications. Surgery usually consists of ORIF of the fracture. Fixation is accomplished by

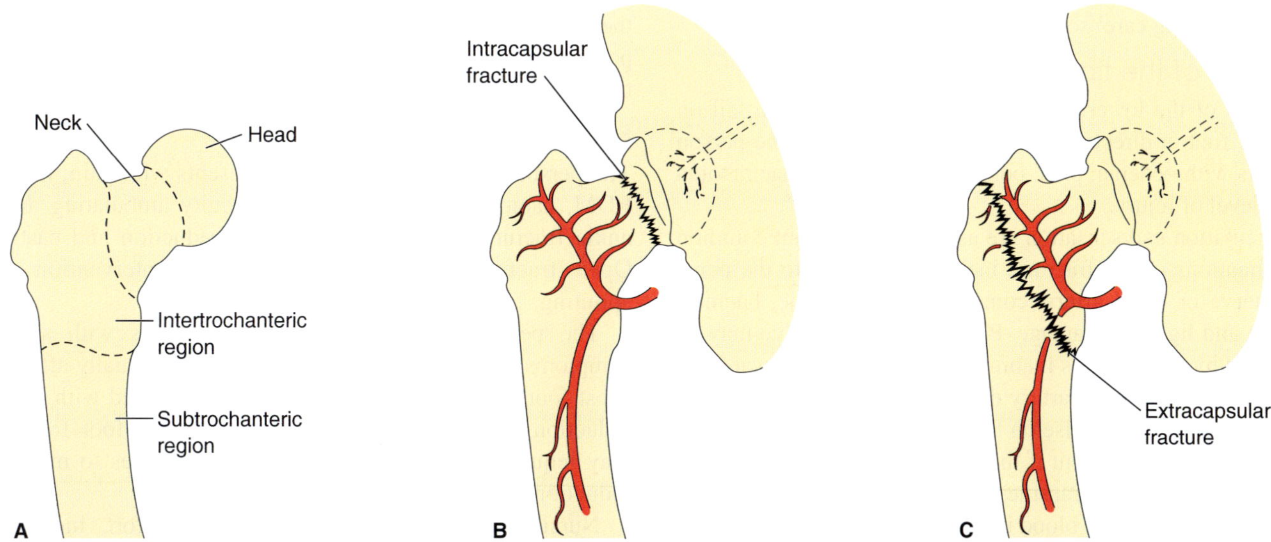

FIGURE 38.8 ***Regions where hip fractures may occur: A, The head of the femur, the neck of the femur and the trochanteric regions of the femur. B, Intracapsular fractures occur across the head or neck of the femur. C, Extracapsular fractures occur across the trochanteric regions. Note how both intracapsular and extracapsular fractures disrupt the blood supply to the bone***

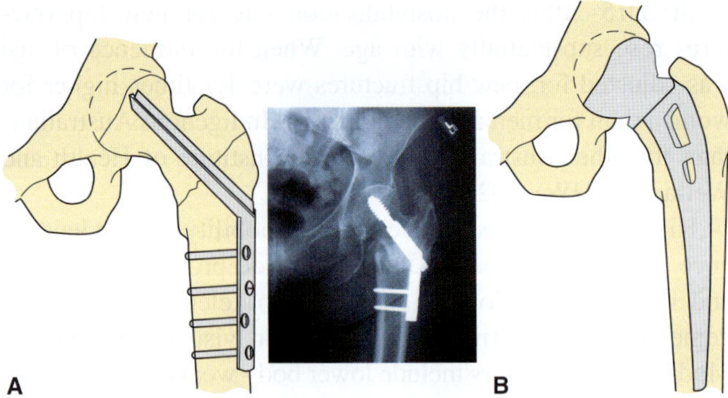

FIGURE 38.9 ***Surgical fixation of hip fractures. A, A surgical nail or screw used to stabilise an intertrochanteric fracture. B, Use of a hip prosthesis (artificial hip) to replace a damaged femoral head***

Source: Image from Linda Gilliland/123RF.

securing the femur in place with pins, screws, nails or plates (see Figure 38.9A). An ORIF works well for fractures in the trochanteric area. Fractures of the femoral neck frequently disrupt blood supply to the femoral head. If blood supply is disrupted, the surgeon will replace the femoral head with a prosthesis (see Figure 38.9B). If the acetabulum has been damaged, the surgeon may insert a metal cup. Replacement of either the femoral head or the acetabulum with a prosthesis is called a *hemiarthroplasty*. Replacement of both the femoral head and the acetabulum is a *total hip arthroplasty (THA)*, discussed in the chapter 'Nursing care of people with musculoskeletal disorders'.

Nursing care for a person with a hip fracture focuses on maintaining skin integrity, preventing infection, alleviating pain, maintaining circulation to the injured extremity and increasing mobility, and is discussed in more detail in the following 'Nursing care' section.

Fracture of the tibia and/or fibula

Fractures of the lower extremities often result from a fall on a flexed foot, a direct blow or a twisting motion. The person presents with oedema, pain, bony deformity and a haematoma at the level of injury.

Circulation and sensation are assessed to rule out common complications of the fracture, including damage to the peroneal nerve or tibial artery, compartment syndrome, haemarthroses and ligament damage. Peroneal nerve damage may be indicated by the person's inability to point the toe upwards on the affected side. Tibial artery damage may be the cause of an absent dorsalis pedis pulse on the affected side. Compartment syndrome may be present if the person develops pain on passive movement and paraesthesias. An oedematous knee may indicate a collection of blood in the knee joint. Ligament damage may be present if the person cannot move the knee and/or ankle.

If the fracture is closed, a closed reduction and casting are frequently performed. A long leg cast that allows for partial weight bearing is used. Partial weight bearing usually is prescribed by the doctor within 10 days of the fracture. A short leg cast will be applied in 3 to 4 weeks. If the fracture is open, either external fixation or ORIF will be performed. After surgery, a cast may be applied and weight bearing begins according to the doctor's orders, usually in about 6 weeks.

Nursing care is designed to increase comfort, monitor neurovascular status and prevent complications. The nurse instructs the person in cast care, on the use of assistive devices, how to perform neurovascular assessment and when to follow up with the doctor.

Fracture in the ankle and foot

The person with an ankle fracture presents with pain, limited ROM, haematoma, oedema and difficulty ambulating. Most ankle fractures are treated by closed reduction and casting. Open fractures are treated by surgical intervention and splinting.

The person with a foot fracture presents with similar symptoms; however, ROM of the ankle is not usually affected. Most foot fractures are non-displaced and treated with closed reduction and casting. More severe displaced foot fractures may require surgery and the placement of wires to maintain reduction of the fracture.

Nursing care focuses on increasing comfort, increasing mobility and educating the person. Analgesia is given for pain. The extremity should be elevated and ice can be applied. The person is taught cast care, neurovascular assessment and crutch walking.

FAST FACTS

Hip fracture in older adults

- Almost 1 in 3 older Australians have a fall each year.
- Over 40% have multiple falls.
- Over 30% require medical attention after a fall.
- Hip fracture in older adults is most often the result of a fall; in contrast, car crashes are the most common cause of a hip fracture in young and middle-aged adults.
- The risk of a fractured hip increases with each decade of life, especially in Caucasian postmenopausal women, who have the highest incidence of osteoporosis. Women have about 80% of all hip fractures. Women who smoke are at greater risk because smoking reduces bone density in menopausal women.
- Complications are related both to the fracture and to the resulting treatment. Only a small number of people retain their previous mobility, while about 20% require nursing home care.
- Half of all older adults hospitalised for a hip fracture cannot return home or live independently after the fracture.

Sources: Data from ACSQHC (2015); Burns, Stevens & Lee (2016); Queensland Health (2016).

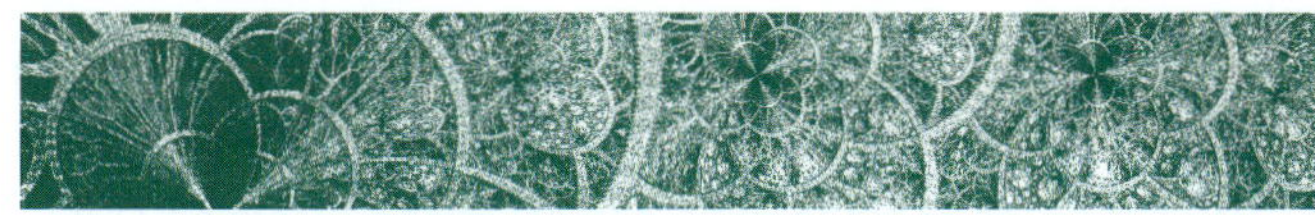

Nursing care

In planning and implementing nursing care for the person with fractures, the nurse should consider the person's response to the traumatic experience. Although each person has individual needs, nursing care commonly focuses on the person's problems with pain, impaired physical mobility, impaired tissue perfusion and neurovascular compromise.

Health promotion

Trauma prevention can save lives. Many communities are educating people of all ages, from primary school students to older adults, in trauma prevention. Young adults face a high risk of sustaining trauma. They need to be taught the importance of safety equipment—such as automobile seat belts, bicycle and motorised vehicle helmets, shin guards, proper footwear, protective eyewear and hard hats—in preventing or decreasing the severity of injury from trauma. Older adults should have regular screenings for osteoporosis (with a bone density test), activity levels, cognitive and affective disorders, vision impairments and risk of falls. Older adults can reduce their risk of falling by increasing lower body strength and balance through regular physical activity and by asking their healthcare provider or pharmacist to review their medications. Educational programs about workplace and farm safety, including information about ergonomic principles, can also help prevent musculoskeletal injuries.

Having a regular exercise program and avoiding obesity are important factors in maintaining good bone health in all adults. An adequate intake of calcium is essential to ensure proper growth, development and maintenance of strong bones throughout life. It is important that women ensure good bone health prior to menopause, because a decrease in oestrogen during and after menopause drops calcium use and retention, and increases the risk of osteoporosis. Strong bones are formed by calcium intake and weight-bearing exercise, both of which are equally important in the postmenopausal woman.

Older people are at higher risk of musculoskeletal trauma due to falls. For older people, home assessments must be performed and potential hazards removed. Specific teaching topics for preventing falls in older adults are outlined in the 'Nursing care of the older adult' box.

Assessment

Collect the following data through the health history and physical examination (see the chapter 'A person-centred approach to assessing the musculoskeletal system').

- *Health history*: age, history of traumatic event, history of chronic illnesses, history of prior musculoskeletal injuries, medications. (Ask the older adult specifically about anticoagulants and calcium supplements.)
- *Physical assessment*: pain with movement, pulses, oedema, skin colour and temperature, deformity, range of motion, touch. These assessments include the 5 Ps of neurovascular assessment, in both the initial assessment and ongoing focused assessments.

Nursing diagnoses and interventions

Nursing care for people with fractures ranges from teaching for home care treatments provided in the emergency or urgent care department (such as manual reduction and cast application) to providing interventions to maintain health and decrease the risk of complications in people with complex or multiple fractures. Teaching is also necessary for caregivers of the older adult who is discharged home or to a long-term care or rehabilitation facility following a fractured hip. See the accompanying nursing care plan.

NURSING CARE OF THE OLDER ADULT **Teaching older adults to prevent falls**

- Begin a regular exercise program; lack of exercise leads to weakness and an increased chance of falling. Low-impact exercises that improve balance and coordination (such as Tai Chi) are the most helpful.
- Make your home safer:
  - Remove any items in your pathway, including from stairways, to avoid tripping.
  - Remove small throw rugs or use double-sided tape to keep rugs from slipping.
  - Place frequently used items within easy reach to avoid use of a step-ladder.
  - Install grab bars next to your toilet and in the bath or shower.
  - Use non-slip mats in the bathtub and on shower floors.
  - Improve lighting, using lamp shades or frosted bulbs to reduce glare.
  - Install handrails and lights in all staircases or steps.
  - Wear shoes that give good support and have thin, non-slip soles. Avoid wearing slippers and athletic shoes with deep treads.
- Ask your doctor to review your medications, including prescriptions and over-the-counter medications. Some medications, or a combination of medications, may cause dizziness or drowsiness, contributing to falls.
- Have your vision checked frequently (every 6 months) by an eye specialist. Your glasses may no longer have the correct prescription or you may have developed an eye condition such as cataracts or glaucoma that limits your vision.

NURSING CARE PLAN A person with a hip fracture

Barbara Wallace, aged 74, has a history of osteoporosis. She is a widow and lives alone in a two-storey terrace house. Mrs Wallace is retired and depends on a pension and social security for her income. She takes pride in making all her own meals from scratch.

While walking to the shopping centre one day, Mrs Wallace trips and falls up the gutter and fractures her left hip. She is transported by ambulance to the nearest hospital emergency department.

ASSESSMENT

During the initial assessment at the ED, abnormal findings are that Mrs Wallace's left leg is shorter than her right leg and is externally rotated. Distal pulses are present and bilaterally strong; both legs are warm. Mrs Wallace complains of severe pain in her hip but states that no numbness or burning is present. She is able to wiggle the toes on her left leg and has full movement of her right leg. Initial vital signs are as follows: T 36.6°C, P 100 and regular, R 18, BP 120/58. Diagnostic tests include FBC, blood chemistry, crossmatch and x-ray studies of the left hip and pelvis. The FBC reveals a haemoglobin of 11.0 g/dL and a normal WBC count. Blood chemistry findings are within normal limits. The x-ray reveals a fracture of the left femoral neck. Mrs Wallace is admitted to the hospital. She is given a femoral block and ordered regular analgesia. An open reduction and internal fixation (ORIF) is planned for the following day.

DIAGNOSES

- *Acute pain* related to fractured left femoral neck and muscle spasms.
- *Impaired physical mobility* related to bed rest and fractured left femoral neck.
- *Risk of ineffective tissue perfusion* related to unstable bones and swelling.
- *Risk of disturbed tactile sensory perception* related to the risk of nerve impairment.

PLANNING

- Identify and manage pain.
- Monitor changes in neurovascular status.
- Monitor postoperative complications.

Expected outcomes

- Mrs Wallace will verbalise a decrease in pain.
- Improved comfort for Mrs Wallace.
- Maintain normal neurovascular status.
- Prevention of postoperative complications including DVT, pressure areas, atelectasis, urinary stasis and constipation.

IMPLEMENTATION

- Assess pain on a scale of 0 to 10 before and after implementing measures to reduce pain.
- Administer medications (e.g. narcotics/stool softeners) as per the doctor's order.
- Position Mrs Wallace so as to reduce pain.
- Perform neurovascular assessment every 2 to 4 hours and document findings.
- Encourage deep breathing and relaxation techniques.
- Demonstrate postoperative exercises.
- Teach the purpose of and the procedure for performing isometric and flexion/extension exercises.

EVALUATION

Three days after surgery, Mrs Wallace is out of bed and in a chair. She verbalises a decrease in pain. There have been no abnormal neurovascular assessments. She is able to independently perform isometric and flexion/extension exercises in both lower extremities. She has used her bowels and is voiding as before the fall. Safe discharge planning includes explaining the benefits to Mrs Wallace of going to a rehabilitation facility before going directly home, and referrals for home care. A community nurse will visit and the discharge planner at the hospital has organised review by the physiotherapist and the occupational therapist to order a trapeze for her bed, an elevated toilet seat, an elevated cushion for her chair and a walker.

CRITICAL THINKING IN THE NURSING PROCESS

1. What factors placed Mrs Wallace at risk of a hip fracture?
2. Identify the preoperative management and how you can explain this to Mrs Wallace. Explain the reason for the femoral block and why she needs to remain in bed.
3. Describe how each of the following, if manifested by Mrs Wallace, would increase her risk of postoperative complications: urinary incontinence; weight more than 20% under normal for her height; chronic constipation. Which nursing diagnoses and interventions would you include in her plan of care to decrease the risk?

REFLECTION ON THE NURSING PROCESS

1. Outline what you have learned from this case study that you will take into your future practice.
2. Which education requirements for Mrs Wallace would the nurse need to implement prior to her being discharged?

Acute pain

Pain is caused by soft tissue damage and is compounded by muscle spasms and swelling.

- Monitor vital signs. *Some analgesics decrease respiratory effort and blood pressure.*
- Ask the person to rate the pain on a scale of 0 to 10 (with 10 as the most severe pain) before and after any intervention. *This facilitates objective assessment of the effectiveness of the chosen pain relief strategy. Pain that increases in intensity or remains unrelieved with analgesics can indicate compartment syndrome.*
- For the person with a hip fracture, apply Buck's traction as per doctor's orders. Keep the traction weights hanging freely. *Buck's traction immobilises the fracture and decreases pain and additional trauma.*

- Move the person gently and slowly. *Gentle moving helps prevent the development of severe muscle spasms.*

CONSIDERATION FOR PRACTICE

Do not let weights lie on the bed or the floor. The weights can be removed long enough to move the person up or down in bed to ensure freely hanging weights.

- Elevate the injured extremity above the level of the heart. *Elevating the extremity promotes venous return and decreases oedema, which decreases pain.*
- Encourage distraction or other non-invasive methods of pain relief, such as deep breathing and relaxation. *Distraction, deep breathing and relaxation help decrease the focus on the pain and may lessen the intensity of pain.*
- Administer pain medications as prescribed. For home care, explain the importance of taking pain medications before the pain is severe. *Analgesics alleviate pain by stimulating opiate receptor sites.*

CONSIDERATION FOR PRACTICE

In the case of fracture in an extremity, supporting the extremity above and below the fracture can also decrease pain and muscle spasms.

Risk of peripheral neurovascular dysfunction

In the person with a fracture, compartment syndrome or deep venous thrombosis can impair circulation and, in turn, reduce tissue perfusion.

- Assess the 5 Ps every 1 to 2 hours. Report abnormal findings immediately. *Unrelenting pain, pallor, diminished distal pulses, paraesthesias and paresis are strong indicators of compartment syndrome.*

CONSIDERATION FOR PRACTICE

Pulses may remain strong, even in the presence of compartment syndrome.

- Assess nail beds for capillary refill. If nails are too thick or discoloured, assess the skin around the nail. *Delayed capillary refill may indicate decreased tissue perfusion.*

CONSIDERATION FOR PRACTICE

It may not be possible to accurately assess capillary refill in older adults, who often have thickened, discoloured nails. If so, test nearby skin.

- Monitor the extremity for oedema and swelling. *Excessive swelling and haematoma formation can compromise circulation.*
- Assess for deep, throbbing, unrelenting pain. *Pain that is not relieved by analgesics may indicate neurovascular compromise.*

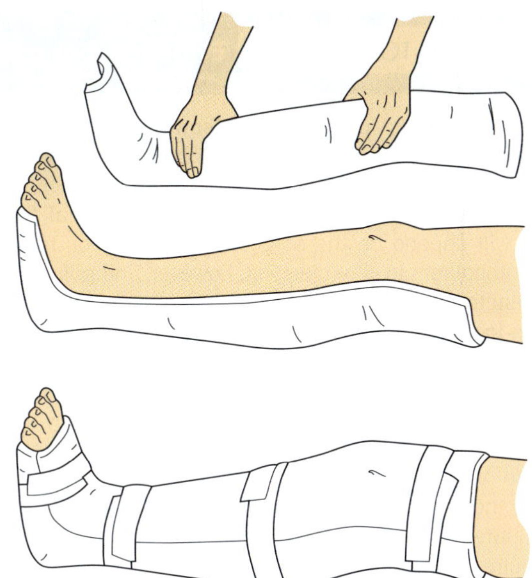

FIGURE 38.10 ***Bivalving is the process of splitting the cast down both sides to alleviate pressure on or allow visualisation of the extremity***

- Monitor the tightness of the cast. *Oedema can cause the cast to become tight; a tight-fitting cast may lead to compartment syndrome or paralysis.*
- If cast is tight, be prepared to assist the doctor with bivalving (see Figure 38.10). *Bivalving, the process of splitting the cast down both sides, alleviates pressure on the injured extremity.*
- If compartment syndrome is suspected, assist the doctor in measuring compartment pressure. Normal compartment pressure is 10 to 20 mmHg. *Compartment pressure greater than 30 mmHg indicates compartment syndrome.*
- Elevate the injured extremity above the level of the heart. *Elevating the extremity increases venous return and decreases oedema.*
- Administer anticoagulant per doctor's order. *Prophylactic anticoagulation decreases the risk of clot formation.*

Risk of infection

The person who undergoes surgical repair will have a postoperative wound. Any break in skin integrity must be monitored for infection. Wound healing in an orthopaedic person is affected by the cause of the wound, as well as by the therapies used to repair musculoskeletal structures. It is important for nurses to understand normal wound healing processes; characteristics of musculoskeletal wounds, contamination and drainage; and potential complications, in order to plan for and implement appropriate interventions.

- For people with skeletal pins, follow established guidelines for skeletal pin site care, as outlined in the 'Translation to practice' box. *Pins or wires attached to traction, casts or external fixators stabilise a segment of bone so that optimal healing can occur. However, pin infections of varying severity do occur.*

TRANSLATION TO PRACTICE Evidence-based practice for the person with skeletal pins

Clinical guidelines for specific person care interventions, such as skeletal pin care, should be based on research in order to provide the most appropriate evidence-based practice. Management of people with an external fixation device will depend on the surgeon. Each surgeon has their own protocol for pin care cleaning; however, unit policy should be consulted.

- Pins located in areas with considerable soft tissue should be considered at greater risk of infection.
- People and their families should be taught pin site care before discharge from the hospital. They should be required to demonstrate whatever care needs to be done and should be provided with written instructions that include signs and symptoms of infection—such as exudate, erythema, tenderness and pain—which may require removal of the pins.

IMPLICATIONS FOR NURSING

While the preference of the surgeon may determine the care required for external pin sites, unit policy should also be consulted.

CRITICAL THINKING IN PERSON-CENTRED CARE

1. List the factors that may increase the risk of infection of skeletal pin sites. Describe the nursing interventions that may be used to reduce this risk.
2. You are caring for a person with skeletal pins for external fixation of a fracture of bones of a lower extremity. There is dried yellow drainage around the pin site. Based on clinical decision making, would you remove the crusts? Why or why not?
3. You are teaching a person how to undertake pin care at home. Make a list of manifestations of infection the person may experience. What would you recommend if any of these manifestations occur?

Source: Data from Lethaby, Temple & Santy-Tomlinson (2013). Pin site care for preventing infections associated with external bone fixators and pins. *Cochrane Database of Systematic Reviews, 12*, CD004551.

- Monitor vital signs and lab reports of WBCs. *Increases in pulse rate, respiratory rate, temperature and WBCs may indicate infection.*
- Use a sterile technique for dressing changes. *The initial postoperative dressing will be changed by the surgeon. The nurse must change all subsequent dressings without introducing organisms into the operative site.*
- Assess the wound for size, colour and the presence of any drainage. *Redness, swelling and purulent drainage indicate infection.*
- Administer antibiotics per doctor's orders. Prophylactic antibiotic administration inhibits bacterial reproduction and thereby helps prevent skin flora from entering the wound. *In the case of 'dirty wounds', such as those occurring from vehicular crashes, antibiotics are routinely administered.*

Impaired physical mobility

The person who has experienced a fracture requires immobilisation of the fractured bone(s). Immobilisation alters normal gait and mobility. The person will need to use assistive devices such as crutches, canes, slings or walkers.

- Teach or assist the person with *ROM exercises for the unaffected limbs. ROM exercises help prevent muscle atrophy and maintain strength and joint function. Flexion and extension exercises prevent the development of foot drop, wrist drop or frozen joints.*
- Teach isometric exercises and encourage the person to perform them every 4 hours. *Isometric exercises help prevent muscle atrophy and force synovial fluid and nutrients into the cartilage.*
- Encourage ambulation when able; provide assistance as necessary. *Ambulation maintains and improves circulation, helps prevent muscle atrophy and helps maintain bowel function.*
- Teach and observe the person's use of assistive devices (such as canes, crutches, walkers, slings) in conjunction with the physical therapist. *Proper use of devices is necessary for safe ambulation and helps prevent the loss of joint function secondary to complications and falls.*
- Turn the person on bed rest every 2 hours. If the person is in traction, teach the person to shift his or her weight every hour. *Turning and shifting weight increase circulation and help prevent skin breakdown.*

Risk of disturbed tactile sensory perception

The person who has sustained a fracture is at risk of nerve injury from the initial trauma, as well as from complications such as compartment syndrome.

- Assess the ability to differentiate between sharp and dull touch and the presence of paraesthesias and paralysis every 1 to 2 hours. *Paraesthesias develop as a result of pressure on nerves and may indicate compartment syndrome.*

CONSIDERATION FOR PRACTICE

Paralysis is a late sign of nerve entrapment and requires that the healthcare provider be notified immediately.

- Elevate the injured extremity above the level of the heart. *Elevating the extremity decreases swelling and the risk of compartment syndrome and nerve entrapment.*
- Check the cast for fit. *A tightly fitting cast can decrease blood flow to distal tissues, compress nerves and cause compartment syndrome.*

- Support the injured extremity above and below the fracture site when moving the person. *Such support helps prevent displacement of bony fragments and decreases the risk of further nerve damage.*

Community-based care

Person and family teaching focuses on individualised needs. The type of fracture and its location determine how much teaching the person and family will require. For example, a person who has a simple non-displaced tibial fracture may need to be taught only cast care and crutch walking. An older person who has sustained a hip fracture and requires surgical intervention, by contrast, has a wider array of teaching needs, including the use of an abduction pillow, proper bending and proper sitting. Address the following topics for home care of the person who has fractured a hip:

- Encourage independence in ADLs:
  - Explain that the person should sit only on high chairs to prevent excess flexion of the hip; a high toilet seat can be added to a regular toilet seat.
  - Encourage the person and family to equip the shower with a rail to aid stability and prevent falls.
  - If a walker is needed, teach the person its proper use: do not carry the walker but lift it, advance the walker and then take two steps, or use a rolling walker.
  - If a walking stick is needed, instruct the person to use it on the affected side.
  - Stress the importance of well-balanced meals and explain all prescribed medications.
  - Be conscious (especially with younger people) that sexuality and need for sexual expression may not be diminished as a result of injury. Finding suitable and appropriate avenues for people to express their sexual needs should be a topic of conversation and care planning as required.

People who have experienced a fracture or have had orthopaedic surgery often have a cast and require an extended period of immobilisation or limited activities. Address the following topics for home care:

- Do not try to scratch under a cast with a sharp object.
- Do not get a plaster cast wet.
- Follow the doctor's order for weight bearing.
- Physiotherapy departments or offices can often evaluate the home environment for safety and suggest modifications as needed. Physiotherapists also teach crutch walking, limited weight bearing, transferring and other activities.
- Home care agencies can teach wound care and provide ongoing monitoring of wound healing.
- Local medical equipment and supply sources rent or sell durable equipment such as crutches, walkers, wheelchairs, overhead trapeze units, shower chairs, elevated toilet seats, grab bars and bedside commodes. Slings or braces may be purchased through medical equipment dealers.
- Local pharmacies are good resources for dressing supplies such as antiseptic solutions or ointments, dressings and tape.
- Fitness equipment suppliers may be able to provide rehabilitation equipment such as hand or ankle weights for strengthening exercises.

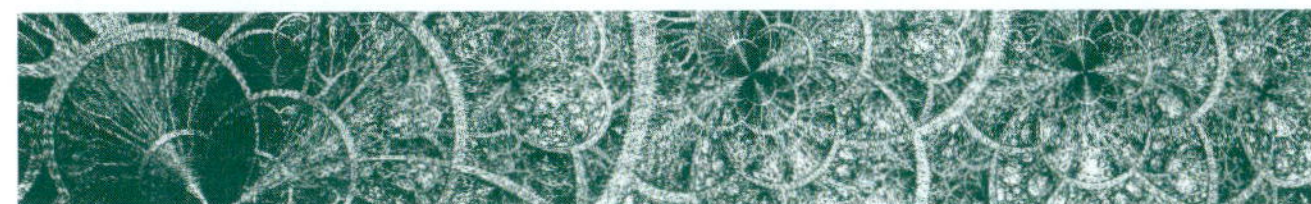

THE PERSON WITH AN AMPUTATION

An **amputation** is the partial or total removal of an extremity. Amputation may be the result of an acute process, such as a traumatic event, or a chronic condition, such as peripheral vascular disease or diabetes mellitus. Regardless of the cause, an amputation is devastating to the person.

The loss of all or part of an extremity has a significant physical and psychosocial effect on the person and family. Adaptation may take a long time and require much effort. Interprofessional healthcare is always important, but is especially necessary to meet the person's physical, spiritual, cultural and emotional needs after either an unexpected or planned amputation.

Causes of amputation

Peripheral vascular disease (PVD) is the major cause of amputation of the lower extremities (see the chapter 'Nursing care of people with vascular and lymphatic disorders'). Common risk factors for the development of PVD include hypertension, diabetes, smoking and hyperlipidaemia. Peripheral neuropathy also places the person with diabetes at risk of amputation. In peripheral neuropathy, loss of sensation frequently leads to unrecognised injury and infection. Untreated infection may lead to gangrene and the need for amputation. These risks are discussed in the chapter 'Nursing care of people with diabetes mellitus'.

The incidence of traumatic amputations is highest in young men. Most amputations in this group result from motor vehicle crashes or accidents involving machinery at work. The person presents to the trauma centre with an injury that may be life threatening; significant loss of blood and tissue may have already occurred and shock may develop. (See the chapter 'Nursing care of people experiencing trauma and shock' for a discussion of shock and trauma.) Other traumatic events that may necessitate an amputation are frostbite, burns or electrocution.

Amputations result from or are necessitated by interruption in blood flow, either acute or chronic. In acute trauma situations, the limb is partially or completely severed and tissue death ensues. However, replantation of fingers, small body parts and entire limbs has been successful. In chronic disease processes, circulation is impaired, venous pooling begins, proteins leak into the interstitium and oedema develops. Oedema increases the risk of injury and further decreases circulation. Stasis ulcers develop and readily become infected because impaired healing and altered immune processes allow bacteria to proliferate. The presence of progressive infection further compromises circulation and ultimately leads to gangrene (tissue death), which requires amputation.

FAST FACTS

- Males are at higher risk of amputations and are three times more likely to suffer an amputation than females.
- The middle and older age groups have the highest incidence of amputation. This is generally due to peripheral vascular disease, atherosclerosis and changes due to diabetes mellitus. In Australia, the most common causes of lower extremity amputations are disease, trauma and thermal injuries, congenital or birth defects, and tumours.
- Upper extremity amputation is usually due to trauma or birth defect.
- Demographics show that amputees represent 1 per 1,000 individuals across Australia, and subsequently there are in excess of 20,000 amputees living in Australia.

Source: Australian Physiotherapists in Amputee Rehabilitation (2018). Retrieved from https://www.aopa.org.au/.

Levels of amputation

The level of amputation is determined by local and systemic factors. Local factors include ischaemia and gangrene; systemic factors include cardiovascular status, renal function and severity of diabetes mellitus. The goals are to alleviate symptoms, to maintain healthy tissue and to increase functional outcome. When possible, the joints are preserved because they allow greater function of the extremity. Figure 38.11 illustrates common sites of amputation.

Types of amputation

Amputations may be open (*guillotine*) or closed (*flap*). Open amputations are performed when infection is present. The wound is not closed but remains open to drain. When infection is no longer present, surgery is performed to close the wound. In closed amputations, the wound is closed with a flap of skin that is sutured in place over the stump. Terms used to refer to amputations are defined in Table 38.3.

Amputation site healing

For the prosthesis to fit well, the amputation site must heal properly. To promote healing, a rigid or compression dressing is applied to prevent infection and minimise oedema. A compression bandage is usually applied immediately after surgery to support the soft tissues. The bandage may be elastic and is applied to the residual limb. The compression bandage is worn at all times, except for showering and physiotherapy. Bandages are reapplied several times a day to ensure a snug fit, but not to interfere with circulation.

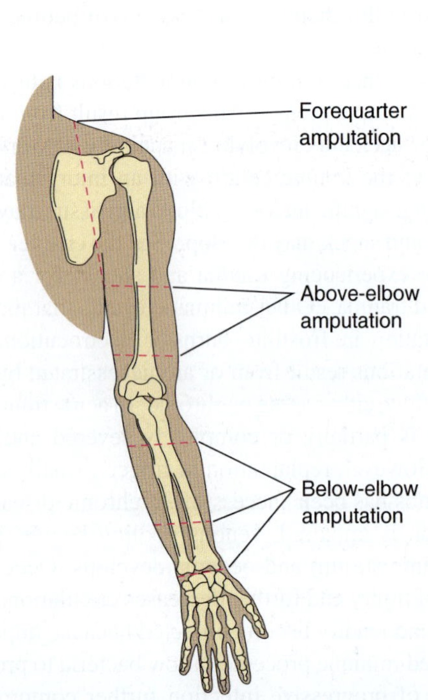

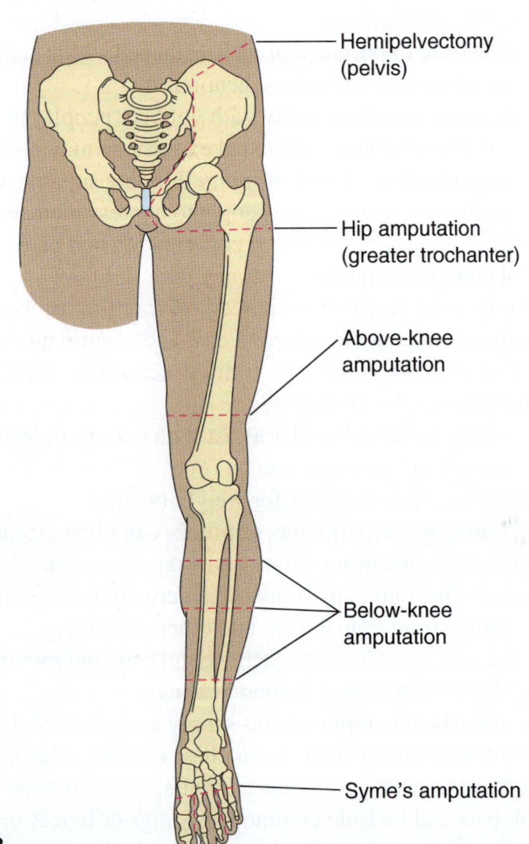

FIGURE 38.11 ***Common sites of amputation. A, The upper extremities. B, The lower extremities. The surgeon determines the level of amputation based on blood supply and tissue condition***

TABLE 38.3 Amputation terms

TERM	MEANING
Arm	Amputation of a portion of the arm, either above or below the elbow
Disarticulation	Amputation through a joint
Forequarter	Removal of the entire arm and disarticulation of the shoulder
Closed (flap)	Amputation in which a flap of skin is formed to cover the end of the wound
Open (guillotine)	Perpendicular cutting of the extremity in which the wound is left open; used when infection is present
Leg	Amputation below the knee (BK)
Thigh	Amputation above the knee (AK)
Finger or toe	Amputation of one or all of the fingers or toes
Syme	Modified disarticulation of the ankle
Foot	Amputation of part of the foot and toes

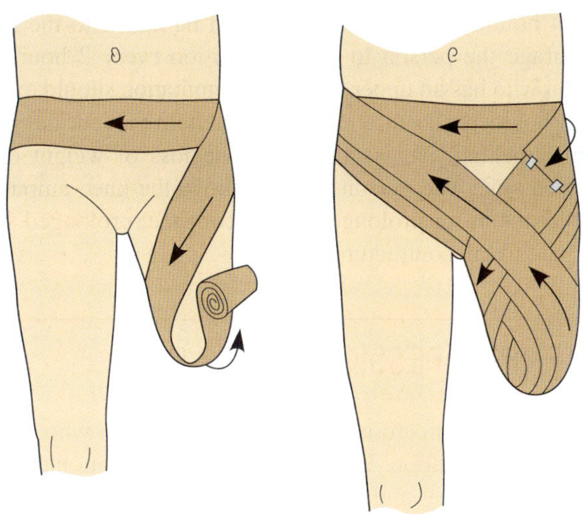

FIGURE 38.12 ***Stump dressings increase venous return, decrease oedema and help shape the stump for a prosthesis. With an above-knee amputation, a figure-eight bandage is started by bringing the bandage down over the stump and back up around the hips***

Once the wound has healed, the compression bandage need only be worn when the prosthesis is not worn. The bandage is applied from the distal to the proximal extremity (see Figure 38.12).

Complications

Complications that may occur after an amputation include infection, delayed healing, chronic stump pain and phantom pain, and contractures.

Infection

Generally, the person who suffers a traumatic amputation has a greater risk of infection than the person who has a planned amputation. However, even planned amputations carry a risk of infection. The person who is older, has diabetes mellitus or suffers peripheral neurovascular compromise is at a particularly high risk of infection. Infection may present itself locally or systemically. Local manifestations of infection include drainage, odour, redness and increased discomfort at the suture line. Systemic manifestations include fever, an increased heart rate, a decrease in blood pressure, chills and positive wound or blood cultures.

Delayed healing

If infection is present, or if the circulation remains compromised, delayed healing (occurring at a slower rate than expected) will result. In older people, pre-existing conditions can increase the risk of delayed healing. In people of any age, electrolyte imbalances can contribute to delayed healing processes, as can a diet that lacks the proper nutrients to meet the body's increased metabolic demands during healing. Smoking compromises healing by causing vasoconstriction and decreasing blood flow to the stump. Deep venous thrombosis and compromised venous return, which may result from prolonged immobilisation, are other potential factors. Decreased cardiac output decreases blood flow and thus also delays healing.

Chronic stump pain and phantom pain

Chronic stump pain is the result of neuroma formation, causing severe burning pain. Interventions to relieve this pain include medications, nerve blocks, transcutaneous electrical nerve stimulation (TENS) and surgical stump reconstruction. Phantom limb pain is not the same as phantom limb sensation. A majority of amputees experience phantom limb sensation (sensations such as tingling, numbness, cramping or itching in the phantom foot or hand) early in the postoperative period. It is often self-limiting but may last for decades in some people. When phantom limb sensation is painful, it is referred to as **phantom limb pain**. Although various theories have been proposed, the exact cause of this experience is unknown. Treatments include pain management, TENS and a variety of surgical procedures. The management of phantom limb pain is difficult for both people and healthcare professionals. People with phantom limb pain often benefit from referral to a pain clinic for a comprehensive pain management program.

Mirror therapy, or mirror box therapy, is a physical therapy technique that may be used to increase movement and decrease pain in limbs. It is suitable for complex regional pain and phantom limb pain, stroke and other chronic pain conditions. Its initiation as a therapy should be guided by an experienced physical therapist, occupational therapist or physiotherapist.

Contractures

A contracture is an abnormal flexion and fixation of a joint caused by muscle atrophy and shortening. Contracture of the joint above the amputation is a common complication. The person needs to be taught to extend the joint. The person with an above-the-knee amputation should lie prone for periods throughout the day. The person with a below-the-knee amputation should elevate the stump, keeping the knee extended. The same principles apply to the upper extremities. All joints should receive either active or passive ROM exercises every

2 to 4 hours. A trapeze frame should be added to the bed to encourage the person to change position every 2 hours. The person who has an upper extremity amputation should exercise both shoulders. Postural exercises can help prevent the person from hunching over secondary to the loss of weight on the affected side. The person with an above-the-knee amputation should not sit for prolonged periods of time; prolonged sitting can lead to hip contracture.

INTERPROFESSIONAL CARE

Interprofessional care is essential for the person who has sustained an amputation. Physiotherapy and occupational retraining are necessary and the person may also benefit from the presence of spiritual support. The entire healthcare team must view both the positive and the negative effects of amputation; that is, they must see amputation as a means to increase the person's independence and to relieve symptoms. The person should be able to become familiar with the members of the healthcare team and their roles; this allows the person greater control over their care and rehabilitation and promotes independence.

Diagnosis

Preoperatively, the person has routine laboratory and diagnostic tests (see the chapter 'Nursing care of people having surgery' for care of the person having surgery). Preoperative tests, including Doppler flowmetry, segmental blood pressure determination, transcutaneous partial pressure oxygen readings and angiography, are performed to assess the circulation present in the limb at different levels and to determine the level of viable tissue. Postoperative tests include FBC to monitor for haemorrhage, WBC count to monitor for infection, blood chemistries to evaluate electrolytes and fluid balance, and a vascular Doppler ultrasonography if a DVT is suspected.

Medications

The person receives medications preoperatively, intraoperatively and postoperatively. Preoperatively, the doctor may prescribe intravenous antibiotics. Intraoperatively, anaesthetic agents are administered. It also may be necessary to administer agents to control blood pressure during the surgery. Postoperatively, the person resumes any routinely prescribed medications and in addition may receive antibiotics and analgesics. Steroids may be administered to decrease swelling. A protein pump inhibitor (PPI) antagonist may also be ordered to decrease the risk of peptic ulcer formation. Stool softeners may be administered to prevent constipation.

Prosthesis

The type of prosthesis selected for the person with an amputation depends on the level of the amputation as well as the person's occupation and lifestyle. Each prosthesis is based on a detailed prosthetic prescription and is custom made for the person based on the specific characteristics of the stump. Most are made of plastic and foam materials. Many factors influence the person's use of the prosthesis, including the status of the remaining limb, cognitive status, cardiovascular status, preoperative activity level and motivation to use the prosthesis.

People with a lower extremity amputation are often fitted with early walking aids. Pneumatic devices that fit over the stump are used in the immediate postoperative period to allow early ambulation, decreased postoperative swelling and improved morale. People may begin weight bearing as soon as 2 weeks after surgery. People with upper extremity amputations may be fitted for a prosthesis immediately after surgery. While rehabilitation of the person with an amputation is a team effort, involving the person, nurse, doctor, physical therapist, occupational therapist, social worker, prosthetist and vocational counsellor, it is commonly lead by a physiotherapist (Australian Physiotherapists in Amputee Rehabilitation, 2018).

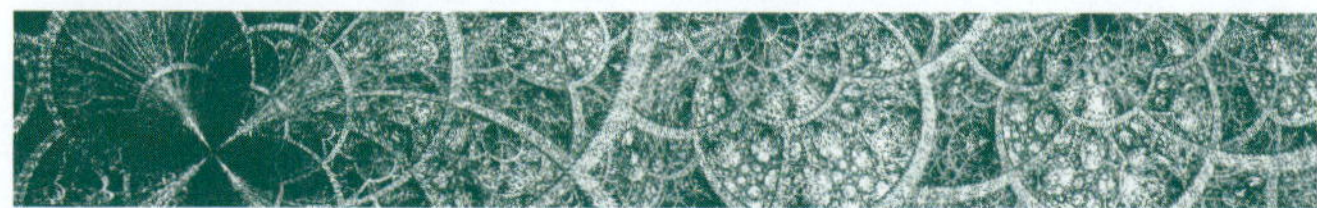

Nursing care

Health promotion

The goals of health promotion activities focus on preventing the progression of chronic diseases such as peripheral vascular disease and diabetes mellitus and on safety. People with PVD from any cause need education about foot care and early recognition of decreased circulation. Education within both urban and rural populations should provide knowledge about working safely with lawn care equipment as well as farm and occupational machinery.

In addition, it is important that the public know what to do if a traumatic amputation occurs in the home, community or workplace. The following guidelines may help preserve the amputated part until it can be surgically reattached:

- Keep the person in a prone position with the legs elevated.
- Apply firm pressure to the bleeding area, using a towel or article of clothing.
- Wrap the amputated part in a clean cloth. If possible, soak the cloth in saline (such as contact lens solution).
- Put the amputated part in a plastic bag and put the bag on ice. Do not let the amputated part come into direct contact with the ice or water.
- Send the amputated part to the emergency department with the injured person and be sure the emergency personnel know what it is.

Assessment

Collect the following data through the health history and physical examination. Further focused assessments are described in the following nursing interventions sections.

- *Health history*: mechanism of injury, current and past health problems, pain, occupation, ADLs, changes in sensation in the feet, cultural and/or religious guidelines for handling the amputated part.

- *Physical examination*: bilateral neurovascular status of the extremities, bilateral capillary refill time, skin over the lower extremities (discolouration, oedema, ulcerations, hair, gangrene).

Nursing diagnoses and interventions

The goals of nursing care for a person with an amputation are to relieve pain, promote healing, prevent complications, manage comorbidities, support the person and family during the process of grieving and adaptation to alterations in body image, and restore mobility. Care is individualised and the circumstances that led to the amputation (e.g. traumatic injury or disease) must also be addressed. (See the accompanying nursing care plan.) Applying rehabilitation principles to nursing care is also important.

Acute pain

Pain from the surgical procedure can be compounded by muscle spasms, swelling and phantom limb pain.

- Ask the person to rate the pain on a scale of 0 to 10 (with 10 as the most severe pain) before and after any intervention. *This facilitates objective assessment of the effectiveness of the chosen pain relief strategy. Pain that increases in intensity or remains unrelieved with analgesics can indicate compartment syndrome.*

NURSING CARE PLAN A person with a below-the-knee amputation

John Rocke is a 55-year-old divorcee with no children (preferred pronoun 'he'). He has a history of type 2 diabetes mellitus and poor control of blood glucose levels. Mr Rocke is unemployed and currently receives unemployment benefits. He lives alone in a second-floor unit. Mr Rocke had developed gangrene in the foot and failed to seek prompt medical attention; as a result, a left below-the-knee amputation was necessary.

Mr Rocke is in his second postoperative day and his vital signs are stable. The stump is splinted and has a soft dressing. The wound is approximating well without signs of infection. He has not performed ROM exercises or turning since his surgery, complaining of severe pain. When the nurse goes into the room, he yells, 'Get out! I don't want anyone to see me like this.' No one has visited him since his hospitalisation. He is tolerating a diabetic diet and is using a urinal independently. He has an order for morphine, 5 mg IM/SC every 4 hours prn for pain and cephazolin, 1 g IV every 8 hours. He is on blood glucose coverage with regular insulin subcutaneously.

ASSESSMENT

Jane Simmons, RN, has just come on duty. She notes that Mr Rocke is upset and angry. He will not let anyone enter the room to give him medication or assess his vital signs.

DIAGNOSES

- *Disturbed body image* related to amputation of left lower leg.
- *Dysfunctional grieving* related to anger and loss of left lower leg.
- *Situational low self-esteem* related to appearance.
- *Risk of injury from infection and contractures* related to refusal of care.
- *Acute pain* related to surgery.

PLANNING

- Assess and manage Mr Rocke's pain related to the amputation.
- Ask a social worker to consult with Mr Rocke. Utilising a social worker may assist the person to discuss his current feelings about the amputation.
- Manage risk of contractures and infection.

Expected outcomes

- Verbalise his feelings about the amputation.
- Able to control his own analgesia and be pain free.
- Be allowed to control his pain with a PCA pump.
- Verbalise a decrease in pain.
- Verbalise the importance of turning.
- Turn every 2 hours.
- Allow the staff to monitor his vital signs and administer medications.

IMPLEMENTATION

- Actively listen to the person.
- Offer to arrange a visit with a fellow amputee.
- Assess pain and effectiveness of analgesia.
- Ask the doctor if the person can be placed on a PCA pump.
- Teach the person the importance of turning every 2 hours to prevent contractures.
- Encourage turning and lying prone.
- Teach the importance of antibiotics in preventing and treating infection.

EVALUATION

One week after his surgery, Mr Rocke is actively participating in his care. He has apologised for his behaviour and has explained to Ms Simmons that he was angry about the loss of his leg. He states, 'I thought I knew what to expect, but I didn't.'

CRITICAL THINKING IN THE NURSING PROCESS

1 Once Mr Rocke is ready to assist with his stump care, how would you proceed? Would you give him full responsibility for care and dressings, or would you gradually increase his participation? Why?
2 Which factors in Mr Rocke's home environment and medical history may make self-care more difficult? Do you expect Mr Rocke to follow up on care after his discharge? Why or why not?
3 Mr Rocke states, 'Why should I exercise this leg—it was already cut off!' How would you respond? What is the purpose of exercising the stump?

REFLECTION ON THE NURSING PROCESS

1 Identify the issues regarding the care of Mr Rocke that will be able to assist you with your future nursing care.
2 Looking back at the care you have given Mr Rocke, identify any issues that you feel that you could have seen earlier to improve Mr Rocke's outcome.

- Splint and support the injured area. *Splinting prevents additional injury by immobilising the stump and decreasing oedema while moulding the stump for a good prosthetic fit.*
- Unless contraindicated, elevate the stump on a pillow for the first 24 hours after surgery. *Elevating the stump promotes venous return and decreases oedema, which will decrease pain.*
- Move and turn the person gently and slowly. *Gentle moving and turning prevents the development of severe muscle spasms.*
- Administer pain medications as prescribed. A PCA pump may be ordered by the doctor. *Analgesics alleviate pain by stimulating opiate receptor sites. PCA pumps increase person control over and allow early relief of pain before it intensifies.*
- Encourage deep breathing and relaxation exercises. *These techniques increase the effectiveness of analgesics and modify the pain experience.*
- Reposition the person every 2 hours; turn from side to side and onto abdomen. *Repositioning alleviates pressure from one area and distributes it throughout the body, and helps prevent cramping of muscles.*

CONSIDERATION FOR PRACTICE

Lying prone prevents hip contracture.

Risk of infection

The person who has an amputation is at risk of wound infection. Early recognition of infection can lead to early treatment and prevent wound dehiscence.

- Assess the wound for redness, drainage, temperature, oedema and suture line approximation. *Redness is normal in the immediate postoperative period; if it persists, however, it can indicate infection. A hot area that is palpated over the incision or increased drainage may also indicate infection.*
- Take the person's temperature every 4 hours. *Increased body temperature may indicate infection.*
- Monitor WBC count. *The WBC count rises in the presence of infection.*
- Use aseptic technique to change the wound dressing. *Aseptic technique prevents contamination of the wound with bacteria.*
- Administer antibiotics as ordered. Antibiotics *inhibit bacterial cell replication and help prevent or eradicate infection.*
- Teach the person stump-wrapping techniques. *Correctly wrapping the stump from the distal to the proximal extremity increases venous return and prevents pooling of fluid, thereby reducing the chance of infection.*

Risk of impaired skin integrity

Stump care is essential, not only in the postoperative healing period but also throughout life with a prosthesis. A variety of skin problems may be caused by a prosthesis, including epidermoid cysts, abrasions, blisters and hair follicle infections. The person must be taught stump care prior to discharge.

- Each day, preferably at night, wash the stump with soap and warm water, and dry thoroughly. *Inspect the stump for redness, irritation or abrasions. It is essential to maintain intact skin to ensure successful use of the prosthesis.*
- Massage the end of the stump, beginning 3 weeks after surgery. *Massage helps desensitise the remaining part of the limb and prevents scar tissue formation. If the skin adheres to the underlying tissue, it will tear when stressed from wearing a prosthesis.*
- Expose any open areas of skin on the remaining part of the limb for 1 hour four times a day. *Air exposure promotes healing.*
- Change stump socks and elastic wraps each day. Wash these in mild soap and water and allow to completely dry before using again. *Stump socks and elastic wraps must be kept clean and dry to prevent skin breakdown.*

Risk of dysfunctional grieving

The person who has lost an extremity is at risk of dysfunctional grieving. Denial of the need for surgery and the inability to discuss feelings compound this risk.

- Encourage verbalisation of feelings, using open-ended questions. *Asking open-ended questions allows the person to discuss feelings and communicates the listener's willingness to listen.*
- Actively listen and maintain eye contact. *Active listening and eye contact communicate respect for what the person is expressing.*
- Reflect on the person's feelings. *Reflection statements such as 'You seem angry' allow the person to recognise feelings and perhaps develop a plan for resolution.*
- Allow the person to have unlimited visiting hours, if possible. *Unlimited visiting hours allow increased social support.*
- If desired by the person, provide spiritual support by encouraging activities such as visits from a spiritual leader, prayer and meditation. *These activities often provide support during the grieving process.*

Disturbed body image

Although amputation is a reconstructive surgery, the person's body image will be disturbed. Risk of body image disturbance is higher in young people, in whom body image is a particularly important component of self-image.

- Encourage verbalisation of feelings. *This allows the person to communicate concerns and fears and lets the person know the nurse is willing to listen.*
- Allow the person to wear clothing from home. *Familiar clothing provides emotional comfort and helps the person retain a sense of his or her own identity.*
- Encourage the person to look at the stump. *Looking at and touching the stump helps the person face their fear of the unknown and move from denial to acceptance.*

- Encourage the person to care for the stump. *Active participation in care increases self-esteem and independence.*
- Offer to have a fellow amputee visit the person. *A support person who has experienced the same change gives the person the hope that they too can regain independence.*
- Encourage active participation in rehabilitation. *Active participation in rehabilitation increases independence and mobility.*

Impaired physical mobility

If time allows, the person should begin strengthening muscles preoperatively. If the amputation is the result of an emergency, exercises begin within 24 to 48 hours of surgery. The return of independent mobility boosts self-esteem and promotes adaptation to amputation.

- Perform ROM exercises on all joints. *ROM exercises help prevent the development of joint contractures that limit mobility.*
- Maintain postoperative stump shrinkage devices. These may be elastic bandages, shrinker socks, an elastic stockinette or a rigid plaster cast. *In order for the prosthetic limb to fit properly and as the wound heals, therapists will work with the person to wrap the stump with elastic wraps or stockings that minimise swelling and shape the stump for the best fit possible into a prosthetic limb.*
- Turn and reposition the person every 2 hours. The person with a lower extremity amputation should lie prone every 4 hours, for up to 2 hours. *Repositioning increases blood flow to muscles, forces synovial fluid into joints and helps prevent contractures.*
- Reinforce teaching by the physical therapist in crutch walking or the use of assistive devices. *These devices increase mobility by balancing the person and facilitating ambulation.*
- Encourage active participation in physical therapy. *Physical therapy will fatigue the person in the early stage of healing. Encouragement may increase the person's participation in the physical therapy regimen and thereby increase activity tolerance.*

Community-based care

Person and family teaching includes stump care, prosthesis fitting and care, medications, assistive devices, exercises, rehabilitation, counselling, support services and follow-up appointments. The depth of teaching depends on the cause and site of the amputation and the needs of the person. See the 'Meeting individualised needs' box.

Holistic nursing care is especially important for the older person with an amputation. The normal ageing process

MEETING INDIVIDUALISED NEEDS The person with an amputation

Amputation of a limb has significant long-term consequences for the person. The person will grieve the loss of a body part and must adjust to a new self-image. The person's ability to perform normal ADLs and to maintain their usual family and social roles may be significantly affected, at least initially. Depending on the person's occupation, job performance may be affected, necessitating a change of career.

The nurse may be responsible for involving multiple members of the healthcare team in the person's care and rehabilitation, and for coordinating their activities. Following an amputation, the person may need the services of any or all of the following:

- social services to help with rehabilitative and financial arrangements
- physiotherapists to teach ambulation techniques and to provide deep heat or massage
- occupational therapists to assist the person in developing adaptive techniques to deal with the loss of a limb
- prosthetists to develop a prosthesis for the missing limb that will meet the person's needs for ADLs and other activities
- home nursing services for nursing care such as assessments and wound care
- support group services to assist in adapting to the body image change and effects of amputation on ADLs.

ASSESSING FOR HOME CARE

Preparing the amputee for home care includes a careful assessment of the person's family and support services, and of the home for possible barriers to the person's safety, mobility and independence.

Assess the person's acceptance of the amputation and knowledge base about care needs, any activity restrictions or special needs and resources for home care. Discuss home management (i.e. who is responsible for household activities such as cleaning and cooking). Enquire about arrangements that have been made for home care activities and ADLs. Evaluate the person's use of prescription and non-prescription medications, paying particular attention to possible interactions and drugs that may affect the person's balance, mental alertness or appetite. Ask about social habits, such as cigarette smoking, alcohol use or other drug use, that may affect healing or the person's ability to provide self-care.

Assess the person's home environment for possible safety hazards or barriers to ambulation, such as:

- scatter rugs
- stairs between living areas of the house
- presence of grab bars to facilitate toileting and bathing
- access to clean water and other needs for wound care.

HEALTH EDUCATION FOR THE PERSON AND FAMILY

The new amputee needs a great deal of teaching to learn to adapt to loss of a limb, whether it is an upper or lower extremity that has been lost. Because the person must be ready to learn before teaching can be effective, use therapeutic communication techniques to encourage the person to verbalise feelings about the amputation and its effects. Use active listening and educate the person about ways to reduce anxiety and deal with feelings of helplessness and loss. Encourage the person to participate

(continued)

MEETING INDIVIDUALISED NEEDS The person with an amputation (continued)

in care of the stump to build self-esteem and reinforce teaching. Include the following in teaching for home care:

- Teach the person to wrap the stump appropriately in preparation for fitting the prosthesis.
- Discuss positioning of the stump. Contractures are a particular problem for people with an above-knee amputation and can interfere with the ability to use a prosthesis effectively.
- Teach the person how to perform stump exercises to maintain joint mobility and muscle tone of the affected limb.
- Encourage the person to resume physical activities as soon as possible. This improves the person's health and wellbeing, as well as the person's self-esteem.
- Discuss household modifications to promote independence, such as grab bars in the bathroom, taps with single-handle controls for water flow and temperature, and handheld shower heads and shower chairs for bathing.

In addition, suggest the following resources:

- Limbs 4 Life: https://www.limbs4life.org.au
- Limbkids: www.limbkids.asn.au
- Healthdirect—Amputation: https://www.healthdirect.gov.au/amputation
- Amputees Federation of New Zealand Inc: https://www.amputee.co.nz

decreases renal and liver function; hence, medications have longer half-lives. Altered circulation prolongs wound healing, and slowing of reflexes and alterations in gait may disrupt balance. A walker may be more appropriate than crutches because older people have less strength in the upper extremities. Safety issues, such as decreasing the risk of recurrent falls, must be addressed. The nurse should also assess the person's need for in-home assistance and make appropriate referrals to visiting nurses and home health aides.

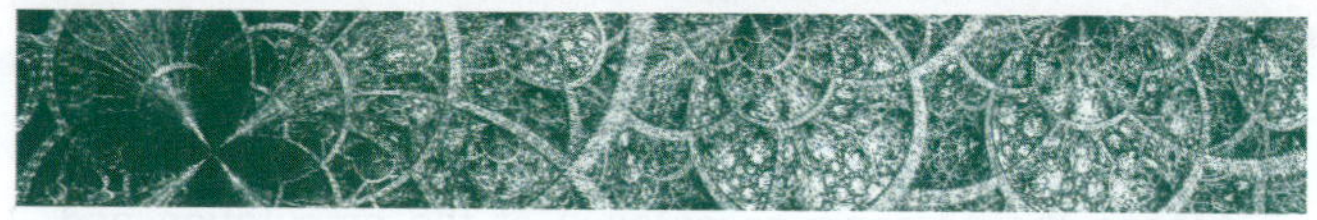

THE PERSON WITH A REPETITIVE USE INJURY

Repeatedly twisting and turning the wrist, pronating and supinating the forearm, kneeling or raising arms over the head can result in repetitive use injuries. People with repetitive use injuries pose a challenge to the healthcare team. Often these people appear puzzled as they relate a history of manifestations that have worsened over time. They deny abrupt trauma and often worry about the ability to return to work. Repetitive use injuries are common. The number of workers' compensation claims for repetitive use injuries is steadily growing. The increase is believed to be a result of technology advances in the workplace.

Pathophysiology

Common repetitive use injuries include carpal tunnel syndrome, bursitis and epicondylitis.

Carpal tunnel syndrome

The carpal tunnel is a canal through which flexor tendons and the median nerve pass from the wrist to the hand. The syndrome develops from narrowing of the tunnel and irritation of the median nerve. Carpal tunnel syndrome involves compression of the median nerve as a result of inflammation and swelling of the synovial lining of the tendon sheaths. The person complains of numbness and tingling of the thumb, index finger and lateral ventral surface of the middle finger. The person may also complain of pain in this area that interferes with sleep and is alleviated by shaking or massaging the hand and fingers. The affected hand may become weak and the person may be unable to hold utensils or perform activities that require precision.

Carpal tunnel syndrome is one of the three most common work-related injuries. The incidence is believed to be related directly to the number of people using computers. The incidence of carpal tunnel syndrome is higher in women, especially postmenopausal women.

Bursitis

Bursitis is an inflammation of a bursa. A bursa is an enclosed sac found between muscles, tendons and bony prominences. The bursae that commonly become inflamed are in the shoulder, hip, knee and elbow. Constant friction between the bursa and the musculoskeletal tissue around it causes irritation, oedema and inflammation. Manifestations develop as the sac becomes engorged. The area around the sac is tender and extension and flexion of the joint near the bursa produce pain. The inflamed bursa is hot, red and oedematous. The person guards the joint to decrease pain and may point to the area of the bursa when identifying joint tenderness.

Epicondylitis

Epicondylitis is inflammation of the tendon at its point of origin into the bone. Epicondylitis is also referred to as *tennis elbow* or *golfer's elbow*. The exact pathophysiology of epicondylitis is unknown. Current theories attribute inflammation of the tendon to microvascular trauma. Tears, bleeding and oedema are thought to cause avascularisation and calcification of the tendon. Manifestations of epicondylitis include point tenderness, pain radiating down the dorsal surface of the forearm and a history of repetitive use.

INTERPROFESSIONAL CARE

Medical management of repetitive use disorders focuses on relieving pain and increasing mobility. Once the diagnosis is made, treatment can range from conservative measures, such as rest and pharmacological agents, to aggressive measures such as surgery.

Diagnosis

Carpal tunnel syndrome is diagnosed by the person's history and physical examination. The history may reveal an occupation that involves areas such as computer work, jackhammer operation, mechanical work or gymnastics. History of a radial bone fracture or rheumatoid arthritis also increases the risk of carpal tunnel syndrome. Tests specific for carpal tunnel include Phalen's test (see the chapter 'A person-centred approach to assessing the musculoskeletal system'). Bursitis and epicondylitis are diagnosed by history and physical examination.

Medications

The person with a repetitive use injury usually receives NSAIDs. Narcotics may also be administered for acute flare-ups and severe pain. For the person who has epicondylitis or carpal tunnel syndrome, corticosteroids may be injected into the joint.

Treatments

Treatment of repetitive use injuries is performed first by conservative management, followed, if necessary, by surgery.

CONSERVATIVE MANAGEMENT The first steps in the care of all repetitive use injuries are to immobilise and rest the involved joint. The joint may be splinted and ice may be applied (as described in Table 38.1) in the first 24 to 48 hours to decrease pain and inflammation. Ice application may be followed by heat application every 4 hours.

SURGERY Surgery is usually reserved for the person who does not obtain relief with conservative treatment. Surgery for carpal tunnel syndrome includes resection of the carpal ligament to enlarge the tunnel. In epicondylitis and bursitis, calcified deposits may be removed from the area surrounding the tendon or bursa.

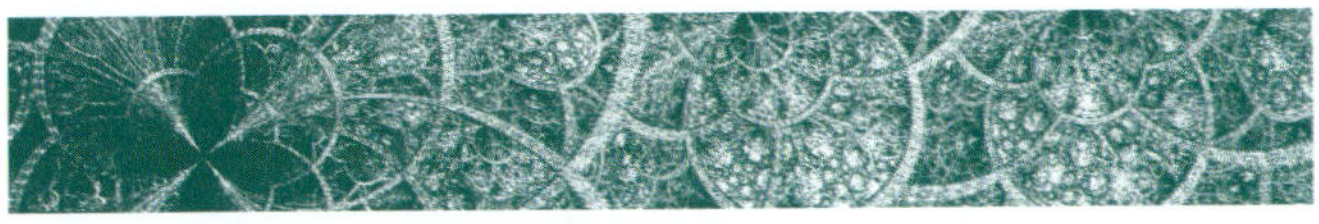

Nursing care

The nursing care of a person with a repetitive use injury focuses on relieving pain, teaching about the disease process and treatment, and improving physical mobility.

Nursing diagnoses and interventions

Acute pain

Swelling and nerve inflammation cause pain in the person with a repetitive use injury.

- Ask the person to rate the pain on a scale of 0 to 10 (with 10 being the most severe pain) before and after any intervention. *This facilitates objective assessment of the effectiveness of the chosen pain relief strategy.*
- Encourage the use of immobilisers. *Splinting maintains joint alignment and prevents pain due to movement of inflamed tissues.*
- Teach the person to apply ice and/or heat as prescribed. *Ice causes vasoconstriction and decreases the pooling of blood in the inflamed area. Ice may also numb the tender area. Heat decreases swelling by increasing venous return.*
- Encourage use of NSAIDs as prescribed. *NSAIDs decrease swelling by inhibiting prostaglandins.*
- Explain why treatment should not be abruptly discontinued. *Abrupt discontinuation of treatment may cause reinflammation of the injured area.*

Impaired physical mobility

Joint pain and swelling can impair mobility.

- Suggest interventions to alleviate pain (such as using an immobiliser and taking pain medications). *If the joint is pain free, the person will be more likely to take an active role in therapy.*
- Refer to a physiotherapist for exercises. *The physiotherapist can assist the person with exercise to prevent joint stiffness.*
- Suggest consultation with an occupational therapist. *Occupational therapy can help the person learn new ways to perform tasks to prevent recurring symptoms.*

Community-based care

Address the following topics for home care:

- Causes of and treatments for repetitive use injury.
- Rehabilitation to allow the person to return to a state of independence.
- Ways to avoid unnecessary exposure to the activities that increase risk of redeveloping the injury. Suggest evaluation of the person's work environment by an environmental risk manager who can prescribe measures to reduce the risk of repetitive use injuries. Wrist supports or an ergonomic keyboard may be useful for the person who uses a computer extensively. Appropriate desk and chair height also are important in maintaining the correct anatomical position while working.
- Information about sources for braces or other assistive devices.

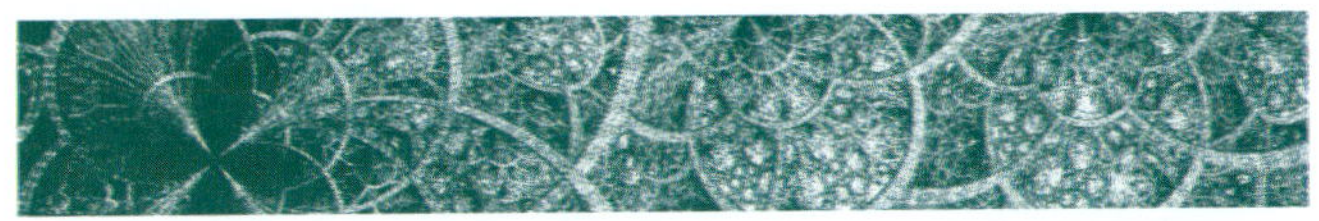

CHAPTER HIGHLIGHTS

- The most commonly reported musculoskeletal injuries are contusions, strains and sprains. Immediate treatment includes RICE (rest, ice, compression, elevation) therapy.
- Dislocations may be congenital, traumatic or pathological. Nursing assessments include monitoring neurovascular status by assessing for increased pain, decreased or absent pulses, pale skin, inability to move a body part or extremity, and changes in sensation.
- Any of the 206 bones of the body may sustain a fracture. Fractures are closed or simple (skin is intact) or open or compound (skin integrity is interrupted); open fractures are at risk of infection. Other fracture descriptors include oblique or spiral, avulsed, comminuted, compressed, impacted or depressed.
- Fractures heal through three phases: inflammatory, reparative and remodelling. Healing is influenced by the age and physical condition of the person and by the type of fracture.
- Fracture complications include compartment syndrome, fat embolism syndrome, deep venous thrombosis, infection, delayed union and non-union, and reflex sympathetic dystrophy.
- Fractures are treated with surgery, traction and/or casts to stabilise the fractured bone, maintain bone immobilisation, prevent complications and restore function.
- Fractures of the hip are most often sustained by older adult women and are usually the result of a fall. They are the most common injury in the older population, resulting in the greatest number of deaths, and cause the most serious health problems of all fractures for people aged 65 years and older.
- Nursing care for the person with a fracture focuses on interventions for acute pain, risk of peripheral vascular dysfunction, risk of infection, impaired physical mobility and risk of disturbed tactile sensory perception.
- An amputation is the partial or total removal of an extremity. This loss has a significant physical and psychosocial effect on the person and the family. The most common cause for amputation of a lower extremity is peripheral vascular disease. Trauma is the most common cause for upper extremity amputation.
- Complications that may follow an amputation include infection, delayed healing, chronic stump pain, phantom pain and contractures. Stump care is necessary to prevent complications and to prepare the stump for a prosthesis.
- Nursing care for the person with an amputation is provided as part of the interprofessional team and is focused on a return to functional health, with interventions to meet needs for acute pain, impaired skin integrity, grieving, disturbed body image and impaired physical mobility.
- Repetitive use injuries, especially common in the workplace, include carpal tunnel syndrome, bursitis and epicondylitis.

CONCEPT CHECK

1 You are teaching a young adult how to provide self-care for a sprained ankle. You explain that the reason for applying ice immediately after the injury is based on the principle that ice:
1 increases the diameter of blood vessels
2 decreases the diameter of blood vessels
3 is helpful in increasing white blood cells
4 lowers the blood pressure and pulse

2 A person with a compound, open fracture has been admitted to the emergency department and is scheduled for immediate surgery. Which of the following nursing diagnoses would be most appropriate in the immediate postoperative period?
1 *Risk of post-traumatic stress disorder (PTSD)*
2 *Impaired transfer ability*
3 *Risk of infection*
4 *Risk of falls*

3 While providing care to an older woman with a cast on her left lower arm (from below the elbow to above the fingers), you perform a neurovascular assessment. Which of the following assessments indicates a possible complication?
1 slightly oedematous fingers
2 warm, pink skin above the cast
3 pale, cold fingers
4 pain rating of 2 on a 1 to 10 scale

4 Which of the following minerals is essential to bone healing?
1 potassium
2 magnesium
3 sodium
4 calcium

5 You are assessing a young man with a newly applied long leg cast. He complains of extreme pain in his leg and his toes are cyanotic and lack sensation. What is your priority intervention?
1 Document the assessments carefully and accurately.
2 Notify the healthcare provider who applied the cast.
3 Elevate the leg on at least three pillows.
4 Apply an ice bag over the painful area.

6 Your assigned person has been diagnosed with DVT of the left lower extremity. Which body system would require very careful monitoring?
1 haematological
2 respiratory
3 digestive
4 renal

7 Although nursing diagnoses are always individualised, what is one nursing diagnosis common to all musculoskeletal injuries?
1 Disturbed body image
2 Acute pain
3 Chronic pain
4 Risk of infection

8 Indicate the position you would place the remaining extremity following a below-the-knee amputation during the first 24 hours after surgery.
1 elevated above the level of the heart
2 lower than the rest of the body
3 crossed over the intact extremity
4 level with the rest of the body

9 The day following a below-the-knee amputation, the person you are caring for tells you that he feels as though his toes are cramping in the amputated foot. What is this experience called?
1 chronic stump pain
2 contractures
3 attention seeking
4 phantom limb pain

10 A friend is cutting wood with a circular saw. He suddenly screams that he has cut off his finger. What would you do with the amputated finger?

1 Don't worry about it; the important thing is to get him to the hospital.
2 Put it in a storage bag filled with warm water.
3 Tape it to his hand so the emergency personnel will know where it is.
4 Wrap it in a towel, put it in a plastic bag and lay it on ice.

BIBLIOGRAPHY

Australian Commission on Safety and Quality in Health Care (ACSQHC) (2015). *Preventing falls and harm from falls in older people: Best practice guidelines for Australian hospitals*. Retrieved from https://www.safetyandquality.gov.au/

Australian Commission on Safety and Quality in Health Care (ACSQHC) (2016). *Hip Fracture Care Clinical Care Standard*. Sydney: ACSQHC.

Australian Institute of Health and Welfare (AIHW) (2022). *Hip fracture incidence and hospitalisations in Australia 2015–16*. Retrieved from https://www.aihw.gov.au/

Australian Physiotherapists in Amputee Rehabilitation (2018). Retrieved from https://www.aopa.org.au/

Burns, E. R., Stevens, J. A. & Lee, R. (2016). The direct cost of fatal and non-fatal falls among older adults—United States. *Journal of Safety Research*, *58*, 99–103. Retrieved from https://www.sciencedirect.com/

Guzon-Illescas, O., Perez Fernandez, E., Crespí Villarias, N. et al. (2019). Mortality after osteoporotic hip fracture: Incidence, trends, and associated factors. *Journal of Orthopaedic Surgery and Research*, *14*, 203. https://doi.org/10.1186/s13018-019-1226-6

Hoffman, M. (2020). Compartment syndrome. *WebMD*. Retrieved from https://www.webmd.com/

Lethaby, A., Temple, J. & Santy-Tomlinson, J. (2013). Pin site care for preventing infections associated with external bone fixators and pins. *Cochrane Database of Systematic Reviews*, *12*, CD004551.

Mayo Clinic (2022). *Dislocation: First aid*. Retrieved from https://www.mayoclinic.org/

National Institute of Arthritis and Musculoskeletal and Skin Diseases (2022). *Sports injuries*. Retrieved from https://www.niams.nih.gov/

Norris, T. L. (2018). *Porth's pathophysiology: Concepts of altered health states* (10th ed.). Philadelphia: Lippincott Williams & Wilkins.

Perth Children's Hospital (2021). *Pulled elbow*. Retrieved from https://pch.health.wa.gov.au/

Queensland Health (2016). *Falls professional resources—Stay on your feet*. Retrieved from https://www.health.qld.gov.au/

Stevens, H., Tran, H. & Gibbs, H. (2019). Venous thromboembolism: Current management. *Australian Prescriber*, *42*, 123–126.

Tiziani, A. (2017). *Harvard's nursing guide to drugs* (10th ed.). Chatswood, NSW: Elsevier.

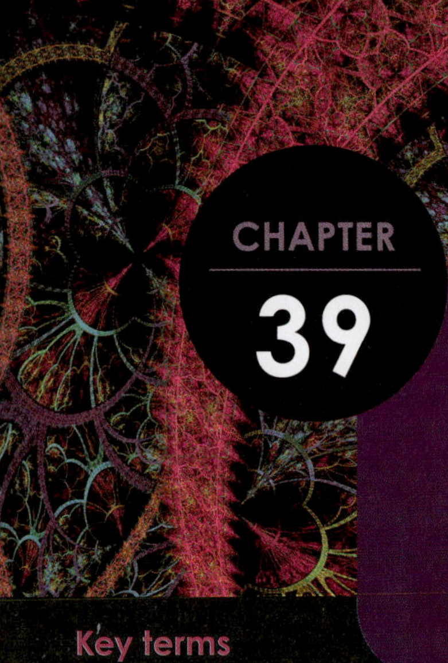

CHAPTER 39

Nursing care of people with musculoskeletal disorders

David Stanley

Key terms

ankylosing spondylitis (AS) 1449
arthritis 1411
fibromyalgia 1466
gout 1422
muscular dystrophy (MD) 1437
osteoarthritis (OA) 1429
osteomalacia 1426
osteomyelitis 1456
osteoporosis 1411
Paget's disease 1419
polymyositis 1455
reactive arthritis (ReA) 1449
rheumatic disorders 1411
rheumatoid arthritis (RA) 1438
scleroderma 1464
septic arthritis 1460
Sjögren's syndrome 1466
systemic lupus erythematosus (SLE) 1450
tophi 1422

Learning outcomes

- Explain the pathophysiology, manifestations, complications, interprofessional care and nursing care of metabolic, degenerative, autoimmune, inflammatory, infectious, neoplastic, connective tissue and structural musculoskeletal disorders.
- Compare and contrast the pathophysiology, manifestations, diagnosis and treatments for osteoporosis, osteoarthritis, Paget's disease and rheumatoid arthritis.
- Discuss the purposes, nursing implications and health education for the person and family regarding medications used to treat osteoporosis, Paget's disease, gout, osteomalacia, osteoarthritis, rheumatoid arthritis, systemic lupus erythematosus, osteomyelitis, bone tumours, scleroderma and lower back pain.
- Describe the surgical procedures used to treat people with arthritis.

Clinical competencies

- Assess functional status of people with musculoskeletal disorders and monitor, document and report abnormal manifestations.
- Use evidence-based research to assess people at risk of osteoporosis and to evaluate the effectiveness of internet use to teach older adults with rheumatoid arthritis.
- Determine priority nursing diagnoses, based on assessed data, to select and implement individualised nursing interventions for people with musculoskeletal disorders.
- Administer topical, oral and injectable medications used to treat musculoskeletal disorders knowledgeably and safely.
- Provide skilled care to people having a surgical debridement for osteomyelitis and a total joint replacement.
- Integrate interprofessional care into care of people with musculoskeletal disorders.
- Provide teaching appropriate for community-based self-care of musculoskeletal disorders.
- Revise the plan of care as needed to provide effective interventions to promote, maintain or restore functional health status to people with musculoskeletal disorders.

Various metabolic, degenerative, autoimmune, inflammatory, infectious, neoplastic, connective tissue and structural disorders may affect the musculoskeletal system. Many of these diseases have significant physical, psychosocial and financial consequences. When these problems occur, people experience a variety of individualised responses to their altered health status. Nursing care is directed towards meeting physiological needs, providing education and ensuring psychological support for the person and family.

In 2012–2013, 20% of Australian First Nations people reported having a musculoskeletal disease. The rate of total burden due to musculoskeletal conditions was generally similar across the states and territories, although the rate in Tasmania was 20% higher than the national rate. The rate was also higher among people living in very remote areas and inner regional areas compared with other remote areas, and higher among people living in areas of the lowest socioeconomic group compared with other socioeconomic groups. As well, the musculoskeletal conditions were higher among Aboriginal and Torres Strait Islander people compared with non-Indigenous Australians, with the exception of burden of back pain and problems, which was lower among Indigenous Australians (Australian Institute of Health and Welfare (AIHW), 2020a).

Arthritis refers to inflammation of the joints, while **rheumatic disorders** refer to diseases of the muscles and bones as well as the joints. These diseases affect not only the joints but also the connective tissues of the body. The various types of arthritis are discussed in this chapter in different sections, depending on the primary aetiology of the disorder. Approximately 12.5% of all Australians had arthritis in 2021–2022, and 70.7% of people with arthritis had at least one other chronic condition (Australian Bureau of Statistics (ABS), 2022). According to the ABS, rates of arthritis increase with age and are more prevalent in females (ABS, 2022). Women are more likely than men to have arthritis, particularly those over the age of 55 (ABS, 2022). People living in areas of most disadvantage are more likely than those living in areas of least disadvantage to have arthritis (15.3% compared to 9.5%) (ABS, 2022).

There are more than 100 different types of arthritis, but the most common are osteoarthritis, rheumatoid arthritis, systemic lupus erythematosus, ankylosing spondylitis and gout (Arthritis Australia, 2017). The aetiology of most rheumatic disorders is not clear; in many cases, the pathophysiological processes involved are often complex and poorly understood. Many are primary disorders; others occur as secondary processes associated with another disease. The wear and tear of ageing, autoimmune processes, metabolic disorders, genetic factors and infection are also implicated as causative factors in some forms of rheumatic disease.

Arthritic disorders are a leading cause of disability; however, their very prevalence may lead the public and healthcare professionals to treat them as normal ageing processes or to discount the validity of the pain and disability experienced by the person with arthritis.

Metabolic bone disorders

Metabolic bone disorders originate in the bone remodelling process, which normally involves a sequence of events of bone reabsorption and formation. In the adult, this process is primarily internal remodelling through replacement of trabecular bone. Adults replace about 25% of trabecular bone every 4 months through reabsorption of old bone by osteoclasts and formation of new bone by osteoblasts (Norris, 2018). Metabolic bone disorders may result from a variety of factors, including ageing, calcium and phosphate imbalances, genetics and changes in levels of hormones.

THE PERSON WITH OSTEOPOROSIS

Osteoporosis, literally defined as 'porous bones', is a metabolic bone disorder characterised by loss of bone mass, increased bone fragility and an increased risk of fractures. The reduced bone mass is caused by an imbalance of the processes that influence bone growth and maintenance. Although osteoporosis may result from an endocrine disorder or malignancy, it is most often associated with ageing.

In Australia, the number of people suffering from osteoporosis is increasing. Women over the age of 50 are at greatest risk of developing a fracture, with the risk being four times greater than for men (AIHW, 2018a). An estimated 924,000 Australians and 20% of people aged 75 years and over have osteoporosis (ABS, 2019). This includes people who have osteoporosis or osteopenia. Osteoporosis is more common in women than men. In 2017–2018, 29% of women aged 75 and over had osteoporosis compared with 10% of men. Older age groups also tend to be affected. The proportion of women with osteoporosis increases with age, with those aged 75 and over being most affected (AIHW, 2020b).

Risk factors

The risk of developing osteoporosis depends on how much bone mass is achieved between ages 25 and 35 and how much is lost later. Certain diseases, lifestyle habits and ethnic backgrounds increase the risk of developing osteoporosis (see the 'Focus on cultural diversity' box). Different variables affect one's risk of osteoporosis: some can be modified and others cannot. The risk factors are summarised in Box 39.1.

Unmodifiable risk factors

Both men and women are susceptible to osteoporosis as they age because the osteoblasts and osteoclasts undergo alterations that diminish their activity. Those with smaller stature and low body weight are more susceptible. Women have a significantly higher risk of manifestations and complications of osteoporosis because their peak bone mass is 10–15% less than that of men. In addition, age-related bone loss begins earlier and proceeds more rapidly

FOCUS ON CULTURAL DIVERSITY The person with osteoporosis

- Significant risk is reported for people of all cultural backgrounds, but the highest percentage of cases are in European and Asian women aged 50 or older, with 20% estimated to have osteoporosis and 52% estimated to have low bone mass.
- The prevalence of osteoporosis among Aboriginal and Torres Strait Islander people is 2.3%, affecting about 18,900 people, including about 1,000 who live in remote areas (0.7% of the remote Indigenous population). After adjusting for age, twice as many females (5.1%) than males (2.5%) are affected by the condition. The prevalence in Indigenous Australians (3.9%) and non-Indigenous Australians (3.3%) is similar overall for females but is 1.9 times higher for Indigenous males than non-Indigenous males (see Figure 39.1).

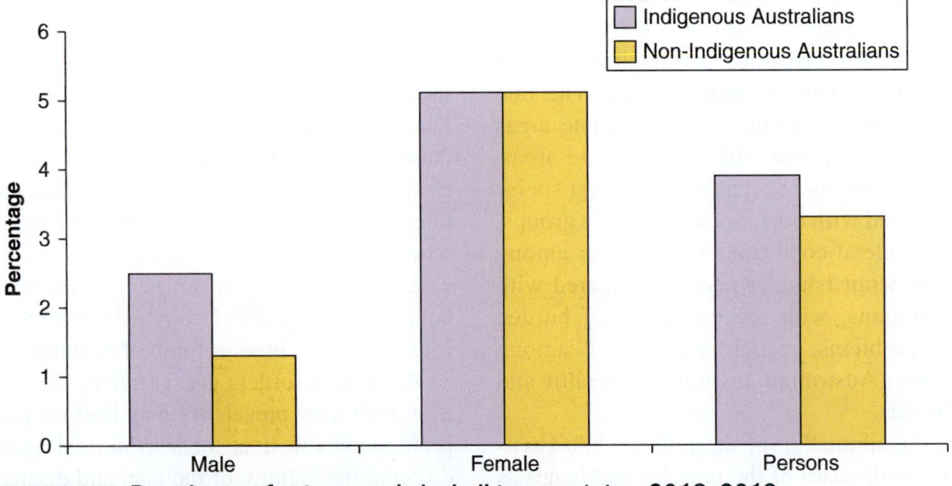

FIGURE 39.1 ***Prevalence of osteoporosis by Indigenous status, 2018–2019***

Note: Rates are age-standardised to the Australian population as at 30 June 2001.

Source: AIHW (2020b). *Osteoporosis*. Retrieved from https://www.aihw.gov.au/reports/chronic-musculoskeletal-conditions/osteoporosis/contents/what-is-osteoporosis. Licensed under the Creative Commons Attribution 4.0 International License, https//creativecommons.org/licenses/by/4.0.

BOX 39.1 Risk factors for osteoporosis

- A family history of osteoporosis
- Personal history of fracture after age 50
- Current low bone mass
- History of fracture in a first-degree relative
- Being female, especially Caucasian or Asian
- Being thin and/or having a small frame
- Menopause-associated low oestrogen levels
- Low testosterone levels in men
- Dietary: low lifetime calcium intake, vitamin D deficiency
- Medication use: anticonvulsants, corticosteroids
- Lifestyle: inactivity, cigarette smoking, excess alcohol
- Presence of certain chronic diseases

in women, beginning in their thirties and accelerating before menopause. Oestrogen in women and testosterone in men appear to help prevent bone loss; decreasing levels of these hormones associated with ageing contribute to bone loss. Age-related bone loss in men occurs 15 to 20 years later than in women and at a slower rate.

Premature osteoporosis is increasing in female athletes, who have a greater incidence of eating disorders and amenorrhoea. Poor nutrition and intense physical training can result in a deficient production of oestrogen. Decreased oestrogen, combined with a lack of calcium and vitamin D, results in a loss of bone density (Norris, 2018).

People who have an endocrine disorder such as hyperthyroidism, hyperparathyroidism, Cushing's syndrome or diabetes mellitus are at high risk of osteoporosis. These disorders affect the metabolism, in turn affecting nutritional status and bone mineralisation.

Modifiable risk factors

Modifiable risk factors include behaviours that place a person at risk of developing osteoporosis, as well as physical changes such as menopause whose contribution to osteoporosis can be modified by preventive strategies. Calcium deficiency is an important modifiable risk factor contributing to osteoporosis. Calcium is an essential mineral in the process of bone formation and other significant body functions. When there is an insufficient intake of calcium in the diet, the body compensates by removing calcium from the skeleton, weakening bone tissue. Acidosis, which may result from a high-protein diet, contributes to osteoporosis in two ways. Calcium is withdrawn from the bone as the kidneys attempt to buffer the excess acid. Acidosis also may directly stimulate osteoclast function.

A high intake of diet drinks with a high phosphate content also can deplete calcium stores.

With menopause and decreasing oestrogen levels, bone loss accelerates in women. Oestrogen promotes the activity of osteoblasts, increasing new bone formation. In addition, oestrogen enhances calcium absorption and stimulates the thyroid gland to secrete calcitonin, a hormone that suppresses osteoclast activity and increases osteoblast activity.

Both cigarette smoking and excess alcohol intake are risk factors for osteoporosis. Smoking decreases the blood supply to bones. Nicotine slows the production of osteoblasts and impairs the absorption of calcium, contributing to decreased bone density. Alcohol has a direct toxic effect on osteoblast activity, suppressing bone formation during periods of alcohol intoxication. In addition, heavy alcohol use may be associated with nutritional deficiencies that contribute to osteoporosis. Interestingly, moderate alcohol consumption in postmenopausal women actually may increase bone mineral content, possibly by increasing levels of oestrogen and calcitonin.

Sedentary lifestyle is another modifiable risk factor that can cause osteoporosis. Weight-bearing exercise, such as walking, influences bone metabolism in several ways. The stress of this type of exercise causes an increase in blood flow to bones, which brings growth-producing nutrients to the cells. Walking causes an increase in osteoblast growth and activity.

Prolonged use of medications that increase calcium excretion, such as aluminium-containing antacids and anticonvulsants, increase the risk of developing osteoporosis. Heparin therapy increases bone resorption and its prolonged use is associated with osteoporosis. Antiretroviral therapy for people with AIDS or HIV infection and androgen-suppressing drug treatments used for prostate cancer may cause decreased bone density and osteoporosis (Marieb & Keller, 2021; Norris, 2018). Anyone who takes a glucocorticoid medication for more than 3 months is at risk of glucocorticoid-induced osteoporosis. These medications, often prescribed to control many rheumatic diseases, include prednisolone (Prednisone) and dexamethasone (Decadron, Hexadrol). They can directly affect bone cells, slowing the rate of bone formation. They also interfere with how the body uses calcium and affect levels of sex hormones, leading to bone loss. Problems that result, such as an increased possibility of fractures, can be prevented by taking a daily regimen of calcium supplements with added vitamin D and one multivitamin. Hormone replacement therapy can also assist in slowing osteoporosis, but there are risks involved with this treatment. Bisphosphonates can assist, and selective oestrogen receptor modulators and statins can increase bone density (Marieb & Keller, 2021).

Pathophysiology

Although the exact pathophysiology of osteoporosis is unclear, it is known to involve an imbalance of the activity of osteoblasts that form new bone and osteoclasts that resorb bone. Until age 35, when peak bone mass occurs, formation occurs more rapidly than does reabsorption. After peak bone mass is achieved, slightly more is lost than is gained (about 0.3–0.5% per year); this loss is accelerated if the diet is deficient in vitamin D and calcium. In women, bone loss begins to increase to 1–2% per year from the age of 45 years, increases to 2–4% per year at the onset of menopause (with loss of oestrogen), then slows but does not stop at about age 60. In men, bone density tends to remain relatively stable until middle age, decreasing by about 0.5–1.0% per year from the age of 45–55 years (Osteoporosis Australia, 2022).

Osteoporosis affects the diaphysis (shaft of the bone) and the metaphysis (portion of the bone between the diaphysis and the epiphysis). The diameter of the bone increases, thinning the outer supporting cortex. As osteoporosis progresses, trabeculae are lost from cancellous bone (the spongy tissue of bone) and the outer cortex thins to the point that even minimal stress will fracture the bone (Norris, 2018).

Manifestations

The most common manifestations of osteoporosis are loss of height, progressive curvature of the spine, lower back pain and fractures of the forearm, spine or hip. Osteoporosis is often called the 'silent disease' because bone loss occurs without symptoms.

The loss of height occurs as vertebral bodies collapse. Acute episodes generally are painful, with radiation of the pain around the flank into the abdomen. Vertebral collapse can occur with little or no stress; minimal movements such as bending, lifting or jumping may precipitate the pain. In some people, vertebral collapse may occur slowly, accompanied by little discomfort. Along with loss of height, characteristic dorsal kyphosis and cervical lordosis develop, accounting for the 'dowager's hump' often associated with ageing. The abdomen tends to protrude and the knees and hips to flex as the body attempts to maintain its centre of gravity (see Figure 39.2).

Complications

The most common fractures are vertebral, hips and wrists. There may be no obvious manifestations of osteoporosis until fractures occur. Some fractures are spontaneous; others may result from everyday activities. While wrist and vertebral fractures have not been shown to increase disability or mortality, persistent pain and associated posture changes may restrict the person's activities or interfere with activities of daily living (ADLs).

INTERPROFESSIONAL CARE

Care of the person with osteoporosis focuses on stopping or slowing the process, alleviating the symptoms and preventing complications. Proper nutrition and exercise are important components of the treatment program.

Diagnosis

The manifestations of osteoporosis can mimic those of other bone disorders, so diagnostic tests are needed to differentiate osteoporosis from other problems.

A bone mineral density (BMD) scan assesses the mass of bone per unit volume—how tightly the bone is packed.

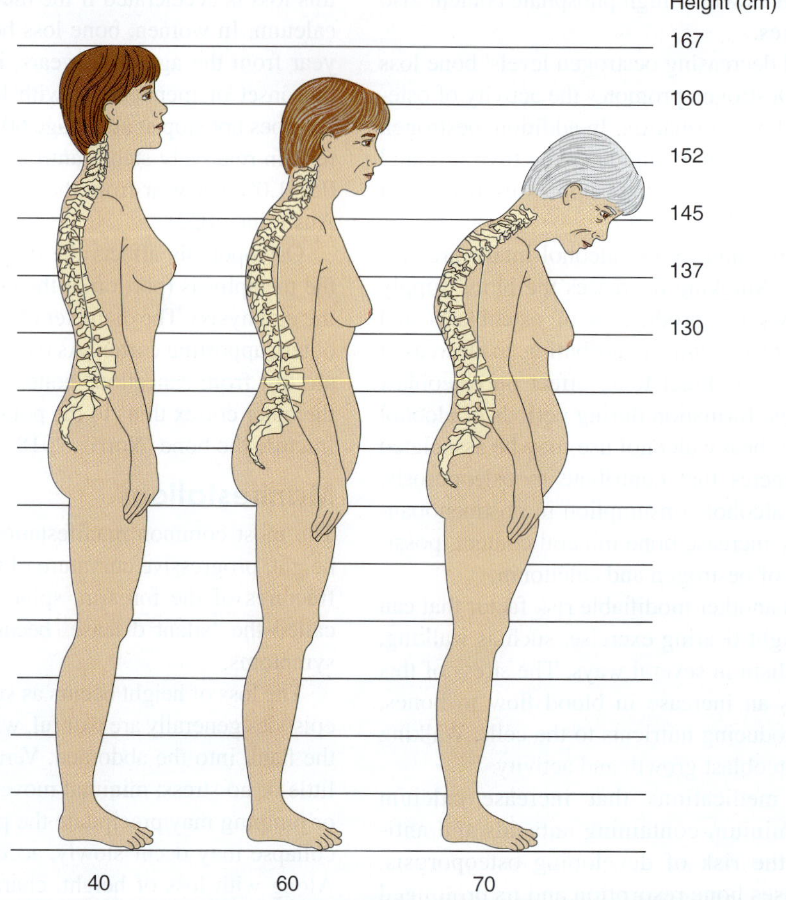

FIGURE 39.2 ***Spinal changes caused by osteoporosis. As the condition progresses, height can be reduced by as much as 17 cm***

Dual-energy x-ray absorptiometry (DEXA) measures bone density in the lumbar spine or hip and is considered to be highly accurate. Ultrasound transmits painless sound waves through the heel of the foot to measure bone density. This 1-minute test is not as sensitive as DEXA but is accurate enough for screening purposes. These tests are described in the chapter 'A person-centred approach to assessing the musculoskeletal system'. Quantitative computed tomography (QCT) and quantitative ultrasound (QUS) are also used in diagnosis.

Laboratory tests include alkaline phosphatase (AST), which may be elevated following a fracture, and serum bone Gla protein (osteocalcin), which can be used as a marker of osteoclastic activity and therefore is an indicator of the rate of bone turnover. This test is most useful to evaluate the effects of treatment, rather than as an indicator of the severity of the disease. A comparison of laboratory test results for metabolic bone diseases is outlined in Table 39.1.

Medications

Oestrogen replacement therapy reduces bone loss, increases bone density in the spine and hip, and reduces the risk of fractures in postmenopausal women. It is particularly recommended for women who have undergone surgical menopause before age 50 and is often prescribed for women with other osteoporosis risk factors. Oestrogen therapy alone is associated with an increased risk of endometrial cancer, so it usually is prescribed in combination with progestin (hormone replacement therapy, or HRT). The choice of using HRT to prevent osteoporosis is one that must be made between the woman and her healthcare provider.

Raloxifene (Evista) is a selective oestrogen receptor modulator (SERM) that appears to prevent bone loss by mimicking oestrogen's beneficial effects on bone density in postmenopausal women. It does not have the risks of oestrogen. Hot flushes are a common side effect and this drug should not be taken by a woman with a history of blood clots.

Alendronate (Fosamax) and risedronate (Actonel) are from the class of drugs known as bisphosphonates. Bisphosphonates are potent inhibitors of bone resorption that may be used to prevent and treat osteoporosis. They inhibit bone breakdown, preserve bone mass and increase bone density in the hip and vertebrae. Alendronate is especially useful for men and young adults and to prevent or treat glucocorticoid-induced osteoporosis. The nursing implications of bisphosphonates are found in the 'Medication administration: the person with Paget's disease' box. Teriparatide (Forteo) is a synthetic parathyroid hormone, administered subcutaneously to stimulate new bone formation and mass. It is used to decrease the risk of bone fracture from osteoporosis in postmenopausal women and in men with primary or secondary hypogonadism.

TABLE 39.1 Differential features of osteoporosis, osteomalacia and Paget's disease

DIFFERENTIATING FEATURES	OSTEOPOROSIS	OSTEOMALACIA	PAGET'S DISEASE
Pathophysiology	Resorption greater than bone formation	Inadequate mineralisation of bone matrix	Excessive osteoclastic activity and formation of poor-quality bone
Calcium level (serum)	Normal	Low or normal	Normal or elevated (especially in immobilised people)
Phosphate level (serum)	Normal	Low or normal	Normal
Parathyroid hormone level (serum)	Normal	High or normal	Normal
Alkaline phosphatase level (serum)	Normal	Elevated	Increased; not a reliable test for people who have liver disease or are pregnant
Hydroxyproline (urine)	Not applicable	Not applicable	Increased
Radiographic findings	Osteopenia, fractures	Decreased bone density, radiolucent bands known as Looser's zones or pseudofractures	'Punched-out' appearance of bone, increase in bone thickness, linear fractures, mosaic pattern of bone matrix

Ibandronate sodium (Boniva) is the first monthly osteoporosis medication. It is used for both treatment and prevention of postmenopausal osteoporosis and reduces the number of vertebral fractures in women with osteoporosis, as well as increasing bone density in women who do not have the disease (Bone Health and Osteoporosis Foundation, 2022). Ibandronate sodium needs to be taken on the same day of each month.

Calcitonin is a hormone that increases bone formation and decreases bone resorption. Calcitonin increases spinal bone density and reduces the risk of compression fractures; it may reduce the risk of hip fracture as well. Calcitonin usually is prescribed as a nasal spray, although it also is available in parenteral form. Because calcitonin is a protein, it can precipitate anaphylactic-type allergic responses.

Sodium fluoride stimulates osteoblast activity, increasing bone formation. When used to treat osteoporosis, bone mass of the spine increases and the risk of spinal fractures may be reduced. Fluoride therapy may, however, be associated with an increased risk of hip and other non-vertebral fractures.

Medications being investigated include vitamin D metabolites and other bisphosphonates. See the 'Medication administration' box for information about calcium, calcitonin and fluoride.

MEDICATION ADMINISTRATION The person with osteoporosis

CALCIUM

Postmenopausal women, regardless of whether they take replacement oestrogen, are encouraged to take calcium to prevent osteoporosis.

Nursing responsibilities

- Help the person to maintain an adequate dietary intake of calcium. The best dietary source is milk and other dairy products, including yoghurt.
- Postmenopausal women who take oestrogen need 1,000 mg of calcium daily. Those who do not take oestrogen need about 1,500 mg daily to minimise osteoporosis.
- Identify alternative sources, such as skim milk and low-fat yoghurt, oysters, canned sardines or salmon, beans, cauliflower and dark-green leafy vegetables.

Health education for the person and family

- Take calcium carbonate in divided doses 30 to 60 minutes before meals to allow for absorption.
- Take calcium citrate with meals to minimise gastrointestinal distress.

CALCITONIN

Calcitonin–salmon injection, synthetic Calcimar
Miacalcin (injection or nasal spray)

In postmenopausal osteoporosis, calcitonin prevents further bone loss and increases bone mass if the person consumes adequate amounts of calcium and vitamin D. Calcitonin may be used in postmenopausal women who cannot or will not take oestrogen.

Nursing responsibilities

- Calcitonin is protein in nature; both the parenteral form and the nasal spray forms may cause an anaphylactic-type allergic response. Observe the person for 20 minutes after administration; have appropriate emergency equipment and drugs available to treat anaphylaxis.
- Alternate nostrils daily when administering calcitonin nasal spray.
- Review medical history for conditions that contraindicate use of calcitonin products: hypersensitivity to salmon calcitonin and lactation (calcitonin is secreted in breast milk and may inhibit lactation).
- Observe for side effects: nausea and vomiting, anorexia, mild transient flushing of the palms of the hands and the soles of the feet, and urinary frequency.
- Teach the person the proper technique for handling and injecting the drug at home.

Health education for the person and family

- Take the medication in the evening to minimise side effects.
- Warm nasal spray to room temperature before using.
- Rhinitis (runny nose) is the most common side effect with calcitonin nasal spray. Other possible side effects include

(continued)

MEDICATION ADMINISTRATION The person with osteoporosis (continued)

sores, itching or other nasal symptoms. Report nosebleeds to your healthcare provider.

- Nausea and vomiting may occur during initial stages of therapy; they disappear as treatment continues.
- While taking the medication, be sure to consume adequate amounts of calcium and vitamin D.

FLUORIDE

Fluoride is a mineral long recognised as essential for the normal formation of dentine and tooth enamel. Fluoride appears to decrease the solubility of bone mineral and therefore the rate of bone reabsorption. Its use in preventing and treating osteoporosis is relatively new but promising.

Nursing responsibilities

- Monitor serum fluoride levels every 3 months.
- Have bone mineral density studies conducted at 6-month intervals to document progress of bone growth.

Health education for the person and family

- Take sodium fluoride tablets after meals and avoid milk or dairy products; these reduce gastrointestinal absorption of the medication.
- While taking fluoride, be sure to maintain an adequate calcium intake.
- Use fluoride mouth rinse immediately after brushing teeth and just before retiring at night. Do not swallow the rinse and avoid eating or drinking for at least 30 minutes after use.
- Notify the healthcare provider if teeth become stained or mottled after repeated use of fluoride mouth rinse.

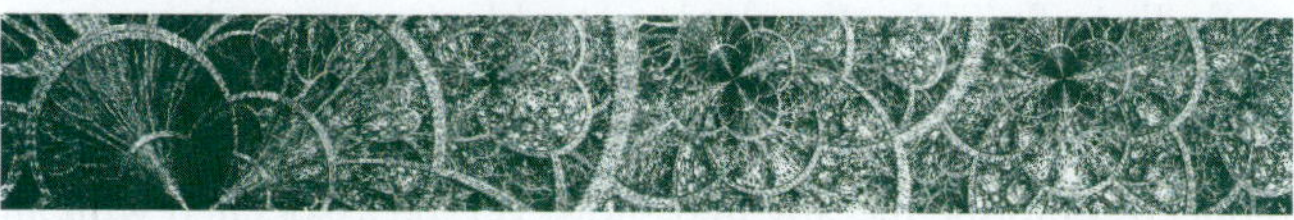

Nursing care

Osteoporosis is both preventable and treatable; therefore, nursing care focuses primarily on planning and implementing interventions to prevent the disease, its manifestations and the resulting injuries. An important aspect of preventing osteoporosis is educating people under age 35. See the accompanying nursing care plan for a person with osteoporosis.

Health promotion

Health promotion activities to prevent or slow osteoporosis focus on calcium intake, exercise and health-related behaviours.

NURSING CARE PLAN A person with osteoporosis

Nancy Bauer is a 53-year-old school teacher. She has been married for 36 years and has two children. Mrs Bauer is 165 cm tall. She has smoked one packet of cigarettes a day for 30 years and drinks one to two glasses of wine with dinner each evening. She does not routinely exercise. Mrs Bauer has had symptoms of menopause for 8 years, including hot flushes in the early years and mood swings of late. She has never been on hormone replacement therapy.

Mrs Bauer is currently seeking medical advice for continuous lower back pain. The pain is not relieved with an over-the-counter analgesic and she frequently wakes up during the night because of the pain. She is diagnosed with osteoporosis.

ASSESSMENT

The nurse practitioner notes that Mrs Bauer's vital signs are within normal limits. She has full range of motion of all extremities and is able to stand and bend over, but she reports discomfort when returning to the upright position. Mrs Bauer has a slightly pronounced 'hump' on her upper back and is 2.5 cm shorter than her stated height on admission. Her muscle strength is symmetrical and strong.

DIAGNOSIS

- *Acute pain* of the lower spine related to vertebral compression.
- *Deficient knowledge* related to osteoporosis and treatment to prevent further damage.
- *Imbalanced nutrition: less than body requirements* related to inadequate intake of calcium.
- *Risk of injury* related to effects of change in bone structure secondary to osteoporosis.

PLANNING

Ensure Mrs Bauer is able to manage her pain and educate her regarding her osteoporosis and associated issues.

Expected outcomes

- Verbalise a decrease in back pain.
- Be able to describe ways to treat her osteoporosis and prevent further complications.
- Verbalise an understanding of the current research and treatment regarding osteoporosis.
- Verbalise safety precautions to prevent fractures due to falls.
- Seek consultation for supplements and medications to prevent further bone loss.
- Verbalise how stopping smoking can help prevent further progression of osteoporosis.
- Design a program of physical activity and weight-bearing exercise to prevent complications of osteoporosis.

IMPLEMENTATION

- Teach back-strengthening exercises.
- Refer to an osteoporosis support group, if available.
- Assess current knowledge base and correct misconceptions regarding treatment of osteoporosis.
- Provide current educational literature regarding treatment of osteoporosis.

NURSING CARE PLAN A person with osteoporosis (continued)

- Review safety and fall precautions and provide literature regarding how to create a safe home environment.
- Instruct in dietary and calcium supplements that help prevent effects of osteoporosis.
- Provide realistic, yet optimistic, feedback about loss of height and bone integrity and the potential outcomes of treatment.
- Discuss physical exercises that help prevent complications due to osteoporosis.

EVALUATION

On her return visit 6 months later, Mrs Bauer reports that she feels much better. She is no longer irritable and does not experience mood swings because she has been taking her prescribed hormone replacements for 6 months. She is eating products rich in calcium and taking a daily supplement of calcium with vitamin D. Mrs Bauer has reduced her wine intake to one glass in the evening and now drinks decaffeinated coffee and tea. She also states that since she stopped smoking, she has been walking 30 to 45 minutes every day.

CRITICAL THINKING IN THE NURSING PROCESS

1 What is the rationale for stopping smoking and limiting caffeine and alcohol intake in the treatment of osteoporosis?
2 Which foods would you encourage for people at high risk of osteoporosis whose serum cholesterol and LDL/HDL ratios indicate a high risk of cardiovascular disease?
3 Which physical activities would you consider beneficial in helping to prevent the effects of osteoporosis in the female person who is wheelchair bound or has limited mobility?
4 Develop a care plan for Mrs Bauer for the nursing diagnosis *Risk of trauma.*

REFLECTION ON THE NURSING PROCESS

1 Reflecting on the care for Mrs Bauer, identify the main issues you have learned from this case study that you will able to apply in future practice.
2 What type of health education is required for Mrs Bauer prior to discharge, and how would this be best delivered to her?

Nutrition

For people of all ages, stress the importance of maintaining a daily calcium intake that meets recommendations of the National Institutes of Health (for Australia and New Zealand) and the National Health and Medical Research Council (NHMRC) & Ministry of Health (MoH) (2015). This is particularly important for adolescent girls and young adult women who may avoid eating many high-calcium foods such as dairy products because of concerns about weight. Optimal calcium intake before ages 30 to 35 probably increases peak bone mass. Emphasise that low-fat (or non-fat) dairy products also contain calcium, although some fat in the product may enhance calcium absorption.

Milk and milk products are the best sources of calcium. The lactose in milk facilitates calcium absorption as well. Other food sources of calcium include sardines, clams, oysters and salmon, as well as dark-green leafy vegetables such as broccoli, bok choy and spinach. For people who avoid dairy products because of lactose intolerance or a vegan diet, suggest alternative sources.

Calcium supplements are available in many forms. Most supplements provide calcium carbonate in the range of 200 to 600 mg per tablet. Other forms of calcium, including citrate, gluconate and lactate, generally provide a lower amount of elemental calcium per tablet. A combination of calcium with vitamin D is recommended (e.g. Ostelin), particularly for older adults who may have a vitamin D deficiency that impairs their ability to absorb and use calcium.

Exercise

Teach people the importance of physical activity and weight-bearing exercises in preventing and slowing bone loss. Suggest that people participate in regular exercise, such as walking for at least 20 minutes four or more times a week. Inform people that swimming and pool aerobic exercises are not as beneficial for maintaining bone density because of the lack of weight-bearing activity.

Healthy behaviours

Behaviours that help prevent osteoporosis include not smoking, avoiding excessive alcohol intake and limiting caffeine intake to two or three cups of coffee each day.

Assessment

Collect the following data through the health history and physical examination:

- *Health history*: age, risk factors, history of fractures, smoking history, alcohol intake, medications, usual diet, menstrual history including menopause, usual exercise/activity level, lower back pain (see the following 'Translation to practice' box).
- *Physical examination*: height, spinal curves.

Nursing diagnoses and interventions

Nursing care of people who have osteoporosis focuses on teaching about the disease process, helping maintain physical mobility and nutrition, and solving problems associated with pain and injury.

Health-seeking behaviours

At multiple points in the person's lifetime, nurses can provide vital information that will help people use self-care strategies to reduce their risk of developing osteoporosis:

- Assess the person's health habits, including diet, exercise, smoking and alcohol use. *The risk of developing osteoporosis in later life is affected by such things as diet, regular participation in weight-bearing exercise and personal habits such as smoking and alcohol consumption.*
- Teach women and men of all ages the importance of maintaining an adequate calcium intake. Provide a list of calcium-rich foods and discuss the use of calcium supplements with people who do not consume adequate dietary calcium. *Calcium needs vary during the course of a*

TRANSLATION TO PRACTICE Evidence-based practice for the person with osteoporosis

Osteoporosis is a major health problem in Australia and New Zealand. Risk factors for osteoporosis include being Caucasian, having a small body frame, not doing weight-bearing exercises and having a family history of osteoporosis. Nursing can do much to prevent the development of osteoporosis by assessing risk factors and teaching about diet, exercise and lifestyle.

IMPLICATIONS FOR NURSING

Assessment is a critical component of the nursing process, enabling nurses to identify people at risk of diseases, to monitor ongoing interventions and to design teaching specific to a person's needs. The risk factors for osteoporosis are genetics, calcium and vitamin D status, body mass index, previous fractures, recurrent falls, medical conditions such as malabsorption disorders, thyroid disease, diabetes, chronic kidney or liver disease, and medications such as antiepileptic drugs, antidepressants and long-term glucocorticoids (AIHW, 2022).

CRITICAL THINKING IN PERSON-CENTRED CARE

1 At what age do women develop maximum bone mass? (Review information in a text or on the internet.) Based on this information, what type of teaching would be most effective?
2 Compare and contrast your teaching for a 24-year-old Indigenous Australian woman who has a calcium-poor diet but is a non-smoker, and a thin, Caucasian, 64-year-old woman who is postmenopausal and smokes.
3 While screening people in a clinic for health risks, including osteoporosis, a man in his seventies says, 'Oh, I can't have bad bones... I'm a man!' How would you respond?

lifetime; however, many people never consume adequate amounts of calcium. This affects their peak bone mass and the rate of bone loss with ageing. Calcium in foods is more completely absorbed than that supplied by calcium supplements.

- Discuss the importance of maintaining a regular schedule of weight-bearing exercise, either through an exercise program or regular physical activity. *Weight-bearing exercise promotes osteoblast activity, helping maintain bone strength and integrity.*
- Refer people to smoking-cessation programs and alcohol treatment programs as appropriate. *Smoking interferes with oestrogen's protective effects on bones, promoting bone loss. Excess alcohol intake affects the nutritional status of the person, increasing the risk of calcium and vitamin D deficiency.*
- Refer people with significant risk factors for osteoporosis to primary care providers or clinics for bone-density evaluation. *Early identification and treatment of osteoporotic changes in bones can reduce the risk and possible long-term consequences of falls and fractures.*

Risk of injury

Falls that would result in little or no injury in the healthy adult may cause fractures in the person with osteoporosis. Even normal movements such as twisting, bending, lifting or rising from bed can precipitate a vertebral fracture.

- Implement safety precautions as necessary for the person who is hospitalised or in a long-term care facility. Maintain the bed in a low position; use side rails if indicated to prevent the person from getting up alone; provide night-time lighting to toilet facilities. *Most falls are preventable, particularly in hospitals and long-term care facilities.*
- Avoid using restraints (if hospitalised or a resident in a long-term care facility) if at all possible. *Restraints may actually increase the person's risk of falling, as well as the risk of injury associated with a fall.*

CONSIDERATION FOR PRACTICE

People may fracture osteoporotic bones when pulling against restraints.

- Teach people who are able to participate in weight-bearing exercises to perform exercises at least three times a week for a sustained period of 30 to 40 minutes. *The mechanical force of weight-bearing exercises promotes bone growth. Bones weaken and demineralise without exercise. Walking is an easy, low-impact form of exercise. Swimming (including walking on the bottom of the pool) does not provide the needed weight-bearing activity.*
- Encourage older adults to use assistive devices to maintain independence in ADLs. *Walking sticks, frames and other assistive devices encourage independence and support activities that promote bone growth.*
- Teach older people about safety and fall precautions. *An assessment of the person's home for safety and fall risks may reduce the risk of fractures and, in turn, the cost of hospitalisation and potential disability and/or death.*

Imbalanced nutrition: less than body requirements

Most Australians do not maintain their recommended daily intake of calcium. People must therefore be made aware of the relationship between an adequate calcium intake and maintaining strong bones. The recommendations for Australia and New Zealand are:

- 1,300 mg/day for girls and boys aged 12 to 18 years
- 1,000 mg/day for pregnant and lactating women over 19; 1,300 mg/day for pregnant and lactating women under 18
- 1,000 mg/day for women aged 19 to 50
- 1,000 mg/day for men aged 19 to 70
- 1,300 mg/day for women over 50 and men over 70 (NHMRC & MoH, 2015).

Teach people taking calcium supplements the importance of taking the medication at the proper time and the side effects that may occur. Free hydrochloric acid is needed for calcium absorption. Vitamin D is used to assist absorption. Calcium carbonate supplement should be taken 30 to 60 minutes before meals to allow adequate absorption. Calcium citrate supplements should be taken with meals to prevent gastrointestinal distress.

> **CONSIDERATION FOR PRACTICE**
> **Calcium supplements should be taken in divided doses (two to three times daily) for improved distribution.**

Acute pain

Advanced stages of osteoporosis can result in pain and immobilisation. Acute pain usually results from a complicating fracture, especially a compression fracture of the vertebrae.

- Suggest anti-inflammatory pain medications for treatment of both acute and chronic phases of pain. People should be instructed in the amount and frequency as noted on the manufacturer's labels. Opioids can cause increased risk of osteoporosis. *Continuous administration of ibuprofen or other non-steroidal anti-inflammatory drugs (NSAIDs) can be useful to provide relief from pain, but people must be cautioned not to exceed dosage recommendations.*

> **CONSIDERATION FOR PRACTICE**
> **Teach people on long-term anti-inflammatory medications to watch for bright-red bleeding from the stomach (in vomitus) or black bowel movements.**

- Suggest the application of heat to relieve pain. A heating pad may offer temporary pain relief. To avoid the 'rebound effect', the heat should be removed every 20 to 30 minutes.

Community-based care

The person who has osteoporosis needs education on safety and preventing falls. In addition to home safety, outdoor safety is important too. People should be taught to use assistive devices for added stability, to wear rubber-soled shoes for traction and to walk on the grass when footpaths are slippery, avoiding uneven surfaces to reduce risk of tripping.

Address the following topics when discussing home care:

- resources for medical supplies and assistive devices
- diet, exercise and medications
- pain management
- maintaining good posture to help prevent stress on the spine
- helpful resources:
  - Arthritis Australia: https://arthritisaustralia.com.au
  - Department of Health and Aged Care: www.health.gov.au
  - Bone Health & Osteoporosis Foundation: https://www.bonehealthandosteoporosis.org/
  - Osteoporosis and Related Bone Diseases National Resource Center (NIH): https://www.bones.nih.gov/health-info/bone/osteoporosis/overview
  - Healthy Bones Australia: https://healthybonesaustralia.org.au/
  - Osteoporosis New Zealand: https://osteoporosis.org.nz.

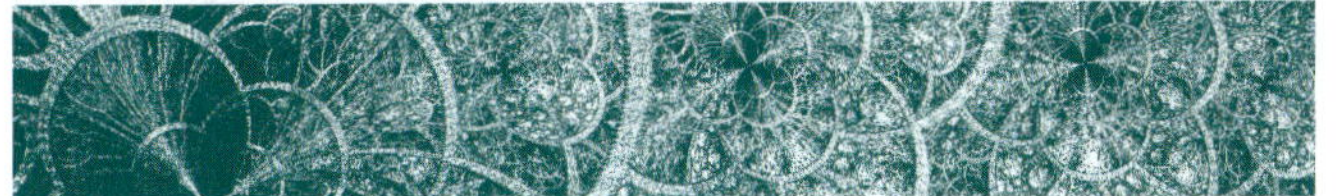

THE PERSON WITH PAGET'S DISEASE

Paget's disease, also called *osteitis deformans*, is a progressive metabolic skeletal disorder that results from excessive metabolic activity in bone, with excessive bone resorption followed by excessive bone formation. This chronic remodelling results in the affected bones being larger and softer, with manifestations of bone pain, arthritis, obvious skeletal deformities and fractures. The disorder affects bones of the axial skeleton, especially the femur, pelvis, vertebrae and skull. The disease may affect one bone or multiple bones. The cause is unknown; however, several theories have been proposed, including hormonal imbalance, vascular disorder, neoplasm, autoimmune disorder and inborn error of connective tissue. Australia historically has the highest prevalence of Paget's disease outside the UK (Britton et al., 2017).

Paget's disease occurs in both men and women, affecting 4% of the population over the age of 50 in Australia. It is less common in people of Asian, Indian and Scandinavian descent. It is more common in men—2:1 compared to women—and up to 40% of all people with Paget's disease have at least one other relative with the disorder. It has a familial tendency as a result of mutations in several genes. The measles virus has been found in bone lesions and the relevance of that finding is under investigation (Paget's Association, 2022).

Pathophysiology

Paget's disease progresses slowly. It usually follows a two-stage process: an excessive amount of osteoclastic bone resorption followed by excessive osteoblastic bone formation. The initial phase presents with an abnormal increase in osteoclasts. The bones increase in size and thickness because of the acceleration in bone resorption and regeneration, resulting in a thick layer of coarse bone with a rough and pitted outer surface (Norris, 2018). Resorption of cancellous bone occurs rapidly. As new bone tissue tries to replace the loss, fibrous tissue forms in the bone marrow. The bone is at first hyperaemic and soft, and bowing occurs. When this excessive bone cell activity decreases, the result is a gain in bone mass, but the newly formed bone becomes hard and brittle. This brittleness may lead to fractures.

Manifestations

Most people with Paget's disease are asymptomatic for years and the disease often is discovered when typical changes are seen on an incidental x-ray. Manifestations are often vague and depend on the specific area involved (see the 'Manifestations' box). The most common manifestation is localised pain of the long bones, spine, pelvis and cranium. The pain is described as a mild to moderate deep ache that is aggravated by pressure and weight bearing. It is more noticeable at night or when the person is resting. The pain usually is due to metabolic bone activity, secondary degenerative osteoarthritis, fractures or nerve impingement. Because of the increase in blood flow to pagetic bone, flushing and warmth of the overlying skin may be apparent.

Complications

Complications of Paget's disease are as follows:

- nerve palsy syndromes from involvement of the upper extremities

MANIFESTATIONS Paget's disease

MUSCULOSKELETAL EFFECTS
- Pain (in the long bones of lower extremities or joints)
- Deformity (enlargement of skull, bowing of lower extremities and deformity of elbows and knees)
- Fractures of lower extremities
- Pathological fractures (especially of the tibia)
- Compression fractures
- Collapse of the vertebrae, resulting in kyphosis and loss of height
- Muscle weakness

NEUROLOGICAL EFFECTS
- Hearing loss
- Spinal cord injuries
- Dementia
- Pain from spinal stenosis
- Bladder and/or bowel dysfunction

CARDIOVASCULAR EFFECTS
- Congestive heart failure

METABOLIC EFFECTS
- Symptoms of hypercalcaemia in immobilised people
- Hypercalciuria and renal calculi
- Increased skin temperature over affected extremities

- pathological fractures from loss of bone structure
- mental deterioration from compression of the brain when the skull is involved
- compression of the spinal cord from affected cervical vertebrae causing quadriplegia
- cardiovascular disease, resulting from vasodilation of the vessels in the skin and subcutaneous tissues overlying the affected bones
- osteogenic sarcoma, seen in 5–10% of people with severe disease (Norris, 2018).

INTERPROFESSIONAL CARE

Care of the person with Paget's disease focuses on relieving pain, suppressing bone cell activity if necessary and preventing or minimising the effects of complications. Many people with Paget's disease are asymptomatic and do not require treatment. For more severely affected people, pharmacological agents are usually effective. Occasionally, surgery may be required.

Diagnosis

Many of the diagnostic tests that are useful for the diagnosis of osteoporosis are equally useful for people with Paget's disease (see Table 39.1). These include x-rays and bone scans to illustrate localised areas of demineralisation in the early stages, seen as 'punched-out' areas that lend a coarse, irregular appearance to the bone. In the later phase, x-rays show enlargement of the bones, tiny cracks in the long bones, and/or bowing of the weight-bearing bones. Computed tomography (CT) scans and magnetic resonance imaging (MRI) help identify possible causes of pain, including degenerative problems, spinal stenosis or nerve root impingement. Diagnostic tests are described in the chapter 'A person-centred approach to assessing the musculoskeletal system'.

Laboratory tests used in diagnosis include a plasma alkaline phosphatase, which will show a steady rise as the disease progresses; the normal level (30 to 115 international units (IU)/L) may be elevated from high normal to more than 3,000 international units/L. A urinary collagen pyridinoline test is a sensitive indicator of the rate of bone resorption. Liver function tests, isotope bone scans and vitamin D levels are also useful diagnostic tools (Paget's Association, 2022).

Medications

People who have mild symptoms often find relief using aspirin or NSAIDs such as ibuprofen and indomethacin. People who are experiencing manifestations and whose diagnostic test results are elevated are usually treated with an agent that retards bone resorption, such as calcitonin or a bisphosphonate.

Bisphosphonates such as alendronate, pamidronate and risedronate are the primary treatments used for severe Paget's disease. These drugs inhibit bone resorption, possibly by attaching to the surface of the calcium/phosphate phase of bone and inhibiting osteoclast activity. They are safe and usually are well tolerated by the person. Alendronate is available as an oral preparation and pamidronate is available for intravenous administration. Oral preparations are poorly absorbed from the GI tract and may cause gastric or oesophageal irritation. Alendronate should be given with a full glass of water on an empty stomach, at least 30 minutes before other medications or food. Pamidronate is given as an intravenous infusion in 5% dextrose or 0.9% sodium chloride. It is given for 3 successive days, generally promoting a rapid response with reduced urinary excretion of hydroxyproline and pyridinium and a fall in alkaline phosphatase. Intravenous pamidronate may cause flu-like symptoms, but these generally are brief. Calcium supplements also are prescribed for people receiving bisphosphonates. After bisphosphonate treatment, people often experience remission of symptoms for a year or more. See the 'Medication administration' box for nursing implications.

CALCITONIN Calcitonin inhibits osteoclastic resorption of bone and is secreted by the thyroid gland. It also works as an analgesic for bone pain. The two derivatives of this medication are salmon (fish) and human. Salmon calcitonin (Calcimar/salcatonin/calcitriol) is generally preferred because it is inexpensive and widely available. Human calcitonin (Cibacalcin) is derived from human thyroid glands, which makes it more expensive and difficult to obtain. The parenteral form of calcitonin is used in treating Paget's disease (50–100 units daily). (See the 'Medication administration: the person with osteoporosis' box for nursing implications.)

Surgery

Different surgical interventions may be used to treat people with Paget's disease, such as repairing a complete fracture through pagetic bone, realigning a knee through tibial osteotomy to

MEDICATION ADMINISTRATION **The person with Paget's disease**

BISPHOSPHONATES
Alendronate
Etidronate
Pamidronate
Risedronate
Tiludronate

The bisphosphonates inhibit bone resorption, increasing the mineral density of bones and reducing the incidence of fractures. They are also used in both the prevention and treatment of osteoporosis. When used for Paget's disease, bisphosphonates slow the accelerated bone turnover associated with this disease. Bone pain is relieved and the incidence of pathological fractures is reduced. Cardiac and vascular manifestations of the disease also improve.

Nursing responsibilities

- Administer alendronate with water 30 minutes before food or other medications due to its common side effect of nausea.
- Do not give foods high in calcium, vitamins with mineral supplements or antacids within 2 hours of administering alendronate as this may interfere with the absorption of the drug.
- Instruct the person to avoid lying down for 30 minutes after taking the drug to facilitate delivery of the dose to the stomach, as alendronate causes GI tract irritation (Bryant et al., 2018).
- Assess renal function studies before initiating therapy; alendronate is not recommended for use in people with renal insufficiency.
- Dilute the prescribed dose of pamidronate in 1,000 mL of 5% dextrose or 0.9% sodium chloride; infuse over at least 4 hours. Do not add to calcium-containing solutions such as Hartmann's solution.
- Monitor the IV site for signs of thrombophlebitis.
- Assess the person for signs of electrolyte imbalance or other adverse responses such as a drug fever.

Health education for the person and family

- Take the medication as directed with clear water only. Consuming other beverages or food within 30 minutes of taking alendronate may interfere with its absorption and effectiveness.
- Do not lie down until after the person has eaten. Alendronate can irritate the oesophagus.
- Report symptoms such as new or worsening heartburn, difficulty swallowing or painful swallowing.
- Fever with or without chills may occur while receiving intravenous pamidronate; this will subside without treatment. Flu-like symptoms also may occur; these will subside within a week or so.
- Report any abnormal symptoms such as tingling around the mouth or numbness and tingling of the fingers or toes, which may indicate an imbalance of electrolytes in the blood.
- Take calcium and vitamin D supplements as instructed by the person's primary care provider.
- Response to these medications is gradual and continues for months after the drug is stopped.

decrease pain or replacing a hip and/or knee for osteoarthritis. Because increased bleeding is a manifestation of Paget's disease, it is important to administer a potent bisphosphonate prior to surgery to decrease hypervascularity and reduce the risk of increased operative blood loss (Singer, 2016).

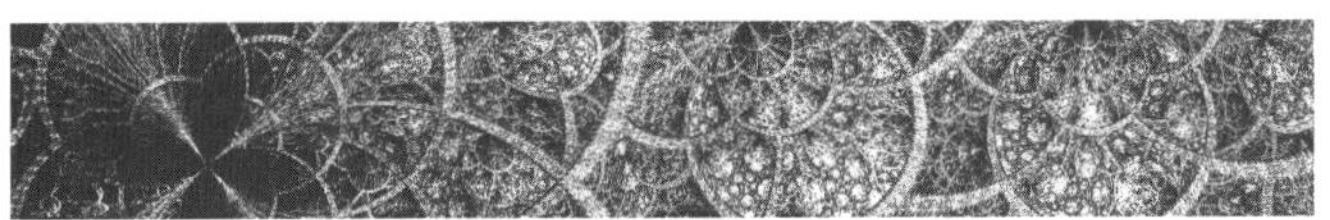

Nursing care

Nursing diagnoses and interventions

The nursing interventions for the person with symptomatic Paget's disease focus on pain control, prevention of injury or fractures, and education regarding the disease process and prescribed therapies.

Chronic pain

The most common manifestation of Paget's disease is bone pain. This usually is the manifestation that prompts the person to seek healthcare.

- Assess the location and extent of the pain to determine the bone areas involved. *Bone pain in Paget's disease is poorly localised and is frequently described as 'aching and deep'.*
- Teach the person to take NSAIDs or aspirin on a regular basis as prescribed. *Pain is most noticeable at night or when the person is resting. The pain can become evident when it is aggravated by pressure and weight bearing.*
- Ensure correct placement of prescribed brace or corset. *The person may be required to wear a light brace or corset to relieve back pain and provide support when assuming an upright position. The person may need instruction in the correct application of the device and in the evaluation of pressure areas that may result from wearing the device.*
- Suggest referral for heat therapy and massage. *Heat therapy and massage can alleviate mild discomfort. Care should be taken when applying massage over areas prone to pathological fractures.*

Impaired physical mobility

People with Paget's disease need to maintain or improve mobility so that they can perform necessary self-care activities and prevent complications of immobility.

- Provide an assistive device for use when ambulating. *During the active phase of Paget's disease, the person is prone to fractures. Bone deformities, activity intolerance, fear of falling and pain are all factors that may make the person more prone to falls. An assistive device can provide both physical and psychological support during ambulation, permit the person to ambulate further and provide a device for resting during ambulation.*

> **CONSIDERATION FOR PRACTICE**
> **Activities as seemingly simple as lifting a heavy box may result in a fracture in the person with Paget's disease.**

- Teach good body mechanics. *The person with bone deformities should avoid activities that require lifting and twisting.*
- Reinforce information about exercise protocols and activity regimens. *Exercise and activity protocols should be planned carefully to prevent injury and to minimise fatigue.*

Community-based care

A diagnosis of Paget's disease can be frightening for the person and family. It is important that they understand that this is a treatable disease and that many manifestations of the disease will be relieved with treatment. Inform the person that remissions of the disease often last for a year or more after effective treatment. The Paget Foundation should be suggested as a resource. Discuss the following topics:

- the importance of following the prescribed treatment regimen and keeping scheduled follow-up appointments
- because it may take several weeks to notice a response to treatment, the importance of continuing therapy during this time and after a response is obtained
- if bisphosphonates such as alendronate or pamidronate are ordered, the importance of taking supplemental calcium to prevent low blood calcium levels
- the importance of remaining active
- safety in the home and outdoor environment to prevent falls
- the need to report to the primary care provider any sudden pain or disability, even if no trauma has occurred, because pathological fractures are possible.

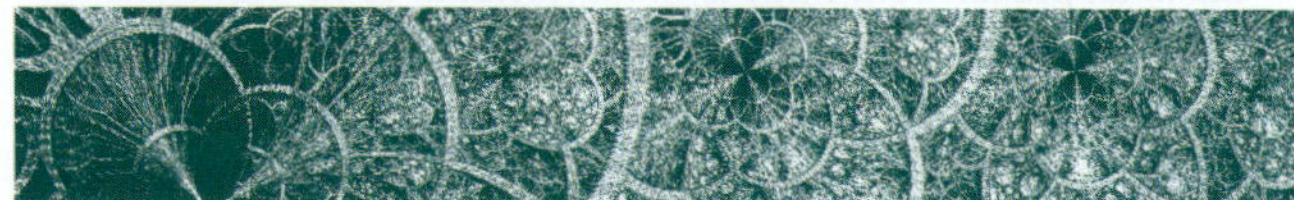

THE PERSON WITH GOUT

Gout is a metabolic disease that occurs from an inflammatory response to the production or excretion of uric acid resulting in high levels of uric acid in the blood (hyperuricaemia) and in other body fluids, including synovial fluid. The disorder is characterised by deposits of urates (insoluble precipitates) in the connective tissues of the body. Gout has an acute onset, usually at night, and often involves the first metatarsophalangeal joint (great toe). The initial acute attack is usually followed by a period of months or years without manifestations. As the disease progresses, urates are deposited in various other connective tissues. Deposits in the synovial fluids cause acute inflammation of the joint (*gouty arthritis*). Over time, urate deposits in subcutaneous tissues cause the formation of small white nodules (called **tophi**). Deposits of crystals in the kidneys can form urate kidney stones and result in kidney failure.

Gout may occur as either a primary or a secondary disorder. Primary (inherited) gout is characterised by elevated serum uric acid levels resulting from either an inborn error of purine metabolism or a decrease in renal uric acid excretion due to an unknown cause. Purines are part of the structure of the nuclear compounds DNA and RNA; they also may be synthesised by the body. Impaired uric acid excretion leads to hyperuricaemia in the majority of people with primary gout. In secondary gout, hyperuricaemia occurs as a result of another disorder or treatment with certain medications. Disorders associated with rapid cell turnover, such as some malignancies (leukaemia, in particular), haemolytic anaemia and polycythaemia, can increase purine metabolism. Chronic renal disease, hypertension, starvation and diabetic ketoacidosis can interfere with uric acid excretion, as can certain drugs, including some diuretics (such as frusemide, ethacrynic acid and chlorothiazide), pyrazinamide, cyclosporin, ethambutol and low-dose salicylates. Alcohol ingestion appears to interfere with uric acid excretion and to accelerate its synthesis.

Gout occurs more often in men, usually after the age of 40. Self-reported data shows that an estimated 4.5% of Australians have gout and it is more common in males than females—almost 8 in 10 (79%) people with gout are males (ABS, 2019). A number of risk factors for gout have been identified (see Box 39.2). Of these, male gender and ageing cannot be modified; the others can be. Consumption of a diet rich in meat and seafood is associated with a higher risk of developing gout, whereas total protein intake and consumption of purine-rich vegetables have not been shown to contribute to its development (AIHW, 2019; Mayo Clinic, 2021). While alcohol intake has long been known to increase the risk of hyperuricaemia and gout, recent studies have shown that consumption of soft drinks sweetened with sugar or fructose (corn syrup) also increases the risk of gout in men. Obesity and metabolic syndrome (abdominal obesity, hyperlipidaemia, hypertension and insulin resistance) are strongly correlated with hyperuricaemia and gout (Mayo Clinic, 2021).

Pathophysiology

Uric acid is the breakdown product of purine metabolism. Normally, a balance exists between its production and its excretion, with approximately two-thirds of the amount produced each day excreted by the kidneys and the rest in the faeces. The normal serum urate levels for men and women vary, the normal range being 2–7 mg/dL (120–420 μmol/L) for men and 2–6 mg/dL (120–360 μmol/L) for women, although these figures may differ between laboratories or populations. Hyperuricaemia is therefore defined as serum urate levels > 7 mg/dL (> 420 μmol/L) for men and > 6 mg/dL (> 360 μmol/L) for women. Higher levels of uric acid are associated with increased incidence and prevalence rates for gout. Men have higher concentrations of uric acid and therefore a higher prevalence of gout, whereas premenopausal women and children have lower concentrations and therefore a lower prevalence of gout (ABS, 2019).

> **BOX 39.2 Risk factors for gout**
>
> - Male gender
> - Age
> - Diet: higher consumption of meat and seafood
> - Alcohol intake, beer in particular
> - Consumption of sugar- or fructose-sweetened soft drinks
> - Obesity
> - Medications: diuretics, aspirin

At levels greater than 7.0 mg/dL, the serum is saturated and monosodium urate crystals may form. It is not known exactly how monosodium urate crystals are deposited in joints. Several mechanisms may be involved:

- Crystals tend to form in peripheral tissues of the body, where lower temperatures reduce the solubility of the uric acid.
- A decrease in extracellular fluid pH and reduced plasma protein binding of urate crystals are evident.
- Tissue trauma and a rapid change in uric acid levels may also lead to crystal deposition. A rapid increase in uric acid may occur with tissue trauma and release of cellular components.

The monosodium urate crystals may form in the synovial fluid or in the synovial membrane, cartilage or other joint connective tissues. They may also form in the heart, earlobes and kidneys. These crystals stimulate and continue the inflammatory process, during which neutrophils respond by ingesting the crystals. The neutrophils release their phagolysosomes, causing tissue damage, which perpetuates the inflammation.

Manifestations

The manifestations of gout are hyperuricaemia, recurrent attacks of inflammation of a single joint, tophi, kidney disease and kidney stones. Unless treated, the manifestations of gout appear in three stages: asymptomatic hyperuricaemia, acute gouty arthritis and tophaceous gout (see the 'Manifestations' box).

Asymptomatic hyperuricaemia

The first stage is asymptomatic hyperuricaemia, with serum levels averaging 9 to 10 mg/dL. Most people with hyperuricaemia do not progress to further stages of the disease.

Acute gouty arthritis

The second state is acute gouty arthritis. The acute attack (called a 'flare'), usually affecting a single joint, occurs unexpectedly, often beginning at night. It may be triggered by trauma, alcohol ingestion, dietary excess or a stressor such as surgery. It is often precipitated by an abrupt or sustained increase in uric acid levels. The affected joint becomes red, hot, swollen and exquisitely painful and tender.

Approximately 50% of initial attacks of acute gouty arthritis occur in the metatarsophalangeal joint of the great toe. Other sites for acute attacks include the instep of the foot, ankles, heels, knees, wrists, fingers and elbows. The pain, often intense, peaks within several hours and may be accompanied by fever and an elevated white blood cell (WBC) count and erythrocyte sedimentation rate (ESR). The affected joints are swollen and the skin over the joint is warm and dusky red.

Acute attacks of gouty arthritis last from several hours up to several weeks and typically subside spontaneously. There are no long-lasting sequelae and the person enters an asymptomatic period called the intercritical period. The intercritical period may last up to 10 years; however, approximately 60% of people experience a recurrent attack within 1 year. Successive attacks tend to last longer, occur with increasing frequency and resolve less completely than the initial attack.

Tophaceous (chronic) gout

Tophaceous (or chronic) gout occurs when hyperuricaemia is not treated. The urate pool expands and monosodium urate crystal deposits (tophi) develop in cartilage, synovial membranes, tendons and soft tissues. They are seen most often in the helix of the ear; in tissues surrounding joints and bursae (especially around the elbows and knees); along tendons of the fingers, toes, ankles and wrists; on ulnar surfaces of the forearms; along the shins of the legs; and on other pressure points. The skin over tophi may ulcerate, exuding chalky material containing inflammatory cells and urate crystals. Tophi can also develop in the tissues of the heart and spinal epidura. Although tophi themselves are not painful, they may restrict joint movement and cause pain and deformities of the affected joints. Tophi may also compress nerves and erode and drain through the skin.

Complications

Kidney disease may occur in people with untreated gout, particularly when hypertension is also present. Urate crystals are deposited in renal interstitial tissue. Uric acid crystals also form in the collecting tubules, renal pelvis and ureter, forming stones. The stones can range in size from a grain of sand to a massive structure filling the spaces of the kidney. Uric acid stones can potentially obstruct urine flow and lead to acute kidney failure.

MANIFESTATIONS **Gout**

ACUTE GOUTY ARTHRITIS

- Usually monoarticular, affecting metatarsophalangeal joint of great toe, instep, ankle, knee, wrist or elbow
- Acute pain
- Red, hot, swollen and tender joint
- Fever, chills, malaise
- Elevated WBC and erythrocyte sedimentation rate

TOPHACEOUS (CHRONIC) GOUT

- Tophi evident on joints, bursae, tendon sheaths, pressure points, helix of ear
- Joint stiffness, limited ROM and deformity
- Ulceration of tophi with chalky discharge

INTERPROFESSIONAL CARE

The classic presentation of acute gouty arthritis is so distinctive that the diagnosis can often be based on the person's history and physical examination. Treatment is directed towards terminating an acute attack, preventing recurrent attacks and reversing or preventing complications resulting from crystal deposition in tissues and formation of uric acid kidney stones.

Diagnosis

Diagnostic testing is performed to establish an accurate diagnosis and direct long-term therapy. Diagnostic tests are described in the chapter 'A person-centred approach to assessing the musculoskeletal system'.

Serum uric acid is nearly always elevated (usually above 480 mmol/L). The WBC count shows significant elevation, reaching levels as high as 20,000/mm^3 during an acute attack. The ESR is elevated during an acute attack from the acute inflammatory process that accompanies deposits of urate crystals in a joint. In addition, a 24-hour urine specimen is analysed to determine uric acid production and excretion, and analysis of fluid aspirated from the acutely inflamed joint or material aspirated from a tophus shows typical needle-shaped urate crystals, providing the definitive diagnosis of gout.

Medications

Medications are used to terminate an acute attack, prevent further attacks and reduce serum uric acid levels to prevent long-term sequelae of the disease. It is important to treat the acute attack of gouty arthritis before initiating treatment to reduce serum uric acid levels, because an abrupt decrease in serum uric acid may lead to further acute manifestations. Pharmacological therapy is a mainstay of treatment in achieving these goals.

ACUTE ATTACK NSAIDs and colchicine are the treatment of choice for an acute attack of gout. Colchicine has known anti-inflammatory effects but no analgesic properties. That is why it is combined with an NSAID for analgesic effects. Indomethacin (Indocid) is the most frequently used NSAID for gout, although others are equally effective. Other NSAIDs that may be prescribed include ibuprofen (Nurofen), naproxen (Naproxyn, Anaprox), diclofenac (Voltaren) or ketorolac (Toradol). Although extremely effective, NSAIDs are contraindicated for people with active peptic ulcer disease, impaired kidney function or a history of hypersensitivity reactions to the drugs. As with other anti-inflammatory drugs, people should be aware of possible risks and follow recommended doses carefully.

Colchicine can dramatically affect the course of an acute attack. Joint pain begins to diminish within 12 hours of the initiation of treatment and disappears within 2 days. Colchicine apparently acts by interrupting the cycle of urate crystal deposition and inflammation in an acute attack of gout. It has no anti-inflammatory effect in other forms of arthritis and its use is limited to gout. The use of colchicine is limited by significant side effects. When administered orally, many people develop abdominal cramping, diarrhoea, nausea or vomiting. Intravenous administration is limited by potential toxic effects, including local pain, tissue damage if extravasation occurs during injection, bone marrow suppression and disseminated intravascular coagulation (DIC). It is contraindicated for people who have significant gastrointestinal, kidney, hepatic or cardiac disease.

Corticosteroids may also be prescribed for the person with acute gouty arthritis. If possible, the intra-articular route is preferred for monoarticular arthritis to avoid the multiple systemic effects of steroid therapy. When gout is polyarticular, corticosteroids may be administered either orally or intravenously.

Analgesics may also be prescribed during an acute episode of gouty arthritis. Either codeine or pethidine may be administered to manage the person's pain. Aspirin is avoided because it may interfere with uric acid excretion.

PROPHYLACTIC THERAPY In people at high risk of future attacks of acute gout, prophylactic therapy with daily colchicine may be initiated. Prophylaxis is particularly useful during the first 1 to 2 years of treatment with antihyperuricaemic agents. Although colchicine does not affect the serum uric acid directly, it reduces the frequency of attacks by preventing crystal deposition within the joint. The doses required to achieve this effect are small and few side effects are associated with therapy.

Treatment to reduce serum uric acid levels is typically initiated for people with recurring gout, tophi or renal damage. Asymptomatic hyperuricaemic people require no treatment. Uricosuric agents are used for people who do not eliminate uric acid adequately; allopurinol is prescribed for people who produce excessive amounts of uric acid. Uricosuric drugs block the tubular reabsorption of uric acid, promoting its excretion and reducing serum levels. These drugs reduce the frequency of acute attacks, particularly when administered with colchicine. Probenecid lowers the serum concentration of uric acid by competitively inhibiting the reabsorption of urate at the proximal renal tubule, thus increasing urinary excretion of uric acid (Bryant et al., 2018).

Allopurinol (Zyloprim) is a xanthine oxidase inhibitor that lowers plasma uric acid levels and facilitates the mobilisation of tophi. Because of its effectiveness in lowering serum uric acid levels, it may trigger an attack of acute gout. Febuxostat (Adenuric) is a non-purine selective xanthine oxidase inhibitor used when allopurinol is contraindicated.

The nursing implications for medications used to treat gout are included in the 'Medication administration' box.

Complementary and alternative therapy

A variety of nutritional and herbal supplements may be used to help prevent gout or decrease the onset of manifestations. These include:

- Vitamin E and selenium may decrease tissue inflammation.
- Amino acids (alanine, aspartic acid, glutamic acid and glycine) increase the ability of the kidneys to excrete uric acid.
- Dark reddish-blue berries (such as cherries and blackberries) are good sources of flavonoids, which help lower uric acid levels, decrease inflammation and prevent or repair joint tissue damage.
- Acupuncture can provide pain relief.

Treatments

Treatments for gout, in addition to medications, include dietary management and rest.

NUTRITION Dietary purines contribute only slightly to uric acid levels in the body and no specific diet may be recommended. If a low-purine diet is recommended, the person should be taught that high-purine foods include all meats and seafood, yeast, beans, peas, lentils, oatmeal, spinach, asparagus, cauliflower and mushrooms (although plant-based, high-purine diets do not have as much effect). The obese person is advised to lose weight but fasting is contraindicated for people with gout. Alcohol intake and specific foods that tend to precipitate attacks are avoided.

MEDICATION ADMINISTRATION The person with gout

COLCHICINE

Colchicine is used to terminate an acute attack of gouty arthritis and to prevent recurrent episodes of the disease. Colchicine does not alter serum uric acid levels, but appears to interrupt the cycle of urate crystal deposition and inflammatory response. It may be administered either by mouth or intravenously. Colchicine is also available as a fixed-dose combination with a uricosuric agent, probenecid. Only plain colchicine is used to treat an acute attack of gout; combination therapy is employed to prevent further attacks.

Nursing responsibilities

- Assess for possible contraindications to colchicine therapy, including serious gastrointestinal, renal, hepatic or cardiac disease.
- Administer the following as ordered:
  - *Intravenous doses*: give undiluted or diluted in up to 20 mL sterile 0.9% sodium chloride for injection. Administer over a period of 2 to 5 minutes.
  - *Oral doses*: give on an empty stomach to facilitate absorption.
- Evaluate for adverse effects, including abdominal cramping, nausea, vomiting and diarrhoea, and report promptly, because these side effects may necessitate discontinuation of the drug.

Health education for the person and family

- Drink 3 to 4 L of liquid per day.
- Report adverse responses, including gastrointestinal problems, fatigue, bleeding, easy bruising or recurrent infections, to the healthcare provider.
- Do not drink alcohol.

URICOSURIC DRUGS

Probenecid (Benemid)

Sulfinpyrazone (Anturane)

Probenecid inhibits the tubular reabsorption of urate, promoting the excretion of uric acid and decreasing serum uric acid levels. Sulfinpyrazone potentiates the renal excretion of uric acid, reducing serum uric acid levels. It is used to prevent recurrent attacks of acute gouty arthritis and to treat chronic gout.

Nursing responsibilities

- Assess for prior hypersensitivity responses to this drug.
- Administer after meals or with milk to minimise gastric distress.
- Increase fluid intake to at least 3 L/day to prevent the formation of uric acid kidney calculi.
- Administer sodium bicarbonate or potassium citrate as ordered to maintain an alkaline urine.
- Do not administer aspirin to people receiving probenecid because salicylates interfere with the action of the drug.
- Monitor people receiving the following drugs concurrently with probenecid for increased or toxic effects: penicillin and related antibiotics, indomethacin, paracetamol, naproxen, ketoprofen, lorazepam and rifampin.
- Monitor for possible adverse effects of probenecid, including headache, dizziness, hepatic necrosis, nausea and vomiting, renal colic, bone marrow depression, anaphylaxis, fever, hives and pruritus.
- Administer sulfinpyrazone with meals or antacid to minimise gastric distress.
- Monitor people taking sulfinpyrazone with other sulfa drugs for increased or toxic effects; monitor for hypoglycaemia when receiving insulin or oral hypoglycaemics concurrently; and monitor for bleeding or increased anticoagulant effect when receiving warfarin concurrently.
- Assess for contraindications to therapy with sulfinpyrazone, including active peptic ulcer disease, a history of hypersensitivity to phenylbutazone or other pyrazoles or blood dyscrasias.

Health education for the person and family

- Do not take aspirin or products containing aspirin while taking probenecid. Use paracetamol for relief of mild pain.
- Drink at least 3 L of fluids per day to minimise the risk of kidney stone formation.
- Take sulfinpyrazone with meals to minimise gastric distress and report epigastric pain, nausea or black stools to the healthcare provider promptly.

ALLOPURINOL (ZYLOPRIM)

Allopurinol acts on purine metabolism, reducing the production of uric acid and decreasing serum and urinary concentrations of uric acid. It is used for people with manifestations of primary or secondary gout, including acute attacks, tophi, joint destruction, urinary stones and nephropathy. It is not indicated for use in the treatment of asymptomatic hyperuricaemia.

Nursing responsibilities

- Monitor intake and output and increase fluid intake to approximately 3 L/day.
- Monitor for desired effect of decreased serum uric acid levels and for adverse effects such as nausea, diarrhoea and rash.
- Assess blood urea nitrogen (BUN) and creatinine levels prior to the initiation of and during treatment with allopurinol. Report signs of impaired kidney function such as an elevated BUN and creatinine, decreased urine output, and dilute or frothy urine to the healthcare provider.
- Administer with meals to minimise gastric distress.
- Monitor FBC periodically because allopurinol therapy may cause bone marrow depression.
- In people receiving warfarin concurrently, monitor prothrombin times and be alert to evidence of bleeding, because allopurinol prolongs the half-life of warfarin.
- Monitor people receiving chlorpropamide, cyclophosphamide, hydantoin, theophylline, vidarabine or ACE inhibitors concurrently for increased drug effects.
- Discontinue the drug and notify the healthcare provider immediately if the person develops a rash. Rash and hypersensitivity responses occur more frequently in people receiving ampicillin, amoxicillin or thiazide diuretics.

Health education for the person and family

- Stop taking the drug and report any skin rash, painful urination, blood in the urine, eye irritation or swelling of the lips or mouth to the healthcare provider immediately.
  Take the medication after meals to minimise gastric distress.
- Drink 3 to 4 L of fluid daily to maintain a urinary output greater than 2 L/day.
- Acute gouty attacks may occur during the initial stages of allopurinol therapy; continue therapy prescribed for attacks (such as colchicine) to minimise acute episodes.
- Do not take a double dose of medication if you miss a dose.

A liberal fluid intake to maintain a daily urinary output of 2,000 mL or more is recommended to increase urate excretion and reduce the risk of urinary stone formation. Urinary alkalinising agents, such as sodium bicarbonate or potassium citrate, may be prescribed as well to minimise the risk of uric acid stones. It is important to monitor people receiving these preparations carefully for signs of fluid and electrolyte or acid–base imbalances.

REST During an acute attack of gouty arthritis, apply ice and seek bed rest (Musculoskeletal Australia, 2022). It is continued for approximately 24 hours after the attack has subsided because early ambulation may bring about recurrence of acute manifestations (Papadakis, McPhee & Rabow, 2022). The affected joint may be elevated and hot or cold compresses may be applied for comfort.

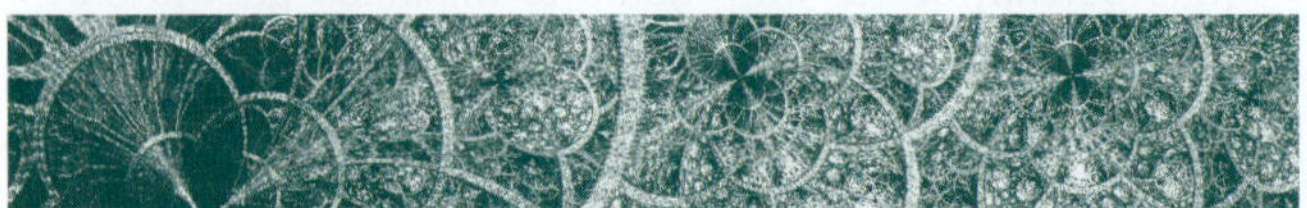

Nursing care

People with gout provide self-care at home. Teaching focuses on self-management of pain and altered mobility.

Nursing diagnoses and interventions

Pain is a primary focus for nursing interventions in the person experiencing an acute attack of gout. The person's mobility is also impaired during an acute attack, because of both pain and prescribed activity limitations.

Acute pain

The pain associated with an attack of acute gouty arthritis is intense and accompanied by exquisite tenderness of the affected joint. Measures to alleviate the pain are vital in the initial period until anti-inflammatory medications become effective and the acute inflammatory response is relieved. The following are important in teaching about pain relief:

- Position the affected joint for comfort. Elevate the joint or extremity (usually the foot) on a pillow, maintaining alignment. *Elevation and normal body alignment facilitate blood return from the affected joint, alleviating some of the oedema.*
- Protect the affected joint from pressure, placing a foot cradle on the bed to keep bed covers off the foot. *A foot cradle keeps bed linen from applying pressure on the affected joint.*

CONSIDERATION FOR PRACTICE

The affected joints are so painful that even the weight of a sheet can be unbearable.

- Take anti-inflammatory and anti-gout medications as prescribed. In the initial period, colchicine may be given hourly. *These medications reduce the acute inflammatory response, gradually relieving discomfort.*
- Take analgesics as prescribed. *Supplemental analgesia may be necessary in the acute period until the inflammatory response is mediated.*
- Maintain bed rest. *It is important to immobilise the affected joint and promote rest to prevent exacerbation of joint inflammation.*

Community-based care

Discuss the following topics with the person:

- The disease and its manifestations. Tell the person that initial attacks cause no permanent damage but that recurrent attacks can lead to permanent damage and joint destruction. Discuss other potential effects of continued hyperuricaemia, including tophaceous deposits in subcutaneous and other connective tissues. Discuss the potential for kidney damage and kidney stones.
- The rationale for and use of prescribed medication. Stress the need to continue the medication until the healthcare provider discontinues it, even though the person is free of manifestations of gout. Tell the person to avoid drugs that increase uric acid blood levels: hydrochlorothiazide (Dithiazide), cyclosporin (Neoral), frusemide (Lasix) and high doses of aspirin. People who need to reduce their risk of heart attacks may safely take one low-dose aspirin each day.
- The importance of a high intake of fluids each day and avoiding the use of alcohol.

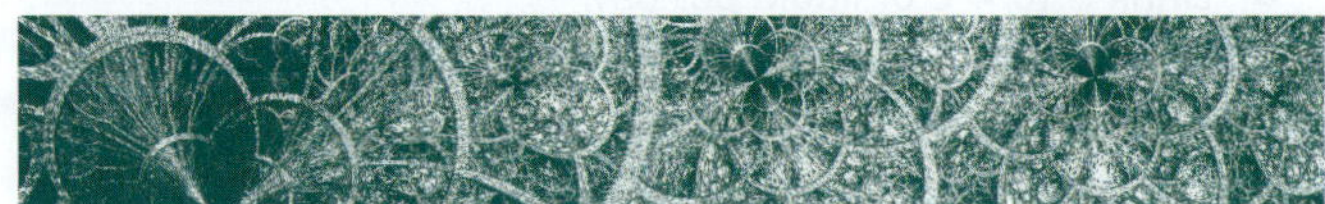

THE PERSON WITH OSTEOMALACIA

Osteomalacia, often referred to as *adult rickets*, is a metabolic bone disorder characterised by inadequate or delayed mineralisation of bone matrix in mature compact and spongy bone, resulting in softening of bones. Bone mineralisation requires adequate calcium and phosphate ions in extracellular fluid. When either of these ions is insufficient due to: (1) inadequate calcium intake or decreased calcium absorption from the intestines because of insufficient vitamin D, or (2) increased renal losses or decreased intestinal absorption of phosphate, the bone matrix is not mineralised and cannot sustain weight bearing. Marked deformities of weight-bearing bone and pathological fractures occur. The primary causes of osteomalacia are vitamin D deficiency and hypophosphataemia. Osteomalacia can be corrected with treatment.

Osteomalacia has been almost non-existent in Australia and New Zealand because many foods are fortified with vitamin D, but its incidence is increasing among older adults and people who adhere to strict vegetarian diets. It is a significant health problem in cultures whose diets tend to be deficient in calcium and vitamin D. Women in northern China, Japan and northern India have a higher incidence of the disorder (Cohen & Drake, 2022; Norris, 2018).

The main risk factors for vitamin D deficiency are a diet low in vitamin D, decreased endogenous production of vitamin D because of inadequate sun exposure, impaired intestinal absorption of fats (vitamin D is a fat-soluble vitamin) and disorders that interfere with the metabolism of vitamin D to its active forms. Gastrectomy and small-bowel disorders may reduce the absorptive surface of the bowel to the extent that nutrients are not completely or adequately absorbed. Both vitamin D and calcium absorption may be affected. Hepatobiliary disorders that interfere with bile production and release and chronic pancreatic insufficiency with inadequate pancreatic enzyme production can affect the absorption of fats and vitamin D from the bowel. Once absorbed, vitamin D is metabolised in the liver and the kidney to its active form; therefore, liver disorders such as cirrhosis and kidney disorders can affect this activation. Certain drugs, such as isoniazid, rifampicin and anticonvulsants, accelerate vitamin D metabolism, resulting in less availability to the tissues. Renal excretion of vitamin D is increased in some kidney disorders such as nephrotic syndrome. (See Box 39.3.)

Hypophosphataemia can be the result of insufficient dietary intake, excessive losses through the urine or stool, or a shift into the cells. Alcohol abuse is the most common cause of hypophosphataemia because of related dietary deficiencies, vomiting, antacid use and increased renal excretion of phosphate. Ingesting large amounts of non-absorbable antacids causes increased phosphate losses in the stool. Several acquired and genetic disorders cause increased losses of phosphate in the urine.

BOX 39.3 Causes of osteomalacia

Vitamin D deficiency

- Inadequate dietary intake
- Lack of sun exposure
- Malabsorption from intestines: gastrectomy, small-bowel disorders, gallbladder disease, chronic pancreatic insufficiency
- Kidney or liver disorders
- Drug effects: isoniazid, rifampicin, anticonvulsants

Phosphate depletion

- Inadequate intake
- Impaired absorption due to chronic antacid use
- Impaired renal tubular reabsorption due to either acquired or genetic disorders

Systemic acidosis

- Renal tubular acidosis
- Ureterosigmoidostomy
- Fanconi's syndrome

Mineralisation inhibitors

- Hypophosphatasia
- Sodium fluoride or disodium etidronate (Didronel)
- Aluminium intoxication

Chronic kidney failure

- Calcium malabsorption

Pathophysiology

The two main causes of osteomalacia are insufficient calcium absorption in the intestine due to a lack of calcium or resistance to the action of vitamin D, and increased losses of phosphorus through the urine (Norris, 2018). In its natural form, vitamin D is obtained from certain foods and ultraviolet radiation of the sun. Vitamin D maintains adequate serum levels of calcium and phosphate for normal mineralisation of the bone. Vitamin D deficiency, or resistance to its action, disrupts the normal mineralisation of the bone, causing softening of the bone.

Vitamin D is inactive when it is absorbed from the intestine or synthesised from exposure to ultraviolet light. For vitamin D to become active, a two-step process must occur: (1) vitamin D (and its metabolites) is transported in the blood to the liver, where it is converted to calcidiol, and (2) calcidiol is then transported to the kidney and transformed to an active form, calcitriol.

The active form of vitamin D is needed for optimal absorption of calcium and phosphorus from the intestine. Calcium and phosphorus are transported in the blood to the bones for normal mineralisation. If there is a lack of vitamin D, calcium and phosphorus are not absorbed from the intestine and serum calcium and phosphorus levels therefore fall. A deficiency in these minerals in turn activates the parathyroid glands, with loss of calcium and phosphorus from bone. The continued loss of calcium and phosphate in the bone disrupts bone mineralisation.

Impaired bone mineralisation causes abnormalities in both spongy and compact bone. The osteoid (the soft, non-calcified part of the matrix) continues to be produced but is not mineralised. This abnormal build-up of demineralised bone leads to gross deformities of the long bones, spine, pelvis and skull, because the bone is soft and unable to bear the weight and stress of body movement.

Manifestations

The manifestations of osteomalacia include bone pain and tenderness (see the 'Manifestations' box). As the disease progresses, fractures occur. In contrast to osteoporosis, osteomalacia is not associated with a significant occurrence of hip fractures. Instead, pathological fractures occur in the commonly weakened areas (e.g. distal radius and proximal femur).

MANIFESTATIONS Osteomalacia

- Bone pain: may be vague and generalised at first, becoming more intense with activity as the disease progresses; occurs most frequently in the pelvis, long bones of the extremities, spine and ribs.
- Difficulty changing from lying to sitting position and sitting to standing position.
- Muscle weakness: frequently an early sign in severe cases.
- Waddling gait: may be due to pain and muscle weakness.
- Dorsal kyphosis: may occur in severe cases.
- Pathological fractures.

INTERPROFESSIONAL CARE

Osteomalacia may be difficult to differentiate from osteoporosis because the manifestations are very similar; however, once the specific cause is determined, appropriate therapy will correct the disorder.

Diagnosis

A history of inadequate dietary intake, kidney failure or some malabsorption states may suggest osteomalacia. Diagnostic tests are described in the chapter 'A person-centred approach to assessing the musculoskeletal system'. Table 39.1 compares the diagnostic findings of osteomalacia with those of osteoporosis and Paget's disease. X-rays demonstrate the effects of generalised bone demineralisation: trabecular bone loss, cyst formation, compression fractures, bowing and bending deformities of the long bones, and osteoid deposits, particularly in the vertebral bodies and pelvis.

Laboratory tests include serum calcium, parathyroid hormone and alkaline phosphatase levels. Calcium may be normal or low, depending on the cause of the disease. Calcium levels may be reduced when calcium absorption is impaired or in severe vitamin D deficiency. Secondary hypoparathyroidism may shift calcium from the bone into extracellular fluid, maintaining a normal serum calcium level. Parathyroid hormone is frequently elevated as a compensatory response to hypocalcaemia in kidney failure or vitamin D deficiency. Alkaline phosphatase is usually elevated.

Medications

Therapeutic management of osteomalacia depends on the cause of the disease. Because the causes are so diverse, it is difficult to generalise treatment. Most people are placed on vitamin D therapy. Calcium and phosphate supplements may be indicated. Radiological evidence of healing is often apparent within weeks of initiating therapy.

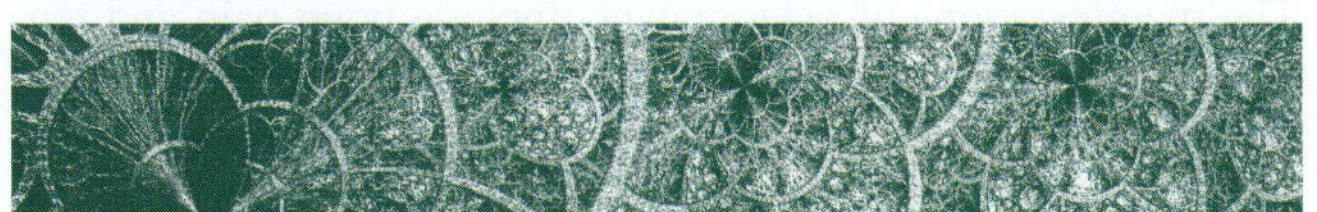

Nursing care

Managing the person with osteomalacia includes assessing the person's current dietary intake of vitamin D, calcium and phosphorus, and exposure to ultraviolet light. It also includes managing the person's responses to bone pain and tenderness, fractures and muscle weakness.

Community-based care

Teaching is important not only for the person with osteomalacia, but also for people at risk of developing the disease. When milk and other dairy products began to be fortified with vitamin D, the incidence of childhood rickets decreased dramatically. Now many people are unaware of the importance of vitamin D, calcium and phosphorus to bone health.

Older adults as a group are at high risk of osteomalacia because of dietary deficiencies, age-related intestinal malabsorption and possible physical mobility limitations that restrict their exposure to sunlight. Teaching includes the importance of maintaining an adequate intake of milk and other dairy products that are not only rich in calcium and phosphorus, but also are fortified with vitamin D. Few other food sources provide enough vitamin D to meet recommended levels. Cod liver oil may be used as a supplement because it contains significant amounts of vitamin D. Supplements are not recommended, however, for people who get adequate vitamin D through dietary sources and sun exposure, because this fat-soluble vitamin may become toxic at high levels. Instruct people who are taking supplements to report to their healthcare provider symptoms such as anorexia, nausea and vomiting, frequent urination, muscle weakness and constipation that may be indicative of hypervitaminosis D.

Teach the person with osteomalacia about safety measures to prevent falls, such as removing trip hazards, having adequate lighting and installing aids such as grab rails as required.

Teach people with bone pain and muscle weakness to use assistive devices such as walkers, canes or crutches when ambulating. Provide referrals to physical therapy for teaching people how to safely use these devices. Participating in a supervised exercise program such as water aerobics or Tai Chi can improve muscle strength and balance.

Degenerative disorders

Degenerative disorders, especially degenerative joint disease, are the most common forms of arthritis in the older adult. Both primary and secondary forms are seen in adults of all ages. Primary or idiopathic osteoarthritis, the most common type, occurs without a clear precipitating factor. Secondary osteoarthritis is associated with an identifiable cause. For instance, it may be related to trauma to a joint, inflammation, skeletal disorders such as congenital hip dysplasia or metabolic disorders. Regardless of cause, degenerative disorders of the joints and muscles can lead to impaired mobility and chronic pain. These problems may in turn cause disability, especially in the performance of ADLs by older adults.

FOCUS ON CULTURAL DIVERSITY The person with osteoarthritis

- Indigenous Australians are more likely than other Australians to report having arthritis but are much less likely to have hip or knee replacements.
- People in the most disadvantaged areas of Australia are less likely than those in the least disadvantaged areas to have a total hip replacement, but more likely to have a total knee replacement.
- People in regional and remote areas are more likely than those living in major cities to have hip or knee replacements.

Source: AIHW (2022). *Osteoarthritis*. Retrieved from https://www.aihw.gov.au/reports/chronic-musculoskeletal-conditions/osteoarthritis/contents/what-is-osteoarthritis. Licensed under the Creative Commons Attribution 4.0 International License, https//creativecommons.org/licenses/by/4.0.

THE PERSON WITH OSTEOARTHRITIS

Osteoarthritis (OA) (also labelled *degenerative joint disease*) is the most commonly occurring of all forms of arthritis and a leading cause of pain and disability in older adults (Norris, 2018). This disease is characterised by loss of articular cartilage in articulating joints and hypertrophy of the bones at the articular margins. OA may be idiopathic (without known cause) or secondary (associated with known risk factors). OA affects more than 1.8 million Australians (1 in 13, or over 8% of the total population) over the age of 45 years. Men are affected more than women at an earlier age, but the rate of OA in women exceeds men by the middle adult years. The joints most affected are in the hand, wrist, neck, lower back, hip, knee, ankle and feet. Men are more likely than women to have hip OA, whereas postmenopausal women more often have hand OA.

The cultural and ethnic effects on the development of OA are outlined in the 'Focus on cultural diversity' box.

Localised OA affects only one or two joints. Generalised OA affects three or more joints. It may also be classified as nodal (involving the hand) or non-nodal (no hand involvement). Nodal OA may also affect the knees, hips, cervical spine and lumbar spine. Idiopathic OA most commonly affects the terminal interphalangeal joints (*Heberden's nodes*) and less often the proximal interphalangeal joints (*Bouchard's nodes*) (see Figure 39.3), the joints of the thumb, the hip, the knee, the metatarsophalangeal joint of the big toe and the cervical and lumbar spine. Secondary OA may occur in any joint from an articular injury.

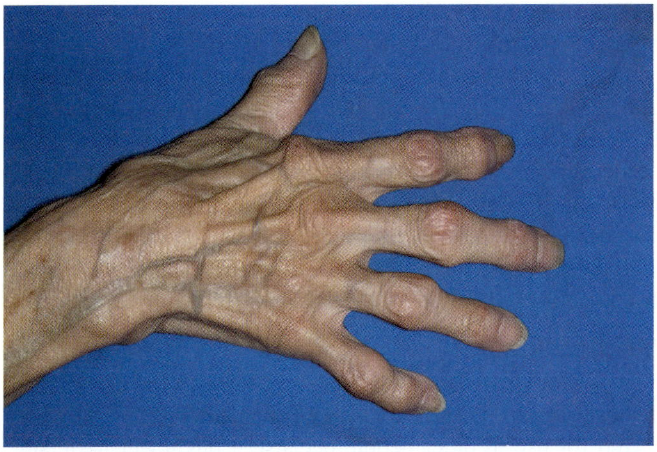

FIGURE 39.3 ***Typical interphalangeal joint changes associated with osteoarthritis***

Source: Scott Camazine/AlamyStockPhoto.

Risk factors

Idiopathic OA is associated with increasing age. It has been suggested that OA may be inherited as an autosomal recessive trait, with genetic defects causing premature destruction of the joint cartilage. The causes of secondary OA include trauma, mechanical stress and inflammation of joint structures, joint instability, neurological disorders, endocrine disorders and selected medications.

Excessive weight contributes to the development of OA, especially in the hip, ankle and knee. Excess fat may have a direct metabolic effect in the development of the disease. Primary OA of the knee is almost four times more common in obese women and five times more common in obese men (AIHW, 2022). Inactivity is another risk factor. Moderate recreational exercise has been shown to decrease both the chance of developing OA and the progression of manifestations when OA is present. People involved in strenuous, repetitive exercise (such as participating in sports) have an increased risk of developing secondary OA.

Other risk factors that are linked to OA are hormonal factors such as decreased oestrogen in menopausal women, excessive growth hormone and increased parathyroid hormone.

Pathophysiology

The cartilage that lines joints provides a smooth surface, so that the bones of the joint glide over one another without friction, and it distributes the load from one bone to the next, dissipating the mechanical stress that occurs with joint loading. This cartilage normally contains more than 70% water. More than 90% of its dry weight is collagen, which provides strength, and proteoglycans, which provide elasticity and stiffness to compression. Cartilage cells, the chondrocytes, nest in this meshwork of collagen and proteoglycans. Normal articular cartilage exudes some of its water with compression, providing lubrication for joint surfaces. This water is reabsorbed during relaxation of the joint.

In OA, proteoglycans and collagen are lost from the cartilage as a result of enzymatic degradation. The water content of the cartilage increases as the collagen matrix is destroyed. With the loss of proteoglycans and collagen fibres, the cartilage becomes yellow or brownish grey and loses its tensile strength. Surface ulcerations occur and fissures develop in deeper layers of the cartilage. Eventually, large areas of articular cartilage are lost and underlying bone is exposed. The bone thickens in exposed areas, reducing its ability to absorb energy in joint loading. Cysts can also develop in the bone. *Cartilage-coated osteophytes* (bony outgrowths often called 'joint mice') change the anatomy of the joint. As these spurs or projections enlarge, small pieces may break off, leading to mild synovitis (inflammation of the synovial membrane).

Manifestations

The onset of OA is usually gradual and insidious, and the course slowly progressive. Pain and stiffness in one or more joints (usually weight bearing) are the first manifestations of OA. The pain is localised to the affected joints and may be described as a deep ache. It is typically aggravated by use or motion of the joint and relieved by rest, although it may become persistent as the disease progresses. Pain at night may be accompanied by paraesthesias (numbness, tingling). Pain may also be referred to other parts of the body; for example, OA of the lumbosacral spine may cause severe pain along the path of the sciatic nerve. Following periods of immobility, such as sleeping all night or sitting for an extended period, involved joints may stiffen. Usually only a few minutes of activity are necessary to relieve the stiffness. Range of motion (ROM) of the joint decreases as the disease progresses and grating or crepitus may be noted during movement. Bony overgrowth may cause joint enlargement and flexion contractures may occur because of joint instability. In OA, enlarged joints are characteristically bony hard and cool on palpation. Manifestations specific to affected joints are outlined in the 'Manifestations' box.

MANIFESTATIONS Osteoarthritis

AFFECTED SITE	MANIFESTATIONS
Interphalangeal joints	■ *Heberden's nodes*—bony enlargements of distal joints; may cause pain, redness, swelling ■ *Bouchard's nodes*—bony enlargement of proximal joints
First carpometacarpal	■ Swelling, tenderness at base of thumb ■ Crepitus with movement ■ 'Squared' appearance of joint
Spine	■ Localised pain and stiffness ■ Muscle spasm ■ Limited range of motion ■ Nerve root compression with radicular pain and motor weakness
Hips	■ Pain referred to inguinal area, buttock, thigh or knee ■ Loss of internal rotation ■ Limited extension, adduction and flexion
Knees	■ Pain and bony enlargement ■ Effusions ■ Crepitus ■ Instability and deformity with advanced disease

Complications

OA of the spine may involve the vertebral bodies and intervertebral discs, diarthrodial joints, or both. *Spondylosis* is degenerative disc disease. As the intervertebral discs degenerate, disc space between the vertebrae is lost. Degenerative disc disease may be complicated by herniation, the protrusion of the nucleus pulposus of the disc. Herniation usually occurs in a lateral direction, potentially compressing nerve roots and causing radicular (distributed along the nerve) pain and muscle weakness. See the chapter 'Nursing care of people with cerebrovascular and spinal cord disorders' for further discussion of disc disorders.

Disc degeneration and joint space narrowing alter the mechanics of the spinal column, promoting osteoarthritic changes in the articular processes (the facet joints) of the vertebrae. The cartilage covering the inferior and superior articular processes degenerates, causing localised pain, stiffness, muscle spasm and limited range of motion. Osteophytes may form on articular processes, further contributing to pain and muscle spasm.

The presentation of OA in older people is similar to that in younger adults. However, in this population, the risk of debilitation is greater and the disease may progress faster. In addition, pain, stiffness and limited ROM increase the risk of falls and fractures in the older adult.

INTERPROFESSIONAL CARE

At this time, no treatment is available to stop the process of joint degeneration. It is important to relieve pain and maintain the person's function, mobility, self-care and quality of life. Research is also ongoing on a new class of medications called disease-modifying osteoarthritis drugs (DMOADs) and gene therapy, although this is still unclear as to effect (Persson et al., 2018). Vitamin D and chondroitin can slow the rate of degeneration of joints, especially knees (Arthritis Foundation, 2022).

Diagnosis

The diagnosis of OA is generally based on the person's history, physical examination and x-rays of affected joints. Diagnostic tests are described in the chapter 'A person-centred approach to assessing the musculoskeletal system'.

Characteristic changes of OA are visible in x-ray studies of affected joints. Initially, irregular joint space narrowing is seen. Progressive changes include increased density of subchondral (under cartilage) bone, osteophyte formation at the joint periphery and the formation of cysts in the bone. In some cases, MRI or CT scan may be done to determine the extent of joint damage.

Examination of synovial fluid from involved joints can help rule out other types of arthritis such as inflammatory arthritis and gout.

Medications

The pain of OA often can be managed through the use of analgesics such as aspirin. Paracetamol (Panadol) is generally preferred for use in older people because it has fewer toxic side effects. NSAIDs such as ibuprofen (Nurofen), naproxen (Naprosyn), indomethacin (Indocid) and diclofenac (Voltaren) may also be prescribed, but side effects and contraindications must be considered.

Topical medications include counterirritants, salicylates and capsaicin, sold without prescription as creams, gels, sprays, patches or ointments to relieve pain. Capsaicin, a topical heat-sensation-producing agent, used alone or in conjunction with paracetamol is beneficial. The person should be taught to keep the medications away from their eyes, nose, mouth or any open skin, and not to bandage or apply heat to the treated area. The products should be used no more than three or four times a day and discontinued immediately if severe irritation occurs.

Medications that are effective in decreasing the pain and stiffness of OA are the NSAID COX-2 inhibitors. However, because of the increased risk of adverse cardiovascular (hypertension, heart attack and strokes) and gastrointestinal (bleeding) effects of most drugs in this category, several were recalled by the Therapeutic Goods Administration (TGA) in 2004 (TGA, 2014); for example, celecoxib (Celebrex) and more recently etoricoxib (Arcoxia). Dangerous contraindications remain despite new developments.

Potent anti-inflammatory medications, such as systemic corticosteroids, are seldom prescribed for people with OA, although intra-articular corticosteroid injections may be used. With intra-articular injections, a long-acting corticosteroid medication, often mixed with a local anaesthetic such as lignocaine, is injected directly into the joint space of the affected joints. Although this procedure may provide marked pain relief, it can hasten the rate of cartilage breakdown if performed more frequently than every 4 to 6 months.

Treatments

OA is initially treated conservatively, but as pain increases and joint function decreases, further treatments may be recommended. Exercise and weight loss will assist in the first instance, followed by pharmacological and non-pharmacological treatments, and the possibility of surgery if warranted (National Institute for Health and Care Excellence, 2017).

CONSERVATIVE TREATMENT The goals of OA treatment are to relieve pain and maintain as much normal joint function as possible. Conservative treatment may include any or all of the following:

- ROM exercises, muscle-strengthening exercises, aerobic exercises
- heat and ice
- a balance between exercise and rest
- use of a cane, crutches or a walker
- weight loss, if indicated
- analgesic and anti-inflammatory medications.

VISCOSUPPLEMENTATION Viscosupplementation is a new treatment for OA of the knee. Hyaluronan, a natural component of synovial fluid, is injected directly into the knee joint. The injection may provide pain relief and improvement in knee function for up to 1 year, but its long-term effects are unknown (Hunter, 2015; NHMRC, 2009).

SURGERY Surgical procedures can provide dramatic results for people with significant chronic pain and loss of joint function. Although elective surgical procedures are frequently avoided in the older adult, even older people can benefit Significantly if they do not have a chronic medical condition that contraindicates surgery.

ARTHROSCOPY An *arthroscopy* is a surgical procedure in which an arthroscope (a thin tube that is lit and has a camera in one end) is inserted into a joint. It may be done to diagnose the type of arthritis or to perform debridement by smoothing rough cartilage and flushing out the joint to remove debris. Although arthroscopic debridement and lavage of involved joints have been used, arthroscopy has not proven effective in the treatment of knee OA. It may be useful to remove large pieces of debris or repair a torn cartilage (Mayo Clinic, 2020).

OSTEOTOMY An *osteotomy*, an incision into or transection of the bone, may be performed to realign an affected joint, particularly when significant bony overgrowth or osteophyte formation has occurred. This procedure may also be used to shift the joint load towards areas of less severely damaged cartilage. Although osteotomy does not halt the process of OA, it may have a beneficial effect on joint function and pain, delaying the need for a joint replacement by several years.

JOINT ARTHROPLASTY A *joint arthroplasty* is the reconstruction or replacement of a joint. Arthroplasty is usually indicated when the person has severely restricted joint mobility and pain at rest. Pain is virtually eliminated and the function of the joint is generally improved. Arthroplasty may involve partial joint replacement or reshaping of the bones of a joint. For most people with OA, both surfaces of the affected joint are replaced with prosthetic parts in a procedure known as a *total joint replacement*. Joints that may be replaced include the hip, knee, shoulder, elbow, ankle, wrist and joints of the fingers and toes.

There has been a 38% increase in hip and knee replacements from 2005–2006 to 2015–2016. There were 50,600 knee replacements (181/100,000) and 30,900 knee replacements 112/100,000) in 2015–2016 (AIHW, 2018b).

In a total joint replacement, some or all of the synovium, cartilage and bone on both sides of the joint are removed. A metallic prosthesis is inserted to replace one joint surface (generally the load-end or distal portion of a weight-bearing joint). The other joint surface is replaced by a silicone-lined ceramic or plastic prosthesis.

Most prosthetic joints are uncemented; that is, made of porous ceramic and metal components inserted so that they fit tightly into existing bone. The implant is secured by new bone growth into the prosthesis, a process that requires approximately 6 weeks. Although a longer non-weight-bearing period is necessary initially until the prosthesis is fixed in place by the bony growth, the implant appears to have a longer useful lifespan than cemented prostheses. In a cemented joint replacement, methyl methacrylate (a pliable polymer that hardens to hold the prosthesis in place) is used to secure the prosthesis to existing bone. Although the person is able to resume normal activities more rapidly following a cemented joint replacement, methyl methacrylate initiates an inflammatory response and the joint eventually loosens.

- In a *total hip replacement*, the articular surfaces of the acetabulum and femoral head are replaced. The entire head of the femur and part of the femoral neck are removed and replaced with a prosthesis (see Figure 39.4). The acetabulum is remodelled and a prosthesis of high-molecular-weight polyethylene is inserted. The success rate for total hip replacement is reported to be greater than 90%. Most hip replacements last 10 to 15 years, after which a second joint replacement, called a revision, can be performed. Potential problems associated with a total hip replacement include blood clots in leg veins, dislocation within the prosthesis, loosening of joint components from surrounding bone and infection. If recurrent or ineffectively treated, these complications may necessitate removal of the prosthesis, resulting in severe shortening of the extremity and an unstable hip joint. It is vital to have sufficient guided rehabilitation after any replacement to ensure safety and range of movement with the new prosthetic.
- *Total knee replacement* is performed if the person has intractable pain and x-ray films show evidence of arthritis of the knee. Several prosthetic devices involving removal of varying amounts of bone are available for knee joint replacement (see Figure 39.5). The femoral side of the joint is replaced with a metallic surface and the tibial side with polyethylene. More than 80% of people obtain significant or total relief of pain with a total knee replacement. Again, they must engage in a vigorous program of rehabilitation to achieve the best results. Joint failure is more common with knee replacement than with a total hip replacement. Loosened joint components, often on the tibial side, are the most common cause of failure. The possible complications following a total knee replacement are the same as for a total hip replacement.
- *Total shoulder replacement* is indicated for unremitting pain and marked limitation of range of motion because of arthritic involvement of both the humeral and glenoid joint surfaces of the shoulder. The joint is immobilised in a sling or abduction splint for 2 to 3 weeks following arthroplasty. Dislocation, loosening of the prosthesis and infection are potential problems associated with total shoulder replacement.

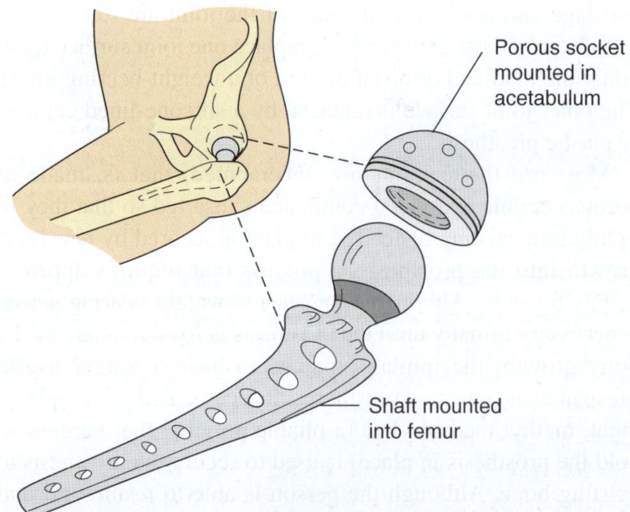

FIGURE 39.4 ***Total hip prosthesis***

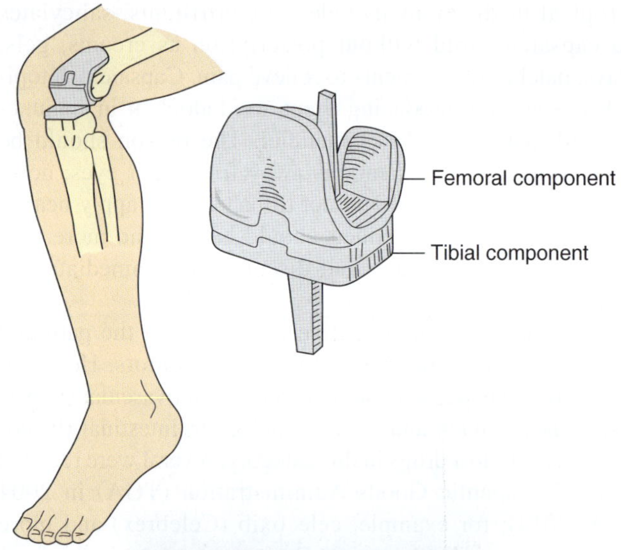

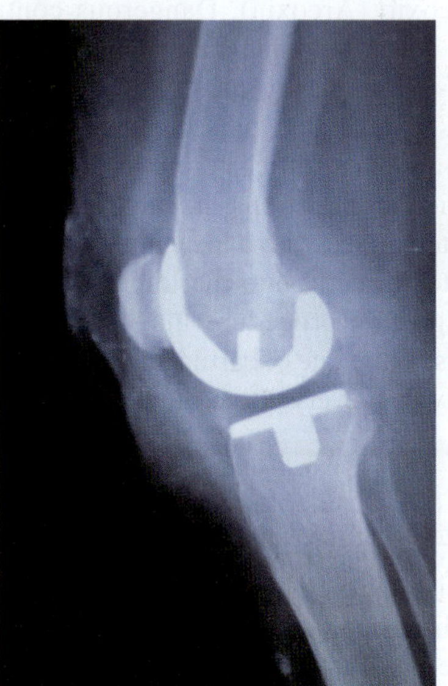

FIGURE 39.5 ***Total knee replacement***

Source: Image Edward Olive/123RF.

- *Total elbow replacement* involves replacement of the humeral and ulnar surfaces of the elbow joint with a metal and polyethylene prosthesis. Pain and disabling stiffness of the joint are indications for an elbow arthroplasty. Complications, including dislocation, fracture, tricep weakness, loosening and infection, occur frequently.

Infection is the main complication associated with total joint replacement. Not only does infection interfere with healing and prolong recovery, but it may also necessitate removal of the prosthesis and may lead to loss of joint function. Other potential complications include circulatory impairment to the affected limb, thromboembolism, nerve damage and dislocation of the joint.

Nursing care for the person undergoing total joint replacement is outlined in the accompanying box. Refer to the chapter 'Nursing care of people having surgery' for further discussion of care for the person undergoing surgery.

NURSING CARE OF THE PERSON having total joint replacement

PREOPERATIVE CARE

- Assess the person's knowledge and understanding of the planned operative procedure. Provide further explanations and clarification as needed. *It is important that the person has a clear and realistic understanding of the surgical procedure and expected results. Knowledge decreases anxiety and increases the person's ability to assist with postoperative care procedures.*
- Obtain a health history and physical assessment, including range of motion of the affected joints. *This information allows nurses to tailor care to the needs of the individual and serves as a baseline for comparison of postoperative assessment data.*
- Explain necessary postoperative activity restrictions. Teach how to use mobility assistance devices such as the overhead trapeze for changing positions. *The person who learns and practises moving techniques before surgery can use them more effectively in the postoperative period.*
- Provide or reinforce teaching of postoperative exercises specific to the joint on which surgery is to be performed. *Exercises are prescribed postoperatively to: (a) strengthen muscles providing joint stability and support, (b) prevent muscle atrophy and joint contractures, and (c) prevent venous stasis and possible thromboembolism.*
- Teach respiratory hygiene procedures such as the use of incentive spirometry, coughing and deep breathing, and the purpose of using these techniques. *Adequate respiratory hygiene is imperative for all people undergoing joint replacement to prevent respiratory complications associated with immobility and the effects of anaesthesia. In addition, many people undergoing total joint replacement are older and may have reduced mucociliary clearance.*
- Discuss postoperative pain control measures, including use of patient-controlled analgesia (PCA) or epidural infusion as appropriate. *It is important for the person to understand the purpose and use of postoperative pain control measures to allow early mobility and reduce complications associated with immobility.*
- Teach or provide prescribed preoperative skin preparation such as shower, shampoo and skin scrub with antibacterial solution if ordered; these are often used in surgeries when implantable devices are inserted. *These measures help reduce transient bacteria that may be introduced into the surgical site.*
- Administer prophylactic antibiotics as ordered. *Antibiotic therapy is initiated before or during surgery and continued postoperatively to further reduce the risk of infection.*

POSTOPERATIVE CARE

- Monitor vital signs, including temperature and level of consciousness, every 4 hours or more frequently as indicated, particularly in the first 24 to 48 hours, and if using a PCA. Report significant changes to the healthcare provider. *These routine assessments provide information about the person's cardiovascular status and can give early indications of complications such as excessive bleeding, fluid volume deficit and infection.*
- Perform neurovascular checks (colour, temperature, pulses and capillary refill, movement and sensation) on the affected limb hourly for the first 12 to 24 hours, then every 2 to 4 hours. Report abnormal findings to the healthcare provider immediately. *Surgery can disrupt the blood supply to or innervation of the affected extremity. If so, rapid intervention is important to preserve the function of the extremity.*
- Monitor incisional bleeding by emptying and recording suction drainage every 4 hours and assessing the dressing frequently. *Significant blood loss can occur with a total joint replacement, particularly a total hip replacement.*
- Reinforce the dressing as needed. *The dressing is usually changed 24 to 48 hours after surgery but may need reinforcement if excess bleeding occurs.*
- Maintain intravenous infusions and accurate intake and output records during the initial postoperative period. *The person is at risk of fluid volume deficit in the initial postoperative period because of blood and fluid loss during surgery, as well as the effects of the anaesthetic.*
- Maintain bed rest and/or prescribed positioning of the affected extremity using a sling, abduction splint, brace, immobiliser or other prescribed device. *Proper positioning of the affected extremity is vital in the initial postoperative period so that the joint prosthesis does not become dislocated or displaced.*
- Help the person shift position at least every 2 hours while on bed rest. Ensure that movements are supported so as not to displace the affected joint. *Shifting of position helps prevent pressure ulcers and other complications of immobility.*
- Remind the person to use the incentive spirometer, to cough and to breathe deeply at least every 2 hours. *These measures are important to prevent respiratory complications such as orthostatic pneumonia.*
- Assess the person's level of comfort frequently. Maintain PCA, epidural infusion or other prescribed analgesia to promote comfort. *Adequate pain management promotes healing and mobility.*
- Help the person get out of bed as soon as allowed. Teach and reinforce the use of techniques to prevent weight bearing on the affected extremity, such as the overhead trapeze, pivot turning and toe touch. *Early mobility prevents complications such as pneumonia and thromboembolism, but appropriate techniques must be used to prevent injury to the operative site.*
- Initiate physical therapy and exercises as prescribed for the specific joint replaced, such as quadriceps setting, leg raising and passive and active ROM exercises. *These exercises help prevent muscle atrophy and thromboembolism and strengthen the muscles of the affected extremity so that it can support the prosthetic joint.*
- Use sequential compression devices or anti-embolism stockings, as prescribed. *This helps prevent thromboembolism and pulmonary embolus for the person who must remain immobile following surgery.*
- For the person with a total hip replacement, prevent hip flexion of greater than 90 degrees or adduction of the affected leg. Provide a seat riser for the toilet or commode. *These measures prevent dislocation of the joint.*
- Assess the person with a total hip replacement for signs of prosthesis dislocation, including pain in the affected hip, or shortening and internal rotation of the affected leg.

(continued)

NURSING CARE OF THE PERSON having total joint replacement (continued)

- For the person with a total knee replacement, use a continuous passive range-of-motion (CPM) device or ROM exercises as prescribed. *Dislocation is not a problem with a knee replacement and more emphasis is placed on ROM exercises in the early postoperative period.*
- Maintain fluid intake and encourage a high-fibre diet. Administer stool softeners or rectal suppositories as needed. *Immobility and some analgesics contribute to the potential problem of constipation; these measures help maintain regular faecal elimination.*
- Encourage consumption of a well-balanced diet with adequate protein. *Adequate nutrition promotes tissue healing.*
- Teach or reinforce post-discharge exercises and activity restrictions. Emphasise the importance of scheduled follow-up physician visits. *People are discharged from the acute care facility before healing is complete. Exercises are prescribed and activities are resumed gradually to protect the integrity of the joint replacement and prevent contractures.*
- For those people needing additional direct care after discharge, arrange placement in a long-term care or rehabilitation facility. *Activity restrictions may preclude discharge to home for some people.*
- Make referrals as needed to community nursing and physiotherapy. *People often require home healthcare for both nursing care needs and continued physiotherapy following discharge from acute or long-term care.*

PHYSICAL THERAPY AND REHABILITATION Recovery from all types of joint replacement requires postoperative physical therapy, focusing on building strength and regaining joint flexibility. Rehabilitation begins in the hospital, most often the day following surgery, and may be continued during home care. Recovery from a hip replacement is 80% complete in 4 weeks and 100% complete in 6 months. Recovery from a knee replacement is 80% complete in 4 weeks and 100% complete after 1 year. During rehabilitation, the person must follow a regimen of exercise, rest and medication (AIHW, 2022).

COMPLEMENTARY AND ALTERNATIVE THERAPIES The following complementary therapies are examples of those that may be used by people with OA to relieve pain and stiffness. These same therapies are also used by people with rheumatoid arthritis:

- biomagnetic therapy
- rest and joint protection
- weight loss
- acupuncture
- eliminating nightshade foods (from the Solanaceae family of foods), such as potatoes, tomatoes, capsicum and eggplant, and tobacco
- taking nutritional supplements, such as glucosamine and chondroitin
- herbal therapy
- massage therapy
- osteopathic manipulation
- vitamin therapy
- yoga.

Nursing care

Osteoarthritis is a chronic process for which there is no cure. The focus of nursing care for the person with OA is providing comfort, helping maintain mobility and ADLs, and assisting with adaptations to maintain life roles. See the accompanying nursing care plan for a person with OA.

Health promotion

Although OA cannot be prevented, maintaining a normal weight and having a program of regular, moderate exercise will reduce risk factors. Glucosamine and chondroitin are nutritional supplements for OA that are increasingly popular and have been found to be of benefit in reducing manifestations. People should discuss these supplements with their healthcare provider before using them.

Assessment

Collect the following data through the health history and physical examination (see the chapter 'A person-centred approach to assessing the musculoskeletal system'):

- *Health history*: family history of OA, occupation, recreational activities, joint pain and stiffness, ability to carry out ADLs and self-care activities. Medications, analgesia regimen and comorbidities are also important.
- *Physical assessment*: height/weight; gait; joints: symmetry, size, shape, colour, appearance, temperature, pain, crepitus, range of motion, Heberden's nodes, Bouchard's nodes.

Nursing diagnoses and interventions

The priority nursing interventions for people with OA are directed towards managing chronic pain, facilitating physical mobility and improving ability to provide self-care.

Chronic pain

Pain is a primary manifestation of OA. As joint tissues degenerate and changes in joint structure occur, the amount of discomfort generally increases. The pain associated with OA increases with activity and tends to be relieved with rest. Non-pharmacological comfort measures are appropriate, with mild analgesics used to supplement these as needed.

- Monitor the level of pain, including intensity, location, quality and aggravating and relieving factors. *Accurate assessment of pain provides a basis for evaluation of the effect of interventions.*

NURSING CARE PLAN A person with osteoarthritis

Raymond Nasso is a 72-year-old retired commercial fisherman who has experienced arthritic pain in his hips for the past 10 to 15 years. During the past year, the pain in his right hip has become severe, prompting him to seek medical attention. Significant degenerative changes in both hip joints are noted on x-ray films. The physician recommends a total replacement of the right hip and total replacement of the left hip to follow in 6 to 12 months. Mr Nasso has preoperative teaching and tests the afternoon prior to his surgery, scheduled for 0800 the following morning.

ASSESSMENT

Christie Phlaugh, RN, completes a health history and examination of Mr Nasso on admission. Reviewing his medical record, she notes that Mr Nasso has mild Parkinson's disease and is taking carbidopa/levodopa (Sinemet 25-100) four times a day to control his symptoms. No other chronic medical conditions have been reported. Mr Nasso says he has been essentially healthy his entire life. He has no known allergies to medications, has never smoked and consumes only small amounts of alcohol.

On examination of Mr Nasso, Ms Phlaugh notes that he is alert and oriented. His vital signs are BP 116/64, P 68 regular, R 18, T 36.3°C PO. Peripheral pulses are strong and equal in the upper extremities and slightly weaker but equal in the lower extremities. His feet are cool to the touch but have immediate capillary refill. He has full ROM of his shoulders, elbows and wrists. The ROM of both hips is significantly restricted. Hip flexion beyond 90 degrees prompts pain on both sides. Both flexion and extension of the knees are limited slightly. Mr Nasso walks with a limp, favouring his right hip, and has a shuffling gait.

Preoperative laboratory studies including FBC, coagulation studies, chemistry panel and urinalysis show a serum creatinine of 1.7 mg/dL and BUN of 30 mg/dL, with no other abnormal values noted. His skin swabs, ECG and chest x-ray show no apparent pathologies. Cephazolin 500 mg is to be administered intravenously at 0600 prior to surgery and Mr Nasso is to shower and shampoo with antibacterial soap at bedtime. The physical therapist meets with Mr Nasso to evaluate his mobility and begin teaching him about postoperative weight-bearing restrictions.

DIAGNOSES (POSTOPERATIVE)

- *Acute pain* related to surgical incision.
- *Impaired physical mobility* related to activity and weight-bearing restrictions.
- *Risk of infection* related to disruption in skin integrity.
- *Risk of ineffective right leg tissue perfusion* related to vascular disruption and oedema.

PLANNING

Ensure Mr Nasso is able to manage his pain and prevent postoperative complications.

Expected outcomes

- Maintain an adequate level of comfort postoperatively as demonstrated by verbal expressions of comfort and the ability to move easily within restrictions.
- Remain free of infection.
- Maintain adequate perfusion of affected leg.
- Remain free of injury postoperatively.
- Comply with instructions to cough and breathe deeply.
- Remain free of adverse consequences of immobility such as pneumonia, pressure areas, thromboembolism or contracture.

IMPLEMENTATION

- Assess pain at least hourly during first 24 to 48 hours postoperatively and as needed thereafter.
- Instruct in the use of PCA and monitor its effectiveness.
- Help change position at least every 2 hours; encourage the use of the overhead trapeze to shift position frequently.
- Assess the surgical site frequently; report signs of excess bleeding or inflammation.
- Monitor temperature every 4 hours.
- Maintain sequential compression device and anti-embolic stocking as ordered; remove for 1 hour daily.
- Assist out of bed three times a day after the first 24 hours, according to physiotherapy instructions and ability.
- Maintain abduction of the right hip with pillows.
- Perform passive ROM exercises of unaffected extremities every shift.
- Encourage frequent quadriceps-setting exercises and plantar and dorsiflexion of feet.
- Assess pulses, colour, movement and sensation of right foot hourly for the first 24 hours, then every 2 hours for 24 hours, then every 4 hours.
- Encourage the use of the incentive spirometer hourly for first 24 hours, then at least every 2 hours while awake.

EVALUATION

Mr Nasso returns to the orthopaedic unit from the recovery ward. For the first 36 hours after surgery, he is confused and disoriented, but his orientation and thought processes gradually clear. His family has stayed with him and he has not experienced injury or other adverse consequences from his confusion. Otherwise, Mr Nasso has had an uneventful postoperative recovery. Six days after surgery, he is transferred to an extended care rehabilitation facility for further therapy until he is able to ambulate with partial weight bearing on his affected leg. He returns home 5 weeks after surgery, able to use a walker for ambulation. Arrangements are made for an over-bed trapeze, elevated toilet seat and shower chair in his home. A community nurse and physiotherapist visit Mr and Mrs Nasso weekly for a month following his discharge. During this time Mr Nasso gradually resumes full weight bearing. Mr Nasso expresses pleasure with the relief of his hip pain and says he has no fear of having his left hip replaced in the future.

CRITICAL THINKING IN THE NURSING PROCESS

1. Mr Nasso's preoperative laboratory work showed a modest elevation in his serum creatinine and BUN. What do these studies indicate? How might these changes affect nursing responsibilities related to medication administration for Mr Nasso?
2. Mr Nasso became confused postoperatively. Which factors in his history might have alerted the nurses to this possibility? How might anaesthesia and postoperative analgesics have contributed to his confusion?
3. Develop a care plan for Mr Nasso using the nursing diagnosis of *Acute confusion*.

REFLECTION ON THE NURSING PROCESS

1. From caring for Mr Nasso, identify two key issues that you will be able to utilise for future practice.
2. Which health education and teaching techniques are required prior to Mr Nasso's discharge?

- Teach people to take prescribed analgesic or anti-inflammatory medication as needed. Analgesics reduce the perception of pain and may decrease muscle spasm as well. *Anti-inflammatory medication may be ordered to decrease local inflammatory response in affected joints.*
- Encourage rest of painful joints. *The pain of OA is often relieved by joint rest.*
- Suggest applying heat to painful joints using the shower, a tub or sitz bath, warm packs, hot wax baths, heated gloves or diathermy, which uses high-frequency electrical currents to generate heat. *Heat application reduces accompanying muscle spasm, relieving pain. Moist heat penetrates deeper than dry heat; diathermy delivers heat directly to lesions in deeper body tissues.*
- Emphasise the importance of proper posture and good body mechanics for walking, sitting, lifting and moving. *Good body mechanics and posture reduce stress on affected joints.*
- Encourage the overweight person to reduce weight. *Excess weight places abnormal stress on joints, particularly the knees.*
- Encourage the use of non-pharmacological pain relief measures such as progressive relaxation, meditation, visualisation and distraction. *These adjunctive pain relief measures can reduce the person's reliance on analgesics and increase comfort.*

Impaired physical mobility

As intra-articular cartilage degenerates and joint structures are altered, the person with OA experiences pain, stiffness and decreased range of motion in affected joints. When the spine, large weight-bearing joints of the hips and knees, or the ankles and feet are affected, physical mobility can be significantly reduced.

- Assess the range of motion of affected joints. *Assessing joint mobility is important as a basis for planning appropriate interventions.*
- Perform a functional mobility assessment, evaluating gait, ability to sit and rise from sitting position, ability to step into and out of the tub or shower, and negotiation of stairs. Home visits by occupational therapists can be useful to assess function and hazards within the home, as well as organising what assistance measures could be put in place. *The functional assessment provides vital data about the person's ability to maintain ADLs.*
- Teach active and passive ROM exercises as well as isometric, progressive resistance and low-impact aerobic exercises. *Active ROM exercises help maintain muscle tone and mobility of affected joints and prevent contractures. Isometric and progressive resistance exercises improve muscle tone and strength; aerobic exercise improves endurance and cardiovascular fitness.*

> **CONSIDERATION FOR PRACTICE**
> **The older woman with OA may be more willing to take part in weight-bearing exercises if she does so as part of a group or organised activity.**

Self-care deficit

Just as OA of the lower extremities can reduce the person's mobility, OA of the upper extremities (the wrist, hand and finger joints, in particular) can significantly interfere with performance of ADLs such as cooking and brushing the hair. When the lower extremities are affected, bathing and toileting can be difficult.

- Perform a functional assessment of the upper and lower extremities. For upper extremities, assess the ability to touch the back of the head and to hold and use small items such as eating utensils. *The functional assessment provides important data about the person's ability to provide self-care.*
- Assess the home setting to determine the need for assistive devices such as handrails, grab bars, walk-in shower stall or shower chair, and handheld showerhead. *Many assistive devices are relatively easy and inexpensive to obtain and can significantly improve the person's independence in performing ADLs.*
- Assist in obtaining other assistive devices such as long-handled shoehorns, zipper grabbers, long-handled tongs or grippers for retrieving items from the floor, jar openers and special eating utensils. *These devices can prolong independence in performing ADLs.*

Community-based care

Because of the chronicity of OA, people and their families need appropriate teaching to manage the disease and its consequences effectively. Much of the teaching focus is on preservation of joint function and mobility. Discuss the following topics:

- Safeguard against hazards to safe mobility, such as scatter rugs. Encourage installation of safety devices such as handrails and grab bars.
- Understand the disease process and its chronic degenerative nature.
- Learn exercise techniques, including ROM, isometric, postural, stretching and strengthening, to maintain healthy cartilage, preserve ROM and develop supportive muscles and tendons. A walking program is beneficial for people with OA of the knee.
- Do not overuse or stress affected joints with heavy lifting, excessive stair climbing or bending, or other repetitive actions.
- Sit in a straight chair without slumping; avoid soft chairs or recliners, and sleep on a firm mattress or use a bed board.
- Use pain relief measures including prescribed or over-the-counter analgesic medications and non-pharmacological pain relief measures such as heat, rest, massage, relaxation and meditation.

For the person who has had a total joint replacement, discuss the following:

- use and weight bearing of the affected limb
- appropriate environmental modifications, such as an overhead trapeze for getting out of bed, elevated toilet seats and types of chairs to use and avoid when sitting
- prescribed exercises
- use of assistive devices for ambulation, such as crutches or a walker

- possible complications, including signs of infection or dislocation, and the need to notify the physician promptly if these occur.

Make referrals to home care, physical or occupational therapy, or other community agencies as indicated, and suggest the following resources:

- Arthritis Australia: https://arthritisaustralia.com.au
- Australian Rheumatology Association: https://rheumatology.org.au/.

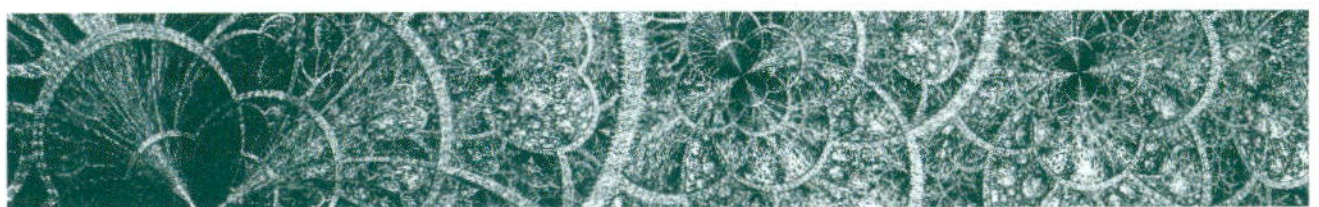

THE PERSON WITH MUSCULAR DYSTROPHY

Muscular dystrophy (MD) is a group of inherited muscle diseases that cause progressive muscle degeneration and wasting. The differences in the types of MD relate to the age at onset, the gender affected by the disorder, the muscles involved and the rate at which the disease progresses. These factors are summarised in Table 39.2. In the majority of cases of MD, there is a positive family history.

The most common form of MD, Duchenne muscular dystrophy, is inherited as a recessive single gene defect on the X chromosome (a sex-linked recessive disorder) and is transmitted from the mother to male children. This disorder affects males exclusively and occurs in 1 of 3,500 live male births. It can be recognised early in pregnancy in about 95% of cases by genetic studies or in late pregnancy through amniocentesis. Genetic counselling cannot be reliably used to prevent this disease because there is no way to determine if the woman carries the defective gene. The manifestations appear in early childhood, with the average lifespan being about 15 years after onset (Norris, 2018). Those with Duchenne MD will have a raised creatinine phosphokinase (CK) (muscle enzyme) in blood results. It can be raised in other forms of MD also, but particularly with Duchenne MD (Muscular Dystrophy Australia, 2018).

Other types of MD have an onset at any age and a slow progression with a normal lifespan.

Pathophysiology

The basic defect in MD is unknown; however, three theories have been proposed. The *vascular* and *neurogenic theories* suggest that the cause is a lack of blood supply to the muscle or a disturbance in the interaction between the nerve and muscle. The *membrane theory* suggests that an alteration in the cell membranes of the muscle causes them to degenerate. Recent genetic studies have shown a deficiency in the amount of dystrophin, a muscle membrane protein, in people with Duchenne MD. Dystrophin plays an important role in protecting the muscle against mechanical stresses.

Manifestations

All forms of MD exhibit manifestations of muscle weakness. The specific muscles involved depend on the type of MD. As the disease progresses, the person develops difficulty with ambulation and eventually becomes wheelchair bound and finally bed bound. Cardiac abnormalities, decreased lung function, endocrine abnormalities and mental retardation may also occur.

INTERPROFESSIONAL CARE

Because there is no cure or specific treatment for MD, care focuses on preserving and promoting mobility. An interdisciplinary approach, involving many members of the healthcare team, is necessary to meet the physical and psychological

TABLE 39.2 Types of muscular dystrophy

TYPE	SEX AND AGE AT ONSET	CLINICAL MANIFESTATIONS	PROGRESSION
Duchenne	Males Ages 3 to 5	Weakness of pelvic and shoulder girdles Waddling gait Toe walking Lordosis Cardiac abnormalities Low IQ in 50% of cases	Rapid; person usually confined to wheelchair by age 15; death occurs by age 20
Myotonic	Males and females Any age	Myotonia of hand muscles Muscular weakness of arms and legs Cardiac abnormalities Endocrine abnormalities Mental retardation (common)	Slow; death usually occurs in early fifties
Becker's	Males Ages 5 to 20	Weakness of pelvic and shoulder girdles	Slow; person usually confined to wheelchair at 25 years after onset; normal lifespan
Facio-scapulohumeral	Males and females Ages 10 to 20	Weakness of face and shoulder girdles	Slow; normal lifespan
Limb-girdle	Males and females Ages 20 to 40	Weakness of shoulder and pelvic girdles	Extremely variable; usually slow

needs of these people and their families. Diagnosis and classification of the muscular dystrophies are most often based on the manifestations and the pattern of muscle involvement. Biochemical examination, muscle biopsy and electromyography confirm the diagnosis. Diagnostic tests are described in the chapter 'A person-centred approach to assessing the musculoskeletal system'.

Tests include measuring creatine kinase (CK-MM, the isoenzyme found in skeletal muscle), which is elevated in the person with suspected MD; performing a muscle biopsy to identify fibrous connective tissue and fatty deposits that displace functional muscle fibres; and conducting an electromyogram (EMG), which will show a decrease in amplitude in MD.

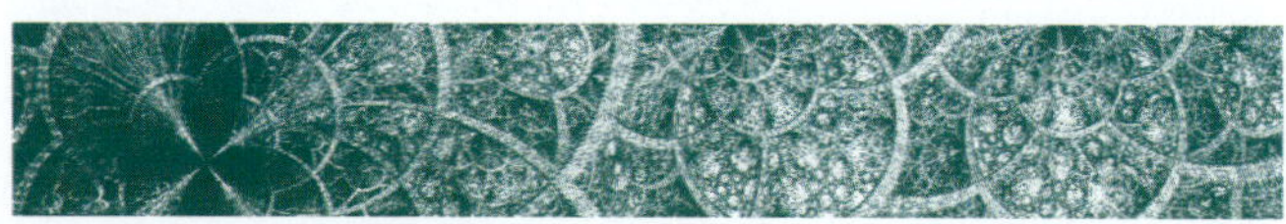

Nursing care

Nursing care for a person with MD focuses on promoting independence and mobility and providing psychological support for both the person and family. A holistic approach is essential in planning and implementing care.

Nursing diagnoses and interventions

Self-care deficit

The progressive muscle weakness that is associated with MD impairs the person's ability to perform self-care.

- Provide the person and their family with supportive care during the progress of the disease. The goal of treatment is to prolong each functional stage and delay or prevent deformity. *When transition from ambulation to a wheelchair occurs, depression and grief may occur.*
- Promote independence. Encourage tasks that can be accomplished rather than letting the person struggle with tasks that may prove frustrating. Energy conservation techniques are beneficial. *All forms of MD result in progressive muscle weakness. Management of the disease is directed towards keeping the person as functional as possible while preventing any deformities.*

Community-based care

Education of the person with MD focuses on maintaining function and independence and preventing deformities. Teach prescribed exercises such as stretching and counterposturing exercises. For the person with braces, discuss skin care and ways to prevent irritation under the brace. Because the person may have weakness involving muscles of respiration, teach the person how to prevent respiratory infections, such as avoiding crowds during flu season and being immunised against pneumococcal pneumonia and influenza. Provide information about support services and organisations such as the Muscular Dystrophy Association.

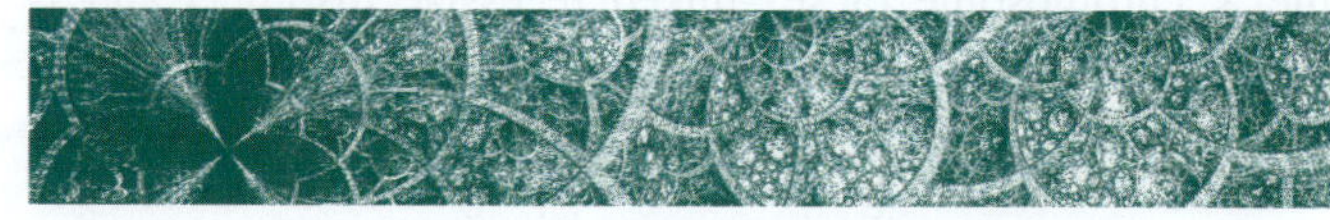

Autoimmune and inflammatory disorders

Autoimmune and inflammatory disorders of the musculoskeletal system are chronic systemic rheumatic disorders, characterised by diffuse inflammatory lesions and degenerative changes in connective tissues. The disorders have similar clinical features and may affect many of the same structures and organs.

THE PERSON WITH RHEUMATOID ARTHRITIS

Rheumatoid arthritis (RA) is a chronic systemic autoimmune disease that causes inflammation of connective tissue, primarily in the joints. Its course and severity are variable and the range of manifestations is broad. Manifestations of RA may be minimal, with mild inflammation of only a few joints and little structural damage, or relentlessly progressive, with multiple inflamed joints and marked deformity. Most people exhibit a pattern of symmetrical involvement of multiple peripheral joints and periods of remission and exacerbation.

The cause of RA is unknown. A combination of genetic, environmental, hormonal and reproductive factors is thought to play a role in its development. It is speculated that infectious agents, such as bacteria, mycoplasmas and viruses (especially Epstein–Barr virus), may play a role in initiating the autoimmune processes present in RA. Several studies have found that heavy smokers are at increased risk of developing RA. It is known that the incidence of RA has decreased during the past 40 years, supporting the theory that environmental factors may change and either promote or protect against RA (Arthritis Foundation, 2022; Norris, 2018). In 2014–2015, 405,900 Australians reported having RA, affecting 2% of women and 1.6% of men (AIHW, 2018b).

The course of RA is variable and fluctuating. Remissions are most likely to occur in the first year of the disease. The rate at which joint deformities develop is not constant. Disease progression is fastest during the first 6 years, slowing thereafter. RA contributes to disability and has a tendency to shorten life expectancy. About 10% of people with RA go into long-term remission within 1 year; and another 50–60% go into remission within 2 years (Arthritis Foundation, 2022; Norris, 2018).

The incidence of RA increases with age up to about 70 years. Although the onset and manifestations of RA are much

FAST FACTS
- RA is found worldwide, affecting 0.3–2% of the total population and all races.
- RA affects three times as many women as men.
- The onset of RA occurs most frequently between the ages of 30 and 50 years.
- RA is less common than OA: in 2014–2015, 1.8% of Australians reported having RA, whereas 9% of Australians reported having OA (AIHW, 2018b).

the same in older and younger people, differentiating between RA and OA in the older adult may be difficult at times. It is important to establish an accurate diagnosis, however, because the management of these disorders differs significantly. Clinical features distinguishing RA from OA are listed in Table 39.3.

For older people, RA is managed much as it is for younger people. However, prolonged bed rest or inactivity is not prescribed for acute episodes because it may result in irreversible immobility in the older adult. Also, medications are used with greater caution because of the increased risk of toxicity. In many cases, emphasis is placed less on preventing joint deformity and more on maintaining functional status for the older person with RA.

Pathophysiology

It is believed that long-term exposure to an unidentified antigen causes an aberrant immune response in a genetically susceptible host. As a result, normal antibodies (immunoglobulins) become autoantibodies and attack host tissues. These transformed antibodies, usually present in people with RA, are called *rheumatoid factors (RFs)*. The self-produced antibodies bind with their target antigens in blood and synovial membranes, forming immune complexes. (See the chapter 'Nursing care of people with altered immunity' for further information about autoimmune processes.)

The damage to cartilage that occurs in RA is the result of at least three processes:

1. Neutrophils, T cells and other synovial fluid cells are activated and degrade the surface layer of the articular cartilage.
2. Cytokines, especially interleukin-1 (IL-1) and tumour necrosis factor alpha (TNF-α), cause the chondrocytes to attack the cartilage.
3. The synovium digests nearby cartilage, releasing inflammatory molecules containing IL-1 and TNF-α.

Leucocytes are attracted to the synovial membrane from the circulation, where neutrophils and macrophages ingest the immune complexes and release enzymes that degrade synovial tissue and articular cartilage. Activation of B and T lymphocytes results in increased production of rheumatoid factors and enzymes that increase and continue the inflammatory process.

The synovial membrane is damaged by the inflammatory and immune processes. It swells from infiltration of the leucocytes and thickens as cells proliferate and abnormally enlarge. The inflammation spreads and can then involve synovial blood vessels. Small venules are occluded and vascular flow to the synovial tissue decreases. As blood flow decreases and metabolic needs increase (from the increased number and size of cells), hypoxia and metabolic acidosis occur. Acidosis stimulates synovial cells to release hydrolytic enzymes into surrounding tissues, starting erosion of the articular cartilage and inflammation of the supporting ligaments and tendons.

The inflammation also causes haemorrhage, coagulation and deposits of fibrin on the synovial membrane, in the intracellular matrix and in the synovial fluid. Fibrin develops into *granulation tissue (pannus)* over denuded areas of the synovial membrane. The formation of pannus leads to scar tissue formation that immobilises the joint (see Figure 39.6).

Joint manifestations

The onset of RA is typically insidious, although it may be acute (precipitated by a stressor such as infection, surgery or trauma). Joint manifestations are often preceded by systemic manifestations of inflammation, including fatigue, anorexia, weight loss and non-specific aching and stiffness. People report joint swelling with associated stiffness, warmth, tenderness and pain. The pattern of joint involvement is typically polyarticular (involving multiple joints) and symmetrical. The proximal interphalangeal (PIP) and metacarpophalangeal (MCP) joints of the fingers, wrists, elbows, knees, ankles and toes are most frequently involved, although RA can affect any joint. Stiffness is most pronounced in the morning, lasting more than 1 hour. It may also occur with prolonged

TABLE 39.3 Comparison of the manifestations of rheumatoid arthritis and osteoarthritis

FEATURE	RHEUMATOID ARTHRITIS	OSTEOARTHRITIS
Onset	Usually insidious, may be abrupt	Insidious
Course	Generally progressive, characterised by remissions and exacerbations	Slowly progressive
Pain and stiffness	Predominant on arising, lasting > 1 hour; also occurs after prolonged inactivity	Pain with activity; stiffness following periods of immobility generally relieved within minutes
Affected joints	Appear red, hot, swollen; 'boggy' and tender to palpation; decreased ROM, weakness Multiple joints affected in symmetrical pattern; PIP, MCP, wrists, knees, ankles and toes often involved	Affected joints may appear swollen; cool and bony hard on palpation; decreased ROM One or several joints affected including hips, knees, lumbar and cervical spine, PIP and DIP, wrist and 1st MTP joint
Systemic manifestations	Fatigue, weakness, anorexia, weight loss, fever; rheumatoid nodules; anaemia	Fatigue

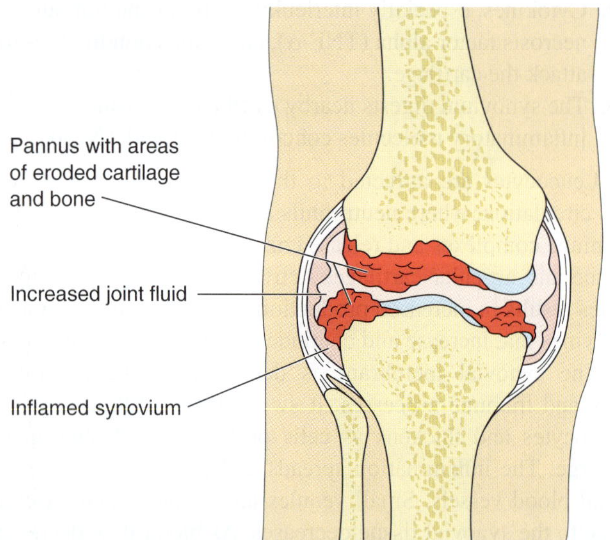

FIGURE 39.6 ***Joint inflammation and destruction in rheumatoid arthritis. Note synovial inflammation with pannus formation and the erosion of cartilage and underlying bone***

rest during the day and may be more severe following strenuous activity. Swollen inflamed joints feel 'boggy' or sponge-like on palpation because of synovial oedema. Range of motion is limited in affected joints and weakness may be evident.

The persistent inflammation of RA causes deformities of the joint itself and supporting structures such as ligaments, tendons and muscles. As the joint is destroyed, ligaments, tendons and the joint capsule are weakened or destroyed. Joint cartilage and bone are also destroyed. Weakening or destruction of these supporting structures results in lack of opposition to muscle pull, causing deformity.

Characteristic changes in the hands and fingers include ulnar deviation of the fingers and subluxation at the MCP joints. Swan-neck deformity is characterised by hyperextension of the PIP joint with compensatory flexion of the distal interphalangeal (DIP) joints (see Figure 39.7). A flexion deformity of the PIP joints with extension of the DIP joint is called a

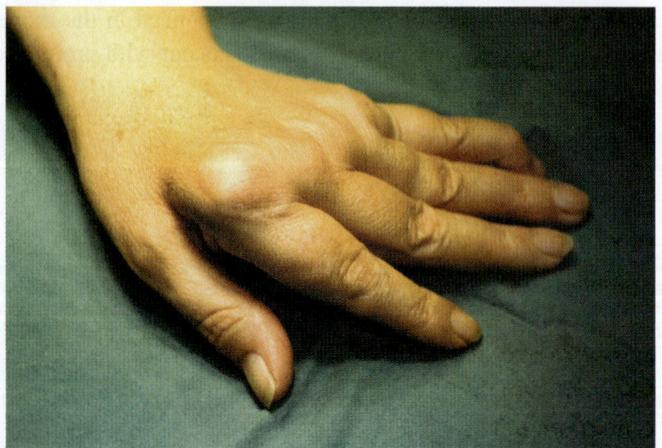

FIGURE 39.7 ***Typical hand deformities associated with rheumatoid arthritis***

Source: Mediscan/Alamy Stock Photo.

boutonnière deformity. The ability to effect a pinch is limited by hyperextension of the interphalangeal joint and flexion of the MCP joint of the thumb.

Wrist involvement is often in all areas of the joint, leading to limited movement, deformity and carpal tunnel syndrome. Inflammation of the elbows often causes flexion contracture.

The knees are frequently affected in RA, with visible swelling often obliterating normal contours. Instability of the knee joint along with quadriceps atrophy, contractures and valgus (knock-knee) deformities can lead to significant disability. Ambulation may be limited by pain and deformities when the ankles and feet are involved. Typical deformities of the feet and toes include subluxation, hallux valgus (deviation of the great toe towards the other digits of the foot), lateral deviation of the toes and cock-up toes (turned-up toes).

Spinal involvement is usually limited to the cervical vertebrae. Neck pain is common and neurological complications can occur.

Extra-articular manifestations

RA is a systemic disease with a variety of extra-articular manifestations. These are seen particularly in people with high levels of circulating rheumatoid factor. Fatigue, weakness, anorexia, weight loss and low-grade fever are common when the disease is active. Anaemia resistant to iron therapy frequently affects people with RA. Skeletal muscle atrophy is common, usually most apparent in the musculature around affected joints.

Rheumatoid nodules can develop in about 20% of people with RA, usually in subcutaneous tissue in areas subject to pressure: on the forearm, olecranon bursa, over the MCP joints and on the toes. Rheumatoid nodules are granulomatous lesions that are firm and either movable or fixed. They may also be found in viscera, including the heart, lungs, intestinal tract and dura.

Other possible extra-articular manifestations of RA include subcutaneous nodules, pleural effusion, vasculitis, pericarditis and splenomegaly (enlargement of the spleen). See 'Multisystem effects of rheumatoid arthritis'.

Increased risk of coronary heart disease

People with rheumatoid arthritis have an increased risk of developing coronary heart disease (CHD). In turn, CHD increases the risk of myocardial infarction and death; in fact, RA is associated with a shortened life expectancy (Arthritis Foundation, 2022; Norris, 2018). RA affects the heart by:

- direct effects on the blood vessels, with measures of C-reactive proteins (inflammatory markers) being more predictive of future cardiovascular disease than low-density lipoprotein (LDL) levels
- increased risk of having low high-density lipoprotein, high cholesterol and triglyceride levels, high blood pressure and high levels of homocysteine—all of which increase the risk of CHD
- the damaging side effects that many medications, such as methotrexate and steroids, often have on coronary vessels.

Multisystem effects of rheumatoid arthritis

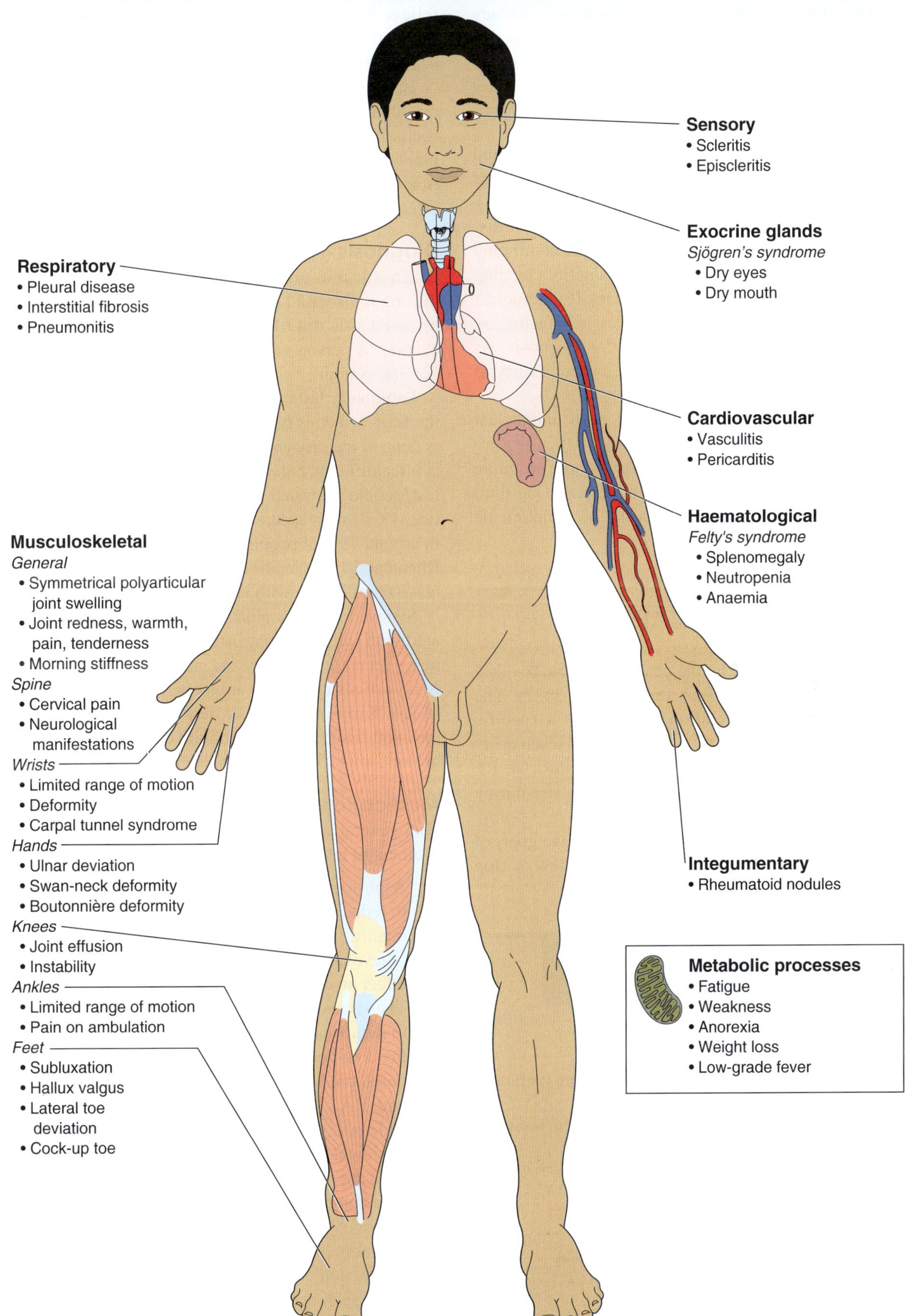

Lymphadenopathy can also occur around affected joints. Splenomegaly can also occur as a result. Blood vessels can display an inflammatory response, leading to thromboses. Kidney damage can also exist as a result of the autoimmune response and intermittent peripheral vascular compromise can occur (Raynaud's phenomenon).

Juvenile rheumatoid arthritis

Juvenile rheumatoid arthritis can be found in children and accounts for around 5% of RA cases. It can occur in three stages: (1) oligoarthritis (less than three joint involvement), (2) polyarthritis (more than three joints), and (3) Still's disease (systemic involvement). Large joints are more commonly involved, as well as inflammation around the anterior chamber of the eye, which can lead to vision problems if antinuclear antibodies are present. Rheumatoid nodules and factor are not common, but if present can have a worse prognosis. As adolescence occurs, RA can affect growth, and morbidity as an adult.

If children are seronegative, or do not have antinuclear antibodies or rheumatoid factor, the disease will often resolve itself in time. If seropositive, however, these people are more likely to have long-term RA symptoms and effects. One-third to half of those with juvenile arthritis can still be symptomatic 10 years later.

INTERPROFESSIONAL CARE

The diagnosis of RA is based on the person's history, physical assessment and diagnostic tests (Arthritis NSW, 2022). The American Rheumatism Association (2022) uses a specific diagnostic process (see Box 39.4). At least four of seven criteria must be present to establish the diagnosis. Positive RF occurs in approximately 80% of people and levels rise during active phases of the disease.

Once the diagnosis of RA has been established, the goals of therapy are to relieve pain, reduce inflammation, slow or stop joint damage, and improve wellbeing and ability to function. No cure currently exists for RA; the goal of treatment is to relieve its manifestations. An interprofessional approach is used, with a balance of rest, exercise, physical therapy and suppression of the inflammatory processes.

Because a cure is not available and traditional therapies are not always fully effective, many non-traditional treatments, including diets, topical preparations, vaccines, hormones, plant extracts and copper bracelets, have been put forth. These treatments are often costly and none has been shown to be effective.

BOX 39.4 Diagnostic criteria for rheumatoid arthritis

- Morning stiffness lasting for at least 1 hour and persisting for at least 6 weeks
- Arthritis with swelling or effusion of three or more joints persisting for at least 6 weeks
- Arthritis of wrist, MCP or PIP joints persisting for at least 6 weeks
- Symmetrical arthritis with simultaneous involvement of corresponding joints on both sides of the body
- Rheumatoid nodules
- Positive serum rheumatoid factor
- Characteristic radiological changes of rheumatoid arthritis noted in hands and wrists (American Rheumatism Association, 2022).

Diagnosis

Diagnostic tests are used to help establish the diagnosis of RA. Testing is also used to rule out other forms of arthritis and connective tissue disorders. Diagnostic tests are described in the chapter 'A person-centred approach to assessing the musculoskeletal system'.

Laboratory tests are used to measure rheumatoid factors and the ESR, which is typically elevated. A full blood count (FBC) is done to identify anaemia. Diagnosing RA in the early stages is often difficult, but a new test is highly effective. In this blood test, people are tested for antibodies to cyclic citrullinated peptide (CCP) with accurate detection of early RA. CCP is found in around 70% of people with RA (BMJ Best Practice, 2018a). Rheumatoid factor antibodies are also tested and are positive in 60–70% of people with RA.

Synovial fluid examination will demonstrate changes associated with inflammation, including increased turbidity (cloudiness), decreased viscosity and increased protein and WBC levels. X-rays of affected joints are the most specific test for diagnosis of RA. Early in the disease, few changes may be evident other than soft tissue swelling and joint effusions. As the disease progresses, joint space narrowing and erosions are seen.

Medications

Four general approaches are used in the pharmacological management of people with RA:

1. Aspirin and other NSAIDs and mild analgesics are used to reduce the inflammatory process and manage the manifestation of the disease. Although these drugs may relieve manifestations of RA, they appear to have little effect on disease progression.
2. The second approach uses low-dose oral corticosteroids to reduce pain and inflammation. Recent studies suggest that low-dose oral corticosteroids also may slow the development and progression of bone erosions associated with RA.
3. A diverse group of drugs classified as disease-modifying or slow-acting antirheumatic drugs are employed in the third approach to treating RA. These drugs, which include gold compounds, D-penicillamine, antimalarial agents such as hydroxychloroquine, infliximab and sulfasalazine, appear to alter the course of the disease, reducing its destruction of joints. Immunosuppressive and cytotoxic drugs such as methotrexate are included in this category as well.

4. Intra-articular corticosteroids may be used to provide temporary relief in people for whom other therapies have failed to control inflammation.

ASPIRIN Aspirin is often the first drug prescribed in the treatment of RA unless its use is contraindicated for the person. Aspirin is an inexpensive and effective anti-inflammatory and analgesic agent. The dose of aspirin required to achieve a therapeutic blood level of 15 to 30 mg/dL and its full anti-inflammatory effect is approximately 4 g per day in divided doses (three or four 5 g (325 mg) tablets qid). This effective dose is just under the toxic dose, which produces tinnitus and hearing loss. The person may be instructed to increase the dose of aspirin gradually until either maximal improvement or toxicity occurs. If tinnitus develops, the person reduces the dose by two to three tablets per day until the tinnitus stops.

Gastrointestinal side effects and interference with platelet function are the greatest hazards of aspirin therapy. People are instructed to take aspirin with meals, milk or antacids to minimise gastrointestinal distress and reduce the risk of GI bleeding. Enteric-coated forms of aspirin and non-acetylated salicylate compounds produce less gastric distress than plain or buffered aspirin and reduce the risk of gastric ulceration, but they are more expensive. Salsalate (Disalcid, Mono-Gesic, Salflex) and choline magnesium trisalicylate (Trilisate, Tricosal) are examples of non-acetylated salicylate products. All salicylate products are contraindicated for people with a history of aspirin allergy.

OTHER NON-STEROIDAL ANTI-INFLAMMATORY DRUGS A number of other NSAIDs are available for use in the management of RA if aspirin is not tolerated or effective. All NSAIDs act by inhibiting prostaglandin synthesis. Although the efficacy of all NSAIDs, including aspirin, is equivalent, people's responses are individual. Several trials of different NSAIDs may be necessary to find the most effective drug.

Some NSAIDs are considerably more expensive than aspirin but may cause less gastrointestinal distress and require fewer doses per day. Gastric irritation, ulceration and bleeding remain the most common toxic effects of NSAIDs. They can also affect the lower intestinal tract, leading to perforation or aggravation of inflammatory bowel disorders. All NSAIDs can also be toxic to the kidneys.

NSAIDs commonly prescribed for people with RA are listed in Table 39.4. The TGA (2014) has issued planned regulatory actions for both prescription and over-the-counter (OTC) non-selective NSAIDs. These actions include increased label warnings about the potential serious adverse cardiovascular and gastrointestinal effects of these drugs; the non-prescription drugs include those containing ibuprofen, naproxen and ketoprofen. Nursing implications for the administration of NSAIDs are described in the chapter 'Nursing care of people with infections'.

CORTICOSTEROIDS Systemic corticosteroids can dramatically relieve the symptoms of RA and appear to slow the progression of joint destruction. The long-term use of corticosteroids is associated with multiple side effects, such as poor wound healing, increased risk of infection, osteoporosis and gastrointestinal bleeding. Severe rebound manifestations can occur when these medications are discontinued. For these reasons, the use of systemic corticosteroids is limited to low dosages daily. The nursing implications for corticosteroid therapy are discussed in the chapter 'Nursing care of people with altered immunity'.

TABLE 39.4 Examples of non-steroidal anti-inflammatory drugs used to treat rheumatoid arthritis

DRUG	AVERAGE DOSE	COMMENTS AND PRECAUTIONS
Aspirin	600–900 mg 4 to 6 times daily	Least expensive NSAID; associated with risk of GI ulceration, bleeding and possible haemorrhage; may cause hepatotoxicity
Diclofenac (Voltaren)	50 mg tds or qid; or 75 mg bd	Expensive; risk of hepatotoxicity
Celecoxib	100 mg bd	GIT ulceration and bleeding. Adverse renal effects in some individuals
Flurbiprofen (Ansaid)	50–100 mg tds or qid, not to exceed 300 mg/day	Expensive
Ibuprofen (Nurofen, Advil others)	300 mg qid; 400–800 mg tds or qid	Available in prescription and OTC forms; less gastric distress reported than with aspirin or indomethacin; discontinue if visual disturbances develop
Indomethacin (Indocid)	25–50 mg bd or tds	A potent NSAID used for moderate to severe RA and acute episodes of chronic disease; higher incidence of adverse GI effects and CNS effects such as headache, dizziness and depression
Ketoprofen (Orudis)	50–75 mg tds or qid	Expensive; older adults and people with renal insufficiency require lower doses
Ketorolac	10 mg (max 40 mg)	Increased risk of GI bleeding and other severe effects increase with duration of treatment
Naproxen (Aleve, Anaprox, Naprosyn)	250–500 mg bd	Available in prescription and OTC preparations
Piroxicam (Feldene)	20 mg daily in a single or divided dose	Expensive; GI side effects including stomatitis, anorexia and gastric distress may occur more frequently than with other NSAIDs. Contraindicated in people with renal impairment
Sulindac (Clinoril)	150–200 mg bd	May be safer for use than other NSAIDs in people with chronic renal disease; rare fatal hypersensitivity reaction with fever, liver function abnormalities and severe skin reaction

bd = twice daily; qid = four times daily; tds = three times daily.

DISEASE-MODIFYING DRUGS Disease-modifying drugs are a diverse group of medications including drugs that modify immune and inflammatory responses, gold salts, antimalarial agents, sulfasalazine and D-penicillamine (see Table 39.5). They share characteristics that make them useful in the treatment of RA. Although beneficial effects are not apparent for several weeks or months following the initiation of therapy, they can produce not only clinical improvement but also evidence of decreased disease activity. Because their anti-inflammatory effect is minimal, NSAIDs are continued during therapy. As many as two-thirds of people taking disease-modifying drugs show improvement, although these drugs have not been shown to slow bone erosion or facilitate healing. All of these drugs are fairly toxic and close monitoring is necessary during the course of therapy.

Drugs that modify the autoimmune and inflammatory responses in people with RA include leflunomide (Arava) and etanercept (Enbrel). Leflunomide reversibly inhibits an enzyme involved in the autoimmune process and etanercept inhibits the binding of tumour necrosis factor to receptor sites. Infliximab (Remicade) is a biological response modifier and TNF-α receptor antagonist. Given by intravenous infusion, the drug is administered to reduce infiltration of inflammatory cells and TNF-α production. Adalimumab (Humira) is a biological response modifier that is given to people with RA to reduce the inflammatory events of polyarthritis and slow the progression of joint damage. Given by subcutaneous injection, the drug cannot be administered if the person has an acute or chronic infection in any part of the body. Prior to initiating the drug, the person should be tested for tuberculosis.

Gold salts may be administered by mouth, but the intramuscular route is preferred because it is more effective. The mode of action of gold is unknown, but it may produce clinical remission in some people and decrease new bony erosions. Weekly therapy is continued until significant improvement is noted unless toxic reactions occur. People experiencing benefit from gold therapy may be continued on monthly injections for several years. About one-third of people on gold therapy experience toxic reactions, including dermatitis, stomatitis, bone marrow depression and proteinuria. Mild skin reactions do not always necessitate discontinuation of therapy. FBC and urinalysis are monitored throughout treatment with gold to assess for more severe toxic responses.

Hydroxychloroquine (Plaquenil) is an antimalarial agent sometimes employed in the treatment of RA. Three to 6 months of therapy is required to achieve the desired response and many

TABLE 39.5 Disease-modifying drugs used to treat rheumatoid arthritis

CLASS/MEDICATIONS	USUAL DOSE	ADVERSE EFFECTS	COMMENTS/NURSING RESPONSIBILITIES
Gold salts Gold sodium thiomalate (Myochrysine) Aurothioglucose (Solganal) Auranofin (Ridaura Capsules)	Parenteral: 1st dose 10 mg; 2nd dose 25 mg, then 50 mg weekly IM Oral: 6 mg daily	• Pruritus, dermatitis • Stomatitis, metallic taste • Renal toxicity • Blood dyscrasias • Gastrointestinal distress	• Frequent UA and FBC • Monitor the person after injection for flushing, fainting, dizziness, sweating, possible anaphylactic reaction
Antimalarial Hydroxychloroquine (Plaquenil)	200–600 mg daily with meals	• CNS reactions including irritability, nightmares, psychoses • Retinopathy • Alopecia, pruritus • Blood dyscrasias • GI disturbances	• Should not be used during pregnancy • Regular ophthalmological examination required
Other Sulfasalazine (Azulfidine)	2 g/day in divided doses with meals	• Anorexia, nausea, vomiting, gastric distress • Decreased sperm count • Headache • Rash • Blood dyscrasias • Hypersensitivity responses including Stevens–Johnson syndrome • CNS, liver and renal toxicity	• Administer in evenly divided doses • Maintain high fluid intake • May cause yellow-orange skin or urine discolouration • Regular FBC necessary
Penicillamine (Cuprimine, Depen Titratable)	125–250 mg/day initially, slowly increased to a total of 1,000–1,500 mg/day	• Skin rashes • Fever • Gastrointestinal distress • Oral ulcers, loss of taste • Fever • Bone marrow depression with thrombocytopenia, leucopenia, anaemia • Renal toxicity • May induce immune complex disorders such as Goodpasture's syndrome and myasthenia gravis	• Regular FBC and UA necessary • Administer on an empty stomach • Discontinue during pregnancy • May require 2 to 3 months of therapy before benefit is seen

CNS = central nervous system; FBC = full blood count; UA = urinalysis.

people do not experience significant benefit. Although hydroxychloroquine has a relatively low toxicity, it can cause pigmentary retinitis and vision loss. People receiving this drug require a thorough vision examination every 6 months.

Sulfasalazine, a drug regularly prescribed for chronic inflammatory bowel disease, may also be prescribed for RA. See the chapter 'Nursing care of people with bowel disorders' for further discussion of this drug and its nursing implications.

For people not responding to the above preparations, penicillamine may be prescribed. Although this agent may be effective in the management of RA, toxic reactions are common and can be severe, including bone marrow suppression, proteinuria and nephrosis.

IMMUNOSUPPRESSIVE THERAPY Immunosuppressive or cytotoxic drugs are increasingly employed in the management of RA. Indeed, many now consider methotrexate the treatment of choice for people with aggressive RA. Methotrexate may be used along with NSAIDs in the initial treatment plan. A weekly dose can produce a beneficial effect in as few as 2 to 4 weeks. Mild-to-moderate patients are frequently commenced on methotrexate as the first-line disease-modifying antirheumatic drug (DMARD). There are also studies trialling a first-line triple therapy of methotrexate, sulfasalazine and hydroxychloroquine in combination. For more severe RA, methotrexate and a biological agent such as abatacept, a TNF inhibitor, is prescribed. Gastric irritation and stomatitis are the most frequent side effects associated with methotrexate, but side effects may be better controlled if folic acid is taken at the same time. Alcoholism, diabetes, obesity, advanced age and renal disease increase the risk of toxic effects (hepatotoxicity, bone marrow suppression, interstitial pneumonitis).

Other immunosuppressive agents such as cyclosporin, azathioprine and monoclonal antibodies have also been employed in the treatment of people with severe, progressive, crippling disease who have failed to respond to other measures.

There are continuing trials for emerging drugs used to treat RA, such as sarilumab, a human monoclonal antibody, and baricitinib, a janus kinase inhibitor, recently approved as an S4 in Australia.

Care must be taken in pregnancy as some treatments are contraindicated.

Treatments

The primary objectives in treating RA are to reduce pain and inflammation, preserve function and prevent deformity.

REST AND EXERCISE A balanced program of rest and exercise is an important component in the management of people with RA. During an acute exacerbation of the disease, the person may be hospitalised or a short period of complete bed rest may be prescribed. For most people, however, regular rest periods during the day are beneficial to reduce manifestations of the disease. Additionally, splinting of inflamed joints reduces unwanted motion and provides local joint rest. A variety of orthotic devices are available to reduce joint strain and help maintain function.

Rest must be balanced with a program of physical therapy and exercise to maintain muscle strength and joint mobility. ROM exercises are prescribed to maintain joint function and prevent contractures. Isometric exercises are used to improve muscle strength without increasing joint stress. Isotonic exercises also help improve muscle strength and preserve function. Low-impact aerobic exercises, such as swimming and walking, have been shown to benefit people with RA without adversely affecting joint inflammation or prompting acute episodes.

PHYSICAL AND OCCUPATIONAL THERAPY Physical and occupational therapists can design and monitor individualised activity and rest programs.

HEAT AND COLD Heat and cold are used for their analgesic and muscle-relaxing effects. Moist heat is generally the most effective and can be provided by a tub bath. Joint pain is relieved in some people through the application of cold.

ASSISTIVE DEVICES AND SPLINTS Assistive devices, such as a cane, walker or raised toilet seat, are most useful for people with significant hip or knee arthritis. Splints provide joint rest and prevent contractures. Night splints for the hands and/or wrists should maintain the extremity in a position of maximum function. The best 'splint' for the hip is lying prone for several hours a day on a firm bed. In general, splints should be applied for the shortest period needed, should be made of lightweight materials and should be easily removed to perform ROM exercises once or twice a day.

NUTRITION For most people with RA, an ordinary, well-balanced diet is recommended. Some people may benefit from substitution of usual dietary fat with omega-3 fatty acids found in certain fish oils.

SURGERY Surgical intervention may be employed for the person with RA at a variety of disease stages. Early in the course of the disease, synovectomy (excision of synovial membrane) can provide temporary relief of inflammation, relieve pain and slow the destructive process, helping to preserve joint function. Arthrodesis (joint fusion) may be used to stabilise joints such as cervical vertebrae, wrists and ankles. Arthroplasty, or total joint replacement, may be necessary in cases of gross deformity and joint destruction. Total joint replacement and nursing care of people undergoing this surgery are discussed in the preceding section on OA.

OTHER THERAPIES Several newer treatments that are not yet in widespread use may be employed in people with progressive RA. Plasmapheresis has been used to remove circulating antibodies, moderating the autoimmune response. Total lymphoid irradiation decreases total lymphocyte levels, although serious adverse effects are associated with this treatment and its continued efficacy has not been established.

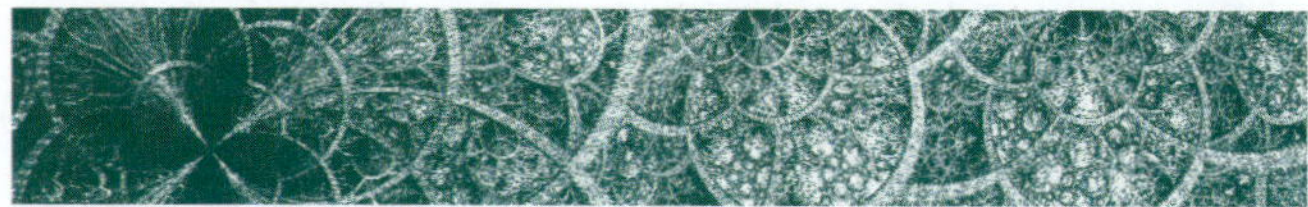

Nursing care

People with chronic, progressive, systemic disorders such as RA have multiple nursing care needs involving many functional health patterns. Physical manifestations of the disease often result in acute and chronic pain, fatigue, impaired mobility and difficulty performing routine tasks. The disease also has many psychosocial effects. The person has an incurable chronic disease that may lead to severe crippling. Pain and fatigue can interfere with the person's ability to perform expected roles, such as home maintenance or job responsibilities. Even though the person's hands may appear swollen or deformed, other people may not understand the systemic nature of the disease or appreciate the difference between RA and OA. See the accompanying nursing care plan for a person with RA.

NURSING CARE PLAN A person with rheumatoid arthritis

Joanne James is a 42-year-old high school science teacher who began noticing vague joint pain, fatigue, poor appetite and general malaise, which she initially attributed to a case of the flu. However, her symptoms continued and she reports feeling very stiff in the mornings, often taking until 10 or 11 am to begin to feel 'normal'. She then began to notice aching in her hands and wrists, which she attributed to the quilting she loves to do in the evenings. She made an appointment with her family GP when she noticed that her knuckles and finger joints were not just achy but also swollen and hot. Noting that Mrs James has lost 5 kg since her last visit and has mild anaemia and a significantly elevated ESR, the GP referred her to the rheumatology clinic for further evaluation. Following examination, laboratory and radiological testing, the rheumatologist established a diagnosis of rheumatoid arthritis and initiated a multidisciplinary team conference to plan the management of Mrs James's condition.

ASSESSMENT

Cathy Greenstein, RN, completes an assessment of Mrs James. She notes that Mrs James is well groomed and answers questions readily but appears fatigued and ill. Mrs James relates that her job has been extremely stressful because teacher layoffs have resulted in larger class sizes and fewer teaching assistants. Despite her symptoms, she continues to teach full time, but says she feels unable to keep up with all her responsibilities due to her fatigue.

Mrs James states that she is allergic to penicillin. Her past medical history reveals only the usual childhood diseases and three uncomplicated pregnancies, resulting in the births of her children, aged 14, 11 and 9. Physical assessment findings include BP 124/78, P 82 regular, R 18, T 37.8°C PO. Hands: swelling of the proximal interphalangeal (PIP) and metacarpophalangeal (MCP) joints of both hands; second and third PIP and second MCP joints on right hand are red, shiny, hot, spongy and tender to palpation; able to extend fingers to 180 degrees but cannot make a complete fist with either hand, with flexion limited to less than 90 degrees; grip strength is weak bilaterally; wrist ROM is limited in all directions. Knees are swollen and flexion is slightly limited; positive bulge sign in the right knee. Diagnostic findings are an ESR of 52 mm/hr, a haematocrit of 30% and positive for rheumatoid factor. Few changes other than soft tissue swelling are evident on hand and wrist x-rays.

DIAGNOSES

- *Chronic pain* related to joint inflammation.
- *Impaired home maintenance* related to fatigue.
- *Activity intolerance* related to the effects of inflammation.
- *Deficient knowledge of therapeutic regimen.*

PLANNING

Manage Mrs James's pain and educate her in relation to how to manage her condition and continue to undertake her usual activities.

Expected outcomes

- Verbalise effective pain management strategies:
  - Verbalise a plan to reduce responsibilities for home maintenance.
  - Express a willingness to plan rest breaks during the day.
- Demonstrate understanding of the prescribed therapeutic regimen and its importance for both short- and long-term benefit.

IMPLEMENTATION

- Use assistive devices to minimise joint stress with ADLs.
- Teach techniques for relieving pain and morning stiffness, including:
  - Schedule NSAIDs at equal intervals throughout the day.
  - Take morning NSAID dose with milk and crackers approximately 30 minutes before rising.
  - Perform ROM exercises in shower or bathtub.
  - Apply local heat with paraffin dip or compress, use cold packs as needed.
  - Teach techniques to minimise joint stress while performing ADLs.
- Discuss ways to delegate household tasks to other family members.
- Explore ways to incorporate 30-minute rest breaks into work schedule.
- Provide arthritis literature and information.
- Provide information about the disease process and its manifestations, prescribed medications with desired and adverse effects, and the importance of balancing rest and activity.

EVALUATION

The initial treatment regimen of aspirin, rest, exercise and physical therapy succeeded in partially relieving the acute manifestations of rheumatoid arthritis in Mrs James. However, complete remission has not been achieved. Her specialist is looking to

NURSING CARE PLAN **A person with rheumatoid arthritis (continued)**

commence her on DMARDS. She has had difficulty scheduling rest periods at work and has had to struggle to delegate household tasks. 'I don't look sick to the kids and they seem to think housecleaning is a terrible imposition on their time. It's often easier to just do it myself than to fight about it. Besides, that way it gets done right.' Mrs James has faithfully followed the prescribed medication regimen and exercise routines and she has kept her scheduled appointments and maintained contact with the treatment team.

CRITICAL THINKING IN THE NURSING PROCESS

1 Mrs James is 42 years old. Would your nursing interventions differ if she were 72 years old? If so, how?
2 Rheumatoid arthritis is a chronic illness. What are the physical, emotional and economic implications of a chronic illness that results in chronic pain and deformity?
3 Develop a nursing care plan for Mrs James using the nursing diagnosis of *Ineffective role performance*.

REFLECTION ON THE NURSING PROCESS

1 Identify issues from this case study that would enable you to care for people with rheumatoid arthritis in your future practice.
2 For a person newly diagnosed with rheumatoid arthritis, which education strategies would be appropriate when caring for this person?

Health promotion

People with RA have control of their lives by becoming arthritis self-managers. They can help prevent deformities and the effects of arthritis by following prescriptions for exercise, rest, weight management, posture and positioning. The following suggestions are recommended:

- Respect pain as a warning signal. When pain is experienced, change the method of doing things, use equipment or tools if necessary and take intermittent rest periods. Prolonged rest may lead to decreased range of motion.
- A structured exercise program greatly improves the wellbeing of RA sufferers. Stretching, strengthening and aerobic conditioning are all important in the rehabilitation of RA.
- Superficial heat has great effect on hands and feet due to less subcutaneous tissues in these areas. Heat packs and hydrotherapy are excellent for prevention of pain.
- Use adaptive equipment to assist with functional independence (Johns Hopkins Arthritis Center, 2016).

Assessment

Collect the following data through the health history and physical examination (see the chapter 'A person-centred approach to assessing the musculoskeletal system'):

- *Health history*: pain, stiffness, fatigue, joint problems: location, duration, onset, effect on function, fever, sleep patterns, past illnesses or surgery, ability to carry out ADLs and self-care activities.
- *Physical assessment*: height/weight; gait; joints: symmetry, size, shape, colour, appearance, temperature, range of motion, pain; skin: nodules, purpura; respiratory: cough, crackles; cardiovascular: pericardial friction rub, apical bradycardia, S_3.

Nursing diagnoses and interventions

Many nursing diagnoses may be appropriate for the person with RA. This section focuses on those related to its predominant manifestations and their effect on the person's life.

Chronic pain

Pain is a constant feature of RA when the disease is active. Pain accompanies both acute inflammation and lower levels of chronic inflammation. Some people say the pain in joints and surrounding tissue is like a deep, constant toothache. Pain can significantly affect the person's ability to provide self-care and maintain daily activities. It also contributes to the person's fatigue.

- Monitor the level of pain and duration of morning stiffness. *Pain and morning stiffness are indicators of disease activity. Increased pain may necessitate changes in the therapeutic treatment plan.*
- Encourage the person to relate pain to activity level and adjust activities accordingly. Teach the importance of joint and whole-body rest in relieving pain. *Pain is an indicator of excess stress on inflamed joints. Increasing pain indicates a need to decrease activity levels.*
- Teach the use of heat and cold applications to provide pain relief. The person may apply heat by showering or taking tub baths or using warm compresses or other local applications such as paraffin dips, but care must be taken not to burn the skin. *For people who find that heat increases pain and swelling during periods of acute inflammation, cold packs may be more effective. Both heat and cold have analgesic effects and can help relieve associated muscle spasms.*
- Teach about the use of prescribed anti-inflammatory and other medications and the relationship of pain and inflammation. *Anti-inflammatory agents reduce chemical mediators of inflammation and swelling, relieving pain.*
- Encourage using other non-pharmacological pain relief measures such as visualisation, distraction, meditation and progressive relaxation techniques. *These techniques can reduce muscle tension and help the person focus away from the pain, decreasing the intensity of the pain experience.*

Fatigue

The pain and chronic inflammatory processes associated with RA lead to fatigue. Other factors contribute as well. Discomfort often disrupts the person's sleep patterns. Anaemia, muscle atrophy and poor nutrition also play a role in the development of fatigue. The person with RA may experience depression or hopelessness, with associated manifestations of fatigue.

- Encourage a balance of periods of activity with periods of rest. *Both joint and whole-body rest are important to reduce the inflammatory response.*
- Stress the importance of planned rest periods during the day. *Rest is vital during acute exacerbations of the disease but also important to maintain the person in remission.*
- Help in using energy-conserving techniques and prioritising activities, performing the most important ones early in the day. *Assigning priorities helps the person avoid performing relatively unimportant activities at the expense of more meaningful and important ones.*
- Encourage regular physical activity in addition to prescribed ROM exercises. *Aerobic exercise promotes a sense of wellbeing and restful sleep patterns.*
- Refer to counselling or support groups. *Counselling and support groups can help the person develop effective coping strategies and deal with depression and hopelessness.*

Ineffective role performance

Fatigue, pain and the crippling effects of RA can interfere with the person's ability to pursue a career and fill other life roles, such as parent, spouse or homemaker. As the person's role changes, so must the roles of other family members. This can contribute to changes in family processes, increased stress in the family and further difficulty coping with the effects of the disease.

- Discuss the effects of the disease on the person's career and other life roles. Encourage the person to identify changes brought on by the disease. *Discussion helps the person to accept the changes and begin to identify strategies for coping with them.*
- Encourage the person and family to discuss their feelings about role changes and grieve lost roles or abilities. *Verbalisation allows family members to validate and accept feelings about losses and changes, thus helping them to move into new roles.*
- Listen actively to concerns expressed by the person and family members; acknowledge the validity of concerns about the disease, prescribed treatment and the prognosis. *Demonstrating acceptance of these feelings and concerns promotes trust and validates their reality.*

CONSIDERATION FOR PRACTICE

Remember that grief resolution takes time and that people may respond to loss with anger.

- Help the person and family identify strengths they can use to cope with role changes. *Identifying strengths helps the person and family to consider role changes that maintain self-esteem and dignity.*
- Encourage the person to make decisions and assume personal responsibility for disease management. *People who assume a personal and active role in managing their disease maintain a greater sense of self-control and self-esteem.*

Disturbed body image

The acute and long-term effects of RA can affect the person's body image, leading to feelings of hopelessness and powerlessness, social withdrawal and difficulty adapting to changes. When inflammation and joint deformity occur despite compliance, the person may have difficulty accepting the need to continue therapeutic measures, particularly those that have side effects or are costly or time consuming. In addition, unproven alternative treatment strategies may become increasingly attractive to the person, who may feel that they have limited alternatives.

- Demonstrate a caring, accepting attitude towards the person. *This attitude helps the person accept the physical changes brought on by the disease.*
- Encourage the person to talk about the effects of the disease—both physical effects and effects on life roles. *Verbalisation helps the person identify feelings and gives the nurse an opportunity to validate these feelings.*
- Encourage the person to maintain self-care and usual roles to the extent possible. *Discuss the use of easy-dress clothing and adaptive devices that promote independence. Independence enhances the person's self-esteem.*
- Provide positive feedback for self-care activities and adaptive strategies. *Positive reinforcement encourages the person to continue adaptive measures and maintain independence.*
- Refer to self-help groups, support groups and other agencies that provide assistive devices and literature. *These groups and agencies can help the person develop adaptive strategies to cope with the effects of RA, enhancing the person's self-concept, body image and independence.*

Community-based care

RA is typically a chronic, progressive disease. As with most diseases of this nature, involvement of the person and family in its management is vital. Education is an important nursing role in caring for people with RA and their families. Address the following topics for home care of the person and for family members:

- disease process and treatments, including rest and exercise
- medications
- management of stiffness and pain
- energy conservation
- use of assistive devices to maintain independence, including self-care aids such as handheld showers, long-handled brushes and shoehorns, and eating utensils with oversized or special handles
- clothing options such as elastic waist pants without zippers, Velcro closures, zippers with large pull-tabs and slip-on shoes
- how to apply splints and take care of skin
- home and equipment modifications, such as a raised toilet seat, grab bars in the bathroom, a bath chair or adapted counter heights for people in a wheelchair
- physical therapy, occupational therapy, community services and home care services

- helpful resources:
  - Arthritis Australia: https://arthritisaustralia.com.au
  - Australian Rheumatology Association: https://rheumatology.org.au
  - National Institute of Arthritis and Musculoskeletal and Skin Diseases: https://www.niams.nih.gov
  - New Zealand Rheumatology Association: https://www.rheumatology.org.nz.

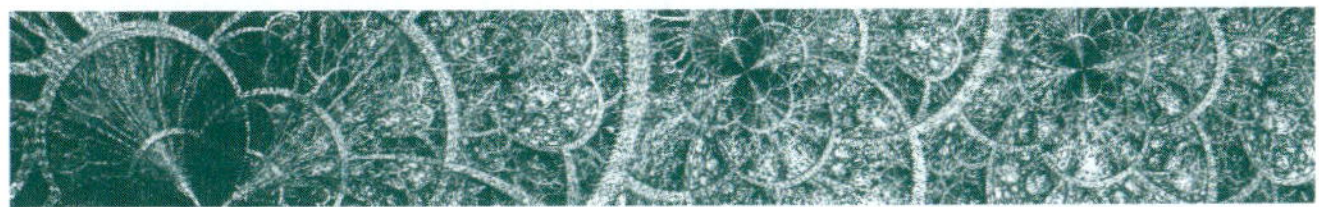

THE PERSON WITH ANKYLOSING SPONDYLITIS

Ankylosing spondylitis (AS) is a chronic inflammatory arthritis that primarily affects the axial skeleton, leading to pain and progressive stiffening and fusion of the spine. The typical age of onset is between 15 and 45. The incidence is greater in men than women and men have more severe disease. AS is difficult to diagnose in the early stages but may be a major cause of persistent back pain in young adults.

The cause of ankylosing spondylitis is unknown. As with the other spondyloarthropathies, there is a strong genetic component. Approximately 90% of people with AS have the HLA-B27 antigen; about 8% of the general population have this antigen (Norris, 2018). AS affects 1–2% of the Australian population.

Pathophysiology

Early inflammatory changes are often first noted in the sacroiliac joints. As the cartilage erodes, joint margins ossify and are replaced by scar tissue. The joints of the spine are also affected, with inflammation of the cartilaginous joints and gradual calcification and ossification that leads to ankylosis or joint consolidation and immobility. Other organ systems may be affected as well, including the eyes, lungs, heart and kidneys.

Manifestations

The onset of ankylosing spondylitis is usually gradual and insidious. People may have persistent or intermittent bouts of lower back pain. The pain is worse at night, followed by morning stiffness that is relieved by activity. Pain may radiate to the buttocks, hips or down the legs. As the disease progresses, back motion becomes limited, the lumbar curve is lost and the thoracic curvature is accentuated. In severe cases, the entire spine becomes fused, preventing any motion. People with AS may also experience peripheral arthritis, primarily affecting the hip, shoulders and knee joints. Systemic manifestations include anorexia, weight loss, fever and fatigue. Many people develop uveitis (inflammation of the iris and the middle, vascular layer of the eye).

For most people with AS, the disease is intermittent with mild to moderate acute episodes. These people have a good prognosis with little risk of severe disability.

INTERPROFESSIONAL CARE

Diagnostic testing shows an elevated ESR during periods of active disease and typically a positive HLA-B27 antigen. The diagnosis of ankylosing spondylitis is usually confirmed with x-ray examination of the sacroiliac joints and spine. The sacroiliac joint becomes blurred and gradually obliterated. As the disease progresses, vertebrae become squared and disc spaces narrow.

As with other forms of arthritis, the management of AS is multidimensional. Physiotherapy and daily exercises are important to maintain posture and joint ROM. NSAIDs relieve pain and stiffness and allow the person to perform necessary exercises. Indomethacin (Indocid) is the NSAID most commonly used to treat AS. It may, however, have many adverse effects, including headache, nausea and vomiting, depression and psychosis. Other drugs that may be prescribed include sulfasalazine (Azulfidine) and topical or intra-articular corticosteroids. Severe hip joint arthritis may necessitate total hip arthroplasty.

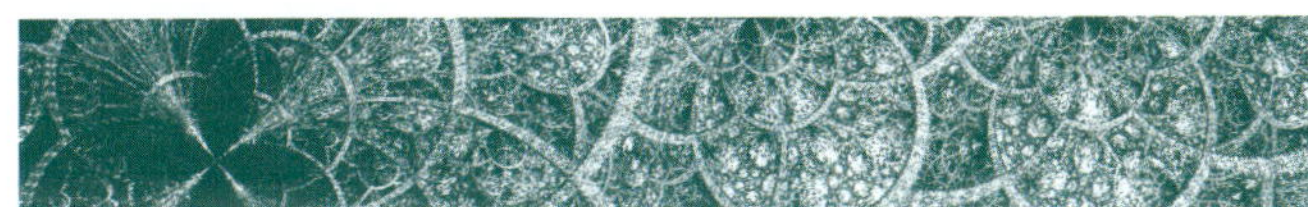

Nursing care

The primary nursing role in ankylosing spondylitis is to provide supportive care and education. To promote mobility, teach the person to take NSAIDs at regular intervals throughout the day with food, milk or antacid. Encourage the person to maintain a fluid intake of 2,500 mL or more per day. Suggest that the person utilise hot showers when exercising because warm, moist heat prompts mobility. Stress the importance of following the prescribed physical therapy and exercise program to maintain mobility.

Teach the person that proper positioning and posture are important. When sleeping, a bed board may be used to provide firmness and the person should sleep in the supine position using either no pillow or only one small pillow. Other important self-care activities include losing weight if applicable, using muscle-strengthening exercises and avoiding smoking. Suggest occupational counselling if pain and deformity are severe enough to cause work-related problems.

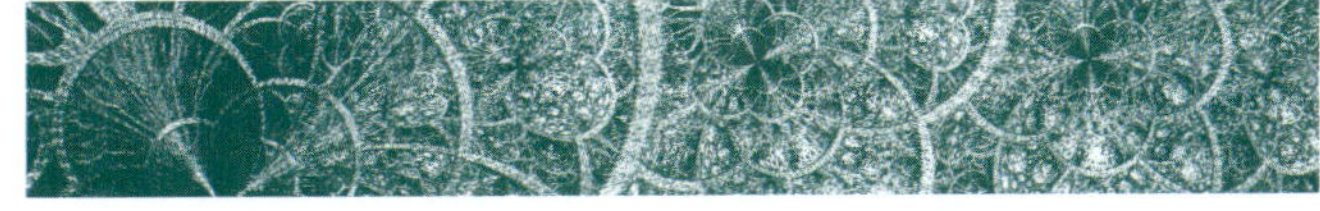

THE PERSON WITH REACTIVE ARTHRITIS

Reactive arthritis (ReA) (*Reiter's syndrome*) is an acute, non-purulent inflammatory arthritis that is believed to be a response to an exposure to or infection with certain types of bacteria, including *Chlamydia* (a bacterium contracted during sexual activity) or *Salmonella*, *Shigella*, *Yersinia* or *Campylobacter* (which cause dysentery from contaminated or spoiled food). This type of arthritis most often affects young men who have an inherited HLA-B27 antigen. Reactive arthritis is often found in people with HIV infection, although the reason for the association is not clear. Reactive arthritis is typically self-limited, although it can be recurrent or progressive. About 15–20% of people with ReA develop a chronic arthritis or spondylitis (Spondylitis Association of America, 2022).

Manifestations

Non-bacterial urethritis is often the initial manifestation of Reiter's syndrome. In women, urethritis and cervicitis may be asymptomatic. Conjunctivitis and inflammatory arthritis follow. The arthritis is usually asymmetric, affecting large weight-bearing joints such as the knees and ankles, the sacroiliac joints or the spine. Mouth ulcers, inflammation of the glans penis and skin lesions may occur. The heart and aorta may also be affected.

INTERPROFESSIONAL CARE

The diagnosis of reactive arthritis is based on the person's history and presenting symptoms. Manifestations of ReA typically occur 2 to 4 weeks after the infection and subside in 3 to 12 months. The condition has a tendency to recur. No test is specific for the disorder. Urethral or cervical cultures are obtained to rule out gonococcal infection. When *Chlamydia* is suspected, the person and sexual partner are treated with tetracycline or erythromycin. Reactive arthritis is treated symptomatically, usually with NSAIDs.

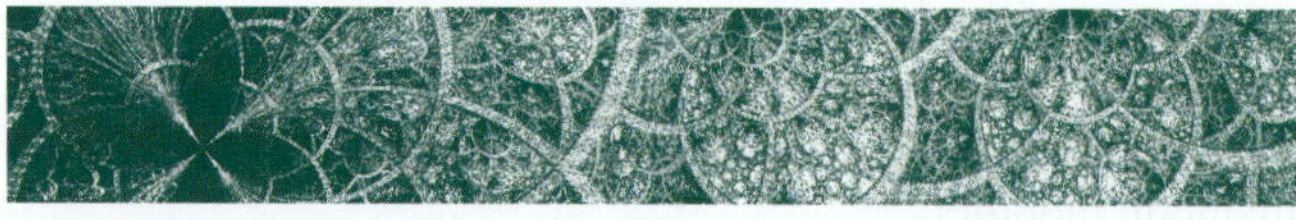

Nursing care

People with reactive arthritis usually are seen in primary care settings such as a clinic or GP's office, making the nursing role primarily one of education. Teach the person about the association of the arthritis with the precipitating infection (if identified). Stress the importance of treating the infection effectively if it is still present. Use this opportunity to provide information about sexually transmitted infections and protective measures to prevent their transmission (see the chapter 'Nursing care of people who have sexually transmitted infections'). Discuss the usual self-limiting nature of ReA, the appropriate use of prescribed NSAID preparations and symptomatic relief measures such as application of heat and rest.

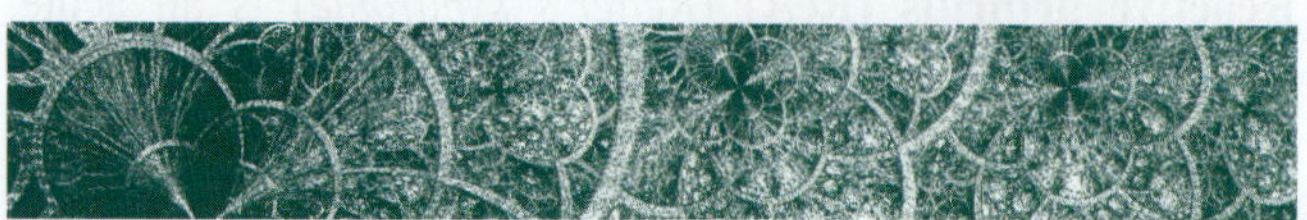

THE PERSON WITH SYSTEMIC LUPUS ERYTHEMATOSUS

Systemic lupus erythematosus (SLE) is a chronic inflammatory connective tissue disease. It affects almost all body systems, including the musculoskeletal system. The manifestations of SLE are widely variable and are thought to result from cell and tissue damage caused by deposition of antigen–antibody complexes in connective tissues. SLE affects multiple body systems and can range from a mild, episodic disorder to a rapidly fatal disease process.

Although the exact aetiology of SLE is unknown, genetic, environmental and hormonal factors play a role in its development. Twin studies and a familial pattern of the disease point to a genetic component, as does an increased incidence of other connective tissue diseases in relatives of people with SLE. Certain human leucocyte antigen (HLA) genes are seen more frequently in people with SLE. Environmental factors such as viruses, bacterial antigens, chemicals, drugs or ultraviolet light may play a role in activation of the pathological mechanisms of the disease. In addition, it is felt that sex hormones may influence the development of SLE. Women with SLE have reduced levels of several active androgens that are known to inhibit antibody responses. Oestrogens have been shown to enhance antibody responses and have an adverse effect in people with SLE.

The course of SLE is mild in most people, with periods of remission and exacerbation. The number and severity of exacerbations tend to decrease with time. In some people, however, SLE is a virulent disease with significant organ system involvement.

People with active disease have an increased risk of infections, which are often opportunistic and severe. Infections such as pneumonia and septicaemia are the leading cause of death in people with SLE, followed by the effects of renal or central nervous system (CNS) involvement. See 'Multisystem effects of systemic lupus erythematosus'.

FAST FACTS

- More than 20,000 people are affected by SLE in Australia and New Zealand, with women predominating by a ratio of 9:1 over men.
- SLE is more common in Polynesians in New Zealand (3.5 times greater than Europeans), with similar numbers in Indigenous Australians (Australasian Society of Clinical Immunology and Allergy, 2019).
- SLE usually affects women of childbearing age (when the incidence is 30 times greater than in men) but it can occur at any age.
- The incidence of SLE is higher in some families (Norris, 2018).

Pathophysiology

The pathophysiology of SLE involves the production of a large variety of autoantibodies against normal body components such as nucleic acids, erythrocytes, coagulation proteins, lymphocytes and platelets. Autoantibody production results from hyperreactivity of B cells (humoral response) because of disordered T-cell function (cellular immune response). The most

Multisystem effects of systemic lupus erythematosus

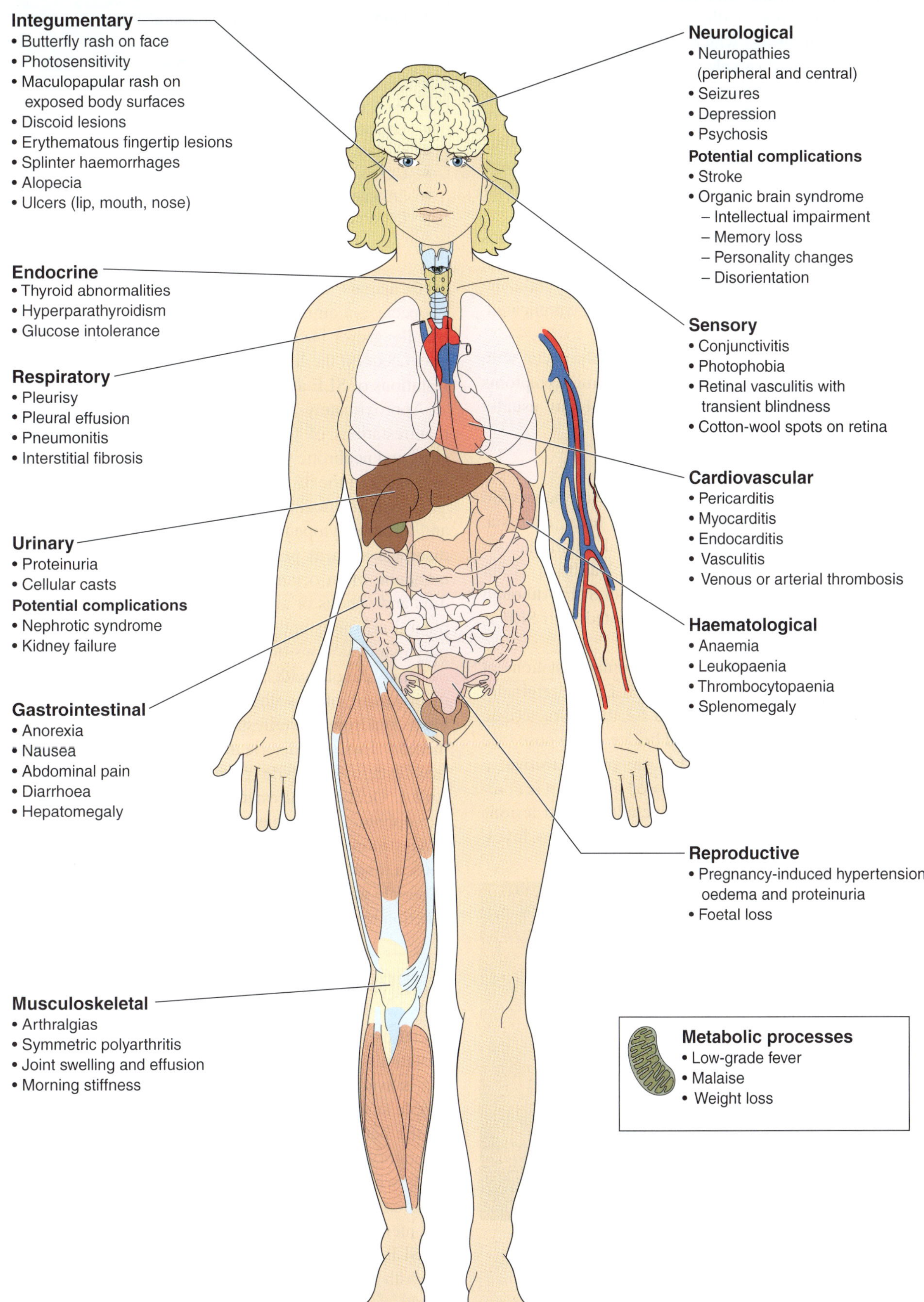

characteristic autoantibodies in SLE are produced in response to nucleic acids, including DNA, histones, ribonucleoproteins and other components of the cell nucleus.

SLE autoantibodies react with their corresponding antigen to form immune complexes, which are then deposited in the connective tissue of blood vessels, lymphatic vessels and other tissues. The deposits trigger an inflammatory response leading to local tissue damage. The kidneys are a frequent site of complex deposition and damage; other tissues affected include the musculoskeletal system, brain, heart, spleen, lung, GI tract, skin and peritoneum. The autoantibodies produced and their target tissue determine the manifestations of SLE.

A number of drugs can cause a syndrome that mimics lupus in people with no other risk factors for the disease. Procainamide (e.g. Procan-SR, Pronestyl) and hydralazine (Apresoline, Hydralyn) are the most common drugs implicated, along with isoniazid (INH).

Renal and CNS manifestations of SLE rarely occur with drug-induced lupus, but arthritic and other systemic symptoms are common. Manifestations of drug-induced lupus usually resolve when the medication is discontinued.

Manifestations

Typical early manifestations of SLE mimic those of rheumatoid arthritis, including systemic manifestations of fever, anorexia, malaise and weight loss, and musculoskeletal manifestations of multiple arthralgias and symmetric polyarthritis. Joint symptoms affect more than 90% of people with SLE. Although synovitis may be present, the arthritis associated with SLE is rarely deforming.

Most people affected by SLE have skin manifestations at some point during their disease. In fact, SLE was originally described as a skin disorder and named for the characteristic red butterfly rash across the cheeks and bridge of the nose (see Figure 39.8). Many people with SLE are photosensitive; a diffuse maculopapular rash on skin exposed to the sun is common. Other cutaneous manifestations include discoid lesions (raised, scaly, circular lesions with an erythematous rim), hives, erythematous fingertip lesions and splinter haemorrhages. Alopecia is common in people with SLE, although the hair usually grows back. Painless mucous membrane ulcerations may occur on the lips or in the mouth or nose. Common manifestations of SLE are listed in the 'Manifestations' box.

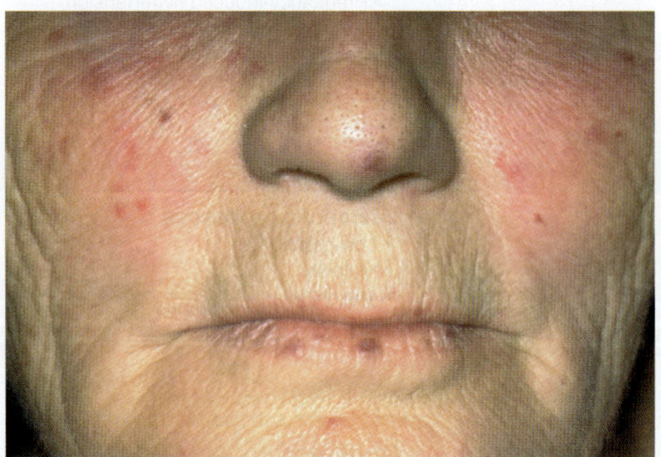

FIGURE 39.8 ***The butterfly rash of systemic lupus erythematosus***

Source: Mediscan/Alamy Stock Photo.

MANIFESTATIONS SLE

- Painful or swollen joints and muscle pain
- Unexplained fever
- Red rash, especially on the face
- Unusual loss of hair
- Pale, cyanotic fingers or toes
- Sensitivity to the sun
- Oedema in legs and around eyes
- Ulcers in the mouth
- Enlarged glands
- Extreme fatigue

Approximately 50% of people with SLE experience renal manifestations of the disease, including proteinuria, cellular casts and nephrotic syndrome. Up to 10% develop renal failure as a result of the disease.

Haematological abnormalities such as anaemia, leucopenia and thrombocytopenia are common with SLE. Cardiovascular disorders such as pericarditis, vasculitis and Raynaud's phenomenon often occur. Less frequently, myocarditis, endocarditis and venous or arterial thrombosis may develop. Pleurisy, pleural effusions and lupus pneumonitis are common pulmonary manifestations of SLE.

Many people with SLE develop transient nervous system involvement, often within the first year of the disease. Organic brain syndrome manifestations include decline in intellect, memory loss and disorientation. Other possible neurological manifestations include psychosis, seizures, depression and stroke. Ocular manifestations of SLE include conjunctivitis, photophobia and transient blindness due to retinal vasculitis.

Gastrointestinal manifestations of SLE, such as anorexia, nausea, abdominal pain and diarrhoea, may affect up to 45% of people with the disease. The liver may be enlarged and liver function tests may yield abnormal results.

INTERPROFESSIONAL CARE

Because of the diversity of organ system involvement and manifestations of SLE, diagnosis can be difficult. No one specific test is available to confirm the presence of this disease in all people suspected of having it. Instead, the diagnosis is based on the person's history and physical assessment, as well as laboratory studies.

As with rheumatoid arthritis, effective management of SLE requires teamwork, with active participation by both the person and members of the healthcare team. Although there is no cure for SLE, the 10-year survival rate is greater than 70% for people with this disease, which was once considered fatal in most cases.

Diagnosis

The multiple autoantibodies produced in SLE cause a number of abnormalities in laboratory tests. Diagnostic tests for the musculoskeletal system are described in the chapter 'A person-centred approach to assessing the musculoskeletal system'.

- *Anti-DNA antibody testing* is a more specific indicator of SLE, because these antibodies are rarely found in any other disorder.
- *ESR* is typically elevated, occasionally to > 100 mm/h.
- *Serum complement levels* are usually decreased as complement is consumed or 'used up' by the development of antigen–antibody complexes.
- *FBC* abnormalities include moderate to severe anaemia, leucopenia and lymphocytopenia, and possible thrombocytopenia.
- *Urinalysis (UA)* shows mild proteinuria, haematuria and blood cell casts during exacerbations of the disease when the kidneys are involved. Renal function tests including *serum creatinine* and *blood urea nitrogen (BUN)* may also be ordered to evaluate the extent of kidney disease.
- *Kidney biopsy* may be performed to assess the severity of renal lesions and guide therapy (see the chapter 'A person-centred approach to assessing the renal system').

Medications

The person with mild or remittent SLE may need little or no therapy other than supportive care. Arthralgias, arthritis, fever and fatigue can often be managed with aspirin or other NSAIDs. Aspirin is particularly beneficial for people with SLE because its antiplatelet effects help prevent thrombosis. It may, however, cause liver toxicity and hepatitis.

Skin and arthritic manifestations of SLE may be treated with antimalarial drugs such as hydroxychloroquine (Plaquenil). Hydroxychloroquine has also been shown to be effective in reducing the frequency of acute episodes of SLE in people with mild or inactive disease. Retinal toxicity and possibly irreversible blindness are the primary concerns with this drug. For this reason, the person taking hydroxychloroquine undergoes ophthalmological exam every 6 months.

People with severe and life-threatening manifestations of SLE (such as nephritis, haemolytic anaemia, myocarditis, pericarditis or CNS lupus) require corticosteroid therapy in high doses. Such people may require 40 to 60 mg of prednisone per day initially. The dosage is tapered as rapidly as the person's disease allows, although lowering the dosage may precipitate an acute episode. Some people with SLE require long-term corticosteroid therapy to manage symptoms and prevent major organ damage. These people are at increased risk of corticosteroid side effects, such as cushingoid effects, weight gain, hypertension, infection, accelerated osteoporosis and hypokalaemia.

Immunosuppressive agents such as cyclophosphamide or azathioprine may be used, alone or in combination with corticosteroids, to treat people with active SLE or lupus nephritis (see the 'Medication administration' box). When these agents are used in combination, lower, less toxic doses of each drug can be

MEDICATION ADMINISTRATION Immunosuppressive agents for SLE

CYTOTOXIC AGENTS

Azathioprine (Imuran)
Cyclophosphamide (Cytoxan)
Cyclosporin (Sandimmune)

Certain cytotoxic or antineoplastic drugs are effective as immunosuppressive agents. They act by decreasing the proliferation of cells within the immune system and are widely used to prevent rejection following a tissue or organ transplant. They are usually administered concurrently with corticosteroid therapy, allowing lower doses of both preparations and resulting in fewer side effects.

Nursing responsibilities

- Monitor blood count, with particular attention to the WBC and platelet counts. Notify the healthcare provider if WBCs fall below 4,000 or platelets below 75,000.
- Monitor kidney and liver function studies, including BUN, creatinine, creatinine clearance and liver enzyme levels. Report any abnormal levels to the healthcare provider.
- Oral preparations should be administered with food to minimise gastrointestinal effects. Antacids may be ordered.
- Increase fluids to maintain good hydration and urinary output.
- Monitor intake and output.
- Monitor for signs of abnormal bleeding: bleeding gums, bruising, petechiae, joint pain, haematuria and black or tarry stools.
- Use meticulous handwashing and other appropriate measures to protect the person from infection. Assess for signs of infection.
- Pulmonary fibrosis is a potential adverse effect of cyclophosphamide. Therefore, monitor the results of pulmonary function studies and be alert to clinical signs of dyspnoea or cough.

Health education for the person and family

- Avoid large crowds and situations where you might be exposed to infections.
- Report signs of infection such as chills, fever, sore throat, fatigue or malaise to the healthcare provider.
- Use contraceptive measures to prevent pregnancy while you are taking these drugs because they cause birth defects.
- Avoid the use of aspirin or ibuprofen while taking these drugs. Report any signs of bleeding to the healthcare provider.
- You may stop menstruating while you are taking cyclophosphamide. The menses will resume after the drug is discontinued.
- If you are taking cyclophosphamide, be sure to report difficulty breathing or cough to the healthcare provider.

used. The person receiving immunosuppressive agents is at increased risk of infection, malignancy, bone marrow depression and toxic effects specific to the drug prescribed.

Treatments

Because of the photosensitivity associated with SLE, the person should be cautioned to avoid sun exposure. People should use sunscreens with a sun protection factor (SPF) rating of 15 or higher when outdoors. Topical corticosteroids may be used to treat skin lesions. Some healthcare providers recommend avoiding the use of oral contraceptives, because oestrogen can trigger an acute episode.

People with lupus nephritis who progress to develop end-stage kidney disease are treated with dialysis (haemodialysis or peritoneal dialysis) and kidney transplantation.

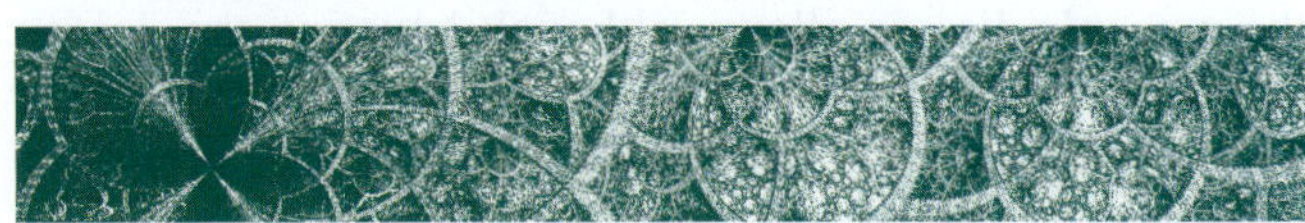

Nursing care

Nursing care for the person with mild SLE may be limited to teaching and trying to reduce exacerbations by reducing stress and infections. The person with severe disease, however, has many diverse nursing needs, which vary according to the organ systems involved. Because of the close link between rheumatoid arthritis and SLE, many of the nursing diagnoses and interventions identified for the person with arthritis may be appropriate for the person with lupus. The person with lupus nephritis or end-stage kidney disease has the nursing care needs related to glomerulonephritis and chronic kidney failure. This section focuses on the needs of the person related to the dermatological manifestations of lupus, an increased risk of infection and health maintenance.

Nursing diagnoses and interventions

The priority nursing interventions for the person with SLE are focused on problems with impaired skin integrity, ineffective protection and impaired health maintenance.

Impaired skin integrity

Skin lesions are a common manifestation of SLE. A rash or discoid lesion interrupts the integrity of the skin and the first line of protection against infection, increasing the person's already high risk of infection. These lesions, which usually appear on exposed parts of the skin, can also be disfiguring and cause the person emotional distress.

- Assess knowledge of SLE and its possible effects on the skin. *Assessment allows the nurse to base teaching and information on the person's existing knowledge, improving learning and retention.*
- Discuss the relationship between sun exposure and disease activity, both dermatological and systemic. *It is important for the person to understand that sun exposure may not only cause dermatological manifestations but also trigger an acute episode.*
- Suggest the following strategies to limit sun exposure:
  - Avoid being outdoors during hours of greatest sun intensity (10 am to 3 pm).
  - Use sunscreen with an SPF of 15 or higher when sun exposure cannot be avoided. Apply it 30 minutes before going out into the sun.
  - Reapply sunscreen after swimming, exercising or bathing.
  - Wear loose clothing with long sleeves and wide-brimmed hats when outdoors.

  These strategies can help the person maintain a normal lifestyle while helping to prevent acute episodes.
- Keep skin clean and dry; apply therapeutic creams or ointments to lesions as prescribed. *These measures promote healing and reduce the risk of infection.*

Ineffective protection

Ineffective protection can be a problem for the person with SLE, who is at increased risk of infection and multiple organ system problems because of the disease. In addition, treatment with corticosteroids or immunosuppressive agents further impairs immune responses and the ability to fight infection. The following interventions are for the person who is hospitalised.

- Wash hands before and after providing direct care. *Handwashing removes transient organisms from the skin, reducing the risk of transmission to the person.*

> **CONSIDERATION FOR PRACTICE**
> **Hands must be washed before and after providing direct care, even if gloves are worn. A decrease in this type of medical asepsis is contributing to the increasing number of hospital-acquired infections that are resistant to antibiotics.**

- Use strict aseptic technique in caring for intravenous lines and indwelling urinary catheters or performing any wound care. *Aseptic technique offers protection against external and resident host microorganisms.*
- Assess frequently for infection. Monitor temperature and vital signs every 4 hours. Assess for signs of cellulitis, including tenderness, redness, swelling and warmth. Report signs of infection to the healthcare provider promptly. *Therapy can suppress usual responses, such as elevated temperature and inflammation. The fever of infection may be mistaken for the fever commonly associated with lupus. The person receiving immunosuppressive therapy for the disease has an even higher risk of infection.*
- Monitor laboratory values, including FBC and tests of organ function; report changes to the healthcare provider. *An elevation in the WBC count with a shift to the left (increased numbers of immature leucocytes in the blood) may be an early indication of infection. Changes in liver function studies, renal function studies, myocardial enzymes or other laboratory values may indicate organ system involvement.*
- Initiate reverse or protective isolation procedures as indicated by the person's immune status. *These procedures provide further protection from infection for the severely immunocompromised person.*

- Ensure an adequate nutrient intake, offering supplementary feedings as indicated or maintaining parenteral nutrition if necessary. *Adequate nutrition is important for healing and immune system function.*
- Teach the person the importance of good handwashing after using the bathroom and before eating. *Handwashing reduces the risk of infection with endogenous organisms.*
- Monitor for potential adverse effects of medications, including thrombocytopenia and possible bleeding, fluid retention with oedema and possible hypertension, loss of bone density, osteoporosis and possible pathological fractures, renal or hepatic toxicity, and cardiac effects, particularly in the person with fluid retention and hypervolaemia. Medications used to treat SLE have many potential adverse effects that can impair normal protective and homeostatic mechanisms.

Impaired health maintenance

As with other chronic diseases, much of the responsibility for maintaining optimal health rests with the person. Disease manifestations such as fatigue, arthralgias, arthritis and increased risk of infection can interfere with the person's ability to maintain health. Psychosocial issues can also be a significant factor in health maintenance for the person with lupus. These issues may include denial of the significance of the disease, poor coping, lack of financial and other resources, and an inadequate support system.

- Assess the ability to maintain optimal health, identifying physical and psychosocial factors that may affect health maintenance. *Before intervening to improve the person's health maintenance, the nurse must identify and understand factors affecting it.*
- Provide care and teaching in a non-judgmental manner. *To intervene effectively, the nurse must accept the person and family as they are.*
- Encourage the person and family members to discuss the effect of the disease on their lives. *Open discussion helps the person and the nurse identify barriers to health maintenance and begin exploring alternative strategies.*
- Initiate an interprofessional care conference with the person and family. *In this care conference, a number of perspectives can be expressed, improving the planning of strategies for health maintenance activities.*
- Refer the person and family to counselling as needed. *Counselling may help the person and family develop the necessary coping skills to accept and deal with the disease.*
- Refer the person and family to community and social service agencies and local support groups. *These groups and agencies are valuable resources for the person and family.*

Community-based care

Teaching is a critical factor in preparing people with SLE for self-care at home. Address the following topics:

- the disease and its potential effects. Promote an optimistic outlook, stressing that the majority of people do not require long-term corticosteroid therapy and that the disease may improve over time
- the importance of skin care
- the importance of avoiding exposure to infection
- the need to follow the prescribed treatment plan, including rest and exercise, medications and follow-up appointments. Discuss manifestations of an acute episode (often called a flare) and stress the importance of contacting the healthcare provider promptly if any of these manifestations occur

> **CONSIDERATION FOR PRACTICE**
>
> **Warning signs of a flare-up**
>
> - Increased fatigue
> - Pain, abdominal discomfort
> - Rash
> - Headache
> - Fever
> - Dizziness

- the significance of wearing a MedicAlert® tag identifying the condition and therapy such as corticosteroids or immunosuppressives
- family planning with the person and spouse. The use of oral contraceptives may be contraindicated for the person; if appropriate, provide information about alternative means of birth control. Pregnancy is not contraindicated for most women with lupus. However, the pregnant person requires close monitoring because acute episodes sometimes accompany pregnancy
- the need for preventive healthcare for both men and women with SLE. Women should have gynaecological and breast examinations, and men should have prostate examinations, each year. Both men and women should have regular screenings for cholesterol and blood pressure. Annual influenza vaccinations are important, as is pneumococcal vaccinations for older people. If people are taking corticosteroids or antimalarial medications, annual eye examinations should be conducted to screen for and treat any eye problems
- helpful resources:
    - Arthritis Australia: https://arthritisaustralia.com.au
    - Lupus Association of NSW Inc.: https://lupusnsw.org.au.

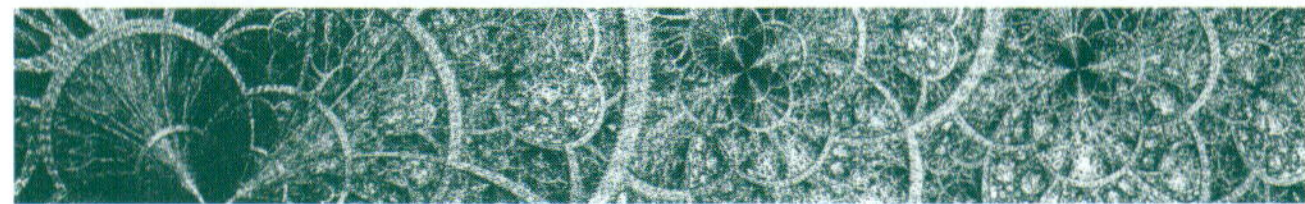

THE PERSON WITH POLYMYOSITIS

Polymyositis is a systemic connective tissue disorder characterised by inflammation of connective tissue and muscle fibres leading to muscle weakness and atrophy. When muscle fibre inflammation is accompanied by reddened skin lesions, this disease is known as dermatomyositis, which is comparable to polymyositis and the two are often grouped together as they have similar symptoms and treatments. Polymyositis is an autoimmune disorder of unknown cause that affects more women than men. The onset of the disease typically occurs between the ages of 40 and 60 years, although a childhood-onset form is also seen.

The immune mechanism causing the inflammatory response in polymyositis is not clear, but autoantibodies can be identified in the majority of people with the disease. The activation of complement is thought to contribute to the inflammatory process. Inflammation leads to muscle fibre necrosis and degeneration.

Manifestations

Initial manifestations of polymyositis include muscle pain, tenderness and weakness; rash; arthralgias; fatigue; fever; and weight loss. Skeletal muscle weakness is the predominant manifestation. Its onset may be either insidious or abrupt. Muscle weakness tends to progress over weeks to months. Muscles of the shoulder and pelvic girdles are particularly affected, making it difficult for the person to get out of chairs, climb stairs and reach overhead. Weakness of neck flexor muscles may make it difficult to raise the head from a pillow. Affected muscles may also be tender and painful. In dermatomyositis, a characteristic dusky red rash may be present on the face and upper trunk. Other manifestations include Raynaud's phenomenon, dysphagia, dyspnoea and cough (due to interstitial pneumonitis). The risk of malignancy is increased, particularly in people with dermatomyositis.

INTERPROFESSIONAL CARE

There is no specific test to diagnose polymyositis. Autoantibodies may be identified in blood serum. Serum levels of muscle enzymes are elevated, particularly creatine kinase (CK) and aldolase levels. Biopsy of involved muscle shows patchy muscle fibre necrosis and the presence of inflammatory cells.

A combination of rest and corticosteroid therapy is prescribed for the person with polymyositis. Long-term corticosteroid therapy may be necessary to manage the disease. Immunosuppressive agents such as methotrexate, cyclophosphamide and azathioprine may be used for people who do not respond well to treatment with corticosteroids.

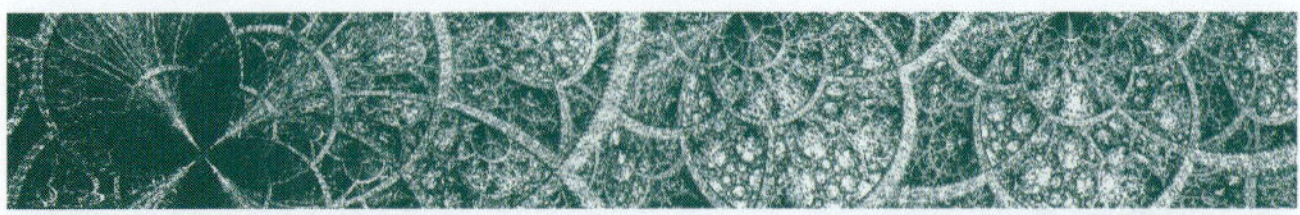

Nursing care

The nursing role in caring for the person with polymyositis is supportive. Measures to promote comfort are important. Muscle weakness may interfere with the person's ability to provide self-care and manage health and home. The person may have difficulty with speech because of pharyngeal muscle weakness. Provide alternate means of communication as needed and use patience in listening. Observe closely while the person eats, because aspiration is a potential problem. Modify the person's diet as needed to maintain nutrition and safety.

Educating the person and their family is an important component of care. Emphasise the need to balance periods of rest and activity. Discuss skin care to prevent dryness and infection. Teach the person about prescribed medications and their short- and long-term side effects. Provide information about safety measures while eating. Encourage family members to become trained in performance of CPR. Discuss signs of respiratory infection and other possible complications of polymyositis, including kidney failure and malignancy.

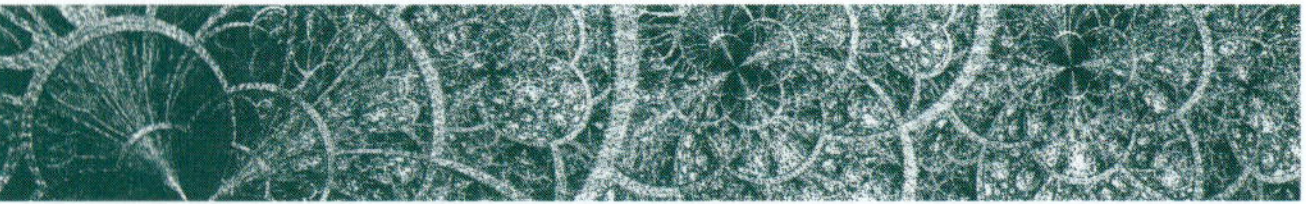

THE PERSON WITH OSTEOMYELITIS

Osteomyelitis is an infection of the bone. It may be an acute, subacute or chronic process. It occurs as a consequence of bacteraemia (haematogenous osteomyelitis) or invasion from a contiguous focus of infection or skin breakdown near the site of the osteomyelitis, where there may be vascular insufficiency.

Osteomyelitis can occur at any age, but adults over age 50 are more commonly affected. The older adult is at risk of osteomyelitis for several reasons. Immune function tends to decline with ageing; the older adult also is more likely to have a chronic disease process that affects immune function. Circulatory status in older adults often is compromised by atherosclerotic processes, impairing blood flow to the bone. Older adults have a higher risk of pressure ulcers because of circulatory, skin, sensation and mobility changes associated with ageing. Pressure ulcers that cannot be staged and treated because of eschar formation pose a particular risk. In addition, the older adult may not demonstrate the typical signs of infection and inflammation, thus allowing an infectious process to become well established before it is detected.

Pathophysiology

The cause of osteomyelitis is usually bacterial; however, fungi, parasites and viruses can also cause bone infection. *Staphylococcus aureus* is the most common infecting organism (BMJ Best Practice, 2018b). Other organisms include *Escherichia coli*, *Pseudomonas*, *Klebsiella*, *Salmonella* and *Proteus*.

Direct contamination of bone from an open wound, such as an open fracture or a gunshot or puncture wound, is the most common cause of osteomyelitis; osteomyelitis also may occur as a complication of surgery. The third mode of entry for micro-organisms that invade bone tissue is the extension from adjacent soft tissue infection. People with venous stasis or arterial ulcers of the lower extremities or long-term complications of diabetes mellitus are at risk of this type of bacterial invasion.

After entry, bacteria lodge and multiply in the bone, resulting in the inflammatory and immune system response. Phagocytes attempt to contain the infection, releasing enzymes in the process that destroy bone tissue. Pus forms, followed by oedema and vascular congestion. The Haversian canals in the medullary (marrow) cavity of the bone allow the infection to travel to other segments of the bone. If the infection reaches the outer margin of the bone (see Figure 39.9), it raises the periosteum of the bone, spreading along the surface. Lifting of the periosteum from the

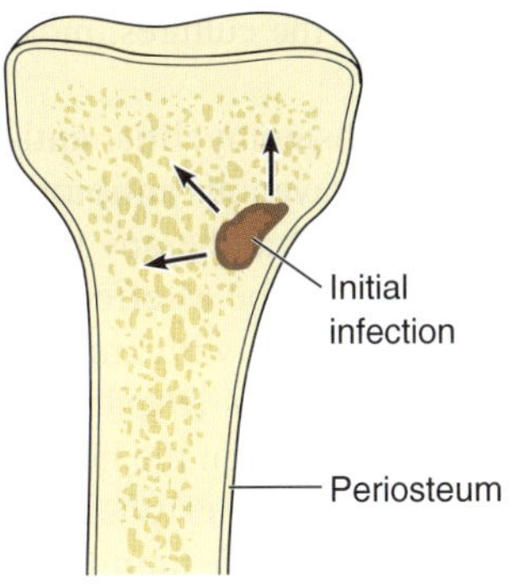

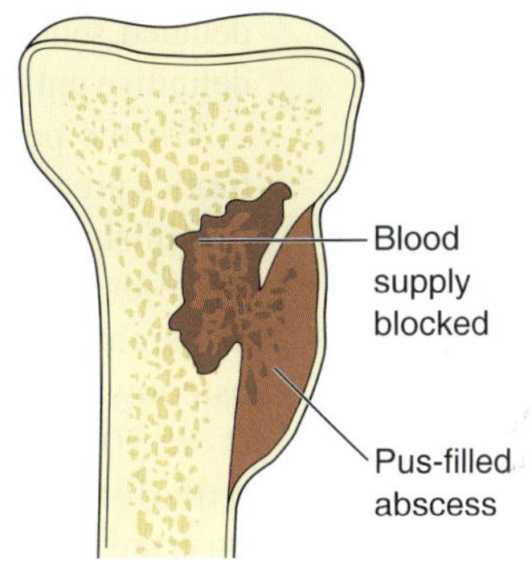

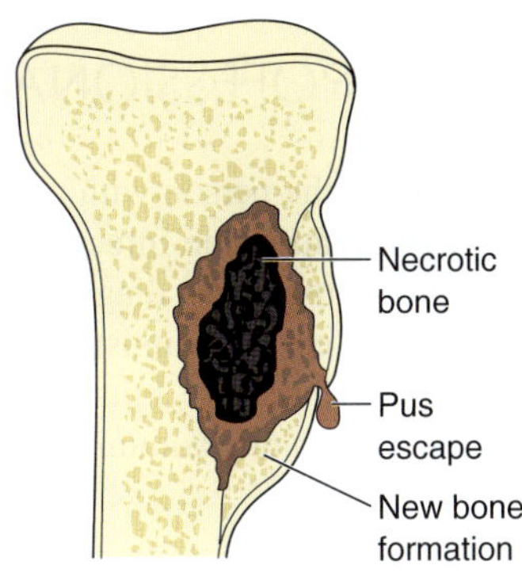

FIGURE 39.9 ***Osteomyelitis. A, Site of initial infection. Bacteria enter and multiply in the bone and the inflammatory response is initiated. B, Acute phase, in which infection spreads to other parts of the bone. Pus forms, oedema occurs and the vascular supply is compromised. If the infection reaches the outer margin of the bone, the periosteum is lifted and ischaemia and necrosis eventually occur. C, Chronic phase. Necrotic bone separates, a new layer of bone forms around the necrotic bone and a sinus develops to allow the wound to drain***

cortex disrupts the blood vessels that enter the bone. Pressure increases, further compromising the vascular supply and leading to ischaemia and eventual necrosis of the bone. Blood and antibiotics cannot reach the bone tissue once the pressure compromises the vascular and arteriolar systems. In addition, bacteria adhere to damaged bone, coating the underlying bone with a protective film that further impedes host defences.

Haematogenous osteomyelitis

Haematogenous infections are caused by pathogens that are carried in the blood from sites of infection elsewhere in the body. Haematogenous osteomyelitis primarily affects older adults, people with sickle cell anaemia and intravenous drug users. The spine is the usual site of infection in adults. Pathogens enter the well-perfused vertebral bodies of adults via the spinal arteries. From there, the infection spreads into the disc space. The lumbar spine is involved more frequently than the thoracic or cervical spine. Urinary tract infections, soft tissue infection, endocarditis and infected intravenous sites are sources of pathogens.

People with acute haematogenous osteomyelitis experience an acute onset of pain, tenderness and fever. Soft tissue swelling over the affected bone may be noted. The course of vertebral osteomyelitis in intravenous drug users often is subacute, with vague, dull pain in the affected region and a normal or low-grade fever. The pain intensifies over 2 to 3 months and is accompanied by tenderness, muscle spasm and limited range of motion.

Osteomyelitis from a contiguous infection

Infections caused by an extension of infection from adjacent soft tissues fall into this category of osteomyelitis. The infection is a result of or a complication of direct penetrating wounds, joint replacements, decubitus ulcers and neurosurgery. This is the most common cause of osteomyelitis in adults.

The diagnosis of osteomyelitis often is not made until the infection has become chronic because the signs of acute infection may be masked by local tissue inflammation. Failure to heal a surgical wound or fracture or a developing sinus tract may be initial indicators of a bone infection.

Osteomyelitis associated with vascular insufficiency

People with diabetes and peripheral vascular disease are at risk of developing osteomyelitis involving the feet. Diabetic neuropathy exposes the foot to trauma and pressure ulcers. The person may be unaware of the infection as it spreads into the bone. When tissue perfusion is poor, normal inflammatory responses and wound healing are impaired. The infection often is diagnosed when the person seeks treatment for a non-healing sore, swollen toe or acute cellulitis.

Manifestations

Manifestations of osteomyelitis vary according to the age of the person, the cause and site of involvement, and whether the infection is acute, subacute or chronic (see the 'Manifestations' box).

MANIFESTATIONS **Osteomyelitis**

CARDIOVASCULAR EFFECTS
- Tachycardia

GASTROINTESTINAL EFFECTS
- Nausea and vomiting
- Anorexia

MUSCULOSKELETAL EFFECTS
- Limp in involved extremity
- Localised tenderness, especially in epiphyseal area

INTEGUMENTARY EFFECTS
- Drainage and ulceration at involved site
- Swelling, erythema and warmth at involved site
- Lymph node involvement, especially in the involved extremity

OTHER EFFECTS
- High temperature with chills
- Abrupt onset of pain
- Malaise

INTERPROFESSIONAL CARE

The care of the person with osteomyelitis focuses on relieving pain, eliminating the infection and preventing or minimising complications. Early diagnosis is important to prevent bone necrosis by early administration of the appropriate antibiotic. Most people require both debridement of bone and a long period of antibiotic administration.

Diagnosis

The diagnosis of osteomyelitis is based on bone scans, MRI, blood tests and biopsy. As described in the chapter 'A person-centred approach to assessing the musculoskeletal system', an MRI, CT scan and bone scan may be conducted to identify abscesses, sinus tracts and bone changes. An ultrasound can detect subperiosteal fluid collections, abscesses and periosteal thickening and elevation associated with osteomyelitis. During an acute infection, ESR and WBC are elevated. Blood and tissue cultures (from affected bone or soft tissue) are obtained to identify the infecting organism and direct antibiotic therapy.

Medications

Antibiotic therapy is mandatory to prevent acute osteomyelitis from progressing to the chronic phase. Parenteral antibiotic therapy begins as soon as cultures (blood and/or wound) are obtained. A penicillinase-resistant semisynthetic penicillin may be given until the culture and sensitivity results are known. These antibiotics are used initially because many cases of osteomyelitis are caused by *Staphylococcus aureus*. When the detailed sensitivity report is obtained from the cultures, more definitive antibiotics are prescribed.

For the person with acute or chronic osteomyelitis, antibiotics are continued for 4 to 6 weeks. Intravenous antibiotic administration or oral therapy is common. Oral therapy with twice-daily ciprofloxacin has been shown to be as effective as parenteral therapy for treating adult people with chronic osteomyelitis caused by susceptible organisms (Papadakis et al., 2022). People can be treated as 'hospital in the home' with long-term IV antibiotics via PICC (peripherally inserted central venous catheter) for up to 6 months if needed.

Surgery

Surgical debridement is the primary treatment for the person with chronic osteomyelitis. The periosteum is excised and the cortex is drilled to release the pressure from accumulated pus. During this procedure, cultures may be obtained and sent to the laboratory for analysis. The wound holes are irrigated and the wound is then closed. The cavity may be kept clean by inserting drainage tubes that are connected to an irrigation and suction system. Postoperatively, the nurse is responsible for instilling and removing diluted antibiotic solutions through the drainage tubes. See the accompanying nursing care box for related nursing care.

A musculocutaneous (myocutaneous) flap is another approach used for the treatment of the dead space caused by extensive debridement of the infected site. The procedure involves moving or rotating a muscle and the section of skin fed by the arteries from that muscle into the cavity created by the surgery. A skin graft is performed later.

NURSING CARE OF THE PERSON undergoing surgical debridement for osteomyelitis

PREOPERATIVE CARE

- Discuss the impending surgery, the person's concerns regarding surgery and its risks, and what steps will be taken if surgery is ineffective. *Open discussion and active listening are important means of gaining the person's trust and encouraging the person to express concerns about the outcome of the surgery. Surgery is frequently performed when 36 to 48 hours of antimicrobial therapy yields no improvement and when prolonged bacteraemia and evidence of an abscess formation are present. The periosteum is excised, allowing access to the purulent material in the infected area. If pus is not apparent, several holes may be drilled into the bone. In some cases, irrigation tubes are inserted and connected to an elaborate system for postoperative antimicrobial therapy.*
- People may need extensive antimicrobial treatment postoperatively if an irrigation system is surgically implanted. Before the procedure, explain to the person that bed rest and an extended period of treatment in the hospital are imperative. *People who understand the events that may occur postoperatively may be more accepting of the required restrictions.*

POSTOPERATIVE CARE

- Provide meticulous care of the dressing and/or irrigation setup. Frequently, the irrigation tubes are connected to a three-way stopcock, which allows irrigation and drainage of the debrided area without separating the tube from the collection device. *Nurses need to be extremely cautious and adhere to strict sterile technique and universal precautions.*
- Assess the person for manifestations of further infection. *Although the person will receive antimicrobial agents, it is important to monitor the person continually for sudden spikes in temperature, pain at the involved site and other indications of superinfection. There is increased risk while the bone is more exposed.*

HEALTH EDUCATION FOR THE PERSON AND FAMILY

- While receiving antimicrobial agents, be sure to drink adequate amounts of fluid and eat a high-kilojoule diet to minimise the risks of damage to the kidneys, yeast infection and adverse gastrointestinal effects. Adequate nutrition will also help in the healing process.

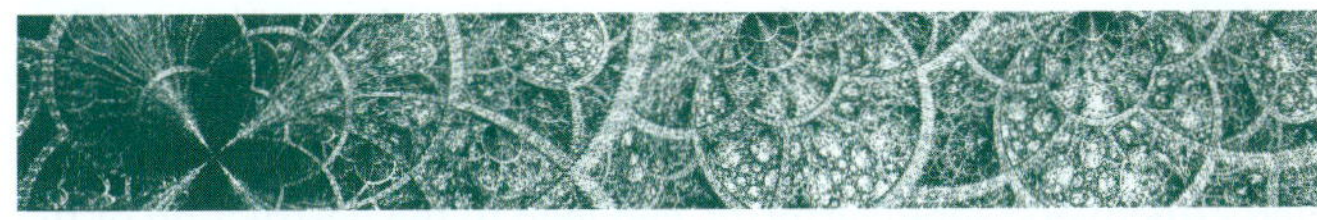

Nursing care

The person with chronic osteomyelitis faces frequent and lengthy hospitalisations and/or treatment modalities. The prognosis is uncertain and functional deficits and amputation are a constant concern. The ongoing financial implications, possible inability to work and role changes within the family are also concerns for the person.

Nursing diagnoses and interventions

Nursing diagnoses associated with acute osteomyelitis focus on preventing the transmission of infection and problems due to immobility. Providing comfort and person teaching are also very important.

Risk of infection

Compromised immune status places the person with osteomyelitis at risk of superinfection. An inadequate kilojoule intake is an additional factor that contributes to the risk.

- Maintain strict handwashing practices. *Meticulous handwashing helps prevent the spread of infection by minimising the entry of organisms into susceptible people.*

> **CONSIDERATION FOR PRACTICE**
> **Careful handwashing before and after direct care is essential even if gloves are worn.**

- Administer antimicrobial therapy at specified time intervals. *Optimal blood levels of antibiotic therapy are mandatory in people with infectious processes.*
- Maintain the person's optimal dietary kilojoule and protein intake. *High kilojoule and protein intake provides the person with sufficient nutritional support for the body's needs during the stressful event of the inflammatory process.*

Hyperthermia

The infection and associated inflammatory process can cause fever in the person with osteomyelitis.

- Monitor temperature every 4 hours and when the person reports chills and/or fever. *Blood cultures are frequently ordered when an acute elevation of temperature occurs. A sudden rise in temperature in people with either acute or chronic osteomyelitis may indicate inadequate antimicrobial management.*
- Maintain a cool environment and provide light clothing and bedding during temperature elevation. *Proper environmental conditions and clothing enhance the evaporative process during acute temperature elevation and promote comfort.*
- Ensure a daily fluid intake of 2,000 to 3,000 mL. *Dehydration may result from evaporative fluid losses during acute temperature elevations. Furthermore, people taking large doses of antibiotic therapy may experience fluid loss through excessive diarrhoea as a side effect of the therapy. Fluid replacement is necessary during this time to prevent further dehydration.*

Impaired physical mobility

Pain, infection, inflammation and the use of immobilisers and braces can all impair movement and mobility of the person with osteomyelitis.

- Maintain the affected limb in functional position when immobilised. *The person may hesitate to move the involved extremity because of continuous pain; therefore, the extremity must be maintained in functional position to avoid flexion contracture.*
- Maintain rest and avoid subjecting the affected extremity to weight-bearing activities. *The involved extremity must be immobilised to avoid pathological fractures caused by stress on the weakened bone.*
- Ensure active or passive ROM exercises every 4 hours. *Flexion contracture occurs when the person remains immobile or when there is only minimal joint movement. Consult a physical therapist for a plan of exercises to avoid contractures.*

Acute pain

The person with osteomyelitis experiences pain due to swelling.

- Use a splint or immobiliser when the person experiences acute pain from swelling. *Splinting or immobilising the involved extremity provides support and reduces pain caused by movement. Watch for skin breakdown or rubbing on areas of swelling and bony prominences, which can cause pressure ulcers.*
- Ask the doctor to order scheduled administration of narcotic and non-narcotic analgesics on a 24-hour basis rather than as needed. *The use of 24-hour administration allows blood levels of pain-relieving medications to remain constant. PCA via syringe pumps or long-acting medications may be useful.*

> **CONSIDERATION FOR PRACTICE**
> **People are often reluctant to ask for a prn pain medication, allowing the pain to reach a level that is difficult to manage.**

- Use non-pharmacological strategies (e.g. heat, distraction, relaxation techniques) for pain management. *Pain of the muscles and joints may be controlled through non-pharmacological interventions. Warm moist packs, warm baths or heating pads to the involved extremity provide comfort due to vasodilation.*
- Avoid excessive manipulation of the involved area; handle the area gently. Carefully assess the person for guarding, limping or unwillingness to move the affected part. Communicate to other healthcare professionals the person's preferences for assistive devices and means of manipulating the involved area. *Gentle handling and minimal manipulation help reduce pain.*

Community-based care

Although people may be hospitalised for acute treatment and surgery, most care is provided at home. Community health services can provide intravenous medications, if prescribed. Discuss the following topics for home care:

- the importance of careful handwashing, especially after toileting and dressing changes
- the importance of taking all antibiotics as prescribed. Include information about helping prevent the yeast infections (of the mouth or vagina) often associated with prolonged antibiotic therapy by daily ingestion of live-culture yoghurt or probiotics
- the need to take pain medications on a regular basis to prevent pain from becoming severe. Provide information about how to deal with side effects, such as constipation, by increasing fluid and fibre intake
- how to perform wound care effectively if needed, how to maintain a clean wound and how to prevent further infection
- sources for needed equipment and supplies as well as access and referral to community wound care specialists and nurses as required
- the importance of regular check-ups to watch for further infection
- rest or limited weight bearing for the affected extremity or body part. Teach how to avoid complications associated with prolonged immobilisation, such as frequently shifting position; maintaining optimal skin care and integrity; keeping linen clean, dry and wrinkle free; and doing active ROM exercises for unaffected joints
- the importance of maintaining good nutrition. An adequate supply of kilojoules, protein and other nutrients is necessary for immune function and healing. Suggest frequent small meals and using nutritional supplements such as Ensure to help maintain nutritional intake.

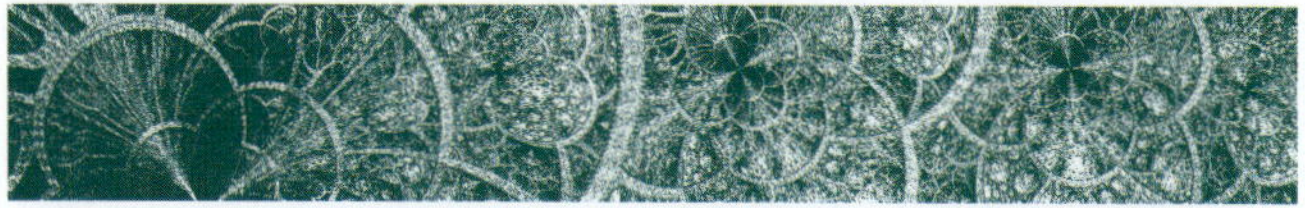

THE PERSON WITH SEPTIC ARTHRITIS

Septic arthritis can develop if a joint space is invaded by a pathogen. The primary risk factors for septic arthritis are persistent bacteraemia (bacteria in the blood) (e.g. due to use of injectable drugs, endocarditis) and previous joint damage (e.g. due to trauma or rheumatoid arthritis). Arthroscopic surgery and total joint replacements that allow potential direct contamination of the joint are additional risk factors (Papadakis et al., 2022).

Pathophysiology

The most common bacteria implicated in septic arthritis include *gonococci*, *S. aureus* and *streptococci*. Infections by Gram-negative bacteria such as *E. coli* and *Pseudomonas* are seen with increasing frequency, particularly in people who inject recreational drugs or are immunocompromised.

Infection of the joint leads to inflammation with resulting synovitis and joint effusion. Abscesses may form in synovial tissues or bone underlying joint cartilage. If not treated promptly and effectively, septic arthritis can lead to the destruction of the affected joint. A single joint, often the knee, is usually affected. Septic arthritis may also affect other joints such as the shoulder, wrist, hip, fingers or elbow.

Manifestations

The onset of septic arthritis is typically abrupt, marked by pain and stiffness of the infected joint. The joint appears red and swollen and is hot and tender to the touch. Effusion (increased fluid within the joint space) is usually present. Systemic manifestations of infection, such as chills and fever, often accompany local manifestations, although these may be muted if the person is taking anti-inflammatory medications.

INTERPROFESSIONAL CARE

Septic arthritis is a medical emergency requiring prompt treatment to preserve joint function. When it is suspected, fluid from the affected joint is aspirated and sent for Gram stain and culture. Cultures also are obtained from all likely sources of the infection, including blood, sputum or wounds. The synovial fluid culture is always positive in non-gonococcal septic arthritis but often is negative for bacteria in early gonococcal arthritis. Infected synovial fluid usually is cloudy, with a high WBC count and a low glucose level. Joint x-ray films are often normal in the initial stages, but soon show demineralisation, bony erosions and joint space narrowing.

The infected joint is treated with rest, immobilisation, elevation and systemic antibiotics. Treatment with a broad-spectrum parenteral antibiotic is initiated before the results of culture are obtained. The medication may be changed or adjusted once the organism has been identified. Antibiotic therapy is continued for at least 2 weeks after inflammatory manifestations have abated. Frequent joint aspirations may be performed to remove excess fluid and pus and to monitor for the continued presence of bacteria. Surgical drainage may be performed if the hip joint is involved (because of the difficulty of aspirating this joint) or when medical therapy does not rapidly eliminate bacteria from the synovial fluid. Physical therapy is implemented during the recovery period to ensure maintenance of optimal joint function.

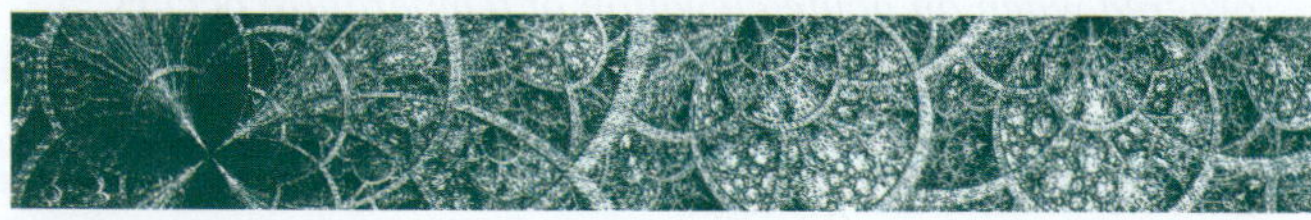

Nursing care

Septic arthritis can be frightening to the person who experiences a sudden onset of joint pain and swelling and is faced with the possibility of rapid functional loss of movement. Nursing care is both supportive and educative. People may be hospitalised for initial treatment with intravenous antibiotics. It is important to monitor the person's response to therapy, including systemic manifestations such as fever. Position the affected joint appropriately, using pillows to elevate it as needed. Splints or traction may be used to immobilise the joint. Warm compresses may be ordered for comfort. Active ROM exercises preserve joint mobility and should be initiated as soon as the doctor allows, with referral to a physiotherapist for exercise regimens appropriate for the individual.

The person with septic arthritis needs information about the disorder, its aetiology and its treatment. Teach the person how organisms may gain entry into the joint space. Discuss the role that the use of injected drugs and sexually transmitted infections play in septic arthritis and means to prevent infection if this is appropriate (e.g. using clean needles, practising safer sex). Refer the person to a drug treatment program if necessary. Emphasise the importance of complying with all aspects of the treatment plan to prevent joint destruction and disability.

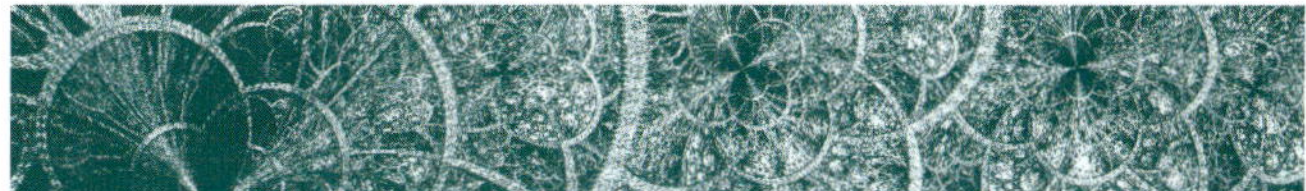

Neoplastic disorders

Bone tumours may be either primary (arising in the bone itself) or metastatic (seeded from a tumour elsewhere in the body). Like other tumours, bone tumours can be either benign or malignant.

THE PERSON WITH BONE TUMOURS

Benign bone tumours tend to grow slowly and do not often destroy surrounding tissues. Primary malignant tumours of the bone are rare, accounting for only about 1% of all adult cancers, with about 250 Australians diagnosed each year—secondary bone cancer is diagnosed more commonly (Cancer Council, 2019). Malignant tumours grow rapidly and metastasise. Virtually every malignant tumour can metastasise to bone. However, the most common metastatic bone tumours originate from primary tumours of the prostate, breast, kidney, thyroid and lung.

Primary bone tumours arise from bone tissue itself—that is, cartilage (chondrogenic), bone (osteogenic), collagen (collagenic) and bone marrow cells (myelogenic). The tissue type, neoplasm classification, sites and incidence of the most common primary bone tumours are summarised in Table 39.6. The focus for discussion in this section is care of the person with a primary bone tumour.

Pathophysiology

The aetiology of bone tumours is unknown but there is a connection between increased bone activity and the development of primary bone tumours. Bone tumours frequently occur when primary bone growth is at its peak in adolescence or is overstimulated during disease, such as Paget's disease.

Primary tumours cause bone breakdown, called *osteolysis*, which weakens the bone, resulting in bone fractures. Normal bone

TABLE 39.6 Description of common primary bone tumours

TISSUE TYPE	BENIGN	MALIGNANT	SITE	INCIDENCE
Chondrogenic (cartilage-forming tumours)	Osteochondroma—most common benign tumour		Pelvis, scapula, ribs	Higher in males
	Chondroma		Hands, feet, ribs, spine, sternum or long bones	Ages 30 to 50 Higher in males
		Chondrosarcoma	Femur, pelvis, ribs, head (epiphysis) of long bones	13% of malignant bone tumours Middle age and older Higher in males
Osteogenic (bone-forming tumours)	Osteoid Osteoma		Shaft (diaphysis) of long bones (i.e. femur, tibia)	Ages 20 to 30 Higher in males
		Osteosarcoma—most common malignant tumour	Long bones, knee	38% of malignant bone tumours Predominant in adolescents and people aged 50 to 60
Collagenic (collagen-forming tumours)		Fibrosarcoma	Femur, tibia	4% of malignant bone tumours Wide age distribution, but usually occurs in people aged 40 to 50 Higher in females
Myelogenic (tumours of bone marrow cells)	Giant cell tumour		Shaft (diaphysis) of long bones (i.e. femur, tibia, radius, humerus)	4–5% of bone tumours Wide age distribution Higher in females

adjacent to the tumour responds to tumour pressure by altering its normal pattern of remodelling. The bone's surface then becomes altered and the contours enlarge in the area of the tumour growth.

Malignant bone tumours invade and destroy adjacent bone tissue by producing substances that promote bone resorption or by interfering with a bone's blood supply. Benign bone tumours, unlike malignant ones, have a symmetrical and controlled growth pattern. As they grow, they push against neighbouring bone tissue. This weakens the bone's structure until it becomes unable to withstand the stress of ordinary use and frequently causes pathological fracture.

Manifestations

The three main manifestations of bone tumours are pain, a mass, and impaired function. Bone pain usually comes on slowly and lasts for as long as a week, is constant or intermittent, and may be worse at night. The mass is described as a swelling or lump on the bones that is firm, slightly tender and may be felt through the skin. The mass may interfere with normal movement and/or may cause the bone to break. The mass or swelling may go undetected due to slow growth and may be diagnosed as a result of another injury to the affected limb or surrounding area. Manifestations of bone tumours are listed in the 'Manifestations' box.

INTERPROFESSIONAL CARE

Treatment and care of the person with a bone tumour focuses on prompt diagnosis, removal of the tumour, prevention of complications and education.

Diagnosis

The diagnosis of a bone tumour is critical to the survival of the person and possible preservation of the affected limb. Diagnostic tests are described in the chapter 'A person-centred approach to assessing the musculoskeletal system'.

Radiological studies include x-rays, CT scans and MRI. X-rays show the location of the tumours and the extent of bone involvement. Benign tumours are characterised by sharp margins that are clearly separate from the surrounding normal bone. Metastatic bone destruction has a characteristic 'moth-eaten' pattern in which the growth has a less defined margin that cannot be separated from the normal bone. CT scan and MRI are useful in evaluating the extent of tumour invasion into bone, soft tissues and neurovascular structures. Percutaneous needle biopsy or needle biopsy at the time of surgery is used to determine the exact type of bone tumour.

Laboratory tests include an alkaline phosphatase (elevated with malignant bone tumour) and calcium levels (increased with massive bone destruction).

Treatments

As with other malignant tumours, bone tumours are treated with chemotherapy, radiation therapy and surgery.

CHEMOTHERAPY Chemotherapeutic agents are administered to shrink the malignant tumour before surgery, to control recurrence of tumour growth after surgery or to treat metastasis of the tumour. Chemotherapeutic agents used to treat bone tumours are listed in Box 39.5. See the chapter 'Nursing care of people with cancer' for further discussion of chemotherapy and its nursing implications.

MANIFESTATIONS Neoplasms of the musculoskeletal system

	MANIFESTATIONS
BONY SARCOMAS SITE	
Upper or lower extremity or pelvis	■ Worsening deep bony pain ■ Pain at night or during rest that may radiate and become severe ■ Muscular weakness or atrophy
Metaphysis of distal femur, proximal tibia, proximal humerus and pelvis	■ Soft tissue mass extending from bone with erythematous or warm skin over tissue mass ■ Change in ability to perform ADLs ■ Fever
SOFT TISSUE SARCOMAS SITE	
Upper or lower extremity and pelvis	■ Enlarging firm mass with irregular borders, which causes pain in surrounding soft tissue structures
Thigh; shoulder and pelvis	■ Erythema or warmth and venous dilation over skin ■ Muscular weakness and atrophy with limited range of motion change in ability to perform ADLs and change in gait ■ Paraesthesia with neurological involvement and distal swelling ■ Palpable local lymph nodes
Pelvis	■ Altered bowel and bladder habits or pain with intercourse

BOX 39.5 Chemotherapeutic agents used for musculoskeletal neoplasms

Alkylating agents
Ifosfamide
Cyclophosphamide

Antibiotics
Doxorubicin
Bleomycin

Antimetabolites
Methotrexate

Plant alkaloids
Vincristine

Synthetic agents
Cisplatin

RADIATION THERAPY Radiation therapy may be used in combination with chemotherapy. Radiation therapy is frequently applied to metastatic bone carcinomas as a method of pain control. It is also used to eliminate bony tumours or any remaining tumour after a surgical procedure. Radiation therapy is discussed in the chapter 'Nursing care of people with cancer'.

SURGERY The goal of surgery for the treatment of primary bone tumours is to eliminate the tumour completely. Tumours are removed either by excising the tumour itself or by amputating the affected limb. The type of procedure varies: removal of the tumour only, removal of the tumour along with a small margin of normal tissue surrounding the tumour, removal of the tumour and a wide zone of normal tissue, or removal of the tumour and part or all of the bone in which it lies. Cadaver allografts or metal prostheses often are used to replace missing bone, avoiding amputation. Care of the person undergoing amputation is discussed in the chapter 'Nursing care of people with musculoskeletal trauma'.

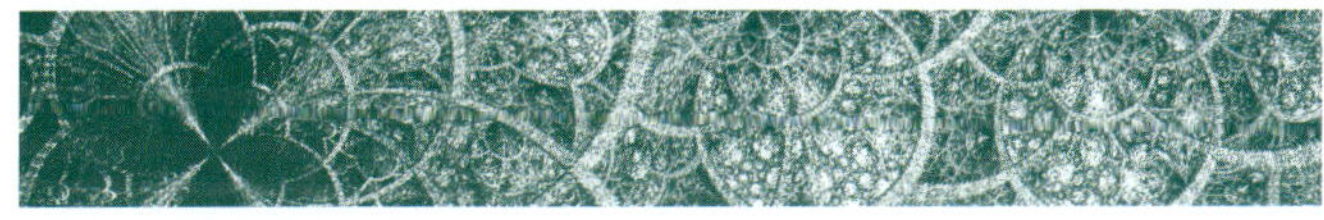

Nursing care

Nursing care for the person with bone tumours requires innovative interventions from the time of diagnosis through the rehabilitation phase. In the acute phase, problems associated with pain, lack of knowledge, immobility, coping and anxiety are foremost. If the person develops complications from treatment or if a malignancy metastasises, problems related to home health maintenance management, self-concept and prevention of further complications take priority. Palliative care and pain and symptom management may also be necessary if the malignancy progresses.

Nursing diagnoses and interventions

The person with a bone tumour requires nursing care to meet many health problems, including prevention of injury, relief of pain, assistance with mobility and teaching about the disease process and treatment.

Risk of injury

In the person with a bone tumour, changes in bone tissue can cause pathological fractures.

- Teach how to avoid falls or injury to the tumour site, such as by using assistive devices when walking and ensuring the home environment is not conducive to falling (e.g. remove throw rugs and use night lights). *Pathological fractures may occur at the tumour site because bone destruction can weaken the area.*
- Provide referral to physical or occupational therapy for fitting of and teaching about assistive devices for ambulating, such as a cane, crutches or a walker. *Assistive devices can reduce the risk of falling when the person has significant weakness of an extremity or when balance has been affected by treatment of the disease.*

Acute and chronic pain

In the person with a bone tumour, pain may be related to direct invasion of the tumour or to pathological fractures. People may experience both acute and chronic pain.

- Develop strategies for controlling both acute pain (from surgery, fracture or inflammation) and chronic pain (from progression of the disease). *Analgesics combined with non-pharmacological methods of pain control provide optimum relief of pain. Chronic pain, when mild in nature, is best managed with NSAIDs or aspirin. Moderate pain is best managed with a combination of codeine and NSAIDs. Severe pain is best relieved with long-acting or sustained-relief narcotic analgesics.*
- Provide assistive devices (e.g. canes, walkers, crutches) when the person ambulates. *Assistive devices lessen the pain by supporting weight bearing during ambulation.*

Impaired physical mobility

Pain, muscle wasting or surgical procedures can impair the physical mobility of the person with a bone tumour.

- Begin muscle-strengthening and active and passive ROM exercises immediately after surgery. A continuous passive motion (CPM) machine may be used after surgical procedures to either upper or lower extremities. *Muscle-strengthening exercises must be encouraged as soon as possible to prevent muscle wasting and shorten the rehabilitation period.*
- Encourage exercises that help strengthen the triceps muscles. *The triceps are major muscles in the arms and must be strengthened to assist in use of crutches or other assistive devices.*
- For the person who has undergone an amputation of a lower extremity, encourage quadriceps and gluteal setting exercises and leg raises. *These exercises will benefit the person when the rehabilitation period begins.*

Decisional conflict

A lack of knowledge about the diagnosis and treatment regimen can impair the person's ability to make informed decisions about the treatment plan.

- Discuss issues related to diagnosis, radiological evaluation, biopsy, surgery, chemotherapy, radiation therapy, potential complications, alternative therapies, risks, benefits, nursing management, discharge plans, home care and long-term treatment and follow up. *The person requires this information in order to make informed decisions about treatment. Support through this stage is imperative.*

Community-based care

The person with a primary bone tumour needs information about the disease, its potential consequences and treatment options. Present information in a matter-of-fact manner, taking time to listen to and address the person's and family's concerns. Discuss expected effects and potential side effects of surgery, chemotherapy and radiation therapy. Provide information about how to minimise side effects. Teach the postsurgical person about wound care, demonstrating dressing changes and stump care (if amputation has occurred). Provide the person with a list of local resources for obtaining supplies. Discuss activity and weight-bearing restrictions. Refer the person to physical therapy for teaching about ambulation and appropriate muscle-group-strengthening exercises. Ensure that the person who has experienced an amputation is working with or has a referral to a prosthetic specialist as required. For the person with metastatic disease, discuss hospice services and support groups for people with cancer.

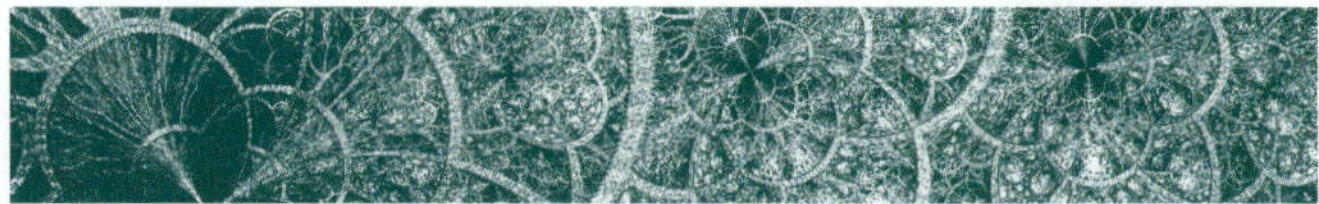

Connective tissue disorders

Connective tissue is the most abundant and widely distributed body tissue. It not only connects body parts but also provides support; forms bones, cartilage and the walls of blood vessels; and attaches muscles to bones. Connective tissue consists of three elements: (1) long fibres embedded in a (2) non-cellular ground substance and (3) cells specific to the class of connective tissue. Fibres made up primarily of collagen, a protein, are the most abundant in connective tissue.

Connective tissue disorders, also known as collagen diseases, are a group of immune-mediated disorders. Although they appear to have a genetic component, their cause is unknown. Because connective tissue and collagen are widely distributed in many varied tissues, these are systemic diseases with diverse manifestations.

THE PERSON WITH SYSTEMIC SCLEROSIS (SCLERODERMA)

Systemic sclerosis, also known as **scleroderma** ('hardening of the skin'), is a chronic disease characterised by the formation of excess fibrous connective tissue and diffuse fibrosis of the skin and internal organs. The cause of scleroderma is unknown, but genetic, immune and environmental factors are thought to play a role. Although this uncommon disease is distributed worldwide, a higher incidence is noted in coal and gold miners and in people exposed to certain chemicals such as polyvinyl chloride, epoxy resins and aromatic hydrocarbons.

Pathophysiology

Abnormalities in cellular immune function and activation of the immune system are believed to contribute to the development of scleroderma. Abnormal proliferation of fibrous connective tissue occurs in affected tissues, including the skin, blood vessels, lungs, kidneys and other organs. Excess collagen is produced and blood vessels can become narrowed.

Scleroderma may be either localised, affecting the skin only, or generalised (systemic sclerosis), with both skin and visceral organ involvement. Localised involvement may occur as irregularly shaped patches of skin (morphea) or a line of disease on the arm, leg or side of the face (linear scleroderma) (More than Scleroderma, 2022). Eighty per cent of people with generalised disease have limited involvement, frequently manifested by CREST syndrome, a combination of calcinosis (abnormal calcium salt deposition in the tissues), Raynaud's phenomenon, oesophageal dysfunction, sclerodactyly (localised scleroderma of the fingers) and telangiectasia (dilated, superficial blood vessels, sometimes called spider veins). The remainder of people with generalised systemic sclerosis have a diffuse form of the disease and a higher risk of visceral organ involvement. Infections and diseases of the cardiovascular, renal, pulmonary and central nervous systems are the most common causes of death in people with systemic sclerosis.

FAST FACTS

- Scleroderma affects over 5,000 people in Australia (Scleroderma Australia, 2020).
- Scleroderma affects women more often than men by a ratio of approximately 3:1.
- Although it can occur at any age from infancy to older adulthood, the onset of scleroderma typically occurs between the ages of 25 and 55 years (Scleroderma Foundation, 2022).

Manifestations

The initial manifestations of systemic sclerosis are usually noted in the skin, which thickens markedly. Diffuse, non-pitting swelling also is noted. As the disease progresses, the skin begins to atrophy, becoming taut, shiny and hyperpigmented (see Figure 39.10). Facial skin tightening leads to loss of skin lines and a pursed-lip appearance. Skin tightness may limit mobility, particularly of the face and hands. Other skin manifestations include telangiectasias (flat, red areas caused by dilation of small blood vessels, usually noted on the face, hands and in the mouth) and calcium deposits, usually noted around joints.

Arthralgias and Raynaud's phenomenon are common early manifestations of systemic sclerosis. Raynaud's phenomenon (intermittent attacks of small-artery vasospasm) is characterised by pallor of the fingers followed by cyanosis and then reactive hyperaemia with redness. Attacks are usually triggered by cold temperatures.

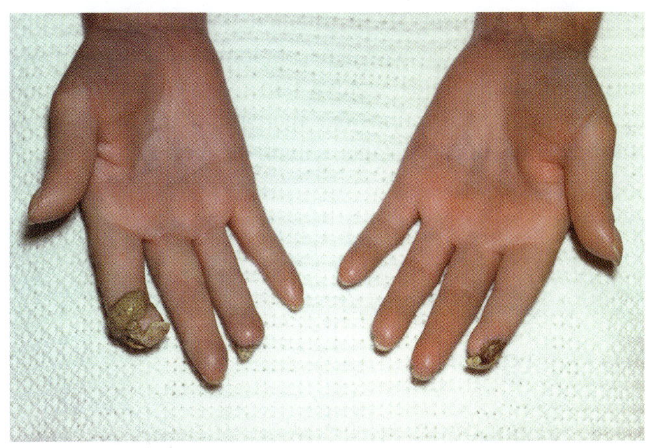

FIGURE 39.10 ***Characteristic skin changes of scleroderma***

Source: Mediscan/AlamyStockPhoto.

The person with visceral organ involvement may have varied symptoms. Dysphagia is common because the motility of the oesophagus is affected. Pulmonary involvement can lead to exertional dyspnoea due to impaired gas exchange and right-sided heart failure due to pulmonary hypertension. Involvement of the heart may cause manifestations of pericarditis and arrhythmias. Diarrhoea or constipation, abdominal cramping and malabsorption can occur when the GI tract is affected. Renal effects can lead to proteinuria, haematuria, hypertension and kidney failure.

The prognosis for localised and limited scleroderma is good; many people have a normal lifespan. The course of diffuse systemic sclerosis is highly variable. This disease is usually progressive; complete remission is rare.

INTERPROFESSIONAL CARE

The manifestations of systemic sclerosis often allow diagnosis with little or no testing. No cure is currently available; treatment is symptomatic and supportive.

Diagnosis

No single diagnostic test is specific for systemic sclerosis, although a titre of 1:40 or higher for antinuclear antibody (ANA) is the most sensitive for diagnosis. Other laboratory studies that are done include an ESR, which is typically elevated from the chronic inflammatory process and an FBC, which will demonstrate anaemia. A skin biopsy may be done to confirm the diagnosis.

Medications

Medications to treat systemic sclerosis are chosen based on the person's symptoms. Immunosuppressive agents and corticosteroids are of limited benefit, but they may be used to slow or prevent pulmonary fibrosis and in life-threatening disease. Penicillamine may be used to treat scleroderma and pulmonary fibrosis. Calcium channel blockers such as nifedipine or alpha-adrenergic blockers such as prazosin (Minipress) or nifedipine (Adalat) may be prescribed for people with Raynaud's phenomenon. When manifestations of oesophagitis accompany systemic sclerosis, H_2-receptor blockers such as cimetidine (Tagamet) or ranitidine (Zantac), antacids or omeprazole (Losec; protein pump inhibitor), which block all gastric secretion, may be ordered. Tetracycline or another broad-spectrum antibiotic may be prescribed to suppress intestinal flora and relieve symptoms of malabsorption. People with kidney disease are usually treated with angiotensin-converting enzyme (ACE) inhibitors such as captopril (Capoten) to control hypertension and preserve kidney function. End-stage kidney disease is managed with dialysis and transplantation.

Physical therapy

Physical therapy is an important part of the management of systemic sclerosis to maintain mobility of affected tissues—the hands and face, in particular. Because the mouth opening, if involved, becomes increasingly smaller as the disease progresses, stretching and strengthening of facial muscles can be vital to maintaining oral food intake.

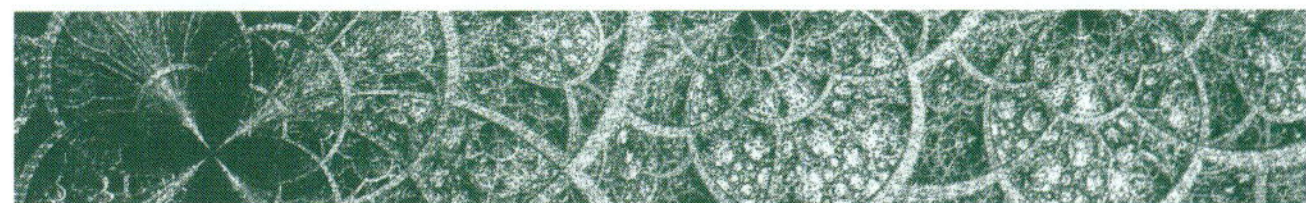

Nursing care

Nursing care needs of people with systemic sclerosis are individualised to the effects and manifestations of the disease, with interventions summarised in the following section.

Nursing interventions

Skin manifestations are present to some degree in nearly all people with scleroderma. Nursing care related to the skin focuses on maintaining skin integrity and flexibility. Measures to maintain supple skin are important because elasticity cannot be regained once it is lost. Apply moisturisers to prevent dryness and cracking. Protect the skin where it is stretched taut over joints or bony prominences. Perform ROM exercises to help prevent joint contractures due to increasingly tight skin.

Difficulty swallowing and recurrent oesophagitis may interfere with the person's nutritional status. Provide small, frequent meals. Consult with the dietitian and the person to determine which foods are easy to swallow. Keep the person in a sitting or Fowler's position after meals and elevate the head of the bed at night to minimise oesophageal reflux.

The dermatological and systemic effects of the disease may have significant psychological effects on the person, leading to feelings of helplessness and hopelessness and self-esteem disturbance. Establish an atmosphere of trust with the person. Listen actively and acknowledge concerns about the disease and its effects on the person's life and appearance. Encourage the person to share these concerns with family members and significant others. Provide referral to social services or counselling as appropriate.

The person with predominant pulmonary disease has nursing care needs similar to those of other people with restrictive respiratory disorders. If the person with systemic sclerosis has impaired renal function, nursing care is similar to that for people with chronic renal failure (see the chapter 'Nursing care of people with kidney disorders').

Community-based care

Teach the person with systemic sclerosis about the disease and introduce measures to help manage its effects. Stress the importance of good skin care and physical therapy exercises to maintain mobility, particularly of the hands and face. Discuss the need to avoid chilling (local and whole body) to prevent episodes of Raynaud's phenomenon. If needed, stress the need to stop smoking because of the vasoconstrictive effect of nicotine and the respiratory effects of the disease. Provide the person with information about manifestations of disease progression and organ involvement. Teach the person to report new or worsening symptoms to the doctor. In addition, suggest the following resources:

- Scleroderma Australia: www.sclerodermaaustralia.com.au
- Scleroderma New Zealand: http://scleroderma.org.nz.

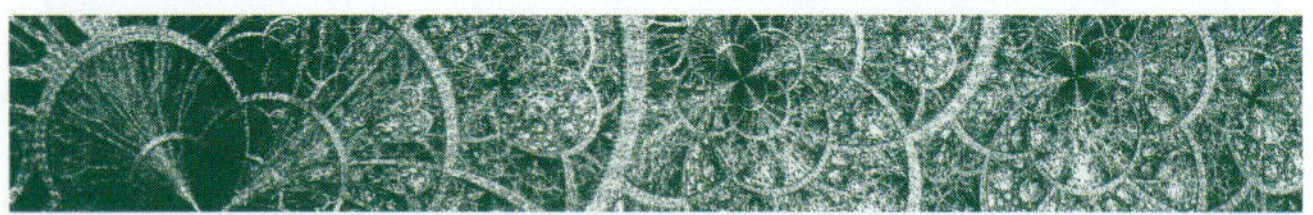

THE PERSON WITH SJÖGREN'S SYNDROME

Sjögren's syndrome is an autoimmune disorder that causes inflammation and dysfunction of exocrine glands throughout the body. Sjögren's syndrome primarily affects women, with a ratio of women to men at 9:1. The highest incidence is between the ages of 40 and 60 years. Although it can occur as a primary disorder, Sjogren's syndrome is often associated with other rheumatic disease, including rheumatoid arthritis, SLE, primary biliary cirrhosis, scleroderma, Hashimoto's thyroiditis and interstitial pulmonary fibrosis (Papadakis et al., 2022).

Pathophysiology

In this disease, exocrine glands in many areas of the body are destroyed by infiltration of lymphocytes and deposits of immune complexes. The salivary and lacrimal glands are particularly affected, leading to the characteristic manifestations of *xerophthalmia* (dry eyes) and *xerostomia* (dry mouth). People often experience dry, gritty-feeling eyes and may develop corneal ulcerations. Mucosal dryness affects taste, smell, chewing and swallowing and leads to increased dental caries. Parotid gland enlargement is common. Excess dryness can also affect the nose, throat, larynx, bronchi, vagina and skin. Systemic effects of Sjögren's syndrome include arthritis, dysphagia, pancreatitis, pleuritis, neurological manifestations including migraine and vasculitis. Nephritis may occur, but kidney failure rarely results. People with Sjögren's syndrome have a greatly increased risk of developing malignant lymphoma.

INTERPROFESSIONAL CARE

The diagnosis of Sjögren's syndrome is often based on the person's history and clinical presentation. A Schirmer's test, which measures the quantity of tears secreted in a 5-minute period in response to irritation, ocular staining and slit-lamp examination of the eye, may be performed. A definitive diagnosis can be made by biopsy of either the lacrimal or the salivary gland.

Treatment is supportive. Artificial tears are used to decrease eye irritation and dryness. The person can keep the mouth moist by drinking fluids, using a saliva substitute and chewing sugarless gum. Medications that increase mouth dryness, such as atropine and decongestants, should be avoided.

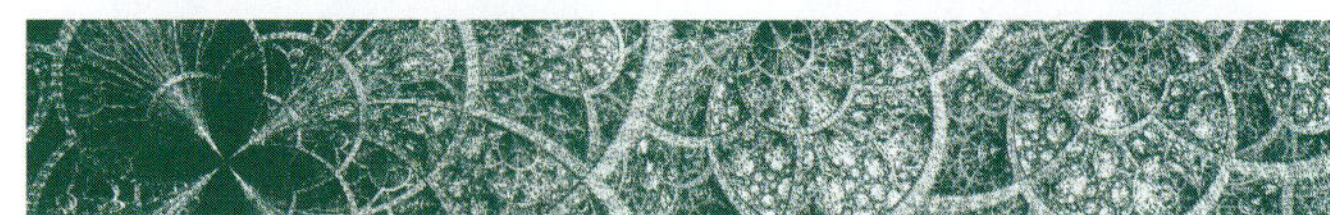

Nursing care

Nurses caring for people with Sjögren's syndrome need to teach measures to protect the person's eyes and oral mucosa. Instil artificial tears as needed. Encourage the person to sip fluids throughout the day. Provide frequent oral hygiene, particularly before and after meals. Ensure that the person has sufficient fluids to drink during meals, because fluids help with chewing and swallowing.

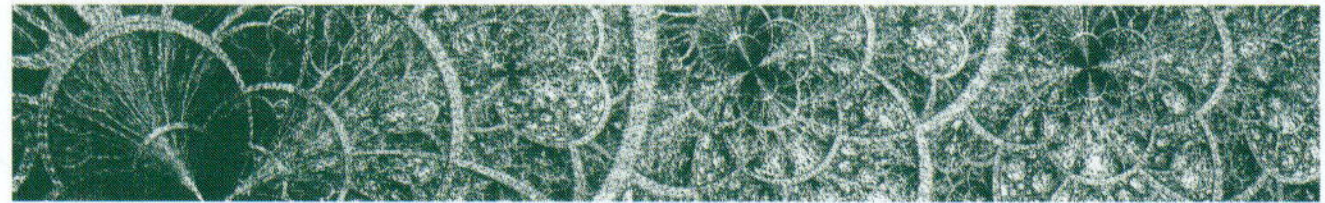

THE PERSON WITH FIBROMYALGIA

Fibromyalgia is a common rheumatic syndrome characterised by musculoskeletal pain, stiffness and tenderness. It affects around 2% of the population, with most being women in middle age. The cause is unknown, but possible aetiologies include sleep disorders, depression, infections and an altered perception of normal stimuli. Fibromyalgia can be a complication of hypothyroidism, rheumatoid arthritis or (in men) sleep apnoea. It closely resembles chronic fatigue syndrome, except that musculoskeletal pain is predominant in fibromyalgia whereas fatigue is a more significant feature of chronic fatigue syndrome.

Pathophysiology

No inflammatory, structural or physiological muscle changes have been demonstrated in fibromyalgia. A connection between fibromyalgia and the central nervous system has been studied, and there may be connections with biochemical, immunoregulation and metabolism abnormalities. Physical trauma such as spinal injury, physical and emotional stress and genetic predisposition have also been linked to the onset of fibromyalgia.

Manifestations

A gradual onset of chronic, achy muscle pain is typical, although the onset may be sudden, occasionally following a viral illness. The pain may be localised or involve the entire body. The neck, spine, shoulders and hips are often affected. Pain is produced by palpating localised 'tender points' (see Figure 39.11). Local tightness or muscle spasm may also occur. Systemic manifestations of fibromyalgia include fatigue, sleep disruptions, headaches, morning stiffness, painful menstrual periods and problems with thinking and memory (called the 'fibro fog'). Pain and fatigue are aggravated by exertion.

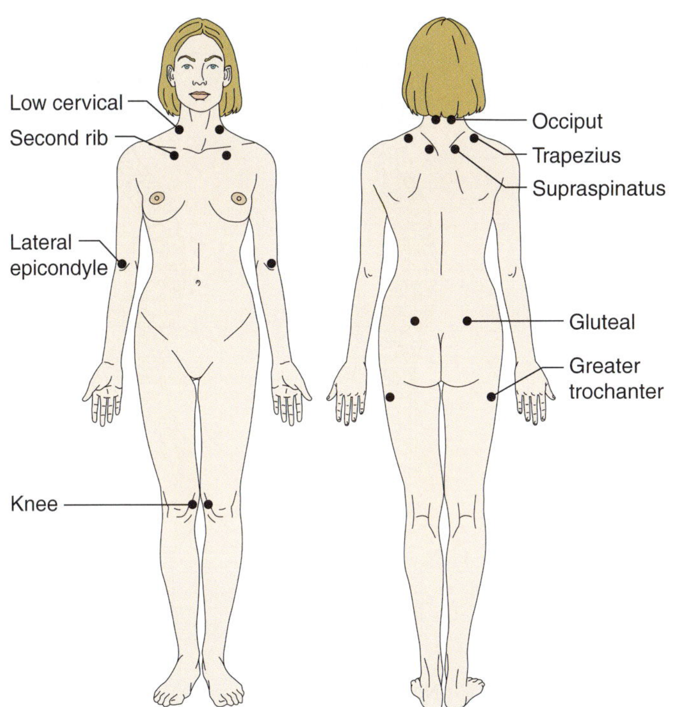

FIGURE 39.11 *Location of 'tender points' in fibromyalgia*

INTERPROFESSIONAL CARE

The diagnosis of fibromyalgia is based on the history and physical assessment. The criteria—developed by the American College of Rheumatology and used in Australia and New Zealand—that are used for diagnosis are a history of widespread pain that has been present for at least 3 months, and pain at 11 of the 18 tender points on palpation. There are no laboratory or diagnostic tests for the disorder, although tests may be performed to rule out other rheumatic disorders, such as rheumatoid arthritis or SLE. Fibromyalgia also may occur as a complication of hypothyroidism, so thyroid function studies are performed.

Acknowledgement of the person's symptoms and the chronic but treatable nature of this disease is important. Therapeutic measures include a program of structured aerobic exercise for conditioning, as well as stretching exercises.

Heated pool treatments with or without exercise have been shown to be beneficial. Evidence to support other treatments, such as cognitive behavioural therapy, hypnotherapy, music therapy, biofeedback, acupuncture and Tai Chi, is mixed (Emerge Australia, 2018).

Medical treatments regularly used in the treatment of fibromyalgia in Australia include tricyclic antidepressants (TCAs), which promote better sleep, paracetamol, non-steroidal anti-inflammatories (NSAIDs), anti-epileptic medications and other pain medications. Milnacipran, a selective serotonin and norepinephrine reuptake inhibitor (SNRI), has been listed for the management of fibromyalgia, assisting in the treatment of chronic pain and fatigue. It is currently listed as a restricted benefit in Australia. Medicinal cannabis has also been trialled for use in fibromyalgia with some positive effect (TGA, 2017).

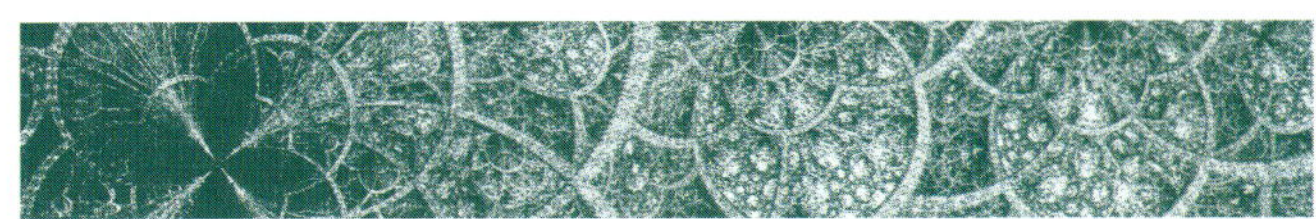

Nursing care

Nursing care for people with fibromyalgia is supportive and educational, and provided in community settings such as clinics and other primary care settings. It is important to validate people's concerns and reassure them that their symptoms are not 'all in the head'. Self-management strategies are important. Provide verbal and written instructions about the use of heat, exercise, stress-reduction techniques and prescribed medications to relieve manifestations. In addition, suggest the following resources:

- Arthritis Australia: https://arthritisaustralia.com.au
- Fibromyalgia Australia: https://fibromyalgiaaustralia.org.au.

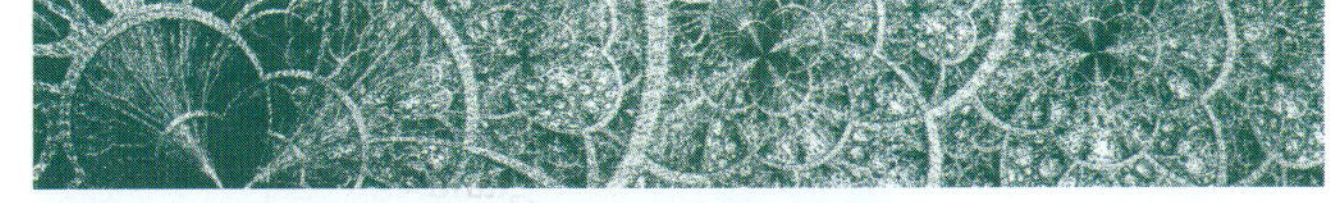

Structural disorders

Structural disorders of the musculoskeletal system most commonly affect the spine. The disorders discussed in this section are spinal deformities and lower back pain.

THE PERSON WITH SPINAL DEFORMITIES

Scoliosis and kyphosis are the two most common deformities of the spinal column. *Scoliosis* is a lateral curvature of the spine. *Kyphosis* is excessive angulation of the normal posterior curve of the thoracic spine. (See Figure 39.12.)

Scoliosis is usually diagnosed in adolescence, with girls more affected than boys by a ratio of 8:1. About 1 in 15 girls develop some scoliosis during their growing period, from about 9 to 14 years. In most cases, the curve is mild and does not need treatment. Only about 3 in 1,000 children have curves large enough to need treatment (Government of Western Australia, Child and Adolescent Health Service/WA Country Health Service, 2018). Idiopathic scoliosis is the most common form of the disorder, accounting for approximately 75% of cases. Congenital and neuromuscular disorders such as cerebral palsy, poliomyelitis and muscular dystrophy account for the rest.

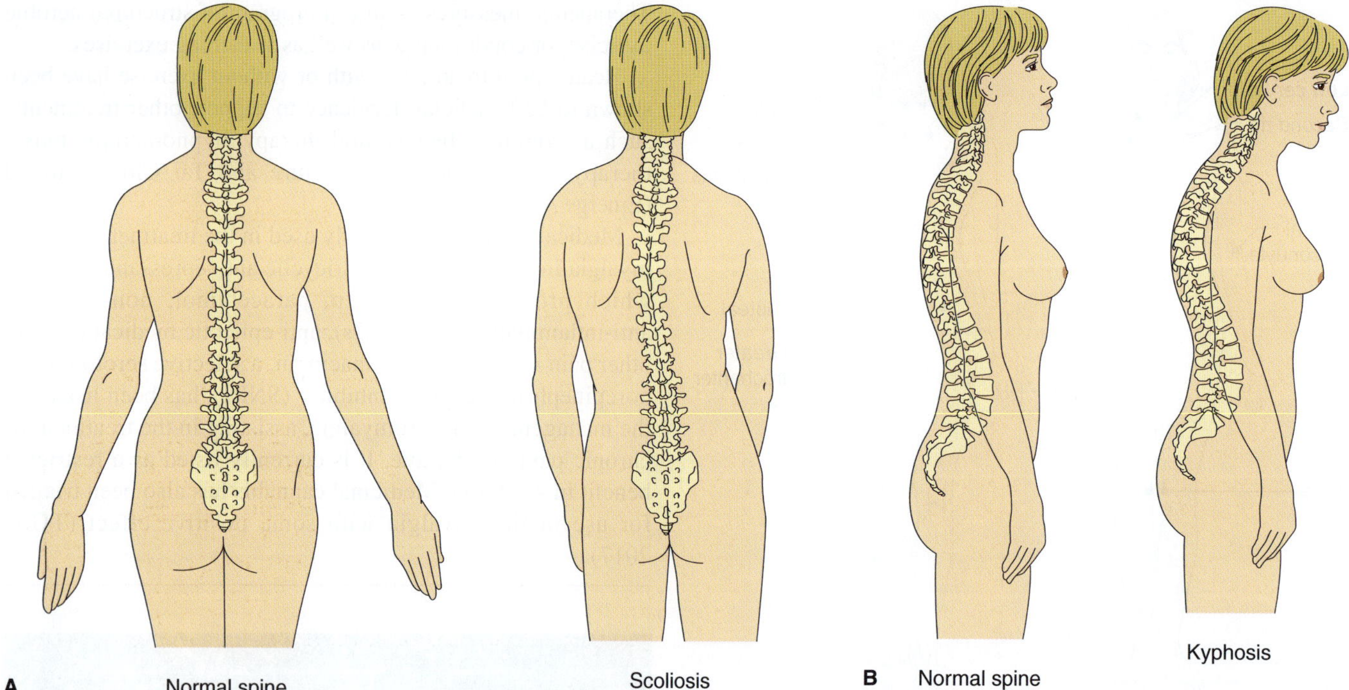

FIGURE 39.12 ***Common deformities of the spinal column. A, Scoliosis is a lateral curvature of the spine. B, Kyphosis is an exaggerated posterior curvature of the thoracic spine***

Pathophysiology

Scoliosis is most often idiopathic, meaning there is no known cause. It is broken down into age of onset: infantile, juvenile, adolescent or early/late onset. Other types are congenital, paralytic and neuromuscular. Detailed discussions of the causes and treatment of scoliosis and kyphosis in younger people can be found in paediatric nursing textbooks. This discussion focuses on the nursing care of adults with these disorders. The manifestations of scoliosis and kyphosis are listed in the 'Manifestations' box.

MANIFESTATIONS Scoliosis and kyphosis

SCOLIOSIS

- Asymmetry of shoulders, scapulae, waist creases
- Prominence of the thoracic ribs or paravertebral muscles on forward bend
- Lateral curvature and vertebral rotation on posteroanterior x-ray film

SEVERE SCOLIOSIS

- Back pain
- Shortness of breath
- Anorexia, nausea

KYPHOSIS

- Posterior rounding at the thoracic level
- Kyphotic curve of over 45 degrees on x-ray film

Scoliosis

Scoliosis is classified as *postural* when the small curve corrects with bending, and *structural* when the curve does not correct with bending. Most people requiring treatment have structural scoliosis, a curve caused by a fixed deformity.

The lateral curve that occurs in scoliosis is usually evident in the thoracic, lumbar or thoracolumbar regions of the spine. The vertebral bodies in these spinal regions can be rotated as well as curved to one side or the other.

As scoliosis emerges, the soft tissues (muscles and ligaments) shorten on the concave side of the curvature. Over time, progressive deformities of the vertebral column and ribs develop, causing one-sided compression of the vertebral bodies. The degree of compression and twisting varies according to the location of each vertebra within the curved portion of the spine.

If the lateral curvature is less than 40 degrees when the person's spine reaches maturity, the risk of further progression during adult life is small. However, the spine becomes unstable if the lateral curvature is greater than 50 degrees and curvature likely will worsen throughout the person's lifetime.

Scoliosis is usually first noted by the deformity it causes, such as one shoulder that is higher than the other, a prominent hip or a projecting scapula. Pain is present in severe cases, usually in the lumbar region. Pain also may be caused by pressure on the ribs or the crest of the ilium. Shortness of breath may result from diminished chest expansion and gastrointestinal disturbances may occur because of crowding of the abdominal organs.

Kyphosis

Like scoliosis, kyphosis is classified as postural or structural. Postural kyphosis is caused by a slumping posture. Structural kyphosis may result from congenital malformations or paediatric disorders such as rickets or poliomyelitis. However, kyphosis also may occur during adulthood from vertebral tuberculosis and Paget's disease, or from metabolic disorders such as osteoporosis and osteomalacia. The condition can also result from disc degeneration, surgical removal or radiation of intervertebral discs for the treatment of spinal cord tumours or cysts.

The manifestations of kyphosis include moderate back pain and increased curvature of the thoracic spine as viewed from the side ('hunchback'). Impaired mobility and respiratory problems may occur in cases of severe curvature.

INTERPROFESSIONAL CARE

Diagnosis of scoliosis and kyphosis is important to prevent severe spinal deformity in the adult. The person stands with the arms relaxed and hanging freely at the sides while the examiner evaluates the person from both the back and the front for symmetry of the shoulders, scapulae, waist creases and the length of the arms. The person then bends forwards and the examiner observes for prominence of the thoracic ribs or vertebral muscles. The person is then viewed from the side while the screener looks for increased thoracic rounding or lumbar swayback.

Diagnosis

Upright posteroanterior and lateral x-rays are used to confirm the diagnosis of curvature of the spine. For the person with scoliosis, the degree of curvature is measured by determining the amount of lateral deviation to the left or right. For the person with kyphosis, anteroposterior and lateral views typically reveal wedging of the vertebrae. MRI, CT scans and nerve and bone density testing may also be used.

Treatments

Scoliosis and kyphosis may be treated conservatively or with surgery.

CONSERVATIVE TREATMENT Braces, electrical stimulation and traction may be used to prevent progression of scoliosis and kyphosis in younger people whose skeletons have not yet matured. Unfortunately, these approaches are ineffective in adults. Conservative treatment for adults with scoliosis and kyphosis may include weight reduction, active and passive exercises and the use of braces for support.

SURGERY The use of surgery to correct spinal deformities depends on factors such as the degree of curvature and the person's overall physical, emotional and neurological status. Even with surgery, it is not possible to correct the abnormal curvature completely. The surgical procedure involves attaching metal reinforcing rods to the vertebrae and is usually performed using an anterior approach, although more severe curvature may require both an anterior and a posterior approach. The types of straightening devices used most frequently use bilateral rods with wire hooks or screws that stabilise the spine and correct the deformity.

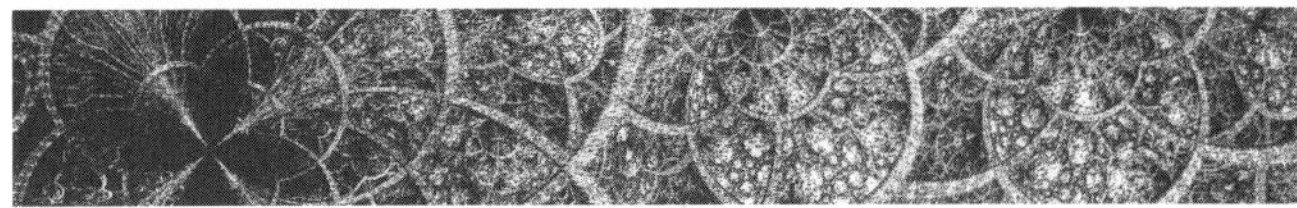

Nursing care

Nursing diagnoses and interventions

Nursing interventions focus on minimising the risk of injury and neurological impairment. Assist the person to minimise further damage by maintaining good posture and using braces as needed for support.

> **CONSIDERATION FOR PRACTICE**
> **Some braces do not allow the person to flex or hyperextend the spinal column.**

- Teach the person ways to reduce irritation of skin surfaces beneath the brace: wearing a smooth cotton T-shirt or cotton tube under the brace at all times, changing undergarments at least once daily and washing them with a mild soap. Undergarments should be changed more frequently in warmer weather. *The person wearing a brace is especially prone to skin breakdown and must take precautions to prevent it.*

> **CONSIDERATION FOR PRACTICE**
> **Teach the person to avoid lotion and body powders; they may irritate the skin.**

- Teach the person to loosen the brace during meals and for the first 30 minutes after each meal. *People have difficulty eating if the brace is tight. Loosening the brace during and after each meal will allow adequate nutritional intake and promote comfort.*
- Teach people how to apply the brace and explain ambulatory restrictions. *People requiring a brace need to learn how to apply the brace prior to ambulating. Ambulation is frequently restricted to walking rather than sitting for long periods.*
- Turn people who have undergone spinal surgery by using the log-rolling technique and ensure all cares are completed without misalignment of the spine. *People require a position change at least every 2 hours. The use of a turn sheet and sufficient assistance allow the nurse to maintain the person's proper body alignment during all turning procedures.*

Risk of peripheral neurovascular dysfunction

Surgical procedures can lead to neurological impairment in the person with a spinal deformity.

- Monitor the movement and sensation of lower extremities every 2 hours for the first 8 hours, then every shift and as needed. *Neurological assessment related to sensation and movement of the lower extremities is necessary because the surgical procedure is in close proximity to spinal nerves. Swelling of the surgical site can impinge on the spinal nerves and cause a loss of sensation and movement.*

Community-based care

People with structural scoliosis or kyphosis need reassurance that the condition was not caused by poor posture. If a brace is prescribed to relieve pain and other symptoms associated with the disorder, provide verbal and written instructions for wearing the brace, such as the number of hours per day it is to be worn and activity restrictions to follow when wearing or not wearing the brace. Teach the person how to protect and care for skin under the brace.

Surgical people need postoperative teaching regarding site care and activities. People who have spinal surgery often are allowed to ambulate fairly soon after surgery, but sitting may be restricted because of the stresses it places on the spine. Instruct the person to notify the healthcare provider if numbness, tingling, pain or weakness of an extremity develops after surgery.

Discuss the importance of not smoking and of avoiding respiratory infections for people with scoliosis or kyphosis that restricts respiratory excursion. Encourage these people to obtain pneumococcal pneumonia and influenza immunisations.

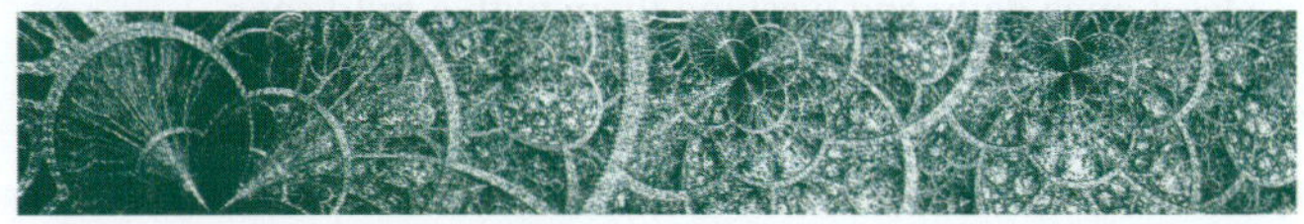

THE PERSON WITH COMMON FOOT DISORDERS

Hallux valgus, hammer toe and Morton's neuroma are common foot disorders that cause pain or difficulty in walking. All three disorders may be caused by wearing poorly fitting or confining shoes. These disorders are more prevalent among women.

Pathophysiology

Hallux valgus

Hallux valgus, commonly called a *bunion*, is the enlargement and lateral displacement of the first metatarsal (the great toe) (see Figure 39.13). Hallux valgus develops often when chronic pressure against the great toe causes the connective tissue in the sole of the foot to lengthen so that the stabilising action of the great toe is gradually lost. This can be caused by long-term wearing of narrow, pointed or high-heeled shoes. It can also be a congenital disorder and juvenile hallux valgus can occur with no history of tight-fitting shoe wear. The toe bends laterally away from the midline of the body and the metatarsophalangeal joint (MTP) is exposed to friction during walking and becomes enlarged. As the deformity progresses, calluses form over the metatarsal head and bursitis develops in the MTP. In severe cases, the lateral displacement of the great toe may approach 70 to 90 degrees and the second toe may be forced upwards, causing hammer toe.

Hallux valgus is obvious on physical examination of the foot. The person may report an inability to fit into shoes. Often, the person may report joint pain or pain around calluses. In advanced or severe cases, the first metatarsal joint may have limited range of motion, particularly in dorsiflexion, and crepitus (crackling or popping) may occur during joint movement.

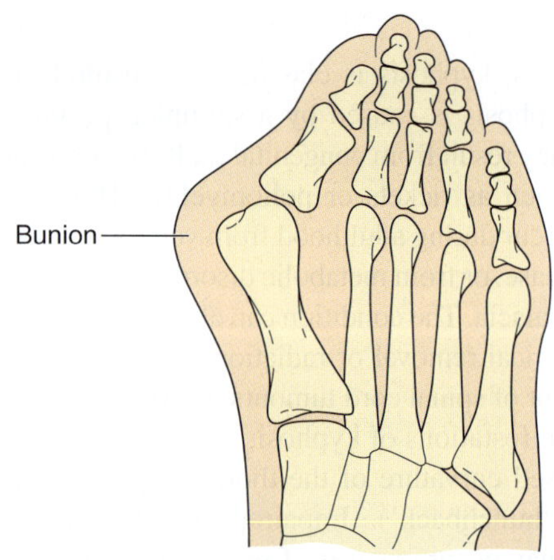

FIGURE 39.13 ***Hallux valgus (bunion)***

Hammer toe

Hammer toe (claw toe) is the dorsiflexion of the first phalanx with accompanying plantar flexion of the second and third phalanges. The condition may affect any toe, but the second toe is most commonly affected. People initially experience mild inflammation of the synovial membranes of the involved joints. As the deformity progresses, the dorsiflexed joint rubs against the overlying shoe, causing painful corns to develop.

Morton's neuroma

Morton's neuroma is a tumour-like mass formed within the neurovascular bundle of the intermetatarsal spaces (see Figure 39.14). The neuromas usually occur in only one foot, most frequently in the third web space. Like other

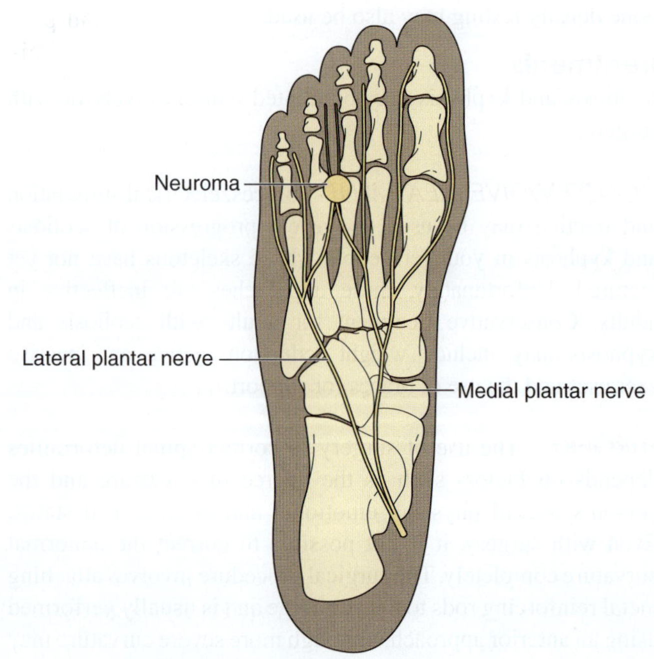

FIGURE 39.14 ***Morton's neuroma***

common foot disorders, Morton's neuroma is usually caused by wearing tight, confining shoes. The condition develops when repeated compression of the toes causes irritation and scarring of tissues surrounding the plantar digital nerve. The affected nerve becomes inflamed and swells. After repeated episodes of inflammation, the nerve fibres become fibrotic and a neuroma forms.

Manifestations include a burning pain at the web space of the affected foot that radiates into the tips of the involved toes. Weight bearing usually worsens any symptoms; removing the shoe and massaging the foot often relieves the pain. The neuroma may present as a palpable mass between the affected toes. The area over the neuroma usually is tender.

INTERPROFESSIONAL CARE

Care of the person with common foot disorders such as hallux valgus, hammer toe and Morton's neuroma focuses on relieving pain, correcting the structural deformity and preventing re-occurrence. In most cases, all three conditions are diagnosed by inspection. X-ray films of the affected foot are taken if the need for surgery arises.

Conservative treatment for common foot disorders usually involves the use of corrective shoes. Orthotic devices that cushion and stretch the affected joints may be placed within shoes or between the person's toes. For Morton's neuroma, metatarsal pads are used to spread the person's toes and decompress the affected nerve. Analgesics may be prescribed to relieve pain and inflammation. In severe cases, corticosteroid drugs may be injected into the affected joints or surrounding tissue to relieve acute inflammation.

Surgery is reserved for people with intractable toe deformities or pain. Hallux valgus is treated with bunionectomy; ligaments are lengthened or shortened as needed, and pins are drilled into place so the toe remains in position. Similarly, the correction of hammer toe also involves straightening the affected toe and inserting pins to retain the correction. A cast may be applied over the foot following surgery to correct toe deformities. Surgery for Morton's neuroma causes loss of sensation to a portion of the foot because removing the neuroma involves cutting out a portion of the plantar nerve.

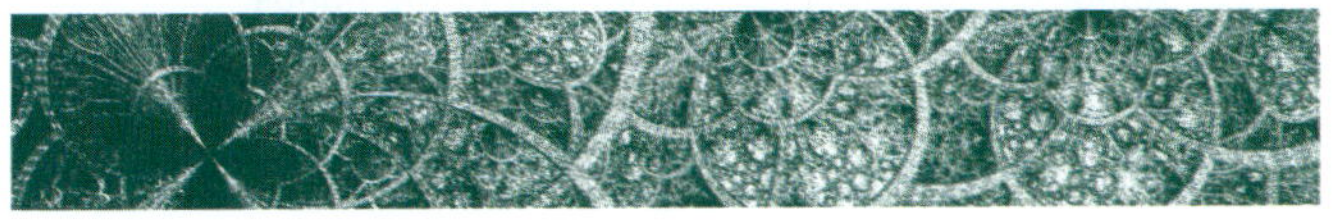

Nursing care

Nursing care for people with these foot deformities focuses on the same areas because the conservative treatment and preoperative and postoperative interventions are similar.

Nursing diagnoses and interventions

Pain relief, prevention of infection and person education are important components of the nursing care of people with foot disorders.

Chronic pain

In the person with a foot deformity, constant pressure of footwear over the involved joint can cause pain.

- Instruct people to wear corrective footwear to assist in the conservative treatment of foot problems. *Pain related to foot problems can result from improper footwear that does not provide proper toe room; in addition, heels higher than 2.5 cm can cause constant flexion and hyperextension problems. In some instances, the person must purchase special shoes or orthotics to ensure correct fit and relief of symptoms.*
- Suggest purchasing appropriate pads to wear over painful bunions, calluses/corns and the ball of the foot. *Protective pads are manufactured for specific foot problems; these include bunion pads, corn pads and metatarsal pads.*
- Instruct people to remove pads and inspect the skin every other day. *People who have difficulty reaching or observing the involved foot should ask another person to do the inspection for them. It is especially important to emphasise the need for inspection to people who have experienced loss of sensation of the feet due to such disorders as diabetes and chronic peripheral vascular disease.*

Risk of infection

Like all surgeries, foot surgery carries a risk of infection. This risk may be increased because of impaired peripheral circulation and exposure of the feet to the environment.

- Teach people proper care and cleaning of exposed pins implanted during the surgical procedure. *Pins inserted into soft tissue of the toes and bones are prone to becoming infected and can potentially result in osteomyelitis.*
- Teach people how to keep pins and casts dry while bathing or ambulating in inclement weather. *People must wear a plastic bag over the cast or pins when bathing or walking in rain or snow. When casts or pins are exposed in water, infection may result.*

Community-based care

For people in all age groups, teach the importance of well-fitting footwear. Discuss the long-term effects of wearing high-heeled shoes with constricting toes, with women in particular. Suggest alternatives for stylish footwear and encourage people to wear supportive and non-restrictive footwear at all times. Discuss the possible effects of bunions on balance and talk about safety measures to prevent falls and injury. Teach people techniques to relieve pressure on affected joints.

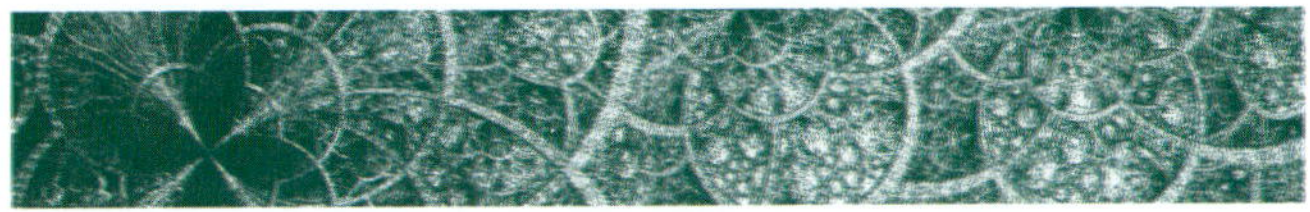

CHAPTER HIGHLIGHTS

- Metabolic bone disorders begin in the bone remodelling process and may result from ageing, calcium and phosphate imbalances, genetics and changes in hormone levels. The disorders include osteoporosis, Paget's disease, gout and osteomalacia.
- Osteoporosis is a major health problem in Australia, with fractures being the most common complication. Health promotion activities to prevent development of the disease include a calcium-rich diet, weight-bearing exercise and a healthy lifestyle.
- Gout is characterised by hyperuricaemia and the deposit of tophi in the subcutaneous tissues. Attacks of the disease typically begin with an acutely painful inflammation of the first joint of the great toe.
- Degenerative musculoskeletal disorders include osteoarthritis (OA) and muscular dystrophy (MD). OA is the most commonly occurring of all forms of arthritis and a leading cause of pain and disability in older adults. The disease is characterised by loss of cartilage in articulating joints and hypertrophy of bone at the articular margins. Pain and inflammation are most often conservatively managed with NSAIDs.
- If pain and disability are not controlled in people with arthritis, total joint replacements may be performed.
- Autoimmune and inflammatory disorders of the musculoskeletal system include rheumatoid arthritis (RA), ankylosing spondylitis (AS), reactive arthritis (ReA), systemic lupus erythematosus (SLE) and polymyositis.
- Although the cause of RA is unknown, it is believed to be a combination of genetic, environmental, hormonal and reproductive factors. RA is a systemic disease, affecting one or many joints with the risk of severe contractures and deformity and also causes fatigue, weakness, anorexia, weight loss and fever. The primary objectives of treatment and care are to reduce pain and inflammation, preserve function and prevent deformity.
- SLE is a chronic inflammatory connective tissue disease, affecting almost all body systems, including the musculoskeletal system. Skin lesions are a common manifestation, exhibited by a characteristic rash on the face. The person with SLE is at increased risk of infection.
- Osteomyelitis and septic arthritis are infectious musculoskeletal disorders. Osteomyelitis may be the result of a blood-borne pathogen, a contiguous infection or a complication of vascular insufficiency. Septic arthritis is a medical emergency, requiring immediate treatment to preserve joint function.
- Bone tumours may be benign or malignant, primary or metastatic. The primary manifestations of a bone tumour are pain, a mass and impaired function. Nursing care is directed towards teaching to prevent injury and interventions to relieve pain.
- Scleroderma is a chronic disease characterised by the formation of excess connective tissue and diffuse fibrosis of the skin and internal organs. It may be either localised or generalised. Other connective musculoskeletal disorders are Sjögren's syndrome and fibromyalgia.
- Structural musculoskeletal disorders affecting the spine are manifested by scoliosis, kyphosis and lower back pain. Those commonly affecting the feet are hallux valgus, hammer toe and Morton's neuroma.

CONCEPT CHECK

1 Although all of the following nursing diagnoses are important when planning care for the person with osteoporosis, which is most significant in terms of long-term disability?
1 *Chronic pain*
2 *Risk of falls*
3 *Activity intolerance*
4 *Acute pain*

2 You are preparing a teaching plan for a woman with osteoarthritis. Which group of medications should you prepare to discuss?
1 opioids
2 antibiotics
3 hormones
4 NSAIDs

3 You are monitoring the laboratory reports for a person with an acute attack of gout. Which of the following measurements would you expect to be increased?
1 haematocrit
2 uric acid
3 alkaline phosphatase
4 creatinine

4 What is a potential complication of both osteoporosis and osteomalacia?
1 infection
2 blood clots
3 fractures
4 contractures

5 You are assessing a woman who has come to an orthopaedic clinic complaining of knee pain. Which of the following assessments you made would indicate an increased risk of osteoarthritis?
1 being overweight by 15 kg
2 having a history of falls
3 eating a diet high in calcium
4 walking 30 minutes each day

6 A postoperative nursing care plan for a person who has had a total knee replacement includes monitoring vital signs and laboratory results. The rationale for these interventions is to:
1 teach the person the importance of these assessments
2 promote rapport between the person and the healthcare providers
3 ensure adequate circulation to the involved extremity
4 prevent the progression of infection

7 When comparing osteoarthritis and rheumatoid arthritis, what assessment finding would be different in the person with rheumatoid arthritis?
1 Health history includes weight loss and fever.
2 Abnormal joint findings are limited to the hands.
3 Stiffness is relieved by activity.
4 Heberden's nodes are located on the finger joints.

8 *Ineffective protection* is an appropriate nursing diagnosis for the person with SLE. What would be your most important intervention for the hospitalised person?
1 Monitor laboratory findings.
2 Provide appropriate skin care.
3 Practise careful handwashing.
4 Administer prescribed medications.

9 Of the different types of arthritis, which one is considered a medical emergency, requiring immediate diagnosis and treatment?
1 osteoarthritis
2 septic arthritis
3 reactive arthritis
4 gouty arthritis

BIBLIOGRAPHY

American Rheumatism Association (2022). *Diagnostic criteria for RA*. Retrieved from https://www.wheelessonline.com/

Arthritis Australia (2017). Retrieved from https://www.arthritisaustralia.com.au/

Arthritis Foundation (2022). *Osteoarthritis treatment*. Retrieved from https://www.arthritis.org/

Arthritis NSW (2022). *Rheumatoid arthritis*. Retrieved from https://www.arthritisnsw.org.au/

Australasian Society of Clinical Immunology and Allergy (2019). *Systemic lupus erythematosus (SLE)*. Retrieved from https://www.allergy.org.au/

Australian Bureau of Statistics (ABS) (2019). *National health survey*. Retrieved from https://www.abs.gov.au/

Australian Bureau of Statistics (ABS) (2022). *Health conditions prevalence*. Retrieved from https://www.abs.gov.au/

Australian Institute of Health and Welfare (AIHW) (2018a). *Osteoporosis snapshot*. Retrieved from https://www.aihw.gov.au/

Australian Institute of Health and Welfare (AIHW) (2018b). *Arthritis snapshot*. Retrieved from https://www.aihw.gov.au/

Australian Institute of Health and Welfare (AIHW) (2019). *What is gout?* Retrieved https://www.aihw.gov.au/

Australian Institute of Health and Welfare (AIHW) (2020a). *Chronic musculoskeletal conditions*. Retrieved from https://www.aihw.gov.au/

Australian Institute of Health and Welfare (AIHW) (2020b). *Osteoporosis*. Retrieved from https://www.aihw.gov.au/

Australian Institute of Health and Welfare (AIHW) (2022). *Osteoarthritis*. Retrieved from https://www.aihw.gov.au/

BMJ Best Practice (2018a). *Rheumatoid arthritis*. Retrieved from https://bestpractice.bmj.com/

BMJ Best Practice (2018b). *Osteomyelitis*. Retrieved from https://bestpractice.bmj.com/

Bone Health and Osteoporosis Foundation (2022). *Ibandronate sodium (Boniva®)*. Retrieved from https://www.bonehealthandosteoporosis.org/

Britton, C., Brown, S., Ward, L., Rea, S. L., Ratajczak, T. & Walsh, J. P. (2017). The changing presentation of Paget's disease of bone in Australia: A high prevalence region. *Calcified Tissue International*, *101*(6), 564–569. doi: 10.1007/s00223-017-0312-1

Bryant, B., Knights, K. Rowland, A. & Darroch, S. (2018). *Pharmacology for health professionals* (5th ed.). Sydney: Elsevier.

Cancer Council (2019). *Bone cancer*. Retrieved from https://www.cancer.org.au/

Cohen, A. & Drake, M. T. (2022). Epidemiology and etiology of osteomalacia. *UpToDate*. Retrieved from https://www.uptodate.com/

Emerge Australia (2018). *Fibromyalgia*. Retrieved from https://emerge.org.au/

Government of Western Australia, Child and Adolescent Health Service/WA Country Health Service (2018). *Scoliosis*. Retrieved from https://loretonedlands.wa.edu.au/

Hunter, D. (2015). Viscosupplementation for osteoarthritis of the knee. *New England Journal of Medicine*, *372*, 1040–1047.

Johns Hopkins Arthritis Center (2016). *Rehabilitation management for rheumatoid arthritis patients*. Retrieved from https://www.hopkinsarthritis.org/

Marieb, E. N. & Keller S. (2021). *Essentials of human anatomy & physiology* (12th ed.). Global edition. Upper Saddle River, NJ: Pearson.

Mayo Clinic (2020). *Arthroscopy*. Retrieved from https://www.mayoclinic.org/

Mayo Clinic (2021). *What is gout?* Retrieved from https://www.mayoclinic.org/

More than Scleroderma (2022). *What in the world is scleroderma?* Retrieved from https://www.morethanscleroderma.com/

Muscular Dystrophy Australia (2018). *Duchenne's muscular dystrophy*. Retrieved from https://www.mda.org.au/

Musculoskeletal Australia (2022). *Understanding gout*. Retrieved from https://msk.org.au/

National Health and Medical Research Council (NHMRC) (2009). *Guideline for the non-surgical management of hip and knee osteoarthritis*. Retrieved from https://www.nhmrc.gov.au/

National Health and Medical Research Council (NHMRC) & Ministry of Health (MoH) (2015). *Nutrient reference values for Australia and New Zealand*. Retrieved from https://www.nrv.gov.au/

National Institute for Health and Care Excellence (2017). *Management of osteoarthritis*. Retrieved from https://pathways.nice.org.uk/

Norris, T. L. (2018). *Porth's pathophysiology: Concepts of altered health states* (10th ed.). Philadelphia: Lippincott Williams & Wilkins.

Osteoporosis Australia (2022). *What you need to know about osteoporosis*. Retrieved from https://www.osteoporosis.org.au/

Paget's Association (2022). *Paget's disease*. Retrieved from https://paget.org.uk/

Papadakis, M., McPhee, S. & Rabow, M. (2022). *Current medical diagnosis and treatment* (61st ed.). New York: McGraw-Hill Education.

Persson, M. S. M., Sarmanova, A., Doherty, M. & Zhang, W. (2018). Conventional and biologic disease-modifying anti-rheumatic drugs for osteoarthritis: A meta-analysis of randomised controlled trials. *Rheumatology*, *57*(10), 1830–1837. https://doi.org/10.1093/rheumatology/key131

Scleroderma Australia (2020). Retrieved from https://www.sclerodermaaustralia.com.au/

Scleroderma Foundation (2022). *What is scleroderma?* Retrieved from https://www.scleroderma.org/

Singer, F. (2016). Paget's disease of bone. In K. R. Feingold, B. Anawalt, A. Boyce et al. (eds), *Endotext*. South Dartmouth (MA): MDText.com, Inc. https://www.ncbi.nlm.nih.gov/books/NBK279033/

Spondylitis Association of America (2022). *Reactive arthritis*. Retrieved from https://spondylitis.org/

Therapeutic Goods Administration (TGA) (2014). *NSAIDs and cardiovascular risks: Questions and answers*. Retrieved from https://www.tga.gov.au/

Therapeutic Goods Administration (TGA) (2017). *Guidance for the use of medicinal cannabis in the treatment of chronic non-cancer pain in Australia*. Retrieved from https://www.tga.gov.au/

UNIT 10 BUILDING CLINICAL COMPETENCE

Responses to altered musculoskeletal function

Clinical scenario

- You have been assigned to work with the following four people for the 0700 shift on an orthopaedic unit. Significant data obtained during report are as follows:
- Barry Drummond is a 70-year-old Indigenous man with type 2 diabetes mellitus who is 3 days postoperative with bilateral below-the-knee amputations. Vital signs are T 37.2°C, P 88, R 24, BP 150/92. He is complaining of feeling pain in his feet.
- Joyce Stevens is an 84-year-old who is 2 days postoperative for hip replacement surgery. Her vital signs are T 37.5°C, P 100, R 30 and shallow, BP 110/86. She is confused when spoken to. Petechiae have been noted on her arms and legs. She is complaining of difficulty breathing.
- James Gunning, a 21-year-old, was admitted with osteomyelitis of the upper right leg. He has a history of a gunshot wound to the leg. Vital signs are T 39.2°C, P 98, R 22, BP 138/80. He is scheduled for surgical debridement of the wound this morning. He is complaining of pain and requesting pain medication.
- Kim Wong is a 30-year-old who was admitted with manifestations of painful and swollen joints, muscle pain, pale and cyanotic fingers and toes and oedema of the legs and periorbital areas. Her vital signs are T 38.1°C, P 78, R 16, BP 108/72. She is complaining of extreme fatigue. She is to have blood drawn for complete blood count (FBC), anti-DNA antibody testing and serum complement levels.

Critical-thinking questions

1 In what order would you visit these people after report?
1.
2.
3.
4.

2 What top two priority nursing diagnoses would you choose for each of the people presented above? Can you explain, if asked, the rationale for your choices?

	Priority Nursing Diagnosis #1	Priority Nursing Diagnosis #2
Barry Drummond		
Joyce Stevens		
James Gunning		
Kim Wong		

3 After the amputation wound is dressed, what is the person taught to do to toughen the stump?
1. Dangle the stump for 20 minutes every hour while awake.
2. Push the stump into soft and then harder surfaces.
3. Elevate the stump on two pillows, keeping the knee straight.
4. Apply prosthesis over the compression dressing.

4 To prevent hip contractures in the person with an above-the-knee amputation, what does the nurse instruct the person to do?
1. Lie supine for short periods throughout the day.
2. Elevate the stump above the level of the heart.
3. Perform active range-of-motion exercises every 8 hours.
4. Avoid sitting in a chair for prolonged periods of time.

5 The nurse explains to the person with gout that a low-purine diet is recommended. The person understands a low-purine diet when which meal is ordered?
1. ham and asparagus casserole
2. chicken and potatoes
3. chilli and spinach salad
4. prawn and scallop pasta

6 The person's laboratory results are haematocrit of 28%, haemoglobin of 8 g/dL, WBC count of 4,000/mm^3, platelet count of 98,000/mL, eosinophil sedimentation rate of 100 mm/h, positive anti-DNA antibodies. What medical diagnosis is supported by these lab values?
1. systemic lupus erythematosus
2. rheumatoid arthritis
3. ankylosing spondylitis
4. polymyositis

7 People who have autoimmune diseases such as systemic lupus erythematosus are at increased risk of developing what disease?
1. chronic renal failure
2. hypertension
3. liver insufficiency
4. coronary heart disease

8 A prescription for ibuprofen (Nurofen) is given on discharge to the person with rheumatoid arthritis. Which toxic effects of the medication does the nurse instruct the person about?
1. diarrhoea, nausea and vomiting
2. blurred vision, tinnitus and headache
3. gastric irritation, ulceration and bleeding
4. dizziness, dry mouth and abdominal cramps

9 When performing a neurovascular assessment, which are included in the initial and focused assessments? (Select all that apply.)
1. pain
2. paroxysm
3. pallor
4. pulses
5. paresis
6. pallaesthesia
7. paraesthesia

10 Which person is at greatest risk of developing osteoporosis?
1. menopausal, Caucasian woman who smokes one packet of cigarettes a day
2. menopausal, Indigenous Australian woman who has diabetes and hypertension
3. premenopausal, underweight Asian woman who is allergic to dairy products
4. premenopausal, obese Indigenous woman who has a sedentary lifestyle

11 An older adult sprained an ankle after tripping on an uneven footpath. Which is the most important intervention?
1. Use a walker when ambulating.
2. Take anti-inflammatory and pain medications to reduce ankle pain.
3. Follow a regimen of rest, ice, compression and elevation.
4. Immobilise the ankle with an air splint.

12 Which actions by the nurse need to be followed when caring for the person with osteomyelitis?

1. Place the person in a private room and use gloves and gown with wound care and good handwashing.
2. Place the person in a semiprivate room with another infected person and use isolation precautions for both people.
3. Place the person near the nurse's station and use standard precautions when caring for the person.
4. Place the person at the end of the hall away from other people to prevent spread of infection and teach the person to use good handwashing.

Case study

William Comfort is a 24-year-old Caucasian male admitted with a compound fracture of the left femur. He states he was quad biking on a hillside footpath and was thrown from the vehicle. He slid approximately 30 metres down the hill on his left side. His fall was stopped when his foot became tangled in some bushes. On admission, his vital signs were T 37.7°C, P 100 and thready, R 24, BP 116/70. His height is 1.88 m and weight is 89 kg. Assessment revealed an open fracture of the left leg with bleeding and oedema around the open site and severe pain on movement of the leg. Popliteal and pedal pulses are difficult to palpate. His left leg is pale and cool to touch with a capillary refill of 4 seconds. He states his leg feels numb. Multiple lacerations and abrasions are noted on his left trunk and arm. He states he does not have any medical problems and has not seen a doctor in the past 5 years. He is employed as a computer technician. He lives in an apartment with two friends.

Blood is drawn for a baseline complete blood count (FBC) and urine is obtained for a urinalysis. An intravenous line is started in the right arm with Hartmann's solution infusing at 150 mL/h. He is given a tetanus toxoid immunisation and is medicated with morphine sulfate for pain. X-rays are taken of the left leg, left arm and abdomen. The wounds are cleansed with an antibacterial solution and antibiotic ointment is applied. He went to surgery for an open reduction of the left leg fracture and has been placed in skeletal traction to separate the bony fragments and reduce and immobilise the left leg fracture.

The pathophysiology of a femur fracture is a large amount of force applied to the shaft of the femur, resulting in breaking of the bone. An open fracture is diagnosed when the bone is broken with bone fragments protruding through the skin. Manifestations of a femur fracture are oedema and a deformed and painful thigh. The person is unable to move the hip or knee. Popliteal and pedal pulses are difficult to palpate. Capillary refill time is increased. Pallor and coolness indicate arterial compromise. Sensations to the leg may be burning, numbness, prickly feeling or stinging. Complications of a femur fracture include hypovolaemia, fat embolism, dislocation of the hip or knee, muscle atrophy and ligament damage.

Skeletal traction is the application of a pulling force through placement of pins into the bone. Pins are inserted under sterile conditions into the bone. One or more pulling forces may be applied to maintain alignment of the femur fracture. The disadvantages of skeletal traction are increased anxiety, increased risk of infection and increased discomfort.

When planning nursing care for Mr Comfort, the nursing diagnosis of *Impaired physical mobility* related to fracture of the left femur with skeletal traction is appropriate for implementing nursing interventions.

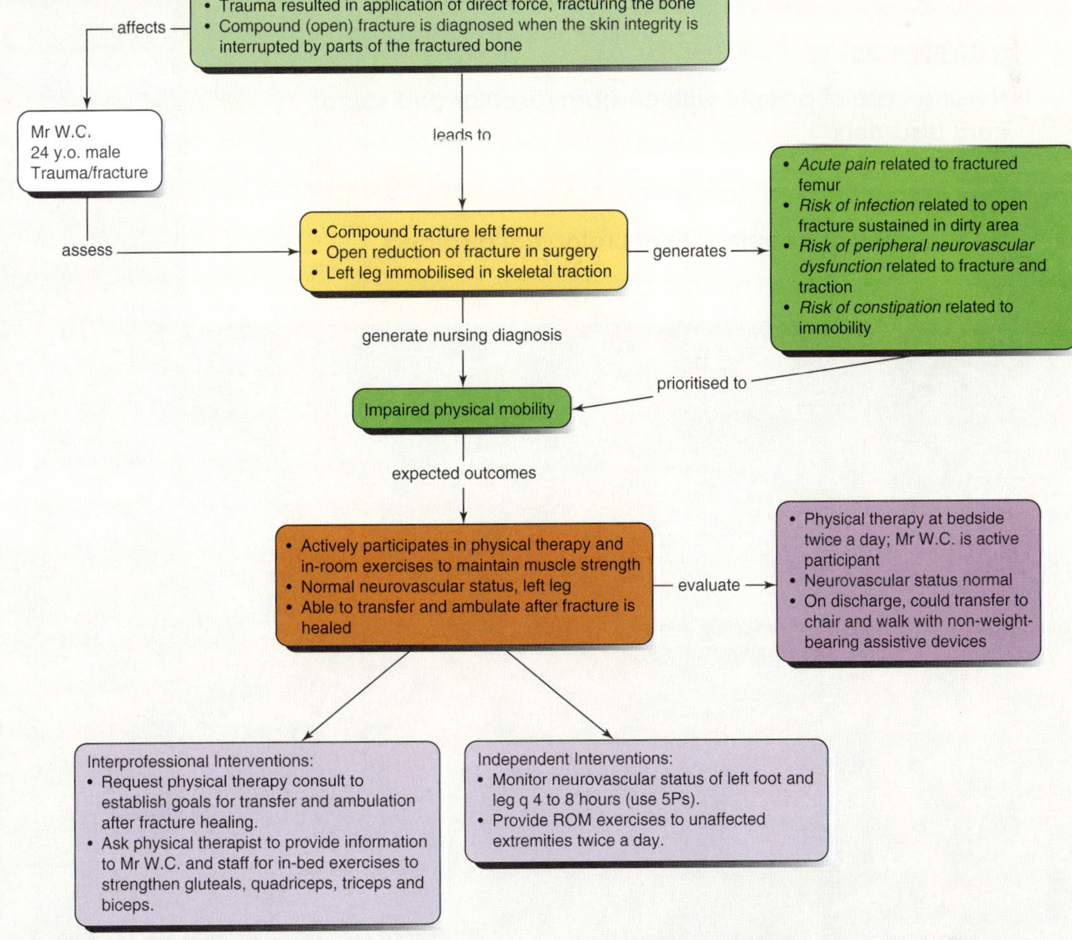

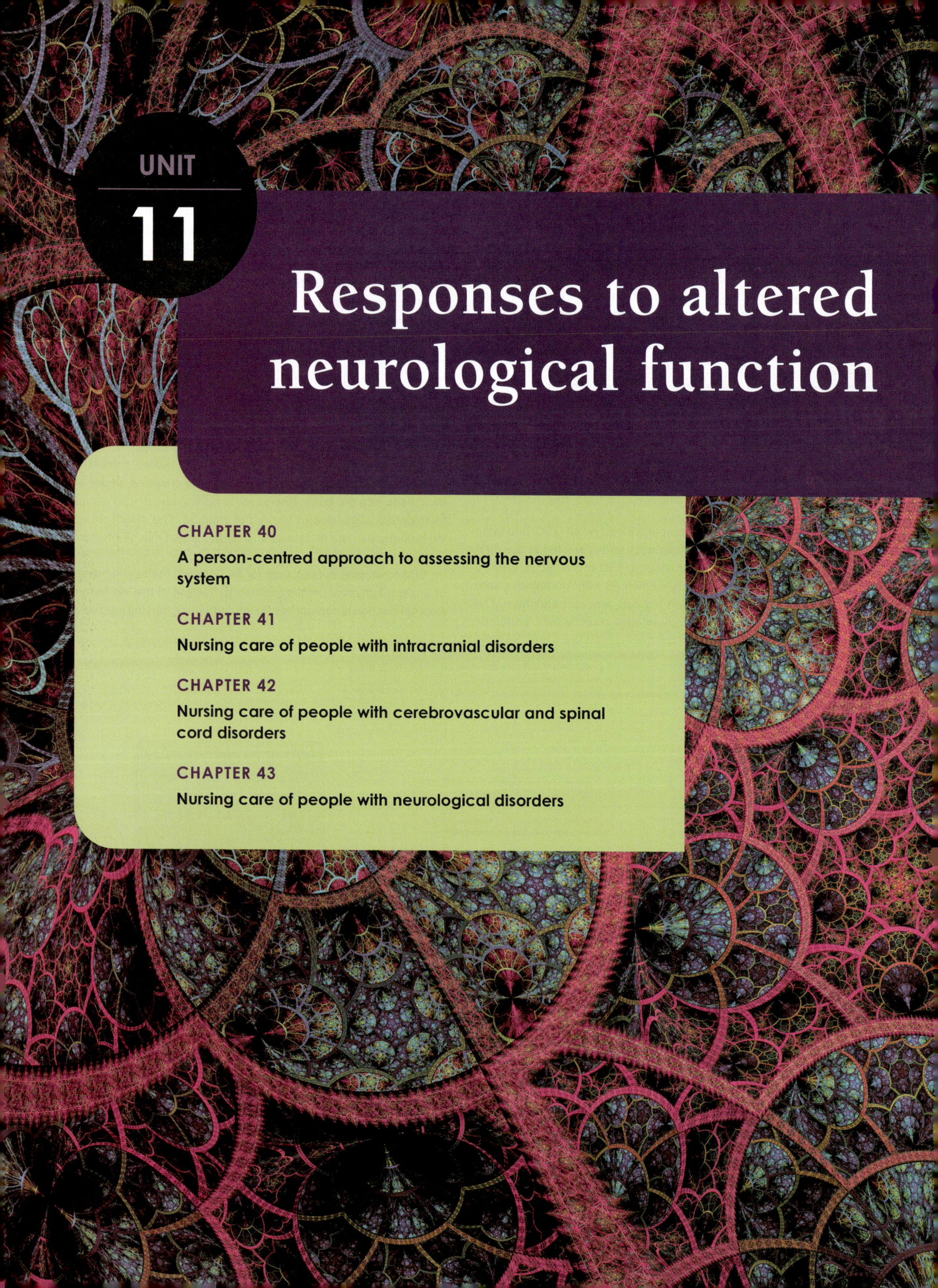

UNIT 11

Responses to altered neurological function

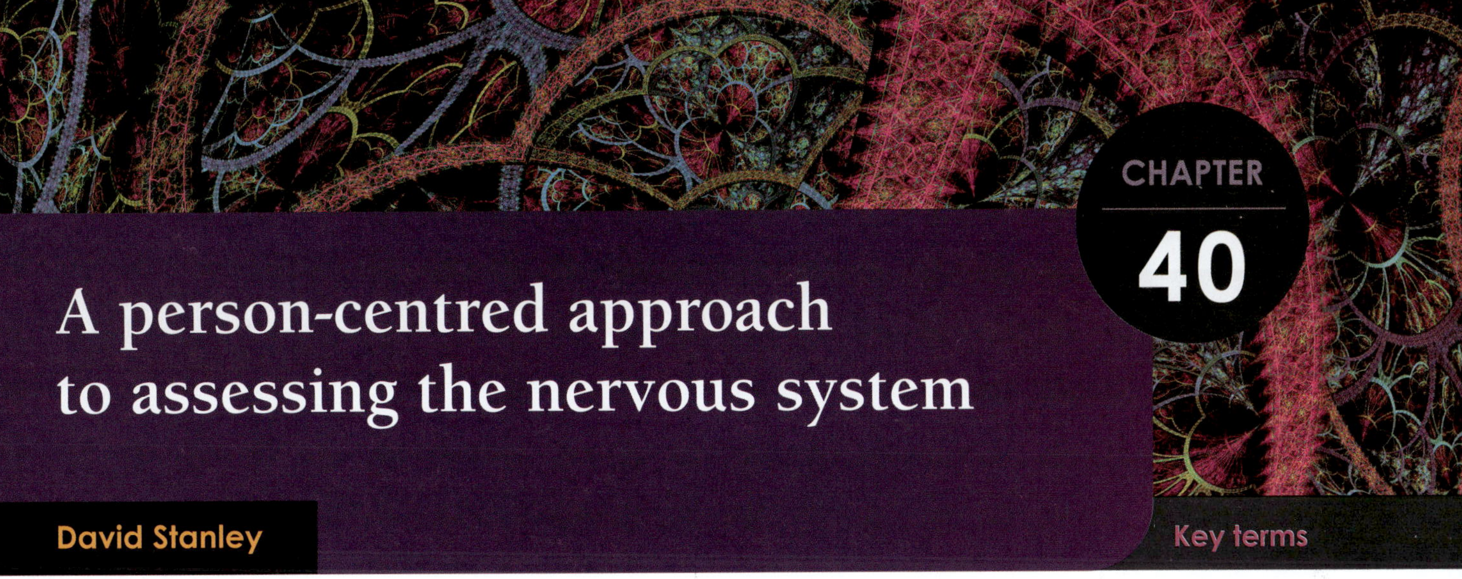

CHAPTER 40

A person-centred approach to assessing the nervous system

David Stanley

Key terms

anosmia 1495
aphasia 1494
ataxia 1499
decerebrate posturing 1501
decorticate posturing 1501
diaphoresis 1486
dysarthria 1494
dysphonia 1494
fasciculations 1497
flaccidity 1498
kinaesthesia 1497
spasticity 1498
tremors 1498

Learning outcomes

- Describe the anatomy, physiology and functions of the nervous system.
- Identify specific topics for consideration during a health history assessment interview of a person with a neurological disorder.
- Explain techniques for assessment of neurological function, including examinations of mental status, cranial nerves, sensory nerves, motor nerves, cerebellar function and reflexes.
- Identify manifestations of impairment of neurological function.
- Describe normal variations in assessment findings for the older adult.

Clinical competencies

- Conduct and document a health history for a person with or at risk of alterations in the neurological system.
- Conduct and document a physical assessment of neurological structures and functions.
- Perform specific neurological assessments for people with suspected meningeal irritation and for people who are disoriented or comatose.
- Monitor the results of diagnostic tests and report abnormal findings.

Equipment needed

- Cotton balls
- Safety pin
- Tongue depressor
- Tuning fork
- Reflex hammer
- Pencil and paper
- Penlight
- Printed materials
- Substances to test the senses of smell and taste

The nervous system coordinates body functions, muscle movements, senses, mental abilities and emotions. It collects information from the internal and external environments as sensory input, processes and interprets the input and causes responses that are manifested as motor or sensory output.

Anatomy, physiology and functions of the nervous system

The nervous system is divided into two regions: the central nervous system (CNS), which consists of the brain and spinal cord; and the peripheral nervous system (PNS), which consists of the cranial nerves, the spinal nerves and the autonomic nervous system.

Nerve cells, action potentials and neurotransmitters

The CNS and PNS are highly integrated and consist of only two types of cells: neurons, which receive impulses and send them on to other cells; and neuroglia, which protect and nourish the neurons.

Neurons

Each neuron consists of a dendrite, a cell body and an axon (see Figure 40.1). The dendrite is a short process (projection) from the cell body that conducts impulses towards (afferent) the cell body. Cell bodies, most of which are located within the CNS, are clustered in ganglia or nuclei. The cell bodies and dendrites comprise what is often called the grey matter of the CNS. The axon, a long process, conducts impulses away (efferent) from the cell body. Many axons are covered with a myelin sheath, a white lipid substance. It is interrupted at intervals in unmyelinated areas called nodes of Ranvier, which allow movement of ions between the axon and the extracellular fluid. The myelin sheath serves to increase the speed of nerve impulse conduction in axons and is essential for the survival of larger nerve processes. Myelinated nerve fibres comprise the white matter of the brain and spinal cord.

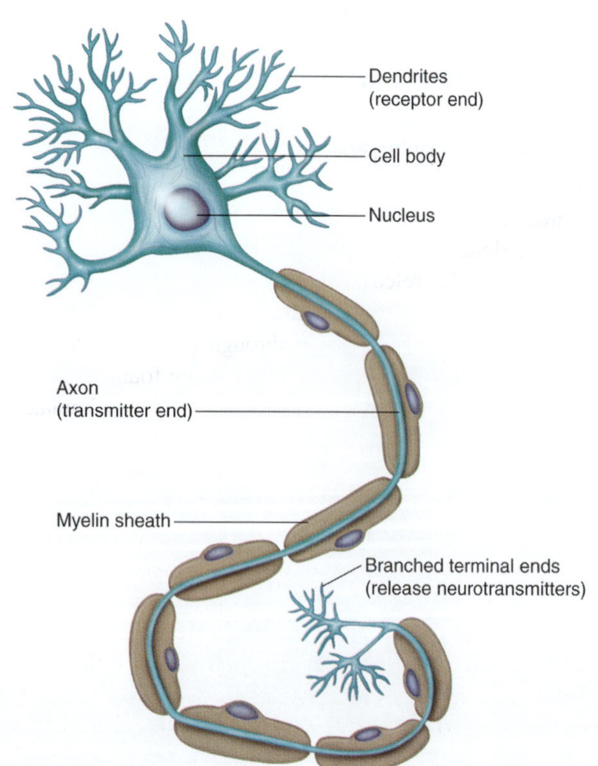

FIGURE 40.1 *A typical neuron*

Neuroglia

Neuroglia or glia cells are divided into seven types. Three types are found in the PNS: *enteric cells* which perform a number of functions within the enteric system related to both homeostasis and digestive processes; *satellite cells* which surround neuron cell bodies with ganglia; and *Schwann cells* which surround and form myelin sheaths around the larger nerve fibres in the PNS. The four types of neuroglia cells in the CNS are: *astrocytes* which support and bind and nourish the neurons; *oligodendrocytes* that produce myelin that surrounds axons within the CNS forming the myelin sheath; *ependymal cells* that line the central cavities of the brain and the spinal cord and function in the production of cerebral spinal fluid (CSF); and *microglia* which have a phagocytic function and assist in the removal of microorganisms or neuronal debris (see Figure 40.2).

Action potentials

Action potentials are movements of electrical charge along an axon membrane that allow neurons to communicate with other neurons and body cells. These movements are also referred to as impulses. They are initiated by stimuli and propagated by the rapid movement of charged ions through the cell membrane. When a neuron reaches a certain level of stimulation, an electrical impulse is generated and conducted along the length of its axon. The movement of impulses to and from the CNS is made possible by afferent and efferent neurons. Afferent neurons are also called sensory neurons and have receptors in skin, muscles and other organs and relay impulses to the CNS. Efferent, or motor, neurons transmit impulses from the CNS to cause some type of action or movement.

Nerve impulses occur when a stimulus reaches a point great enough to generate a change in electrical charge across the cell membrane of a neuron. A neuron that is not involved in impulse conduction is in a resting, or polarised, state, in which the number of positive ions in the fluid outside the cell membrane is greater than the number within the fluid of the cell. The chief regulators of membrane potential are sodium and potassium: sodium is the main positive ion in the extracellular fluid and potassium is the main positive ion in the intracellular fluid. In response to an electrical stimulus, the cell membrane becomes permeable to

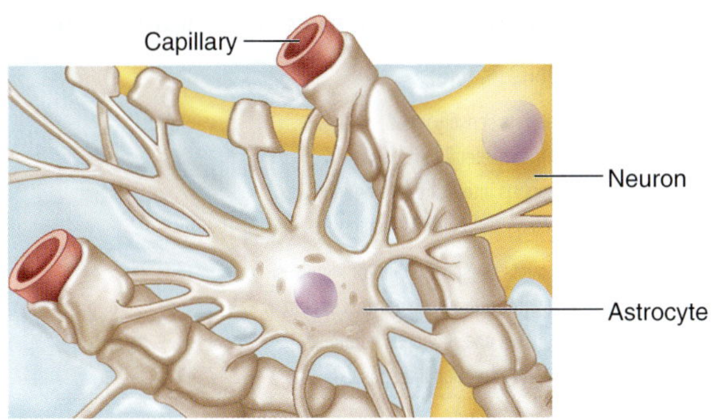

(A) Astrocytes are the most abundant CNS neuroglia

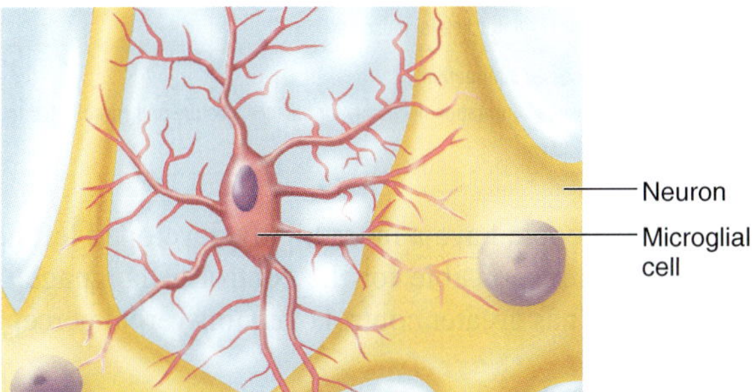

(B) Microglial cells are defensive cells in the CNS

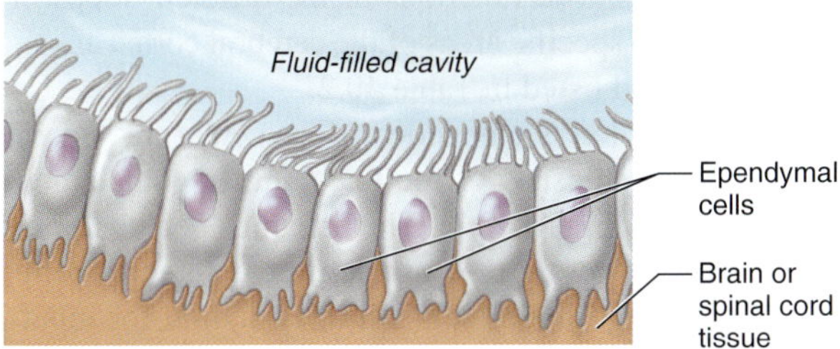

(C) Ependymal cells line cerebrospinal-fluid-filled cavities

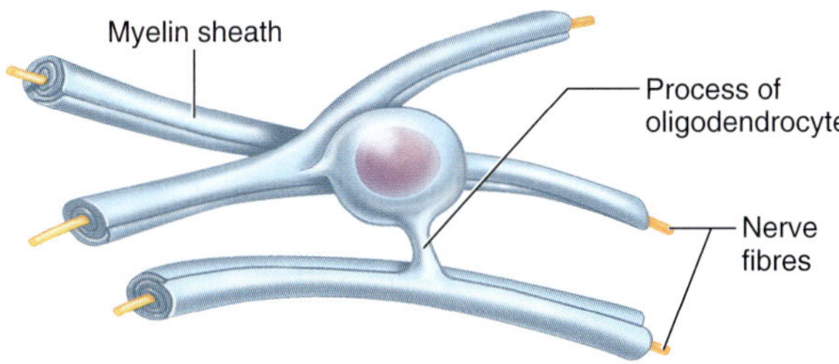

(D) Oligodendrocytes have processes that form myelin sheaths around CNS nerve fibres

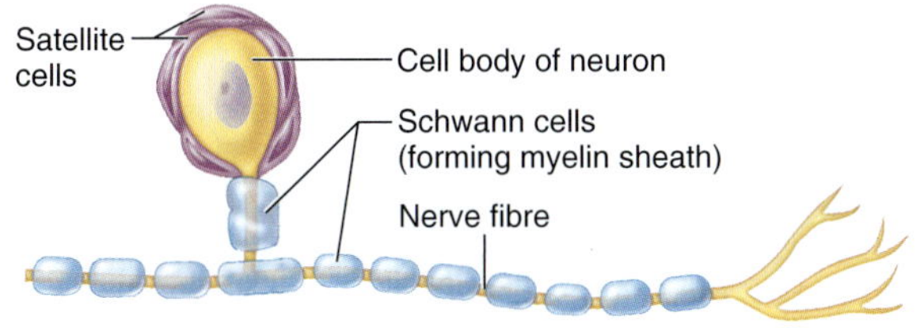

(E) Satellite cells and Schwann cells (which form myelin) surround neurons in the PNS

FIGURE 40.2 ***Neuroglia. A–D, Supporting cells of the CNS. E, Supporting cells of the PNS***

Source: Marieb & Hoehn (2010). *Human anatomy & physiology* (8th ed.), Figure 11.3, p. 388. Upper Saddle River, NJ: Pearson Education. © 2010. Printed and electronically reproduced by permission of Pearson Education, Inc.

sodium, which moves into the cell. This changes the polarity of the cell membrane and the neuron is said to depolarise. This event stimulates a nerve impulse to travel down the axon. When the charges and ions return to their original resting state, the neuron is repolarised. The events in an action potential are as follows:

1. Initially, sodium permeability increases. As the membrane is depolarised, sodium channels open and sodium rushes into the cell to a point of depolarisation. In other words, the charge inside of the cell becomes less negative in comparison to the outside of the cell.
2. This is followed by a decrease in sodium permeability, lasting only about 1 millisecond. The sodium gates close and the sodium influx stops.
3. The final event is an increase in potassium permeability. The potassium gates open, potassium rushes out of the cell and the cell interior becomes progressively less positive. The membrane potential moves back to its resting state and is repolarised.

The action potential is generated only at the point of the stimulus; but, once generated, it is propagated along the entire length of the axon regardless of whether the stimulus continues. Conduction of the impulse is faster in myelinated fibres, with the action potential rapidly moving from one node of Ranvier to the next. The conduction of the impulse is slower in unmyelinated fibres.

Neurotransmitters

Neurotransmitters are the chemical messengers of the nervous system. When the action potential reaches the end of the axon at the presynaptic terminal, a neurotransmitter is released and travels across the synaptic cleft to bind with receptors in the postsynaptic neuron dendrite or cell body. The neurotransmitter may either be inhibitory or excitatory. The excitatory neurotransmitter is almost always acetylcholine (ACh), which is rapidly degraded by the enzyme acetylcholinesterase. Noradrenaline (NA), which may be either excitatory or inhibitory, is another major neurotransmitter.

Nerves that transmit impulses through the release of ACh are called *cholinergic*. Receptors that bind ACh are found in the viscera, skeletal muscle cells and the adrenal medulla (where they stimulate the release of adrenaline). The effect of ACh binding may be either to stimulate or to inhibit a response.

Nerves that transmit impulses through the release of NA are called *adrenergic*. Receptors that bind NA are found in the heart, lungs, kidneys, blood vessels and all target organs stimulated by the sympathetic division except the heart. Adrenergic receptors are further divided into alpha and beta types. Alpha-adrenergic receptors help control such varied functions as arterial vasoconstriction and pupil dilation. Beta-adrenergic fibres may be either beta$_1$- or beta$_2$-receptors. Beta$_1$-receptors are found in the heart, where they regulate the rate and force of contraction. Beta$_2$-receptors are found in receptor cells of the lungs, arteries, liver and uterus; they help regulate bronchial diameter, arterial diameter and glycogenesis. Generally, binding of NA to alpha-receptors stimulates a response, whereas binding to beta-receptors inhibits a response.

Other major neurotransmitters include gamma aminobutyric acid (GABA), which inhibits CNS function; dopamine, which may be inhibitory or excitatory and helps control fine movement and emotions; and serotonin, which is usually inhibitory and controls sleep, hunger and behaviour and also affects consciousness.

The central nervous system

The central nervous system consists of the brain and spinal cord, highly evolved clusters of neurons that act to accept, interconnect, interpret and generate a response to nerve impulses originating throughout the body.

The brain

The brain is the control centre of the nervous system and also generates thoughts, emotions and speech. Males and females have equivalent brain sizes, averaging 1,450 g in weight for a female and 1,600 g for a male. The brain is surrounded by the skull, a bony structure that provides support and protection. There are four main regions of the brain: the cerebrum, the diencephalon, the brainstem and the cerebellum (see Figure 40.3). The general functions of these regions are summarised in Table 40.1.

The two hemispheres of the cerebrum account for almost 60% of brain weight. The surface of the cerebrum is folded into elevated ridges of tissue called gyri, which are separated by shallow grooves called sulci. Deep grooves, called fissures, further divide the surface of the cerebrum. The longitudinal fissure separates the hemispheres and the transverse fissure separates the cerebrum from the cerebellum. In addition, each cerebral hemisphere is divided into frontal, parietal, temporal and occipital lobes (see Figure 40.4).

The cerebral hemispheres are connected by the corpus callosum, a thick band of nerve fibres that allows communication between the two hemispheres. Each hemisphere receives sensory and motor impulses from the opposite side of the body. One of the cerebral hemispheres tends to develop more than

TABLE 40.1 General functions of the four regions of the brain

REGION	FUNCTIONS
Cerebrum	Interprets sensory input. Controls skeletal muscle activity. Processes intellect and emotions. Contains and controls memory.
Diencephalon	Conducts sensory and motor impulses. Regulates autonomic nervous system. Regulates and produces hormones. Mediates emotional responses.
Brainstem	Serves as conduction pathway. Serves as site of decussation of tracts. Contains respiratory nuclei. Helps regulate skeletal muscles.
Cerebellum	Processes information. Provides information necessary for balance, posture and coordinated muscle movement.

the other. Most people have a more highly developed left hemisphere, which is responsible for the control of language. The right hemisphere has greater control over non-verbal perceptual functions.

The cerebral cortex is the outer surface of the cerebrum. It consists of neuron cell bodies, unmyelinated fibres, neuroglia and blood vessels. The functions of the different lobes of the cerebrum and the specific areas of the cerebral cortex are shown in Figure 40.4 and listed in Table 40.2.

The diencephalon is embedded in the cerebrum superior to the brainstem. It consists of the thalamus, hypothalamus and epithalamus (see Figure 40.3). The thalamus begins to process sensory impulses before they ascend to the cerebral cortex. It serves as a sorting, processing and relay station for input into the cortical region. The hypothalamus, located inferior to the thalamus, regulates temperature, water metabolism, appetite, emotional expressions, part of the sleep–wake cycle and thirst. The epithalamus forms the dorsal part of the diencephalon and

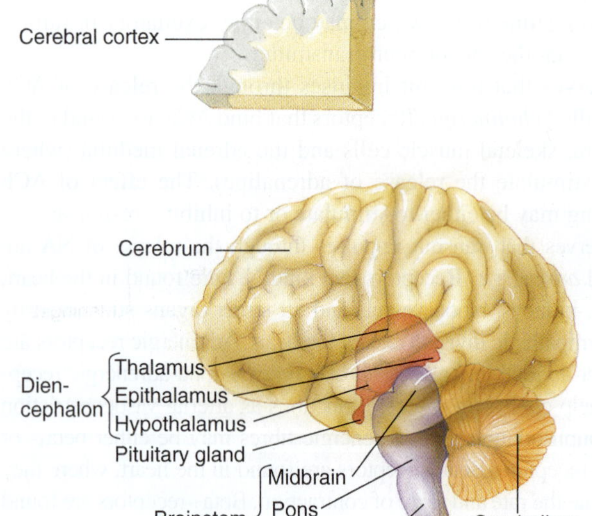

FIGURE 40.3 ***The four main regions of the brain***

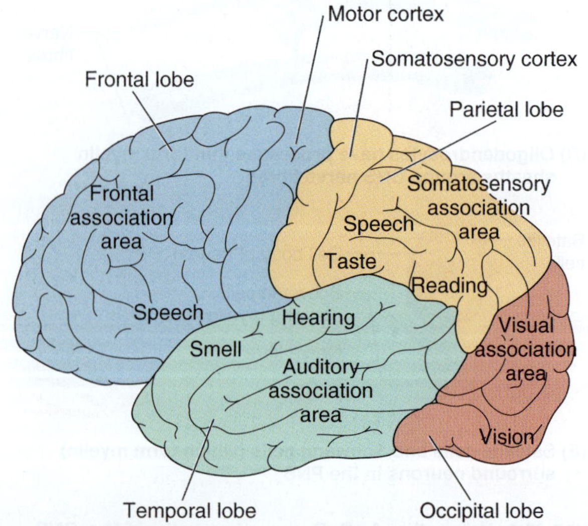

FIGURE 40.4 ***Lobes of the cerebrum and functional areas of the cerebral cortex***

TABLE 40.2 Functions of lobes of the cerebrum and areas of the cerebral cortex

AREA	FUNCTIONS
Parietal lobe (somatic sensory area of cerebral cortex)	Promotes recognition of pain, temperature and light touch. The left side receives input from the right side of the body, and vice versa.
Occipital lobe	Receives and interprets visual stimuli.
Temporal lobe	Receives and interprets olfactory and auditory stimuli.
Frontal lobe	Controls movements of voluntary muscles.
Primary motor area	Facilitates voluntary movement of skeletal muscles.
Speech area	Promotes understanding of spoken and written words.
Motor speech area (Broca's area)	Promotes vocalisation of words.

includes the pineal body, which is part of the endocrine system that affects growth and development.

BRAINSTEM The brainstem consists of the midbrain, pons and medulla oblongata (see Figure 40.3). The midbrain is a centre for auditory and visual reflexes. In addition, it functions as a nerve pathway between the cerebral hemispheres and lower brain. The pons is located just below the midbrain. It consists mostly of fibre tracts, but it also contains nuclei that control respiration. The medulla oblongata, located at the base of the brainstem, is continuous with the superior portion of the spinal cord. Nuclei of the medulla oblongata play an important role in controlling cardiac rate, blood pressure, respiration and swallowing.

The cerebellum is connected to the midbrain, pons and medulla. Its functions include coordinating skeletal muscle activity, maintaining balance and controlling fine movements.

VENTRICLES The ventricles are a network of four interconnecting cavities and are filled with cerebrospinal fluid (CSF). They are linked by ducts that allow the CSF to circulate. One lateral ventricle is located within each hemisphere. These communicate with the third ventricle through the foramen of Monro. The third ventricle communicates with the fourth ventricle through the cerebral aqueduct that runs through the midbrain. The cerebral aqueduct is continuous with the central canal of the spinal cord.

CEREBROSPINAL FLUID Cerebrospinal fluid is formed by the choroid plexus, which are groups of specialised capillaries located in the brain ventricles. Derived from blood plasma, CSF is a clear and colourless liquid consisting of 99% water and contains protein, sodium, chloride, potassium, bicarbonate and glucose in tightly controlled values (see Table 40.3). The usual amount of CSF ranges from 80 to 200 mL, averaging about 150 mL, and is replaced several times each day. CSF is normally produced and absorbed in equal amounts. CSF circulates from the lateral ventricles of the cerebral hemispheres into the third ventricle, through the midbrain and into the fourth ventricle. Some CSF flows down the centre of the spinal cord as the rest of it circulates into the subarachnoid space and returns to the blood through

TABLE 40.3 Normal laboratory values for cerebrospinal fluid

COMPONENT	NORMAL VALUE
Appearance	Clear and colourless
pH	7.35
Specific gravity	1.007
WBCs	0-8 mm^3
Protein	0.15-0.45 g/L
Glucose	2.8-4.4 mmol/L
Chloride	118-132 mEq/L
Pressure	< 200 mmH_2O

the arachnoid villi. CSF forms a cushion for the brain tissue, protects the brain and spinal cord from trauma, helps provide nourishment for the brain and removes waste products of cerebrospinal cellular metabolism.

MENINGES The brain and spinal cord are covered and protected by connective tissue membranes called meninges. The meninges form divisions within the skull, enclose venous sinuses and contain CSF. There are three layers to the meninges (see Figure 40.5). The outermost double layer, the dura mater, is attached to the inner surface of the skull. The middle layer is the arachnoid mater, which encloses the entire CNS and forms the subarachnoid space that contains CSF. The innermost layer, the pia mater, clings to the brain, spinal cord and segmental nerves and is filled with small blood vessels.

CEREBRAL CIRCULATION AND THE BLOOD–BRAIN BARRIER The brain receives about 750 mL of blood each minute and uses 20% of the body's total oxygen uptake. The large amount of oxygen is necessary for metabolism of glucose, which is the brain's sole source of energy. Blood flow to the brain is mostly controlled by autoregulatory or local

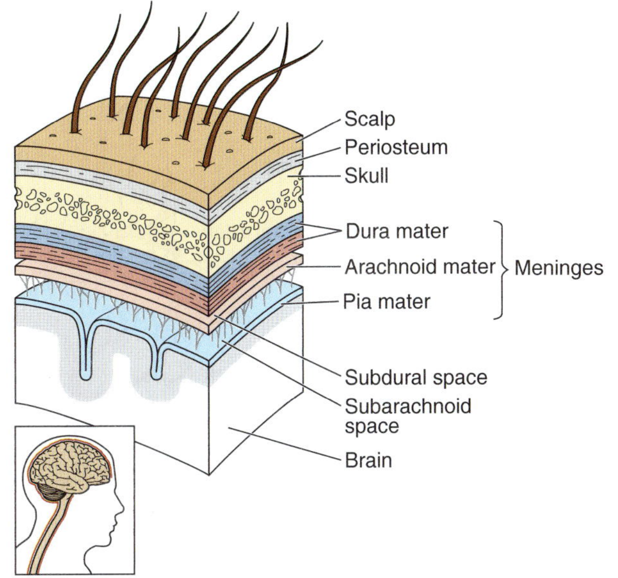

FIGURE 40.5 ***Anatomy of the meninges***

mechanisms that respond to the brain's metabolic needs. Autoregulation is defined as the ability of the brain to maintain constant cerebral blood flow despite changes in systemic blood pressure. At least three metabolic factors affect cerebral blood flow: carbon dioxide, hydrogen ion and oxygen concentrations. Of these, increased carbon dioxide is the main stimulus for vasodilation with resultant increased cerebral blood flow.

The anterior part of the brain is supplied with blood by the two internal carotid arteries, and the posterior part of the brain is supplied with blood by the vertebral arteries. The internal carotid artery branches into further arteries: the ophthalmic, posterior communicating, anterior choroidal, anterior cerebral and middle cerebral. The brainstem and cerebellum receive their blood supply from the basilar artery. These main arteries are connected by small anterior and posterior communicating arteries, which form a circle of connected blood vessels called the circle of Willis (see Figure 40.6). This circle serves as a protective device, providing alternative routes for brain tissues to receive their blood supply.

The capillaries in the brain have low permeability because the cells that compose their walls join at very tight junctions and are surrounded by a basement membrane and by the processes of supporting cells in the brain (called astrocytes). As a result, the brain is protected from many harmful substances in the blood. This blood–brain barrier allows lipids, glucose, some amino acids, water, carbon dioxide and oxygen to pass through it, thus maintaining a controlled environment. Substances such as urea, creatinine, proteins, some toxins and most antibiotics generally cannot pass this barrier and enter brain tissue. However, injury to or infection of the brain may cause increased permeability of the blood–brain barrier, altering concentrations of proteins, water and electrolytes.

THE LIMBIC SYSTEM AND THE RETICULAR FORMATION The limbic system and the reticular formation are functional brain systems. These systems, made of networks of neurons, communicate across areas of the brain.

The limbic system consists of structures that form a ring of tissue in the medial side of each hemisphere, surrounding the upper portion of the brainstem and corpus callosum. The limbic system integrates and modulates input to make up the affective part of the brain, providing emotional and behavioural responses to environmental stimuli.

The reticular formation is located through the central core of the medulla oblongata, pons and midbrain. This system has widespread connections throughout the brain and relays sensory input from all body systems to all levels of the brain. The reticular formation includes the reticular activating system (RAS). The RAS is a stimulating system for the cerebral cortex, keeping it alert and responsive to incoming sensory stimuli while filtering out repetitive or unwanted stimuli. The sleep centre inhibits activity of the RAS, and drugs and alcohol may depress it. Other parts of the reticular formation include motor nuclei that help maintain muscle tone and coordinated movements through interconnections with spinal nerves and the vasomotor and cardiovascular regulatory centres, which are part of autonomic regulation of the cardiovascular system.

The spinal cord

The spinal cord extends from the medulla to the level of the first lumbar vertebra (see Figure 40.7). It serves as a centre for conducting messages to and from the brain and as a reflex centre. The spinal cord is about 42 cm long and 1.8 cm thick. The cord is protected by the vertebrae, the meninges and CSF. The grey matter of the cord is on the inside and the white matter is on the outside, the reverse of the arrangement in the brain.

The spinal cord is surrounded and protected by 33 vertebrae: 7 cervical, 12 thoracic, 5 lumbar, 5 sacral and 4 fused vertebrae, which form the coccyx. Each vertebra consists of a body and a vertebral arch. This arch encloses a space called the vertebral

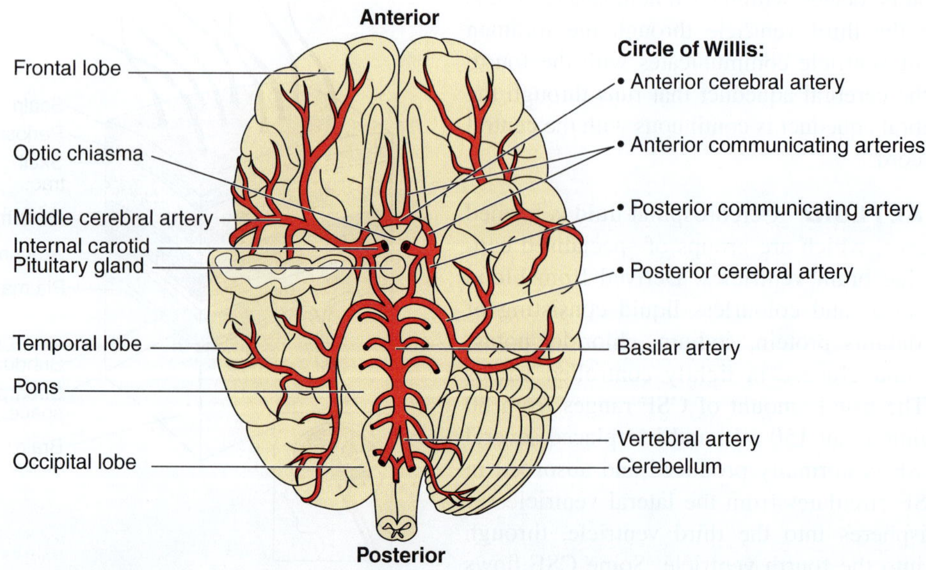

FIGURE 40.6 ***The main arteries serving the brain and the circle of Willis***

foramen. The vertebral foramina of all the vertebrae form the vertebral canal through which the spinal cord passes. Intervertebral foramina are spaces between the vertebrae through which spinal nerve roots pass as they exit the vertebral column.

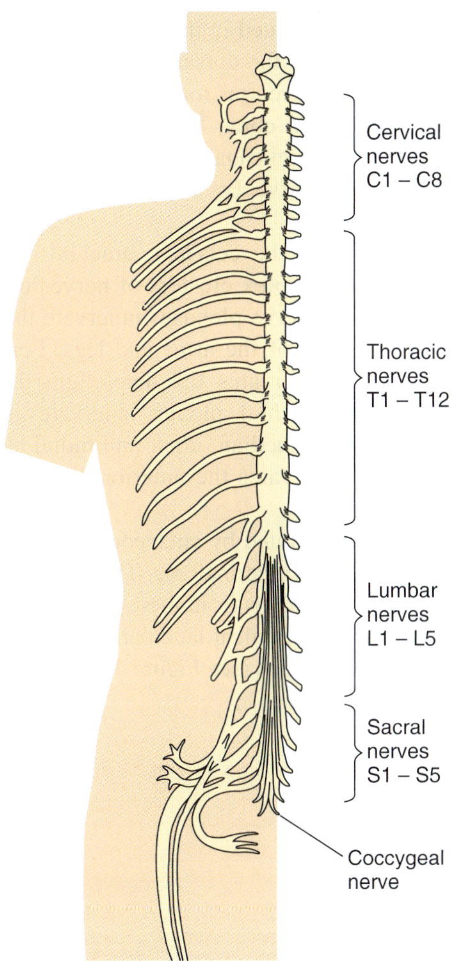

FIGURE 40.7 *Distribution of spinal nerves*

Intervertebral discs are located between each of the movable vertebrae. Each disc is made of a thick capsule surrounding a gelatinous core called the nucleus pulposus. Ligaments surround the vertebral column and provide mobility and protection.

The roots of 31 pairs of spinal nerves, divided into the cervical, thoracic, lumbar, sacral and coccygeal nerves, arise from the cord (see Figure 40.7). Each separates into posterior (sensory) and anterior (motor) roots. Damage to the posterior roots results in loss of sensation, whereas damage to the anterior roots results in flaccid paralysis.

FUNCTIONS OF THE SPINAL CORD AND SPINAL ROOTS Messages to and from the brain are conducted via ascending (sensory) pathways and descending (motor) pathways (see Figure 40.8). The main ascending tracts are the lateral and anterior spinothalamic tracts, which carry sensations for pain, temperature and crude touch; and the posterior tracts, which carry sensations for fine touch, position and vibration. The lateral and anterior corticospinal (pyramidal) tracts are descending tracts consisting of fibres that originate in the motor cortex of the brain and travel to the brainstem and then down the spinal cord. They mediate voluntary purposeful movements and stimulate certain muscular actions while inhibiting others. They also carry fibres that inhibit muscle tone. The rubrospinal, anterior and lateral reticulospinal and tectospinal (extrapyramidal) tracts include the pathways between the cerebral cortex, basal ganglia, brainstem and spinal cord outside the pyramidal tract. They maintain muscle tone and gross body movements.

UPPER AND LOWER MOTOR NEURONS Upper motor neurons, such as those of the corticospinal and extrapyramidal tract, carry impulses from the cerebral cortex to the anterior grey column of the spinal cord. Damage to upper motor neurons results in increased muscle tone, decreased muscle strength, decreased coordination and hyperactive reflexes. Lower motor neurons begin in the anterior grey column of the spinal cord

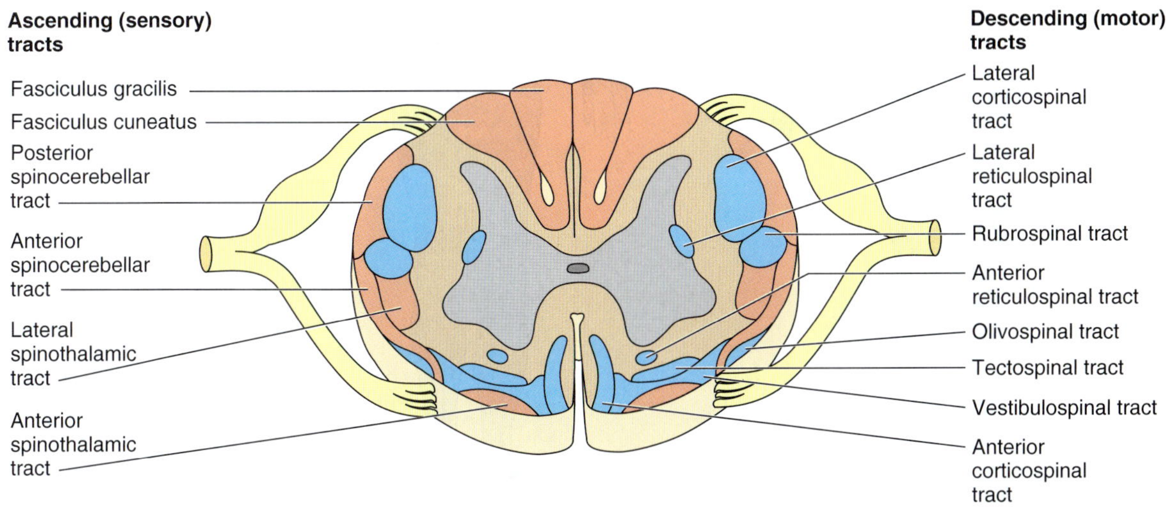

FIGURE 40.8 *Ascending and descending tracts of the spinal cord*

and end in the muscle. Damage to lower motor neurons results in decreased muscle tone, muscle atrophy, fasciculations and loss of reflexes.

The peripheral nervous system

The peripheral nervous system links the CNS with the rest of the body. It is responsible for receiving and transmitting information from the external environment. It consists of nerves, ganglia (groups of nerve cells) and sensory receptors located outside—or peripheral to—the brain and spinal cord. The PNS is divided into a sensory (afferent) division and a motor (efferent) division. Most nerves of the PNS contain fibres for both divisions and all are classified regionally as either spinal nerves or cranial nerves.

Spinal nerves

The 31 pairs of spinal nerves (see Figure 40.7) are named by their location:

- cervical nerves: 8 pairs
- thoracic nerves: 12 pairs
- lumbar nerves: 5 pairs
- sacral nerves: 5 pairs
- coccygeal nerves: 1 pair.

Spinal nerves exit the vertebral column through intervertebral foramina to travel to the body regions they serve. The spinal cord does not reach the end of the vertebral column; as a result, the lumbar and sacral nerve roots travel inferiorly through the vertebral canal for some distance before exiting the vertebral column through their associated intervertebral foramina. This collection of descending nerve roots is called the cauda equina.

Each spinal nerve contains both sensory and motor fibres. The sensory fibres are located in the dorsal root and their cell bodies are located within the dorsal root ganglion. The motor fibres are located in the ventral root and their cell bodies are located within the spinal cord. The dorsal and ventral roots merge outside the vertebral canal just past the dorsal root ganglion, forming a spinal nerve. Each spinal nerve further divides into branches called rami.

The ventral rami of the cervical, brachial, lumbar and sacral regions form complex clusters of nerves called plexuses. The main spinal nerve plexuses innervate the skin and the underlying muscles of the arms and legs. For example, the cervical plexus innervates the diaphragm through the phrenic nerve; the brachial plexus innervates the upper extremities through the median, ulnar and radial nerves; and the lumbar plexus innervates the anterior thigh through the femoral nerve.

An area of skin innervated by cutaneous branches of a single spinal nerve is called a dermatome. The dorsal roots of the spinal nerves carry sensations from these specific dermatomes. Dermatomes provide anatomical landmarks that are useful for locating neurological lesions (see Figure 40.9).

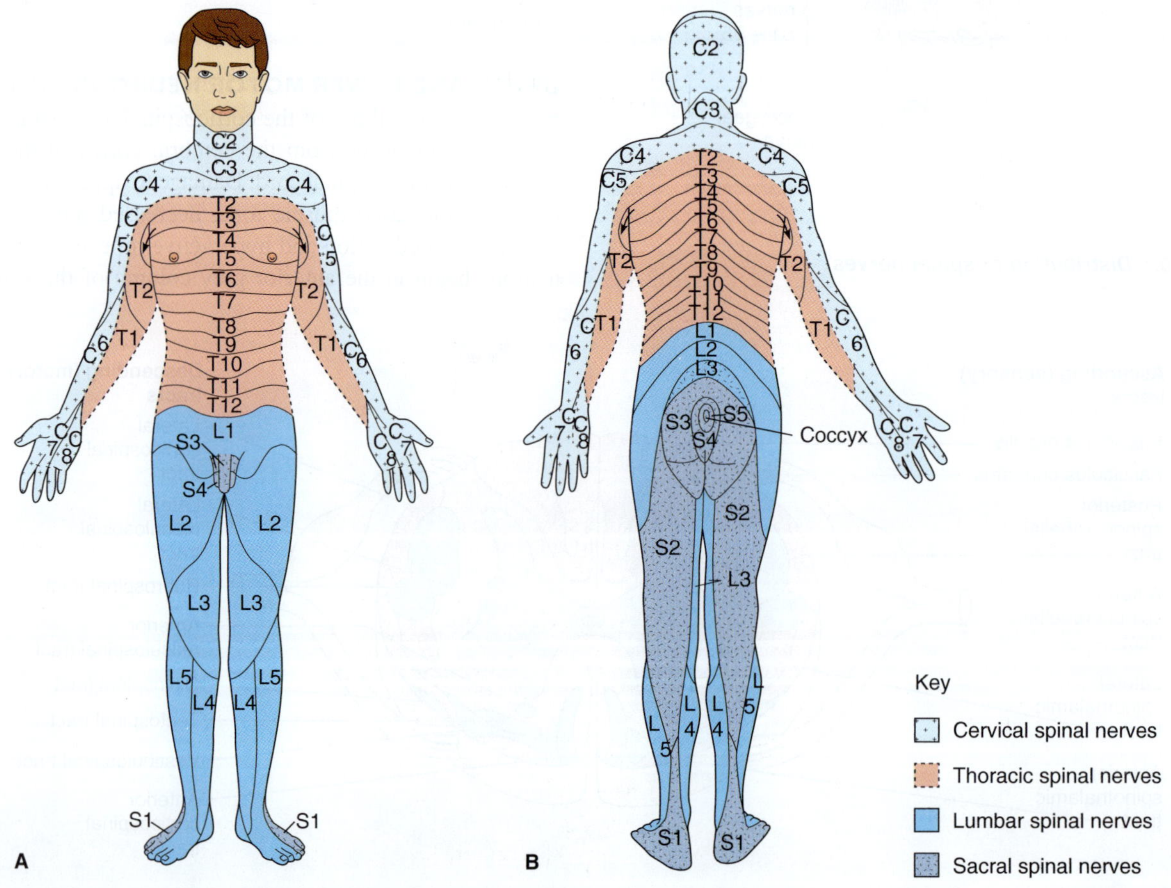

FIGURE 40.9 *A, Anterior and B, posterior dermatomes of the body*

Cranial nerves

Twelve pairs of cranial nerves originate in the forebrain and brainstem (see Figure 40.10). The vagus nerve extends into the ventral body cavity, but the 11 other pairs innervate only head and neck regions. Five of the pairs are solely motor function, three pairs are solely sensory and the remaining four nerves are mixed function, serving as both motor and sensory. The cranial nerves and their related functions are listed in Table 40.4.

Reflexes

A reflex is a rapid, involuntary, predictable motor response to a stimulus. Reflexes are categorised as either somatic or autonomic. Somatic reflexes result in skeletal muscle contraction. Autonomic reflexes activate cardiac muscle, smooth muscle and glands. A reflex occurs over a pathway called a reflex arc.

The essential components of a reflex arc are a receptor, a sensory neuron to carry afferent impulses to the CNS, an integration centre in the spinal cord or brain, a motor neuron to carry efferent impulses and an effector, which is the tissue that responds by contracting or secreting (see Figure 40.11).

Somatic reflexes mediated by the spinal cord are called *spinal reflexes*. Many spinal reflexes occur without impulses travelling to and from the brain, with the cord serving as the integration centre, whereas others require brain activity and modulation. *Deep tendon reflexes (DTRs)* occur in response to muscle contraction and cause muscle relaxation and lengthening. DTRs depend on intact sensory and motor nerve roots, functional synapses in the spinal cord, a functional neuromuscular junction and a competent muscle. Thus, an abnormal DTR could indicate a variety of health problems, including a lesion of a spinal nerve. Flexor, or withdrawal, reflexes are caused by actual or perceived painful stimuli and result in withdrawal of the part of the body that is threatened. Superficial responses result from gentle cutaneous stimulation. These responses depend on functional upper motor pathways and on an intact reflex arc.

The autonomic nervous system

The autonomic nervous system (ANS) is a division of the PNS that regulates the internal environment of the body. It is also called the general visceral motor system because it consists of motor neurons that innervate the body's viscera. Skeletal muscle activity and reflexes are regulated by a division of the PNS called the somatic nervous system; the ANS regulates the activity of cardiac muscle, smooth muscle and glands.

The ANS is primarily controlled by the reticular formation in the brainstem. Stimulation of centres in the medulla initiates reflexes that regulate cardiac rate, blood vessel diameter and gastrointestinal function.

The ANS has sympathetic and parasympathetic divisions. Although fibres from both divisions affect the same structures, the actions of the two divisions are opposite in effect and they serve to counterbalance each other. The main neurotransmitters for impulse transmission in the ANS are acetylcholine and noradrenaline. Acetylcholine is the primary neurotransmitter of the parasympathetic division. Noradrenaline is the primary neurotransmitter of the sympathetic division.

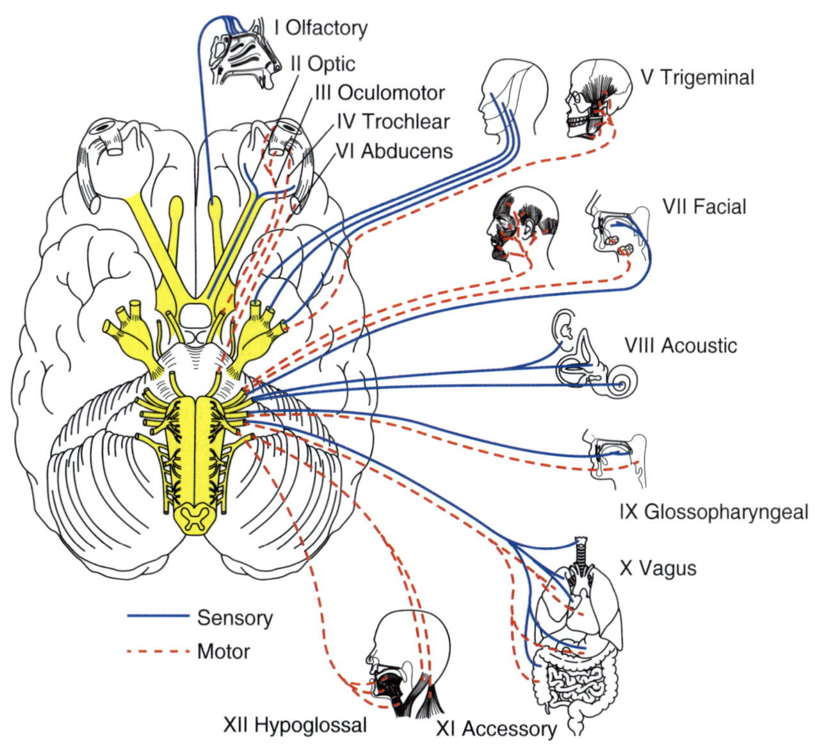

FIGURE 40.10 ***Cranial nerves***

TABLE 40.4 Cranial nerves

NAME	FUNCTION
I Olfactory	Sense of smell
II Optic	Vision
III Oculomotor	Eyeball movement Raising of upper eyelid Constriction of pupil Proprioception
IV Trochlear	Eyeball movement
V Trigeminal	Sensation of the upper scalp, upper eyelid, nose, nasal cavity, cornea and lacrimal gland Sensation of the palate, upper teeth, cheek, top lip, lower eyelid and scalp Sensation of the tongue, lower teeth, chin and temporal scalp Chewing
VI Abducens	Lateral movement of the eyeball
VII Facial	Movement of facial muscles Secretions of lacrimal, nasal, submandibular and sublingual glands Sensation of taste
VIII Acoustic	Sense of equilibrium Sense of hearing
IX Glossopharyngeal	Swallowing Gag reflex Secretions of parotid salivary gland Sense of taste Touch, pressure and pain from pharynx and posterior tongue Pressure from carotid arteries Receptors to regulate blood pressure
X Vagus	Swallowing Regulation of cardiac rate Regulation of respirations Digestion Sensation from thoracic and abdominal organs Proprioception Sense of taste
XI Accessory	Movement of head and neck Proprioception
XII Hypoglossal	Movement of tongue for speech and swallowing

Sympathetic division

The sympathetic division of the ANS prepares the body to handle situations that are perceived as harmful or stressful and to participate in strenuous activity. Cell bodies for this division arise in the lateral horns of the spinal cord in the area from T1 to L2. The fibres separate after leaving the cord and form a chain of ganglia that extends from the neck to the pelvis. Long fibres then extend to the organs that are supplied by the sympathetic division. Stimulation of the sympathetic division can exert the following effects on target organs or tissues:

- dilated pupils
- inhibited secretions
- copious production of sweat (**diaphoresis**)
- increased rate and force of heartbeat
- vasodilation of the coronary arteries

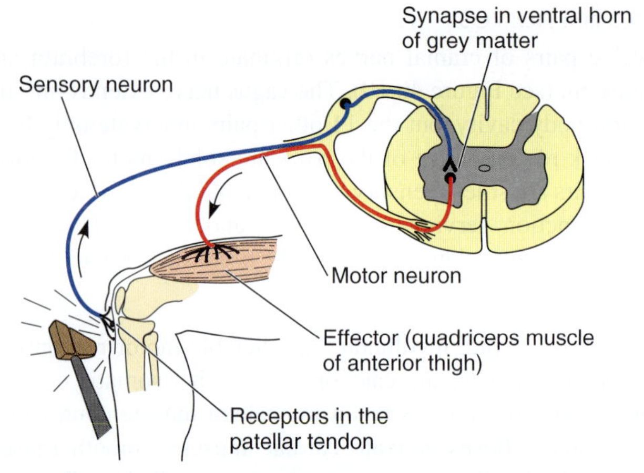

FIGURE 40.11 ***A typical reflex arc of a spinal nerve. In the two-neuron reflex arc, the stimulus is transferred from the sensory neuron directly to the motor neuron at the point of synapse in the spinal cord***

- dilation of the bronchioles
- decreased digestion
- increased release of glucose by the liver
- decreased urine output
- vasoconstriction of arteries
- vasoconstriction of abdominal and skin blood vessels
- increased blood clotting
- increased metabolic rate
- increased mental alertness.

Parasympathetic division

The parasympathetic division of the ANS operates during non-stressful situations. Cell bodies for this division are located in the brainstem (for the cranial nerves) and in the lateral grey matter of S2 to S4. Other than the fibres supplying the cranial nerves III, VII, IX and X, the fibres are carried by the vagus nerve to body tissues, thoracic organs and visceral organs. Stimulation of the parasympathetic division of the ANS produces the following effects:

- constriction of pupils
- stimulation of glandular secretions
- decreased heart rate
- vasoconstriction of coronary arteries
- constriction of the bronchioles
- increased peristalsis and secretion of gastrointestinal fluid.

ASSESSING NEUROLOGICAL FUNCTION

Structures and functions of the neurological system are assessed by findings from a health assessment interview to collect subjective data, a physical assessment to collect objective data and diagnostic tests. Sample documentation of an assessment of the neurological system is included in the 'Sample documentation' box.

SAMPLE DOCUMENTATION

Assessment of the neurological system

11/5/2023 NURS 1000 hrs

45-year-old male having annual physical examination. No history of injury or infection involving the head or spine. No reported history of seizures, dizziness, headaches, memory loss or problems with speaking or swallowing. Alert, oriented to person, place and time. Able to follow directions, explain simple proverbs and compare unlike objects. Cranial nerve testing results:

I = Identifies scents correctly.

II = Vision 40/20 in both eyes. Has full visual fields bilaterally.

III, IV, VI = Bilateral full extraocular movements, pupils are equally round, react to light and accommodation. No ptosis present in either eye.

V = Able to identify sharp, dull and light touch to forehead, cheek and chin.

VII = Equality of facial expressions. Able to smile, frown, wrinkle forehead, show teeth, puff out cheek, purse lips, raise eyebrows and close eyes against resistance.

VIII = Air conduction and bone conduction present bilaterally.

IX, X = Vocal control and gag reflex present. Swallows without difficulty.

XI = Equal strength when shrugging both shoulders.

XII = Able to protrude tongue midline without tremors.

All extremities have full range of motion with no noted tremors, tics or weakness. No atrophy of muscles noted. Can perform repetitive alternating movements without difficulty. Gait is steady. Negative Romberg test. All reflexes are 2 + bilaterally. Abdominal reflex present. No Babinski's present.

D Sassir
(DAVID SASSIR, RN)

Health assessment interview

A health assessment to determine problems with neurological structure and/or function may be conducted during a health screening, may focus on a chief complaint (such as headaches) or may be a component of a total health assessment. Health problems affecting the neurological system may manifest as problems with musculoskeletal function, mental health, endocrine function or a number of other systems, and as such, a holistic assessment is necessary. If the person's level of consciousness is altered, the nurse may need to rely on family members for information. One assessment tool for assessing a person's level of consciousness is the Glasgow Coma Scale (see Table 40.5).

TABLE 40.5 Glasgow Coma Scale

ASSESSMENT	RESPONSE	SCORE*
Eyes open	Spontaneously	4
(Record C if eyes are closed by	To speech	3
swelling.)	To pain	2
	No response	1
Best motor response	Obeys commands	6
(Record best upper arm response.)	Localises pain	5
	Flexion withdrawal	4
	Abnormal flexion	3
	Abnormal extension	2
	No response	1
Best verbal response	Oriented	5
(Record T if an endotracheal or	Confused	4
tracheostomy tube is in place.)	Inappropriate words	3
	Incomprehensible sounds	2
	No response	1
Total score:		____

*A higher score indicates a higher level of consciousness.

If the person has problems with neurological structure or function, analyse its onset, characteristics, course, severity, precipitating and relieving factors, and any associated symptoms, noting the time and circumstances.

Questions about present health status include information about numbness, tingling sensations, tremors, problems with coordination or balance, or loss of movement in any part of the body. Ask the person about difficulty with speaking, seeing, hearing, tasting or detecting odours. In addition, elicit information about memory, emotional state (such as anxiety or depression), recent changes in sleep patterns, ability to perform self-care and activities of daily living, sexual activity and weight. If the person is taking prescribed medications, over-the-counter medications or herbal supplements, ask about the type and purpose, as well as the frequency and duration of use. Information about use of illicit substances, especially psychoactives, is also important.

The health assessment should also include questions about any past history of seizures, fainting, dizziness, headaches and any trauma, tumours or surgery of the brain, spinal cord or nerves. Discuss illnesses that may cause neurological manifestations, including cardiac disease, strokes, pernicious anaemia, sinus infections, liver disease and/or kidney failure. Also ask the person about family history of neurological health problems, diabetes mellitus, hypertension, seizures or mental health problems.

Question the person about occupational hazards, such as exposure to toxic chemicals or materials, use of protective headgear and the amount of time spent performing repetitive motions (e.g. data entry and assembly). Ask questions about self-care to assess the person's diet and use of tobacco, drugs or alcohol, and ask whether they wear a helmet when riding a bike or motorcycle or participating in contact sports, or use a seat belt when driving a vehicle.

Interview questions categorised by functional health patterns are listed in the 'Functional health pattern interview' table.

Physical assessment

Physical assessment occurs when the nurse first meets the person and then on an ongoing basis, and involves making a holistic evaluation of the person's mental, social and physical status. The mental status examination is conducted with both the nurse and the person seated in a conversational manner. The rest of the neurological examination may be performed with the person either sitting or standing. A thorough neurological examination is discussed below, but in many instances the nurse will conduct a focused assessment specific to the person's health status.

The neurological system is assessed through inspection, palpation and percussion (with a reflex hammer). When conducting the mental status and cognitive portions of the examination, it is important to be aware that fatigue or illness may alter findings. Provide rest periods for the person as needed. When interpreting findings, consider the person's age, educational background and cultural orientation. It is essential to be aware of normal agerelated findings for the older adult (see Table 40.6).

FUNCTIONAL HEALTH PATTERN INTERVIEW Neurological system

FUNCTIONAL HEALTH PATTERN	INTERVIEW QUESTIONS AND LEADING STATEMENTS
Health perception–Health management	■ Have you ever had surgery, injury or illness of the neurological system, such as seizures, stroke, tumour, meningitis? If so, describe the problem and how it was treated.
	■ Do you have high blood pressure? If so, how is it treated?
	■ Have you ever had problems with the ability to move body parts? Describe.
	■ Would you say you think clearly? If not, how and when did the change occur?
	■ Are you having any problems with the ability to see, hear, taste or smell? Explain.
	■ Have you ever had any diagnostic tests for a neurological problem, such as an MRI or spinal tap? If so, what were the results?
	■ Do you take medications for seizures, headaches or other neurological problems? If so, what are they and how often do you take them?
	■ Do you now or have you ever smoked, used street drugs or drunk alcohol? If so, what type, how much and for how long?
	■ Where were you born and raised as a child?
Nutritional–Metabolic	■ Describe your usual food and fluid intake for a 24-hour period.
	■ Have you noticed any problems with chewing or swallowing your food?
	■ Do you have trouble with coughing when you eat or drink?
Elimination	■ Has there been any change in your urinary or bowel elimination? If so, describe the change.
	■ Do you use laxatives, suppositories or enemas to assist with bowel elimination? If so, what type and how often?
	■ Are you able to go to the bathroom without assistance? If not, describe your usual routine.
Activity–Exercise	■ Describe your usual activities in a 24-hour period.
	■ Do you have any problems with balance, coordination or walking? Do you use any assistive device when you walk, such as a cane or walker?
	■ Have you noticed any weakness in your arms or legs? If so, describe.
	■ Are you able to move all of your body parts? If not, explain.
	■ Do you trip or fall easily?
	■ Have you experienced any shakiness or tremors? Where?
	■ If you have seizures, what type do you have? Can you tell when they are going to happen? Does anything specific make you have a seizure? How do you feel after the seizure is over?
Sleep–Rest	■ Does this health problem interfere with your ability to sleep and rest? If so, how?
	■ Do you take any medication to help you sleep? If so, what?
	■ Describe your energy level. Do rest and sleep restore your energy?
Cognitive–Perceptual	■ Describe any headaches you experience, including frequency, type, location and precipitating/relieving factors.
	■ Do you ever feel dizzy or have you fainted? Do you ever feel the room is spinning? Explain.
	■ Do you ever experience any numbness, burning or tingling sensations? If so, where and when?
	■ Do you have any visual problems, such as double vision, blurring or blind spots?

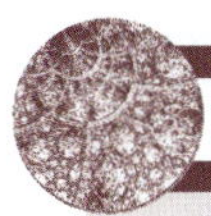

FUNCTIONAL HEALTH PATTERN INTERVIEW **Neurological system (continued)**

FUNCTIONAL HEALTH PATTERN	INTERVIEW QUESTIONS AND LEADING STATEMENTS
	■ Do you have any problems with hearing? Explain.
	■ Has there been any change in your ability to taste or smell? If so, explain.
	■ Do you have any difficulty remembering things? If so, describe what you do.
Self-perception–Self-concept	■ How does having this condition make you feel about yourself?
Role–Relationships	■ How has having this condition affected your relationships with others?
	■ Has having this condition interfered with your ability to work? Explain.
	■ Has anyone in your family had problems with neurological disease? Explain.
Sexuality–Reproductive	■ Has this condition interfered with your usual sexual activity?
Coping–Stress–Tolerance	■ Has having this condition created stress for you? If so, does your health problem seem to be more difficult when you are stressed?
	■ Have you experienced any kind of stress that makes the condition worse? Explain.
	■ Describe what you do when you feel stressed.
Value–Belief	■ Describe how specific relationships or activities help you cope with this problem.
	■ Describe specific cultural beliefs or practices that affect how you care for and feel about this problem.
	■ Are there any specific treatments that you would not use to treat this problem?

TABLE 40.6 Age-related changes in the neurological system

AGE-RELATED CHANGE	SIGNIFICANCE
• ↓ number of brain cells, cerebral blood flow and metabolism • Slower nerve conduction velocity	Delayed response to multiple stimuli and slower reflexes; may need additional time to process and respond to verbal stimuli
• Slower retrieval of information from long-term memory	There is some age-related forgetfulness, which can be improved by using memory aids such as making lists
• Slower response to changes in balance	May contribute to increased risk of falls
• May exhibit less readiness to learn and depend on prior experiences to solve problems • Is more easily distracted and has a decrease in the ability to maintain attention	Learning new skills or knowledge is improved when they are related to previously learned information and when limits are set on times for learning (e.g. no more than 30 minutes at one time).

The assessment should take place in a private, comfortable setting. Ask the person to remove outer clothing, shoes and stockings. Provide a gown for the person to wear. It is important to explain that the neurological examination is lengthy and may consist of questions and requests that seem strange to the person. Explain the rationale for each part of the examination.

A brief version of this physical assessment, often referred to as a *neuro check*, may be performed in a shorter time period when a person requires frequent ongoing assessments of neurological status (see Box 40.1).

BOX 40.1 Abbreviated neurological assessment

1. Assess level of consciousness (response to auditory and/or tactile stimulus).
2. Obtain vital signs (BP, P, R).
3. Check pupillary response to light.
4. Assess strength of hand grip and movement of extremities bilaterally.
5. Determine ability to sense touch/pain in extremities.

Diagnostic tests

The results of diagnostic tests of neurological structure and function are used to support the diagnosis of a specific injury or disease, to provide information to identify or modify the appropriate medications or therapy used to treat the disease, and to help nurses monitor the person's responses to treatment and nursing care interventions. Diagnostic tests to assess the structures and functions of the neurological system are described below and summarised in the following bulleted list. More information is included in the discussion of specific injuries or diseases in the following chapters.

- Radiological examinations of the skull and spine include standard x-rays, computed tomography (CT) scans, magnetic resonance imaging (MRI), magnetic resonance angiography (MRA) and magnetic resonance spectroscopy (MRS). Findings from these examinations are used to diagnose and evaluate fractures, vertebral displacements, tumours, haemorrhage, aneurysms, cysts, oedema, ischaemia, atrophy, necrosis, seizures, multiple sclerosis, Alzheimer's disease, coma and vascular lesions.

- Both positron emission tomography (PET) and single-photon emission computed tomography (SPECT) are used to assess brain function and blood flow, to differentiate types of dementia, to evaluate the stage of a brain tumour and to identify brain tumours, strokes and seizure disorders.
- Occlusion of the carotid arteries is evaluated by measuring velocity of blood flow with a carotid duplex study; and extracranial blood vessels are evaluated with a transcranial Doppler study.
- Electrical activity of the brain is measured with an electroencephalogram (EEG) to diagnose brain disease and brain death. A magnetoencephalogram (MEG) measures electrical activity of neurons to pinpoint the area of the brain affected by a stroke, brain trauma, brain disorders or seizures.
- Cerebrospinal fluid, removed through a lumbar puncture (LP), is examined in the laboratory to diagnose a variety of brain diseases and infections.
- A myelogram is used to identify lesions of the spinal cord, such as tumours or herniated intervertebral discs.

Regardless of the type of diagnostic test, the nurse is responsible for explaining the procedure and any special preparation needed, assessing for medication use that may affect the outcome of the tests, supporting the person during the examination as necessary, documenting the procedures as appropriate and monitoring the results of the tests.

Genetic considerations

When conducting a health assessment interview and a physical assessment, it is important for the nurse to consider genetic influences on the health of the adult. Several neurological diseases that directly affect the nervous system have a genetic component; some are due to mutation of a single gene while others have a more complex method of inheritance (Andreoletti et al., 2019). During the health assessment interview, it is important to ask about family members with health problems affecting neurological structure or function. In addition, ask about a family history of problems with muscular coordination, Parkinson's disease, narcolepsy, tremor, seizures, Alzheimer's disease or motor neurone disease. During the physical assessment, assess for any manifestations that might indicate a genetic disorder (see the 'Genetic considerations' box). If data are found to indicate genetic risk factors or alterations, ask about genetic testing and refer for appropriate genetic counselling and evaluation.

DIAGNOSTIC TESTS The neurological system

NAME OF TEST X-rays of skull and spine

PURPOSE AND DESCRIPTION Standard x-rays of the skull and spine are done to identify fractures, displacement of vertebrae, spinal curves and tissue displacement (as by tumours).

RELATED NURSING CARE No special preparation is needed.

NAME OF TEST Computed tomography (CT) scan

PURPOSE AND DESCRIPTION Used to identify intracerebral haemorrhage, tumours, cysts, aneurysms, oedema, ischaemia, atrophy and tissue necrosis. May also be used to evaluate a shift in intracranial contents and differentiate type of stroke. Involves computer-assisted x-rays of several levels of cross-sections of the body part being examined; may be done with or without contrast.

PREPARATION

- Ensure a signed consent form. Check specific policy on withholding food and fluids. Medications may be required to be given up to 2 hours before test.

RELATED NURSING CARE

- Assess for possible reaction to iodine dye (by asking about allergy to seafood). Document any allergy and inform the physician and radiology department.
- Remove metal hairpins, clips and earrings.

HEALTH EDUCATION FOR THE PERSON AND FAMILY

- If applicable, instruct the person not to drink or eat anything before the test except for the ordered medications.
- Inform them that they may be given an intravenous infusion. When the contrast dye is injected, they may feel warm and have a metallic taste in the mouth. The test will last from 30 to 90 minutes and their head will be positioned in a cradle.
- The CT scanner is circular with a round opening. Inform the person that they will be secured to a table and the scanner will revolve around the body part to be examined. The scanner will make a clicking noise. The test is painless and someone will always be immediately available during it.

DIAGNOSTIC TESTS The neurological system (continued)

NAME OF TEST Magnetic resonance imaging (MRI), Functional MRI

PURPOSE AND DESCRIPTION An MRI is done to identify and monitor conditions of the brain and spinal cord, including stroke, tumours, trauma, seizures and multiple sclerosis. It uses magnetic energy to provide images. Gadolinium contrast media may be used to enhance visualisation. A functional MRI may be ordered to evaluate metabolic or blood flow responses of the brain to specific tasks, such as activity and rest.

RELATED NURSING CARE Assess for metal implants (such as a pacemaker or defibrillator), body piercings and shrapnel, which would contraindicate tests.

NAME OF TEST Magnetic resonance angiography (MRA)

PURPOSE AND DESCRIPTION Can provide information about the blood vessels of the brain and identify vascular lesions. The MRA uses the signals from blood vessels to reconstruct only those vessels with blood flow. It can also be done using contrast media.

RELATED NURSING CARE Assess for metal implants, as for an MRI, which would contraindicate tests.

NAME OF TEST Magnetic resonance spectroscopy (MRS)

PURPOSE AND DESCRIPTION Identifies biochemical changes in the brain that may be used to confirm the presence of Alzheimer's disease, determine the extent of head injury from trauma or stroke, and identify the causes of coma.

RELATED NURSING CARE Assess for metal implants, as for an MRI, which would contraindicate tests.

NAME OF TEST Positron emission tomography (PET), Single-photon emission computed tomography (SPECT)

PURPOSE AND DESCRIPTION When used to study the brain, a PET can assess normal brain function and cerebral blood flow and volume; can differentiate different types of dementia; and can identify stages of brain tumours. A substance containing a radionuclide is administered and cross-sections of tissue are detected and displayed by computer. A SPECT is similar to a PET but uses different radioactive dyes that are indicated for different uses. It can be used to diagnose strokes, brain tumours and seizure disorders.

RELATED NURSING CARE Tell the person not to drink coffee or alcohol or to smoke for 24 hours before the test. Assess blood glucose levels pre test as dyes may impact on functioning. Post test, encourage oral fluids to facilitate excretion of the radioactive substance.

NAME OF TEST Cerebral angiogram

PURPOSE AND DESCRIPTION The cerebral angiogram is the definitive diagnostic procedure for aneurysms, arteriovenous malformations, blood vessel patency and stenosis, thrombosis, vasospasm and space-occupying lesions (such as tumours or haematomas). May be performed either as part of a surgical procedure or with local anaesthesia. In radiology, a contrast medium is injected and films are taken at various time intervals.

RELATED NURSING CARE Inform about need to remain NBM for 8 hours prior to the procedure and explain that a burning sensation may be felt for a few (4 to 6) seconds behind the eyes or in the jaw, teeth, tongue or lips. Bed rest is maintained for 8 hours after the procedure, vital signs are monitored and fluids are forced to clear the contrast medium.

NAME OF TEST Carotid duplex study, Transcranial Doppler study

PURPOSE AND DESCRIPTION A carotid duplex study evaluates the velocity of blood flow through the carotid arteries and identifies occlusive disease. Uses sound waves produced by the blood flow to produce an image. A transcranial Doppler study follows the same procedure but is used to evaluate intracranial blood vessels.

RELATED NURSING CARE No special preparation is needed.

(continued)

DIAGNOSTIC TESTS The neurological system (continued)

NAME OF TEST Electroencephalogram (EEG), Magnetoencephalogram (MEG)

PURPOSE AND DESCRIPTION An EEG is used to measure the electrical activity of the brain to diagnose brain disease and brain death. Electrodes are applied to the scalp with skin clips and a graphic picture is obtained (similar to an ECG of the heart). An MEG can identify the area of the brain affected by a stroke, brain disorders or trauma, or seizures. MEG detects magnetic fields generated by activity of neurons.

RELATED NURSING CARE Withhold fluids, foods and medications (as prescribed) that may stimulate or depress brain waves. These include anticonvulsants, tranquillisers, depressants and caffeine-containing foods. Many medications are withheld for 24 to 48 hours before the test. Help the person to wash their hair before the test.

HEALTH EDUCATION FOR THE PERSON AND FAMILY

- Inform the person that the test takes about 1 hour. It is painless and will be performed while sitting in a comfortable chair or lying on a stretcher. The electrodes are applied to the scalp with a thick paste.
- During the test, the person will first be asked to breathe in and out deeply for a few minutes. Then, they will close their eyes while a light is flashed on them and, finally, they will lie quietly with the eyes closed. After the test, the nurse will help the person wash the paste out of their hair.

NAME OF TEST Evoked potentials

PURPOSE AND DESCRIPTION Measures nerve conduction along pathways to evaluate evoked potential of muscle contractions. Used to diagnose and evaluate neuromuscular diseases and identify nerve damage. Transcutaneous or percutaneous electrodes are applied to the skin and provide recordings.

RELATED NURSING CARE No special preparation is needed.

NAME OF TEST Electromyogram (EMG)

PURPOSE AND DESCRIPTION Measures the electrical activity of skeletal muscles at rest and during contraction; useful in diagnosing neuromuscular diseases. Needle electrodes are inserted into skeletal muscle (as on the legs) and electrical activity can be heard, viewed on an oscilloscope and recorded on graph paper. Normally, there is no electrical activity at rest.

RELATED NURSING CARE Tell the person not to drink fluids containing caffeine or to smoke for 3 hours before the test and not to take medications such as muscle relaxants, anticholinergics and cholinergics.

NAME OF TEST Lumbar puncture (LP)

PURPOSE AND DESCRIPTION The lumbar puncture is used to measure CSF pressure and to obtain a sample of CSF to use in diagnosis of multiple sclerosis or increased intracranial pressure from meningitis, subarachnoid haemorrhage, brain tumour, brain abscess, encephalitis and viral infections. A needle is inserted in L3–L4 or L4–L5 and fluid is aspirated.

RELATED NURSING CARE

- Ask the person to empty their bladder before the procedure begins.
- Help the person to assume a lateral recumbent position near the side of the bed. The person should assume the fetal position, with their hands clasped around their knees.
- The person should drink fluids so that their body can replace the fluid that was withdrawn. If they have a headache or backache, they can take medications for pain. The person should notify their healthcare provider if they notice increased pain or drainage from the area where the procedure was done.
- Post procedure, take and record vital signs as indicated by organisational standards. Monitor neurological status at least every 4 hours for 24 hours. Monitor the puncture site for leakage of cerebrospinal fluid or haematoma formation.
- Ensure that the person voids within 8 hours of the procedure. Encourage increased intake of fluids (up to 3,000 mL in 24 hours).

DIAGNOSTIC TESTS The neurological system (continued)

HEALTH EDUCATION FOR THE PERSON AND FAMILY

- Inform the person that a local anaesthetic will be injected into the skin over the area of the needle insertion. This medication may cause a burning sensation. A long, thin needle will then be inserted into the lower back below the level of the spinal cord. Cerebrospinal fluid will be withdrawn.
- Inform the person that there may be slight pain down one leg during the procedure and that it is important to remain still during the procedure.
- A small dressing will be used to cover the place where the needle was inserted. After the procedure, the person must remain flat in bed for the number of hours prescribed by the doctor. (This ranges from 4 to 24 hours.) The nurses will take their vital signs and look under the small dressing at regular intervals.

NAME OF TEST Myelogram

PURPOSE AND DESCRIPTION Used to identify lesions of the spinal cord, such as tumours or herniated intervertebral disc. A lumbar puncture is done, a contrast medium is injected into the subarachnoid space and x-rays are taken.

RELATED NURSING CARE

- The meal prior to the procedure is usually omitted. The person should be well hydrated.
- Administer prescribed pretest medications, such as a sedative or diazepam (Valium).
- Inform the person that they must stay in bed with the head of the bed elevated for at least 6 to 12 hours. The nurse will check their blood pressure, pulse and respirations. The nurse will also check their ability to feel and move at least every 4 hours (or more often) after the examination.
- Post procedure, take and record vital signs and assess neurological status as prescribed (and at least every 4 hours) for 24 hours and report any changes. Assess the site of the lumbar puncture for leakage of cerebrospinal fluid or bleeding every 4 hours. Notify the physician of leakage or bleeding.
- Encourage increased intake of oral fluids to replace that withdrawn during the examination. (This may also help decrease a post-myelogram headache.) Make sure that the person voids within 8 hours after the examination. Notify the physician if the person has not voided within 8 hours.
- Administer analgesics as prescribed for post examination pain, headache or muscle spasms. Keep the person's head elevated at least 30 degrees (in bed or in a chair) for 12 hours or as ordered.
- Administer prescribed medications for nausea. Do not give any phenothiazine derivatives for 48 hours (to reduce the possibility of seizures).
- Resume diet if there is no nausea or vomiting.

HEALTH EDUCATION FOR THE PERSON AND FAMILY

- Inform the person that they will remain NBM several hours before the test.
- The examination will last about 1 hour. The person may have to lie on their stomach, sit and lean forward, or sit with the knees to the chest. A strap may be used to prevent falls and the table will be tilted during the examination.
- A lumbar puncture will be performed to inject the dye. A local anaesthetic will be used where the needle will be inserted. There may be a feeling of pressure during needle insertion. The needle will be inserted below the level of the spinal cord. Tell the physician if you experience pain.

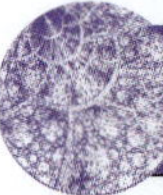

GENETIC CONSIDERATIONS Neurological disorders

- In all types of spinocerebellar ataxia, there is degeneration of the spinal cord and cerebellum, resulting in loss of muscular coordination and spasticity.
- One risk factor for Parkinson's disease is a positive family history of the disease. This neurodegenerative disease affects about 40,000 people in Australia, and is manifested by tremor, muscular stiffness, and difficulty with balance and walking (Brain Foundation, 2022a).
- There are a number of genetic factors that may influence a predisposition to multiple sclerosis as well as the severity and course of the disease.
- Narcolepsy, a sleep disorder, does have a familial connection.
- Huntington's disease is an inherited degenerative disorder that leads to dementia. In Australia, it currently affects 6 or 7 people in every 100,000.
- Friedreich's ataxia is a rare inherited disease that causes a progressive loss of voluntary muscle coordination and enlargement of the heart.
- Essential tremor (ET) can develop at any age, including childhood, but becomes increasingly common with advancing age, affecting up to 10–25% of older people. ET is familial in 50% of cases and the cause is unknown in the remainder. If ET runs in the family, each child with an affected parent will have a 50% chance of inheriting the disorder (Brain Foundation, 2002b). In more than half of cases, ET is inherited as an autosomal dominant trait, meaning that children of an individual with the disease have a 50% chance of also developing the disorder.
- Epilepsy is one of the most common neurological diseases, characterised by abnormal cell firing in the brain that causes recurring seizures. The majority of people with epilepsy are able to live normal lives with few restrictions on their activities (Brain Foundation, 2022c).
- Charcot–Marie–Tooth syndrome is the most common inherited peripheral neuropathy in the world, characterised by a slowly progressive degeneration of the muscles of the foot, lower leg, hand and forearm.
- Alzheimer's disease (AD) is a leading cause of death in adults, increasing in incidence with age and more common in women. AD tends to run in families, with mutations in four genes believed to be responsible for the disease.
- Motor neurone disease (MND) is a neurological disease that causes progressive degeneration of motor neurons in the brain and spinal cord, resulting in paralysis and death. Chromosome abnormalities have been linked to familial MND.

NEUROLOGICAL ASSESSMENTS

Technique/normal findings	Abnormal findings
Mental status	
Assess appearance, including dress, hygiene, grooming, gait and posture. *The person should be appropriately dressed and clean, with normal gait and posture.*	■ Unilateral neglect (inattention to one side of the body) may occur with some strokes. Poor hygiene and grooming may be seen in people with dementing disorders. ■ Abnormal gait and posture may be seen in transient ischaemic attacks (TIAs), strokes and Parkinson's disease.
Assess behaviour, including actions and affect, content and quality of speech and level of consciousness (LOC). Use the Glasgow Coma Scale (see Table 40.5) to document findings. *A score of 15 on the Glasgow Coma Scale indicates the person is alert and oriented.*	■ Emotional swings or changes in personality may be observed in people who have had a stroke. ■ The face appears mask like (very little expressive movement of facial muscles) in people with Parkinson's disease. ■ Apathy is seen in people with dementing disorders. ■ **Aphasia** (defective or absent language function) may occur in TIAs and strokes. Aphasias are seen with damage to the left cerebral cortex. Aphasias are more often seen with strokes of the left hemisphere than the right hemisphere. ■ **Dysphonia** (change in the tone of the voice) is common in strokes. Dysphonia is seen with paralysis of the vocal cords (cranial nerve X). ■ **Dysarthria** (difficulty speaking) is seen with lesions of upper and lower motor neurons, the cerebellum and the extrapyramidal tract. ■ Damage to the brainstem and/or cerebral cortex may alter LOC. ■ Drowsiness and decreased LOC may be associated with brain trauma, infections, TIAs, stroke and brain tumours. ■ Level of consciousness, ranging from confusion to coma, is usually altered with a stroke.
Assess cognitive function. **Note orientation to time, place and person.** **Note attention span and recent and remote memory.**	■ Disorientation to time and place may occur in people with stroke of the right cerebral hemisphere. ■ Memory deficits are often seen in people with a stroke. ■ Perceptual deficits may be seen in strokes. These same deficits may occur following brain trauma and in dementing disorders. ■ Impaired cognition is often noted with strokes, cerebral trauma and brain tumours.

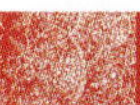

NEUROLOGICAL ASSESSMENTS (continued)

Technique/normal findings	Abnormal findings
Ask the person to: ■ repeat five to seven numbers ■ recall three items after 5 minutes ■ recall their address, breakfast or birthday.	
Assess thought processes (both content and perceptions) by noting responses to questions. Note ability to understand what is said and to express thoughts. Note ability to make logical and safe judgments. *The person should be oriented to time, place and person; demonstrate attention and ability to remember recent and past events; respond appropriately to questions; and be able to make judgments.*	
Cranial nerves	
Test CN I (olfactory). Note the person's ability to smell scents (e.g. soap, coffee) with each nostril. *Sense of smell should be equal in both nostrils.*	■ **Anosmia** (an inability to smell) may be seen with lesions of the frontal lobe and may also occur with impaired blood flow to the middle cerebral artery. Altered sense of smell is associated with a number of neurological conditions.
Test CN II (optic). Assess vision in each eye with Snellen chart (see the chapter 'A person-centred approach to assessing the eye and ear' for guidelines). *Based on previous ability to see and use of visual aids, the person should be able to see with both eyes.*	■ Blindness in one eye may be seen with strokes or with other cerebral vascular accidents (CVAs). Impaired vision or blindness in one side of both eyes (homonymous hemianopia) is associated with stroke. ■ Impaired vision may be seen with strokes and brain tumours. ■ Blindness or double vision may be noted with stroke and TIAs.
Test CN III, IV and VI (oculomotor, trochlear and abducens).	■ Nystagmus (involuntary eye movement) may be seen with strokes.
Assess extraocular movements by asking the person to follow your finger as you write an H in the air (see the chapter 'A person-centred approach to assessing the eye and ear'). Assess pupil response by covering one eye at a time and shining a bright light directly into the uncovered eye (use a penlight or the ophthalmoscope). See the chapter 'A person-centred approach to assessing the eye and ear' for more detailed assessment guidelines. *Extraocular movements should be present bilaterally and pupils should be equally round and reactive to light.*	■ Constricted pupils are associated with impaired blood flow from a stroke. ■ Sluggish pupil response is associated with increased cranial pressures such as following traumatic brain injury (TBI).

(continued)

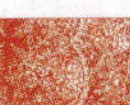

NEUROLOGICAL ASSESSMENTS (continued)

Technique/normal findings	Abnormal findings
Assess for ptosis (drooping eyelids). *Eyelids should not droop.*	■ Ptosis (also called Horner syndrome) occurs with strokes, myasthenia gravis and palsy of CN III.
Test CN V (trigeminal). **Assess ability to feel light, dull and sharp sensations on the face. With the person's eyes closed, check whether sensation is the same on both sides of the face. Stroke the cheek with a wisp of cotton for light touch, with a closed safety pin for dull touch and with a tongue depressor for sharp touch. If the sharp point of a safety pin is used to assess sharp touch, be sure to avoid scratching the surface of the skin and discard the pin after it is used.** *Ability to feel light, dull and sharp sensations should be intact.*	■ Changes in facial sensations are noted with impaired blood flow to the carotid artery. ■ Decreased sensations to the face and cornea on the same side of the body, as well as numbness of the lip and mouth, occur with strokes. ■ Loss of facial sensation or contraction of the masseter and temporal muscles is seen with lesions of CN V. ■ Severe facial pain is seen with trigeminal neuralgia (tic douloureux).
Test CN VII (facial). **Assess ability to taste sweet, sour and salt on the anterior two-thirds of the tongue by asking the person to stick out their tongue and applying a sweet, sour or salty substance.** **Assess ability to frown, show teeth, blow out cheeks, raise eyebrows, smile and close eyes tightly.** *Ability to taste sweet, sour and salt is intact. Should be able to frown, show teeth, blow out cheeks, raise eyebrows, smile and close eyes tightly. Muscle movement should be equal bilaterally.*	■ Loss of ability to taste may occur with brain tumours or with nerve impairment. ■ Asymmetry or decreased movement of facial muscles is noted with lesions of the upper and lower motor neurons. ■ Paralysis of the lower motor neurons from injury to CN VII results in the inability to close eyes, a flat nasolabial fold, paralysis of lower face and inability to wrinkle forehead. ■ Paralysis of the upper motor neurons from a stroke results in weakness of eyelids and paralysis of lower face. ■ Pain, paralysis and sagging of facial muscles is seen on the affected side in Bell's palsy.
Test CN VIII (acoustic). **Assess ability to hear whispered and spoken words.** *The person should be able to hear with both ears.*	■ Decreased hearing or deafness may occur with strokes and/or tumours of CN VIII.
Test CN IX and X (glossopharyngeal and vagus). **Assess gag reflex by touching back of the person's throat with a tongue depressor.** **If gag reflex is intact, observe the person swallowing a small drink of water.** **Observe for a symmetrical rise of the soft palate and uvula as the person says 'ah'.** *The person should be able to swallow without difficulty, have symmetrical rise of the soft palate, have intact gag reflex.*	■ Dysphagia (difficulty swallowing) is common with impaired blood flow to the brain. ■ Unilateral loss of the gag reflex occurs with lesions of CN IX and X.

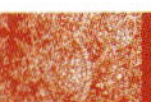

NEUROLOGICAL ASSESSMENTS (continued)

Technique/normal findings	Abnormal findings
Test CN XI (spinal accessory). Assess the person's ability to turn their head and shrug their shoulders against resistance: ask the person to turn their head to one side against the resistance of your hand; ask them to shrug their shoulders while you exert downward pressure. Observe symmetry, strength and size of muscles. *The person should be able to turn their head and shrug their shoulders against resistance.*	■ Muscle weakness is noted with lower motor neuron disease. Contralateral hemiparesis is seen with strokes.
Test CN XII (hypoglossal). Assess the person's ability to stick out their tongue and move it from side to side against resistance of a tongue depressor. *The person should be able to stick out tongue and move it from side to side against resistance.*	■ Atrophy and **fasciculations** (twitches) of the tongue are seen in lower motor neuron disease. The tongue may deviate towards the involved side of the body.
Sensory function	
Assess ability to perceive various sensations. **Touch both sides of various parts of the body (the chest, abdomen, arms and legs) with one or more of the following:** ■ **cotton wisp** ■ **sharp object** ■ **dull object** ■ **vibrating tuning fork placed on bony prominences.** *The person can differentiate between soft and sharp and can feel vibrations appropriately.*	■ Decreased sensation of pain occurs with injury to the spinothalamic tract. ■ Decreased vibratory sensations are seen with injuries to the posterior column tract. ■ Transient numbness of face, arm or hand is seen with TIAs. ■ Sensory loss on one side of the body is seen with lesions of higher pathways to the spinal cord. ■ Bilateral sensory loss is seen in polyneuropathy (a disease in which multiple peripheral nerves are affected, such as Guillain–Barré syndrome or diabetes mellitus). Sensations are impaired with strokes, brain tumours and spinal cord trauma or compression.
Assess sense of position (kinaesthesia). **Move the person's finger or big toe up or down. Ask the person to describe the movement.** *The person can accurately describe position of their finger or toe when moved up or down.*	■ Lesions of the posterior column of the spinal cord may affect sense of position.

(continued)

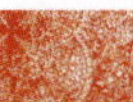

NEUROLOGICAL ASSESSMENTS (continued)

Technique/normal findings	Abnormal findings
Assess ability to discriminate fine touch. **Ask the person to identify:** ■ **object in hand, such as a coin or key (tests stereognosis)** ■ **number written on hand (tests graphaesthesia) (see Figure 40.12)** ■ **two points of simultaneous pinpricks on the hand (tests two-point discrimination) (see Figure 40.13)** ■ **where they are being touched (tests localisation).** *The person can identify and discriminate fine touch.*	■ Inability to discriminate fine touch (stereognosis, graphaesthesia, two points, point localisation and extinction) may occur with injury to the posterior columns or sensory cortex.

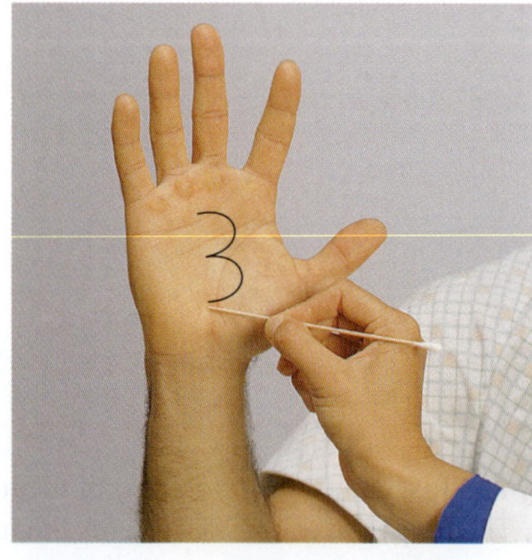

FIGURE 40.12 *Testing graphaesthesia*

Source: Pearson Education.

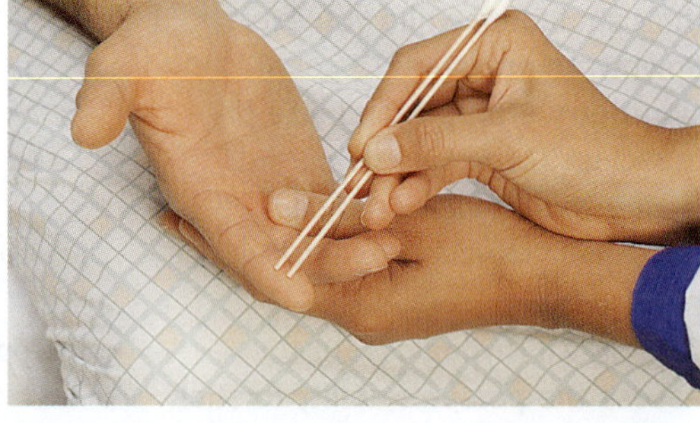

FIGURE 40.13 *Testing two-point discrimination*

Source: Pearson Education.

Motor function

Technique/normal findings	Abnormal findings
Assess bilateral symmetry and size of muscles.	■ Atrophy of muscles is seen with disease of the lower motor neurons.
Assess for tremors (rhythmic movements) and fasciculations (irregular movements). Observe movements as the person is at rest (not making a purposeful movement) and with activity (making a purposeful movement, such as reaching for a glass of water). *Muscles are bilaterally symmetrical and of equal size. Tremors or fasciculations are not present.*	■ Tremors that occur with activity are seen in multiple sclerosis and diseases of the cerebellar system. ■ Tremors that occur at rest and disappear with movement are common in Parkinson's disease. ■ Fasciculations occur in disease or trauma to the lower motor neurons, as a side effect of medications, in fever, in sodium deficiency and in uraemia.
Assess muscle tone. *Muscle tone is appropriate.*	■ Muscle tone is decreased (**flaccidity**) in disease or trauma of the lower motor neurons and early stroke. ■ Muscle tone is increased (**spasticity**) in disease of the corticospinal motor tract. ■ Muscles are rigid in disease of the extrapyramidal motor tract. ■ Muscles move in small, regular jerky movements (cogwheel rigidity) in Parkinson's disease.
Assess bilateral muscle strength and movement. **Ask the person to:** ■ **squeeze your hands** ■ **push their feet against the resistance of your hands** ■ **raise both legs off the bed.** *Muscle strength and movement are bilaterally equal and strong.*	■ Weakness of the arms, legs or hands is often seen with TIAs. ■ Hemiplegia (paralysis of one-half of the body vertically) is noted with strokes. ■ Flaccid paralysis is noted with strokes. ■ Paralysis or decreased movement is seen in multiple sclerosis and myasthenia gravis. ■ There is total loss of motor function below the level of injury in complete spinal cord transection and in injuries to the anterior portion of the spinal cord. ■ Spasticity of muscles may occur as a result of incomplete spinal cord injuries.

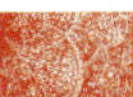

NEUROLOGICAL ASSESSMENTS (continued)

Technique/normal findings	Abnormal findings
Cerebellar function	
Assess the gait. Ask the person to walk normally, then in a heel-to-toe fashion, then on toes and finally on heels. *The person has appropriate gait and can walk heel-to-toe, on toes and on heels.* **Perform Romberg's test. Ask the person to stand with their feet together and eyes closed. (Stand close to the person to prevent falling.)** *There should be minimal swaying for up to 20 seconds.*	▪ **Ataxia** is a lack of coordination and a clumsiness of movements, with staggering, wide-based and unbalanced gait. Ataxia is often seen with strokes and cerebellar tumours. Swaying and falling are seen in cerebellar ataxia. Inability to walk on toes, then heels, may indicate disease of the upper motor neurons. ▪ Spastic hemiparesis is often associated with strokes or upper motor neuron disease. The person walks with one leg stiffly dragging while the other leg circles out and forwards. One arm is held flexed and close to the side. ▪ Steppage gait is noted with disease of the lower motor neurons. The person drags or lifts their foot high, then slaps the foot on to the floor. The person cannot walk on their heels. ▪ Sensory ataxia may be associated with polyneuropathy or damage to the posterior columns. The person walks on their heels before bringing down their toes and the feet are held wide apart. Gait worsens with the eyes closed. ▪ Parkinsonian gait is often seen in Parkinson's disease. The person stoops over while walking and shuffles their feet. Their arms are held close to the side. ▪ A positive Romberg's test may be seen in cerebellar ataxia.
Assess coordination. **Observe ability to pat knees, alternating front and back of hands and increasing speed.** **Observe ability to touch each finger of one hand to the thumb.** **Observe ability to touch the nose, then one of your fingers, then the nose again.** **Observe ability to run each heel down each shin, while in a supine position (see Figure 40.14).** *The person demonstrates coordinated movements.*	▪ Ataxic movements are apparent in cerebellar disease.

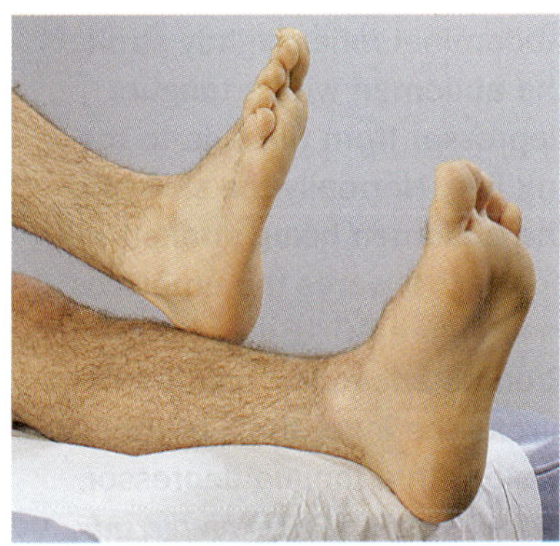

FIGURE 40.14 ***Heel-to-shin test***

Source: Pearson Education.

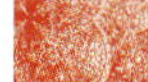

REFLEX ASSESSMENTS

A reflex hammer is used to strike the tendon of various reflex sites. To test deep tendon reflexes, ask the person to lock the fingers of both hands together and then pull; this encourages relaxation and promotes reflexes of lower extremities. Superficial reflexes are assessed by lightly stroking the area with the end of a tongue depressor. The following criteria for recording reflexes are often used:

0 = absent or no response
1 = hypoactive; weaker than normal (+)
2 = normal (++)
3 = stronger than normal (+++)
4 = hyperactive, sustained clonus (++++)
A score of 2 is considered normal.

Technique/normal findings	Abnormal findings
Assess the patellar, biceps, brachioradialis, triceps and Achilles deep tendon reflexes (see Figure 40.15).	▪ Hyperactive reflexes are present with lesions of upper motor neurons. ▪ Decreased reflexes are present with lower motor neuron involvement.

(continued)

REFLEX ASSESSMENTS (continued)

Technique/normal findings	Abnormal findings

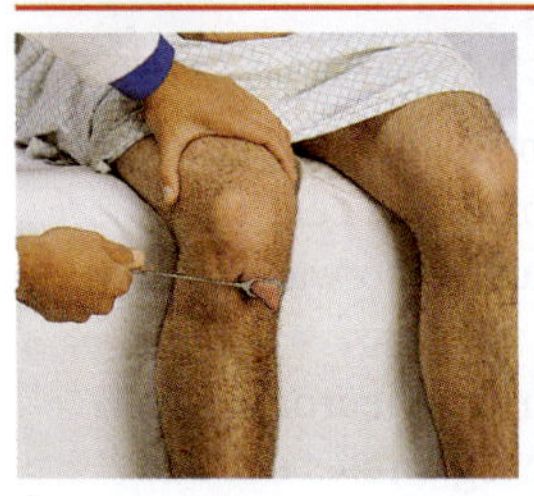
A

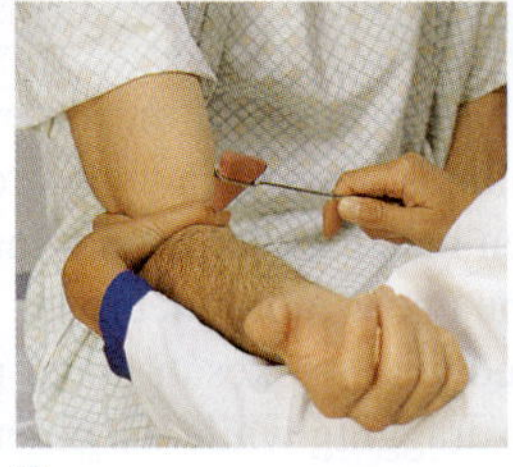
B

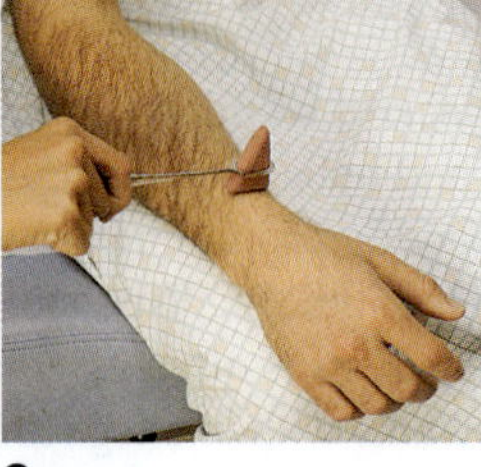
C

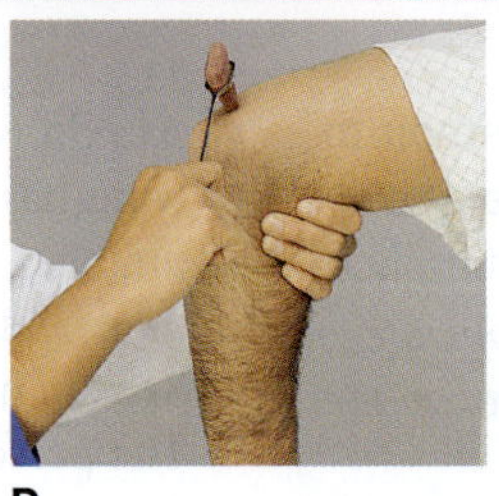
D

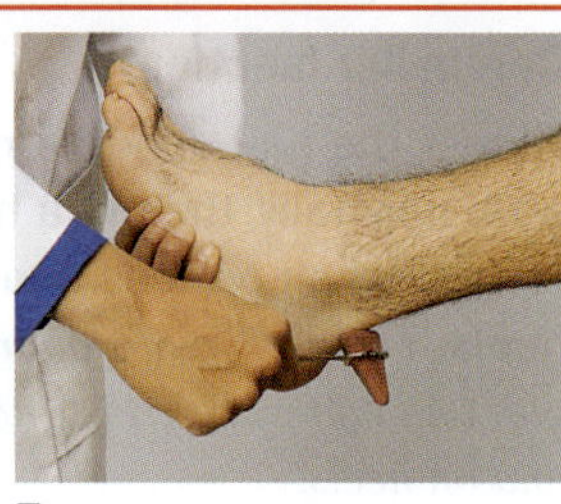
E

FIGURE 40.15 ***Deep tendon reflexes A, Using reinforcement technique to test the patellar reflex. B, Biceps reflex. C, Brachioradialis reflex. D, Triceps reflex. E, Achilles reflex***

Source: Pearson Education.

Assess for clonus by dorsiflexing the person's foot.

- Clonus, a hyperactive, rhythmic dorsiflexion and plantar flexion, is noted with upper motor neuron disease.

Assess the superficial abdominal and cremasteric reflexes.

- Superficial reflexes may be absent with disease of the lower and upper motor neurons.

Abdominal reflex: lightly stroke the abdomen with a tongue depressor from the side to the midline. Normally the side of the abdomen being stroked will contract towards the umbilicus (see Figure 40.16).
Cremasteric reflex: lightly stroke the inner thigh of the male with a tongue depressor. *Normally, the testicle on the side being stroked will rise.*

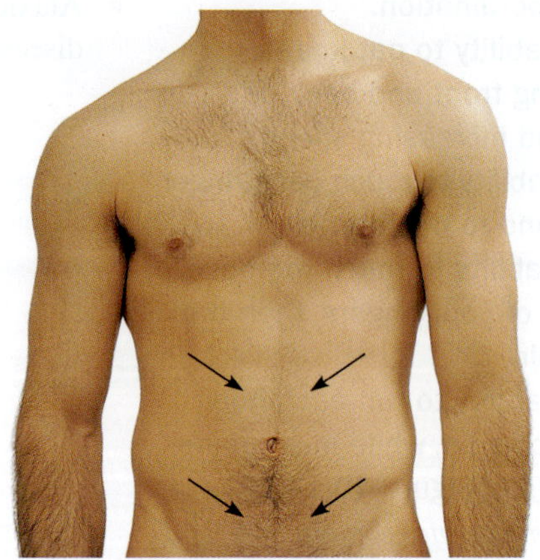

FIGURE 40.16 ***Location of superficial abdominal reflexes***

Source: Pearson Education.

Assess the Babinski reflex (see Figure 40.17).

- Dorsiflexion of the big toe and fanning of the other toes is seen with upper motor neuron disease of the pyramidal tract.

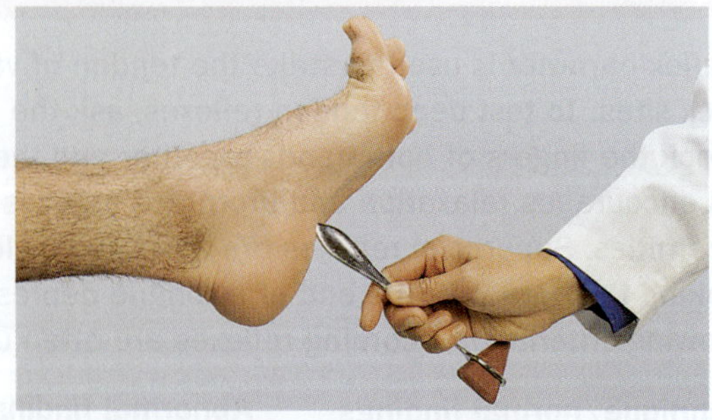

FIGURE 40.17 ***Assessing the Babinski reflex***

Source: Pearson Education.

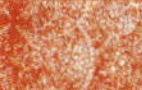

SPECIAL NEUROLOGICAL ASSESSMENTS

Technique/normal findings	Abnormal findings
Assess for Brudzinski's sign. With the person in the supine position, flex their head to their chest (see Figure 40.18). *There should be no pain, resistance or flexion of the hips or knees.*	▪ Pain, resistance and flexion of hips and knees occur with meningeal irritation.
Assess for Kernig's sign. With the person supine, flex their knees and hips, then straighten their knee (see Figure 40.19). *There should be no pain or resistance.*	▪ Excessive pain and/or resistance occurs with meningeal irritation.

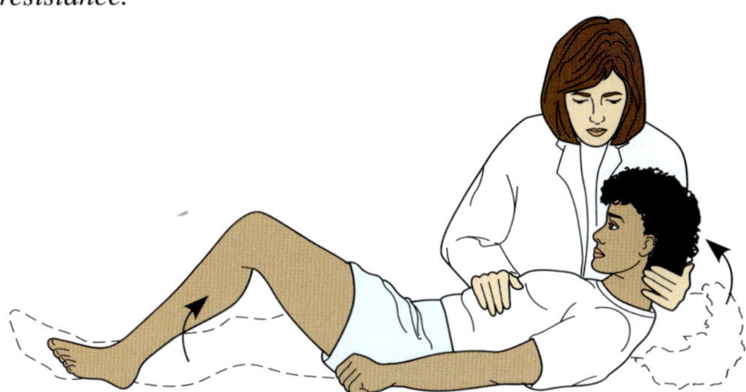

FIGURE 40.18 ***Assessing for Brudzinski's sign***

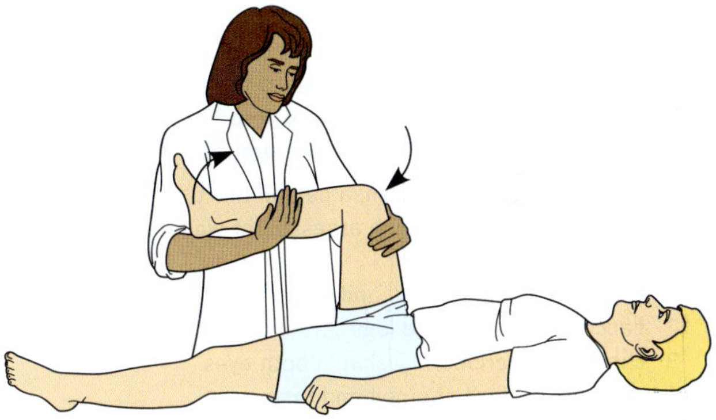

FIGURE 40.19 ***Assessing for Kernig's sign***

Assess for abnormal postures in people who are unconscious. *There should be no abnormal posturing.*	Observe for **decorticate posturing**, in which the upper arms are close to the sides; the elbows, wrists and fingers are flexed; the legs are extended with internal rotation; and the feet are plantar flexed (see Figure 40.20). Decorticate posturing occurs with lesions of the corticospinal tracts. Observe for **decerebrate posturing**, in which the neck is extended, with the jaw clenched; the arms are pronated, extended and close to the sides; the legs are extended straight out; and the feet are plantar flexed (see Figure 40.21). Decerebrate posturing occurs with lesions of the midbrain, pons or diencephalon.

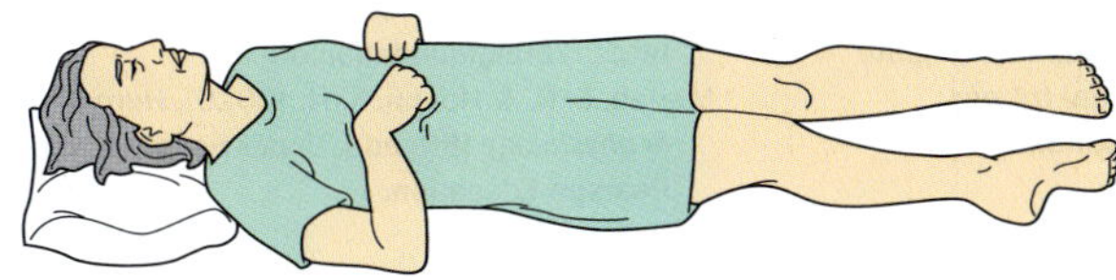

FIGURE 40.20 ***Decorticate posturing***

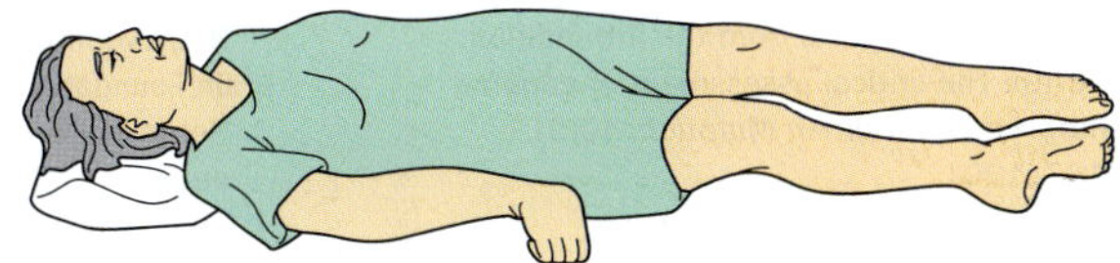

FIGURE 40.21 ***Decerebrate posturing***

CONCEPT CHECK

1 Which component of the brain protects it from harmful substances?
1 the circulation of cerebrospinal fluid
2 the large oxygen demand
3 the structure of neurons
4 the blood–brain barrier

2 Which pathophysiology results from damage to the lower motor neurons?
1 loss of cognitive ability
2 inability to communicate verbally
3 loss of reflexes
4 decreasing levels of consciousness

3 Which of the following statements about cerebrospinal fluid (CSF) is true?
1 If CSF contains glucose, the person has a metabolic disorder.
2 CSF circulates through the brain via the meninges.
3 CSF protects the brain and spinal cord from trauma.
4 A lumbar puncture is done to withdraw CSF from the brain.

4 Following a motorcycle crash, a person has damage to the posterior spinal roots. Which assessment would you expect to find?
1 loss of sensation to dull and sharp
2 flaccid paralysis of the legs
3 changes in peripheral vision in both eyes
4 decreased sense of smell and taste

5 You narrowly miss having a car crash while merging on to the freeway. Your body's responses to this stress are caused by which division of the autonomic nervous system?
1 sympathetic
2 parasympathetic
3 cholinergic
4 adrenergic

6 Which of the physical assessment techniques is not used in the neurological examination?
1 inspection
2 auscultation
3 percussion
4 palpation

7 What would you need to assess function of cranial nerve V (trigeminal)?
1 cotton ball and safety pin
2 stethoscope with bell and diaphragm
3 measuring tape and pencil
4 various scents, such as coffee and vanilla

8 In which of the following cases would assessing the corneal reflex be appropriate?
1 anyone over the age of 50
2 people who wear contact lenses
3 a person with spinal cord trauma
4 an unconscious person

9 You have been asked to assess a person's gag reflex. What equipment would you need to do this?
1 safety pin
2 cotton ball
3 tongue depressor
4 stethoscope

10 Which position best describes decorticate posturing?
1 neck extended, arms extended and pronated, feet plantar flexed
2 arms close to sides, elbows and wrists flexed, legs extended
3 in prone position with arms and knees sharply flexed
4 in supine position, spine extended, legs extended

BIBLIOGRAPHY

Andreoletti, G., Pal, L. R., Moult, J. & Brenner, S. E. (2019). Reports from the fifth edition of CAGI: The critical assessment of genome interpretation. *Human Mutation*, *40*(9), 1197–1201.

Brain Foundation (2022a). *Parkinson's disease*. Retrieved from https://brainfoundation.org.au/

Brain Foundation (2022b). *Essential tremor*. Retrieved from https://brainfoundation.org.au/

Brain Foundation (2022c). *Epilepsy*. Retrieved from https://brainfoundation.org.au/

Marieb, E. N. & Hoehn, K. N. (2010). *Human anatomy & physiology* (8th ed.). Upper Saddle River, NJ: Pearson Education.

CHAPTER 41

Nursing care of people with intracranial disorders

David Stanley

Key terms

brain death 1508
cerebral oedema 1513
concussion 1536
consciousness 1504
encephalitis 1541
epidural haematoma 1535
epilepsy 1524
hydrocephalus 1513
increased intracranial pressure (IICP) 1511
intracerebral haematoma 1535
locked-in syndrome 1507
meningitis 1540
persistent vegetative state 1507
seizure 1524
subdural haematoma 1535
traumatic brain injury (TBI) 1531

Learning outcomes

- Compare and contrast the pathophysiology, manifestations, interprofessional care and nursing care of people with alterations in level of consciousness and increased intracranial pressure.
- Explain the pathophysiology, manifestations, complications, interprofessional care and nursing care of intracranial disorders, including headaches, epilepsy, traumatic brain injury, central nervous system infections and brain tumours.
- Describe criteria for diagnosing persistent vegetative state and brain death.
- Discuss the purposes, nursing implications and health education for the person and their family in relation to medications used to treat altered cerebral function, headaches, epilepsy, traumatic brain injury, central nervous system infections and brain tumours.
- Discuss surgical options for the treatment of increased intracranial pressure, epilepsy, traumatic brain injury and brain tumours.

Clinical competencies

- Assess functional status of people with intracranial disorders and monitor, document and report abnormal manifestations.
- Determine priority nursing diagnoses, based on assessed data, to select and implement individualised nursing interventions for people with intracranial disorders.
- Safely administer oral and injectable medications used to treat intracranial disorders knowledgeably and safely.
- Provide skilled care to people having intracranial pressure monitoring, tonic–clonic seizures and intracranial surgery.
- Integrate interprofessional care into the care of people with intracranial disorders.
- Provide appropriate teaching and evidence-based practice to facilitate community-based care to promote safety and prevent injury, and to provide information and support necessary for long-term care of people with intracranial disorders.
- Revise the plan of care as needed to provide effective interventions to promote, maintain or restore functional health status to people with intracranial disorders.

The person with an intracranial disorder presents a unique nursing challenge. Problems the person experiences in the acute stage of the disorder are often a prelude to long-term problems requiring ongoing management. These long-term problems range from alterations in the body's basic functioning to dysfunctions in the complex processes of the individual's mind. Systemic problems may accompany or develop secondary to an intracranial disorder. Intracranial disorders may affect both the person's quality of life and that of the person's family. This chapter discusses altered level of consciousness and increased intracranial pressure, followed by discussion of intracranial disorders that may manifest these and other health problems.

Altered cerebral function

The manifestations of altered cerebral function occur as a result of illness or injury. Assessment of the patterns of those manifestations helps determine the extent of the cerebral dysfunction and the improvement or deterioration of cerebral function. Except in the case of direct damage to the brainstem and reticular activating system (RAS), brain function deterioration usually follows a predictable progression; that is, a pattern in which higher levels of function are impaired initially, progressing to impairment of more primitive functions. Altered level of consciousness (LOC) and behaviour changes are early manifestations of the deterioration of the function of the cerebral hemispheres. Structures in the midbrain and brainstem are affected sequentially, with characteristic changes in LOC; patterns of respiration, pupillary and oculomotor responses; and motor function. Manifestations of predicted progressive deterioration of cerebral function are outlined in Table 41.1. However, there may be deviation from this in some individuals.

THE PERSON WITH ALTERED LEVEL OF CONSCIOUSNESS

Consciousness is a condition in which the person is aware of self and environment and is able to respond appropriately to stimuli. Full consciousness requires both normal rousal, often referred to as alertness, and full cognition.

- Rousal is the state of wakefulness and awareness in which the individual functions and depends on the RAS, a diffuse system of neurons in the thalamus and upper brainstem.
- Cognition is a complex process involving the entirety of an individual's mental activities and is controlled by the cerebral hemispheres, including thought processes, memory, perception, problem solving and emotion.

These two components of consciousness depend on the normal physiological functions of and connections between the rousal mechanisms of the reticular formation and the cognitive functions of the cerebral hemispheres. Because rousal and cognition are independent components of consciousness, each can act separately on stimuli. For example, the RAS reacts to the discomfort caused by a full bladder by waking the person in the middle of the night. Once awake, however, the frontal cortex alerts the person that the bladder is full and prompts the person to go to the toilet and empty it.

Conditions that affect either the RAS or the function of the cerebral hemispheres can interfere with the normal LOC. Terms describing LOC are listed and defined in Table 41.2. Nurses should remember that consciousness is a dynamic state: a person may pass from full consciousness to coma quiet suddenly or experience a slow diminishment of consciousness that does not become evident for weeks or months. The nurse can

TABLE 41.1 Progression of deteriorating brain function

LEVEL OF CONSCIOUSNESS	PUPILLARY RESPONSE	OCULOMOTOR RESPONSES	MOTOR RESPONSES	BREATHING
Alert; oriented to time, place and person	Brisk and equal; pupils regular	Eyes move as head turns; caloric testing (ear irrigation) produces nystagmus	Purposeful movement; responds to commands	Regular pattern with normal rate and depth
Responds to verbal stimuli; decreased concentration; agitation, confusion, lethargy; disoriented	Small and reactive	Roving eye movements; doll's eyes positive, with gaze fixed straight ahead; eye deviation away from cold caloric stimulus and towards warm stimulus	Purposeful movement in response to pain stimulus	Yawning, sighing respirations
Requires continuous stimulation to rouse			Decorticate posturing with upper extremity flexion	Cheyne–Stokes respirations with crescendo–decrescendo pattern in rate and depth followed by period of apnoea
Reflexive positioning to pain stimulus	Pupils fixed (non-reactive) in midposition	Caloric testing produces nystagmus	Decerebrate posturing with adduction and rigid extension of upper and lower extremities	Central neurogenic hyperventilation with rapid, regular and deep respirations; apneustic breathing with prolonged inspiration and pauses at full inspiration and following expiration
No response to stimuli	Pupils fixed in midposition	No spontaneous eye movement or nystagmus	Extension of upper extremities with flexion of lower extremities; flaccidity	Cluster or ataxic breathing with irregular pattern and depth of respirations; gasping respirations or apnoea

TABLE 41.2 Terms used to describe level of consciousness

TERM	CHARACTERISTICS OF PERSON
Full consciousness	Alert; oriented to time, place and person; comprehends spoken and written words
Clouding of consciousness	Mild form of altered mental status characterised by reduced wakefulness and inattention
Confusion	Unable to think rapidly and clearly; easily bewildered, with poor memory and short attention span; misinterprets stimuli; judgment is impaired
Disorientation	Not aware of or not oriented to time, place or person
Drowsy	Lethargic, somnolent; responsive to verbal or tactile stimuli but quickly drifts back to sleep
Stupor	Generally unresponsive; may be briefly roused by vigorous, repeated or painful stimuli; may shrink away from or grab at the source of stimuli
Semicomatose	Does not move spontaneously; unresponsive to stimuli, although vigorous or painful stimuli may result in stirring, moaning or withdrawal from the stimuli, without actual rousal
Coma	Unrousable; will not stir or moan in response to any stimulus; may exhibit non-purposeful response (slight movement) of area stimulated but makes no attempt to withdraw
Deep coma	Completely unrousable and unresponsive to any kind of stimulus, including pain; absence of brainstem reflexes, corneal, papillary and pharyngeal reflexes, and tendon and plantar reflexes

help provide effective care for a person with an altered LOC by looking beyond the diagnostic labels of consciousness and accurately assessing the person's behaviour and response to stimuli.

Pathophysiology

Level of consciousness may be altered by processes that affect the rousal functions of the brainstem, the cognitive functions of the cerebral hemispheres, or both. The main causes are: (1) trauma, injuries or disease processes that affect the cerebral hemispheres directly and widely, or that compress or destroy the neurons of the RAS, and (2) metabolic disorders.

Rousal and cognition

The physiological seat of consciousness, the reticular formation, is a mass of nerve cells and fibres that make up the core of the brainstem, extending from the medulla to the midbrain. The axons of reticular neurons are exceptionally long and branch outwards to cells in the hypothalamus, thalamus, cerebellum and spinal cord. A system of reticular neurons within the RAS passes steady streams of impulses through thalamic relays in order to stimulate the cerebral cortex into wakefulness. The body's sensory tracts interact with RAS neurons; this interrelationship helps control the strength of the RAS's rousing effect on the cerebrum.

Damage to the RAS impairs the person's ability to maintain wakefulness and rousal. Cerebral vascular accidents, or strokes, are the most common cause of RAS destruction. Other causes include demyelinating diseases, tumours, abscesses and head injury. Function of the RAS may also be suppressed by compression of the brainstem, which produces oedema and ischaemia. Pressure and compression of the brainstem may be due to tumours, increased intracranial pressure, haematomas, haemorrhage or aneurysm. Although it is possible to assess LOC or rousal in the person with RAS damage, the impairment in rousal may make it impossible to accurately assess cognitive function.

The function of the brain, especially the cerebral hemispheres, depends on continuous blood flow with unimpeded supplies of oxygen, glucose and key electrolytes. Processes that disrupt this flow of blood and nutrients may cause widespread damage to the cerebral hemispheres, impairing rousal and cognition. Bilateral hemispheric lesions (such as global ischaemia) or metabolic disorders (such as hypoglycaemia) are the most common causes of altered LOC related to cerebral dysfunction of the hemispheres. Localised masses, such as a haematoma or cerebral oedema, which displace normal structures and cause direct or indirect pressure on the opposite hemisphere or brainstem, can also affect LOC. The person who has widespread damage to the cerebral hemispheres but an intact RAS has sleep–wake cycles and may rouse in response to stimuli; the person cannot be said to be alert, however, because cognition is impaired.

Both localised neurological processes and systemic disorders can alter LOC. Processes occurring within the brain, which may directly destroy or compress neurological structures, include the following:

- increased intracranial pressure
- stroke
- haematoma
- intracranial haemorrhage
- tumours
- infections
- injury from excitatory amino acids
- demyelinating disorders.

Any systemic condition that affects the delivery of blood, oxygen and glucose to the brain or alters cell membranes may also alter LOC. If cerebral blood flow is impaired or the person becomes hypoxic or hypoglycaemic, cerebral metabolism is impaired and LOC declines rapidly. Severe hypoxia quickly leads to ischaemia. Ischaemia may be focal (e.g. following a stroke), resulting in a level of altered consciousness, or global (as from cardiac arrest or hypovolaemic shock), which causes almost immediate unconsciousness (Norris, 2018). Individuals at particular risk of developing ischaemia include those with poorly controlled diabetes and those with cardiac or respiratory failure.

Other metabolic alterations that can affect LOC include fluid and electrolyte imbalances, such as hyponatraemia, and acid–base alterations, such as hypercapnoea (an elevated arterial carbon dioxide level). Accumulated waste products and toxins from liver or kidney failure can affect neuronal and neurotransmitter function, altering LOC. Drugs that depress the central nervous system (e.g. alcohol, analgesics, anaesthetics) suppress metabolic and membrane activities in the RAS and cerebral hemispheres, thereby affecting LOC. Furthermore, glutamate (the main excitatory neurotransmitter in the brain) may accumulate during prolonged ischaemia, resulting in acute glutamate toxicity and cell death.

Seizure activity, with abnormal electrical discharges from a local area of the brain or from the entire brain, commonly affects LOC. It appears that the spontaneous, disordered discharge of activity that occurs during a seizure exhausts energy metabolites and also produces locally toxic molecules, altering LOC for a time after the seizure. This period of time is referred to as the post-ictal phase. Consciousness returns when the metabolic balance of the neurons is restored.

As the impairment of brain function progresses, more stimuli are required to elicit a response from the person. Initially, the person may rouse to verbal stimuli and respond appropriately to questions, remaining oriented to time, place and person. With deterioration of neurological function, the person becomes more difficult to rouse and may become agitated and confused when awakened. Generally, orientation to time is lost first, followed by orientation to place and then to person. Continuous stimulation or vigorous shaking is required to maintain wakefulness as LOC decreases. Eventually, the individual becomes nonresponsive, even with deep painful stimuli.

Patterns of respirations

Progressive impairment of neural function also causes predictable changes in respiratory patterns as respiratory centres are affected. In normal respirations, a rhythmic pattern is maintained by neural centres in the pons and medulla that respond to changes in arterial levels of oxygen (PaO_2) and carbon dioxide ($PaCO_2$). When there is damage to the RAS or cerebral hemispheres, neural control of these centres is lost and lower brainstem centres regulate breathing patterns by responding only to changes in $PaCO_2$, resulting in irregular respiratory patterns. The initial manifestations of deteriorating brain function are yawning and sighing. As outlined in Table 41.1, and illustrated in Table 41.3, progressive deterioration in brain function is accompanied by decreasing LOC and changes in breathing patterns. The types of respirations, by area of cerebral damage, are as follows:

- diencephalon: *Cheyne–Stokes respirations* (alternating regular periods of deep, rapid breathing followed by periods of apnoea)
- midbrain: *neurogenic hyperventilation* (may exceed 40 per minute), the result of uninhibited stimulation of the respiratory centres
- pons: *apneustic respirations*, characterised by sighing on mid-inspiration or prolonged inhalation and exhalation; results from excessive stimulation of the respiratory centres
- medulla: *ataxic/apnoeic respirations* (totally uncoordinated and irregular), probably as a result of the loss of responsiveness to CO_2.

Pupillary and oculomotor responses

The brainstem areas that control rousal are adjacent to areas that control the pupils. A predictable progression of pupillary and oculomotor responses occurs as the LOC deteriorates towards coma (see Table 41.1). If the lesion or process affecting neurological function is localised, effects may initially be seen in the ipsilateral pupil (the pupil on the same side as the lesion). With generalised or systemic processes, pupils are affected equally. If the pupils are small and equally reactive, metabolic processes affecting LOC may be present. With compression of cranial nerve III at the midbrain, the pupils may become oval or eccentric (off centre). As the level of functional impairment progresses, the pupils become fixed (unresponsive to light) and, eventually, dilated.

In deteriorating LOC and coma, spontaneous eye movement is lost and reflexive ocular movements may be altered. Normally, both eyes move simultaneously in the same direction; injury to the cranial nerve nuclei in the midbrain and pons can impair normal movement. Doll's eye movements are reflexive movements of the eyes in the opposite direction of head rotation; they are an indicator of brainstem function (see Figure 41.1). As a result of the oculocephalic reflex, the eyes move upwards with passive flexion of the neck and downwards with passive neck extension. As brainstem function deteriorates, this reflex is lost. The eyes fail to turn together and, eventually, remain fixed in the midposition as the head is turned.

TABLE 41.3 Breathing patterns characteristic of altered level of consciousness

PATTERN		DESCRIPTION
Cheyne-Stokes respirations	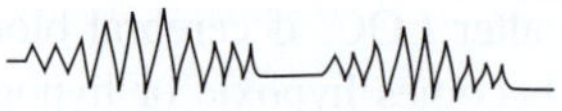	A regular crescendo-decrescendo pattern with increasing, then decreasing, rate and depth of respirations followed by a period of apnoea
Central neurogenic hyperventilation	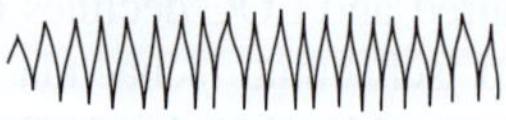	A sustained pattern of rapid, regular, deep respirations (hyperapnoea)
Apneustic breathing	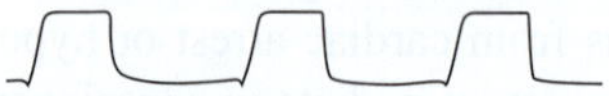	Prolonged inspiration with a pause at full inspiration followed by expiration and a possible pause following expiration
Cluster breathing	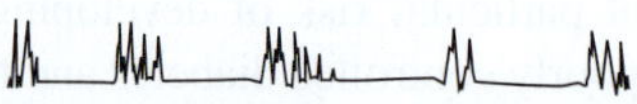	Clusters of several breaths with irregular periods of apnoea between clusters
Ataxic respirations	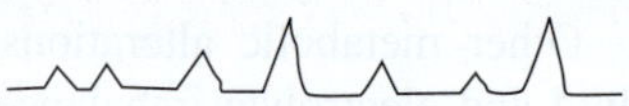	Respirations that are completely irregular in pattern and depth with irregular periods of apnoea

Head in neutral position

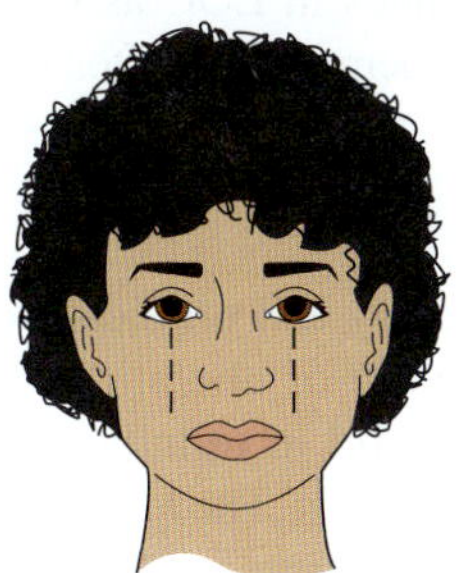

Eyes midline

Head rotated to person's left

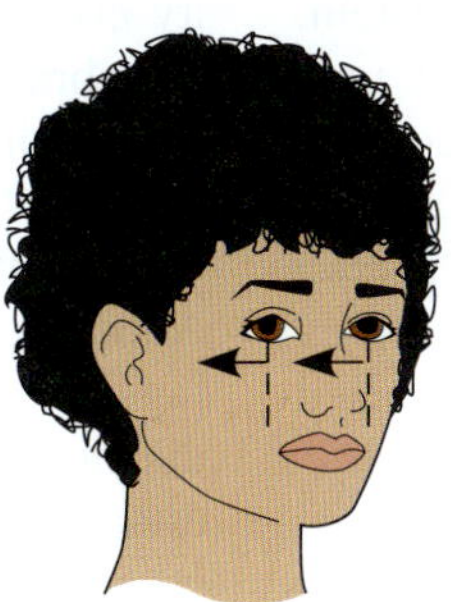

Doll's eyes present:
Eyes move right in relation to head.

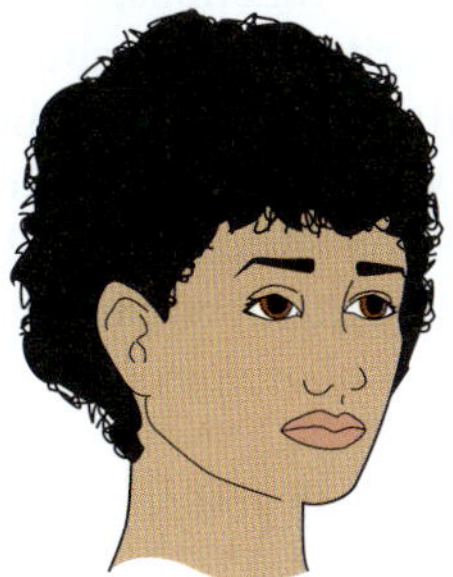

Doll's eyes absent:
Eyes do not move in relation to head.
Direction of vision follows head to left.

FIGURE 41.1 *Doll's eye movements characteristic of altered LOC*

Motor responses

The level of brain dysfunction and the side of the brain affected may be assessed by motor responses. These responses are the most accurate identifier of changes in mental status. In altered LOC, motor responses to stimuli range from an appropriate response to a command (e.g. 'squeeze my hand' or 'push my hands away with your feet') to flaccidity (see Table 41.1). Initially, the person may be able to move purposefully; for example, to brush the examiner's hand away from the face. As function declines, movements become more generalised (withdrawal, grimacing) and less purposeful. Reflexive motor responses may occur, including decorticate posturing with flexion of the upper extremities accompanied by extension of the lower extremities. With further decline, decerebrate posturing is seen, with adduction and rigid extension of the upper and lower extremities. Without intervention, the person eventually becomes flaccid, with little or no motor response to stimuli.

Coma states and brain death

Possible outcomes of altered LOC and coma include full recovery with no long-term residual effects, recovery with residual damage (such as learning deficits, emotional difficulties or impaired judgment) or more severe consequences, such as persistent vegetative state (cerebral death) or brain death. Resources for families are listed in Box 41.1.

BOX 41.1 Organisations providing information for families of people in a coma

Brain Injury Australia
Ph: 1800 BRAIN1
(1800 272 461)
https://www.braininjuryaustralia.org.au

Carers Australia
Ph: (02) 6122 9900
www.carersaustralia.com.au

National Disability Insurance Scheme
Ph: 1800 800 110
https://www.ndis.gov.au

Brain Foundation
Ph: 1300 886 660 or
(02) 9437 5967
https://brainfoundation.org.au

PERSISTENT VEGETATIVE STATE **Persistent vegetative state** (also called irreversible coma) is a permanent condition of complete unawareness of self and the environment and loss of all cognitive functions. Usually, the result of severe brain trauma or global ischaemia, this condition results from death of the cerebral hemispheres with continued function of the brainstem and cerebellum. While the homeostatic regulatory functions of the brain continue, the ability to respond meaningfully to the environment is lost. The diagnosis of persistent vegetative state requires that the condition has continued for at least 1 month (Norris, 2018).

The person has sleep–wake cycles and retains the ability to chew, swallow and cough, but cannot interact with the environment. When awake, the eyes may wander back and forth across the room, but they cannot track an object or person. In a minimally conscious state, the person is aware of the environment and can follow simple commands, manipulate objects, gesture or verbalise to indicate 'yes/no' responses and make meaningful movements (such as blinking or smiling) in response to a stimulus. With appropriate interventions and support, the individual may remain in this state for years.

LOCKED-IN SYNDROME **Locked-in syndrome** is distinctly different from persistent vegetative state in that the person is alert and fully aware of the environment and has intact cognitive abilities, but is unable to communicate through speech or movement because of blocked efferent pathways from the brain. Motor paralysis affects all voluntary muscles, although in some cases, the upper cranial nerves (I to IV) may remain intact, allowing some communication through eye movements and blinking. In essence, the person is 'locked' inside a paralysed body while remaining fully conscious of self and environment. Infarction or haemorrhage of the pons that disrupts outgoing nerve tracts but spares the RAS is the usual cause of locked-in syndrome. This condition may also result when the corticospinal tracts between the midbrain and pons are interrupted. Disorders of the lower motor neurons or muscles, such as acute polyneuritis, myasthenia gravis or motor neurone disease, may also paralyse motor responses, leading to locked-in syndrome.

BRAIN DEATH **Brain death** is the cessation and irreversibility of all brain functions, including the brainstem. Although the exact criteria for establishing brain death may vary, it is generally agreed that brain death has occurred when there is no evidence of cerebral or brainstem function for an extended period (usually 6 to 24 hours) in a person who has a normal body temperature and is not affected by a depressant drug or alcohol poisoning. Generally recognised criteria are:

- unresponsive coma with absent motor and reflex movements
- no spontaneous respiration (apnoea)
- pupils fixed (unresponsive to light) and dilated
- absent ocular responses to head turning and caloric stimulation (caloric stimulation is performed by irrigating the ear with ice-cold water to test the oculovestibular reflex, a reflex controlled by the brainstem. Normally, the cold causes the eyes to move first towards the irrigated side, followed by a return to midline)
- flat electroencephalogram (EEG) and no cerebral blood circulation present on angiography (if performed)
- persistence of these manifestations for 30 minutes to 1 hour and for 6 hours after onset of coma and apnoea.

Apnoea in the comatose person is determined by the apnoea test. The ventilator is removed while maintaining oxygenation by tracheal cannula and allowing the PCO_2 to increase to 60 mmHg or higher. This level of carbon dioxide is high enough to stimulate respiration if the brainstem is functional. An EEG may be used to establish the absence of brain activity when brain death is suspected. A flat (isoelectric) EEG over a period of 6 to 12 hours in a person who is not hypothermic or under the influence of drugs that depress the central nervous system (CNS) is generally accepted as an indicator of brain death.

Prognosis

The prognosis for people with altered levels of consciousness and coma varies according to the underlying cause and pathological process. Age and general medical condition also play a role in determining outcome. Young adults may fully recover following deep coma from head injury, drug overdose or other cause. Recovery of consciousness within 2 weeks is associated with a favourable outcome. In general, the prognosis is poor for people who lack pupillary reaction or reflex eye movements 6 hours after the onset of coma.

INTERPROFESSIONAL CARE

Management of the person with an altered LOC must begin immediately. The focus of management is to identify the underlying cause, preserve function and prevent deterioration if possible. During this period, the A–E primary assessment is essential in preventing further negative outcomes. Airway and breathing must be maintained during the initial acute stage until the diagnosis and prognosis can be established. Intravenous fluids are used to support circulation and to correct fluid, electrolyte and acid–base imbalances. Treatment protocols to reduce increased intracranial pressure or control seizure activity may be initiated. Changes in LOC associated with craniocerebral trauma, such as haematomas, often require immediate surgical intervention.

Diagnosis

Although the person's history and physical examination findings often indicate the cause of alterations in LOC, several diagnostic tests may be useful in ruling out differentials and establishing the formal diagnosis. The tests used to evaluate for possible metabolic, toxic or drug-induced disorders include both radiological and laboratory tests.

CT and MRI scanning are performed in order to detect neurological damage due to haemorrhage, tumour, cyst, oedema, myocardial infarction or brain atrophy. These tests may also identify displacement of brain structures by large or expanding lesions. Radioisotope brain scan is performed to identify abnormal lesions in the brain and evaluate cerebral blood flow. Cerebral angiography allows radiographic visualisation of the cerebral vascular system. This exam can identify lesions such as aneurysms, occluded vessels or tumours, and may also be used to determine cessation of cerebral blood flow and brain death. Transcranial Doppler studies use an ultrasound velocity detector that records sound waves reflected from RBCs in blood vessels to assess cerebral blood flow. Lumbar puncture with cerebrospinal fluid (CSF) analysis is performed when infection and possible meningitis are suspected as a cause of altered LOC. EEG is used to evaluate the electrical activity of the brain. (See the chapter 'A person-centred approach to assessing the nervous system' for further information and nursing implications of specific neurological tests.)

Laboratory tests are used to identify and monitor altered LOC. These may include any or all of the following:

- *Blood glucose* is measured immediately when coma is of unknown origin and hypoglycaemia is suspected or possible. When the blood glucose falls to less than 2.2 to 2.7 mmol/L, cerebral function declines rapidly. The person with type 1 diabetes is at particular risk of hypoglycaemia-induced coma.
- *Serum electrolytes*—sodium, potassium, bicarbonate, chloride and calcium, in particular—are measured to assess for metabolic disturbances and to guide intravenous therapy. Hyponatraemia, in which serum sodium levels are below 115 mmol/L (normal level: 135 to 145 mmol/L), is associated with coma and convulsions, especially if it develops rapidly.
- *Serum osmolality* is evaluated. Both hyperosmolar and hypo-osmolar states may be associated with coma. Hyperosmolality (above 320 mOsm/kg H_2O) causes cellular dehydration of brain tissue as fluid is drawn into the vascular system by osmosis. Hypo-osmolality (less than 250 mOsm/kg H_2O), by contrast, leads to cerebral oedema, increasing intracranial pressure and impairing consciousness.
- *Arterial blood gases* (ABGs) are drawn to evaluate arterial oxygen and carbon dioxide levels, as well as acid–base balance. Hypoxaemia is a frequent cause of altered LOC;

increased levels of carbon dioxide are also toxic to the brain and can induce coma, particularly when the onset of hypercapnoea is acute.

- *Liver function tests*, including bilirubin, aspartate transaminase (AST), alanine transaminase (ALT), lactate dehydrogenase (LDH), serum albumin and serum ammonia levels, are determined to evaluate hepatic function. High ammonia levels seen in hepatic failure interfere with cerebral metabolism and neurotransmitters, affecting LOC.
- Toxicology screening of blood and urine is done to determine if altered LOC is the result of acute drug or alcohol toxicity. Serum alcohol levels are measured and the blood is assessed for the presence of substances such as barbiturates, carbon monoxide or lead.

Medications

Medications are used to support homeostasis and normal function for the person with altered LOC, as well as to treat specific causes and underlying disorders. As decreased consciousness often results in an impaired airway, intravenous medications may be preferred. An intravenous catheter is inserted and fluid balance is generally maintained using isotonic, such as normal saline or Hartmann's solution. The person's response to fluid administration is monitored carefully for evidence of increased cerebral oedema.

If hypoglycaemia is present, glucose-containing solutions are administered intravenously to restore cerebral metabolism rapidly. Conversely, insulin is administered to the person with hyperglycaemia to reduce the blood glucose level and thus the serum osmolality. With narcotic overdose, naloxone is administered. Naloxone is a narcotic antagonist that competes for narcotic receptor sites, effectively blocking the depressant effect of the narcotic. Thiamine may be administered with glucose, particularly if the person is malnourished or known to abuse alcohol, to prevent exacerbation of Wernicke's encephalopathy, a haemorrhagic encephalopathy due to thiamine deficiency that is associated with chronic alcoholism (Papadakis, McPhee & Rabow, 2022).

Any underlying fluid and electrolyte imbalance is corrected by administering medications or appropriate electrolytes. For the person who is hyponatraemic and has a low serum osmolality, frusemide (Lasix) or an osmotic diuretic may be administered to promote water excretion. In cases of infection, such as a person with suspected or confirmed meningitis, appropriate antibiotics will need to be administered intravenously.

Surgery

Although surgery is not indicated for most people with altered LOC, it may be necessary if the cause of coma is an intracerebral tumour, haemorrhage or haematoma. Surgical intervention is discussed later in this chapter, in the section on brain tumours. When there is a risk of increased intracranial pressure, the person is monitored continuously. These measures are discussed in the section on increased intracranial pressure that follows.

Other treatments

Support of the airway and respirations is vital in the person with an altered LOC. The person who is drowsy but rousable may need little more than a nasal or oral pharyngeal airway. With more severe alterations in consciousness, the person may need endotracheal intubation to maintain airway patency, particularly if the cough and gag reflexes are absent. Mechanical ventilation is indicated when hypoventilation or apnoea is present. Unless a not-for-resuscitation (NFR) order is in effect, mechanical ventilation should be initiated even if it has not been established that the disorder is reversible; without ventilatory support, cerebral anoxia develops rapidly and brain death may ensue. ABGs are monitored frequently to determine the adequacy of ventilation. Cautious hyperventilation may be used to reduce $PaCO_2$ and promote cerebral vasoconstriction to reduce cerebral oedema.

Nutrition

In people with long-term alterations in consciousness, such as vegetative state or locked-in syndrome, measures to maintain nutritional status are essential. Enteral feedings with a gastrostomy tube are preferred if the person is unable to take enough food by mouth without aspirating. In some cases, total parenteral nutrition (TPN) may be used.

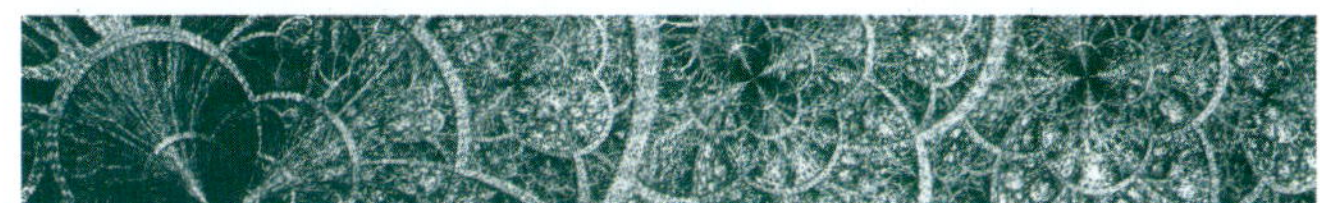

Nursing care

Nursing care of the person with an altered LOC is planned and implemented for a variety of responses of both the person and their family.

Support of the family

Family members of a person with an altered LOC are often very anxious. It is difficult for the family to deal with the person's uncertain prognosis. The family may experience various conflicting emotions, such as guilt and anger. It is important for the nurse to be able to reinforce information provided by the doctor and encourage the family to talk to the person as though they are able to understand. Explain that this communication may initially seem awkward, but in time it will feel appropriate. Evaluate the family's readiness to receive explanations regarding the person's treatment and care. The presence of many medical devices (e.g. intravenous line, catheter, ventilator) may be overwhelming to the family. Despite this, family may not perceive the seriousness of the situation if a thorough explanation is not given. It is important to include family members in the person's care as much as they wish to be involved.

Where possible, the person's significant others should be allowed to stay close to the person. Reinforce the need for family members to care for themselves by encouraging adequate meals and rest. Offer to contact support services such as friends, neighbours and social services that the hospital may provide. Ask family members to leave a telephone number where they can be reached and assure them that they will be called if any significant changes occur. Encourage family members to call if they have questions or concerns.

Nursing diagnoses and interventions

Nursing diagnoses and interventions discussed in this section are directed towards the unconscious person and focus on problems with airway maintenance, skin integrity, contractures and nutrition.

Ineffective airway clearance

Ineffective airway clearance related to loss of the cough reflex and the inability to expectorate is a major problem for the unconscious person. The cough reflex may be absent or impaired when conditions that produce coma depress the function of the medullary centres.

- Assess ability to clear secretions. Monitor breath sounds, rate and depth of respirations, dyspnoea, pulse oximeter and the presence of cyanosis. *The person's ability to clear secretions serves as the initial assessment base for developing further interventions.*
- In unconscious people or those without an intact cough reflex, maintain an open airway by periodic suctioning, limiting the time of suctioning to 10 to 15 seconds or less. Regular suctioning may be necessary to clear the airway of mucus or other drainage. *Suctioning for more than 15 seconds in the person with increased intracranial pressure may cause hypercapnia, which in turn vasodilates cerebral vessels, increases cerebral blood volume and increases intracranial pressure.*

> **CONSIDERATION FOR PRACTICE**
> **If the person has a base-of-skull fracture or CSF draining from the ears or nose, never suction nasally.**

- Assist with repositioning every 2 hours and maintain a side-lying position with the head of the bed elevated approximately 30 degrees. Do not position the unconscious person on the back. *Turning the person from side to side facilitates respirations, prevents the tongue from obstructing the airway and helps prevent pooling of secretions in one area of the lungs (thus decreasing the risk of pneumonia).*
- If the person has a tracheostomy, provide tracheostomy care every 4 hours and suction when secretions are present. *Tracheostomy care is important to maintain an open airway and protect the stoma.*
- Monitor the results of arterial blood gas analysis and pulse oximetry. Maintain records of trends. *ABGs and pulse oximetry directly measure the oxygen content of blood and are good indicators of the lungs' ability to oxygenate the blood.*

Risk of aspiration

The unconscious person with a depressed or absent gag and swallowing reflex is at high risk of aspiration. Drainage, mucus or blood may obstruct the airway and interfere with oxygenation. Aspiration and pooling of secretions in the lungs also increases the risk of pneumonia.

- Assess swallowing and gag reflexes every shift as appropriate to the person's LOC. *Deepening levels of unconsciousness may cause a loss in swallow and gag reflexes.*
- Monitor for and report manifestations of aspiration: crackles and wheezes, dullness to percussion over an area of the lungs, dyspnoea, tachypnoea and cyanosis. *Early recognition facilitates prompt intervention.*
- Provide interventions to prevent aspiration:
  - Maintain NBM status.
  - Place in the side-lying position.
  - Provide oral hygiene and suctioning as needed.

  The side-lying position allows secretions to drain from the mouth rather than into the pharynx. Oral hygiene and suctioning remove secretions that might otherwise be aspirated.

> **CONSIDERATION FOR PRACTICE**
> **Never give oral food and fluids to people with a decreased LOC because of the risk of aspiration.**

Risk of impaired skin integrity

The unconscious person is at risk of impaired skin integrity as a result of immobility and the inability to provide self-care. On average, healthy people change positions during sleep every 11 minutes; the unconscious person often cannot maintain the movement needed to prevent pressure on the skin, especially over bony prominences. As a result, the skin and subcutaneous tissues may become ischaemic and prone to develop pressure injury. Perspiration and incontinence of urine and stool may exacerbate the problem. Nursing interventions are directed at maintaining the integrity not only of the skin but also of the lips and mucous membranes.

- Assess skin every shift, especially over bony prominences, the back of the scalp and around genitals and buttocks. *The large surface area of the skin bears weight and is in constant contact with the surface of the bed. The skin, subcutaneous tissue and muscles, especially those tissues over bony prominences, undergo constant pressure. This impairs normal capillary blood flow, which interferes with the exchange of nutrients and waste products. Tissue ischaemia and necrosis may result and lead to the development of pressure injury.*
- Provide proper positioning. Reposition bed-bound people at least every 2 hours if this is consistent with the overall treatment goals. Keep the head of the bed elevated no higher than 30 degrees unless prescribed differently. Provide interventions that distribute weight more evenly (e.g. alternating pressure air mattresses, egg-crate foam cushions, turning frames). Consider requesting/using a special therapeutic bed that automatically turns the person at regular intervals. Lift the person instead of dragging the person across the sheet. *When the head of the bed is elevated above 30 degrees, the person's torso tends to slide down towards the foot of the bed. Friction and perspiration cause the skin and superficial fascia to remain fixed against the bed linen while the deep fascia and skeleton slide downwards. When a person is pulled rather than lifted,*

Links to National Patient Safety Standards

NSQHS: Comprehensive Care Standard

Implementing this standard is achieved by the establishment of systems that ensure adequate care, including the management of pressure injuries, poor nutrition and cognitive impairment. Caring for individuals with decreased LOC will require vigilant care to achieve expected outcomes.

Source: Australian Commission on Safety and Quality in Health Care (ACSQHC) (2021). *National Safety and Quality Health Service Standards* (2nd ed.). Sydney: ACSQHC.

the skin remains fixed to the sheet while the fascia and muscles are pulled upwards. These shearing forces promote tissue breakdown.

- Provide interventions to prevent breakdown of the skin and mucous membranes:
  - Keep bed linen clean, dry and wrinkle free.
  - Provide daily bath with mild soap.
  - Cleanse the skin after urine and faecal soiling with a mild cleansing agent.
  - Provide oral care and lubricate the lips every 2 to 4 hours.
  - Maintain accurate intake and output records.
  - Keep the cornea moist by instilling appropriate lubricating eye drops and apply protective eye shields or close the eyelids with adhesive strips if the corneal reflex is absent.

  Keeping linen clean, dry and wrinkle free decreases the risk of injury from the shearing force of bed rest and protects against environmental factors that cause drying. Adequate hydration of the stratum corneum appears to protect the skin against mechanical insult. Preventing dehydration maintains circulation and decreases the concentration of urine, thereby minimising skin irritation in people who are incontinent. Proper eye care prevents corneal abrasion and irritation.

Impaired physical mobility

People who are unconscious are unable to maintain normal musculoskeletal movement; as a result, they are at high risk of contractures related to decreased movement. Flexor and adductor muscles are stronger than the extensors and abductors, resulting in the rapid development of flexor and adductor contractures without preventive measures. Passive ROM exercises must be performed routinely to maintain muscle tone and function, to prevent additional disability and to help restore impaired motor function.

- Maintain extremities in functional positions by providing proper support devices. Remove support devices every 4 hours for skin care and passive ROM exercises. Provide pillows for the axillary region; rolled washcloths may be placed in elevated hands; use splints to prevent plantar flexion (foot drop). *Pillows in the axillary region help prevent adduction of the shoulder. Rolled washcloths help decrease oedema and flexion contracture of the fingers. Splints are useful in preventing plantar flexion.*
- Collaborate with a physiotherapist to develop and implement passive range-of-motion (ROM) exercises (unless contraindicated, as for the person with increased intracranial pressure) at least four times a day, keeping the following principles in mind:
  - Place one hand above the joint being exercised. The other hand gently moves the joint through its normal range of motion.
  - Move the body part to the point of resistance and stop.

  Placing one hand above the joint provides support against gravity and prevents unwanted movement. ROM exercises help prevent contractures by stretching muscles and tendons and maintaining joint mobility.

Risk of imbalanced nutrition: less than body requirements

The unconscious person is at risk of an alteration in nutrition related to a reduced or complete inability to eat. This is especially true for the person who is unconscious as the result of an infection or trauma, both of which increase metabolic requirements.

- Monitor nutritional status through daily weights (on bed scales) and laboratory data. For accuracy, weigh the person at the same time each day, using the same scales. Ensure that the person wears the same clothing. *Changes in laboratory data with decreased nutrition include a decrease in the levels of serum prealbumin and serum transferrin.*
- Assess the need for alternative methods of nutritional support (tube feeding or total parenteral nutrition) through collaboration with a dietitian. People unable to take oral food require parenteral nutrition or liquid feedings through a nasogastric, gastrostomy or jejunostomy tube. *Needs for protein, kilojoules, zinc and vitamin C increase during wound healing.*

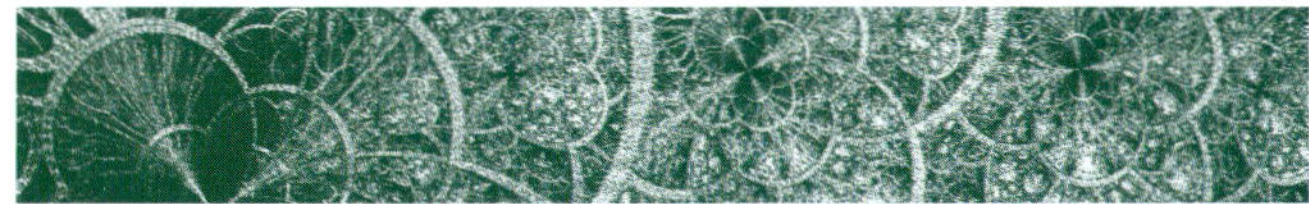

THE PERSON WITH INCREASED INTRACRANIAL PRESSURE

Increased intracranial pressure (IICP) (also called *intracranial hypertension*) is sustained elevated pressure within the cranial cavity (Hickey, 2019). Transient increases in intracranial pressure (ICP) occur with normal activities such as coughing, sneezing, straining or bending forward. These transient increases are not harmful; however, sustained increases in ICP can result in significant tissue ischaemia and damage to delicate neural tissue. Cerebral oedema is the most frequent cause of sustained increases in ICP. Other causes include head trauma, tumours, abscesses, stroke, inflammation and haemorrhage.

Pathophysiology

In the adult, the rigid cranial cavity created by the skull is normally filled to capacity with three essentially non-compressible elements: the brain (80%), cerebrospinal fluid (8%) and blood (12%). A state of dynamic equilibrium exists; if the volume of any of the three components increases, the volume of the others must decrease to maintain normal pressures within the cranial cavity. This is known as the *Monro–Kellie hypothesis*. The normal intracranial pressure is 5 to 10 mmHg (measured intracranially with a pressure transducer while the person is lying with the head elevated 30 degrees) or 60 to 180 cm H_2O (measured with a water manometer while the person is lying in a lateral recumbent position).

Cerebral blood flow and perfusion are important concepts for understanding the development and effects of IICP. Whereas blood and cerebrospinal fluid contribute roughly an equal percentage to normal intracranial volume, vascular factors account for twice the amount of increase in ICP that cerebrospinal fluid does. The brain requires a constant supply of oxygen and glucose to meet its metabolic demands; 15–20% of the resting cardiac output goes to the brain to meet its metabolic needs. Interruption of the cerebral blood flow leads to ischaemia and disruption of the cerebral metabolism.

Pressure and chemical autoregulation are compensatory mechanisms in which cerebral arterioles change diameter to maintain cerebral blood flow when ICP increases. In pressure autoregulation, stretch receptors within small blood vessels of the brain cause smooth muscle of the arterioles to contract. Increased arterial pressure stimulates these receptors, leading to vasoconstriction; when arterial pressure is low, stimulation of these receptors decreases, causing relaxation and vasodilation. Chemical, or metabolic, autoregulation works in much the same way as pressure autoregulation. In this case, the stimulus is a build up of metabolic by-products of cell metabolism, including lactic acid, pyruvic acid, carbonic acid and carbon dioxide. Carbon dioxide and increased hydrogen ion concentration are potent cerebral vasodilators that may act locally or systemically to increase cerebral blood flow. Conversely, a fall in $PaCO_2$ causes cerebral vasoconstriction. Arterial oxygen tension (PaO_2) also affects cerebral blood flow, although it is a less powerful mechanism than that exerted by carbon dioxide and hydrogen ions.

Increases to ICP may result from an increase in intracranial contents from a space-occupying lesion, hydrocephalus, cerebral oedema (swelling), excess CSF or intracranial haemorrhage. Displacement of some CSF to the spinal subarachnoid space and increased CSF absorption are early compensatory mechanisms. The low-pressure venous system is also compressed and cerebral arteries constrict to reduce blood flow. Brain tissue's ability to accommodate change is relatively restricted. The relationship between the volume of the intracranial components and intracranial pressure is known as *compliance*. When the capacity to compensate for pressure in the cranium is exceeded, increased intracranial pressure (hypertension) develops.

Autoregulatory mechanisms have a limited ability to maintain cerebral blood flow. When autoregulation fails, cerebrovascular tone is reduced and cerebral blood flow becomes dependent on changes in blood pressure. Autoregulation may be lost either locally or globally because of several factors, including increasing intracranial pressure, local or diffuse cerebral tissue ischaemia or inflammation, prolonged hypotension and hypercapnoea or hypoxia.

Manifestations

With loss of autoregulation, intracranial pressure continues to rise and cerebral perfusion falls. Cerebral tissue becomes ischaemic and manifestations of cellular hypoxia appear.

Level of consciousness

Because the neurons of the cerebral cortex are most sensitive to oxygen deficit, changes in cortical function are the earliest manifestations of increasing ICP (Norris, 2018). Behaviour and personality changes occur; the person may become irritable and agitated. Memory and judgment are impaired and speech pattern changes may be noted. The person's LOC decreases. As cerebral hypertension and hypoxia progress, the LOC continues to decrease in a predictable pattern to coma and unresponsiveness.

Motor responses

Pressure on the pyramidal tract often causes weakness (hemiparesis) on the contralateral side during the early stages of increased ICP. As ICP continues to increase, hemiplegia and abnormal motor responses, such as decorticate or decerebrate posturing, develop. (See the chapter 'A person-centred approach to assessing the nervous system' for an illustration of these postures.)

Vision and pupils

Altered vision is an early manifestation of changes to ICP; it is caused by pressure on the visual pathways and cranial nerves. Blurred vision, decreased visual acuity and diplopia are common. Pupillary and oculomotor responses are affected as well. Because the cause of IICP is often localised at first, pupillary changes, including gradual dilation and sluggish response to light, may initially be limited to the ipsilateral side.

Vital signs

Ischaemia of the vasomotor centre in the brainstem triggers the CNS ischaemic response, a late sign of IICP. Neuronal ischaemia in the vasomotor centre causes a marked increase in the mean arterial pressure (MAP), with a significant increase in systolic blood pressure and increased pulse pressure. The increased MAP causes reflexive slowing of the cardiac rate. This trio of manifestations (increased MAP, increased pulse pressure and bradycardia) is known as *Cushing's response* (or triad) and represents the brainstem's final effort to maintain cerebral perfusion (Norris, 2018). The respiratory pattern also changes, often in the predictable progression outlined earlier in

MANIFESTATIONS Increased intracranial pressure

- Decreased LOC: early—confusion; restlessness, lethargy; disorientation, first to time, then to place and person; late—comatose with no response to painful stimuli.
- Pupillary dysfunction: sluggish response to light progressing to fixed pupils; with a localised process, pupillary dysfunction is first noted on the ipsilateral side.
- Oculomotor dysfunction: inability to move eye(s) upwards; ptosis (drooping) of the eyelid.
- Visual abnormalities: decreased visual acuity, blurred vision, diplopia.
- Papilloedema: may be a late sign.
- Motor impairment: early—hemiparesis or hemiplegia of the contralateral side; late—abnormal responses such as decorticate or decerebrate positioning; flaccidity.
- Headache: uncommon but may occur with processes that slowly increase ICP; worse on rising in the morning and with position changes.
- Projectile vomiting without nausea.
- Cushing's response: increased systolic blood pressure, widening pulse pressure, bradycardia.
- Respirations: altered respiratory pattern related to level of brain dysfunction.
- Temperature: may be significantly elevated as compensatory mechanisms fail.

Table 41.1. Although the temperature is usually normal in early stages, as ICP continues to increase, hypothalamic function is impaired and the temperature may rise dramatically.

Other manifestations

Additional manifestations of IICP include headache, particularly on rising, that worsens with position changes. Headache is more common with slowly developing ICP changes and occurs because of pressure on pain-sensitive structures, such as the middle meningeal arteries, the venous sinuses and the dura at the base of the skull. Papilloedema (oedema and swelling of the optic disc) may be noted on funduscopic examination. Vomiting, often projectile and occurring without warning, may develop.

Cerebral oedema

Cerebral oedema is an increase in the volume of brain tissue due to abnormal accumulation of fluid. Cerebral oedema is often associated with IICP; it may occur as a local process in the area of a tumour or injury, or it may affect the entire brain. Two types of cerebral oedema have been identified and are described as follows (Norris, 2018):

1. *Vasogenic oedema*, an increase in the capillary permeability of cerebral vessels, occurs with impairment of the blood–brain barrier, allowing diffusion of water and protein into the interstitial spaces of the brain. A variety of pathologies, such as ischaemia, haemorrhage, brain tumours and injuries and infections (such as meningitis), may cause the increase in capillary permeability. The site of the brain injury, the level of increase in capillary permeability and the person's systemic blood pressure influence the rate and extent of the oedema's spread. Vasogenic oedema is manifested by focal (localised) neurological deficits, altered levels of consciousness and severe intracranial hypertension.
2. *Cytotoxic oedema*, actual swelling of the brain cells from an increase in intracellular fluid, involves changes in the functional or structural integrity of cell membranes due to pathologies such as water intoxication (such as from the syndrome of inappropriate secretion of antidiuretic hormone (SIADH)) or severe ischaemia, intracranial hypoxia, acidosis and brain trauma. With abnormally low cerebral perfusion, oxygen and nutrients are depleted, intracranial cells switch to anaerobic metabolism and the sodium–potassium pump in the cell walls is impaired. Sodium diffuses into the cells, pulling fluid with it. The cells swell and intracranial pressure rises. Accumulated metabolic waste products, such as lactic acid, contribute to a rapid deterioration of cell function. Cytotoxic oedema is a slowly progressive process that results in altered consciousness. The oedema may be so severe that it causes cerebral infarction with brain tissue necrosis.

Cerebral oedema tends to be proportional to the extent of the pathology precipitating it. Brain function is not disrupted by cerebral oedema unless the oedema causes an increase in ICP. When it does, a vicious cycle can ensue: cerebral oedema increases ICP, which in turn decreases cerebral blood flow. Brain tissue becomes hypoxic and ischaemic, increasing toxic metabolic by-products, hydrogen ion concentration and carbon dioxide levels in the tissue. Autoregulatory mechanisms cause vasodilation and increase cerebral blood flow, further increasing cerebral oedema and intracranial pressure. Without effective intervention, the person's condition can deteriorate rapidly; ICP increases to the point where brain structures herniate.

Hydrocephalus

Hydrocephalus refers to a progressive dilation of the ventricular system, which becomes dilated as the production of CSF exceeds its absorption (Hickey, 2019). Hydrocephalus may increase ICP when it develops acutely. It is generally classified as either non-communicating or communicating hydrocephalus. Non-communicating hydrocephalus occurs when CSF drainage from the ventricular system is obstructed. It may develop when a mass or tumour, inflammation or haemorrhage, or congenital malformation obstructs the ventricular system. Communicating hydrocephalus is a condition in which CSF is not effectively reabsorbed through the arachnoid villi. It may occur secondarily to subarachnoid haemorrhage or scarring from infection. In *normal pressure hydrocephalus*, seen most often in adults aged 60 or older, ventricular enlargement causes cerebral tissue compression but the CSF pressure on lumbar puncture is normal. This condition may follow cerebral trauma or surgery, or the cause may not be known.

Manifestations of hydrocephalus depend on the rate of its development. They may be mild and insidious in onset, presenting as progressive cognitive dysfunctions, gait disruptions and urinary incontinence. If the process causing hydrocephalus is an acute one, the manifestations are those of IICP.

Brain herniation

If increasing ICP is not treated, cerebral tissue is displaced towards a more compliant area. This can result in brain herniation, the displacement of brain tissue from its normal compartment under dural folds of the falx cerebri or through the tentorial notch or incisura of the tentorium cerebelli (Norris, 2018). Herniation of the cerebellum through the tentorium exerts pressure on the brainstem, with subsequent herniation through the foramen magnum. This is a lethal complication of IICP because it puts pressure on the vital centres of the medulla.

Brain herniation syndromes are generally categorised as supratentorial or infratentorial, depending on their location above or below the tentorium cerebelli (see Figure 41.2). Supratentorial herniation syndromes include cingulate herniation, central or transtentorial herniation, uncal or lateral transtentorial herniation, and infratentorial herniation.

- *Cingulate herniation* (see Figure 41.2A) occurs when the cingulate gyrus is displaced under the falx cerebri. Local blood supply and cerebral tissue are compressed, resulting in ischaemia and further increases in intracranial pressure.
- *Central*, or *transtentorial, herniation* is the downward displacement of brain structures, including the cerebral hemispheres, basal ganglia, diencephalon and midbrain through the tentorial incisura (see Figure 41.2B). The person's neurological signs may deteriorate rapidly, with decreased LOC progressing to coma, Cheyne–Stokes respirations progressing to central neurogenic hyperventilation and pupils progressing from small and reactive to midsized and fixed. The person may demonstrate abnormal motor responses with unilateral decorticate posturing.
- *Uncal*, or *lateral, transtentorial herniation* occurs when a lateral mass displaces cerebral tissue centrally, forcing the medial aspect of the temporal lobe under the edge of the tentorial incisura (see Figure 41.2C). The oculomotor nerve (cranial nerve III) often becomes trapped between the uncus and the tentorium, causing ipsilateral pupillary dilation. Other manifestations include alterations in LOC, motor deficits (which may occur on the same side as the herniation because of compression of the cerebral peduncle on the opposite side), decreased sensation, respiratory changes, abnormal positioning and eventual respiratory arrest.
- *Infratentorial herniation* results from increased pressure within the infratentorial compartment. Herniation may occur either upwards, with structures displaced through the tentorial incisura, or downwards, with displacement through the foramen magnum (see Figure 41.2D). Downward displacement compresses the medulla, including its centres for controlling vital functions. Manifestations associated with medullary compression include coma, altered respiratory patterns, fixed pupils, and decorticate or decerebrate posturing. Respiratory or cardiac arrest may occur.

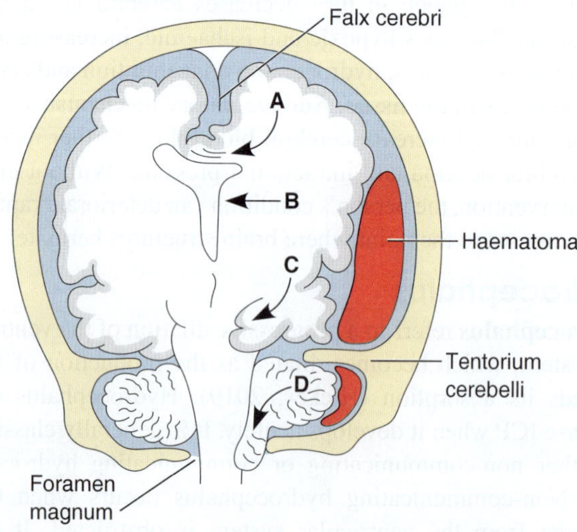

FIGURE 41.2 ***Forms of brain herniation due to intracranial hypertension. A, Cingulate herniation occurs when the cingulate gyrus is compressed under the falx cerebri. B, Central herniation occurs when a centrally located lesion compresses central and midbrain structures. C, Lateral herniation occurs when a lesion at the side of the brain compresses the uncus or hippocampal gyrus. D, Infratentorial herniation occurs when the cerebellar tonsils are forced downwards, compressing the medulla and top of the spinal cord***

INTERPROFESSIONAL CARE

Management of the person with IICP is directed towards identifying and treating the underlying cause of the disorder and controlling ICP to prevent herniation syndrome. IICP is a medical emergency and there is little time to complete lengthy diagnostic tests. The diagnosis must be made on the basis of observation and neurological assessment; even subtle changes may be clinically significant.

Diagnosis

Diagnostic tests focus on identifying the presence and significance of IICP and its underlying cause. A CT scan or MRI is generally the initial test used to identify the possible causes (such as space-occupying lesions or hydrocephalus) and to evaluate therapeutic options. In general, a lumbar puncture is not performed when IICP is suspected because the sudden release of the pressure in the skull may cause cerebral herniation.

In addition to the diagnostic tests listed in the previous section for altered LOC, the following specific tests are usually ordered and their results closely monitored:

- Serum osmolality is an indicator of hydration status in the person with increasing ICP. The test measures the number of dissolved particles (electrolytes, urea, glucose) in the serum. The normal range for the adult is 280 to 300 mOsm/kg H_2O. In addition to the restriction of fluids in the person with IICP, serum osmolality is maintained at a slightly elevated level (325 mOsm/kg H_2O) to draw excess intracellular fluid into the vascular system.
- ABGs are monitored frequently to assess pH and levels of oxygen and carbon dioxide. Hydrogen ions and carbon dioxide are both potent vasodilators; hypoxaemia also causes vasodilation, although to a lesser degree.

Medications

Medications play an important role in the management of ICP changes. Diuretics, particularly osmotic diuretics, are commonly used to reduce ICP and are the mainstays of pharmacological treatment. Nursing implications for these medications are described in the 'Medication administration' box.

Osmotic diuretics work by increasing the osmolarity of the blood, thereby drawing water out of oedematous brain tissue and into the vascular system for elimination via the kidneys. The effects of these drugs vary with the type of injury. Regardless of the agent used, the aim is for the lowest dose that

MEDICATION ADMINISTRATION Increased intracranial pressure

Note: Because the person with IICP often has an altered LOC, education of the person and their family is not discussed here.

OSMOTIC DIURETICS

Mannitol

Urea

Osmotic diuretics (hyperosmotic agents) draw fluid out of brain cells by increasing the osmolality of the blood. The effects of these drugs vary with the type of injury. Mannitol therapy is often initiated if the person's ICP exceeds 15 to 20 mmHg for at least 10 minutes. Both intravenous bolus and continuous infusion techniques are used. Repeated use of mannitol can lead to continual elevations in serum osmolality, with attendant risk of seizures and serious fluid and electrolyte imbalance. Urea is seldom administered intravenously because a severe local reaction may result if leakage occurs at the injection site. Mannitol and urea are used cautiously if renal disease is present.

Nursing responsibilities

- Monitor vital signs, urinary output, central venous pressure (CVP) and pulmonary artery pressures (PAP) before and every hour throughout administration.
- Assess person for manifestations of dehydration.
- Assess person for muscle weakness, numbness, tingling, paraesthesia, confusion and excessive thirst.
- Assess person for pulmonary oedema while administering the medication.
- Monitor neurological status and intracranial pressure readings.
- Monitor renal function and serum electrolytes throughout therapy.
- Follow administration guidelines in regards to preparation of solution and process of administration.
- Do not discontinue medication abruptly. Rebound migraine headaches may occur.

LOOP DIURETICS

Frusemide

Ethacrynic acid

Loop diuretics such as frusemide and ethacrynic acid inhibit sodium and chloride reabsorption at the ascending loop of Henle. They cause a reduction in the rate of CSF production, thus reducing the ICP.

Nursing responsibilities

- Monitor vital signs and electrolytes closely.
- Assess fluid status throughout therapy.
- Monitor blood pressure and pulse before and during administration.
- Monitor renal laboratory studies closely.
- Use an infusion pump to ensure accurate dosage.

INTRAVENOUS FLUIDS

Keeping the person moderately dehydrated to maintain serum osmolality can be effective in reducing cerebral oedema. When giving intravenous fluids, closely monitor the osmolality of the solutions; if people with increased ICP are given hypo-osmolar solutions, increased cerebral oedema can occur. Preferred solutions include 0.45–0.9% sodium chloride solutions.

Nursing responsibilities

- Monitor fluid status closely.
- Monitor neurological status closely.
- Avoid administering hypo-osmolar solutions, such as 5% dextrose.
- 0.45% sodium chloride is considered a suitable fluid for a person who has IICP.
- Take care not to restrict fluids excessively in people receiving dehydrating agents (such as osmotic or loop diuretics).

OTHER PHARMACOLOGICAL INTERVENTIONS FOR IICP

- Antipyretics, such as paracetamol, are used to reduce hyperthermia, thereby decreasing the high cerebral metabolism that contributes to IICP.
- Antihypertensive agents, such as beta-adrenergic blocking agents, may be used if the mean arterial pressure (MAP) is high.
- Vasopressors may be used if the MAP is low.
- Anticonvulsants may be given to prevent or treat seizures associated with changing ICP.

reduces ICP. Mannitol is the most commonly employed osmotic diuretic. Urine output by indwelling catheter is monitored. Electrolyte levels are carefully assessed and potassium is replaced as indicated.

Loop diuretics, such as frusemide (the drug of choice) and ethacrynic acid, may also be prescribed for some people with IICP. These diuretics act on the renal tubule and are extremely effective in promoting diuresis. Additionally, loop diuretics may be used to manage the rebound effect that may occur with mannitol administration.

Sedation and paralysis are used as chemical restraints to control restlessness and agitation because these movements increase blood pressure, ICP and cerebral metabolism. Paralysis with neuromuscular blockage is most often accomplished with pancuronium. Close monitoring during treatment for residual muscle weakness and signs of respiratory distress are essential. A peripheral nerve stimulator may be used for this purpose.

Antipyretics, such as paracetamol, are used alone or in combination with a hypothermia blanket to treat hyperthermia. Hyperthermia increases the cerebral metabolic rate and exacerbates an existing increase in ICP. Anticonvulsants are often required to manage seizure activity associated with brain injury and IICP. Gastrointestinal prophylaxis with intravenous histamine H_2 antagonists or proton pump inhibitors are often used, because people with IICP are at increased risk of developing stress gastritis (Papadakis et al., 2022).

Intravenous fluids are usually necessary to maintain the person's fluid and electrolyte balance as well as vascular volume. If the person's blood pressure is unstable, vasoactive medications may be administered to maintain the MAP in a range that supports cerebral perfusion while minimising increases in ICP. When enteral feeding is not possible, total parenteral nutrition (TPN) may be administered.

Surgery

People with IICP may undergo various intracranial surgical techniques to treat the underlying cause (see the discussion in the later section on brain tumours). In addition, infarcted or necrotic tissue may be resected to reduce brain mass. A drainage catheter or shunt may be inserted laterally via a burr hole into a ventricle to drain excess CSF and reduce hydrocephalus. The removal of even a small amount of CSF may dramatically reduce ICP and restore cerebral perfusion pressure.

ICP monitoring

Critical to preserving brain function and preventing secondary brain damage from altered ICP are careful assessments and monitoring with ICP monitors, measuring cerebral blood flow and cerebral perfusion pressure, and measuring oxygen levels of brain tissue. Intracranial pressure monitors facilitate continual assessment of ICP and the effects of medical therapy and nursing interventions on ICP. In addition, cerebral perfusion pressure (the difference between MAP and ICP) can be readily calculated, allowing more precise manipulation of therapeutic measures to maintain cerebral perfusion and thereby prevent ischaemia. The criteria for ICP monitoring depends on the person, but in general, people who are comatose and have a deteriorating Glasgow Coma Score (described in the chapter 'A person-centred approach to assessing the nervous system') should be monitored.

Basic monitoring systems include an intraventricular catheter, subarachnoid bolt or screw, and epidural probe (see Figure 41.3). Intraventricular fluid-filled catheters are placed in the anterior horn of the lateral ventricle (most often in the right side). Ventricular catheters can both drain CSF and measure ICP. The ICP value is measured deep in the brain and is considered the most reflective of the whole brain pressure. Subarachnoid devices are placed in the subarachnoid space. A fibre-optic transducer-tipped catheter can be placed in the epidural, subdural or parenchymal space, with ICP values considered very accurate. Once the intracranial sensor is implanted, it is connected to a transducer that converts the impulses to a signal that the recording device can translate into an oscilloscope tracing, digital value or graphic recording. Factors that increase the risk of infection during ICP monitoring are listed in Table 41.4.

Transcranial blood flow is monitored with transcranial Doppler studies (TCD) to measure the velocity of blood flow in the cerebral vessels. Cerebral perfusion pressure (CPP) is the pressure required for the heart to provide the brain with

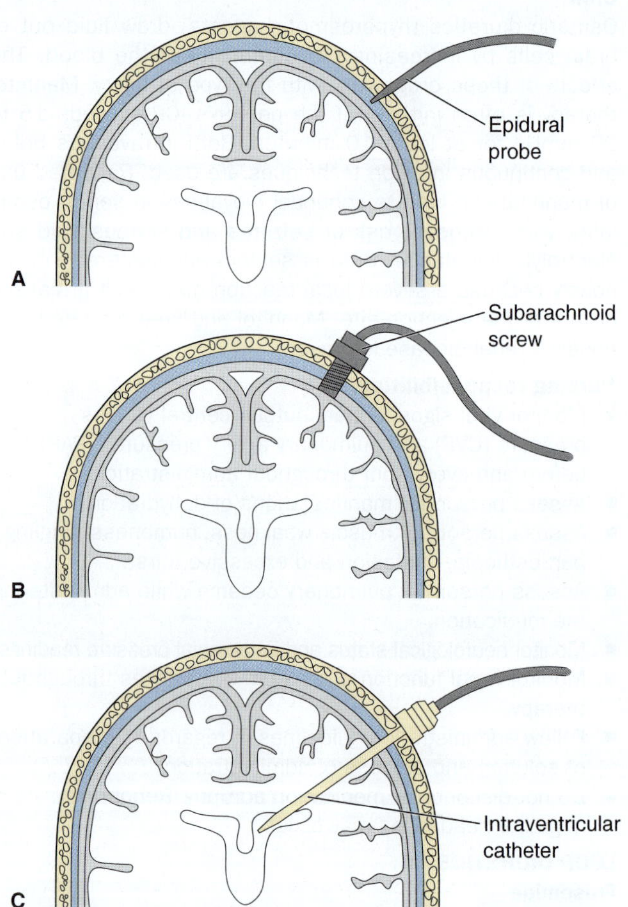

FIGURE 41.3 ***Types of intracranial pressure monitoring. A, Epidural probe. B, Subarachnoid screw. C, Intraventricular catheter***

TABLE 41.4 Risk factors for infection with intracranial pressure monitoring

FACTOR	ASSOCIATED RISK
Intraventricular catheter	Is more invasive than other monitoring devices
Open head trauma or neurosurgery	Disrupts protective skin and skeletal barriers
Intracranial haemorrhage	Necessitates frequent flushing of catheter to maintain patency
Older adult	Tends to have impaired immune defences
Monitoring for more than 3 to 5 days; or open system or frequent irrigation	Offers increased opportunity for pathogens to enter and grow

blood, calculated by subtracting ICP from MAP. (Normal CPP is 70 to 95 mmHg.) Brain oxygenation monitoring may be conducted by using a jugular bulb oxygen saturation (SjO_2) monitor connected to a small fibre-optic catheter inserted into the jugular vein. (Normal SjO_2 is 50–75%.) Another device used to monitor brain tissue oxygenation is the LICOX system, which includes information about ICP, oxygen status and temperature status within the brain tissue itself (Patchana et al., 2020). In addition, cerebral microdialysis catheters can provide information about the nature of the cerebral interstitial fluid.

Mechanical ventilation

People with extreme ICP often require intubation and are placed on a ventilator for respiratory management. Mechanical ventilation may be used to maintain partial pressure of oxygen and carbon dioxide, thus preventing hypoxaemia and hypercapnoea, both of which can increase intracranial pressure. It is important to maintain adequate oxygenation with a partial pressure of arterial oxygen at about 100 mmHg and a partial pressure of arterial carbon dioxide of about 35 mmHg. The person with IICP and signs of impending herniation may be judiciously hyperventilated to cause cerebral vasoconstriction; however, it is important to note that this also increases cerebral ischaemia.

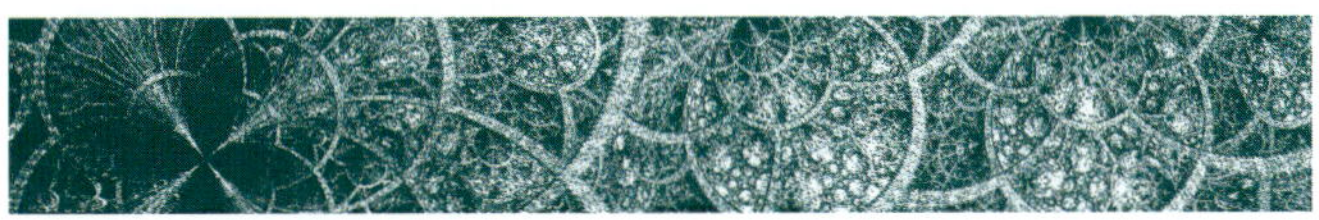

Nursing care

The nursing care of people with IICP involves identifying those at risk and managing factors known to increase intracranial pressure. A major focus is protecting the person from sudden increases in ICP or a decrease in cerebral blood flow.

Nursing diagnoses and interventions

Nursing interventions for people with altered ICP include performing neurological assessments, maintaining the patency of the airway, ensuring adequate ventilation, positioning and moving, instituting seizure precautions and monitoring fluids and electrolytes. Additionally, both the person and their family need emotional support during this period. The person with IICP has varied responses to actual or potential changes in physiological processes and is at a significant risk of deterioration.

Ineffective tissue perfusion: cerebral

A number of disorders may lead to IICP, including cerebral oedema, hydrocephalus, space-occupying lesions and haemorrhage, herniation syndromes and changes in carbon dioxide concentrations. Increasing intracranial pressure alters cerebral perfusion and oxygenation of brain cells. The person with altered ICP requires intensive care and often needs ventilator assistance.

- Assess for and report manifestations of increasing ICP every 15 minutes to 1 hour and as necessary. Assessment areas include LOC, behaviour, motor/sensory functions, pupillary size and reaction to light, and vital signs, including temperature. Look for trends, because vital signs alone do not correlate well with early deterioration. *Assessment of neurological status establishes the person's clinical condition and provides a baseline for measuring changes. Sudden changes in neurological signs often indicate deterioration. An elevated temperature with increased oxygen consumption further increases intracranial pressure. Pupillary responses mirror the status of the midbrain and pons. Pressure on the brainstem may compromise the function of cranial nerves IX and X and protective mechanisms, such as the gag and cough reflexes.*

> **CONSIDERATION FOR PRACTICE**
> **Often, the earliest manifestations of a change in intracranial pressure are alterations in the LOC and respirations.**

- For the person on a ventilator: maintain patency of the airway; pre-oxygenate with 100% oxygen before suctioning; limit suctioning to 10 seconds; suction gently. *Pre-oxygenation helps maintain oxygen levels during suctioning. Suctioning stimulates the cough reflex and Valsalva manoeuvre. Correct suctioning minimises the risk of hypoxaemia.*
- Monitor ABGs. *ABGs provide a reliable indicator of oxygen and carbon dioxide levels. If oxygen concentration is low, oxygen may be given or increased.*
- Elevate head of the bed to 30 degrees or keep flat, as prescribed; maintain the alignment of the head and neck to avoid hyperextension or exaggerated neck flexion; avoid prone position. *Keeping the head of the bed elevated facilitates venous drainage from the cerebrum. Obstruction of jugular veins can impede venous drainage from the brain.*
- Monitor bladder distension and constipation. Administer stool softeners and use the Credé technique (applying pressure to the suprapubic region with the fingers of one or both hands) to empty the bladder. If the Credé technique is not effective, evaluate the pros and cons of urinary catheterisation if the bladder remains distended. *Constipation and bladder distension increase intrathoracic or intra-abdominal pressure and place the person at risk of impaired venous drainage from the brain.*

- If alert, assist the person in moving up in bed. Do not ask the person to push with heels or arms or push against a footboard. Avoid a footboard and restraints. *Moving up in bed requires pushing. Helping the person move prevents initiation of the Valsalva manoeuvre, which increases intracranial pressure.*
- Plan nursing care so that activities are not clustered together; avoid turning the person, getting the person on the bedpan or suctioning within the same time period. Schedule nursing care to provide rest periods between procedures. *Multiple procedures, including certain nursing care activities, can increase ICP. Constant stimulation tends to increase ICP. Individualised nursing care ensures optimal spacing of activities and rest.*
- Provide a quiet environment, limiting noxious stimuli. Avoid jarring the bed. Try to limit situations that cause emotional upset; maintain a calm, reassuring manner; caution family members to refrain from unpleasant conversations or conversations that may be emotionally stimulating to the person. *Noxious stimuli and emotional upsets cause an elevation in ICP.*
- Maintain fluid limitations, if prescribed. *Restricting fluids helps decrease cerebral oedema by reducing total body water.*

Risk of infection

Although any person with an open head wound is at risk of infection, the interventions discussed here are for the person with an intracranial monitoring device. Clinical settings that employ these interventions should have written protocols for managing these systems, and as such, the following nursing actions serve only as a general guide.

- Keep dressings over the catheter dry and change dressings on a prescribed basis (usually every 24 to 48 hours). *Wet dressings are conducive to bacterial growth.*
- Monitor the insertion site for leaking CSF, drainage or infection. Monitor the person for manifestations of infection, including changes in vital signs, chills, increased WBC counts and positive cultures of drainage. *Close monitoring helps detect the earliest signs of infection and helps prevent major complications. Fever in a person with a neurological disorder may be due to infection, but it may also be due to damage to the hypothalamus. Headache, generalised muscle aches, shivering and chills may also be seen in the person with infection.*
- Use strict aseptic technique when in contact with the device. Check drainage system for loose connections. *The use of aseptic technique and monitoring drainage systems for loose connections help prevent hospital-acquired infections. Most such infections are transmitted by healthcare workers who fail to wash their hands properly, to change gloves between patients or to follow aseptic technique protocols. Invasive procedures provide an excellent opportunity for microbes to enter the body.*

Health education for the person and family

Educate the individual at risk of or experiencing increasing ICP (and able to follow instructions) and their family that the person should avoid coughing, blowing the nose, straining to have a bowel movement, pushing against the bed rails or performing isometric (muscle-contracting) exercises. Advise the person to maintain head and neck alignment when turning in bed and to take rest periods.

Encourage the family to talk to the person but maintain a quiet environment with a minimum of stimuli. Inform family members that upsetting the person may increase intracranial pressure and that they should avoid discussions that may distress the person. For people unable to make decisions about treatment and to sign informed consent, the family must carry out these functions.

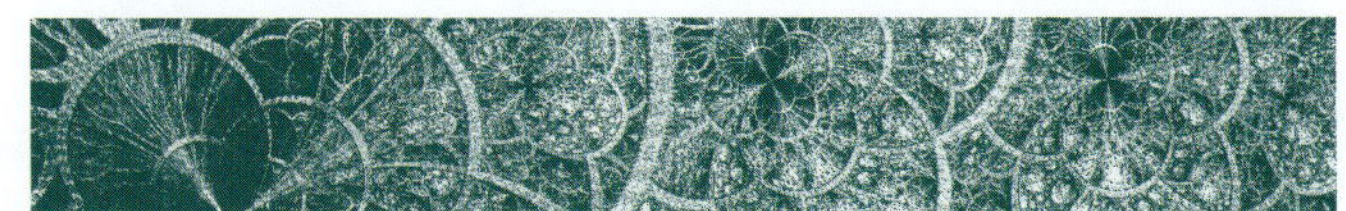

Links to National Patient Safety Standards

NSQHS: Preventing and Controlling Infections Standard

The aim of this standard is preventing healthcare-associated infections and the effective evidence-based management of the infections that do occur. These prevention and management strategies include the development of appropriate infection-control policies and procedures; adhering to infection-control policies and procedures; surveillance of healthcare-associated infection rates; monitoring of staff compliance with infection-control procedures; training and education for all staff; and education for individuals and their families and caregivers.

Caring for individuals with head injuries requires strict adherence to infection-control policies and procedures, particularly for those individuals with open skull fractures or ICP monitors in place. People with head injuries and altered LOC are also at risk of developing pneumonia and urinary tract infections.

Source: ACSQHC (2021). *National Safety and Quality Health Service Standards* (2nd ed.). Sydney: ACSQHC. © Australian Commission on Safety and Quality in Health Care.

THE PERSON WITH A HEADACHE

Headache, one of the most frequent manifestations of a health problem people experience, is pain within the cranial vault. Headaches may occur as a result of benign or pathological conditions, intracranial or extracranial conditions, diseases of other body systems, stress, musculoskeletal tension or a combination of these factors.

Most headaches are mild, transient and relieved by a mild analgesic. However, some headaches are chronic, intense and recurrent. Manifestations of headache vary according to the cause, type and precipitating symptoms.

Pathophysiology

The bones and brain tissue itself lack pain-sensitive nerve fibres, but selected structures within the cranial vault are sensitive to pain. Headache is experienced when there is traction, pressure, displacement, inflammation or dilation of nociceptors (nerve endings that are receptors of noxious stimuli) in areas sensitive to pain (Hickey, 2019). Pain-sensitive structures include supporting structures, such as the skin, muscles and periosteum; the nasal cavities and sinuses; portions of the meninges, cranial nerves II, III, IV, V, VI, IX and X; and cerebral vessels, including extracranial arteries and the venous sinuses. Most facial and scalp structures are sensitive to pain. The most common types of headaches are migraine, cluster and tension headaches (see Table 41.5).

Migraine headache

Migraine headache is a recurring vascular headache lasting from 4 to 72 hours, often initiated by a triggering event and usually accompanied by a neurological dysfunction. It affects 1 in 7 people worldwide and about 4.9 million people within Australia, with three times as many women as men having migraines (Headache Australia, 2021). It is more common between the ages of 12 and 40 years with prevalence declining thereafter. Migraine headaches may occur daily or as infrequently as once a year.

There are two types of migraine headaches: common migraine (without an aura) and classic migraine (with an aura; most often experienced as a visual disturbance prior to the pain). Common migraines occur in 80% of the people who are affected by this disorder. Headaches classified as migraines may differ in intensity, duration and frequency. The exact causes of migraine are not fully understood, but they are believed to be the result of abnormalities in cerebrovascular blood flow, a reduction in brain and electrical activity, or increased release of sensory substances such as serotonin, noradrenaline substance P, nitric oxide or glutamate.

A variety of factors are believed to trigger the onset of a migraine headache. Rapid changes in blood glucose levels, stress, emotional excitement, fatigue, hormonal changes due to menstruation, stimuli such as bright lights, and food high in tyramine or other vasoactive substances (e.g. aged cheese, nuts, chocolate and alcoholic beverages) have been associated with migraine attacks. Hypertension and fever may make the disorder worse.

COMMON MIGRAINE This type is the most common and is associated with hereditary factors. The aura stage is absent; people are aware only that a headache is imminent. The headache develops gradually, lasting hours to days, and may occur in women during periods of premenstrual tension and fluid retention. Chills, nausea and vomiting, fatigue and nasal congestion are often present.

CLASSIC MIGRAINE The classic migraine headache has several stages, as follows:

- The aura stage is characterised by sensory manifestations, usually visual disturbances such as bright spots or flashing lights zigzagging across the visual fields. This stage lasts from 5 to 60 minutes. Less common sensory symptoms include numbness or tingling of the face or hand, weakness of an arm or leg, mild aphasia, confusion, drowsiness and lack of coordination. Additionally, some people experience a premonition the day prior to an attack. They may feel nervous or have other mood changes. The aura period corresponds with the initial physiological change of vasoconstriction.
- The headache stage is characterised by vasodilation, a decline in serotonin levels and the onset of throbbing

TABLE 41.5 Comparison of migraine, cluster and tension headaches

TYPE	RISK FACTORS	FREQUENCY AND DURATION	DESCRIPTION	PRODROMAL AND ASSOCIATED MANIFESTATIONS
Migraine	Female Family history of migraine headache	Episodic: • Tends to occur with stress and crisis • Can last hours to days	Slow onset; pain becomes more severe, involving one side of head more than other	Prodromal manifestations: visual defects, confusion, paraesthesias Associated manifestations: nausea, vomiting, chills, fatigue, irritability, sweating
Cluster	Male Use of alcohol or nitrates May begin in early childhood	Episodes are clustered together in rapid succession for a few days or weeks with remissions that last for months Can last a few minutes to a few hours	May begin in infraorbital region and spread to head and neck; throbbing, deep pain, often unilateral	Prodromal manifestations: uncommon Associated manifestations: flushing, tearing of eyes, nasal congestion, sweating and swelling of temporal vessels
Tension	Related to stress and/or anxiety No family history Often begins in adolescence	Episodic: • Varies with amount of stress • Duration also varies; can be constant	Tight, pressing, vice-like; may involve neck and shoulders	Prodromal manifestations: uncommon Associated manifestations: sustained contraction of neck muscles

headache. It appears that the pain is related to increased vessel permeability and polypeptide exudation by perivascular nerve endings rather than the vasodilation itself. Cerebral arteries are dilated and distended, with walls that are oedematous and rigid. Beginning unilaterally, the headache eventually may involve both sides as it increases in intensity during the next several hours. Nausea and vomiting often occur. The person may be acutely ill and is often extremely irritable. The sensory organs often become hypersensitive and the person withdraws from sound and light. The scalp is tender. The headache may last from several hours to a day or two.

- During the post-headache phase, the headache area is sensitive to touch and a deep aching is present. The person is exhausted. Vessel size and serotonin levels return to normal.

Cluster headache

A *cluster headache* is an extremely severe, unilateral, burning pain located behind or around the eyes. The cluster headache is predominantly experienced by men between the ages of 20 and 40 years. The headaches occur in groups or 'clusters' of one to eight each day for several weeks or months, followed by remission lasting months to years (Hickey, 2019). The physiological mechanism underlying cluster headaches is not well understood, but is thought to involve a vascular disorder, a disturbance of serotonergic mechanisms, a sympathetic defect or deregulation of the hypothalamus.

Although the headache may occur at any time, it typically begins 2 to 3 hours after falling asleep, awakens the person and then lasts from 15 to 180 minutes. Prodromal signs are absent. Intense unilateral pain around or behind one eye is accompanied by rhinorrhoea, lacrimation, flushing, sweating, facial oedema and possible miosis or ptosis on the affected side. The same side of the head is involved in each cluster of attacks.

The headaches often occur in spring and autumn and then disappear for an extended period. Attacks may be triggered by drinking alcohol, eating specific foods or medications such as glyceryl trinitrate (nitroglycerin), or there may be no known precipitating event.

Tension headache

Tension headache is characterised by bilateral pain, with a sensation of a band of tightness or pressure around the head. Sharply localised painful spots (trigger points) may be present. The onset is gradual and the intensity, frequency and duration of the attack vary greatly. This type of headache is caused by sustained contraction of the muscles of the head and neck. It is often precipitated by stressful situations and anxiety. Secondary causes include prolonged computer use and disorders of the eyes, ears, sinuses or cervical vertebrae. Abnormal posture associated with occupations that require bending over a desk (e.g. office workers, students) often precipitates tension-type headache. Additionally, slouching while reading or watching television can lead to muscle contraction. Most headaches are tension-type headaches.

INTERPROFESSIONAL CARE

Identifying the underlying cause(s) of the headache is the initial focus of interprofessional care. If the underlying cause is treatable, the headache will often decrease or disappear. An accurate diagnosis of the type of headache is key to the treatment.

Therapeutic management for migraine headache includes a combination of education, medications and measures to control contributing factors. Dietary changes may be necessary if elements are identified as triggers or if they will otherwise interact with other treatments. Stress management or biofeedback is also part of the overall strategy. Treatment can vary significantly for different forms of headache. Protocols for cluster headache include eliminating aggravating factors (e.g. consumption of alcohol) and using medications and oxygen inhalation. The management of tension headaches is directed towards reducing the person's level of stress and relieving pain with ice and aspirin or non-steroidal anti-inflammatory drugs (NSAIDs).

Diagnosis

Diagnosis and treatment are based on history, identifying triggering or precipitating events, and the type of headache. A thorough history and physical examination are integral parts of the assessment. Neurodiagnostic testing may be done to rule out a structural disease process. Testing may include a brain scan, MRI, x-ray studies of the skull and cervical spine, EEG or lumbar puncture for CSF if inflammation is suspected. Serum metabolic screens and hypersensitivity testing also may be performed if systemic problems are suspected.

Medications

Pharmacological management depends on the type of headache. The goals of treatment are to reduce the frequency and severity of headaches and to limit or relieve a headache that is beginning or in progress.

The management of migraine headache includes administering medications to prevent pain (prophylactic therapy) as well as drugs to stop (or abort) a headache in progress. The person with frequent migraine headaches is a candidate for prophylactic therapy. Drugs used to reduce the frequency and severity of migraine include:

- Methysergide maleate is a serotonin antagonist that competitively blocks serotonin receptors in the CNS and is also a potent vasoconstrictor.
- Propranolol hydrochloride is a beta-blocker that prevents dilation of vessels in the pia mater and inhibits serotonin uptake.
- Topiramate and sodium valproate are CNS agents and anticonvulsants.

When the manifestations of migraine are recognised early, several medications may be used to abort or limit the severity and duration of the headache. Ergotamine tartrate is a complex drug that reduces extracranial blood flow, decreases the amplitude of cranial artery pulsation and decreases basal artery hyperperfusion. Administered at the onset of an attack, ergotamine controls up to 70% of acute attacks. Sumatriptan is available in oral, nasal spray or subcutaneous injection forms. It binds with serotonin receptors and is rapidly effective. Zolmitriptan (Zomig), a selective serotonin receptor agonist, is administered orally and is effective in the treatment of acute headache. Once a migraine is in progress, a narcotic analgesic may be required to manage pain. Anti-emetics may also be prescribed to control nausea and vomiting.

Many of the same medications used for migraine also prevent or treat cluster headache. Because the onset of cluster headaches is abrupt, abortive therapy is not possible. Medications such as ergotamine tartrate may be given in suppository form at bedtime to prevent headache during the episodic attacks. Inhaling 100% oxygen at 7 L/min for 15 minutes at the onset of an attack may relieve a person's headache (Papadakis et al., 2022).

Non-narcotic analgesics such as aspirin or paracetamol may relieve tension headaches. Additionally, tranquillisers such as diazepam may reduce muscle tension, which can contribute to the headache as a causative agent.

Nursing implications for drugs commonly prescribed for headaches are described in the 'Medication administration' box.

MEDICATION ADMINISTRATION Headaches

BETA-BLOCKERS

Propranolol hydrochloride
Pindolol
Atenolol
Timolol

Beta-blockers are effective in the prophylactic treatment of headache. They act by combining with beta-adrenergic receptors to block the response to sympathetic nerve impulses, circulating catecholamines or adrenergic drugs.

Nursing responsibilities

- Before beginning therapy, determine regular and stable pulse and blood pressure.
- Assess baseline and monitor serum glucose level, FBC, electrolytes and liver and renal function studies.
- Note any history of diabetes or impaired renal function.
- Note the rate and quality of respirations; drugs in this category may cause dyspnoea and bronchospasm.
- Administer the drug with meals to prevent gastrointestinal disturbances.
- Be alert that beta-blockers cause bradycardia and the heart rate may not rise in response to stress, such as exercise or fever. Notify the primary healthcare provider if pulse or blood pressure changes significantly.

Health education for the person and family

- Take the medication with meals to provide a coating for the gastrointestinal tract and prevent gastrointestinal disturbances.
- Return for blood work as prescribed.
- Take the last dose of the day at bedtime.
- Rise from a sitting or lying position to a standing position slowly to avoid dizziness and falls.
- Take pulse and blood pressure each day and maintain a record of readings.
- Report any cough, nasal stuffiness or feelings of depression to the healthcare provider.

TRICYCLIC ANTIDEPRESSANTS

Imipramine hydrochloride
Amitriptyline hydrochloride

The tricyclic antidepressants have been successful in the prophylaxis of cluster and migraine headaches. Although the exact mechanism of how they manage these headaches is not known, the medications work by preventing the re-uptake of noradrenaline, or serotonin, or both. They are chemically related to the phenothiazines and as such they exhibit many of the same pharmacological effects (e.g. anticholinergic, antiserotonin, sedative, antihistaminic and hypotensive effects).

Nursing responsibilities

- Assess baseline FBC and liver function studies, heart sounds and neurological status before initiating prescribed therapy.

Health education for the person and family

- Make position changes slowly.
- Chew sugarless gum to relieve dry mouth.
- Do not abruptly quit taking the medication.

ERGOT ALKALOID DERIVATIVES

Methysergide maleate

Methysergide is an ergot alkaloid derivative structurally related to LSD. It acts by stimulating smooth muscle, leading to vasoconstriction. It is thought that methysergide prevents headaches by blocking the effects of serotonin, a powerful vasodilator believed to play a role in vascular headaches. It also inhibits the release of histamine from mast cells and prevents the release of serotonin from platelets.

Nursing responsibilities

- Note any history of kidney or hepatic disease.
- Assess baseline eosinophil and neutrophil counts before beginning therapy.
- Administer the drug with meals to minimise gastrointestinal irritation due to increased hydrochloric acid production.
- Assess for kidney, CNS and cardiovascular complications.
- Drug dosage should be gradually reduced over 2 to 3 weeks to prevent rebound headaches. A drug-free interval of 3 to 4 weeks is required with each 6-month course of therapy to prevent complications.
- Monitor for signs of ergotism, such as coldness or numbness of the fingers and toes, nausea, vomiting, headache, muscle pain and weakness. Vasoconstriction may further impair peripheral circulation and increase blood pressure.

(continued)

MEDICATION ADMINISTRATION Headaches (continued)

Health education for the person and family

- Take the medication with meals to minimise gastrointestinal upset.
- Report to the healthcare provider nervousness, weakness, rashes, hair loss or swelling of the extremities.
- Weigh daily and report any unusual weight gain to the healthcare provider.
- Return to the healthcare provider for a check-up at least every 6 months or as instructed. Do not take the drug on a regular basis for longer than 6 months and do not abruptly stop taking it.
- Return for follow-up blood work as ordered.

SEROTONIN SELECTIVE AGONISTS

Sumatriptan succinate

Zolmitriptan

These agents bind to vascular receptors to vasoconstrict cranial blood vessels and relieve migraine headache.

Nursing responsibilities

- Assess for history of peripheral vascular disease, kidney or hepatic problems, and pregnancy.
- Evaluate relief of migraine headache and assess for side effects of photophobia, sound sensitivity, and nausea and vomiting.

Health education for the person and family

- Do not administer more than two doses in a 24-hour period and allow at least 1 hour between doses.
- If administering as an injectable, instructions for the proper method of giving the injection and disposing of the syringe will need to be given.
- Report wheezing, heart palpitations, skin rash, swelling of the eyelids or face, or chest pain to the healthcare provider immediately.

CALCIUM CHANNEL BLOCKERS

Verapamil

Nifedipine

The calcium channel blockers may have value in controlling cerebral vasospasms by two mechanisms: inhibiting the influx of calcium into the cerebral artery; and interfering with the destruction of erythrocytes and aggregation of platelets.

Nursing responsibilities

- These drugs cause peripheral vasodilation. Therefore, monitor blood pressure and pulse during the initial administration of the drug. Any excessive hypotensive response and tachycardia may precipitate angina. Request written parameters for safe drug administration.
- Monitor intake and output and daily weights. Assess for manifestations of congestive heart failure: weight gain, peripheral oedema, dyspnoea, rales and jugular vein distension.
- Teach the person and family members how to take pulse and blood pressure readings.

Health education for the person and family

- Take the medication with meals to reduce gastrointestinal irritation.
- Take pulse and blood pressure before taking medications each day at the same time and follow instructions regarding when to withhold medication and when to contact the healthcare provider. Keep a record of pulse and blood pressure readings.
- Report any side effects, such as dizziness, vertigo, unusual flushing, facial warmth or headaches, to the healthcare provider.
- Report immediately any swelling of the hands or feet, pronounced dizziness or chest pain accompanied by sweating, shortness of breath or severe headaches.

NON-STEROIDAL ANTI-INFLAMMATORY DRUG (NSAID): SALICYLATE

Acetylsalicylic acid, or aspirin, is a non-narcotic analgesic, antipyretic, anti-inflammatory agent used to relieve headache pain.

Nursing responsibilities

- Determine the type and pattern of pain. If aspirin was used in the past for pain control, note its effectiveness.
- Note any history of peptic ulcers or other conditions that may suggest potential problems with the use of salicylates.
- Assess people receiving anticoagulant therapy for bruises, bleeding of the mucous membranes or blood in the urine or stool.

Health education for the person and family

- Take aspirin after meals or before meals with an antacid and a full glass of water to minimise gastric irritation.
- Report ringing in the ears, unusual bleeding of gums, black tarry stools or other signs of bruising or bleeding to the primary healthcare provider.
- Monitor blood glucose levels carefully (if you have diabetes) and report hypoglycaemia if it occurs.

ERGOTAMINE

Caffeine-ergotamine tartrate combination

Ergotamine tartrate

Ergot alkaloids vasoconstrict the cerebral blood vessels, decreasing the amplitude of the pulsations of the cranial arteries. The major use of ergot alkaloids is for the treatment of migraine headaches. Cafergot has the same actions as Gynergen; in addition, the caffeine it contains provides a vasoconstrictive action, enhancing the effects of ergotamine.

Nursing responsibilities

- Because the drug accumulates in the body and is eliminated slowly, ergotamine poisoning may occur. Sepsis, renal and vascular disease, heavy smoking, malnutrition, pregnancy, contraceptive hormones and fever can increase the risk of ergotamine poisoning.
- These drugs are contraindicated in people with diabetes mellitus, sepsis, hepatic or kidney disease, peripheral and coronary artery disease, hypertension and pregnancy.

Health education for the person and family

- Take the drug immediately at onset of headache.
- Report the following to your healthcare provider: pain in the leg muscles, weakness and coldness or numbness of fingers or toes.
- A dose of Cafergot taken late in the day may prevent sleep because of the effects of caffeine.

Alternative and complementary therapies

The following alternative and complementary therapies are used to relieve the pain of headaches:

- Multivitamin support (vitamin D, elemental calcium, riboflavin (vitamin B) and magnesium)
- acupuncture
- meditation, relaxation, guided imagery
- massage therapies
- melatonin, 5-HTP, CoQ10
- magnetic field therapy
- herbal therapies
- osteopathic manipulation.

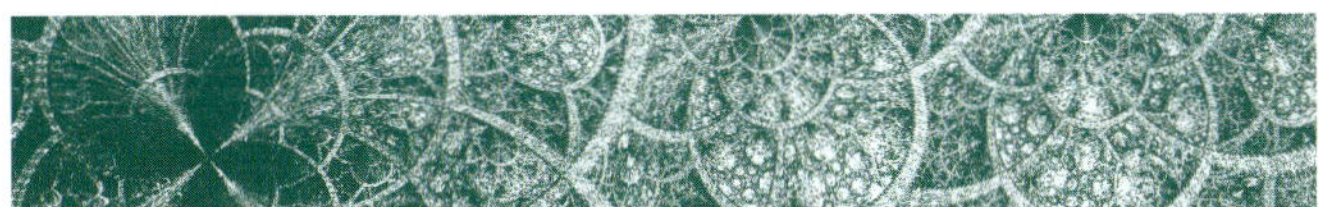

Nursing care

In addition to the nursing care discussed in this section, a nursing care plan for a person with a migraine headache follows.

Health promotion

Teach people with tension headaches relaxation techniques, such as massage and biofeedback. Counselling for chronic anxiety may also be helpful. Triggers for migraine or cluster headache should be identified and, if possible, eliminated. For example, avoiding physical and emotional stress, having regular and consistent sleep patterns, eating meals regularly, and avoiding specific foods or alcohol can be incorporated into daily life and are helpful. Specific suggestions are outlined in Box 41.2.

Assessment

Collect the following data through the health history and physical examination.

- *Health history*: history of intracerebral trauma, tumour or infection; detailed history and description of headache characteristics; family history; triggering factors; usual diet; effects of recurring headaches on lifestyle, activities of daily living (ADLs) and role performance.
- *Physical assessment*: skin (diaphoresis, pallor, flushing), eyes (sensitivity to light, tearing), muscle strength and movement.

BOX 41.2 Suggestions to decrease incidence of migraine headaches

- Wake up at the same time each morning.
- Exercise at least three times a week.
- No smoking or caffeine after 3 pm.
- Identify triggers in the environment and diet and aim to reduce or eliminate these.

Nursing diagnoses and interventions

The primary response of the person requiring nursing interventions is acute pain. Develop nursing interventions to help the person identify strategies for controlling the pain and discomfort of the headache.

Acute pain

Headaches originate from both intracranial and extracranial sources and range in severity from benign, transient discomfort to severe, incapacitating pain. Interventions focus on teaching the person self-care measures to control or relieve the pain and reducing any associated problems, such as nausea and vomiting or anxiety.

- Advise to maintain a diary of headaches, including duration, onset, location, relation to menstruation or food intake and related manifestations such as factors that relieve or intensify the pain. *A thorough assessment of the headache is essential for both the person and the healthcare provider to identify the circumstances and patterns of headache occurrence.*
- Ask the person to rate the pain or discomfort on a scale of 0 to 10 (with 10 being the worst pain). *Using a scale to rate the pain provides an objective measure of the person's subjective experience of the pain or discomfort. The scale can also be used to evaluate the effectiveness of pain relief measures.*
- Advise to minimise light, noise and activity, and to rest in a quiet, non-stimulating environment when experiencing a headache. *Manipulating the environment helps reduce noxious stimuli that may increase pain.*
- Advise to use non-invasive and non-pharmacological pain relief measures such as deep breathing or relaxation to facilitate self-management of pain (see the chapter 'Nursing care of people in pain'). *Alternative strategies to control pain can help to reduce tension and increase the person's sense of control over the pain.*
- Suggest application of cold compresses or dry heat to the head and neck. *The application of cold causes vasoconstriction, which helps reduce pain in vascular headaches. Application of heat can reduce muscle tension and improve circulation.*
- Advise to follow good nutrition guidelines, get regular exercise and sleep, and minimise stress. *Headaches are more likely to occur when ill, tired or under stress.*

Community-based care

In addition to implementing comfort measures, personal education has a high priority. Develop a teaching plan to help the person learn how to limit attacks (e.g. by avoiding precipitating factors) and reduce the effects of the headache. Provide specific information about prescribed medications. Referrals for methods of stress reduction may be necessary for people with long-term or migraine headaches.

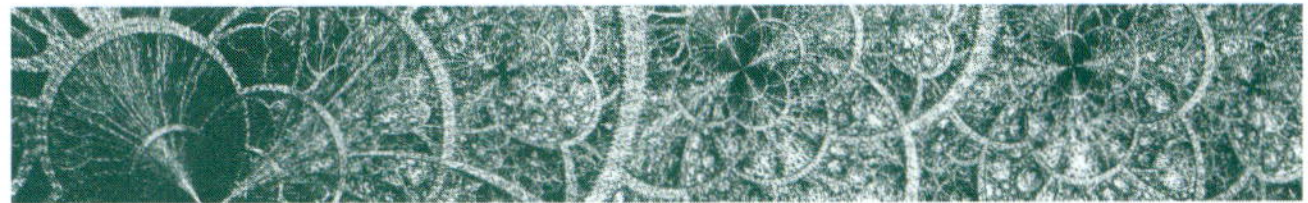

NURSING CARE PLAN A person with a migraine headache

Becky Friedman is a 30-year-old primary school teacher. Her friends and the other teachers regard Ms Friedman as an enthusiastic person who sets high standards for herself and strives for perfection. During the third term (the start of spring), Ms Friedman begins to miss work and sometimes appears very nervous. One day, another teacher notices Ms Friedman running down the hall and into the bathroom; the teacher finds Ms Friedman vomiting. As she washes up, Ms Friedman tells the other teacher that she has been having headaches since she began menstruating, but that they have never been as intense and frequent as during this past year. Ms Friedman agrees to see the Registered Nurse, Jane Schickadanz, at the school clinic for evaluation.

ASSESSMENT

During her health history, Ms Friedman relates that each month before her menstrual cycle she becomes nervous and sees flashing lights. She also has difficulty expressing herself and thinking clearly. The next day she develops a 'sick headache'. She states that the headache can last 1 to 2 days and that afterwards she cannot brush her hair because her scalp hurts. Ms Friedman attributes these symptoms to PMS and adds that she thinks she is allergic to cheese and nuts because she gets sick after eating them. After assessment and in consultation with the doctor, Ms Friedman's problem is diagnosed as a migraine with aura headache. Sumatriptan succinate is prescribed.

DIAGNOSES

- *Acute pain* related to vasodilation of cerebral vessels and a decreased serotonin level manifested by the presence of headaches.
- *Knowledge deficit* related to pain management, evidenced by inadequate use of analgesia.
- *Altered role performance* related to pain, evidenced by an inability to perform occupational tasks.

PLANNING

Provide education about migraine and methods of treatment.

Expected outcomes

- Experience reduced frequency and duration of pain.
- Identify available resources for helping with self-management of pain.

IMPLEMENTATION

- Ask Ms Friedman to keep a diary of her headaches for the next month, noting times of their occurrence, location and duration of pain, and factors that trigger the onset, such as her menstrual period or certain foods.
- Advise Ms Friedman to take medication at the first awareness of an impending attack.
- Suggest an appointment with a counsellor to learn methods of relaxation and stress relief.
- Request a dietary referral for elimination of foods that might precipitate headaches.

EVALUATION

Four weeks after beginning medication therapy with Imitrex and relaxation techniques, Ms Friedman has noted a decrease in the intensity of the headaches. She reports that the medication has stopped the headaches, which, she has noted, tend to occur more frequently immediately before her menstrual period. She is walking for 30 minutes each day and has made changes in her usual diet. Ms Friedman states, 'I feel good about going to work with my kids at school and knowing I can control my pain.'

CRITICAL THINKING IN THE NURSING PROCESS

1. List the questions you would include in a health history that would identify stressors consistent with migraine headaches.
2. Develop a teaching plan for Ms Friedman that includes methods of reducing fluid retention before her menstrual period, as well as a suggested diet based on the food guide pyramid.

REFLECTION ON THE NURSING PROCESS

1. Outline what you have learned from this case study that you will apply to your future nursing practice.
2. Which education strategies could you use to develop a plan of care for Ms Friedman for the nursing diagnosis of *Disturbed sleep pattern* related to pain, evidenced by fatigue?

THE PERSON WITH EPILEPSY

Epilepsy is a chronic disorder of abnormal, recurring, excessive and self-terminating electrical discharge from neurons. Epilepsy is characterised by recurring seizures accompanied by some type of change in behaviour. A **seizure** (sometimes called a convulsion) is a single event of abnormal electrical discharge in the brain resulting in an abrupt and temporary altered state of cerebral function (Hickey, 2019). This abnormal neuronal activity, which may involve all or part of the brain, disturbs skeletal motor function, sensation, autonomic function of the viscera, behaviour and/or consciousness. Epilepsy is categorised as a paroxysmal disorder because its manifestations are discontinuous; that is, minutes, days, weeks or even years may elapse between seizures.

Incidence and prevalence

Epilepsy is one of the most common neurological conditions, affecting an estimated 275,000 people in Australia (Epilepsy Centre, 2022). There is a strong genetic component. Although people of any age may be affected, the prevalence and incidence of epilepsy increases dramatically in older adults (see the 'Meeting individualised needs' box).

The incidence of epilepsy is increasing. Researchers have suggested that the increase may be due to technological advances in obstetric and paediatric care that allow extremely high-risk neonates to survive, and to other technological advances that have improved survival rates after craniocerebral trauma.

Isolated seizure episodes may occur in otherwise healthy people for a variety of reasons, including an acute febrile state,

MEETING INDIVIDUALISED NEEDS **Epilepsy in older adults**

For years, epilepsy was believed to be a disease that only affected children. However, the incidence of epilepsy is higher in adults than in children, and older adults represent 30% of the population with epilepsy. Furthermore, in people aged 65 years and over, there has been a significant increase in the development of new seizure activity (Epilepsy Action Australia, 2020). These data have important implications for nursing assessments and care.

- The most common cause of epilepsy in older adults is arteriosclerosis of the cerebrovascular system (with up to 80% of the older population having arteriosclerosis).
- The manifestations of epilepsy in older adults are different from those in younger adults and children. Although 60% of younger people have generalised tonic–clonic seizures, only 30% of older adults have generalised tonic–clonic seizures. The most common type of seizure in older adults is a complex partial seizure.
- Older adults tend to have longer post-seizure manifestations than younger adults.
- Epilepsy that begins in older adults is often easier to control with anti-epileptic drugs (AEDs) than that in younger people. However, some AEDs decrease the effect of statins used to treat arteriosclerosis (the most common cause of epilepsy in older adults).

infection, metabolic or endocrine disorder (such as hypoglycaemia) or exposure to toxins. Epilepsy may be idiopathic (i.e. it may have no identifiable cause) or it may be secondary to birth injury, infection, vascular abnormalities, trauma or tumours.

FAST FACTS

- Epilepsy affects people of all ages and cultural backgrounds.
- Approximately 275,000 Australians have epilepsy (Epilepsy Centre, 2022).
- Epilepsy is not a mental disorder.

Pathophysiology

Normally, when the mind is actively working, electrical activity in the brain is unsynchronised; when the mind is at rest, electrical activity is mildly synchronised. It is believed that most seizures arise from a few unstable, hypersensitive and hyperreactive neurons in the brain. During a seizure, these neurons produce a rhythmic and repetitive hypersynchronous discharge. Although the exact initiating factor for seizure activity has not been identified, several theories have been proposed (Norris, 2018):

- alterations in the permeability of, or ion distribution across, cell membranes
- alterations in the excitability of neurons resulting from neuroglia (neuroglia are CNS connective or supporting cells; they include astrocytes, oligodendroglia and microglia)
- scarring or decreased inhibition of activity in the cerebral cortex or thalamic region
- imbalances of excitatory and inhibitory neurotransmitters such as acetylcholine (ACh) or gamma aminobutyric acid (GABA).

All people have a seizure threshold; when this threshold is exceeded, a seizure may result. In some people, the seizure threshold may be abnormally low, increasing their risk of seizure activity; in other people, pathological processes may alter the seizure threshold (Norris, 2018). The neurons that initiate seizure activity are called the *epileptogenic focus*. Abnormal neuronal activity may remain localised, causing a partial or focal seizure, or it may spread to involve the entire brain, causing generalised seizure activity.

Seizures may also be provoked or unprovoked. Unprovoked (primary or idiopathic) seizures have no identifiable cause, with multiple episodes diagnosed as a seizure disorder. Provoked (secondary) seizure aetiologies include febrile seizures in children, toxaemia of pregnancy, rapid withdrawal from alcohol or barbiturates, systemic metabolic conditions (such as hypoglycaemia, hypoxia, uraemia and electrolyte imbalances) and pathologies of the brain (such as meningitis, cerebral bleeding or cerebral oedema).

Metabolic needs of the brain increase dramatically during seizure activity. The demand for adenosine triphosphate (ATP), the energy source of the brain, increases by approximately 250%. Consequently, the demand for glucose and oxygen (which are needed to produce ATP) increases and oxygen consumption increases by about 60%. To supply this increased oxygen need and remove carbon dioxide and other metabolic by-products, cerebral blood flow increases to about 2.5 times that of the normal rate. As long as oxygenation, blood glucose levels and cardiac function remain normal, cerebral blood flow can respond to this increased metabolic demand of the brain. If cerebral blood flow cannot meet these needs, however, cellular exhaustion and cellular destruction may result.

Manifestations

Although seizures may be categorised in several ways, the classification developed by the International League Against Epilepsy is the most useful clinically (cited in Papadakis et al., 2022). In this classification, seizures are divided into those that affect only part of the brain (partial seizures) and those that are generalised (affect all of the brain). An individual may have more than one type in what are called mixed seizures.

Partial seizures

Partial (or focal) seizures involve the activation of only a restricted part of one cerebral hemisphere. A partial seizure accompanied by no alteration in consciousness is called a simple partial seizure; one in which consciousness is impaired is called a complex partial seizure.

SIMPLE PARTIAL SEIZURES The manifestations of *simple partial seizures* depend on the involved area of the brain. Manifestations may include alterations in motor function, sensory signs or autonomic or psychic symptoms. Typically, the motor portion of the cortex is affected, causing recurrent muscle contractions of the face or a contralateral part of the body, such as a finger or hand. This motor activity may stay confined to one area or spread sequentially to adjacent parts, a phenomenon known as a *Jacksonian march* or *Jacksonian seizure*. Manifestations of a simple partial seizure involving the sensory portion of the brain may include abnormal sensations or hallucinations. Disruptions in the function of the autonomic nervous system, with resulting tachycardia, flushing, hypotension and hypertension, or psychic manifestations, such as a sense of déjà vu (a feeling that 'this has happened before') or inappropriate fear or anger, may also be experienced during a simple partial seizure.

COMPLEX PARTIAL SEIZURES During a *complex partial seizure*, consciousness is impaired and the person may engage in repetitive, non-purposeful activity, such as lip smacking, aimless walking or picking at clothing. These behaviours are known as automatisms. During the seizure, the person loses conscious contact with the environment; amnesia is common after the seizure and several hours may elapse before the person regains full consciousness. Complex partial seizures usually originate in the temporal lobe and may be preceded by an aura, such as an unusual smell, a sense of déjà vu or a sudden intense emotion.

Generalised seizures

Generalised seizures involve both hemispheres of the brain as well as deeper brain structures, such as the thalamus, basal ganglia and upper brainstem. Consciousness is always impaired with generalised seizures. Absence and tonic–clonic seizures are the common forms of generalised seizure activity; they occur more frequently (especially in children) than partial seizures.

ABSENCE SEIZURES *Absence (petit mal) seizures* are characterised by a sudden brief cessation of all motor activity accompanied by a blank stare and unresponsiveness. Absence seizures are more common in children than in adults. The seizure typically lasts only 5 to 10 seconds, although some may last for 30 seconds or more. Movements such as eyelid fluttering, or automatisms such as lip smacking, may occur during an absence seizure. Seizure activity may vary from occasional episodes to several hundred per day.

TONIC–CLONIC SEIZURES *Tonic–clonic seizures* (grand mal) are the most common type of seizure activity in adults. This type of seizure activity follows a typical pattern. A warning *aura* may precede generalised seizure activity. The aura may be a vague sense of uneasiness or an abnormal gustatory, visual, auditory or visceral sensation (such as a metallic taste in the mouth, a smell of burning rubber or seeing a bright light). Often, however, the seizure occurs without warning.

The seizure begins with a sudden loss of consciousness and sharp tonic muscle contractions (the tonic phase of the seizure). With the muscle contraction, air is forced out of the lungs and the person may cry out. Postural control is lost, and the person falls to the floor in the opisthotonic posture (see Figure 41.4A). Muscles are rigid, with the arms and legs extended and the jaw clenched. Urinary incontinence is common; bowel incontinence may also occur. Breathing ceases and cyanosis develops during the tonic phase of a seizure. The pupils are fixed and dilated. The tonic phase lasts an average of 15 seconds, although it may persist for up to a minute.

The clonic phase, which follows the tonic phase, is characterised by alternating contraction and relaxation of the muscles in all the extremities along with hyperventilation (see Figure 41.4B). The eyes roll back and the person froths at the mouth. The clonic phase varies in duration and subsides gradually. The entire tonic–clonic portion of the seizure generally lasts no more than 60 to 90 seconds.

Following the clonic phase of seizure activity, the person remains unconscious and unresponsive to stimuli. This period is known as the postictal period or phase. The person is relaxed and breathes quietly. The person regains consciousness gradually and may be confused and disoriented on waking. Headache, muscle aches and fatigue often follow the seizure and the person may sleep for several hours. Amnesia of the seizure is usual; the person also may not recall events just prior to the seizure activity.

Because of the lack of warning with tonic–clonic seizures, the person may experience injury. Head injury, fractures, burns or motor vehicle crashes may occur secondarily to seizure activity.

Status epilepticus

Status epilepticus can develop during seizure activity. In this case, the seizure activity becomes continuous, with only very

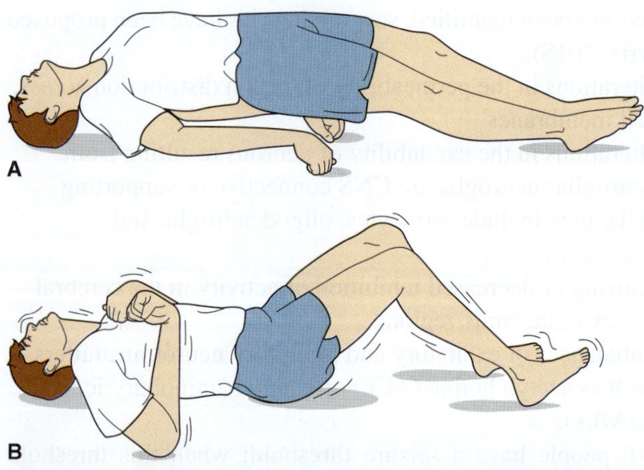

FIGURE 41.4 *Tonic–clonic seizures in grand mal seizures. A, Tonic phase. B, Clonic phase*

short periods of calm between intense and persistent seizures. The repetitive seizures may be of any type, although they are usually generalised tonic–clonic (Norris, 2018). Repeated seizures have a cumulative effect, producing muscular contractions that can interfere with respirations. The person is in great danger of developing hypoxia, acidosis, hypoglycaemia, hyperthermia and exhaustion if the convulsive activity is not halted. Status epilepticus is considered a life-threatening medical emergency that requires immediate treatment.

INTERPROFESSIONAL CARE

Initial treatment focuses on controlling the seizure; the long-term goal is to determine the cause and prevent future seizures. Interprofessional care includes diagnostic testing, medications and, in some cases, surgery.

Diagnosis

Diagnostic testing is performed to confirm the seizure diagnosis and to determine any treatable causes and precipitating factors. (See the chapter 'A person-centred approach to assessing the nervous system' for a description of neurological tests and related nursing care.) Radiological examinations may include an MRI or CT scan to determine abnormalities in the brain and rule out differential diagnoses, and a skull x-ray to identify any bony abnormalities. An electroencephalogram (EEG) helps localise any brain lesions and confirm the diagnosis. A lumbar puncture may be performed to assess spinal fluid for CNS infections (increased WBCs) or tumours (increased protein levels). Blood studies are used to assess blood count, electrolytes, blood urea and blood glucose.

Medications

Anti-epileptic drugs (AEDs) (also called anticonvulsant drugs) can reduce or control most seizure activity. More than 20 drugs are used in the treatment of epilepsy. These medications do not cure the disorder; they only manage its manifestations. AEDs generally act in one of two ways: by raising the seizure threshold or by limiting the spread of abnormal activity within the brain.

The goals of medications for epilepsy are to protect the person from harm and to reduce or prevent seizure activity without impairing cognitive function or producing undesirable side effects. Ideally, the lowest possible dose of a single medication that will control the person's seizures is prescribed; often, however, several medications must be tried before the most effective is identified and a combination of drugs may be needed to manage the person's seizures. Therapy is individualised, based on the type of seizure activity and the person's response to the medication. Some drugs recommended for newly diagnosed adults with either partial or mixed seizures, and commonly used in Australia, are phenytoin, sodium valproate, gabapentin, lamotrigine, oxcarbazepine and topiramate. Examples of and nursing implications for AEDs are described in the 'Medication administration' box; drug interactions are listed in Box 41.3.

BOX 41.3 Drug interactions with AEDs

- *Sodium valproate and phenobarbital.* Blood levels of phenobarbital may rise significantly when sodium valproate is added to the person's medication regimen.
- *Phenobarbital and digoxin.* This combination may increase the metabolism of digoxin, resulting in decreased digoxin levels.
- *Phenobarbital and warfarin.* Phenobarbital may decrease the absorption of warfarin from the gastrointestinal tract and decrease the drug's anticoagulant response.
- *Disulfiram and phenobarbital.* This combination may inhibit the metabolism of the anticonvulsant drug and increase the incidence of side effects associated with the anticonvulsant drug.
- *Carbamazepine and oral contraceptives.* Carbamazepine decreases the effectiveness of oral contraceptives.
- *Other drugs.* Other drugs reported to interact with anticonvulsant drugs include aspirin, certain antibiotics, isoniazid, acetazolamide, antacids, folic acid and narcotics.

If the person has been seizure free for at least 3 years, withdrawal of medications may be considered, with the dose of one drug at a time reduced over weeks or months. There is no way to predict which people can remain seizure free without medication, but if seizures reoccur, the same medications usually provide good control.

Status epilepticus requires immediate intervention to preserve life. Establishing and maintaining the airway is a priority. An intravenous fluid containing dextrose is administered to prevent hypoglycaemia. Diazepam or lorazepam is given intravenously and the dose repeated in 10 minutes if necessary to stop seizure activity. Phenytoin is administered intravenously for longer-term control of seizures. Phenobarbital may also be administered to people in status epilepticus.

Surgery

Resective surgery, with removal of the epileptogenic focus, is an option for the most severe forms of epilepsy. Candidates for this type of surgery include those who are unresponsive to medical management, who have a unilateral focus and who have impaired quality of life from seizures. Resections of the temporal lobe are most commonly performed and are most effective for partial complex seizures. An estimated 5% of people with epilepsy may be candidates for surgery. The goal of surgery is to reduce the person's uncontrollable seizures.

To be selected as a candidate for surgery, the person must be highly motivated and psychologically prepared. A psychological screening is required because the preoperative preparation is extensive and time consuming and the surgery is long and requires that the person remain awake during surgery so that they can cooperate and respond to commands. The EEG is monitored during surgery to identify the epileptogenic focus and evaluate the effect of surgical intervention.

MEDICATION ADMINISTRATION Seizures

ANTI-EPILEPTIC DRUGS (AEDS)

Examples of AEDs are:
Phenytoin
Phenobarbital
Primidone
Carbamazepine
Sodium valproate
Ethosuximide
Clonazepam
Gabapentin
Lamotrigine
Tiagabine hydrochloride
Levetiracetam

AEDs are used to control chronic seizures and involuntary muscle spasms or movements characteristic of certain neurological diseases. These drugs act in the motor cortex of the brain to reduce the spread of electrical discharges from the rapidly firing epileptic foci in this area. These agents control seizures without impairing the normal functions of the CNS. Drugs effective against one type of seizure may not be effective against another; anticonvulsant therapy must be individualised.

Nursing responsibilities

- Monitor blood pressure, pulse and respirations.
- Note evidence of CNS side effects, such as blurred vision, dimmed vision, slurred speech, nystagmus or confusion. Gingival hyperplasia may be noted in people taking phenytoin.
- Recognise that if people are to be on prolonged therapy, they may need a diet rich in vitamin D.
- Monitor the serum calcium level as ordered; phenytoin can contribute to demineralisation of bone.
- When administering anticonvulsants intravenously, monitor closely for respiratory depression and cardiovascular collapse.
- Administer gabapentin 2 hours after antacids.
- Administer tiagabine hydrochloride with food.

Health education for the person and family

- Take the exact dosage prescribed. Do not increase, decrease or discontinue the dosage without discussing this with the healthcare provider; doing so may lead to convulsions.
- Avoid hazardous tasks until the drug has been regulated. AEDs may at first decrease mental alertness and cause drowsiness, headache, dizziness and incoordination of muscles. These effects are usually dose related and may disappear with a change of dosage or continued therapy.
- If you are taking phenytoin, maintain good oral hygiene: use a soft toothbrush, massage the gums and floss daily.
- It is very important to obtain liver function studies regularly as ordered by the healthcare provider. This will help detect early signs of hepatitis and other liver problems. Report for all scheduled laboratory studies, including complete blood count, kidney and liver function studies, and drug levels.
- Carry identification indicating the type of seizures for which you are being treated.
- Do not take gabapentin 1 hour before or less than 2 hours after an antacid.
- If you are taking lamotrigine and develop a rash, tell your healthcare provider.
- Take tiagabine hydrochloride with food.

General postoperative care for the person with intracranial surgery follows the nursing management guidelines outlined later in the chapter. Specific preoperative and postoperative care for a person with a seizure disorder is described in the accompanying box.

Vagal nerve stimulation therapy

Vagal nerve stimulation (VNS) therapy is approved as a treatment for people with partial-onset seizures who do not respond to AEDs. The therapy does not stop the seizures, but rather reduces their number and improves the person's quality of life. It is almost always necessary to continue taking AEDs. The therapy is designed to prevent seizures by sending regular small pulses of electrical energy to the brain via the vagus nerve. A flat, round battery (about the size of a dollar coin) is implanted in the chest wall, and electrodes are threaded under the skin and wound around the vagus nerve in the neck. The battery is programmed to deliver a few seconds of electrical energy every few seconds. If the person feels that a seizure is about to happen, a discharge can be activated by passing a small magnet over the battery. In some people this stops the seizures. Side effects are hoarseness and throat discomfort.

NURSING CARE OF THE PERSON with seizures who is having surgery

PREOPERATIVE CARE

- For most people, AEDs are withheld the morning or evening of the day before surgery. *AEDs may interfere with anaesthetics and perioperative monitoring.*
- For people with frequent and/or severe seizures, however, a partial dose of medication may be administered. *This prevents seizures or status epilepticus during surgery.*

POSTOPERATIVE CARE

- AEDs are administered parenterally until the person can tolerate oral fluids; medications are then continued orally. *It is common for the person to have seizures in the early postoperative period.*
- Steroids may be administered for the first 3 days after surgery and are tapered and then discontinued during the following week. *Steroids are given to decrease cerebral oedema.*

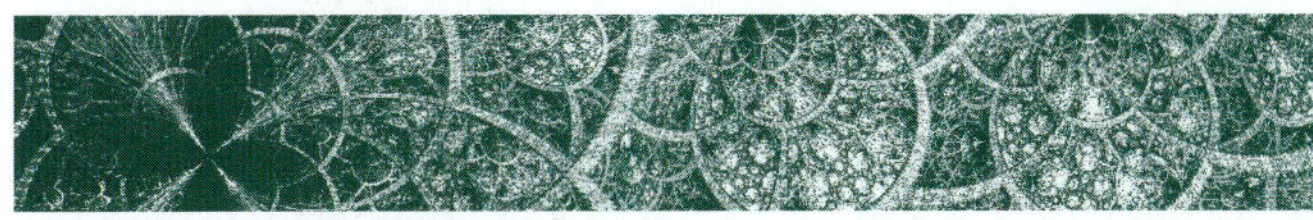

Nursing care

An example nursing care plan for a person with seizures can be seen in the accompanying box.

Health promotion

Health promotion activities for the person with seizures focus on teaching to reduce the incidence of seizure activity and to promote safety. It is important during health promotion to stress the following:

- Know the importance of follow-up care, of keeping medical appointments and of continuing to take AEDs as prescribed even when no seizures are experienced.
- Review any state and local laws that apply to people with seizure disorders. Driving a motor vehicle is usually prohibited for a significant period after a seizure episode. Usually, a driver's licence can be reinstated or obtained after a seizure-free period and a letter from the healthcare provider.
- Know drug interactions with other prescribed drugs, over-the-counter (OTC) drugs, street drugs and alcohol.
- Teach family members first aid for a seizure:
  - Cushion the head.
  - Loosen anything tight around the neck.
  - Turn on the side.
  - Nothing in the mouth.
  - Do not hold down.
- Teach family members to call for medical assistance:
  - if the seizure lasts for more than 5 minutes
  - if there is slow recovery, a second seizure or difficulty breathing after the seizure
  - if there are signs of injury (such as bleeding from the mouth).

NURSING CARE PLAN A person with a seizure disorder

Janet Carlson is a 19-year-old university student who lives with her parents and one younger sister. Although Janet had seizures while she was at high school, they have been controlled with medication. However, she had a tonic–clonic seizure yesterday and immediately made an appointment with her family GP. She is currently taking phenytoin (Dilantin) 300 mg/day as a maintenance medication to prevent seizures.

ASSESSMENT

Evita Farias, RN, completes a health history for Ms Carlson. During the history, she tells Ms Farias that she has been under stress because of difficulties in completing her course requirements this semester. She has not been sleeping as many hours per night and sometimes she forgets to take her medication. Ms Carlson's serum phenytoin level is 8 mg/mL. Therapeutic level is 10 to 20 mg/mL.

DIAGNOSES

- *Risk of injury* related to recurrence of generalised tonic–clonic seizure activity and low serum phenytoin levels, evidenced by increased seizure activity.
- *Deficient knowledge* related to activities that may trigger seizure occurrence, the effect of stress on seizures and medication information manifested by increased seizure activity.

PLANNING

- Improved management of epilepsy through compliance with management regimens and increased knowledge of epilepsy.

Expected outcomes

- Awareness of precipitating and triggering factors related to the onset of seizures.
- Awareness of the relationship between emotional and physical stress and seizures.
- Awareness of the importance of taking AEDs.

IMPLEMENTATION

- Teach Ms Carlson and her family the following:
  - current information about seizures
  - care during and after a seizure
  - medication protocols
  - factors and activities that can trigger seizures
  - the importance of follow-up care.
- Refer Ms Carlson and her family to a local epilepsy support group.
- Recommend that she purchase and wear a MedicAlert® bracelet.

EVALUATION

Ms Carlson is instructed to continue taking Dilantin 300 mg/day. She states the importance of nutrition, rest and measures to reduce stress. She also discusses the importance of maintaining the proper blood levels of her medication, stating that too little or too much of the medication could cause problems. Ms Carlson recognises that the seizures had recurred during a busy time at university during which she had forgotten to take her medication. She is now wearing a MedicAlert® bracelet. Ms Carlson is provided with the telephone number of Epilepsy Action Australia.

CRITICAL THINKING IN THE NURSING PROCESS

1. If you were Ms Carlson's nurse, would your teaching differ if she were living alone? If so, how?
2. Ms Carlson tells you that although she knows she should not drive a car, she often drives her friend to work. How would you approach this problem?

REFLECTION ON THE NURSING PROCESS

1. Which safety strategies could family members implement in the event of a person having a seizure?
2. Outline what you have learned from this case study that you will apply to your future nursing practice.

Assessment

Collect the following data through the health history and physical examination:

- *Health history*: past seizures; age when the first seizure occurred, most recent seizure; factors precipitating a seizure, any warning signs (aura); prophylactic anticonvulsant therapy; and specific concerns the person may have about the seizures.
- *Physical assessment*: important data used in determining an accurate diagnosis describes manifestations obtained from nursing assessments before, during and after a seizure. (Table 41.6 lists nursing assessments with rationale.)

Nursing diagnoses and interventions

Nursing care of people with a seizure disorder focuses on providing care during and immediately after the seizure and on personal/family teaching. The person with seizures has a wide variety of responses to actual or potential changes in health status; interventions discussed in this section focus on facilitating physical and psychological comfort and safety.

Risk of ineffective airway clearance

During a seizure, the tongue may fall back and obstruct the airway, the gag reflex may be depressed, and secretions may pool at the back of the throat. These may put the person at risk of an obstructed airway. Most seizures occur in the home or community; therefore, teach these interventions to the person's family:

- Provide interventions to maintain a patent airway:
  - Loosen clothing around the neck.
  - Turn on the side.
  - Do not force anything into the mouth.
  - If prescribed and available, administer oxygen by mask.
  - Although it was at one time believed that it was necessary to place a padded tongue blade in the person's mouth during a seizure, this is no longer recommended; an improperly placed tongue blade can obstruct the airway. *Turning the person on the side allows secretions to drain from the mouth.*
- Teach family members or significant others how to care for the person during a seizure to prevent airway obstruction. *Family members are often the only people present to provide this emergency intervention.*

Anxiety

The person with a seizure disorder is understandably anxious about the future, with questions about ability to go to school or university, work, have a family and drive a car. Feelings of embarrassment about having a seizure in public and rejection by others are common and also increase the person's anxiety.

- Provide support by explaining that concerns are normal. It is important to be sensitive to the effect of seizures on the person's self-concept and body image; alterations in these areas not only increase anxiety but also cause withdrawal from socialisation with others. *Demonstrating acceptance of the person's concerns allows further discussion.*
- Help identify safe leisure activities. *Worrying about being hurt if a seizure occurs may cause withdrawal from social activities that are pleasurable.*
- Provide information about sources and support groups. *Sharing information with other people with similar health problems allows for a more realistic viewpoint; accurate information can clear up misconceptions that cause anxiety.*
- Provide accurate information about hiring practices and legal limitations on driving or operating heavy or dangerous machinery. *Accurate information decreases anxiety about the unknown. The federal* Disability Discrimination Act *in Australia prohibits discrimination; however, there are legal limitations on driving until the person is proved free of seizures.*

TABLE 41.6 Nursing assessments before, during and after a seizure

ASSESSMENT	RATIONALE
What was the person's level of consciousness? If consciousness was lost, at what point?	Indicates area of brain involved and type of seizure
What was the person doing just before the attack?	May suggest precipitating factors
In which part of the body did the seizure start?	May indicate the site of seizure activity in the brain tissue; for example, if jerking movements were first observed in right hand, the seizure focus may be in left motor cortex
Was there an epileptic cry?	Usually indicates the tonic stage of a generalised tonic-clonic seizure
Were any automatisms such as eyelid fluttering, chewing, lip smacking or swallowing observed?	Often seen in complex, partial and absence seizures
How long did movements last? Did the location or character change (tonic to clonic)? Did movements involve both sides of the body or just one?	Indicates areas in which focal activity originated
Did the head and/or eyes turn to one side and, if so, which side?	Helps localise the focus of the seizure. During the seizure, the head and eyes typically will turn away from the side of the epileptogenic focus
Were there changes in pupillary reactions?	Indicates involvement of the autonomic nervous system
If the person fell, was the head hit?	Skull x-ray studies may be needed to rule out subdural haematoma or fracture
Was there foaming or frothing from the mouth?	Usually indicates a tonic-clonic seizure

Community-based care

Teaching follows a systematic assessment of the needs of both the person and their family. Include family members so that they can learn seizure management, including the care and observations necessary before and during a seizure. Stress the importance of safety and keeping the airway patent.

Help both the person and their family adjust to a diagnosis of epilepsy. Address the following topics:

- the importance of wearing a MedicAlert® bracelet, carrying a medical alert card or using the medical alert feature of a smart device
- taking showers versus baths because of safety issues during a generalised seizure
- factors that may trigger a seizure, such as abrupt withdrawal from medication, constipation, fatigue, excessive stress, fever, menstruation, sights and sounds such as television, flashing video and computer screens
- helpful resources, including:
  - Epilepsy Action Australia: https://www.epilepsy.org.au/about-epilepsy/
  - Epilepsy Foundation: https://www.epilepsyfoundation.org.au.

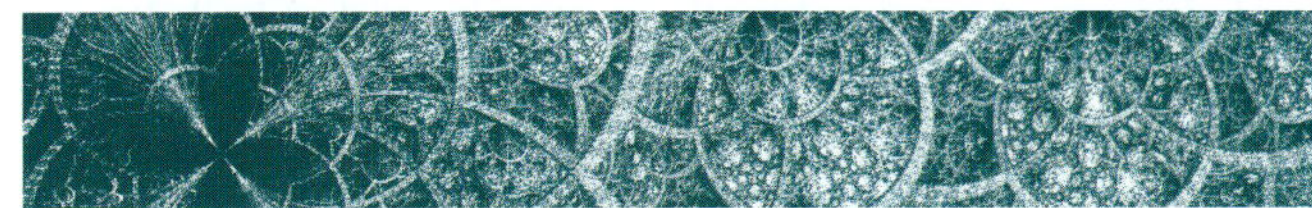

Traumatic brain injury

Traumatic brain injury (TBI) (also called *craniocerebral trauma*) refers to any injury of the scalp, skull (cranium or facial bones) and brain. TBI is the second-largest cause of death and disability in Australia and worldwide, with occurrence three times greater in the Indigenous Australian population, particularly females. TBI may be defined as a traumatic insult to the brain capable of causing physical, intellectual, emotional, social and vocational changes. A TBI may be classified as a penetrating (open) head injury (e.g. resulting from a knife, bullet or baseball bat) or a closed head injury (a blunt injury to the brain that does not result in an open skull fracture). TBI may cause problems with cognition, movement, sensation and emotions. Even mild brain injuries, if repeated over an extended period of time, can result in cumulative neurological and cognitive deficits.

FAST FACTS

- In Australia, there were 23,445 patients aged under 65 who were hospitalised with a traumatic brain injury (TBI) during 2013–2014 or 2014–2015 (Australian Institute of Health and Welfare, 2021).
- Australia's overseas-born population continues to represent the majority (86%) of TB notifications and Australia's Aboriginal and Torres Strait Islander population continues to record TB rates around six times higher than the Australian-born, non-Indigenous population (Department of Health, 2017).

In Australia, the leading causes of TBI are falls (42%), followed by transportation accidents (31%) and assaults (14%). Elevated blood alcohol levels, not wearing motorcycle helmets and not wearing seat belts contribute significantly to crashes and the risk of subsequent injury. Other causes of head injury include sports injuries and occupational and recreational injuries (Brain Injury Australia, 2022). Adults aged 15 to 44 are at the greatest risk, with a male-to-female ratio in the Anglo-Saxon population of 3:1 (Hickey, 2019). Other risk factors include being over the age of 75 and living in a high-crime area.

Specific damage following craniocerebral injuries is related to the mechanism of the injury (how it occurs), the nature of the injury (type) and the location of the injury (where it occurs).

Head injuries may be classified as blunt or penetrating and can occur through several mechanisms:

- Acceleration injury is sustained when the head is struck by a moving object, such as a swinging bat.
- Deceleration injury occurs when the head hits a stationary object, such as a concrete wall.
- Acceleration–deceleration injury (also called a *coup–contrecoup* phenomenon) occurs when the head hits an object and the brain 'rebounds' within the skull (see Figure 41.5). The brain is injured at the point of impact (the coup) and on the opposite side of the impact (the contrecoup). Two or more areas of the brain can be injured as a result of this phenomenon.
- Deformation injuries are those in which the force deforms and disrupts the integrity of the impacted body part (e.g. skull fracture).

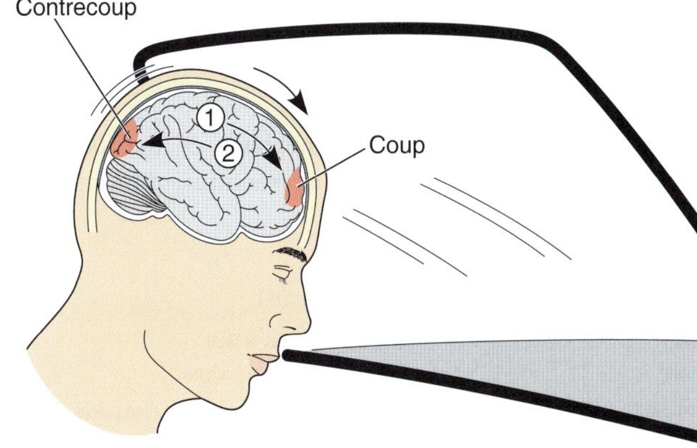

FIGURE 41.5 *Coup–contrecoup head injury. Following the initial injury (coup), the brain rebounds within the skull and sustains additional injury (contrecoup) in the opposite part of the brain*

Types of craniocerebral trauma include injuries to the skull (including fractures), injuries to the brain (including concussion and contusion) and intracranial haemorrhage (including haematomas). Brain injury can result either from the direct effects of the trauma on brain tissue or from secondary responses to trauma, such as cerebral oedema, haematoma (blood clot), swelling or increased intracranial pressure.

THE PERSON WITH A SKULL FRACTURE

A *skull fracture* is a break in the continuity of the skull. It may occur with or without damage to the brain; however, intracranial trauma often results from skull fractures. The considerable force of impact significantly increases the risk of underlying haematoma formation. Disruption of the skull can also cause cranial nerve injury, allow bacteria to enter the cranial vault, and/or allow CSF to leak out.

Pathophysiology

Skull fractures are classified as open or closed depending on whether the dura is torn (open) or not torn (closed). Skull fractures are further classified into one of four categories: linear, comminuted, depressed or basilar (see Table 41.7).

Linear fractures

Linear fractures are the most common, accounting for 80% of all skull fractures. They typically extend from the point of impact towards the base of the skull. Although the risk of infection or CSF leakage is minimal with this type of fracture because the dura usually remains intact, subdural or epidural haematomas (a collection of blood) frequently underlie the fracture. A haematoma (discussed later in this chapter) places pressure on underlying brain tissue, increasing both intracranial pressure and the risk of brain damage.

Comminuted and depressed fractures

Comminuted and depressed skull fractures increase the risk of direct damage to brain tissue from bruising (contusion) and bone fragments. However, the risk of secondary brain injury may be reduced in these fractures, because in breaking the bone, the traumatic impact energy is distributed and dissipated. If the skin overlying the fracture is lacerated or the dura is torn, the risk of infection is increased.

Basilar fractures

Basilar skull fractures involve the base of the skull and usually are extensions of adjacent fractures, although they may occur independently. Although most basilar skull fractures are uncomplicated, they may involve the sinuses of the frontal bone or the petrous portion of the temporal bone (middle ear). If the dura is disrupted, CSF may leak through the tear. CSF leakage may include *rhinorrhoea* (CSF leakage through the nose) or *otorrhoea* (CSF leakage from the ear). Blood may be visible behind the tympanic membrane (haemotympanum) or ecchymosis may be noted over the mastoid process (Battle's sign). Bilateral periorbital ecchymosis ('raccoon eyes') is another possible manifestation. If CSF leakage is present, the risk of infection is high. Other complications of basilar skull fractures include injury to the internal carotid artery and compression of cranial nerve I–V, VII or VIII.

TABLE 41.7 Types of skull fractures

TYPE	DESCRIPTION
Linear (simple)	Simple, clean break in skull Occurs with low-velocity injuries
Comminuted	Bone is crushed into small, fragmented pieces Usually seen with high-impact injuries
Depressed	Inward depression of bone fragments Usually due to a powerful blow to the skull The dura may or may not be intact Bone fragments may penetrate into the brain tissue
Basilar	Occurs at the base of the skull May be linear, comminuted or depressed

INTERPROFESSIONAL CARE

Treatment of the person with a skull fracture depends on the type and location of the fracture. Skull fracture may be only one of several head injuries.

A simple linear fracture generally requires bed rest and observation for underlying injury to brain tissue or haematoma formation. No specific treatment is required unless complications arise. Depressed skull fractures require surgical intervention, usually within 24 hours of the injury, to debride the wound completely and remove bone fragments, which may become embedded in brain tissue or cerebral blood vessels. If depressed deeply, the bone may be elevated. If cerebral oedema is not present, a cranioplasty with insertion of acrylic bone may be performed. Basal skull fractures do not require surgery unless CSF leakage persists. Regular neurological assessments and observation for manifestations of meningitis are required for the hospitalised person. Antibiotics may be administered prophylactically.

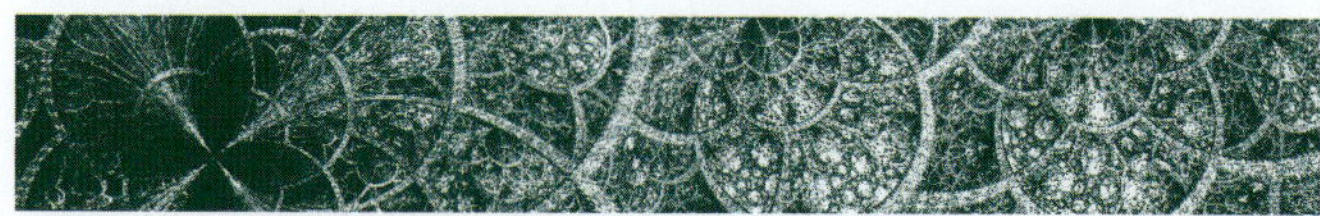

Nursing care

The person with a craniocerebral trauma may have a variety of responses and healthcare needs, depending on the location and extent of the trauma. Many of those problems, with related nursing interventions, are discussed in other sections of this chapter, including seizures, increased intracranial pressure and bleeding within the brain.

Nursing diagnoses and interventions

Risk of infection

The person with a skull fracture is at increased risk of infection related to access to the cranial contents through a tear in the dura. In an open, depressed fracture, the wound may be contaminated by dirt, hair or other debris.

- Monitor for otorrhoea or rhinorrhoea. *Open fractures of the skull increase the possibility of leakage of CSF from the ears or nose.*
- Test drainage of clear fluid from ear and nose for glucose by using a glucose reagent strip, such as Dextrostix. *Clear drainage that tests positive for glucose indicates leakage of CSF; however, be aware that false positives may occur.*
- *Observe blood-tinged fluid for 'halo' sign. CSF dries in concentric rings on gauze or tissues. This sign is suggestive of CSF leakage.*
- Keep the nasopharynx and the external ear clean. Place a piece of sterile gauze in the ear or tape a sterile cotton pad loosely under the nose; change dressings when they become wet. *Wet dressings facilitate movement of organisms.*
- Instruct person not to blow nose, cough or inhibit sneeze; sneeze through open mouth. *Blowing the nose and coughing increase ICP. Withholding a sneeze forces bacteria backwards.*
- Use aseptic technique at all times when changing head dressings or ICP monitor dressings and insertion sites. *Using aseptic technique reduces the possibility of introducing infection.*

Knowledge deficit: skull fracture

The person and their family need to be informed about the degree of injury that has occurred with the skull fracture. The person with a linear fracture, who may not be hospitalised, will need teaching that focuses on the need to monitor progress closely. To prevent complications, advise the person and their family to go to the emergency room if the person experiences any of the following:

- growing drowsiness or confusion
- vomiting (especially if projectile)
- blurred vision
- slurred speech
- prolonged headache
- blood or clear fluid leaking from the ears or nose
- weakness in an arm or leg
- stiff neck
- seizure.

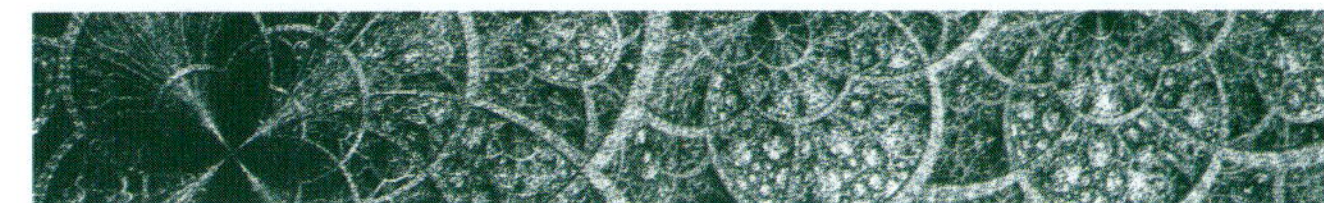

THE PERSON WITH A FOCAL OR DIFFUSE TRAUMATIC BRAIN INJURY

Even when the skull and other structures overlying the brain remain intact, a blow to the head can cause significant brain injury. Closed head injuries may result in either focal or diffuse damage to the brain. They range in severity from mild to severe.

Pathophysiology

Brain injury results from both primary and secondary mechanisms. Primary injury results from the impact. A blow to the head, even with no break in the skull, can cause serious and diffuse brain injury. Injury to axons disrupts oligodendroglia and direct mechanical disruption is caused by debris and leakage. The immediate vascular response to the injury results in increased capillary permeability to solutes.

Secondary injury is the progression of the initial injury resulting from events that affect perfusion and oxygenation of brain cells. These events include intracranial oedema, haematoma, infection, hypoxia or ischaemia. Cerebral ischaemia is the most common cause of secondary brain injury (Norris, 2018). Ischaemia leads to cerebral hypoxia, with consequences of increased glial permeability to sodium (cytotoxic oedema), an influx of calcium with changes in electrophysiology and release of free fatty acids and lactic acidosis.

Acute brain injury affects all body systems as well as the central nervous system. Systemic effects of acute brain injury are listed in Table 41.8.

TABLE 41.8 Systemic effects of acute brain injury

CAUSE	EFFECT
Stimulation of the sympathetic nervous system, which stimulates the adrenal cortex and medulla to increase glucocorticoid and mineralocorticoid levels	• Increased metabolism of carbohydrates, fats and proteins • Retention of sodium and water
Stimulation of the sympathetic nervous system, increasing the serum catecholamine levels	• Hypertension • EEG changes • Arrhythmias (bradycardia, sinus tachycardia)
Altered release of ADH from the posterior pituitary	• Retention of water or diuresis and diabetes insipidus
Neurogenic pulmonary dysfunction	• Abnormal respiratory patterns • Reduced residual capacity with retention of CO_2, vasodilation and increased ICP • Pulmonary oedema
Stress response to trauma	• Hyperglycaemia
Increased platelet, plasma fibrinogen and thromboplastin levels	• Decreased clotting and prothrombin times • Vascular occlusion • Disseminated intravascular coagulation • Anaemia
Immunosuppression	• Infection
Decreased gastric motility and increased gastric acidity	• Gastritis • Gastric ulcers

Focal brain injuries

Focal brain injuries are specific, grossly observable brain lesions confined to one area of the brain. They include contusions, lacerations and intracranial haemorrhage. The force of an impact produces contusions from direct contact with the inside of the skull that in turn may cause epidural haemorrhage and subdural and intracerebral haematomas. The mechanisms of injury are coup and/or contrecoup damage to the brain at the point of the impact and the rebound effect. The damaged brain area is surrounded by oedema, contributing to IICP. Infarction and necrosis, multiple haemorrhages and oedema are found within the contused areas. The maximum effects of the injury peak in 18 to 36 hours.

Intracranial haemorrhage can result directly from the trauma (e.g. beneath a fracture) or from shearing forces on cerebral arteries and veins that occur with acceleration–deceleration. Depending on the site and rate of bleeding, manifestations may appear immediately or may not become evident for hours or even weeks. Intracranial haemorrhages and the haematomas they cause place pressure on surrounding structures, causing manifestations of an expanding focal lesion. They also cause IICP, leading to altered levels of consciousness and potential herniation syndromes. Intracranial haematomas are classified by their location as epidural, subdural or intracerebral. Table 41.9 compares the frequency, locations/common sites, precipitating factors and manifestations of intracranial haematomas; Figure 41.6 illustrates their locations.

CONTUSION A *contusion* is a bruise of the surface of the brain, typically accompanied by small, diffuse venous haemorrhages. Both white and grey matter may have a bruised, discoloured appearance. A decrease in pH, with accumulation of lactic acid and decreased oxygen consumption, may hinder cell function. Contusions (and other focal brain injuries) occur when the brain strikes the inner skull, often with a coup (point of impact) lesion and a contrecoup lesion on the opposite side of the brain. Contusions occur most frequently near bony prominences of the skull. Cerebral oedema can follow contusion, resulting in IICP. Contusions—small, diffuse venous

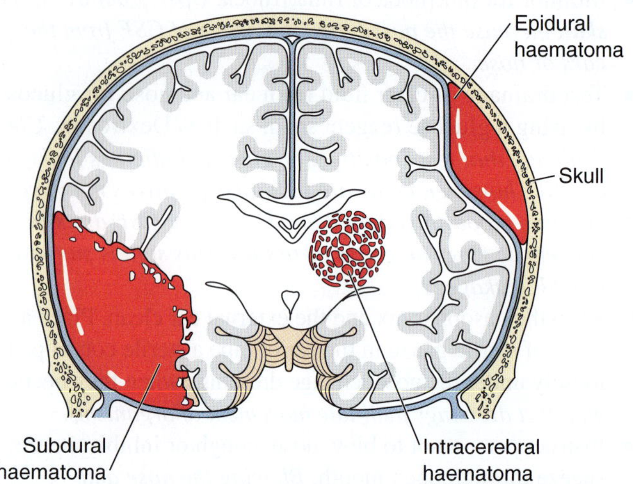

FIGURE 41.6 ***Three types of haematoma: epidural haematoma, subdural haematoma and intracerebral haematoma***

TABLE 41.9 Comparison of intracranial haematomas

TYPE/FREQUENCY	LOCATION/ COMMON SITE	PRECIPITATING FACTORS	MANIFESTATIONS
Epidural haematoma 2–6% of all types of head injuries	Located in the space between the skull and the dura mater Common site: the temporal bone (over the middle meningeal artery)	Skull fractures Contusion	Momentary loss of consciousness followed by a lucid period lasting from a few hours to 1 to 2 days Rapid deterioration in LOC (drowsiness to confusion to coma) Seizures Headache Hemiparesis (may be ipsilateral or contralateral) Fixed dilated ipsilateral pupil Rise in blood pressure, with decreases in pulse and respirations, indicates a rapidly increasing haematoma
Subdural haematoma Approximately 29% of all types of head injuries	Located in the space below the dural surface (between the dura and arachnoid and pia mater layers of meninges) Common site: may occur any place in cranium	Closed head injury Acceleration–deceleration injury Cerebral atrophy (seen in older adults) Chronic alcoholism Use of anticoagulants Contusion	Acute: • headache • drowsiness • agitation • slowed thinking • confusion Subacute: • same as those of acute subdural haematoma but develop more slowly Chronic: • manifestations may not appear until weeks to months after injury • confusion, slowed thinking, drowsiness
Intracerebral haematoma 14–15% of all types of head injuries	Located directly in the brain tissue Common sites: frontal or temporal region	Gunshot wounds Depressed bone fractures Stab injury Long history of systemic hypertension Contusions	Headache Deteriorating consciousness to deep coma Hemiplegia on contralateral side Dilated pupil on the side of the clot

haemorrhages—and brain swelling are at their peak 12 to 24 hours after injury.

Manifestations of the contusion depend on the size and location of the brain injury. An initial loss of consciousness occurs; the LOC may remain altered and behaviour changes such as combativeness may persist for an extended period. Full consciousness may be regained extremely slowly and residual deficits may persist; in some people, full LOC never really returns. Focal effects of the contusion may cause loss of reflexes, hemiparesis (muscular weakness of one-half of the body) or abnormal posturing. Manifestations of IICP may occur if cerebral oedema develops. Regaining full LOC may take an extended period of time and residual deficits may persist.

EPIDURAL HAEMATOMA An **epidural haematoma** (also called an *extradural haematoma*) develops in the potential space between the dura and the skull, which normally adhere to one another. As the blood collects, the expanding haematoma strips the dura away from the skull. Epidural haematomas affect young to middle-aged adults more frequently than older adults, because the dura becomes more tightly attached to the skull with ageing.

Epidural haematomas usually result from a skull fracture that tears an artery, often the middle meningeal artery. Because epidural haematomas are arterial in origin, they tend to develop rapidly. The person may lose consciousness with the initial injury and then have a brief lucid period before the LOC rapidly declines from drowsiness to coma as the haematoma expands, stripping the dura away from the skull and placing pressure on brain tissue. Other manifestations include headache, vomiting, a fixed, dilated pupil on the same side (ipsilateral) as the haematoma, contralateral (opposite side) hemiparesis or hemiplegia and possible seizures. Because epidural haematomas usually develop rapidly, timely intervention is vital to prevent significant increases in ICP and herniation.

SUBDURAL HAEMATOMA **Subdural haematomas**, in which a localised mass of blood collects between the dura mater and the arachnoid mater, are more common than epidural haematomas. Acute subdural haematomas are usually located at the top of the head and develop within 48 hours of the initial head injury. Chronic subdural haematomas develop over weeks or months. The chronic type is seen most often in the older adult and people who have some brain atrophy with subsequent enlarged epidural space. These haematomas are often venous in origin, although they may involve bleeding from small arteries as well. Subdural haematomas may form without direct trauma or contusion; acceleration–deceleration forces may tear the bridging veins that connect veins on the surface of the cerebral cortex to the dural sinuses. As blood collects, it places direct pressure on underlying brain tissue.

Acute subdural haematomas develop rapidly following head injury. Although a lucid period may occur, the person commonly develops drowsiness, confusion and enlargement of the ipsilateral pupil within minutes or hours of the injury. If responsive, the person may complain of a unilateral headache. Hemiparesis and respiratory pattern changes may occur.

Chronic subdural haematomas are often associated with relatively minor trauma such as a fall. Weeks to months may elapse before manifestations of the haematoma occur; the initial trauma may have been forgotten. Chronic subdural haematomas may also occur spontaneously in the older adult or in people with bleeding disorders. Manifestations of the haematoma develop slowly and may be mistaken for the onset of dementia in the older adult. Slowed thinking, confusion, drowsiness, or lethargy are common early manifestations. Other manifestations include headache, dilation and sluggishness of the ipsilateral pupil, and possible seizures.

INTRACEREBRAL HAEMATOMA **Intracerebral haematomas** may be single or multiple and are associated with contusions. They may occur in any location but usually are found in the frontal or temporal lobes. They may result from closed head trauma, particularly contusion or shearing of small blood vessels deep within the hemispheres. Intracerebral haematomas can also accompany other types of head trauma such as lacerations. Older adults are particularly vulnerable to intracerebral haemorrhage because cerebral blood vessels are more fragile and easily torn.

The manifestations of intracerebral haematoma vary according to the location of the haematoma. Headache may develop, along with decreasing LOC, hemiplegia and dilation of the ipsilateral pupil. The expanding clot increases intracranial pressure and herniation may occur.

Diffuse brain injuries

A diffuse brain injury (DBI) affects the entire brain and is caused by a shaking motion, with twisting movement (rotational acceleration) as the primary mechanism of injury. DBIs include concussions and diffuse axonal injuries. Shearing stresses on brain tissue cause axonal damage from shearing, tearing, or stretching of nerve fibres. The most serious axonal injuries are located furthest from the brainstem, with the frontal and temporal axonal tracts being most vulnerable to injury. Physical deficits resulting from DBIs include spastic paralysis, peripheral nerve injury, swallowing disorders, visual and hearing impairments, and taste and smell disorders. Damage decreases the speed of information processing and responding and disrupts attention, resulting in serious cognitive and affective impairments. Cognitive deficits that may result include disorientation and confusion, short attention span, problems with memory and learning, perceptual problems and poor judgment. Possible behavioural deficits include agitation, impulsivity, depression and social withdrawal.

Initially, the damage involves tearing of axons, blood vessels and brain tissue (visible only by electron microscope). The number of damaged axons progressively increases, with pathology involving the nuclei and axons. The damaged axons, which resemble sausage links, regress into round balls called retraction balls (visible with light microscopy). After several weeks, the retraction balls are replaced by clusters of microglia. In the final phase, astrocytosis (equivalent to scarring) occurs at the site of axonal damage, accompanied by demyelination of long axon tracts.

MANIFESTATIONS **Concussion**

- Immediate loss of consciousness (lasting usually no longer than 5 minutes)
- Amnesia regarding events surrounding injury
- Headache
- Drowsiness, confusion, dizziness
- Visual disturbances
- Possible brief seizure activity with transient apnoea, bradycardia, pallor and hypotension

POST-CONCUSSION SYNDROME

- Persistent headache
- Dizziness
- Irritability and insomnia
- Impaired memory and concentration, learning problems

The categories of DBI include mild concussion, classic cerebral concussion and diffuse axonal injury. Manifestations of a concussion are listed in the 'Manifestations' box.

MILD CONCUSSION The word **concussion** means violent shaking. A concussion involves temporary axonal disturbances. It is defined as a momentary interruption of brain function. A concussion is associated with an immediate, brief loss of consciousness on impact. Altered consciousness may last only seconds or may persist for several hours. Amnesia for events immediately preceding (antegrade amnesia) and following (retrograde amnesia) the injury is common. Other manifestations of concussion include headache, drowsiness, confusion, dizziness and visual disturbances such as diplopia or blurred vision.

CLASSIC CEREBRAL CONCUSSION A classic cerebral concussion involves diffuse cerebral disconnection from the brainstem RAS. An immediate loss of consciousness occurs, lasting less than 6 hours. Both retrograde and anterograde amnesia occur. Cerebral contusions may be present. In a severe concussion, a brief seizure and respiratory arrest may occur; transient pallor, bradycardia and hypotension may accompany loss of consciousness.

Following concussion, people may develop post-concussion syndrome with persistent headache, dizziness, irritability, insomnia, impaired memory and concentration, and learning problems. Post-concussion syndrome may last for several weeks or, rarely, up to a year.

DIFFUSE AXONAL INJURY Diffuse axonal injury (DAI) is a brain injury in which a high-speed acceleration–deceleration injury, typically associated with motor vehicle crashes, causes widespread disruption of axons in the white matter. Focal lesions may be found in the corpus callosum, midbrain and brainstem. An immediate loss of consciousness occurs. The prognosis is poor; most people with severe DAI either die or remain in a persistent vegetative state.

DAIs may range from mild to severe. In mild DAI, coma lasts 6 to 24 hours, and cognitive, psychological and sensorimotor deficits may persist. In moderate DAI, injury and impairment is spread throughout the cerebral cortex and diencephalon. There is axonal tearing, coma lasting more than 24 hours and often incomplete recovery. In severe DAI, axonal injury occurs in both cerebral hemispheres, the diencephalon and the brainstem. Immediate autonomic dysfunction occurs and IICP is manifested. Profound cognitive and sensorimotor deficits occur, involving movement, verbal and written communication, ability to learn and reason, and ability to modulate behaviour.

INTERPROFESSIONAL CARE

The person with a brain injury may receive medical and/or surgical treatment. Specific guidelines for the medical management of head injury may depend on local and state policy. Common elements across these guidelines include the following:

- *Concussion.* Following a concussion, the person may be observed for 4 hours in the emergency department (ED) and then discharged home with instructions for further observation to detect manifestations of secondary injury. If the loss of consciousness lasted for more than 2 minutes, the person may be admitted to the hospital for observation.
- *Acute TBI.* Recognition and management of acute TBI with transport to an ED is essential to personal outcomes. Morbidity and mortality increase with hypotension (systolic pressure less than 90 mmHg) and hypoxia (PaO_2 less than 60 mmHg), so fluids are given to support a mean systolic arterial blood pressure at more than 90 mmHg (Hickey, 2019). Assessment of the person's airway, breathing and circulation (ABCs), with management of dysfunction, is necessary to decrease the secondary effects of the brain injury. The fluid of choice for intravenous fluids is hypertonic saline, because it reduces intracranial hypertension. An intracranial pressure monitor probe may be inserted to assess ICP and monitor therapy to reduce cerebral oedema and maintain cerebral perfusion. Osmotic diuretics such as mannitol also may be administered to reduce cerebral oedema. Adequate oxygenation is vital to maintain cerebral metabolism; carbon dioxide is a potent vasodilator, and increased levels may contribute to cerebral oedema and IICP.

On admission to the ICU from the ED, the person may be connected to various monitoring devices. Invasive lines are inserted, including a central venous pressure (CVP) catheter, arterial line, pulmonary catheter, ventriculostomy, ICP monitor and, perhaps, a retrograde jugular catheter. In most instances, an endotracheal tube is inserted and connected to a mechanical ventilator, cardiac monitoring is initiated, bilateral sequential calf compressors are applied, pulse oximetry is started and a rectal temperature probe is inserted. All values are monitored for changes to ensure early detection of cerebral hypoxia and impending ischaemia to prevent secondary brain injury.

Diagnosis

Diagnostic testing may be done to monitor haemodynamic status and detect conditions that may contribute to cerebral oedema. Radiological examinations include skull x-rays (to identify skull fractures and assess penetrating objects) and CT scan or MRI to detect contusions and lacerations associated with diffuse axonal injury. ABGs are analysed, with particular attention to oxygen and carbon dioxide levels.

Managing ICP

ICP is managed (as described in a previous section) to reestablish equilibrium of the intracranial contents and prevent secondary brain damage. Treatments include airway management, hyperventilation (used if signs of herniation appear), fluid resuscitation, positioning, temperature regulation and medications. Medications other than those previously discussed include a category of drugs called neuroprotectants. These drugs are used to treat or alter some of the pathological pathways that occur in ischaemia and must be administered within a short time of the injury to be effective. Classifications of the drugs include lipid peroxidase inhibitors, free radical scavengers, receptor antagonists, calcium channel blockers and gangliosides.

Surgery

Small subdural haematomas can frequently be reabsorbed and may be treated conservatively, with close observation and supportive care. However, the treatment of choice for epidural haematomas and large acute subdural haematomas is surgical evacuation of the clot. This can often be performed through burr holes made into the skull (see Figure 41.7). In an epidural haematoma, the bleeding vessel can also be ligated during this procedure, preventing further bleeding. Further bleeding may occur following evacuation of an acute subdural haematoma in older adults and in people with chronic alcoholism. A craniotomy is necessary to evacuate chronic subdural haematomas because the haematoma tends to solidify, making it difficult or impossible to remove through burr holes. Surgery is less successful in treating intracerebral haematomas because of widespread tissue damage. Supportive care to manage intracranial pressure and prevent complications is provided.

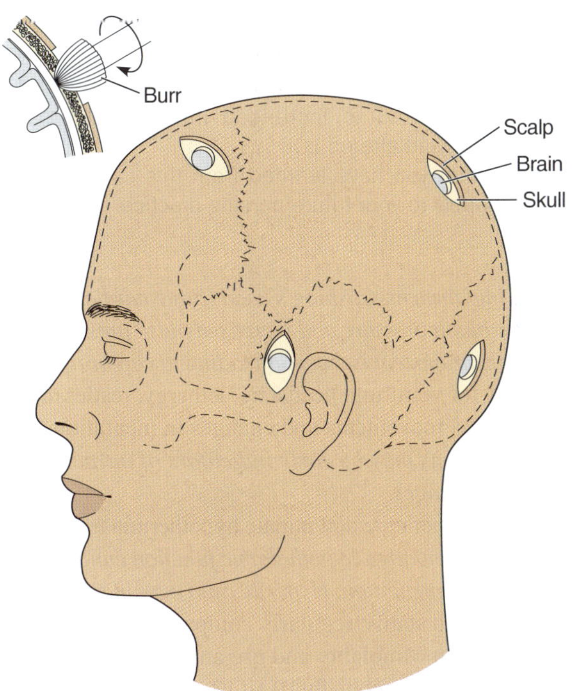

FIGURE 41.7 ***Possible locations of burr holes***

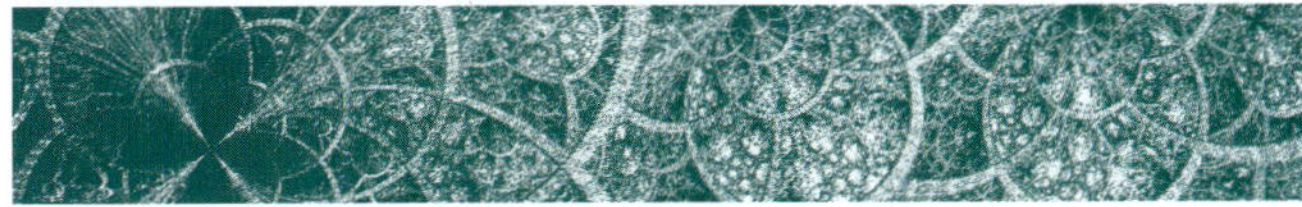

Nursing care

In addition to the nursing care discussed in this section, a nursing care plan for a person with a subdural haematoma follows.

Health promotion

The best way to treat any injury is to prevent it from happening. Public education must continue to stress the importance of safe driving, the dangers of driving under the influence of alcohol or drugs, and the necessity of wearing seat belts and cycle helmets. Legislation changes mandating the use of seat belts, child safety restraints and installation of airbags are all examples of health promotion impacting on policy and legislation. Other behaviours that can reduce the morbidity and mortality associated with TBI are following safety rules during sporting activities, promoting farm safety and teaching older adults about safety (such as preventing falls) in the home.

Assessment

Collect the following data through the health history and physical examination (see the chapter 'A person-centred approach to assessing the nervous system'):

- *Health history*: a history of the injury is helpful in understanding the nature of the craniocerebral trauma; knowledge about loss of consciousness assists the nurse in planning care.
- *Physical examination*: neurological assessment, including pupils, LOC, Glasgow Coma Scale, brainstem reflexes (cornea, cough, gag, extraocular movements), vital signs; skull and face (deformity, lacerations, bruising, bleeding); movement of extremities.

Nursing diagnoses and interventions

Nursing care of the person in the acute care phase initially focuses on maintaining an effective airway and breathing pattern. Nursing care is also directed towards continuous assessment and monitoring of neurological function as well as other body systems. This close monitoring provides early recognition and treatment of problems and complications and initiation of aggressive forms of therapy that may be needed.

Many nursing diagnoses associated with traumatic brain injury correspond with those outlined previously in the sections on the person with altered LOC and IICP. Specific nursing diagnoses discussed in this section focus on problems with intracranial adaptive capacity, airway clearance and breathing patterns.

NURSING CARE PLAN A person with a subdural haematoma

Wong Lee is a 50-year-old boat mechanic who is married and has three sons. Although Mr Lee has been through rehabilitation twice for alcoholism, he has not been able to quit drinking. His doctor has explained the physical consequences and the possible interaction between alcohol and the anticoagulant Mr Lee is taking for chronic atrial fibrillation. While attending a family reunion, during which he eats a large meal and drinks several beers, Mr Lee joins a game of cricket. During Mr Lee's first over the batter hits a ball that strikes Mr Lee in the head. Mr Lee stumbles and drops to the ground, holding his head. He does not lose consciousness and gets up on his own. His sons and wife try to persuade him to go to the hospital, but Mr Lee insists he feels fine.

Two weeks later, after an evening of consuming several mixed drinks, Mr Lee develops a headache. He attributes the headache to a hangover, but instead of improving the next day, the headache becomes steadily worse. He becomes confused and disoriented. His wife, concerned that his drinking is increasing again, calls the doctor, who admits Mr Lee to the detoxification centre at the local hospital. At the hospital, the nursing and medical team becomes concerned about increasing confusion. Eventually a CT scan is performed. The diagnosis of a subdural haematoma is made and Mr Lee is transferred to the neurosurgical ward.

ASSESSMENT

When Saundra Knight, the Registered Nurse on the neurosurgical ward, enters the room, she notices that Mr Lee is sitting in bed, laughing softly and unable to hold himself upright. As she begins to talk to Mr Lee, he states, 'Don't ask me anything—I can't think. My headache is getting worse.' Over the next few hours, the giddiness subsides and Mr Lee becomes drowsy. Ms Knight reports a Glasgow Coma Scale score of 11. An ICP monitor is inserted and reveals increased intracranial pressure. Mr Lee is scheduled to have burr holes and haematoma evacuation that afternoon.

DIAGNOSES

- *Risk of ineffective breathing pattern* related to pressure on the respiratory centre by an intracranial haematoma, evidenced by either an increase or decrease in respiratory rate.
- *Ineffective cerebral tissue perfusion* related to increased intracranial pressure secondary to cerebral oedema, evidenced by a decreased LOC.

PLANNING

Maintain ICP within normal limits through close observation and assessment.

Expected outcomes

- Maintain a respiratory rate and rhythm within normal limits.
- Maintain adequate cerebral perfusion, as evidenced by stable vital signs, stable neurological status and no decrease in LOC.

IMPLEMENTATION

- Perform neurological assessment every 2 hours or as needed.
- Monitor vital signs every 2 hours or as needed.
- Explain to the family the procedure for intracranial surgery.

EVALUATION

The first day postoperatively, Mr Lee begins breathing on his own without ventilatory support. His respiratory rate and rhythm are within normal limits, with no signs of abnormal breath sounds. The ICP monitor readings are appropriate and Mr Lee shows significant improvement in LOC, with a Glasgow Coma Scale score of 15. Mr Lee continues to improve and is discharged home 5 days after surgery.

CRITICAL THINKING IN THE NURSING PROCESS

1. Describe the similarities and differences between Mr Lee's disorder and the manifestations of other types of intracranial haematomas.
2. Mr Lee keeps trying to pull out his ICP line. You know he should not be restrained because pulling against restraints increases restlessness and increases intracranial pressure. What would you do?

REFLECTION ON THE NURSING PROCESS

1. Develop a care plan for the nursing diagnosis of *Acute confusion* related to increased intracranial pressure, evidenced by an altered LOC.
2. Outline what you have learned from this case study that you will apply to your future nursing practice.

Decreased intracranial adaptive capacity

The person with a traumatic brain injury has or is at high risk of IICP. As the mechanisms that normally compensate for changes in intracranial pressure are compromised, intracranial pressure increases in disproportional response to a variety of stimuli. (See the discussion earlier in the chapter for other nursing diagnoses and interventions for the person with increasing ICP.)

- Monitor for manifestations of elevated ICP, including eye opening response, motor response and verbal response. *These responses evaluate the ability to integrate commands with conscious and involuntary movement.*
- Monitor for changes in vital signs: bradycardia or tachycardia, varying breathing patterns, hypertension, and/or widening pulse pressure. *Vital signs vary depending on the site of impairment. Cushing's triad (bradycardia, increased systolic blood pressure and increased pulse pressure) indicates brainstem ischaemia leading to cerebral herniation.*
- Monitor for vomiting, headache, lethargy, restlessness, purposeless movements and changes in mentation. *These manifestations may be early indicators of intracranial pressure changes.*
- Monitor temperature and initiate hypothermia treatment as prescribed. *Impaired hypothalamic function can interfere with temperature regulation. Hyperthermia may increase ICP.*
- Monitor fluid status: regularly compare intake and output, review serum osmolality and use an infusion pump to administer intravenous fluids (if prescribed). *Osmotic diuretics, if used to treat cerebral oedema, may cause hypotension and decreased cardiac output.*

CONSIDERATION FOR PRACTICE

Overhydration from rapid infusion of IV fluids may cause or further increase elevated ICP.

Ineffective airway clearance

The primary objective in the care of any trauma person is maintaining a patent airway to prevent hypoxia. However, in the initial acute care phase, the risk of cervical vertebral fractures and spinal cord injury may complicate the process of establishing a patent airway. In addition, other multisystem injuries may complicate the interpretation of vital signs. In general, all unconscious people with a head injury should be intubated with an endotracheal tube to prevent aspiration. People with head trauma may also require a tracheostomy to provide an airway and may be placed on a ventilator.

- Monitor neurological manifestations on a regular schedule. *Changes in neurological manifestations may indicate increasing ICP, with the risk of further depression of the respiratory system and respiratory arrest.*
- Maintain head and neck in neutral alignment, immobilised until injury is determined. *Head rotation and neck flexion are associated with IICP, decreased jugular venous outflow and localised changes in cerebral blood flow. Immobilisation prevents spinal cord injury in suspected or actual fractures of the cervical spine; spinal cord injury at this level would further impair respiratory function.*
- Clear the nose and mouth of mucus and blood. *This helps maintain patency of the upper airway.*
- Suction the airway as needed, limiting suctioning time to no more than 10 seconds at one time. Do not suction the nasal passages until a dural tear has been ruled out. *Suctioning is usually necessary to maintain a patent airway.*

Ineffective breathing pattern

The person with a traumatic brain injury and haematoma is at high risk *of Ineffective breathing pattern* related to IICP. If ICP increases dramatically, tentorial herniation may occur, leading to sudden respiratory arrest.

- Monitor the respiratory pattern for rate, depth and rhythm every 2 hours or as needed if the person is not on a ventilator. Assess breath sounds, presence of cyanosis, restlessness and use of accessory respiratory muscles. Monitor pulse oximetry and blood gas levels. *Head injuries may cause alterations in respirations. An increased respiratory rate may indicate hypoxia. A decrease in respiratory rate may be the result of depression of the medullary respiratory centre.*
- Monitor ICP readings. *Continuous measurement of ICP is used to diagnose and monitor increased intracranial pressure. As ICP increases, herniation may occur, leading to respiratory arrest and death.*
- If the person is not intubated, prepare for oxygen administration and/or tracheal intubation if respiratory distress occurs. *Supplying oxygen prevents hypoxia until a haematoma can be evacuated, relieving pressure on the respiratory centre.*
- Prepare for cranial surgery if deteriorating respiratory pattern and neurological changes are noted. *Surgical intervention usually consists of placing several burr holes in the skull or performing a craniotomy to remove the haematoma. (Intracranial surgery is discussed later in the chapter.) However, the cerebral oedema and IICP may cause death even if surgery is performed.*

Community-based care

Concussion

Advise the person and their family that a post-concussion syndrome sometimes occurs. If the person experiences persistent headaches and dizziness, is uncharacteristically emotional, seems overly tired or has difficulty paying attention or remembering, the healthcare provider should be notified. Explain that these manifestations may persist for some time. Rehabilitation may help the person compensate for memory impairment and attention deficits.

Acute brain injury

People who survive an acute brain injury will require long-term physical care and rehabilitation. Although recovery is highly individualised, many people who regain consciousness require lifelong care; others remain in a coma or vegetative state. The family often expects the person to recover fully after the coma subsides and they need information about the real possibility of residual deficits in self-care, emotional responses, cognition, communication and movement (see the 'Translation to practice' box).

- The need to encourage self-care and independence as much as possible.
- Information to enhance recovery (Synapse, 2022):
  - Get lots of rest. Don't rush back to work or university.
  - Avoid anything that could cause another blow or jolt to the head.
  - Consult with doctor about when it will be safe to drive a car, ride a bike or use heavy equipment. (Reaction time is often slower after a TBI.)
  - Take only prescribed drugs and don't drink alcohol.
  - Write things down if you are having problems remembering.
  - If the injury was severe, therapy may be needed to learn lost skills, such as speaking, walking or reading.
  - Equipment needs, such as mobility aids and hospital bed.
  - Vocational counselling and services.
  - Referral to community resources and support groups.
  - Helpful resources:
    - Brain Injury Australia: https://www.braininjuryaustralia.org.au
    - Brain Research Institute: Australia: www.brain.org.au
    - Disability Services Australia: www.dsa.org.au.

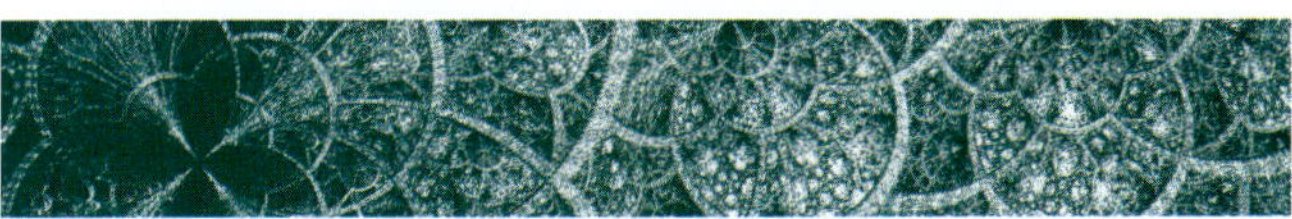

TRANSLATION TO PRACTICE Evidence-based practice: caregivers of young adults with TBI

Traumatic brain injury (TBI) is a leading cause of death and disability across all age groups, but the age group most affected is young adults, especially young men. This is the result of increased risk-taking behaviour in this age group, including drinking alcohol and using drugs while operating a motor vehicle. The population of TBI survivors from this demographic is large and caring for them is expensive. Most research of TBI survivors has focused on problems of the survivor, but few have examined the burden placed on the family. This is especially true for the experience of the survivors' mothers, who are in almost all cases the primary caregiver. A study was conducted by Knox, Douglas and Bigby (2015) to explore the processes by which individuals with severe TBI and their carers make decisions within their life. Both the survivors and the mothers were interviewed and the data were analysed to describe the experience. The individuals with a TBI described the difficulty in wanting to make decisions but being restricted; the carers struggled with a balance of protecting the individual and letting them become independent. The carers struggled to maintain relationships inside and outside of the family. All these experiences resulted in ongoing stress for the both the person with a TBI and their carer.

IMPLICATIONS FOR NURSING

The findings of this study have implications for community-based teaching and interventions for TBI survivors and their caregivers. Each year a significant number of TBI survivors leave the acute care setting and return to their homes, where caregivers are often unprepared for the lifelong multiple disabilities and problems they will face.

Developing an appropriate tool to measure family caregiver burden for those with disabilities from TBI is recommended, so as to be able to design and implement individualised interventions and teaching. The teaching and interventions should be developed as part of a systematic and integrated discharge plan, a community-based program and a follow-up approach to assist TBI survivors and their families to effectively decrease the stressors that are a part of caregiver load.

CRITICAL THINKING IN PERSON-CENTRED CARE

1 You are making a home visit to a 22-year-old woman who has recently been discharged from acute care following a serious car crash resulting in mild diffuse axonal injury. She says to you, 'This is my third year of nursing at university. Will I be able to be a nurse?' How would you respond?
2 On discharge from the hospital, a nursing diagnosis for a young adult TBI survivor who would be cared for at home by his single mother was *Risk of parental role conflict* related to caring for a child with TBI manifested by lack of independence. Do you think this is an appropriate diagnosis? Why or why not?
3 If you were to outline topics for a program to reduce the incidence of TBI in a rural community, how would it differ from one for residents of a large urban city?

Central nervous system infections

THE PERSON WITH A CENTRAL NERVOUS SYSTEM INFECTION

The central nervous system, including the meninges, neural tissues and blood vessels, may be directly affected by bacteria, viruses, fungi, protozoans and rickettsiae. The CNS may also be affected by toxins from bacterial infections. In general, organisms enter the brain in two ways: (1) through the bloodstream by crossing the blood–brain barrier, or (2) by direct invasion through a skull fracture or bullet hole. A CNS infection may also occur as a result of contamination of a surgical field or lumbar puncture. The main CNS infections include meningitis, encephalitis and brain abscesses.

The incidence of pathogenic infections of the CNS increases with the onset of AIDS. People who are HIV positive may have CNS infections caused by toxoplasmosis, cryptococcus, tuberculosis, herpes simplex, cytomegalovirus (CMV) or a polyoma virus (resulting in progressive multifocal leucoencephalopathy).

Pathophysiology

When pathogens enter the CNS and the meninges, an inflammatory process results. The pathology of CNS infections includes the invading pathogens, the subsequent inflammation and the increase in intracranial pressure that may result from the inflammatory processes. Both the pathogenic damage and the IICP may result in brain damage and life-threatening complications.

Meningitis

Meningitis is an inflammation of the pia mater, the arachnoid and the subarachnoid space. Inflammation spreads rapidly throughout the CNS because of the circulation of CSF around the brain and spinal cord. Meningitis may be acute or chronic, and it may be bacterial, viral, fungal or parasitic in origin. Meningococcal meningitis may occur in epidemics among people who are in close contact with one another, such as members of the armed forces and students living in residential colleges. Pneumococcal meningitis, in contrast, primarily affects the very young and very old.

The organism responsible for meningitis must overcome non-specific and specific host defence mechanisms to invade and replicate in the CSF. These defences include the skin barrier, the blood–brain barrier, the non-specific inflammatory response and the immune response. Host response to the particular pathogen is responsible for the manifestations of clinical meningitis. The organisms that initiate the host response in meningitis demonstrate an affinity for the nervous system. They colonise and invade the nasopharyngeal mucosa, survive intravascularly and penetrate the CNS if the blood–brain barrier is damaged, as can happen during surgery.

Infection of the CSF and meninges causes an inflammatory response in the pia, arachnoid and CSF. Because the meninges and subarachnoid space are continuous around the brain, spinal cord and optic nerves, the infection and inflammatory response are always cerebrospinal, involving both the brain and the spinal cord. Inflamed blood vessels in the area leak fluids as cell permeability increases. Purulent exudate infiltrates cranial nerve sheaths and blocks the choroid plexus and subarachnoid villi. IICP occurs as brain tissue responds to the pathogen. With an increase in ICP, cerebral perfusion decreases and cerebral autoregulation is lost.

BACTERIAL MENINGITIS The causative organisms of bacterial meningitis include *Neisseria meningitis*, meningococcus, *Streptococcus pneumoniae, Haemophilus influenzae* and *Escherichia coli*. Risk factors include head trauma with a basal skull fracture, otitis media, mastoiditis, sinusitis, neurosurgery, systemic sepsis or immunocompromise (Norris, 2018). Even when appropriate antibiotics are used, the mortality rate for adults remains at approximately 25%.

Once the pathogen enters the central nervous system, it or its toxic products (free radicals) initiate an inflammatory response in the meninges, CSF and ventricles. Meningeal vessels become engorged and their permeability increases. Phagocytic white blood cells migrate into the subarachnoid space, forming a purulent exudate that thickens and clouds the CSF and interferes with its flow. Rapid exudate formation causes further inflammation and oedema of meningeal cells. Blood vessel engorgement, exudate formation, impaired CSF flow and cellular oedema cause the intracranial pressure to increase.

Manifestations The person with bacterial meningitis typically presents with fever and chills, headache, back and abdominal pain, and nausea and vomiting. (The older adult may not have a high fever but may instead exhibit confusion.) Meningeal irritation causes nuchal rigidity (stiff neck) and positive Brudzinski's sign (flexion of the neck that causes the hip and knee to flex) and positive Kernig's sign (inability to extend the knee while the hip is flexed at a 90-degree angle). Photophobia is present; the person may also experience diplopia. With meningococcal meningitis, a rapidly spreading petechial rash involving the skin and mucous membranes may be noted. The person may also have IICP, manifested by decreased LOC, seizures, changes in vital signs and respiratory pattern, and papilloedema. The manifestations of bacterial meningitis are listed in the 'Manifestations' box.

Complications Complications of bacterial meningitis include arthritis, cranial nerve damage and hydrocephalus. Cranial nerve VIII, the auditory nerve, is frequently affected, with resulting nerve deafness. Thrombophlebitis may develop in cerebral vessels, with infarction of surrounding tissues (Norris, 2018).

MANIFESTATIONS Bacterial meningitis

- Restlessness, agitation and irritability
- Severe headache
- Signs of meningeal irritation:
  - Nuchal rigidity
  - Positive Brudzinski's sign
  - Positive Kernig's sign
- Chills and high fever
- Confusion, altered LOC
- Photophobia (aversion to light), diplopia
- Seizures
- Signs of increased ICP (widened pulse pressure and bradycardia, respiratory irregularity, decreased LOC, headache and vomiting)
- Petechial rash (in meningococcal meningitis)

VIRAL MENINGITIS Acute viral meningitis, also called *aseptic meningitis*, is a less severe disease than bacterial meningitis. It can be caused by numerous viruses, such as herpes simplex, herpes zoster, Epstein–Barr virus or cytomegalovirus (CMV). Viral meningitis most often appears after a case of mumps. Although viral infection also triggers the inflammatory response, the course of the disease is benign and of short duration. Recovery is uneventful.

Manifestations The manifestations of viral meningitis are similar to those of bacterial meningitis, although usually milder. The person may have a mild flu-like illness prior to the onset of meningitis. Headache is intense and is accompanied by malaise, nausea, vomiting and lethargy. Photophobia may be present. The person generally remains oriented, although possibly drowsy. Temperature is mildly elevated. Neck stiffness, positive Brudzinski's sign and positive Kernig's sign are usually present.

Encephalitis

Encephalitis is an acute inflammation of the parenchyma of the brain or spinal cord. It is almost always caused by a virus, but it may also be caused by bacteria, fungi and other organisms. Other less common causes include ingested lead; post-vaccination encephalitis (from vaccines for measles, mumps and rabies) and HIV (Norris, 2018). See Table 41.10 for a list of the most common causes of encephalitis.

VIRAL ENCEPHALITIS Viruses depend on living tissue for reproduction and become highly destructive when they invade brain tissue. The inflammatory response extends over the cerebral cortex, the white matter and the meninges, with degeneration of the neurons. The pathology of encephalitis includes local necrotising haemorrhage, which ultimately becomes generalised, with prominent oedema. There is progressive degeneration of nerve cell bodies. The inflammatory response in encephalitis does not cause exudate formation as it does in meningitis. Certain viruses show a propensity for specific areas of the brain (e.g. herpes simplex virus involves frontal and temporal lobes). The virus gains access to the CNS via the bloodstream or along

TABLE 41.10 Causes of encephalitis

CAUSE	COMMENTS
Arboviruses	Transmitted by bites from ticks and mosquitoes. Bites from ticks occur more frequently in spring. Bites from mosquitoes occur in middle to late summer. Most common type is the Ross River virus. May destroy major parts of the lobe or hemisphere. 20% of people who develop Murray Valley encephalitis die and 40% develop permanent neurological damage (e.g. seizures, blindness, deafness, speech disorders or mental retardation). Young Indigenous children in Western Australia have significantly poor outcomes. The incubation is 5 to 15 days. Mortality rates associated with arboviruses are higher than those associated with enteroviruses.
Enteroviruses, such as echovirus, coxsackievirus, poliovirus, paramyxovirus (the virus that causes mumps), and varicella zoster (the virus that causes chickenpox)	Infection occurs more frequently in summer (except infection by the mumps virus, which occurs more frequently in early winter). Some degree of protection can be afforded by immunisation against measles, mumps and poliomyelitis. Mortality rates are lower than those associated with herpes simplex type 1 virus.
Herpes simplex type 1 virus	Most common non-epidemic encephalitis in Australia. Can occur any time of year and throughout the world. Has an affinity for the frontal and temporal lobes. Prognosis is grave but not hopeless: mortality rate can be as high as 40% and the person may die within 2 weeks.
Amoebic meningoencephalitis due to infection by *Naegleria* and *Acanthamoeba* protozoa	Both protozoa are found in warm freshwater. Enter the nasal mucosa of people swimming in dams or lakes. May also be found in soil and decaying vegetation. Incidence of infection is increasing.
Exogenous poisoning	May occur after ingestion of lead or arsenic or inhalation of carbon monoxide.

peripheral or cranial nerves, or it may already be present in the meninges in the person with meningitis.

The manifestations of viral encephalitis vary, depending on the organism and area of the brain affected. Usual manifestations are similar to those of meningitis, including fever, headache, seizures, stiff neck and altered LOC. The person may be disoriented, agitated and restless, or lethargic and drowsy. As the disease progresses, the LOC deteriorates and the person may become comatose.

ARBOVIRUS ENCEPHALITIS The arboviruses are arthropod (mosquito or tick)-borne agents that infect humans. They include many different types, including dengue, Ross River virus, Barmah Forest virus, Japanese encephalitis, Murray Valley encephalitis and Kunjun. In Australia, adults are most often infected with Ross River virus, with older adults affected more often. The arthropods may live in small mammals and birds or may be carried by horses and deer.

The arthropod-borne agents cause widespread degeneration of nerve cells, and oedema and necrosis—with or without haemorrhage—occur. IICP may develop. Manifestations include fever, malaise, sore throat, nausea and vomiting, stiff neck, tremors, paralysis of extremities, exaggerated deep tendon reflexes, seizures and altered LOC.

Brain abscess

A brain abscess is an infection with a collection of purulent material within the brain tissue. Approximately 80% are found in the cerebrum and 20% are cerebellar.

The causes of a brain abscess include open trauma and neurosurgery; infections of the mastoid, middle ear, nasal cavity or nasal sinuses; metastatic spread from distant foci (such as heart, lungs, skin, abscessed teeth and dirty needles); and arising from other associated areas of infection. The immunocompromised are at increased risk of abscesses. The most common pathogens causing the abscess are streptococci, staphylococci and bacteroids. Yeast and fungi may also cause brain abscess.

A brain abscess results from the presence of microorganisms in the brain tissue. If the abscess is encapsulated, it has the ability to enlarge and, therefore, behave as a space-occupying lesion within the cranium. This predisposes the person not only to the systemic effects of the inflammatory process but also to the serious consequences of increased intracranial pressure. Occasionally, the abscess does not become encapsulated; instead, it spreads through the brain tissue to the subarachnoid space and ventricular system.

Initially, the person exhibits the general symptoms associated with an acute infectious process, such as chills, fever, malaise and anorexia. Because brain abscess generally forms after infection, the person may consider these signs to be an exacerbation of that illness. The person may experience seizures, altered LOC and manifestations of IICP. As the abscess enlarges, specific symptoms are related to location; for example, the person with a frontal lobe abscess may have contralateral hemiparesis, expressive aphasia, focal seizures and frontal headache.

INTERPROFESSIONAL CARE

Bacterial meningitis is a medical emergency that, if not treated immediately, can be fatal within days. Successful management depends on rapid diagnosis and aggressive treatment with antibiotics and corticosteroids to eradicate the infecting organism and support vital functions. The person may be placed in strict or respiratory isolation until the organism has been identified, depending on hospital policy. Universal precautions apply to CSF as well as blood.

Treatment for viral meningitis focuses on managing symptoms and is supportive. Antipyretics and analgesics may provide relief. Antibiotic therapy is not indicated and isolation precautions are not required.

Treatment of the person with a brain abscess focuses on prompt initiation of antibiotic therapy. Other manifestations are treated symptomatically, as with the person diagnosed with meningitis or encephalitis. If pharmacological management is not effective, the abscess may be drained or, if it is encapsulated, removed.

Diagnosis

The diagnosis of meningitis is based on manifestations and diagnostic test results. Gram stain and culture of the CSF are used to determine if a bacterial infection is present and to determine the specific infectious agent. Counterimmunoelectrophoresis (CIE) is a laboratory test that may be ordered to determine the presence of viruses or protozoa. Polymerase chain reaction techniques may be used to detect viral DNA or RNA in spinal fluid. CT scan will show an area of increased contrast surrounding a low-density core with brain abscess.

Lumbar puncture with examination of the CSF is the definitive diagnostic measure for bacterial meningitis. Data that indicate bacterial meningitis include turbid, cloudy fluid; a markedly increased white blood cell (WBC) count and protein content; and a decreased glucose content. The opening pressure on the lumbar puncture is elevated. In contrast, the person with encephalitis may have a normal CSF analysis and pressure or may have some lymphocytes. The person with a brain abscess will have a markedly elevated pressure with elevated protein content and elevated WBC count. Glucose content is normal. (Because a lumbar puncture in the presence of a space-occupying lesion can result in brain herniation and death, a CT scan is performed first if neurological findings support such a lesion.)

Medications

Immediate intravenous administration of a broad-spectrum antibiotic that crosses the blood–brain barrier into the subarachnoid space is instituted in cases of bacterial meningitis. Once culture reports identify the causative organism, drug therapy is continued from 7 to 21 days, using the most effective drug or drugs specific to that bacterium. A major concern in the treatment of CNS infections is penicillin-resistant streptococci. Recommendations for treatment are for a broad-spectrum cephalosporin, such as rifampicin, cefotaxime or vancomycin. However, as the bacteria are killed, the toxins they release increase production of inflammatory cytokines, which are potentially lethal. Steroids such as dexamethasone are often given with the antibiotics to suppress inflammation. The CDC recommends that the person remain on isolation for 24 hours after the start of antibiotic therapy.

Treatment for encephalitis consists of administering specific medications and preventing complications. Fungal meningitis is treated with antifungal agents, such as amphotericin-B, flucytosine and fluconazole. Viral encephalitis is treated with intravenous aciclovir.

Antibiotic therapy is the primary treatment for brain abscess. A combination of broad-spectrum antibiotics is used if the infecting organism is unknown.

Anticonvulsant medications such as phenytoin are often prescribed to prevent or control seizure activity. Antipyretic and analgesic medications may provide symptomatic relief; however, analgesics that have a depressant effect on the CNS (such as opiates) are avoided to prevent masking of early manifestations of deteriorating LOC. The person initially may require anti-emetics to control nausea and vomiting. Fluid and electrolyte status is maintained through intravenous fluid replacement until the person is able to resume oral intake.

Surgery

Surgical drainage of an encapsulated abscess may be necessary. The decision to perform surgery is based on the person's general condition, the stage of abscess development and the site of the abscess.

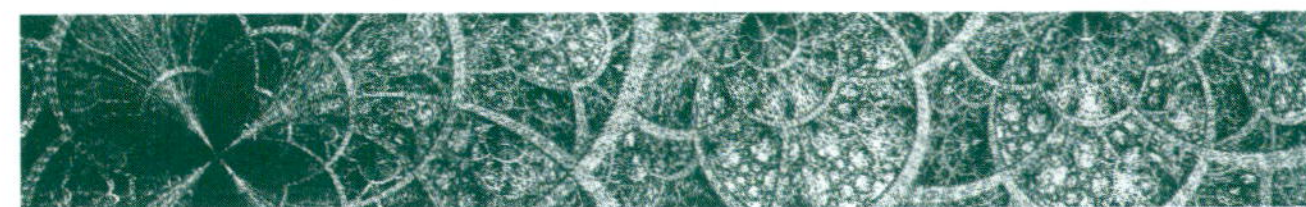

Nursing care

Central nervous system infections are serious illnesses, with potentially life-threatening effects and complications. Nursing assessments and interventions are critical in identifying changes in the person's neurological status and preventing complications from IICP. In addition to the nursing care described in this section, a nursing care plan for a person with bacterial meningitis follows.

Health promotion

As with many other intracranial injuries and disorders, educational activities to promote health by preventing CNS infections are important nursing interventions. The following information should be provided:

- Vaccinations for meningococcal meningitis are recommended or required for members of the armed forces and tertiary students (groups at increased risk of invasive meningococcal meningitis).
- Administration of prophylactic rifampicin is recommended for people exposed to meningococcal meningitis.
- Mosquito control with repellents, insecticides and protective clothing.
- Destruction of the insect larvae and elimination of breeding places, such as pools of stagnant water.
- Vaccination against Japanese B encephalitis (recommended for summer travellers to rural East Asia).
- Prompt diagnosis and treatment of infections of the head, neck and respiratory system.

Assessment

Collect the following data through the health history and physical examination (see the chapter 'A person-centred approach to assessing the nervous system'). Further focused assessments are described with nursing interventions below.

- *Health history*: risk factors (concurrent infections, other illnesses, travel), when manifestations began, severity of manifestations, current nausea and headache, seizures.
- *Physical examination*: Glasgow Coma Scale, LOC, vital signs, motor function, pupillary check, cranial nerves, neck ROM, Brudzinski's sign, Kernig's sign, skin (rash, petechiae, purpura), muscle movement and strength, speech.

Nursing diagnoses and interventions

In planning and implementing nursing care for the person with a CNS infection, the prognosis may depend on the supportive care given. The person is often very ill and the combination of fever, dehydration and cerebral oedema may predispose the person to seizures. Airway obstruction, respiratory arrest or cardiac arrhythmias may occur. Nursing diagnoses and interventions previously discussed for the person with an altered LOC, IICP and seizures are also appropriate for the person with a CNS infection. Nursing interventions in this section focus on *Ineffective protection* and *Risk of fluid volume deficit*.

Ineffective protection

People with CNS infections are less able to protect themselves against insults from both internal and external sources. The effects of the inflammation and resulting pathophysiological processes may include pain, fever, altered LOC, seizures, IICP and cranial nerve dysfunction. In addition, pathophysiological effects on the brain from toxins or thrombosis of a cerebral vessel may lead to permanent neurological deficits, such as loss of motor function or dementia.

- Monitor neurological status on a regular basis. *Many complications are evidenced by changes in neurological manifestations.*

NURSING CARE PLAN A person with bacterial meningitis

Monty Cook is a 22-year-old musician who plays in a local rock band. He is unmarried and lives with his parents. He is known by everyone in the community as a quiet, low-key, easy-going person and an excellent guitar player. During a performance 2 days ago at the local pub, he had difficulty playing his guitar, complaining of bright stage lights blazing in his eyes. When he tried to keep his head down to prevent the lights from hurting his eyes, he noticed his neck was very stiff. After the performance, one of the newest members of the band remarked that it certainly was not their best performance. Monty responded angrily that maybe the new members of the group needed more practice. Then he stomped out and went home to bed.

He wakes at 4 am with a severe headache, sweating and chills; his temperature is 38.9°C and he cannot bend his neck without severe pain. His mother recognises that he is agitated and irritable, which is uncharacteristic. Frightened, she rushes him to the hospital emergency room. A lumbar puncture performed in the emergency room reveals turbid, cloudy fluid; a markedly increased WBC count; and protein with a decreased glucose content. Suspected bacterial meningitis is diagnosed. Mr Cook is admitted to the hospital for treatment and care.

ASSESSMENT

When the Registered Nurse, Aisha Aldi, enters Mr Cook's isolation room, she sees him thrashing about in the bed, talking incoherently and becoming more agitated. On assessment, Ms Aldi notes dry mucous membranes, cracked lips and small petechiae over the upper torso and abdomen. Mr Cook's temperature is 40°C. Kernig's sign is positive. Intravenous broad-spectrum antibiotics are prescribed and initiated. After the first 2 hours of care, Ms Aldi notes a decrease in Mr Cook's level of consciousness.

DIAGNOSES

- *Hyperthermia* related to infection and abnormal temperature regulation by hypothalamus, evidenced by an increased body temperature.
- *Disturbed thought processes* related to intracranial infection, evidenced by confusion, agitation and uncharacteristic behaviours.
- *Risk of injury* related to progression of illness manifested by increased confusion and agitation.

PLANNING

Monitor Mr Cook's condition, provide appropriate nursing care and maintain his safety.

Expected outcomes

- Have a decrease in body temperature.
- Become less restless and agitated.
- Remain free of injury.

IMPLEMENTATION

- Monitor vital signs every 2 hours.
- Provide sponge baths if temperature continues to rise.
- Provide a quiet, non-stimulating environment with the shades drawn.
- Provide oral care every 4 hours.
- Measure and compare intake and output every 2 hours.
- Perform neurological assessments every 2 to 4 hours.
- Monitor for and report seizure activity and decreasing LOC.
- Keep bed in low position with side rails elevated.
- Administer prescribed intravenous antibiotics.

EVALUATION

After 4 days of antibiotic therapy, Mr Cook's temperature has returned to normal ranges. Ms Aldi notes that he has begun opening his eyes and visually tracking her as she moves about the room. Mr Cook responds to a request to squeeze Ms Aldi's fingers and after several hours asks her what had happened. On day 5, Mr Cook states that he feels better and his headache is gone. He asks for sips of juice and begins urinating regularly. Seven days after admission, Mr Cook is discharged and is able to go home with his mother. He has some weakness in his legs, but otherwise has no evidence of neurological deficits.

CRITICAL THINKING IN THE NURSING PROCESS

1. Which strategies should the nurse use to decrease the environmental stimuli for Mr Cook and what is the rationale for doing these?
2. If you were caring for Mr Cook in the initial phase of the illness and he became combative, what would you do?

REFLECTION ON THE NURSING PROCESS

1. Develop a plan of care for the nursing diagnosis of *Acute pain* related to meningitis manifested by headaches. Consider the effect of narcotics on respiratory function in designing the plan.
2. Outline what you have learned from this case study that you will apply to your future nursing practice.

- Monitor vital signs, including temperature, on a regular basis. *The person often has a high temperature throughout the illness, ranging from 38°C to 40.5°C.*
- Monitor levels of consciousness. Assess levels of orientation, memory, attention span and response to stimuli. *Early in the infection, the person often has problems with memory and orientation. There may be problems with following commands, restlessness, irritability and combativeness. As the illness progresses, the LOC decreases to lethargy and finally into deep coma.*

CONSIDERATION FOR PRACTICE

Hyperthermia may result from increased intracranial pressure, while an increased temperature can also increase ICP.

- Monitor for manifestations of seizure activity and institute seizure precautions:
  - Monitor twitching of hands or face and tonic–clonic movements.
  - Have an oral airway and suction equipment readily available.
  - Pad side rails, maintain bed in low position and keep side rails up.

  Irritation of the cerebral cortex secondary to meningeal inflammation may cause seizures. Careful monitoring and seizure precautions are necessary to prevent injury.
- Monitor for manifestations of cranial nerve damage; monitor extraocular movements, facial movement, dizziness, ability to hear, double vision, drooping upper eyelids (ptosis) and pupillary changes. *Cranial nerve dysfunction may result from inflammation or vascular changes in the brain.*
- Monitor for manifestations of IICP: decreased pulse, increased blood pressure, widening pulse pressure, respiratory changes and vomiting. *IICP from infectious or inflammatory exudate, cerebral oedema and hydrocephalus.*
- Administer prescribed medications and maintain prescribed fluid restrictions. *Diuretics are often prescribed to prevent increases in ICP, anticonvulsants are prescribed to prevent or control seizures, and antibiotics are prescribed to eradicate the bacteria. Fluids may be restricted to help prevent IICP.*

Risk of fluid volume deficit

The person is at risk of fluid volume deficit related to increased metabolic rate, diaphoresis and fluid restrictions.

- Monitor for presence or worsening of fluid volume deficit.
- Measure and compare intake and output every 2 to 4 hours.
- Monitor daily body weights.
- Monitor skin turgor.
- Monitor condition of mucous membranes.
- Monitor urine amount, colour and odour.
- Monitor BUN:creatinine ratio.

The elastic property of the skin depends partially on interstitial fluid volume. If there is a fluid volume deficit, skin flattens more slowly after a pinch is released. Mucous membranes are dry. In fluid volume deficit, urine output is decreased, urine is dark in colour and concentrated with a strong odour, and urine specific gravity is greater than 1.020 and BUN will rise out of proportion to serum creatinine.

CONSIDERATION FOR PRACTICE

A weight loss of 0.5 kg represents a fluid loss of approximately 500 mL.

- When administering fluids, either orally or parenterally, consider concurrent illnesses. *People with IICP or kidney failure require complex management.*

See the chapter 'Nursing care of people with altered fluid, electrolyte and acid–base balance' for a further discussion of fluid volume deficit.

Community-based care

The importance of preventive measures, such as recognising predisposing conditions, is a major focus for education. People who have had close contact with the person with meningitis should be monitored for fever, headache or neck stiffness. Some doctors believe that those closest to the person are candidates for antimicrobial prophylaxis. Also address the following topics:

- the need to report any manifestations of ear infection, sore throat or upper respiratory infection
- the names and purposes of all medications that may be prescribed
- the importance of taking all medication until completely gone, because some people may think it is acceptable to stop the medication as soon as they feel better.

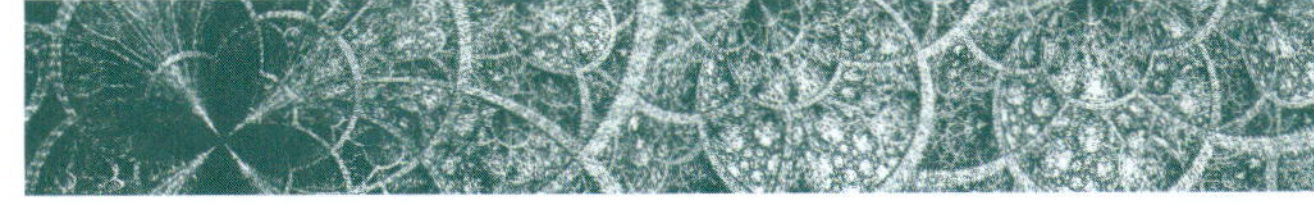

Tumours of the brain

THE PERSON WITH A BRAIN TUMOUR

Brain tumours are growths within the cranium, including tumours in brain tissue, meninges, pituitary gland or blood vessels. Brain tumours may be benign or malignant, primary or metastatic, and intracerebral or extracerebral. Regardless of type or location, brain tumours are potentially lethal as they grow within a closed cranial vault and displace or impinge on CNS structures.

Incidence and prevalence

An estimated 1,400 new cases of malignant brain tumours are diagnosed annually in Australia and approximately 1,200 people die each year (Brain Foundation, 2022). Although brain tumours can occur in any age group, the highest incidence in adults is in those aged 50 to 70. In the adult population, the most common tumour is glioblastoma multiforme, followed by meningioma and cytoma. Glioblastomas represent more than 50% of all primary intracranial lesions (Brain Foundation, 2022).

The cause of many brain tumours is unknown. Although a number of chemical and viral agents can cause brain tumours in laboratory animals, there is no evidence that these agents cause tumours in humans. Other factors associated with brain tumours include heredity, cranial irradiation and exposure to some chemicals (Norris, 2018).

Pathophysiology

Brain tumours may be classified as benign or malignant, based on the tissue type and characteristics of the cells. The use of the term *benign* may be misleading. A tumour that is benign by histological examination but is surgically inaccessible may continue to grow and expand, increasing intracranial pressure and causing neurological deficits, herniation and finally death. In discussions of brain tumours, the term *malignant* is used to describe the lack of cell differentiation, the invasive nature of the tumour and its ability to metastasise.

Brain tumours also may be classified as primary or metastatic, depending on their origin (see Table 41.11). Primary tumours of CNS tissue arise from the cells and structures that are found within the brain; for example, neurons and neuroglia. The primary intracranial tumours that originate in the skull cavity but not from brain tissue itself arise from the supporting

TABLE 41.11 Classification of brain tumours

TUMOUR TYPE	TUMOUR NAME	CHARACTERISTICS
Primary tumours		
Intracerebral tumours:	Glioma	
Account for 40–50% of all brain tumours	• Astrocytoma	Most common glioma
Originate from neuroglia and invade brain tissue		Graded I to IV according to degree of cell differentiation
Most common type of brain tumour	• Glioblastoma multiforme	Most malignant form
	• Ependymoma	Fast-growing tumour that develops from lining of ventricles
		Graded I to IV according to degree of cell differentiation
	• Oligodendroglioma	Slow growing
	• Astroblastoma	Rare, slow growing
		May be encapsulated
		Benign
Extracerebral tumours:	Medulloblastoma	Fast growing and malignant
Tumours arising from the supporting structures of the nervous system		Occurs primarily in children; can occur in adults
		Found in cerebellum
Account for 10–15% of all brain tumours	Meningioma	Slow growing
		Develops in meninges (especially dura)
		Firm and encapsulated
	Acoustic neuroma	Slow growing
		Benign
		Originates from Schwann cells of the cranial nerve XIII
		May also affect cranial nerves V, VII, IX and X
		Also called neurofibromatosis
		Genetic origin due to autosomal dominant Mendelian trait
		Firm, encapsulated lesions attached to nerve
Congenital (developmental) tumours:	Haemangioblastoma	Vascular tumour
Account for 4–8% of all brain tumours	Craniopharyngioma	Slow growing
		Originates from Rathke's pouch
		Solid or cystic tumour
		Compresses pituitary gland
		Presses on the third ventricle and may cause blockage of cerebrospinal fluid (CSF)
Pituitary adenomas:	Chromophobic	Account for 90% of pituitary tumours
Account for 8–12% of all brain tumours		Non-secreting tumour
		Slow growing
	Eosinophilic	Secreting tumours that produce growth hormone
	Basophilic	Secreting tumours that produce adrenocorticotropic hormone
		Fast growing
Secondary tumours		
Metastatic brain tumours:		Slow-growing tumours that arise from other parts of the body
Account for 10% of all brain tumours		Usually well differentiated from the brain
		Spread from tumours of the lung, breast, lower gastrointestinal tract, pancreas, kidney, skin

structures, including the meninges, pituitary gland and pineal gland. Primary brain tumours rarely metastasise outside the CNS. Metastatic brain tumours originate from structures outside the brain, such as the breasts, lungs and prostate gland.

Focal disturbances take place when there is compression of brain tissue and infiltration or direct invasion of brain parenchyma with destruction of neural tissue. As the tumour grows, oedema develops in adjacent tissues. The mechanism is not completely understood, but it is thought that an osmotic gradient causes the tumour to absorb fluid. Some tumours may cause haemorrhage. Venous obstruction and oedema due to breakdown of the blood–brain barrier increase intracranial volume and intracranial pressure. Obstruction of the circulation of CSF from the lateral ventricles to the subarachnoid space causes hydrocephalus.

An estimated 25% of people with a form of cancer will develop brain metastasis. Metastatic brain tumours present in the same way as primary brain tumours, with IICP and focal and/or diffuse cerebral dysfunction. The most common source of intracranial metastasis is cancer of the lung. Other common primary sites are the breast, kidney and gastrointestinal tract. The metastasis reaches the brain through the circulation. In most cases, the tumours are multiple and are scattered through the cerebellum and cerebrum.

Manifestations

Multiple manifestations can develop as a result of the growth of the tumour, while others are related to the location of the lesion. Some of the more common manifestations include changes in cognition or consciousness, a headache that is usually worse in the morning, seizures and vomiting. Compression of brain tissue and the invasion of the brain tumour into the cerebral tissue may lead to changes typically seen with cerebral oedema and IICP. Cerebral blood supply may diminish as the tumour compresses blood vessels. Shifts in brain tissue can occur, leading to brain herniation syndromes and, if untreated, death. See the 'Manifestations' box.

MANIFESTATIONS Brain tumours

FRONTAL LOBE TUMOURS
- Inappropriate behaviour
- Personality changes
- Inability to concentrate
- Impaired judgment
- Recent memory loss
- Headache
- Expressive aphasia
- Motor dysfunctions

PARIETAL LOBE TUMOURS
- Sensory deficits: paraesthesia, loss of two-point discrimination, visual field deficits

TEMPORAL LOBE TUMOURS
- Psychomotor seizures

OCCIPITAL LOBE TUMOURS
- Visual disturbances

CEREBELLUM TUMOURS
- Disturbances in coordination and equilibrium

PITUITARY TUMOURS
- Endocrine dysfunction
- Visual deficits
- Headache

INTERPROFESSIONAL CARE

Treatment for a brain tumour may involve chemotherapy, radiation therapy, surgery or a combination of these interventions. Several variables are considered when selecting the appropriate treatment modality: the size and location of the tumour, the type of tumour, related symptoms (such as neurological deficits) and the person's overall condition.

Diagnosis

The following diagnostic tests may be ordered.

- A CT scan or an MRI with gadolinium enhancement can locate the tumour and define its size, shape, extent to which normal anatomy is distorted and the degree of any associated cerebral oedema.
- Arteriography may show stretching or displacement of cerebral vessels by the tumour, as well as the presence of tumour vascularity.
- EEG provides information about cerebral function, may demonstrate focal or diffuse changes, and is useful if seizures are present.
- Endocrine studies are conducted if a pituitary tumour is suspected.

Medications

The choice of drug for treatment is based on the type of tumour, its location and the person's response to therapy. The use of chemotherapy to treat brain tumours is still emerging. An intraventricular method of medication administration uses an Ommaya reservoir that has been surgically implanted into a lateral ventricle of the brain (see Figure 41.8). Other medications that may be prescribed include corticosteroids and anticonvulsants.

Surgery

Surgery is used to remove tumours, to reduce the size of the tumour or for symptom relief (palliation). The type of procedure, the surgical approach and the timing of surgery (emergency versus planned procedure) influence the overall nursing management of the person having intracranial surgery.

Some of the more common intracranial neurosurgical procedures follow:

- *Burr hole*: a hole made in the skull with a special drill. The hole may facilitate the evacuation of an extracerebral clot or a series of holes may be made in preparation for craniotomy (see Figure 41.7).

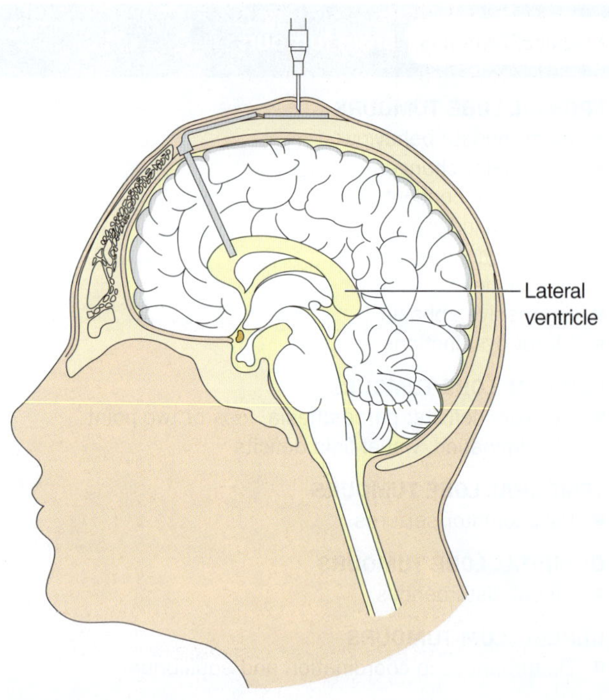

FIGURE 41.8 *Ommaya reservoir for medication administration*

- *Craniotomy*: a surgical opening into the cranial cavity (see Figure 41.9). For a craniotomy, a series of burr holes are made. The bone between the holes is then cut with a special saw called a craniotome. The tumour is excised and the bone flap is returned to the opening. A craniotomy may also be performed to repair defects associated with traumatic head injuries or to repair a cerebral aneurysm.

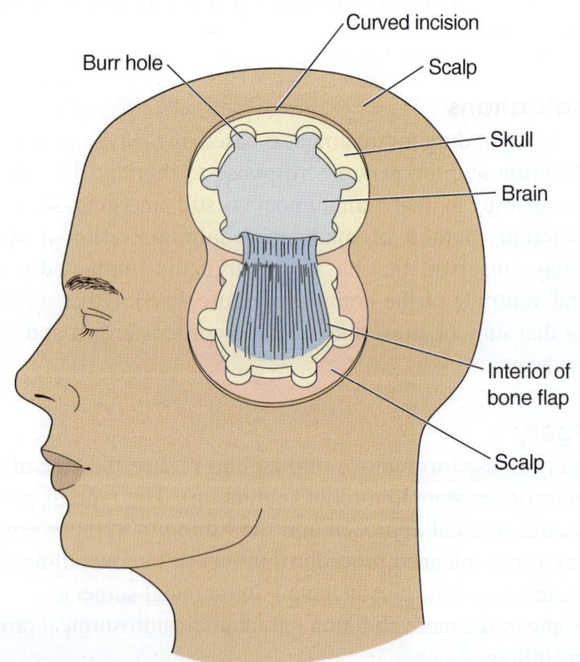

FIGURE 41.9 *In a craniotomy, a portion of the skull and overlying scalp is removed to allow access to the brain*

- A supratentorial craniotomy refers to surgery above the tentorium. It provides access to the frontal, temporal, parietal and occipital lobes. The incision for this procedure is usually within the hairline over the area involved.
- An infratentorial craniotomy refers to surgery below the tentorium. Access is provided to lesions in the cerebellum and the brainstem. The incision is made at the nape of the neck, around the occipital lobe.
- *Craniectomy*: an excision of a portion of the skull and complete removal of the bone flap. This procedure may be done to provide decompression after cerebral oedema. Pressure on the brain structures is lessened by providing space for expansion.
- *Cranioplasty*: plastic repair to the skull in which synthetic material is inserted to replace the cranial bone that was removed. This procedure may be performed after a large craniectomy. The plastic repair restores the contour and integrity of the cranium.

Radiation therapy

Radiation therapy may be administered alone or as adjunctive therapy. Radiation is often the treatment of choice for surgically inaccessible tumours; it may also be used to decrease the size of a tumour prior to surgery. Tumours that were not completely excised by surgery may also be treated with radiation.

Specialty procedures

Technological advances—including the development of special instruments, the use of stereotaxic techniques for localising a specific target and the use of the laser beam—have greatly advanced neurosurgical practice. Microsurgery involves an operating microscope with microinstruments and supportive illumination equipment. Using stereotaxic techniques to precisely locate a specific target point allows for location of discrete areas of the brain that control specific functions and exact locations of deep brain lesions. The use of a laser beam for excision of a tumour results in less damage to surrounding tissue and less postoperative swelling. The gamma knife, which is not actually a knife but a gamma unit, consists of a heavily shielded helmet containing 201 sources of cobalt-60, which is capable of destroying deep and otherwise inaccessible lesions in a single treatment session. A new area of chemotherapy is that of biodegradable anhydrous wafers, which are impregnated with the chemotherapy drug and implanted into the tumour at the time of surgery. The wafers are made so that they slowly release the drug over a period of many months (Norris, 2018).

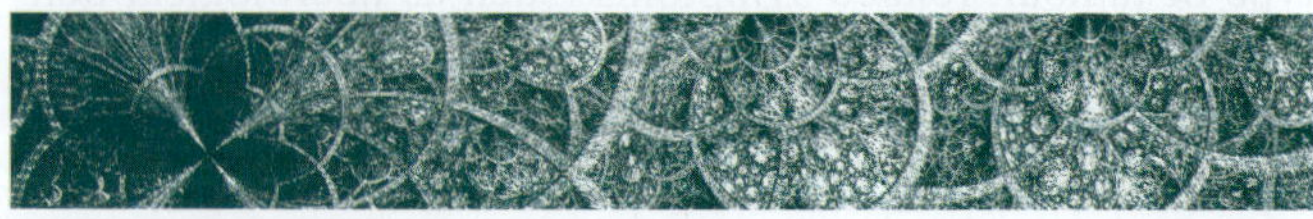

Nursing care

The nursing care of the person with a brain tumour includes support during the diagnostic period and specific management as directed by the selected treatment. The foundation for care is data from the health history and physical assessment, which includes identifying neurological deficits. This information directs planning and implementing care. Many of the alterations in health commonly experienced by the person with a brain tumour have been discussed throughout this chapter, including altered LOC, increased intracranial pressure and seizures. The person will require intensive care in the immediate postoperative period. In addition to the nursing care described in this section, see the accompanying nursing care plan for a person with a brain tumour.

Nursing diagnoses and interventions

This section of the chapter focuses on nursing interventions for the person who has intracranial surgery. The nursing diagnoses discussed are *Anxiety*, *Risk of infection*, *Ineffective protection*, *Acute pain* and *Low self-esteem*.

Anxiety

The diagnosis of a brain tumour brings anxiety and feelings of uncertainty about the future. Both the person and family members are likely to be apprehensive and require education and emotional support.

- Explain routine medical procedures, including blood work and radiological studies. *Baseline laboratory and radiological studies are needed to ensure that the person has no other pre-existing medical condition. Explaining the procedures and assisting the person through this process help decrease anxiety.*
- Reinforce, clarify and repeat information. *Both the person and their family may have limited understanding of the scheduled diagnostic tests, procedures and treatment modalities. The person may be confused or have altered thought processes as a result of the tumour. Information may need to be repeated or re-explained.*
- Encourage the person and their family to verbalise feelings, questions and fears; provide realistic information appropriate to their level of understanding. *Verbalisation helps reduce anxiety and fear.*
- Review the person and their family's strengths and effective coping skills. *Personal strengths, support systems and coping skills can aid in the development of appropriate strategies to reduce anxiety.*
- Arrange for a member of the clergy to visit if desired. *Faith in a higher being is often a strong source of strength and support.*
- Provide preoperative teaching, including the following information:
  - type of anaesthesia and surgery
  - time surgery will begin and expected length of procedure and recovery room stay
  - where the person will be taken after surgery (ICU) (if possible, show the person and their family the ICU and introduce them to the nurse who will be in charge of care after the surgery)
  - where the family can wait during and following surgery
  - appearance of the person after surgery, which may include swollen, bruised eyelids and other facial features; a large dressing covering the head; a partially or fully shaved head; and a tracheostomy or endotracheal tube
  - behaviour of the person after surgery, which will differ depending on the site of surgery, although cognitive and behavioural changes are common.

  Information about what to expect reduces anxiety.
- Allow time for the person and their family to be together. *People need quiet time together with their families to support each other and prepare emotionally for surgery.*

Risk of infection

The person who has had intracranial surgery is at risk of infection from multiple invasive lines, the scalp wound and the risk of introduction of bacteria into the operative area. The nurse provides interventions to monitor for and prevent infection.

- Monitor for leakage of CSF:
  - presence of glucose in clear drainage from ears, nose or wound
  - complaints of 'something dripping down the back of the throat'
  - constant swallowing.

  These manifestations indicate an opening in the dura, which provides an avenue for an ascending infection.
- Provide interventions to prevent contamination of area leaking CSF:
  - If leaking from the nose: keep head of bed elevated 20 degrees unless contraindicated; do not suction nasally; do not clean the nose; tell the person not to put their finger in their nose; do not insert packing.
  - If leaking from the ear: position the person on the side of the leakage unless contraindicated; do not clean the ear; tell the person not to put their finger in their ear; do not insert packing.
  - Place a sterile dressing over the area of drainage and change as soon as it becomes damp.

  Leakage of CSF indicates a break in the dura and increases the risk of an ascending infection. Surgery may be necessary to repair the break; however, the leak usually heals spontaneously in about 1 week.
- Monitor for and report manifestations of infection:
  - Take and record temperature on a regular basis.
  - Assess IV insertion sites for redness, swelling, drainage and pain.
  - Assess scalp wound for redness, swelling, bulging, drainage and pain.
  - Assess for manifestations of meningitis: fever and chills, increasing headache, neck stiffness, positive Kernig's or Brudzinski's sign, photophobia.
  - Monitor laboratory reports for increased WBC count.

  Intact skin is the first line of defence against infection. Any break in the skin increases the risk of infection. Intracranial surgery increases the risk of meningitis, with infectious agents ascending into the brain.
- Implement interventions to prevent infection:
  - Use strict aseptic technique when changing dressings and when caring for wound drains and ICP monitor lines.
  - Keep the person's hands away from drains and dressings; use mitten restraints if necessary.

- Administer prescribed antibiotics.

Sterile technique decreases the risk of introducing infection into a wound. Antibiotics are usually prescribed prophylactically to prevent infection.

Ineffective protection

The person who has intracranial surgery does not have normal human defences against changes in intracranial pressure and is also at risk from cerebral oedema and a shift of intracerebral contents. In addition, the surgery may cause cerebral bleeding or haematoma formation.

- Monitor for manifestations of increased intracranial pressure:
  - restlessness, agitation and decreasing LOC
  - headache
  - vomiting
  - seizures
  - decreasing sensory and motor function
  - changes in pupil size and reaction
  - changes in vital signs: altered respiratory rate or depth, increasing pulse pressure, decreasing pulse rate, increasing blood pressure
  - abnormal posturing.

NURSING CARE PLAN A person with a brain tumour

Claire Lange is a 44-year-old morning television presenter. During a midweek program, she confuses several major news items so badly that her co-anchor tries to correct her. Ms Lange responds angrily that she does not need any help and then rises and storms off the set. As she leaves the camera area, she limps noticeably and appears to drag her left leg. The show's producer asks her what is wrong; she screams that nothing is wrong—she simply has another headache. He follows her to her dressing room and enquires about her headaches. She tells him that they come and go but have been getting worse lately. He then asks her if she has injured her left leg; she responds that the leg was weak because she was tired. As the producer leaves the dressing room, Ms Lange begins to shake and collapses on the floor. The producer recognises that she is having a seizure and calls for an ambulance.

Ms Lange is admitted to the neurology ward of the local hospital for evaluation. A CT scan, MRI and EEG are completed and identify an intracranial mass. A biopsy of the mass is positive for malignant cells. A glioma in the frontal lobe is identified and surgery is scheduled for that week.

ASSESSMENT

When Clara Rosetti, RN, enters Ms Lange's room, she sees Ms Lange looking at her shoulder-length hair in the mirror. Ms Lange tells Ms Rosetti that she has never in her life worn her hair any shorter and 'Now you're going to cut it all off!' She paces the room and makes the statement, 'I guess the hair isn't really important if I survive this situation.' She also says that she has a headache.

DIAGNOSES

- *Acute pain* related to tumour and increase in intracranial pressure manifested by the onset of headaches.
- *Disturbed body image* related to surgery manifested by anxiety surrounding potential hair loss and appearance postoperatively.
- *Anxiety* related to unknown future following surgery, evidenced by emotional distress.

PLANNING

- Reduce anxiety and fear and manage pain effectively.

Expected outcomes

- Verbalise the causes of pain.
- Verbalise an understanding of the changes in body appearance that are associated with the scheduled intracranial surgery (e.g. shaving of the head prior to surgery, cranial incision and facial swelling postoperatively).
- Identify measures that will help minimise the effect of the hair loss.
- Verbalise a reduction in anxiety.

IMPLEMENTATION

- Assess level of discomfort using a rating scale of 0 to 10.
- Provide a quiet, non-stimulating environment.
- Position Ms Lange for comfort, keeping the head of the bed elevated to promote venous drainage.
- Assess LOC for potential increases in ICP.
- Encourage to verbalise feelings about the surgery.
- Suggest measures that may help minimise the impact of hair loss, such as the use of turbans, scarves, hats and wigs.
- Suggest relaxation techniques to decrease anxiety.

EVALUATION

By the time of surgery, Ms Lange has recognised the relationship between the brain tumour and the headache. She states that lying in a flat position and coughing increase the headache. The head of the bed is kept at a 30- to 45-degree angle. Daily activities are spaced to provide periods of rest. Ms Lange demonstrates no significant changes in LOC. She has talked about the effect of the hair loss and her television responsibilities. Ms Lange has learned that the hair preparation would be done in surgery and that the hair would be saved for her. She states she has already consulted her hairdresser and that 'scarves and turbans are on the way'.

CRITICAL THINKING IN THE NURSING PROCESS

1 Outline interventions to decrease intracranial pressure both before and after surgery.
2 When making your initial assessments on the morning of surgery, you find that Ms Lange has a decreased pulse and increased blood pressure. She tells you her headache is worse and suddenly vomits. What do you do now?
3 Ms Lange asks you to be sure that she has absolutely no visitors after surgery because she knows how ugly she will look. How would you respond?

REFLECTION ON THE NURSING PROCESS

1 Which communication and education strategies could you use when caring for people undergoing neurosurgery?
2 Outline what you have learned from this case study that you will apply to your future nursing practice.

Increasing intracranial pressure is manifested by alterations in the functions and centres controlled by the brain.

- Implement interventions to decrease the risk of IICP:
  - Elevate the head of the bed 15 to 30 degrees as prescribed (unless contraindicated).
  - Avoid neck flexion or rotation; keep head in midline position unless a large bone flap or mass was removed; then position the person on unoperated side to decrease venous congestion in the operative area.
  - Do not take rectal temperatures.
  - Avoid clustering activities that increase intracranial pressure: suctioning, turning and bathing.
  - Administer medications to prevent vomiting.
  - Do not suction for more than 10 seconds at one time.
  - Teach the person (if possible) to avoid coughing, sneezing and straining to have a bowel movement.
  - Maintain fluid restrictions as prescribed.
  - For internal shunts: avoid pressure on the shunt, reservoir or tubing. Pump the shunt only if prescribed.
  - For external shunts: avoid kinks in tubing and maintain the drainage collecting device and the person's head at the prescribed levels.

  Keeping the head of the bed slightly elevated facilitates venous drainage from the brain. Neck flexion or rotation disrupts circulation to and from the brain. Rectal stimulation, suctioning, turning, bathing, coughing, sneezing and straining to have a bowel movement all initiate the Valsalva manoeuvre, which constricts the jugular veins and impairs venous return from the brain. Fluid restriction may be prescribed to dehydrate the person slightly and lessen ICP.
- Maintain (as much as possible) a quiet, calm, softly lighted environment. *Avoid excessive sensory stimulation. These interventions promote rest and decrease stimulation, thereby reducing ICP.*
- Implement interventions to prevent seizures or, if they occur, to prevent injury to the person:
  - Pad side rails of the bed.
  - Place bed in lowest position and keep side rails up.
  - Carry out interventions to prevent and treat IICP.
  - Have an oral airway (Guedel's) and suction equipment immediately available.
  - Administer prescribed anticonvulsants.
  - If a seizure occurs: maintain a patent airway; do not restrain the person; do not force anything into the person's mouth; provide physical and emotional support.

  These interventions promote safety and help prevent injury. Anticonvulsants are often prescribed prophylactically to prevent seizures after intracranial surgery.
- Carefully monitor hydration status. Compare trends in intake and output, laboratory results of serum osmolality and urine specific gravity and osmolality. *Changes in fluid balance and osmolality may result from excess intravenous fluids, osmotic diuretics, surgically induced diabetes insipidus or syndrome of inappropriate antidiuretic hormone secretion, fever, diarrhoea, tube feedings or hyperglycaemia.*

Acute pain

The person who has intracranial surgery has pain, manifested as a headache, as a result of either compression or displacement of brain tissue or from increased intracranial pressure. A headache may also be a manifestation of meningitis.

- Assess the location, duration and intensity of the pain, using a scale from 0 (no pain) to 10 (worst pain) in the person who can verbally communicate. *The person is the best source of information about pain.*
- Implement interventions to reduce the pain:
  - Raise the head of the bed slightly.
  - Reduce noise and bright lights in the room.
  - If allowed, loosen head dressing.
  - Administer narcotic analgesics with caution.

  Non-pharmacological measures may be used to reduce IICP and headache.

> **CONSIDERATION FOR PRACTICE**
> **Narcotic analgesics mask changes in eye signs and depress respirations.**

Situational low self-esteem

The person who has intracranial surgery has many alterations that affect self-esteem and body image. Physical changes include a loss of hair on the scalp, swelling and bruising in the eyelids and face, and perhaps an indentation in the skull. The person is no longer independent in self-care but must depend on others to meet basic needs. There are often long-term neurological deficits, affecting areas such as speech, vision, and motor abilities, which require changes in roles and relationships.

- Assess for verbal and non-verbal manifestations of negative self-esteem:
  - denial of changes
  - preoccupation with changes
  - refusal to look in the mirror
  - withdrawal from family and friends
  - expressions of grief and loss (see the chapter 'Nursing care of people experiencing loss, grief and death').

  Low self-esteem can be initiated by stressful situations and changes in body image.
- Provide interventions to improve self-concept:
  - Limit negative self-assessment.
  - Help focus on positive areas of life.
  - Help identify sources of support and strength.
  - Help identify and use helpful coping methods.
  - Encourage significant others to visit.
  - Encourage independence in self-care.

  Self-esteem is derived from one's own perceptions of competence and from the responses of others. When one's self-concept and self-ideal are congruent, self-esteem is enhanced.

Community-based care

The effect of the possible outcomes following the surgery produces fear in both the person and their family, interfering with their ability to retain information. The person may have cognitive or neurological deficits that interfere with learning. Family members also must be assessed for their ability to cope with the stress of the surgery. Information may have to be repeated several times.

People and their families who have experienced intracranial surgery require emotional support. The process of recovery is often extended and may involve adaptation to changes in body image and management of any motor or sensory deficits. The family should be involved in the care of the person. If family members are willing, they may begin to assist with ADLs while the person is in the hospital, such as assisting with personal hygiene and meals. People should also be encouraged to take an active role in their own care. Discharge planning includes a discussion of the following topics: medication information; wound care; the use of wigs, turbans, hats or colourful scarves; and the importance of follow-up visits. In addition, emphasise the importance of reporting manifestations such as stiff neck, increasing headache, elevated temperature, new motor or sensory deficits, vision changes or seizures.

Provide information about the overall treatment plan, management of deficits and/or disabilities, and future needs. Specific teaching topics are as follows:

- safety measures for motor deficits, sensory deficits, lack of coordination, seizures and cognitive deficits
- comfort measures for nausea, vomiting and pain
- measures for communication if aphasia is present
- measures to improve vision if visual deficits are present
- how to buy wigs and hairpieces
- referrals to support groups and community resources
- helpful resources:
  - Brain Foundation: https://brainfoundation.org.au
  - Brain Tumour Alliance Australia: www.btaa.org.au
  - Cancer Council: https://www.cancer.org.au.

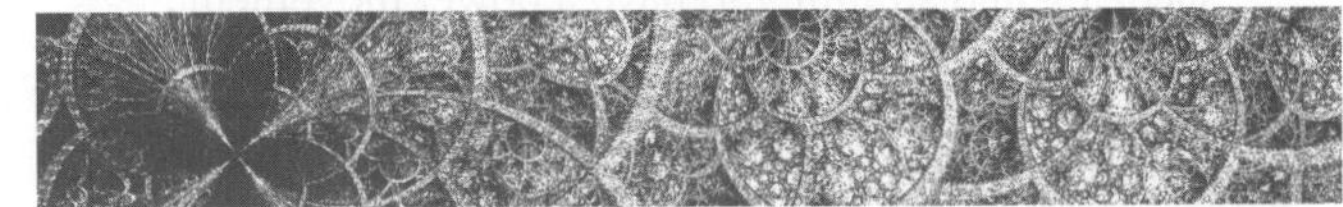

CHAPTER HIGHLIGHTS

- **Altered level of consciousness (LOC) is a common response to intracranial disorders and is an early manifestation of deterioration of the function of the cerebral hemispheres. The alteration in cerebral function occurs in a sequential pattern, with characteristic changes in LOC, respiratory patterns, pupillary and oculomotor responses, and motor function. Coma states include persistent vegetative state and locked-in syndrome.**
- **Increased intracranial pressure (IICP) is a sustained elevated pressure (≥ 10 mmHg) within the cranial cavity. IICP may result from cerebral oedema, hydrocephalus, head trauma, tumours, abscesses, inflammation, haemorrhage or stroke.**
- **The manifestations of IICP include a decreasing LOC, abnormal motor weakness and responses, altered vision, altered vital signs, headache, papilloedema and projectile vomiting. If untreated, IICP causes a displacement (herniation) of cerebral tissue, herniation of the cerebellum through the tentorium, followed by herniation of the brainstem through the foramen magnum. This is a lethal complication of IICP because it puts pressure on the vital centres in the medulla. IICP is primarily managed with osmotic diuretics and monitored with continuous intracranial pressure monitors.**
- **Headaches, a common type of intracranial pain, are categorised as tension, migraine and cluster. A classic migraine is characterised by an aura; a common migraine does not have an aura.**
- **Epilepsy is a chronic disorder of abnormal, recurring, excessive and self-terminating electrical discharges from neurones. A seizure is a single event of abnormal electrical discharge. Seizures are categorised into those that affect only a part of the brain (partial seizures) and those that affect all of the brain (generalised). The most common type of seizure in adults is a tonic–clonic generalised seizure. Seizures are treated medically with anti-epileptic drugs, surgery and/or vagal nerve stimulation therapy.**
- **Traumatic brain injury (TBI) refers to any injury of the scalp, skull or brain and is a leading cause of death and disability. TBIs include skull fractures and focal or diffuse brain injury. An acute brain injury affects all body systems and carries the risk of secondary injury to the brain from hypoxia and ischaemia.**
- **An epidural haematoma develops in the potential space between the dura and the skull. A subdural haematoma collects between the dura mater and the arachnoid mater. Diffuse brain injuries include contusions, concussions and diffuse axonal injury. People with an acute TBI must have immediate transport and treatment in an ED, followed by care in a critical care unit. They will require long-term physical care and rehabilitation.**
- **Central nervous system infections may be caused by bacteria, bacterial toxins, viruses, fungi, protozoans and rickettsiae. Organisms may enter the brain through the bloodstream or by direct invasion. The main CNS infections are meningitis, encephalitis and brain abscess. CNS infections are treated with broad-spectrum antibiotics and antifungal agents.**
- **Brain tumours are growths within the cranium, including on or in brain tissue, the meninges, the pituitary gland or blood vessels. Brain tumours may be benign or malignant, primary or metastatic, and intracerebral or extracerebral. Regardless of the type or location, brain tumours are potentially lethal because they displace or impinge on CNS structures within a closed bony system.**

CONCEPT CHECK

1 Which of the following pathophysiological events results in irregular respiratory patterns as LOC decreases?

1 pressure on the meninges
2 reflexive motor responses
3 loss of the oculocephalic reflex
4 brainstem responses to changes in $PaCO_2$

2 The unconscious person has depressed or absent gag and swallowing reflexes. Which nursing diagnosis would be appropriate?
1 *Decreased intracranial adaptive capacity*
2 *Risk of aspiration*
3 *Imbalanced nutrition: less than body requirements*
4 *Ineffective breathing pattern*

3 What is the rationale for the use of osmotic diuretics to treat IICP?
1 Hyperthermia increases the cerebral metabolic rate and exacerbates IICP.
2 Increased blood osmolality draws oedematous fluid into the vascular system.
3 People with IICP are at increased risk of gastrointestinal haemorrhage.
4 Brain injury and IICP often cause seizures.

4 You are monitoring the neurological status of a person in a coma. Which of the following commands would be most accurate in identifying changes in mental status?
1 'Tell me your name.'
2 'Look at this light when I shine it in your eyes.'
3 'Squeeze my hand.'
4 'Are you having trouble breathing?'

5 On admission to the ED, a person who has altered LOC has a variety of laboratory tests to facilitate the diagnosis of the aetiology of the condition. Which tests would likely be performed? (Select all that apply.)
1 blood glucose
2 serum electrolytes
3 blood and urine toxicology
4 urine for WBCs
5 spinal fluid osmolarity

6 Of the following diagnostic tests, which one is the most accurate indicator of hydration status in the person with altered LOC?
1 FBC
2 urinalysis
3 serum osmolality
4 blood culture

7 Which manifestation is consistently assessed in people with generalised seizures?
1 loss of consciousness
2 repetitive non-purposeful activity
3 tonic movements
4 clonic movements

8 When assessing a person with a head injury, you test fluid dripping from one ear for glucose. What are you assessing for?
1 infection
2 blood
3 CSF
4 serum

9 You are administering an anti-epileptic drug to a person newly diagnosed with seizures. The person asks, 'Will this cure my convulsions?' What would you say?
1 'No, but it will relieve your headache.'
2 'No, but it will help decrease the aura you experience.'
3 'No, not for the first year.'
4 'No, but it may reduce or control them.'

10 Which of the following statements is true of brain tumours?
1 All brain tumours are potentially lethal.
2 Only malignant tumours are lethal.
3 Metastatic brain tumours are benign tumours.
4 Benign brain tumours rarely require treatment.

BIBLIOGRAPHY

Australian Commission on Safety and Quality in Health Care (ACSQHC) (2021). *National Safety and Quality Health Service Standards* (2nd ed.). Sydney: ACSQHC.

Australian Institute of Health and Welfare (2021). *Health service use for patients with traumatic brain injury*. Retrieved from https://www.aihw.gov.au/

Brain Foundation (2022). *Brain tumour/cancer*. Retrieved from http://brainfoundation.org.au/

Brain Injury Australia (2022). Retrieved from https://www.braininjuryaustralia.org.au

Department of Health (2017). *Tuberculosis notifications in Australia, 2014*. Retrieved from https://www.health.gov.au/

Epilepsy Action Australia (2020). *Seniors' issues*. Retrieved from https://www.epilepsy.org.au/

Epilepsy Centre (2022). *What is epilepsy?* Retrieved from https://epilepsycentre.org.au/

Headache Australia (2021). *Migraine—A common and distressing disorder*. Retrieved from https://headacheaustralia.org.au/

Hickey, J. V. (2019). *The clinical practice of neurological and neurosurgical nursing* (8th ed.). Philadelphia: Lippincott Williams & Wilkins.

Knox, L., Douglas, J. M. & Bigby, C. (2015). 'I won't be around forever': Understanding the decision-making experiences of adults with severe TBI and their parents. *Neuropsychological Rehabilitation*, *26*(2), 236–260.

Norris, T. L. (2018). *Porth's pathophysiology: Concepts of altered health states* (10th ed.). Philadelphia: Lippincott Williams & Wilkins.

Papadakis, M., McPhee, S. & Rabow, M. (2022). *Current medical diagnosis and treatment* (61st ed.). New York: McGraw-Hill Education.

Patchana, T., Wiginton, J., Brazdzionis, J. et al. (2020). Increased brain tissue oxygen monitoring threshold to improve hospital course in traumatic brain injury patients. *Cureus*, *12*(2), e7115. doi: 10.7759/cureus.7115

Synapse (2022). *Recovery and rehab*. Retrieved from https://synapse.org.au/

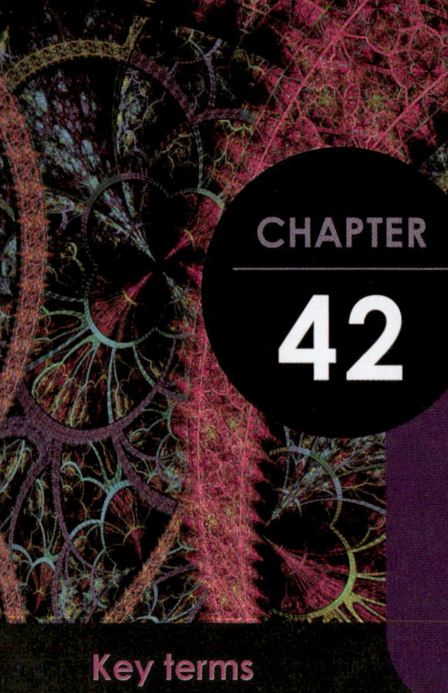

CHAPTER 42

Nursing care of people with cerebrovascular and spinal cord disorders

David Stanley

Key terms

Learning outcomes

- Identify prevalence, incidence and risk factors responsible for disorders of cerebral blood flow and spinal cord structure and function.
- Explain the pathophysiology, manifestations, complications, interprofessional care and nursing care of people with stroke, ruptured intracranial aneurysm, arteriovenous malformation, spinal cord injury, herniated intervertebral disc and spinal cord tumour.
- Compare and contrast the acute treatment and care of the person with a stroke or ruptured intracranial aneurysm and a spinal cord injury.
- Discuss the pathophysiological effects of injuries and tumours of the spinal cord by level of injury.
- Discuss the purposes, nursing implications and health education of the person and family for medications used to treat stroke, ruptured intracranial aneurysm and spinal cord injury.
- Describe the methods used to stabilise and immobilise spinal cord injuries.
- Describe the surgical procedures used to treat cerebrovascular and spinal cord disorders.

Clinical competencies

- Assess functional status of people with cerebrovascular and spinal cord disorders and monitor, document and report abnormal manifestations.
- Use evidence-based research to promote early recognition and treatment of the warning signs of a stroke.
- Determine priority nursing diagnoses, based on assessed data, to select and implement individualised nursing interventions for people with cerebrovascular and spinal cord disorders.
- Administer oral and injectable medications used to treat cerebrovascular and spinal cord disorders knowledgeably and safely.
- Provide skilled care to people having a carotid endarterectomy, halo fixation and a posterior laminectomy.
- Integrate interprofessional care into the care of people with cerebrovascular and spinal cord disorders.
- Provide appropriate teaching to facilitate self-catheterisation, self-care of a ruptured intervertebral disc and community-based self-care of disabilities resulting from cerebrovascular and spinal cord disorders.
- Revise the plan of care as needed to provide effective interventions to promote, maintain or restore functional health status to people with cerebrovascular and spinal cord disorders.

The health problems discussed in this chapter result from alterations in cerebral blood flow and disorders of the spinal cord. People with disorders of cerebral blood flow and the spinal cord experience a wide variety of neurological deficits that affect cognitive and perceptual functional health patterns. They also require treatment and care for both acute and long-term health problems.

Nursing care for people with these disorders is tailored to meet the needs of the person and is individualised according to the person's responses to alterations in intracranial and spinal cord structure and function. This chapter's discussion of nursing care includes consideration of both acute and long-term healthcare needs. The disabilities and long-term effects resulting from cerebrovascular disorders and spinal cord injuries almost always cause loss and grief, not only in the person but also in the family of the person. The chapter 'Nursing care of people experiencing loss, grief and death' provides information about person responses to loss and nursing interventions to help reduce grieving.

Cerebrovascular disorders

THE PERSON WITH A STROKE

A **stroke** (*cerebral vascular accident (CVA)*) is a condition in which neurological deficits result from a sudden decrease in blood flow to a localised area of the brain. Strokes may be *ischaemic* (when blood supply to a part of the brain is suddenly interrupted by a thrombus (blood clot), embolus (foreign matter travelling through the circulation) or stenosis (narrowing)) or *haemorrhagic* (when a blood vessel breaks open, spilling blood into spaces surrounding neurons). The neurological deficits caused by ischaemia and the resultant necrosis of cells in the brain vary according to the area of the brain involved, the size of the affected area and the length of time blood flow is decreased or stopped. A major loss of blood supply to the brain can cause severe disability or death. When the duration of decreased blood flow is short and the anatomical area involved is small, the person may not be aware that damage has been done.

Incidence and prevalence

On average, someone in Australia has a stroke every 10–13 minutes. Stroke is the second leading cause of death in Australia and a major cause of disability: approximately 60,000 people suffer a stroke each year. Of these, many people who survive are left with some type of functional impairment. Although strokes occur in every age group, the highest incidence occurs in people over 75 years of age. Strokes occur more frequently in men than women and Australian men are also more likely to suffer a stroke at a younger age than women (National Stroke Foundation, 2022a). Indigenous Australians are almost twice as likely as non-Indigenous Australians to experience cerebrovascular disease and twice as likely to die as a result (National Stroke Foundation, 2021). In 2018, based on self-reported data, an estimated 387,000 Australians aged 15 and over (1.3% of the population) had experienced a stroke at some time in their lives (Australian Bureau of Statistics (ABS), 2019).

Risk factors

Certain diseases and lifestyle habits increase the risk of a stroke, including the following (National Stroke Foundation, 2022b):

- *Hypertension*. Hypertension is the greatest risk factor for a stroke. Increased systolic and diastolic blood pressure is associated with damage to all blood vessels, including the cerebral vessels. People with hypertension have a four to six times greater risk of stroke than those without hypertension. Thirty per cent of Australian adults over 25 years of age have hypertension.
- *Heart disease*. Atrial fibrillation (AF) is associated with 1 in 4 strokes. It can happen in both men and women, at any age. About 90% of people with AF are under 75 years of age. Most people diagnosed with AF have no family history of it. AF is associated with high blood pressure, heart disease, diabetes and lung cancer (National Stroke Foundation, 2022b). Other cardiovascular problems that increase the risk of a stroke are mitral valve stenosis, patent foramen ovale and cardiac surgery.
- *Diabetes mellitus*. Diabetes leads to vascular changes in both the systemic and cerebral circulation and increases the risk of hypertension. (The prevalence of hypertension is 40% higher in people with diabetes.) The person with diabetes is three times more likely to have a stroke than those without diabetes. Some 7.6% of Australian adults over the age of 25 years have diabetes.
- *High blood cholesterol levels*. Increased blood cholesterol levels contribute to the risk of atherosclerosis, including arteries in the cerebral circulation. Fifty-one per cent of the Australian population over 25 years have an elevated cholesterol level.
- *Smoking*. Cigarette smoking doubles a person's risk of ischaemic stroke and increases the risk of cerebral haemorrhage by up to 3.5%. Smoking is directly responsible for more strokes in young adults. Seventeen per cent of Australians over the age of 14 years smoke daily.
- *Overweight and obesity*. Healthy eating is important for reducing the risk of further stroke. It affects a number of risk factors (e.g. too much salt in the diet increases blood pressure). Obesity, being overweight or having too much body fat can also contribute to high blood pressure, type 2 diabetes, high cholesterol, heart disease, kidney disease and some cancers. The number of Australians who are overweight or obese has steadily increased in recent decades to nearly 2 in 3 adults (63%) and 1 in 4 children (27%) aged 15–17 years. A healthy waist measurement should be less than 80 cm in women and less than 94 cm

FAST FACTS

Estimated cost of stroke in Australia

- Total healthcare cost of stroke was $881 million in 2012–2013.
- The largest portion of the cost is spent on hospital care.
- In 2022, there were more than 475,000 Australians living with the effects of stroke; by 2050, this is predicted to increase to 1 million.

Sources: National Stroke Foundation (2017a, 2018).

in men. These measurements are recommended for people from Caucasian backgrounds; people from different cultural backgrounds should speak with their doctor about their risk (National Stroke Foundation, 2022c).

- *Physical inactivity*. Being inactive can increase the risk of type 2 diabetes, overweight and obesity, high blood pressure and high blood cholesterol. Over half (56%) of Australian adults do not do the recommended amount of physical activity (2.5 hours per week) and 15% do no exercise at all (National Stroke Foundation, 2022d).
- *Substance abuse*. The injection of unpurified substances increases the risk of a stroke and abuse of certain drugs can decrease cerebral blood flow and increase the risk of intracranial haemorrhage. Substances associated with strokes include excessive alcohol intake, marijuana, anabolic steroids, heroin, amphetamines and cocaine.

Other risk factors include a family history of stroke, obesity, a sedentary lifestyle, recent viral and bacterial infections, and previous transient ischaemic attacks. Risk factors specific to women are oral contraceptive use, pregnancy, childbirth, menopause, migraine headaches with aura, autoimmune disorders (such as diabetes and lupus) and clotting disorders.

In addition, having a stroke is a major risk factor for having another stroke (called recurrent stroke); about 25% of people who have a stroke and recover have another stroke within 5 years. The number and rate of stroke deaths declined substantially between 1980 and 2019, with the number dropping by 30%, from around 12,100 to 8,400. The age-standardised stroke death rate declined by three-quarters (76%), falling from 104 to 25 deaths per 100,000 population. Stroke death rates declined in a similar fashion for males and females, with falling stroke death rates being driven by a number of factors, including improvements in risk factors such as lower rates of tobacco smoking, an increased use of blood-pressure-lowering drugs, treatment to prevent blood clots, access to stroke units in hospitals and other advances in medical care (Australian Institute of Health and Welfare (AIHW), 2021).

Pathophysiology

The brain, which makes up only 2% of total body weight, receives approximately 20% of the cardiac output each minute (about 750 mL) and accounts for 20% of the body's oxygen consumption. Cerebral blood flow, especially in the deep cerebral vessels, is largely self-regulated by the brain to meet metabolic needs. This self-regulation (also called *autoregulation*) allows the brain to maintain a constant blood flow despite changes in systemic blood pressure. However, autoregulation is not effective when systemic blood pressure falls below 50 mmHg or rises above 160 mmHg. In the latter case, the increased systemic pressure (as in hypertension) causes an increase in cerebral blood flow with resultant over-distension of cerebral vessels. Cerebral blood flow also increases in response to increased carbon dioxide concentrations, increased hydrogen ion concentrations and decreased oxygen concentrations.

When blood flow to and oxygenation of cerebral neurons are decreased or interrupted, pathophysiological changes at the cellular level take place in 4 to 5 minutes. Cellular metabolism ceases as glucose, glycogen and adenosine triphosphate (ATP) are depleted and the sodium–potassium pump fails. Cells swell as sodium draws water into the cell. Cerebral blood vessel walls also swell, further decreasing blood flow. Even if circulation is restored, vasospasm and increased blood viscosity can continue to impede blood flow. Severe or prolonged ischaemia leads to cellular death. A central core of dead or dying cells is surrounded by a band of minimally perfused cells, called the penumbra. Although cells in the penumbra have impaired metabolic activities, their structural integrity is maintained. The survival of these cells depends on a timely return of adequate circulation, the volume of toxic products released by adjacent dying cells, the degree of cerebral oedema and alterations in local blood flow. The potential survival of cells in the penumbra has led to the use of fibrinolytic agents in the early treatment of ischaemic stroke (Norris, 2018).

The neurological deficits that occur as a result of a stroke can often be used to identify its location. Because the motor pathways cross at the junction of the medulla and spinal cord (decussation), strokes lead to loss or impairment of sensorimotor functions on the side of the body opposite the side of the brain that is damaged. This effect, known as a **contralateral deficit**, causes a stroke in the right hemisphere of the brain to be manifested by deficits in the left side of the body (and vice versa).

A stroke is characterised by a gradual or rapid onset of neurological deficits due to compromised cerebral blood flow. Strokes may result from a variety of problems, including cerebral thrombosis, cerebral embolism and cerebral haemorrhage.

Ischaemic stroke

Ischaemic strokes result from blockage and/or stenosis of a cerebral artery decreasing or stopping blood flow and ultimately causing a brain infarction. This type of stroke accounts for about 80% of all strokes (Cardiac Research Institute, 2022). The blockage may result from a blood clot (either as a thrombus or an embolus) or from stenosis of a vessel resulting from a build up of plaque. Plaque may cause stenosis in large blood vessels (called large vessel disease) or small blood vessels (called small vessel disease). Large vessel disease usually is the result of thrombi. Small vessel strokes, called lacunar infarcts, are small to very small infarcts in the deep, non-cortical areas of the brain or the brainstem. Ischaemic strokes are classified as transient, thrombotic or embolic.

TRANSIENT ISCHAEMIC ATTACK A **transient ischaemic attack (TIA)**, sometimes called a mini-stroke, is a brief period of localised cerebral ischaemia that causes neurological deficits lasting for less than 24 hours (usually less than 1 to 2 hours) (Norris, 2018). The deficits may be present for only minutes or may last for hours. TIAs are often warning signals of an ischaemic thrombotic stroke. One or many TIAs may precede a stroke, with the time between the TIA and a stroke ranging from hours to months. The aetiology of TIA includes inflammatory artery disorders, sickle cell anaemia, atherosclerotic changes in cerebral blood vessels, thrombosis and emboli. Neurological manifestations of a TIA vary according to the location and size of the cerebral vessel involved. Manifestations have a sudden onset and often disappear within minutes or hours. Commonly occurring deficits include contralateral numbness or weakness of the leg, hand, forearm and corner of the mouth (due to middle cerebral artery involvement); aphasia (due to ischaemia of the left hemisphere); and visual disturbances such as blurring (due to involvement of the posterior cerebral artery) (Norris, 2018). The person may also experience a visual disturbance called *amaurosis fugax* (a fleeting blindness of one eye, described as a shade coming down over vision in the affected eye).

THROMBOTIC STROKE A thrombotic stroke is caused by occlusion of a large cerebral vessel by a thrombus (blood clot). Thrombotic CVAs most often occur in older people who are resting or sleeping. The blood pressure is lower during sleep, so there is less pressure to push the blood through an already narrowed arterial lumen and ischaemia may result.

Thrombi tend to form in large arteries that bifurcate and have narrowed lumens as a result of deposits of atherosclerotic plaque. The plaque involves the intima of the arteries, causing the internal elastic lamina to become thin and frayed with exposure of underlying connective tissue. This structural change causes platelets to adhere to the rough surface and release the enzyme adenosine diphosphate. This enzyme initiates the clotting sequence and the thrombus forms. A thrombus may remain in place and continue to enlarge, completely occluding the lumen of the vessel, or a part of it may break off and become an embolus.

The most common locations of thrombi are the internal carotid artery, the vertebral arteries and the junction of the vertebral and basilar arteries. Thrombotic strokes affecting the smaller cerebral vessels are called lacunar strokes, because the infarcted areas slough off, leaving a small cavity or 'lake' in the brain tissue. A thrombotic stroke usually affects only one region of the brain that is supplied by a single cerebral artery.

A thrombotic stroke occurs rapidly but progresses slowly. It often begins with a TIA and continues to worsen over 1 to 2 days; the condition is called a *stroke in evolution*. When maximum neurological deficit has been reached, usually in 3 days, the condition is called a *completed stroke*. At that time, the damaged area of brain tissue is oedematous and necrotic.

EMBOLIC STROKE An embolic stroke occurs when a blood clot or clump of matter travelling through the cerebral blood vessels becomes lodged in a vessel too narrow to permit further movement. The area of the brain supplied by the blocked vessel becomes ischaemic. The most frequent sites of cerebral emboli are at bifurcations of vessels, particularly those of the carotid and middle cerebral arteries. This type of stroke is typically seen in people who are younger than those experiencing thrombotic strokes and occurs when the person is awake and active.

Many embolic strokes originate from a thrombus in the left chambers of the heart, formed during atrial fibrillation. These are referred to as cardiogenic *embolic strokes*. Emboli result when parts of the thrombus break off and are carried through the arterial system to the brain. Cerebral emboli may also be caused by carotid artery atherosclerotic plaque, bacterial endocarditis, recent myocardial infarction, rheumatic heart disease and ventricular aneurysm.

An embolic stroke has a sudden onset and causes immediate deficits. If the embolus breaks down and is absorbed by the body, manifestations will disappear in a few hours to a few days. If the embolus is not absorbed, manifestations will persist. Even if the embolus is absorbed, the vessel wall where the embolus lodges may be weakened, increasing the potential for cerebral haemorrhage.

Haemorrhagic stroke

A **haemorrhagic stroke**, or intracranial haemorrhage, occurs when a cerebral blood vessel ruptures. It occurs most often in people with sustained increase in systolic–diastolic blood pressure. Intracranial haemorrhage usually occurs suddenly, often when the affected person is engaged in some activity. Although hypertension is the most common cause, a variety of factors may contribute to a haemorrhagic stroke, including rupture of a brittle plaque-encrusted artery wall, ruptured intracranial aneurysms, trauma, erosion of blood vessels by tumours, arteriovenous malformations, anticoagulant therapy and blood disorders. Of all forms of stroke, this form is most often fatal and occurs in about 20% of all strokes (Cardiac Research Institute, 2022). There are two types of haemorrhagic strokes: intracerebral haemorrhage and subarachnoid haemorrhage. Haemorrhagic strokes that result from ruptured cerebral aneurysm or an arteriovenous malformation are discussed in the following sections of the chapter.

As a result of the blood vessel rupture, blood enters the brain tissue, the cerebral ventricles or the subarachnoid space, compressing adjacent tissues and causing blood vessel spasm and cerebral oedema. Blood in the ventricles or subarachnoid space irritates the meninges and brain tissue, causing an inflammatory reaction and impairing absorption and circulation of cerebrospinal fluid (CSF).

The onset of manifestations from a haemorrhagic stroke is rapid. Manifestations depend on the location of the haemorrhage, but may include vomiting, headache, seizures, hemiplegia and loss of consciousness. Pressure on the brain tissue from increased intracranial pressure (discussed in the chapter 'Nursing care of people with intracranial disorders') may cause coma and death.

MANIFESTATIONS Stroke by involved cerebral vessel

INTERNAL CAROTID ARTERY
- Contralateral paralysis of the arm, leg and face
- Contralateral sensory deficits of the arm, leg and face
- If the dominant hemisphere is involved: aphasia
- If the non-dominant hemisphere is involved: apraxia, agnosia, unilateral neglect
- Homonymous hemianopia

MIDDLE CEREBRAL ARTERY
- Drowsiness, stupor, coma
- Contralateral hemiplegia of the arm and face
- Contralateral sensory deficits of the arm and face
- Global aphasia (if dominant hemisphere involved)
- Homonymous hemianopia

ANTERIOR CEREBRAL ARTERY
- Contralateral weakness or paralysis of the foot and leg
- Contralateral sensory loss of the toes, foot and leg
- Loss of ability to make decisions or act voluntarily
- Urinary incontinence

VERTEBRAL ARTERY
- Pain in face, nose or eye
- Numbness and weakness of the face on involved side
- Problems with gait
- Dysphagia

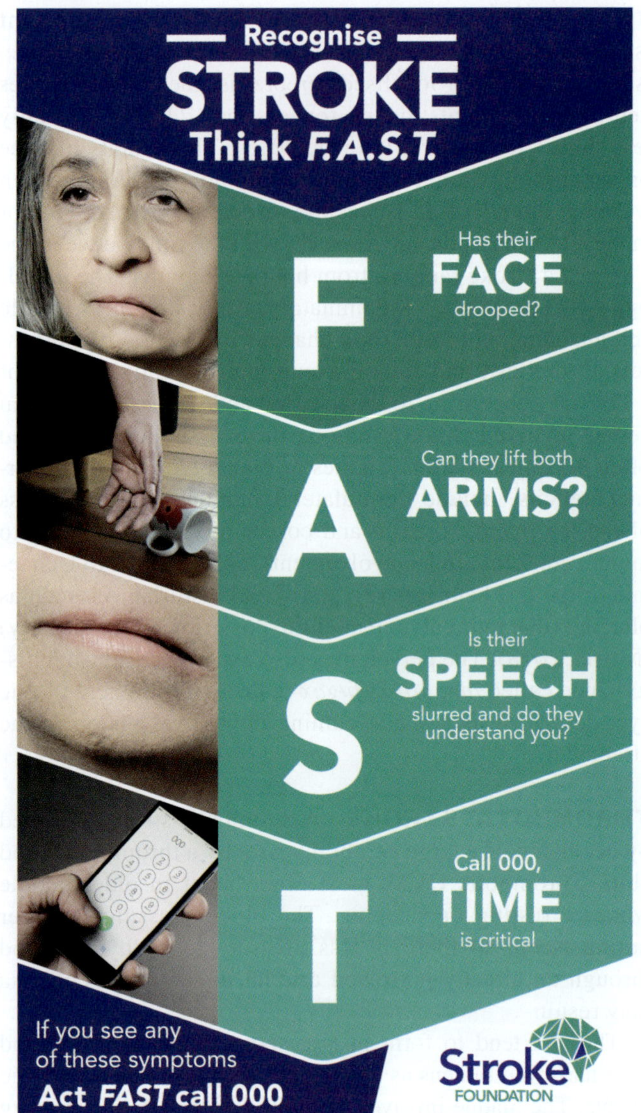

FIGURE 42.1 *Early warning signs of strokes*

Source: National Stroke Foundation (2017b). *Facts and figures about strokes*. Retrieved from https://strokefoundation.org.au/. Courtesy of strokefoundation.org.au.

Manifestations

Manifestations of a stroke vary according to the cerebral artery involved and the area of the brain affected. Manifestations are always sudden in onset, focal and usually one sided. The most common manifestation is weakness involving the face and arm, and sometimes the leg. Other common manifestations are numbness on one side, loss of vision, speech difficulties, a sudden severe headache and difficulties with balance. The various deficits associated with involvement of a specific cerebral artery are collectively referred to as stroke syndromes, although the deficits often overlap, as shown in the 'Manifestations' box.

Early warning signs of strokes are shown in Figure 42.1.

Complications

Typical complications include sensoriperceptual deficits, cognitive and behavioural changes, communication disorders, motor deficits and elimination disorders. These may be transient or permanent, depending on the degree of ischaemia and necrosis as well as time of treatment. As a result of the neurological deficits, the person with a stroke has complications that involve many different body systems (see the 'Manifestations and complications' box). The disabilities resulting from a stroke often cause serious alterations in functional health status.

Sensoriperceptual deficits

A stroke may involve pathological changes in neurological pathways that alter the ability to integrate, interpret and attend to sensory data. The person may experience deficits in vision, hearing, equilibrium, taste and sense of smell. The ability to perceive vibration, pain, warmth, cold and pressure may be impaired, as may proprioception (the body's sense of its position). The loss of these sensory abilities increases the risk of injury. Deficits may include:

- **hemianopia**—the loss of half of the visual field of one or both eyes; when the same half is missing in each eye, the condition is called *homonymous hemianopia* (see Figure 42.2)
- **agnosia**—the inability to recognise one or more subjects that were previously familiar; agnosia may be visual, tactile or auditory
- **apraxia**—the inability to carry out a motor pattern (e.g. drawing a figure, getting dressed) even when strength and coordination are adequate.

MANIFESTATIONS AND COMPLICATIONS Stroke by body system

INTEGUMENT
- Decubitus (pressure) ulcers

NEUROLOGICAL
- Hyperthermia
- Neglect syndrome
- Seizures
- Agnosias
- Communication deficits
  a. Expressive aphasia
  b. Receptive aphasia
  c. Global aphasia
  d. Agraphia
- Visual deficits
  a. Homonymous hemianopia
  b. Diplopia
  c. Decreased acuity
- Cognitive changes
  a. Memory loss
  b. Short attention span
  c. Distractibility
  d. Poor judgment
  e. Poor problem-solving ability
  f. Disorientation
- Behavioural changes
  a. Emotional lability
  b. Loss of social inhibitions
  c. Fear/Anxiety
  d. Hostility
  e. Anger
  f. Depression
- Increased intracranial pressure
- Alterations in consciousness
- Sensory loss (touch, pain, heat, cold, pressure)

RESPIRATORY
- Respiratory centre damage
- Airway obstruction
- Decreased ability to cough

GASTROINTESTINAL
- Dysphagia
- Constipation
- Stool impaction

GENITOURINARY
- Incontinence
- Frequency
- Urgency
- Urinary retention
- Renal calculi

MUSCULOSKELETAL
- Hemiplegia
- Contractures
- Bony ankylosis
- Disuse atrophy
- Dysarthria

Another form of sensory–perceptual deficit is the **neglect syndrome** (or *unilateral neglect*), in which the person has a disorder of attention. In this syndrome, the person cannot integrate and use perceptions from the affected side of the body or from the environment on the affected side and ignores that part. In severe cases, the person may even deny the paralysis. This deficit is more common following a stroke of the right hemisphere where damage to the parietal lobe (a centre for mediation of directed attention) results in perceptual deficits.

Pain and discomfort may accompany a stroke, with the person experiencing acute pain, numbness or strange sensations.

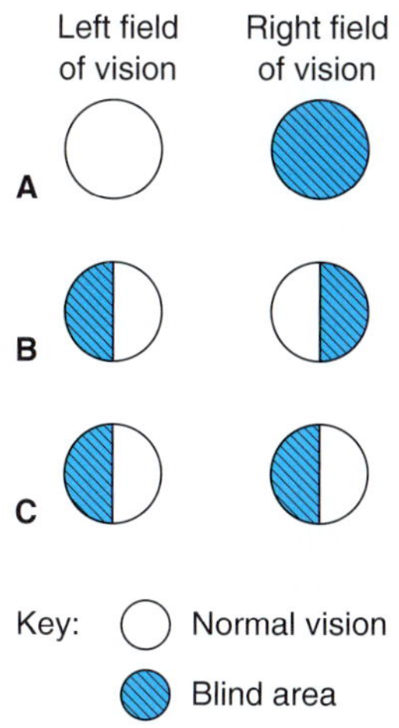

Left field of vision
Right field of vision
A
B
C
Key: Normal vision
Blind area

FIGURE 42.2 ***Abnormal visual fields. A, Normal left field of vision with loss of vision in right field. B, Loss of vision in temporal half of both fields (bitemporal hemianopia). C, Loss of vision in nasal field of right eye and temporal field of left eye (homonymous hemianopia)***

Although not common, damage to the thalamus may cause *central stroke pain*, or *central pain syndrome*. The pain in this syndrome includes hot and cold, burning, tingling and sharp stabbing pain, most often in the extremities. It is worsened by movement and temperature changes. The painful sensations are not relieved by pain medications, nor are there any specific treatments.

Cognitive and behavioural changes

A change in consciousness, ranging from mild confusion to coma, is a common manifestation of a stroke. It may result from tissue damage following ischaemia or haemorrhage involving either the carotid or the vertebral arteries. Altered consciousness may also be the result of cerebral oedema or increased intracranial pressure.

Behavioural changes include emotional lability (in which the person may laugh or cry inappropriately), loss of self-control (manifested by behaviour such as swearing or refusing to wear clothing) and decreased tolerance for stress (resulting in anger or depression). Intellectual changes may include memory loss, decreased attention span, poor judgment and an inability to think abstractly.

Communication disorders

Communication is a complex process, involving motor functions, speech, language, memory, reasoning and emotions. Communication disorders are usually the result of a stroke affecting the dominant hemisphere. The left hemisphere is dominant in about 95% of right-handed people and 70% of left-handed people (Norris, 2018).

Many different impairments may occur and most are partial. Disorders of communication affect both speech (the mechanical act of articulating language through the spoken word) and language (the vocal or written formulation of ideas to communicate thoughts and feelings). Language involves oral and written expression and auditory and reading comprehension. These disorders include:

- aphasia—the inability to use or understand language; aphasia may be expressive, receptive or mixed (global)
- expressive aphasia—a motor speech problem in which one can understand what is being said but can respond verbally only in short phrases; also called *Broca's aphasia*
- receptive aphasia—a sensory speech problem in which one cannot understand the spoken (and often written) word. Speech may be fluent but with inappropriate content; also called *Wernicke's aphasia*
- mixed or global aphasia—language dysfunction in both understanding and expression
- dysarthria—any disturbance in muscular control of speech.

Motor deficits

Body movement results from a complex interaction between the brain, spinal cord and peripheral nerves. The motor areas of the cerebral cortex, the basal ganglia and the cerebellum initiate voluntary movement by sending messages to the spinal cord, which then transmits the messages to the peripheral nerves. A stroke may interrupt the central nervous system (CNS) component of this relay system and produce effects in the contralateral side ranging from mild weakness to severe limitation of any kind of movement.

Depending on the area of the brain involved, strokes may cause weakness, paralysis and/or spasticity. The deficits include:

- **hemiplegia**—paralysis of the left or right half of the body (see Figure 42.3)
- **hemiparesis**—weakness of the left or right half of the body
- flaccidity—absence of muscle tone (hypotonia)
- spasticity—increased muscle tone (hypertonia), usually with some degree of weakness. The flexor muscles are usually more strongly affected in the upper extremities and the extensor muscles are more strongly affected in the lower extremities.

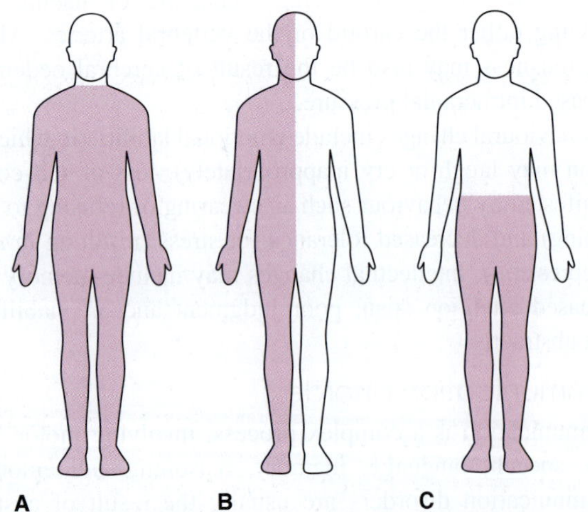

FIGURE 42.3 ***Types of paralysis. A, Quadriplegia is complete or partial paralysis of the upper extremities and complete paralysis of the lower part of the body. B, Hemiplegia is paralysis of one half of the body when it is divided along the median sagittal plane. C, Paraplegia is paralysis of the lower part of the body***

When the corticospinal tract is involved, the affected arm and leg almost always are initially flaccid and then become spastic within 6 to 8 weeks. Spasticity often causes characteristic body positioning: adduction of the shoulder, pronation of the forearm, flexion of the fingers and extension of the hip and knee. There is often foot drop, outward rotation of the leg and dependent oedema in the involved extremities.

The motor deficits may result in altered mobility, further impairing body function. The complications of immobility involve multiple body systems and include orthostatic hypotension, increased thrombus formation, decreased cardiac output, impaired respiratory function, osteoporosis, formation of renal calculi, contractures and decubitus ulcer formation.

Elimination disorders

Disorders of bladder and bowel elimination are common. A stroke may cause partial loss of the sensations that trigger bladder elimination, resulting in urinary frequency, urgency or incontinence. Control of urination may be altered as a result of cognitive deficits. Changes in bowel elimination are common, resulting from changes in level of consciousness (LOC), immobility and dehydration (Hickey, 2019).

INTERPROFESSIONAL CARE

The type of treatment a person with a stroke receives depends on the stage of the disease. In general, there are three treatment stages: stroke prevention, acute care immediately after a stroke and rehabilitation after a stroke. The person with an acute stroke may receive medical and/or surgical treatment. The focus in the acute care phase is on diagnosing the type and cause of the stroke, supporting cerebral circulation and controlling or preventing further deficits. The goals of stroke care are to minimise brain injury and maximise recovery. In Australia, it is recommended that a person suffering from a stroke is cared for in a specialist stroke unit where possible; these units have been shown to decrease morbidity and mortality rates (National Stroke Foundation, 2022e).

Diagnosis

Diagnosis begins with a complete history and careful physical assessment, including a thorough neurological examination. The time of the onset of stroke manifestations is a critical part of assessment. The National Institute of Health (NIH) Stroke Scale is a clinical evaluation tool widely used to assess neurological outcome and degree of recovery. Part of the Scale is detailed in Table 42.1. The tool measures LOC, vision, facial paralysis, motor abilities, ataxia, sensation, language and attention.

Imaging tests are used to identify an increased risk of a stroke or to identify pathophysiological changes after a stroke has occurred.

TABLE 42.1 NIH Stroke Scale: assessment of level of consciousness

INSTRUCTIONS	SCALE DEFINITION	SCORE
1a. *Level of consciousness (LOC)*: the investigator must choose a response, even if a full evaluation is prevented by such obstacles as an endotracheal tube, language barrier, orotracheal trauma/bandages. A 3 is scored only if the person makes no movement (other than reflexive posturing) in response to noxious stimulation.	0 = Alert, keenly responsive. 1 = Not alert, but arousable by minor stimulation to obey, answer or respond. 2 = Not alert, requires repeated stimulation to attend or is obtunded and requires strong or painful stimulation to make movements (not stereotyped). 3 = Responds only with reflex motor or autonomic effects or totally unresponsive, flaccid and flexic.	______
1b. *LOC questions*: the person is asked the month and their age. The answer must be correct. There is no partial credit for being close. Aphasic and stuporous people who do not comprehend the questions will score 2. People unable to speak because of endotracheal intubation, orotracheal trauma, severe dysarthria from any cause, language barrier or any other problem not secondary to aphasia are given a 1. It is important that only the initial answer be graded and that the examiner not 'help' the person with verbal or non-verbal cues.	0 = Answers both questions correctly. 1 = Answers one question correctly. 2 = Answers neither question correctly.	______
1c. *LOC commands*: the person is asked to open and close the eyes and then to grip and release the non-paretic hand. Substitute another one-step command if the hands cannot be used. Credit is given if an unequivocal attempt is made but not completed due to weakness. If the person does not respond to command, the task should be demonstrated to them (pantomime) and the results scored (i.e. follows none, one or two commands). A person with trauma, amputation or other physical impediments should be given suitable one-step commands. Only the first attempt is scored.	0 = Performs both tasks correctly. 1 = Performs one task correctly. 2 = Performs neither task correctly.	______

Note: This is a sample of only one part of the NIH Stroke Scale. The entire scale may be viewed at https://www.mdcalc.com/nih-stroke-scale-score-nihss

Computed tomography (CT) is the first imaging technique used to demonstrate the presence of haemorrhage, tumours, aneurysm, ischaemia, oedema and tissue necrosis. A CT scan can also demonstrate a shift in intracranial contents and is useful in distinguishing the type of stroke (e.g. a haemorrhagic stroke results in an increase in density). Cerebral infarctions usually are visible with a CT scan 6 to 8 hours post stroke; haemorrhage is visible immediately. Other imaging tests that may be used for diagnosis include cerebral arteriogram, transcranial Doppler ultrasound, MRI, MRA, PET and SPECT (see the 'Diagnostic tests' box in the chapter 'A person-centred approach to assessing the nervous system').

A lumbar puncture may be performed to obtain CSF for examination if there is no danger of increased intracranial pressure (ICP). (Removal of CSF when intracranial pressure is increased can result in herniation of the brainstem.) A thrombotic stroke may elevate CSF pressure; after a haemorrhagic stroke, frank blood may be seen in the CSF.

In addition to imaging tests, a blood test has recently been approved to screen for recurrent stroke risk. The PLAC test scans the blood for high levels of lipoprotein-associated phospholipase A2 (Lp-Pla2), found to be more common in a person who has had a stroke.

Medications

Medications are administered to prevent a stroke in a person with a TIA or a previous stroke and to treat the person during the acute phase of a stroke.

PREVENTION Antiplatelet agents are often used to treat a person with a TIA or who has had a previous stroke. Platelets are concentrated in arteries with a high blood flow where they adhere to endothelial tissue damaged by atherosclerosis and occlude the vessel. The drugs used to prevent clot formation and blood vessel occlusion include aspirin, clopidogrel (Plavix), dipyridamole (Persantine) and ticlopidine hydrochloride (Ticlopidine Hexal).

Daily low-dose aspirin reduces TIA occurrence and stroke risk by interfering with platelet aggregation. Ticlopidine hydrochloride is a platelet-aggregation inhibitor that has shown reduction in thrombotic stroke risk.

ACUTE STROKE Medications are used to treat the person during the acute phase of an ischaemic stroke to prevent further thrombosis formation, increase cerebral blood flow and protect cerebral neurons. The type of medication used varies according to the type of stroke.

Anticoagulant drug therapy (discussed in the chapter 'Nursing care of people with haematological disorders') is often ordered for an ischaemic stroke. The most commonly used anticoagulants are warfarin (Coumadin), heparin and enoxaparin (Clexane). Anticoagulants are never administered to a person with a haemorrhagic stroke. Anticoagulants do not dissolve an existing clot but prevent further extension of the clot and formation of new clots. Sodium heparin may be given subcutaneously or by continuous IV infusion, or warfarin sodium (Coumadin) may be given orally.

Fibrinolytic therapy, using a tissue plasminogen activator such as recombinant tissue plasminogen activator alteplase (rt-PA, tPA), sometimes given concurrently with an anticoagulant, is used to treat thrombotic stroke. The drug converts plasminogen to plasmin, resulting in fibrinolysis of the clot. To be effective, it must be given intravenously as soon as possible after the onset of manifestations, after confirming (with a CT scan) that the person has had an ischaemic stroke. Within Australia, current guidelines state the drug must be given within 4.5 hours of onset of symptoms (National Stroke Foundation, 2017a). Antithrombotic drugs, which inhibit the platelet phase of clot formation, have been used as a preventive measure for the person at risk of embolic and thrombotic CVA. Both aspirin and dipyridamole have been used for this purpose. These drugs are sometimes also used in combination with other drugs during acute treatment. Antiplatelet agents are contraindicated in the person with a haemorrhagic stroke.

Management of hypertension is controversial but if the person is eligible for fibrinolytic therapy, blood pressure control is essential to decrease the risk of bleeding. If the blood pressure is sustained at levels 185 mmHg systolic or 110 diastolic, the person cannot be treated with IV tPA (National Stroke Foundation, 2017a).

Corticosteroids, such as prednisone or dexamethasone, have been used to treat cerebral oedema, but the results are not always positive. If the person has an increased ICP, hyperosmolar solutions (such as mannitol) or diuretics (such as frusemide) may be administered. Anticonvulsants, such as phenytoin (Dilantin), and barbiturates may be prescribed if increased ICP causes seizures. Increased ICP is discussed in the chapter 'Nursing care of people with intracranial disorders'.

Treatments

The treatments used in the management of a stroke include surgery and rehabilitation.

SURGERY Surgery may be performed to prevent the occurrence of a stroke, to restore blood flow when a stroke has already occurred or to repair vascular damage or malformations. A carotid endarterectomy at the carotid artery bifurcation may be performed to remove atherosclerotic plaque in the person who has suffered a TIA (see Figure 42.4). Nursing care for the person in the initial postoperative period following a carotid endarterectomy is described in the accompanying box.

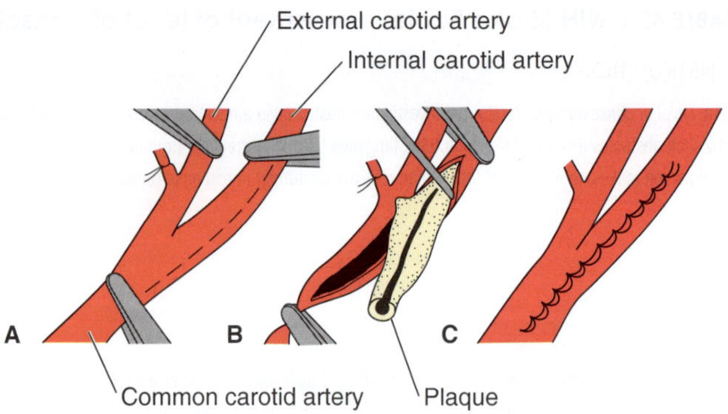

FIGURE 42.4 ***Carotid endarterectomy. A, The occluded area is clamped off and an incision is made in the artery. B, Plaque is removed from the inner layer of the artery. C, To restore blood flow through the artery, the artery is sutured or a graft is completed***

When an occluded or stenotic vessel is not directly accessible, an extracranial–intracranial bypass may be performed. Bypass of the internal carotid, middle cerebral or vertebral arteries may be required. The indications for the bypass are manifestations of ischaemia caused by TIAs or a mild completed stroke. The procedure re-establishes blood flow to the affected area of the brain.

A carotid angioplasty with stenting is a newer option for treating cerebral stenosis. During the procedure an angioplasty balloon catheter is inserted through an artery in the person's arm or leg. Under fluoroscopy, the catheter is advanced to the area of carotid artery stenosis and a small filter is inserted to catch any clots or pieces of debris that might break loose. The balloon is then inflated to widen the artery, followed by insertion of a permanent stent in the area of the angioplasty.

NURSING CARE OF THE PERSON having a carotid endarterectomy

POSTOPERATIVE CARE

- Position on the unoperated side and either maintain a flat position or elevate the head of the bed 30 degrees as prescribed. Maintain head and neck alignment and avoid rotating, flexing or hyperextending the head. *Pressure on the wound is undesirable. Elevating the head decreases oedema in the operative site. Maintaining head and neck alignment prevents additional tension or pressure on the operative side.*
- Support the head when changing position. Teach to support the head with the hands when able to move about. *Supporting the head helps prevent stress on the operative site (which may cause bleeding and haematoma formation); it also helps reduce stress on the suture line.*
- Perform focused assessments to monitor for complications:
  a. *Haemorrhage*. Assess the dressing and the area under the neck and shoulders for drainage. Assess for increased pulse and decreased blood pressure. *The most common cause of respiratory problems is pressure on the trachea from a haematoma formation.*
  b. *Respiratory distress*. Assess respiratory rate, rhythm, depth and effort. Observe for restlessness. Keep a tracheostomy tray at the bedside. *Respiratory distress may result from oedema and haematoma formation, which may compress the trachea.*
  c. *Cranial nerve impairment*. Observe and record any facial drooping, tongue deviation, hoarseness, dysphagia or loss of facial sensation. *Cranial nerves may be stretched during surgery, leading to temporary deficits in cranial nerve function.*
  d. *Hypertension or hypotension*. Take and record blood pressure at least hourly. Report any changes immediately and implement orders for medications to treat hypertension or hypotension. *About one-half of all people having a carotid endarterectomy develop unstable blood pressure related to surgical denervation of the carotid sinus. Uncontrolled hypertension may precipitate a CVA. The most common problem is hypotension, possibly related to stimulation of the carotid body baroreceptors, which are exposed during surgery. Hypotension may result in myocardial ischaemia.*

REHABILITATION Various types of therapy are necessary for post-stroke rehabilitation. Listed below are the types and goals of therapies used:

- Physiotherapy may help prevent contractures and improve muscle strength and coordination. Physiotherapists teach exercises to enable the person to relearn how to walk, sit, lie down and change from one type of movement to another.
- Occupational therapy provides assistive devices and a plan for regaining lost motor skills that greatly improve quality of life after a stroke. These skills include eating, drinking, bathing, cooking, reading, writing and toileting.
- Speech therapy is provided to help the person relearn language and communication skills, as well as improve swallowing.

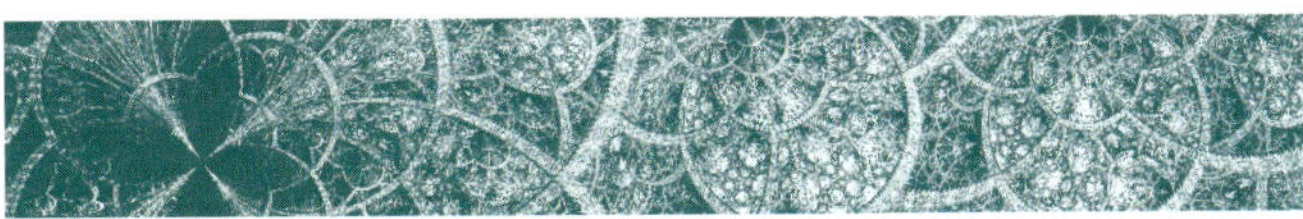

Nursing care

Even though many people who have a stroke recover fully, a substantial number are left with disabilities that affect their physical, emotional, interpersonal and family status. The required nursing care is often complex and multidimensional, requiring consideration of continuity of care for the person in acute care settings, long-term care settings, rehabilitation centres and the home.

Nurses caring for people who have had a stroke require knowledge and skills to meet their needs during both the acute and the rehabilitative phases of care. The person may have multiple losses: loss of mobility, ability to provide self-care, communications, concept of self and interpersonal or intimate relationships with others. Holistic, individualised nursing care is essential in all settings and focuses on promoting the achievement of maximum potential and quality of life.

The person's family is often faced with many changes. The young to middle-aged adult with a family member who has had a stroke may be faced with economic difficulties and social isolation. The middle-aged adult family member may become the caretaker for an older parent—in essence, switching roles with the parent. An older adult may not be able to care for a spouse and may have to accept residential care placement. In addition, the older adult who has no family may have to struggle alone to regain the ability to function independently. Although not all of these problems are amenable to nursing solutions, the nurse is most often the healthcare provider who assesses and identifies the needs of each individual and provides information and referrals to the person and families to help meet those needs.

Because a stroke has the potential to cause many different health problems, a wide variety of nursing diagnoses may be appropriate. It is important to remember that each person will be affected differently, depending on the degree of ischaemia and the area of the brain involved. Nursing diagnoses discussed in this section focus on problems with cerebral tissue perfusion (specific to nursing care during the acute phase), physical mobility, self-care, communication, sensory–perceptual deficits, bowel and urine elimination, and swallowing (specific to prevention of complications and rehabilitation). See the accompanying nursing care plan for a person with a stroke.

Health promotion

Health promotion activities focus on stroke prevention, especially for the person with known risk factors. It is important to discuss, as appropriate, the importance of stopping smoking and drug use with people of all ages. Maintaining a normal weight through diet and exercise can help reduce obesity, which increases the risk of hypertension and type 2 diabetes mellitus. (Both, in turn, increase the risk of a stroke.) Cholesterol levels should be screened regularly to monitor for hyperlipidaemia. Regular healthcare to monitor for and treat cardiovascular disorders and to detect and treat infections such as infective endocarditis is important. It is also important to increase public

NURSING CARE PLAN A person with a stroke

Phillip Boren is a 63-year-old male who had a stroke due to right cerebral thrombosis 1 week ago. He is a history teacher at the local high school. His hobbies are wood carving and gardening. For the past 2 years, Mr Boren has been taking medication for hypertension, but his wife Emily reports that he often forgets to take it and that his blood pressure was high at his last physical examination. Mrs Boren tells the staff that she has never had to worry about her husband's health before and that she wants to learn everything she can to care for him at home. However, she says that her husband was always the one to make the decisions and pay the bills. Mrs Boren adds that all the children, grandchildren and neighbours want to see Mr Boren back at home as soon as possible.

ASSESSMENT

Carol Merck, RN, the nurse assigned to Mr Boren, completes a health history and physical assessment, with Mrs Boren providing information for the history. Mrs Boren reports that her husband did have several spells of dizziness and blurred vision the week before his stroke, but they lasted only a few minutes and he believed them to be due to 'old age and working out in the sun'. On the morning of admission, Mr Boren woke up and could not move his left arm or leg; he also could not speak sensibly. Mrs Boren called 000 and an ambulance took her husband to the hospital.

Physical assessment findings include the following: Mr Boren is drowsy but responds to verbal stimuli. Although he does not respond verbally, he can nod his head to indicate 'yes' when asked questions. Flaccid paralysis is present in his left arm and left leg, with no response noted to touch in those extremities. (He is left-handed.) Visual fields are decreased in a pattern consistent with homonymous hemianopia. A CT scan, negative on admission, is repeated on the day after

(continued)

NURSING CARE PLAN A person with a stroke (continued)

admission and confirms the medical diagnosis of a right-brain stroke due to a thrombus of the middle cerebral artery.

Mr Boren's medical treatment includes heparin sodium administered by continuous intravenous drip, with clotting studies to be performed every 4 hours and the dose adjusted accordingly.

DIAGNOSES

- *Risk of feeding self-care deficit* related to loss of the ability to use the left hand and arm and manifested by a failure to feed self.
- *Risk of impaired physical mobility* related to neurological deficits causing left hemiplegia and manifested by difficulty mobilising.
- *Risk of impaired skin integrity* related to inability to change position and manifested by the development of pressure area sores.
- *Risk of disturbed visual sensory perception* related to changes in visual fields and manifested by difficulty in performing activities of daily living (ADLs).
- *Risk of impaired verbal communication* related to cerebral injury and manifested by slurred or incoherent speech.

PLANNING

- Arrange mealtimes so that Mr Boren is sitting up by the window in a clean and private environment.
- Encourage Mrs Boren to visit at mealtimes, to assist with meals and periodically to bring a favourite food from home.
- Establish and maintain a regular schedule for turning when Mr Boren is in bed.
- Ensure marker and paper or electronic devices are available for alternative communication.

Expected outcomes

- Learn to use his right hand to feed himself.
- Participate in exercises necessary to maintain muscle strength and tone.
- Maintain skin integrity.
- Indicate understanding that visual fields may improve in a few weeks.
- Practise and implement speech therapy activities while at the same time using alternative methods of communication.

IMPLEMENTATION

- Provide adaptive devices (silverware with thick handles and non-slip plates).
- Provide passive ROM exercises for his left arm and leg; schedule active ROM exercises for his right extremities, as well as quadriceps and gluteal sets every 4 hours during waking hours.
- Keep his skin clean and dry at all times.
- Place objects (e.g. call bell, tissues) on unaffected side and approach him from that side.
- Support attempts to communicate verbally; when he is not understood, he may prefer to use a large marker and tablet.

EVALUATION

Mr Boren is discharged to his home after being in the hospital for 10 days. During the first 2 months after discharge, Martha Grimes, RN, the community health nurse, visits Mr and Mrs Boren at home. At the end of 2 months, Mr Boren is using his right hand to feed himself. He has regained partial use of his left arm and leg and is using a walker to move around the house and yard; he is even able to work in his flower garden. His skin has remained intact and his vision is back to normal. He is slowly relearning speech; this has been the most difficult change for him to accept.

CRITICAL THINKING IN THE NURSING PROCESS

1. Hypertension is sometimes referred to as 'the silent killer'. Provide justifications for this statement.
2. What would be your reply if, after you had completed passive ROM on Mr Boren's left arm, he wrote: 'I just ignore that part of my body—it doesn't work anyway.'?
3. Which communication and education strategies would you implement to assist Mr Boren and his family?

REFLECTION ON THE NURSING PROCESS

1. Reflecting on your experience with people who have suffered a stroke, which allied team members should become involved in Mr Boren's care? Why?
2. What information could you provide to Mr Boren's wife to assist her when Mr Boren is discharged home?

awareness of the signs of a TIA or stroke, and of the need to call 000 or mobile 112, or to seek immediate medical care if the following warning signs or symptoms suddenly occur:

- weakness or numbness of the face, arm or leg, especially on one side of the body
- confusion, difficulty speaking or understanding speech
- trouble walking, dizziness, loss of coordination
- difficulty with vision in one or both eyes
- severe headache without a cause.

Information about public awareness of stroke manifestations and the need for immediate treatment are discussed in the 'Translation to practice' box.

Assessment

The following data is collected through the health history and physical examination (see the chapter 'A person-centred approach to assessing the nervous system'). Further focused assessments are described with nursing interventions. Gender-specific questions are required to assess risk factors for stroke; risk factors are different for men and women (see the 'Meeting individualised needs' box).

- *Health history*: risk factors, previous stroke, drug use (prescribed, over-the-counter, street drugs), smoking history, when manifestations began, severity of manifestations, presence of incontinence, LOC, family support system.
- *Physical assessment*: LOC, motor strength, coordination, communication, cranial nerves, sensory function.

Nursing diagnoses and interventions

The acute phase of a stroke is most often the time from admission to the hospital until the person is stabilised, usually 24 to 72 hours after admission (Hickey, 2019). Depending on the severity of the

TRANSLATION TO PRACTICE Evidence-based practice: improved rapid treatment of a stroke

Stroke is the third leading cause of death in Australia and is also a leading cause of severe, long-term disability (ABS, 2020). The risk of disability and death can be reduced in people who experience a sudden ischaemic stroke by the administration of tissue plasminogen activator (tPA). To be effective, tPA must be administered within 4.5 hours of the warning signs of a stroke, but the public's awareness of stroke manifestations and of the need for immediate treatment remains poor. In Australia, 39% of people presenting to hospital with a stroke arrive within 3 hours; however, only 3% of all ischaemic stroke victims receive thrombolytic therapy (National Stroke Foundation, 2017a). Further emphasis on achieving higher rates of thrombolytic treatment is required to improve morbidity and mortality rates.

IMPLICATIONS FOR NURSING

Nurses provide information to the public in a wide variety of health promotion activities, including stroke awareness and the need for immediate treatment to ensure the best outcomes of care. It is important that the programs be geared towards the specific population most at risk as well as people from all socioeconomic and cultural backgrounds. Factors that affect behaviour, such as perceived risk, benefits and barriers of care, readiness to change and self-efficacy, are areas that may be effective in designing educational programs to increase stroke awareness.

CRITICAL THINKING IN PERSON CARE

1. If you were planning a stroke awareness education program, how would you implement it in order to reach the largest population? How would you advertise stroke warning signs to reach the most people?
2. Think of a slogan for the public that increases awareness of the 4.5-hour time limit for treatment with tPA.

MEETING INDIVIDUALISED NEEDS

Risk factors for stroke in women

Some risk factors for stroke apply only to women—most specifically pregnancy, childbirth and menopause. These risks are the result of fluctuations in hormones that occur at different stages of life. However, other risks are also more common for women and information should be collected during a health history. For accurate assessment, ask the following questions, depending on the woman's age:

- How many pregnancies have you had?
- Have you had a miscarriage? If so, how many?
- How many births have you had? When was your last delivery?
- When was your last menstrual cycle?
- Do you take any type of hormone replacement therapy?
- Do you take birth control pills?
- Do you have migraine headaches? If so, do you have an aura?
- Have you ever been diagnosed with diabetes or lupus?
- Have you ever been diagnosed with a clotting disorder? Have you ever had a clot in your leg?

stroke, the person may be admitted to the intensive care unit. Regardless of the hospital setting, the nurse provides interventions to maintain body functions and prevent complications.

Ineffective tissue perfusion: cerebral

The initial assessment and care of the person admitted for intensive care focuses on identifying changes that may indicate altered cerebral perfusion. The person's airway, breathing, circulation and neurological status are monitored, and interventions are provided to maintain cerebral perfusion.

- Monitor respiratory status and airway patency. Auscultate pulmonary sounds and monitor respiratory rate and results of arterial blood gas studies.
- Suction as necessary, using care to suction no longer than 10 seconds at any one time and using sterile technique.
- Place in a side-lying position.
- Administer oxygen as prescribed.
  The person is often unconscious and breathing may be impaired. Suctioning removes secretions that not only obstruct airflow but also pose a risk of aspiration and pneumonia. Suctioning for longer than 10 seconds at a time may increase intracranial pressure (Hickey, 2019). Respiratory complications develop rapidly, as manifested by crackles and wheezes, rapid respirations and respiratory acidosis. The administration of oxygen decreases the risk of hypoxia and hypercapnia, which can increase cerebral ischaemia and intracranial pressure.

CONSIDERATION FOR PRACTICE

Positioning the person on the side allows secretions to drain out of the mouth, helping to prevent aspiration.

- Monitor mental status and use the LOC assessment in the Glasgow Coma Scale: restlessness, drowsiness, lethargy, inability to follow commands, unresponsiveness.
- Monitor strength and reflexes and assess for pain, headache, decreased muscle strength, sluggish pupillary reflexes, absent gag or swallowing reflexes, hemiplegia, Babinski's sign and decerebrate or decorticate posturing. *Frequent monitoring of neurological status is necessary to detect changes. Alterations in mental status, LOC, movement, strength and reflexes indicate increased intracranial pressure, the main cause of death in the acute phase of a stroke.*
- Continuously monitor cardiac status, observing for arrhythmias. *A stroke may cause cardiac arrhythmias, including bradycardia, PVCs (premature ventricular contractions), tachycardia and AV block. Characteristic ECG changes include a shortened PR interval, peaked T waves and a depressed ST segment.*

- Monitor body temperature. *Hyperthermia may develop if the hypothalamus is affected.*
- Maintain accurate intake and output records; measure urinary output via a Foley catheter. *A stroke may damage the pituitary gland, resulting in diabetes insipidus and the possibility of dehydration from greatly increased urinary output.*

CONSIDERATION FOR PRACTICE

Diabetes insipidus is indicated by a large output of dilute urine; dehydration is indicated by scanty amounts of dark, concentrated urine.

- Monitor for seizures. Pad the side rails and administer prescribed anticonvulsants. *Seizures may be the result of cerebral tissue damage or increased intracranial pressure. Padded side rails prevent injury if a seizure occurs. Anticonvulsants prevent or treat seizures.*

Impaired physical mobility

The goals of care for the person with impaired mobility are to maintain and improve functional abilities (by maintaining normal function and alignment, preventing oedema of extremities and reducing spasticity) and to prevent complications.

- Encourage active range-of-motion (ROM) exercises for unaffected extremities and perform passive ROM exercises for affected extremities every 4 hours during day and evening shifts, and once during the night shift. Support the joint during passive ROM exercises. *Active ROM exercises maintain or improve muscle strength and endurance and help to maintain cardiopulmonary function. Passive ROM exercises do not strengthen muscles but do help maintain joint flexibility.*

CONSIDERATION FOR PRACTICE

Both active and passive exercises increase venous return, decreasing the risk of thrombophlebitis.

- Turn every 2 hours around the clock, following a posted schedule for side-to-side and supine-to-prone position changes. (Verify prone positioning with the doctor.) Maintain body alignment and support extremities in proper position with pillows. *Turning on a regular basis, accompanied by proper positioning, maintains joint function, alleviates pressure on bony prominences that can lead to skin breakdown, decreases dependent oedema in hands and feet, and lessens the risk of complications resulting from immobility* (see Figure 42.5).

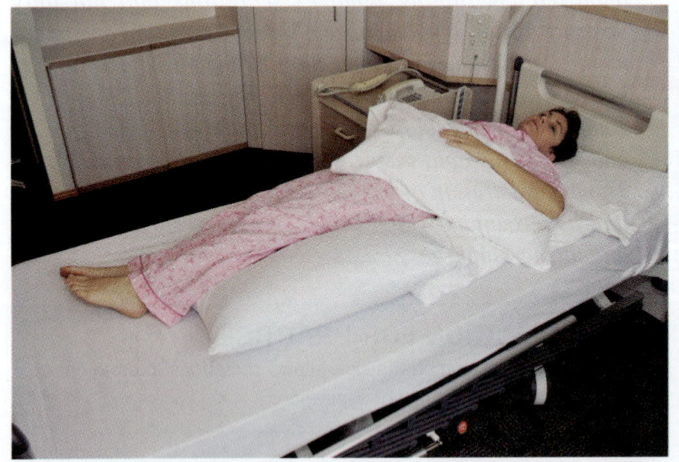
A

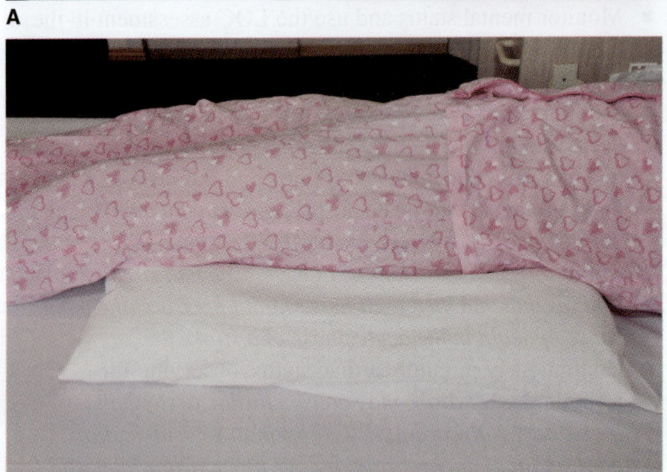
B

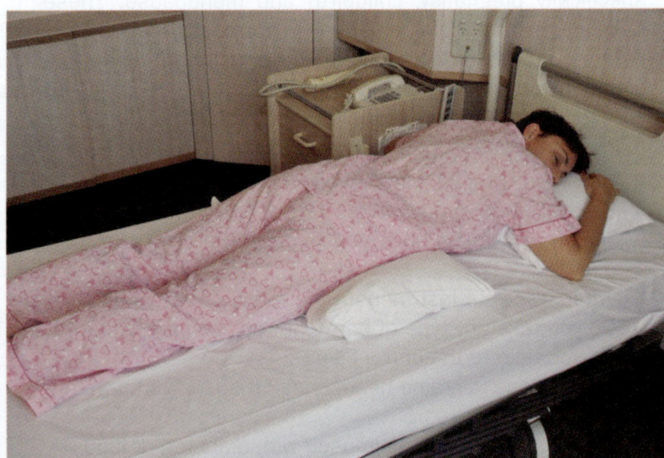
C

FIGURE 42.5 ***Positioning the person with hemiplegia is important in preventing deformity of the affected extremities. A, With the person in a supine position, place a pillow in the axilla (to prevent adduction) and under the hand and arm, with the hand higher than the elbow (to prevent flexion and oedema). B, When the person is lying supine, use a pillow from the iliac crest to the middle of the thigh to prevent external rotation of the hip. C, When the person is in the prone position, place a pillow under the pelvis to promote hip hyperextension***

Source: Courtesy of Trudy Dwyer.

CONSIDERATION FOR PRACTICE

When lying on the affected side, the person may be restless because they do not have normal sensation and feel as if they may fall.

- Monitor the lower extremities each shift for symptoms of thrombophlebitis. Assess for increased warmth and redness in calves; measure the circumference of the calves and thighs. *People on bed rest (especially those with loss of muscle strength and tone) are particularly prone to the development of deep venous thrombosis. Promptly report manifestations of thrombophlebitis.*
- Collaborate with the physiotherapist as the person gains mobility, using consistent techniques to move the person from the bed to the wheelchair and to help the person ambulate. *The use of consistent techniques facilitates rehabilitation.*

Self-care deficit

The person who has had a stroke may have a self-care deficit as a result of impaired mobility or mental confusion. It is important for the person to perform as many of their own ADLs as possible to promote functional ability, increase independence, decrease feelings of powerlessness and improve self-esteem.

Before establishing a plan to increase self-care, determine which hand was dominant before the stroke. If the person's dominant side is affected, self-care will be more difficult.

- Encourage use of the unaffected arm to bathe, brush teeth, comb hair, dress and eat. *Use of the unaffected arm promotes functional ability and independence.*
- Teach the person to put on clothing by first dressing the affected extremities and then dressing the unaffected extremities. *This technique facilitates self-dressing with minimal assistance.*
- Collaborate with the occupational therapist in scheduling times for training for upper extremity functioning necessary for ADLs. Encourage the use of assistive devices (if required) for eating, physical hygiene and dressing. *Following a regular schedule in daily routines promotes learning. The use of assistive devices promotes independence and decreases feelings of powerlessness. Optimal grooming facilitates positive self-concept.*

Impaired verbal communication

The person who loses communication abilities requires intensive speech therapy and emotional support. It is important to determine the specific nature of the impairment when planning interventions and helping family members understand specific problems. Although the speech therapist is usually most involved with speech rehabilitation, nurses must plan interventions to meet communication needs during all phases of care. Use the following guidelines:

- Approach and treat the person as an adult.
- Do not assume that the person who does not respond verbally cannot hear. Do not use a raised voice when addressing the person.
- Allow adequate time for the person to respond.
- Face the person and speak slowly.
- When you do not understand the person's speech, be honest and say so.
- Use short, simple statements and questions.
  Accepting the person and providing dignity and respect enhances the nurse–person relationship. Allowing adequate response time and using short verbal statements or questions while facing the person motivates the person to communicate and decreases frustration.
- Accept frustration and anger as a normal reaction to the loss of function. *Anger represents the person's frustration at the inability to control the loss of function.*
- Try alternative methods of communication, including writing tablets, flash cards and computerised talking boards. *The person who is unable to communicate verbally may use other methods effectively.*

Risk of impaired urinary elimination and constipation

Both urinary and bowel elimination may be altered because of neurological deficits, impaired mobility, cognitive impairment, communication deficits or pre-existing problems (especially if the person is an older adult). Other causes include changes in food and fluid intake and side effects of medications. Urinary incontinence or retention, and constipation and faecal impaction are the usual manifestations.

- Assess for urinary frequency, urgency, incontinence, nocturia and voiding in small amounts. In addition, assess the person's ability to respond to the need to void, to use the call light and to use toileting equipment.

CONSIDERATION FOR PRACTICE

Voiding small amounts of urine frequently may be a manifestation of a bladder dysfunction. Assess for a distended bladder.

- Encourage bladder training by having the person void on schedule, such as every 2 hours, rather than in response to the urge to void.
- Educate the person about Kegel exercises. To perform Kegel exercises, the person contracts the perineal muscles as though stopping urination, holds the contraction for 5 seconds and then releases.
- Use positive reinforcement (verbal praise) for successful management of urinary elimination.
  Voiding every 2 hours or on schedule promotes bladder tone and urine storage. Kegel exercises increase pubococcygeal muscle tone and bladder control, decreasing incontinence. Positive reinforcement can be a useful part of the teaching program.
- Discuss pre-stroke bowel habits, as well as the pattern of bowel elimination since the stroke.
- If the person is able to swallow without difficulty, encourage fluids (up to 2,000 mL per day) and a high-fibre diet.
- Increase physical activity as tolerated.
- Assist in using the toilet facilities at the same time each day (based on usual patterns of bowel elimination), ensuring privacy and having the person sit in an upright position if at all possible.

- Administer prescribed stool softeners if the person is following a bowel elimination routine or is not drinking sufficient fluids.
  Increased fluids, fibre and activity stimulate intestinal motility. Establishing a regular daily time for bowel movements in the upright position and in privacy promotes normal bowel elimination. Stool softeners help prevent the formation of hard stool that is more difficult to expel.

Impaired swallowing

A stroke may impair the ability to swallow. Weakness or lack of coordination of the tongue, attention deficits and deficits involving the swallowing reflex all play a role. Dysphagia (difficulty swallowing) may result in choking, drooling, aspiration or regurgitation. Nursing care focuses on maintaining safety by preventing aspiration and on ensuring adequate nutrition.

- Monitor results of swallowing studies prior to providing oral food and fluids. The speech therapist should be consulted to assess the person for the most appropriate diet.
- Ensure safety when eating:
  - Position in upright sitting position with neck slightly flexed.
  - Order puréed or soft food. Liquids should be of the same consistency as honey.
  - Feed or teach the person to eat by putting food behind the front teeth on the unaffected side of mouth and tilting the head slightly backwards. Teach to swallow one bite at a time.
  - Assess for coughing with eating or drinking. *Coughing may be indicative of dysphagia.*
  - Have suction equipment available at the bedside in case of choking or aspiration.

  Sitting upright with the head and neck first slightly flexed and then tilted back helps the person swallow. The person can usually swallow puréed or soft foods more easily than liquid or solid foods. Using the unaffected side of the mouth helps prevent food from collecting in the mouth and makes swallowing safer; in addition, food is less likely to fall out of the mouth.

> **CONSIDERATION FOR PRACTICE**
> **After eating, check the mouth for 'pocketing' of food, especially in the affected cheek.**

- Monitor lung sounds. *Coarse lung sounds heard in the right upper and/or lower lobes may indicate aspiration as the right bronchus is the first division of the bronchi and where the majority of aspirations occur.*
- Minimise distractions and, if necessary, give step-by-step instructions for eating. *Distractions increase the risk of aspiration. Complex activities are easier to perform when broken down into small steps.*

Community-based care

Throughout the rehabilitation process, it is important to encourage self-care as much as possible but also to involve family members in the plan of care. Stress that ADLs may take twice as long as they did before the stroke. Emphasise that physical function may continue to improve for up to 3 months and speech may continue to improve for even longer. Address the following topics in preparing the person and family for community-based care:

- physical care, medications, physiotherapy, occupational therapy, speech therapy
- realistic expectations
- time off for the caregiver; respite care services
- distributors for equipment and supplies
- home environment conducive to using equipment (e.g. a wheelchair or walker)
- home and equipment modifications (e.g. a raised toilet seat, grab bars in the bathroom, a bath chair, a vice lid opener, a long-handled shoehorn)
- home health services
- community resources, such as Meals on Wheels, senior centres, elder care, large-print telephone buttons, stroke clubs, VitalCall (emergency alerting systems through a local hospital or agency). Financial assistance may be available within the community for housekeeping and personal care assistance
- helpful organisations:
  - Stroke Foundation (with state branches): https://strokefoundation.org.au/
  - Stroke Society of Australasia: https://www.strokesociety.com.au
  - Stroke Association of the ACT: (02) 6269 2636
  - Stroke Association of Queensland (Telephone Peer Support): 1800 673 074
  - Stroke Association of Victoria: http://www.strokeassociation.com.au/
  - StrokeLine: 1800 787 653
  - Stroke Recovery Association of NSW: http://www.strokensw.org.au/
  - The Hospital Research Foundation Group—Stroke (SA): https://www.stroke.org.au.

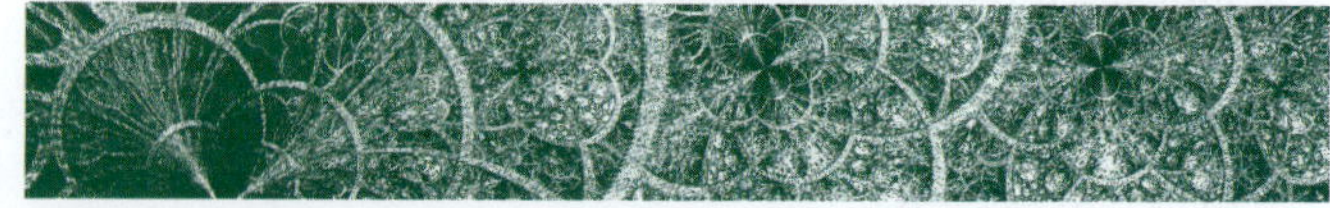

THE PERSON WITH AN INTRACRANIAL ANEURYSM

An **intracranial aneurysm** is a saccular outpouching of a cerebral artery that occurs at the site of a weakness in the vessel wall. The weakness may be the result of atherosclerosis, a congenital defect, trauma to the head, ageing or hypertension. A ruptured cerebral aneurysm is the most common cause of a haemorrhagic stroke.

Incidence and prevalence

Studies suggest the average prevalence of intracranial aneurysms is around 2% of the population; most go through life without any manifestations of bleeding. However, it is estimated that 50–80% of these will never rupture (Brain Aneurysm

Foundation, 2022). Intracranial aneurysms are most common in adults aged 30 to 60 (Hickey, 2019).

The exact aetiology is unknown, but theories of cause include: (1) a developmental defect in the vessel wall, and (2) degeneration or fragility of the vessel wall due to conditions such as hypertension, atherosclerosis, connective tissue disease or abnormal blood flow. Hypertension and cigarette smoking may be contributing factors.

Pathophysiology

Intracranial aneurysms tend to occur at the bifurcations and branches of the carotid arteries, and the vertebrobasilar arteries at the circle of Willis, with most aneurysms (85%) located anteriorly. They range in size from smaller than 15 mm to larger than 50 mm. Intracranial aneurysms tend to enlarge with time, making the vessel wall thin and increasing the probability of rupture.

There are several different types of intracranial aneurysms. A *berry aneurysm* is probably the result of a congenital abnormality of the tunica media of the artery. The aneurysm usually ruptures without warning. A *saccular aneurysm* is any aneurysm with a saccular outpouching which distends only a small portion of the vessel wall. This type of aneurysm is often caused by trauma. In a *fusiform aneurysm*, the entire circumference of a blood vessel swells to form an elongated tube. Most aneurysms of this type occur as a result of the changes of arteriosclerosis. Fusiform aneurysms act as space-occupying lesions. In a *dissecting aneurysm*, the tunica intima pulls away from the tunica media of the artery and blood is forced between the two layers. It may result from atherosclerosis, inflammation or trauma. *Mycotic aneurysms* are caused by emboli from infections such as bacterial endocarditis.

Intracranial aneurysms typically rupture from the dome rather than the base, forcing blood into the subarachnoid space at the base of the brain. The aneurysm may also rupture and force blood into brain tissue, the ventricles or the subdural space. This discussion focuses on intracranial haemorrhages due to rupture of a cerebral aneurysm. See the chapter 'Nursing care of people with intracranial disorders' for further discussion of types of intracranial bleeding and haematomas.

Manifestations

An intracranial aneurysm is usually asymptomatic until it ruptures, although very large aneurysms may cause headache and/or neurological deficits due to pressure on adjacent intracranial structures. Small leakages of blood may occur periodically, causing headache, nausea, vomiting and pain in the neck and back. The person may also have prodromal manifestations before the rupture occurs, such as headache, eye pain, visual deficits and a dilated pupil.

The manifestations of a ruptured intracranial aneurysm (and subsequent subarachnoid haemorrhage) include a sudden, explosive headache; loss of consciousness; nausea and vomiting; a stiff neck and photophobia (due to meningeal irritation); cranial nerve deficits; stroke syndrome manifestations; and pituitary malfunctions (that result primarily from changes in ADH secretion).

The severity of the rupture is often inferred from the manifestations of the subarachnoid haemorrhage. The Hunt–Hess classification of subarachnoid manifestations is frequently used to classify non-traumatic subarachnoid haemorrhages. The grades of severity are:

- grade 1—asymptomatic or minimal headache and slight neck rigidity
- grade 2—moderate to severe headache, neck rigidity, cranial nerve deficits
- grade 3—drowsy, lethargic, mild neurological deficits
- grade 4—stuporous, moderate to severe hemiparesis, early decerebrate rigidity
- grade 5—deep coma, decerebrate rigidity, moribund appearance.

Fibrin and platelets seal off the bleeding point, but the escaped blood forms a clot that irritates the brain tissue. The resulting inflammatory response causes cerebral oedema and both the oedema and the haemorrhage increase intracranial pressure (Hickey, 2019). Bleeding into the subarachnoid space causes meningeal irritation. Hypothalamic dysfunction and seizures are also potential complications.

Complications

The main complications of a ruptured intracranial aneurysm are rebleeding, vasospasm and hydrocephalus.

Rebleeding

The greatest risk of rebleeding is within the first day after the initial rupture and again in 7 to 10 days (when the initial clot breaks down). Rebleeding is manifested by a sudden severe headache, nausea and vomiting, decreasing levels of consciousness and new neurological deficits (Hickey, 2019). The mortality from rebleeding is as high as from the initial rupture.

Vasospasm

Cerebral vasospasm is a common but dangerous complication that occurs between 3 and 10 days after a subarachnoid haemorrhage. It is associated with a large number of deaths and disability. A cerebral vasospasm narrows the lumen of one or more cerebral vessels, causing ischaemia and infarction of tissue supplied by the affected vessels. The actual cause is unknown, but it occurs in blood vessels surrounded by thick blood clots, suggesting that some substance in the clot initiates the spasm. The manifestations vary according to the degree of spasm and the area of brain affected. Regional alterations may cause focal deficits (such as hemiplegia), whereas global alterations cause loss of consciousness.

Hydrocephalus

Hydrocephalus, an abnormal accumulation of CSF within the cranial vault and dilation of the ventricles, is a potential complication of a ruptured intracranial aneurysm. Hydrocephalus is thought to be the result of obstruction of reabsorption of CSF through the arachnoid villi. The obstruction is caused by an increased protein content of the CSF because of lysis of blood in the subarachnoid space (Norris, 2018). The accumulation of CSF increases intracranial pressure. Initial manifestations of hydrocephalus are typically non-specific but commonly include decreasing levels of consciousness.

INTERPROFESSIONAL CARE

The care of the person with a ruptured intracranial aneurysm includes determining the location of the aneurysm, treating the manifestations of the haemorrhage and preventing rebleeding and vasospasm. Interventions using radiology, angiography and a variety of procedures may prevent aneurysm rupture or stop the bleeding. Surgery is usually the treatment of choice to repair the bleeding artery.

Diagnosis

The diagnostic tests conducted to identify the site and extent of a ruptured intracranial aneurysm, as well as rebleeding, are a CT scan and bilateral carotid and vertebral cerebral angiograms. A cerebral angiogram is the gold standard for evaluating cerebral aneurysm; it can demonstrate the source of the aneurysm about 80–85% of the time (Hickey, 2019). A lumbar puncture will reveal blood-tinged spinal fluid. These tests are described in the chapter 'A person-centred approach to assessing the nervous system'.

Medications

Calcium channel blockers, such as nimodipine (Nimotop), are used to improve neurological deficits due to vasospasm following subarachnoid haemorrhage from ruptured intracranial aneurysms. Administered for 21 consecutive days, they have been found to enhance collateral blood flow and reduce the incidence of ischaemic deficits from arterial spasm without side effects (Hickey, 2019).

Other medications that may be prescribed include anticonvulsants, such as phenytoin (Dilantin), to prevent seizures if the person has increased intracranial pressure; analgesics for headache; and stool softeners to prevent constipation and straining with a bowel movement (which increases intracranial pressure and blood pressure and may cause rebleeding).

Procedures used to treat aneurysm

Treatments for an intracranial aneurysm are performed either to prevent rupture or to isolate the vessel to prevent further bleeding. The person with good neurological status may have surgery soon after the rupture. In the person with significant neurological deficits, surgery may be delayed until they are more stable and less at risk of vasospasm; however, the trend is towards surgery as soon as possible.

Several different types of procedures are used to repair a ruptured intracranial aneurysm or to prevent the rupture of an existing large aneurysm. These include:

- The skull is opened (craniotomy) and the aneurysm is located. The neck of the aneurysm may be clipped with a metal clip (preventing the entry of blood into the aneurysm) or the involved artery may be clipped both proximally and distally to the aneurysm to isolate the affected area.
- Endovascular Guglielmi detachable coils (GDCs) are a method used to treat non-ruptured aneurysms. One or more small platinum coils are inserted through a microcatheter and threaded through the carotid or femoral artery to the site of the aneurysm, where they are released and fill the body of the aneurysm. The coils initiate the immune response and the body produces a blood clot inside the aneurysm, strengthening the artery walls and reducing the risk of rupture. After the aneurysm is stabilised, it can be clipped with less risk of haemorrhage and death (Hickey, 2019). However, endovascular coil procedures are also effective without surgery, especially for smaller aneurysms.
- Stents, which are coil or mesh tubes introduced into the body through a catheter, are used to cover the neck of an aneurysm, while coils are deposited within the body of the aneurysm.
- Balloon remodelling is used for large, multiple or surgically inaccessible aneurysms. A balloon is placed across the neck of the aneurysm and coils are inserted into the body of the aneurysm. The balloon prevents the coils from moving out to the aneurysm.
- Parent vessel occlusion is performed to occlude the parent vessel that supplies blood to the aneurysm. Prior to permanent occlusion, the risk of neurological impairment is assessed by monitoring motor, sensory and cognitive functions in an awake person while temporary occlusion is conducted.

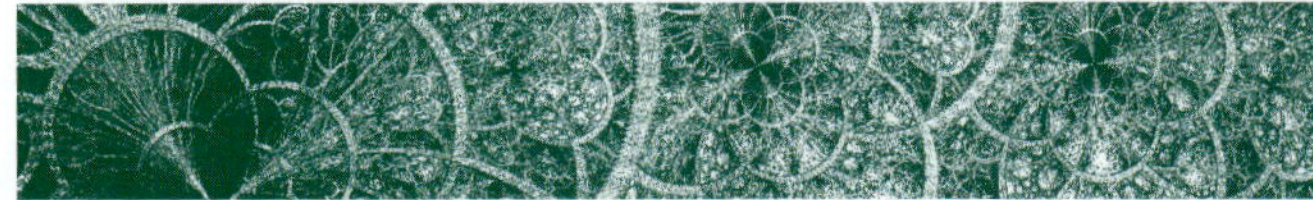

Nursing care

Nursing care is planned and implemented for the person with a ruptured intracranial aneurysm to prevent rebleeding, as well as to meet needs resulting from neurological deficits.

Nursing diagnoses and interventions

Appropriate nursing diagnoses and interventions are described earlier in the chapter in the discussion of nursing care for the person with a stroke. The priority interventions in the acute care stage of a ruptured intracranial aneurysm focus on ineffective cerebral tissue perfusion.

Ineffective tissue perfusion: cerebral

These interventions are for the care of the person immediately after the intracranial aneurysm ruptures. The expected outcome of care is preventing rebleeding and improving cerebral tissue perfusion.

- Institute aneurysm precautions to prevent rebleeding, as follows:
  - Keep the person in a private, quiet, darkened room. Disconnect or remove the telephone. Avoid using bright overhead lights. *A quiet environment helps prevent an increase in blood pressure, which could precipitate rebleeding. The person may experience photophobia (abnormal sensitivity to light) if haemorrhage has damaged the oculomotor nerve.*
  - Elevate the head of the bed 30 to 45 degrees; follow prescribed activity orders (usually complete bed rest, but in some cases bathroom privileges may be approved). *Elevating the head of the bed promotes venous return from the brain and thus decreases intracranial pressure. Decreasing activity reduces the likelihood of increases in blood pressure.*
  - Limit visitors to two family members at any one time and limit the duration of visits. Monitor the person's response to visitors and decrease interactions if the person becomes agitated or upset. *Psychological stress may increase blood pressure and the risk of rebleeding; however, social isolation may increase anxiety and stress. Each person (and family) must be individually evaluated.*
  - Allow reading, watching television or listening to the radio to promote relaxation. *Although these passive activities were previously contraindicated for the person on aneurysm precautions, current therapy is based on the belief that these activities promote relaxation and help control blood pressure.*
- Prevent constipation and straining to have a bowel movement. Administer stool softeners as prescribed. Collaborate with the person and doctor about use of a bedside commode or the bathroom. Do not administer enemas. *The person is at risk of constipation as a result of decreased mobility and the administration of narcotics (such as codeine) for headache. When straining to have a bowel movement, the person uses the Valsalva manoeuvre, which increases intracranial pressure and may precipitate rebleeding.*
- If the person is alert (and depending on doctor preference), allow them to feed self and provide own personal care. *In many instances, self-care causes less anxiety and stress than care provided by the nurse. The extent of care provided varies according to the person's condition and the doctor's preferences. The person who may have to go to theatre will be kept nil by mouth.*

CONSIDERATION FOR PRACTICE

Maintaining a daily stool chart is an important assessment in preventing constipation.

- Monitor vital signs and neurological status as indicated by the person's condition. (Frequency of assessments may range from every 15 minutes to every 4 hours.) *Vital signs and neurological assessments provide ongoing data for evaluation of changes indicative of increasing intracranial pressure and decreasing neurological function. Report any change immediately to the doctor.*

CONSIDERATION FOR PRACTICE

Restlessness and changes in respirations are often early manifestations of increased intracranial pressure.

- Maintain seizure precautions: have suction equipment and an oropharyngeal tube at the bedside, maintain the bed in the low position and keep the side rails padded and raised. *Applying suction and inserting an oropharyngeal airway may be necessary to maintain an open airway in case of seizure. A lowered bed and padded, raised side rails prevent injury if a seizure occurs.*
- Avoid positioning and activities that increase intracranial pressure such as coughing, sneezing, vomiting, sharply flexing the neck, blowing the nose, enemas or moving self up in bed. *These measures help to prevent increasing intracranial pressure and rebleeding.*

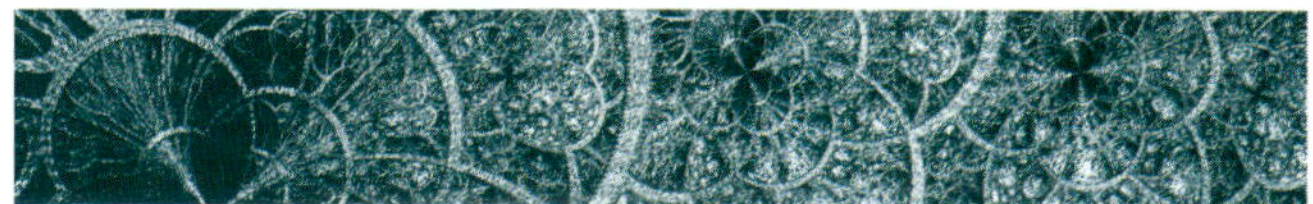

THE PERSON WITH AN ARTERIOVENOUS MALFORMATION

An arteriovenous (AV) malformation is a congenital intracranial lesion, formed by a tangled collection of dilated arteries and veins that allows blood to flow directly from the arterial into the venous system, bypassing the normal capillary network. Most AV malformations (90%) are located in the cerebral hemispheres; the remainder are found in the cerebellum and brainstem.

Rupture of vessels in the malformations accounts for 2% of all strokes. People with this condition develop manifestations before 40 years of age; it affects men and women equally (Norris, 2018). The manifestations are the result of spontaneous bleeding from the lesion into the subarachnoid space or brain tissue.

Pathophysiology

AV malformations displace, rather than encompass, normal brain tissue (Hickey, 2019). The pathophysiological effects of an AV malformation are the result of the shunting of blood from the arterial to the venous system and of altered perfusion of cerebral tissue near the malformation. The shunting of arterial blood directly into the venous system within the malformation transfers the higher arterial pressure directly into the lower-pressure venous system. This increased pressure is likely to cause spontaneous bleeding or progressive expansion and rupture of a blood vessel.

Altered cerebral perfusion results when blood flow through a large, high-flow malformation is diverted from the normal cerebral circulation, causing tissue ischaemia of the area surrounding the malformation. This is sometimes called a vascular 'steal' phenomenon.

AV malformations range in size from very small to very large. Large malformations are usually initially manifested by seizure activity. In contrast, the manifestations of a small malformation are more often due to a haemorrhage that causes neurological deficits. In both instances, the person may have recurrent headaches that do not respond to treatment.

INTERPROFESSIONAL CARE

AV malformations are diagnosed with the same diagnostic tests used to diagnose an intracranial aneurysm.

If the malformation is accessible, the ideal treatment is excision of the malformation and removal of any haematoma. Large malformations may be treated by embolisation. In this procedure, substances such as Gelfoam or metallic pellets are introduced into the involved area of the cerebral circulation, where they form emboli and gradually obstruct blood flow in the malformation. Inaccessible malformations are also treated with radiation therapy or laser therapy to coagulate blood in the malformation and thicken its vascular elements, eventually obstructing it. When the malformation is excised or obstructed, blood flow is no longer shunted and cerebral perfusion improves.

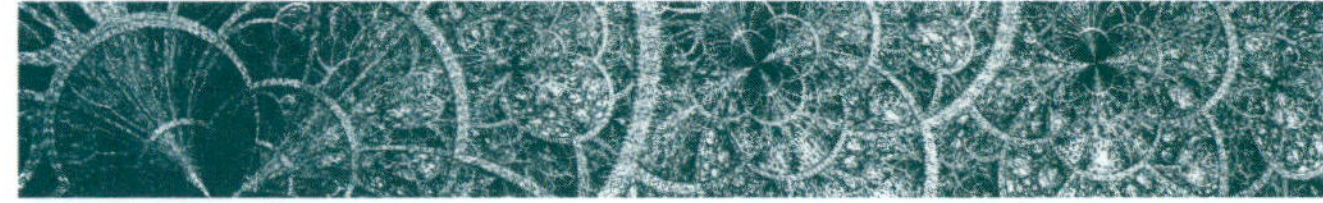

Nursing care

Nursing care depends on the condition of the malformation. If haemorrhage has not occurred, teach the person to avoid activities that raise blood pressure or could cause injury. The person is usually given medications to control blood pressure and prevent seizures.

If the malformation ruptures and causes an intracranial haemorrhage, nursing care is the same as for any person who has had a haemorrhagic stroke (discussed earlier in this chapter).

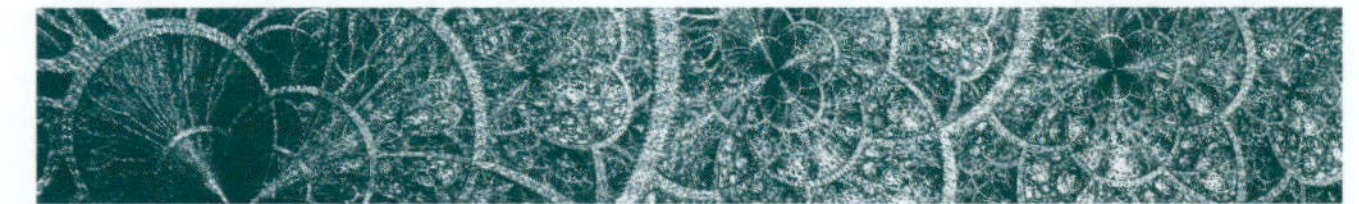

Spinal cord disorders

THE PERSON WITH A SPINAL CORD INJURY

Nursing care of the person with a spinal cord injury takes place from the acute management phase through ongoing rehabilitation in a variety of settings. Although priorities of care may change depending on the person and the setting, care focuses on maximising functional health status to preserve quality of life. The nurse provides care and also collaborates with other healthcare professionals in meeting this goal.

Incidence and prevalence

A **spinal cord injury (SCI)** is usually due to trauma. The main causes of SCI are contusion, laceration, transection, haemorrhage and damage to blood vessels that supply the spinal cord. If vertebrae are fractured and ligaments are torn, bony fragments can damage the cord and make the spinal column unstable. Injury to blood vessels supplying the cord can cause permanent damage. The injury is identified by vertebral level. For example, a C6 spinal cord injury is at the sixth cervical vertebra.

Risk factors

The three main risk factors for SCIs are age, gender and alcohol or drug abuse. Young men are more prone than women to risk-taking behaviours. Older adults are more likely to have a cord injury from even minor trauma as a result of age-related vertebral degeneration. Motor vehicle crashes while under the influence of alcohol or drugs are a major source of trauma to people of all ages.

Pathophysiology

The spinal cord provides a two-way pathway for the conduction of impulses and information to and from the brain and the body, serves as a major reflex centre and (through its attached spinal nerves) is involved in the sensory and motor innervation of the entire body below the head. It consists of an outer region of white matter and an inner region of grey matter. The grey matter comprises the central canal of the cord, the posterior horns, the anterior horns and the lateral horns. It is divided into a sensory half (dorsally) and a motor half (ventrally) and innervates somatic and visceral regions of the body. The white matter consists of tracts or pathways that convey information. The ascending (sensory) pathways carry information about proprioception, fine touch, discrimination, pain, temperature, deep pressure and touch. The descending (motor) pathways carry information about movement. The pyramidal tracts control skilled voluntary movements (such as writing). The extrapyramidal tracts (all tracts other than the pyramidal tracts) bring about all other body movements. See the chapter 'A person-centred approach to assessing the nervous system' for further information.

When the spinal cord is injured, the primary injury causes microscopic haemorrhages in the grey matter of the cord and oedema of the white matter of the cord. These initial pathological changes are followed by the secondary injury, with mechanisms that increase the area of injury. The haemorrhages extend, eventually involving the entire grey matter. Microcirculation to the cord is impaired by oedema and

FAST FACTS

- Approximately 350–400 Australians have an SCI each year.
- In 2015–2016, 80% of cases incurring SCI from traumatic causes were male, with the greatest number in men aged 45–54.
- Falls contributed to approximately 48% of all traumatic SCI cases.
- 39% of traumatic SCI cases were due to land transport crashes involving motor vehicle occupants and unprotected land transport users such as motor cyclists, pedestrians, pedal cyclists and quad bikes. Males accounted for 83% of traumatic SCI due to a land transport crash.
- 5% were water-related, with many traumatic SCI cases caused by being dumped by a wave or diving/jumping into shallow water.
- Football (including rugby codes) accounted for 2% of cases, with three of the four cases sustained during a game of rugby.
- 26% of traumatic SCI cases occurred while the person was engaged in a sport or leisure activity; 89% of these cases were males. The next most common activity when traumatic SCI occurred was while working for income (12%); 87% of these cases were male.
- The total cost of spinal cord injury in Australia is estimated to be $2 billion annually (AIHW, 2019).

haemorrhage. The injured tissue releases noradrenaline, serotonin, dopamine and histamine; these vasoactive substances cause vasospasm and further decrease microcirculation. As a result, vascular perfusion and oxygen tension of the affected area are decreased, which leads to ischaemia.

When ischaemia is prolonged, necrosis of both grey and white matter begins within a few hours and within 24 hours the function of nerves passing through the injured area is lost. Although circulation returns to the white matter of the cord in about 24 hours, decreased circulation in the grey matter continues. Because oedema extends the level of injury for two cord segments above and below the affected level, the extent of injury cannot be determined for up to 1 week.

Tissue repair occurs over a period of 3 to 4 weeks. Phagocytes enter the area 36 to 48 hours after the initial injury. Neurons degenerate and are removed by microphages in the first 10 days after the injury. RBC disintegrate and the haemorrhages are reabsorbed. Eventually the area of injury is replaced by acellular collagenous tissue and the meninges thicken.

Forces resulting in SCI

SCIs are the result of the application of excessive force to the spinal column. The most common causes of abnormal spinal column movements are acceleration and deceleration (forces that are applied to the body; e.g. in motor vehicle crashes and falls). Acceleration occurs when external force is applied in a rear-end collision; the upper torso and head are forced backwards and then forwards. Deceleration occurs in a head-on collision; the external force is applied from the front. The head and body move forwards until they meet a stationary object and then are forced backwards. The following forces and movements (see Figure 42.6) may cause a variety of SCIs, with

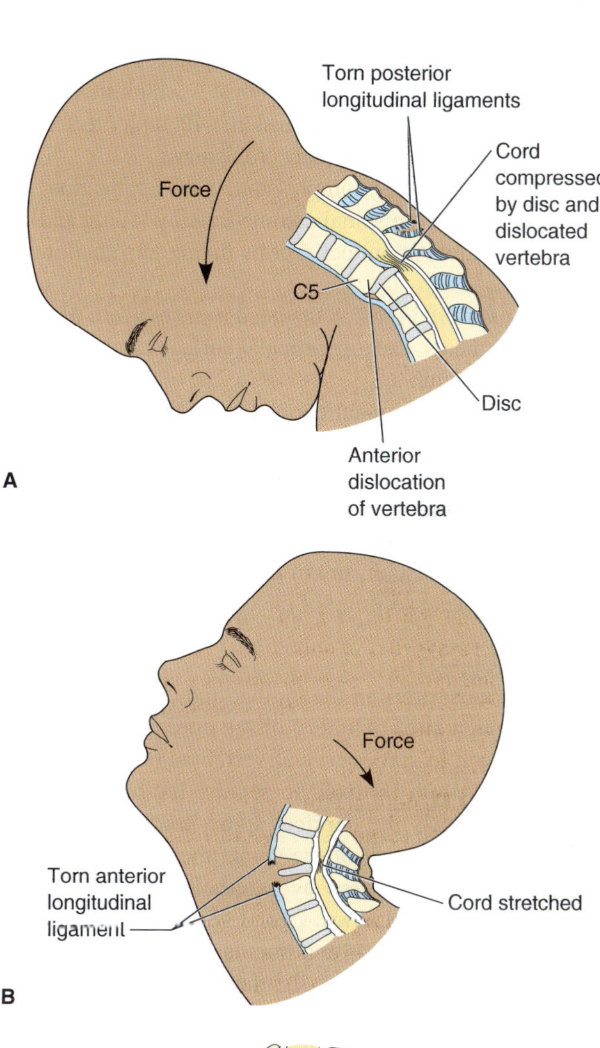

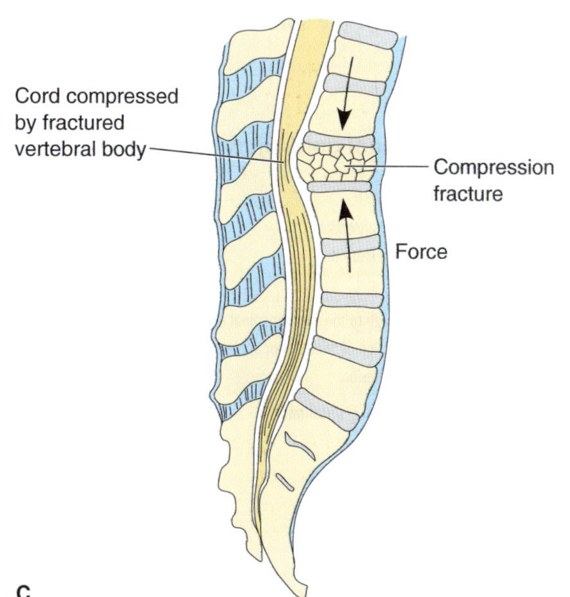

FIGURE 42.6 *Spinal cord injury mechanisms. A, Hyperflexion. B, Hyperextension. C, Axial loading, a form of compression*

the extent of injury depending on the amount and direction of motion and the rate of application of force:

- *Hyperflexion*, or forcible forward bending, may compress vertebral bodies and disrupt ligaments and intervertebral discs.
- *Hyperextension*, or forcible backward bending, often disrupts ligaments and causes vertebral fractures. A whiplash injury is a less severe form of hyperextension, with injury to soft tissues but no vertebral or spinal cord damage.
- *Axial loading*, a form of compression, is the application of vertical force to the spinal column (e.g. by falling and landing on the feet or buttocks, or by diving into shallow water).
- *Excessive rotation*, in which the head is excessively turned, may tear ligaments, fracture articular surfaces and cause compression fractures.

The alteration of the spinal cord and soft tissues caused by these abnormal movements is called deformation.

The spinal cord may be penetrated by bullets and other foreign objects (e.g. sharp objects used as weapons, shrapnel from explosions). Penetrating injuries may cause vertebral fractures, tear ligaments and muscles, or cut through a part or all of the spinal cord. Complete severing of the cord is rare.

Sites of pathology

Injuries occur most often in the lumbar and cervical regions. The most frequent sites of injury of the cord are at the first, second and fourth to sixth cervical vertebrae (C1, C2, C4 to C6); and the eleventh thoracic to second lumbar vertebrae (T11 to L2). Because the cervical spine has a wider range of movement than the rest of the spine, the cervical portion is more likely to be affected by externally applied forces. In addition, the cord fills most of the vertebral canal in the cervical and lumbar regions and thus is more easily injured. Damage to the vertebrae and ligaments causes the spinal column to become unstable, increasing the possibility of compression or stretching of the spinal cord with any further movement.

Classification of SCIs

SCIs are classified according to systems—for instance: (1) as complete or incomplete cord injury, (2) by cause of injury, and (3) by level of injury. In clinical practice, these classifications often overlap. In a *complete SCI* (about 45% of all injuries), the motor and sensory neural pathways are completely interrupted (transected), resulting in total loss of motor and sensory function below the level of the injury. However, 'complete' does not necessarily mean the spinal cord has been severed. In an *incomplete SCI* (about 55% of all injuries), the motor and sensory pathways are only partially interrupted, with variable loss of function below the level of injury. Incomplete SCIs are further classified into syndromes, as outlined in Table 42.2. Both complete and incomplete injuries can occur in paraplegia and quadriplegia. The alterations in function that occur as the result of SCIs vary greatly depending on the amount of tissue damage and the level of injury.

Manifestations

The spinal cord, the vertebrae, the intervertebral discs, the spinal nerves, the ligaments and the surrounding soft tissue structures are in such close anatomical proximity that any condition or injury affecting one structure may well affect any one or all of the other structures. The conditions with the most critical effects are disorders affecting the spinal cord. Disorders and injuries of the spinal cord have the potential to affect movement, perception, sensation, sexual function and elimination. See the 'Manifestations and complications' box.

Spinal shock is the temporary loss of reflex function (called *areflexia*) below the level of injury. This response begins immediately after complete transection of the spinal cord, when connections between the brain and the spinal cord are interrupted and the cord does not function at all. The response also occurs (although in varying degrees) after partial transection, as well as after spinal cord contusions, compression and ischaemia.

Normal activity of the spinal cord is dependent on constant impulses from the higher centres of the brain. When

TABLE 42.2 Incomplete spinal cord injury syndromes

TYPE	CAUSE	LOCATION	DEFICITS
Central syndrome	Cord transection Hyperextension	Cervical	Spastic paralysis of the upper extremities Variable paralysis of the lower extremities Variable effects on the bowel, the bladder and sexual function
Anterior syndrome	Damage to the anterior spinal artery Infarction of the anterior spinal artery Hyperflexion	Anterior two-thirds of the cord	Paralysis below the level of injury Loss of temperature and pain sensation below the level of injury
Posterior syndrome	Vertebral dislocation Herniated disc Compression	Nerve roots	Weakness in isolated muscle groups Tingling, pain Decreased or absent reflexes in the involved area Bowel or bladder dysfunction
Brown-Séquard syndrome	Penetrating trauma	Hemisection of the anterior and posterior cord	Paralysis below the level of injury on the ipsilateral (same) side of the body Contralateral loss of temperature and pain sensation below the level of injury Ipsilateral loss of proprioception below the level of injury
Homer's syndrome	Incomplete cord transection	Cervical sympathetic nerves	Ipsilateral ptosis of the eyelid, constricted pupil and facial anhidrosis (inability to perspire)

MANIFESTATIONS AND COMPLICATIONS **Spinal cord injury by body system**

INTEGUMENT
- Decubitus (pressure) ulcers

NEUROLOGICAL
- Pain
- Areflexia
- Hypotonia
- Autonomic dysreflexia

CARDIOVASCULAR
- Spinal shock
- Paroxysmal hypertension
- Orthostatic hypotension
- Cardiac arrhythmias
- Decreased venous return
- Hypercalcaemia

RESPIRATORY
- Limited chest expansion
- Decreased cough reflex
- Decreased vital capacity

GASTROINTESTINAL
- Stress ulcers
- Paralytic ileus
- Stool impaction
- Stool incontinence

GENITOURINARY
- Urinary retention
- Urinary incontinence
- Neurogenic bladder
- Impotence
- Testicular atrophy
- Inability to ejaculate
- Decreased vaginal lubrication

MUSCULOSKELETAL
- Joint contractures
- Bone demineralisation
- Osteoporosis
- Muscle spasms
- Muscle atrophy
- Pathological fractures
- Paraplegia
- Quadriplegia

damage from an injury stops these impulses, spinal shock follows. There is loss of motor function, tendon reflexes and autonomic function. Spinal shock may begin within 1 hour of the injury. The condition may last from a few minutes to several months (although it usually lasts from 1 to 6 weeks) and then reflex activity returns. Spinal shock ends slowly, with the gradual reappearance of reflexes, hyperreflexia (increased reflex responses), muscle spasticity and reflex bladder emptying.

The manifestations of acute spinal shock (which vary in degree) include the following:

- flaccid paralysis of skeletal muscles below the level of injury
- loss of all spinal reflexes below the level of injury
- loss of sensations of pain, touch, temperature and pressure below the level of injury
- absence of visceral and somatic sensations below the level of injury
- bowel and bladder dysfunction
- loss of the ability to perspire below the level of injury.

A person with a cervical or upper thoracic SCI may also have neurogenic shock, resulting in cardiovascular changes. These changes are due to the inability of higher centres in the brainstem to modulate reflexes. As a result, vascular beds below the level of injury dilate and the cardiac accelerator reflex is suppressed. The person experiences hypotension and bradycardia. Other manifestations may include respiratory insufficiency due to loss of innervation of the diaphragm in C1 to C4 injuries, hypothermia, paralytic ileus, urinary retention and oliguria.

Both bradycardia and hypotension may persist even after the spinal shock resolves. In addition to losing sympathetic control of the heart rate, the person with a high-level SCI experiences decreased peripheral resistance and loss of muscle activity. These changes result in sluggish blood flow and decreased venous return, increasing the risk of thrombophlebitis.

Complications

The complications of an SCI involve many different body systems and result often in permanent disability and loss of functional health status. The complications include, but are not limited to, upper and lower motor neuron deficits, paraplegia and quadriplegia, and autonomic dysreflexia. Other complications, depending on the level and severity of the injury, are ineffective respirations, altered skin integrity, increased risk of thrombosis and alterations in bowel elimination, urinary elimination and sexual pattern.

Upper and lower motor neuron deficits

Injuries to the spinal cord are often classified as either *upper motor neuron lesions* or *lower motor neuron lesions*. Motor neurons are functional units that carry motor impulses. The upper motor neurons (located in the cerebral cortex, thalamus, brainstem and corticospinal and corticobulbar tracts) are responsible for voluntary movement. When these motor pathways are interrupted, the person experiences spastic paralysis and hyperreflexia and may be unable to carry out skilled movement.

Lower motor neurons (located in the anterior horn of the spinal cord, the motor nuclei of the brainstem and the axons that reach the motor end plate of skeletal muscles) are responsible for innervation and contraction of skeletal muscles. Interruption of lower motor neurons results in muscle flaccidity and extensive muscle atrophy, with loss of both voluntary and involuntary movement. If only some of the motor neurons supplying a muscle are affected, the person experiences partial paralysis (paresis); if all motor neurons to a muscle are affected, the person experiences complete paralysis. Hyporeflexia is also present.

Paraplegia and quadriplegia

Two common neurological deficits resulting from an SCI are paraplegia and quadriplegia (see Figure 42.3). **Paraplegia** is paralysis of the lower portion of the body, sometimes involving the lower trunk. Paraplegia occurs when the thoracic, lumbar and sacral portions of the spinal cord are injured, causing loss or impairment of sensory and/or motor function. **Quadriplegia**, also called *tetraplegia*, occurs when cervical segments of the cord are injured, impairing function of the arms, trunk, legs and pelvic organs.

Autonomic dysreflexia

Autonomic dysreflexia (also called *autonomic hyperreflexia*) is an exaggerated sympathetic response that occurs in the person with SCIs at or above the T6 level. This response, which is seen only after recovery from spinal shock, occurs as a result of a lack of control of the autonomic nervous system by higher centres. When stimuli are unable to ascend the cord, mass reflex stimulation of the sympathetic nerves below the level of the injured cord area occurs, triggering massive vasoconstriction. In response, the vagus nerve causes bradycardia and vasodilation above the level of injury. If untreated, autonomic dysreflexia can cause seizures, a stroke or a myocardial infarction, and is potentially fatal (Hickey, 2019).

Autonomic dysreflexia is triggered by stimuli that would normally cause abdominal discomfort (a full bladder is the most common cause), by stimulation of pain receptors and by visceral contractions (Norris, 2018). Causes include faecal impaction, bladder infections or stones, intrauterine contractions, ejaculation, peritonitis and stimulation from pressure injuries or ingrown toenails. The most common precipitating event is a blocked urinary catheter.

The manifestations of this condition include: pounding headache; bradycardia; hypertension (with readings as high as 300/160); flushed, warm skin with profuse sweating above the lesion and pale, cold and dry skin below it; and anxiety (Norris, 2018). Dysreflexia is a neurological emergency and requires immediate treatment.

INTERPROFESSIONAL CARE

The person with an acute SCI requires emergency assessment and care, and medications; sometimes the person also requires immobilisation and surgery. The person is first assessed and stabilised at the scene of the accident, initially treated in the emergency room and then admitted to the hospital's critical care unit.

Emergency care

The danger of death from SCI is greatest when there is damage to or transection of the upper cervical region. When the injury is at the C1 to C4 level, respiratory paralysis is common and the person who survives requires ventilator assistance to breathe. Injuries below C4 may increase the risk of respiratory failure if oedema ascends the cord. It is of critical importance not to complicate the initial injury by allowing the fractured vertebrae to damage the cord further during transport to the hospital. Although at one time injuries to the high cervical cord were almost always fatal, advances in trauma care have greatly improved the survival rate.

All people who have sustained trauma to the head or spine, or who are unconscious, should be treated as though they have a spinal cord injury. Pre-hospital management includes rapid assessment of the ABCs (airway, breathing, circulation), immobilising and stabilising the head and neck, removing the person from the site of injury, stabilising other life-threatening injuries and rapidly transporting the person to the appropriate facility. Guidelines for emergency care are as follows:

- Avoid flexing, extending or rotating the neck.
- Immobilise the neck, placing rolled towels or blankets on each side of the person's neck, or apply a cervical collar before moving the person onto a backboard.
- Secure the head by placing a belt or tape across the forehead and securing it to the stretcher.
- Maintain the person in the supine position.
- Transfer directly from the stretcher with backboard still in place to the type of bed that will be used in the hospital.

Assessment findings at the scene of the accident or in the emergency room vary according to the level of injury. The assessment findings common to the level of injury and spinal shock are outlined in Box 42.1.

The person in the emergency department with a suspected or identified SCI is also treated for respiratory problems, paralytic ileus, atonic bladder and cardiovascular alterations. Respiratory distress in the person with a cervical-level injury is treated by placing the person on a ventilator. Oxygen is administered to the person with a thoracic-level injury. Paralytic ileus (obstruction of the intestines due to lack of peristalsis) is common in the person with a spinal cord injury and is treated by the insertion of a nasogastric tube with connection to suction. To prevent over-distension of an atonic bladder, an indwelling catheter is inserted and connected to dependent drainage. Cardiovascular status is assessed on a continuous basis by inserting invasive monitoring devices, such as a Swan–Ganz catheter, or continuous cardiac output monitoring and attaching the person to a cardiac monitor, or by arterial monitoring to identify hypotension and to draw arterial blood gases (ABGs).

BOX 42.1 Assessment findings in acute SCI

Cervical injury

- Paralysis or weakness of extremities
- Respiratory distress manifested by changes in ABG studies, cyanosis, flaring of the nostrils, use of accessory muscles of respiration and restlessness
- Pulse rate below 60 and systolic BP below 80
- Decreased peristalsis

Thoracic and lumbar injury

- Paralysis or weakness of extremities

Spinal shock

- Loss of skin sensation
- Flaccid paralysis, areflexia
- Absent bowel sounds
- Bladder distension
- Decreasing blood pressure
- Absence of the cremasteric reflex in males (retraction of the left or right testicle in response to stimulation of the skin of, respectively, the inner left or right thigh)

High-dose corticosteroid protocol using methylprednisolone must be implemented within 8 hours of the injury to improve neurological recovery. Clinical research indicates that the use of this adrenocorticosteroid is effective in preventing secondary spinal cord damage from oedema and ischaemia. Treatment with GM1 ganglioside for 3 to 4 weeks is an experimental approach that has been effective for some people (Papadakis, McPhee & Rabow, 2022).

Diagnosis

Diagnostic tests are ordered to identify the level and extent of injury and to detect any complications. The tests include x-ray of the spine, CT or MRI of the spine and somatosensory evoked potential studies to locate the level of spinal cord injury by stimulating peripheral nerves and measuring response times. ABGs are measured to establish a baseline or to identify problems due to respiratory insufficiency.

Medications

The pharmacological treatment of the person with an SCI is symptomatic. It is directed primarily towards decreasing oedema from the injury, treating hypotension and bradycardia, and treating spasticity.

- Corticosteroids, discussed earlier in this section, may be used to decrease or control oedema of the cord.
- Vasopressors are used in the immediate acute care phase to treat bradycardia or hypotension due to spinal and neurogenic shock. Examples of drugs are dopamine to treat hypotension in neurogenic shock and dobutamine to support cardiac function. Atropine should be available at the bedside to treat bradycardia.
- Antispasmodics are used to treat spasticity in the person with SCI. Both baclofen and diazepam may be used. A discussion of nursing implications of treatment with antispasmodics is found in the 'Medication administration' box.
- Analgesics such as non-steroidal anti-inflammatory drugs (NSAIDs) and narcotics are administered to reduce pain.
- Proton pump inhibitors, such as omeprazole, esomeprazole, rabeprazole or pantoprazole, are often administered to prevent stress-related gastric ulcers, a common complication in SCI.
- Unless contraindicated, anticoagulants (heparin or warfarin) may be given to prevent thrombophlebitis.
- Softeners may be administered as part of a bowel retraining program.

Treatments

The treatments used in the management of an SCI include surgery, stabilisation and immobilisation.

SURGERY Early surgical treatment may be necessary if there is evidence of compression of the spinal cord by bone fragments or a haematoma. Surgery may also be done to stabilise and support the spine. However, many people are treated with stabilisation devices and do not require surgery. Surgeries that may be performed include a decompression laminectomy, a spinal fusion and insertion of metal rods. Surgeries of the spine are discussed later in the chapter.

STABILISATION AND IMMOBILISATION As a result of one or more dislocations or fractures of the cervical vertebrae, the person with an SCI may be immobilised in some type of traction or external fixation device to stabilise the vertebral column and prevent any further damage (see Figure 42.7). Traction may also be used to stabilise the spinal column for the person who is not yet in a condition to have surgery or who has severe bleeding and oedema of the injured cord. The doctor applies the traction or fixation device; the nurse is responsible for assessments and interventions following the application.

Although used less frequently today, various devices provide cervical traction. For example, Gardner–Wells tongs may be used (see Figure 42.8). In this type of traction, the doctor applies pins to the skull, approximately 1 cm above each ear and weights are attached to the device.

The halo external fixation device is often used to provide stabilisation if there is no significant involvement of the ligaments

MEDICATION ADMINISTRATION Antispasmodics in spinal cord injury

ANTISPASMODICS
Baclofen
Diazepam
Orphenadrine citrate

These drugs depress the CNS and inhibit the transmission of impulses from the spinal cord to skeletal muscle. They are used to control muscle spasm and pain associated with acute or chronic musculoskeletal conditions. They are not always effective in controlling spasticity resulting from cerebral or spinal cord conditions.

Nursing responsibilities

- Assess the person's spasticity and involuntary movements to obtain baseline data for comparison with results of therapy.
- Do not expect therapy to have effects for 1 week.
- Administer oral medications with food to decrease gastrointestinal symptoms.

Health education for the person and family

- These drugs may cause drowsiness, diplopia and impotence.
- Take your medications with meals to decrease gastric irritation.
- Physical improvement may take several weeks.
- Report slurred speech, drooling or inability to carry out usual functions to the doctor.
- Do not stop taking the medication without consulting your healthcare provider.

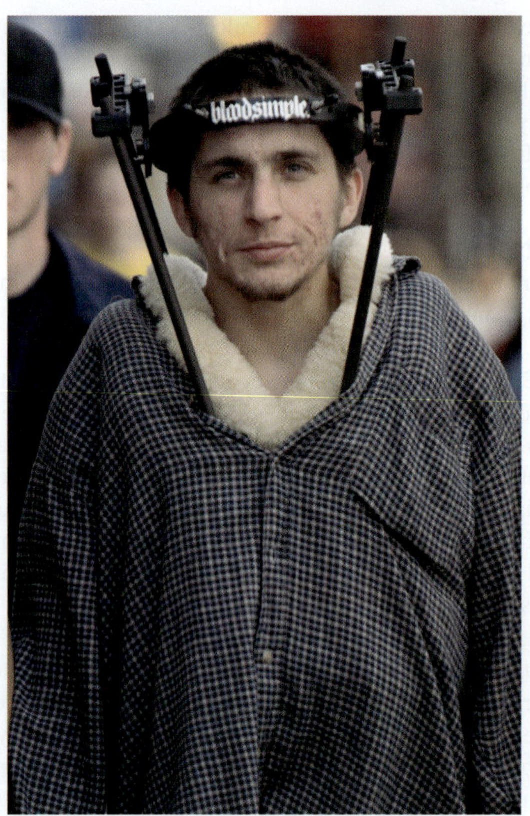

FIGURE 42.7 ***External fixation device***

Source: © Rodolfo Arpia/Alamy Stock Photo.

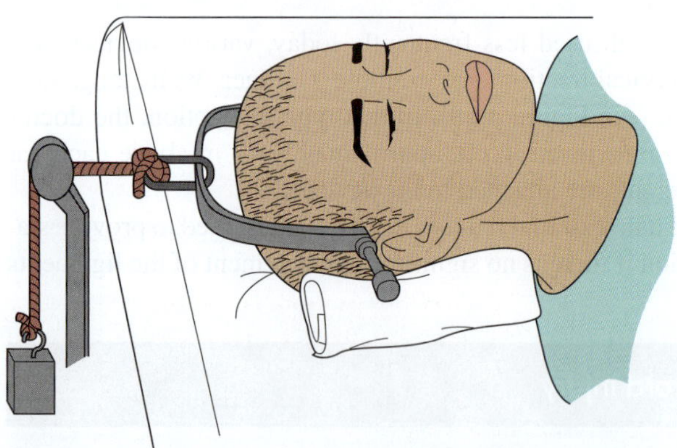

FIGURE 42.8 ***Cervical traction may be applied by several methods, including Gardner–Wells tongs***

(see Figure 42.9). It is most often used to provide stability for fractures of the cervical and high thoracic vertebrae without cord damage. This device allows greater mobility, self-care and participation in rehabilitation programs. The device is secured with four pins inserted into the skull: two in the frontal bone and two in the occipital bone. The halo ring is then attached to a rigid plastic vest lined with sheepskin. See the accompanying box for nursing care of the person using a halo fixation device.

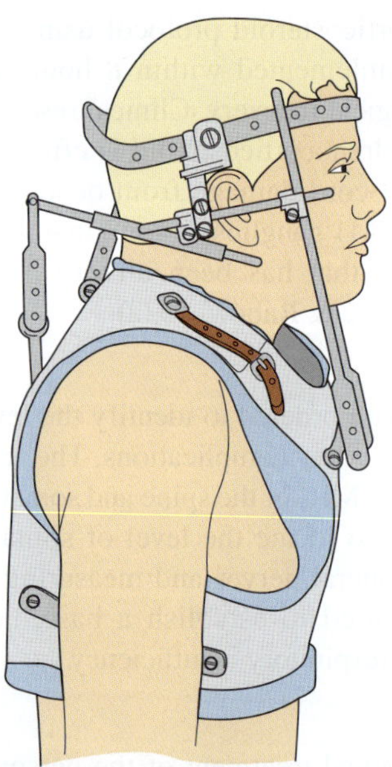

FIGURE 42.9 ***The halo external fixation device***

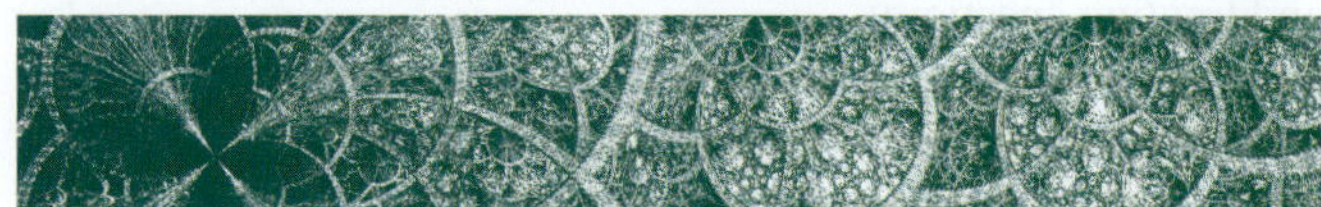

Nursing care

During both the acute phase and the rehabilitative phase, the person with an SCI has complex needs that involve all members of the healthcare team. Because these injuries are more common in younger people, consideration of lifelong effects on both the person and the family is essential. The nurse coordinates person care and develops and implements a care plan that is individualised to each person and family. The focus of the plan is to prevent the secondary complications of immobility and altered body functions, to promote self-care and to educate the person and family. See the accompanying nursing care plan for a person with an SCI.

Health promotion

Health promotion for SCIs primarily involves preventing injuries. Nurses can provide valuable information in the community and in the workplace to prevent SCIs. Programs that focus on wearing seat belts and using approved infant seats and child booster chairs in motor vehicles can do much to help decrease the number of SCIs each year. Education programs that promote workplace safety should include information on preventing falls and using heavy equipment safely.

Assessment

The following data are collected through the health history and physical examination (see the chapter 'A person-centred approach to assessing the nervous system'). Further focused assessments are described with nursing interventions in the next section.

- *Health history*: time, location and type of event causing injury; location, duration, quality and intensity of pain; dyspnoea; sensation; paraesthesia.

NURSING CARE OF THE PERSON in halo fixation

- Maintain integrity of the halo external fixation device.
  a. Inspect pins and traction bars for tightness; report loosened pins to the doctor.
  b. Tape the appropriate wrench to the head of the bed for emergency intervention.
  c. Never use the halo ring to lift or reposition the person.
  Loosening of the apparatus poses the risk of further damage to the cord. It is the responsibility of the nurse to maintain the integrity of the apparatus and the safety of the person.
- Assess muscle function and skin sensation every 2 hours in the acute phase and every 4 hours thereafter.
  a. Assess motor function on a scale of 0 to 5, with 0 being no evidence of muscle contraction and 5 being normal muscle strength with full range of motion.
  b. Assess sensation by comparing touch and pain, moving from impaired to normal areas and testing both the right and left sides of the body.
  Monitoring muscle function and skin sensation allows early identification of potential neurological deficits.
- Monitor pin sites each shift and follow hospital policy for pin care. Some general guidelines are:
  a. Assess pin sites for redness, oedema and drainage.
  b. Depending on policy, clean each pin site with a sterile applicator dipped in hydrogen peroxide, apply a topical antibiotic and cover with sterile 5 cm split gauze squares.
  Organisms can enter the body through the pin-insertion site; assessments and care are provided to detect signs of and prevent infection.
- Maintain skin integrity.
  a. Turn the immobile person every 2 hours.
  b. Inspect the skin around edges of the vest every 4 hours.
  c. Change the sheepskin liner when it is soiled and at least once each week.
  These interventions prevent skin injury and irritation.

NURSING CARE PLAN A person with an SCI

Jim Colins, a 19-year-old university student, is admitted to the hospital by ambulance following a car crash. His family (father, mother and sister) live 200 km away and cannot visit often, although they are very concerned. On admission to the hospital, a CT scan of the spine shows a fracture and partial laceration of the cord at the C7 level. Mr Colins is in halo traction. One night, he tells the nurse, 'I wish I had just died when I got hurt. I don't think I can stand to live like this.'

ASSESSMENT

When Mr Colins is admitted to the critical care unit, he has flaccid paralysis involving all extremities. He has no sensation below the clavicle or in portions of his arms and legs. His bladder is distended and bowel sounds are absent. Other assessment findings include BP 90/56, P 50, T 36.1°C, arterial blood gases PH 7.4, PaO_2 96, $PaCO_2$ 37, SaO_2 96%. Oxygen per nasal prongs is given at 2 L/min and halo traction is applied. A Foley catheter is inserted into his bladder and a nasogastric tube is inserted and attached to low-pressure continuous suction.

After 7 days, Mr Colins is moved from the critical care unit to the neurosurgical unit for continuing care and planning for transfer to a rehabilitation hospital in his home town. His vital signs have stabilised and are normal for his age; respirations and oxygenation are normal. Other neurological assessments remain the same.

DIAGNOSES

- *Risk of impaired physical mobility* related to paralysis of lower and upper extremities and manifested by inability to mobilise independently.
- *Risk of bowel incontinence* related to lack of voluntary sphincter control and manifested by faecal incontinence.
- *Dysfunctional grieving* related to denial of loss and manifested by depression, anger or denial.

PLANNING

- Plan to begin mobilisation and ROM exercises in the morning when Mr Colins is not tired.
- His usual time for a bowel movement is after breakfast; schedule retraining program for that time.
- Discuss the grief process with Mr Colins and his family.

Expected outcomes

- Be actively involved in exercise programs.
- Have a soft, formed stool every second or third day.
- Verbally express his grief to parents and staff.

IMPLEMENTATION

- Conduct passive exercises on all extremities four times a day.
- Provide progressive mobilisation by initially raising the head of the bed 90 degrees (repeat two to three times during the first day of movement); if blood pressure remains normal, dangle the legs for 5 minutes before transferring him to a chair.
- Encourage a diet high in fibre and fluids. Likes wholemeal bread, orange juice and cola; does not like water.
- Promote grief work by providing time to express feelings. Explain to the family that his denial and anger are part of the grieving process.
- Determine food likes and dislikes, and order preferred foods from the menu. Encourage his friends to bring in his favourite foods periodically.
- Take and record weight every third day, using the bed scales.

EVALUATION

By the time Mr Colins is transferred to the rehabilitation hospital he is looking forward to learning how to use special equipment and getting his own motorised wheelchair. He is able to sit up in a chair without dizziness or hypotension. The use of ordered

(continued)

NURSING CARE PLAN A person with an SCI (continued)

stool softeners combined with a high-fibre diet and fluid intake of 2,000 to 3,000 mL per day has maintained bowel elimination. Mr Colins and his parents have spent 3 hours talking about their feelings related to the accident and the future. Although the discussion is emotionally difficult, all three say they now feel much better. Mr Colins still has episodes of angry outbursts and tears, but he is more optimistic about what can be done and believes he can finish university. He selects foods from the menu each day and eats most of his meals, but he especially enjoys the times his friends bring in pizza or Thai takeaway.

CRITICAL THINKING IN THE NURSING PROCESS

1 Considering Mr Colins' age and developmental level, do you think his emotional responses to his injury were appropriate?
2 Issues of sexuality are obviously important to the person with a spinal cord injury. How would you approach Mr Colins about this topic?
3 Which issues in this case study will influence your future practice?

REFLECTION ON THE NURSING PROCESS

1 Design an education strategy to help educate Mr Colins about pressure areas and care needed to prevent them.
2 Outline a nursing discharge program for Mr Colins, incorporating useful information for Mr Colins' family about available resources.

- *Physical examination*: vital signs, motor strength, movement, spinal reflexes, bowel sounds, bladder distension.

Nursing diagnoses and interventions

Because an SCI has many possible effects, many nursing diagnoses may be appropriate. Nursing diagnoses discussed in this section focus on problems with physical mobility, respirations, dysreflexia, bowel and bladder elimination, sexual dysfunction and self-esteem.

Impaired physical mobility

After the initial period of spinal shock and areflexia, the person regains spinal reflex activity and muscle tone that is not under the control of higher centres. The person with injuries above the level of T12 experiences involuntary spastic movements of skeletal muscles. These movements reach a peak about 2 years after the injury and then gradually subside (Norris, 2018). Spasms impair the ability to carry out ADLs and work. In addition, the paraplegia or quadriplegia increases the potential for impaired skin integrity, thrombophlebitis and contractures.

The goals of care for the person with impaired mobility related to an SCI are to reduce the effects of spasticity and to prevent complications involving the skin, the cardiovascular system and joint function.

- Perform passive ROM exercises for all extremities at least twice a day. Identify stimuli that cause spastic movements and either avoid the stimuli (such as certain exercises) or teach the person to expect the movements. *ROM exercises help prevent contractures and stretch spastic muscles, promoting rehabilitation.*
- Maintain skin integrity by turning every 2 hours, assessing pressure points at least once each shift and using a pressure-relieving mattress if necessary. The person may be placed on a regular or special bed, such as a kinetic bed. *Immobility compresses soft tissues and promotes the development of decubitus ulcers. The lack of sensory warning mechanisms and of voluntary motor control of skin dermatomes further increases the risk of altered skin integrity. Special beds allow movement or turning while keeping the spinal column in alignment.*
- Assess the lower extremities each shift for manifestations of thrombophlebitis. Observe for redness and for increased heat every shift; measure thigh and calf circumference daily. If anti-embolic stockings (TEDs) are ordered, remove for 30 to 60 minutes each shift. Assess for skin impairment and provide skin care while TEDs are removed. *The person with neurological deficits is at high risk of deep venous thrombosis (DVT) as a result of immobility, vasomotor dysfunction and decreased venous return with venous stasis. Anti-embolic stockings help to prevent the pooling of blood in the lower extremities and increase venous return, lessening the risk of venous stasis and thrombus formation. Sequential compression devices or calf compressors reduce venous stasis by intermittently squeezing blood from the deep veins in the legs, thereby lessening the risk of DVT.*

CONSIDERATION FOR PRACTICE

Removing TED stockings each shift not only promotes healthy skin but also lets the nurse assess skin integrity.

Impaired gas exchange

Injuries at the level of T1 to T7 leave the phrenic nerve intact, but the innervation of intercostal muscles is affected, compromising respiratory function. In addition, because the abdominal muscles are paralysed, the person cannot expel secretions by coughing. The person with cord injuries at C3 or above has paralysis of the respiratory muscles and cannot breathe without a ventilator.

- Monitor vital capacity and respiratory effectiveness, assessing for tachycardia, restlessness, PaO_2 less than 60 mmHg, $PaCO_2$ greater than 50 mmHg and vital capacity less than 1 L. *People with cervical cord injuries frequently require ventilatory support because of reduced vital capacity and inability to expel secretions by coughing.*

CONSIDERATION FOR PRACTICE
Changes in ABGs and vital capacity signal respiratory insufficiency.

- Monitor for signs of ascending oedema of the spinal cord, including difficulty in swallowing or coughing, respiratory stridor, use of accessory muscles of respiration, bradycardia and increased motor and sensory loss. *Haemorrhage and oedema can further impair respiratory function.*
- Help the person to cough, as follows: place the hand between the umbilicus and xiphoid process and push in and up as the person exhales and coughs. *The person who is unable to cough effectively and has decreased ventilatory capacity may develop atelectasis, pneumonia and respiratory failure.*

Ineffective breathing patterns

Respiratory function is impaired in the person with an SCI in the cervical and thoracic levels if the diaphragm (innervated at C3 to C5), the intercostal muscles (innervated at T1 to T7) and the abdominal muscles are affected. In the person with injury at higher levels, assisted ventilation and a tracheostomy are necessary; when the injury is at lower levels, the person's ability to take a deep breath and cough is diminished. The goal of nursing interventions is to maintain normal respiratory rate (12 to 20 breaths per minute) and to prevent pulmonary complications such as atelectasis and pneumonia.

- Assess respiratory rate, rhythm and depth every 4 hours (or more frequently if needed). Auscultate breath sounds as a part of respiratory assessment. *Injury to the cord in the cervical or thoracic regions can decrease respiratory function and increase the risk of respiratory problems.*

CONSIDERATION FOR PRACTICE
Auscultate the lungs for crackles and wheezes.

- Monitor results of oxygen saturation with pulse oximetry and ABG studies. *ABG studies provide information about gas exchange; decreasing pH, oxygen and oxygen saturation levels, and increasing carbon dioxide levels, signal respiratory acidosis.*
- Administer supplemental oxygen as prescribed. *Oxygen saturation must be maintained at 100% with supplemental oxygen to prevent hypoxaemia and secondary SCI in all acute SCI.*
- Help the person turn, cough and deep breathe at least every 2 hours. Use assisted coughing as necessary. *Paralysis of intercostal or abdominal muscles decreases the ability to expel secretions by coughing; retained secretions increase the risk of pneumonia. The inability to breathe deeply may result in atelectasis.*
- Increase fluids given by mouth to 3,000 mL per day (if oral intake is approved), according to the person's preference for type of liquids and predicated on the person's ability to swallow. *Increased fluid intake thins secretions, which can more easily be expelled and expectorated.*

Dysreflexia

Autonomic dysreflexia is an emergency that requires immediate assessment and intervention to prevent complications of extremely high blood pressure (loss of consciousness, seizure and even death).

- Elevate the head of the person's bed and remove TEDs or sequential compression boots. *These measures increase pooling of blood in the lower extremities and decrease venous return, thus decreasing blood pressure.*
- Assess blood pressure every 2 to 3 minutes while at the same time assessing for stimuli that initiated the response (such as a full bladder, impacted stool or skin pressure). *The most serious danger in dysreflexia is elevated blood pressure, which could precipitate a stroke, myocardial infarction, arrhythmias or seizures. If the person has a Foley catheter, ensure that there are no kinks in the tubing. If the person does not have a Foley catheter, drain the bladder with a straight catheter. If manifestations persist, assess for a faecal impaction. If an impaction is present, insert lignocaine into the anus, wait 10 minutes, and manually remove the impaction.*

CONSIDERATION FOR PRACTICE
Blood pressure readings may be as high as 300/160.

- If blood pressure remains dangerously elevated, the doctor may prescribe intravenous administration of an antihypertensive agent such as diazoxide. Other medications that may be used include nifedipine and hydralazine.

CONSIDERATION FOR PRACTICE
It is important to closely monitor for hypotension following administration of antihypertensive medications, especially if the stimulus for the dysreflexia has been removed.

Impaired urinary elimination and constipation

Depending on the level of the injury, the person with an SCI may have alterations in bowel and bladder function. The person with injuries to the cord at or above the S2 to S4 levels will have a neurogenic bladder, with deficits in control of micturition. Voluntary and involuntary bowel control is affected in the person with a lower motor neuron injury. Both bowel and bladder retraining are possible; if not, some form of assisted elimination is necessary. Although an indwelling catheter may be used in the acute phase of care, the goal is to re-establish a catheter-free state.

- Monitor for manifestations of a full bladder. *Over-distension stretches the bladder and can lead to backflow of urine into the ureters and kidney; stasis of urine in an incompletely emptied bladder increases the risk of infection.*

CONSIDERATION FOR PRACTICE
A distended bladder can be palpated over the lower abdomen above the pubic symphysis.

PROCEDURE 42.1 Self-catheterisation

Self-catheterisation on an intermittent basis (usually as part of self-care at home) is a clean, rather than sterile, procedure. The hands should be washed before and after the procedure and the urinary meatus should be cleaned by washing with soap and water.

Attempt to void. If urine is not of sufficient quantity (at least 100 mL), or if you cannot void at all, perform self-catheterisation. *A large amount of residual urine means that more frequent catheterisations (every 4 to 6 hours) are necessary.*

FEMALE SELF-CATHETERISATION

- While sitting on the wheelchair or the commode, locate the urethra. Visualise the urethra by looking in a mirror or palpate the urethra with a fingertip. *Visualisation or palpation of the meatus is necessary for proper catheter insertion.*
- Lubricate the meatus with a water-soluble lubricant. *Lubrication facilitates the insertion of the catheter and reduces trauma to tissues.*
- Take a deep breath and insert the catheter tip 5 to 7 cm or until urine flows. *The catheter enters the bladder more easily when the sphincter is relaxed. The deep breath relaxes the sphincter. The female urethra is 4 to 6.5 cm long.*
- Hold the catheter securely and allow urine to drain until the flow stops. *Withdrawing and reinserting the catheter increase the risk of infection.*

MALE SELF-CATHETERISATION

- Sit either on the commode or in the wheelchair. Hold the penis with slight upward tension and extend it to its full length. *Extending the penis straightens the urethra.*
- Lubricate the catheter from the tip to about 15 cm downwards. *Lubrication is especially important for male catheterisation because of the length of the urethra.*
- Take a deep breath and insert the catheter 15 to 17 cm or until urine flows. *The catheter enters the bladder more easily when the sphincter is relaxed. The deep breath relaxes the sphincter. The male urethra is about 15 cm long.*
- Hold the catheter securely and allow urine to drain until flow has stopped. *Withdrawing and reinserting the catheter increase the risk of infection.*

FOLLOWING SELF-CATHETERISATION

For both female and male techniques, withdraw the catheter and wash it with soap and water. Store the catheter in a clean container. *The catheter can be reused until it is too soft or too hard to be directed into and through the urinary meatus.*

- Teach the person to use trigger voiding techniques prior to straight catheterisation. These techniques include stroking the inner thigh, pulling the pubic hair, tapping on the abdomen over the bladder and (in females) pouring warm water over the vulva. *These trigger voiding techniques stimulate parasympathetic nerve fibres to cause reflex activity and may facilitate voiding.*
- Teach self-catheterisation to the person who will be able to carry out the procedure alone or with minimal assistance (see Procedure 42.1). *Straight catheterisation at regular intervals is part of bladder training because periodic distension and relaxation of the muscles of the bladder promote reflex bladder activity. In addition, self-care fosters independence.*
- Monitor residual urine throughout the bladder retraining program. *A residual urine amount of less than 80 mL after a triggered voiding is considered satisfactory.*
- Institute a bowel retraining program as follows:
  - Assess usual patterns of bowel elimination to establish best times for an individualised program.
  - Maintain a high-fluid, high-fibre diet.
  - Use stool softeners as prescribed; rectal suppositories and enemas may be used 30 minutes after meals to stimulate stronger peristalsis and facilitate evacuation.
  - Maintain an upright position if at all possible and ensure privacy.
  - If the person is unable to evacuate, digital stimulation or manual removal on a regular basis may be the most effective long-term management.

  A bowel retraining program to regulate the bowel through reflex activity may be instituted in the person with upper motor neuron injuries. The person with a lower motor neuron injury loses the defecation reflex and bowel retraining is more difficult (if not impossible).

Sexual dysfunction

Sexual intercourse is often still possible for the person with an SCI. In men, the general rule is that the higher the level of injury the greater the potential to have reflexogenic erections, although ejaculation or orgasm may not occur and fertility is usually lower as a result of a lack of temperature control of the testes. However, ejaculation may be stimulated and the sperm used to inseminate the person's partner so that fatherhood is a possibility. Men who have sacral-level injuries do not have reflexogenic erections but may have psychogenic erections. They are also more likely to remain fertile.

Women with an SCI generally do not have sensation during sexual intercourse, but pregnancy is possible. However, pregnant women with an SCI are at increased risk of autonomic dysreflexia during labour and delivery. Birth-control options should be discussed prior to discharge from the acute care setting.

A person with an SCI may be deeply concerned about alterations in sexual function. These concerns may lead to lowered self-esteem, altered self-image or changes in feelings about being an attractive and desirable person. Assess concerns and provide a climate that is receptive to discussion about sexuality.

Examples of objectives for sexual counselling for the person with an SCI are that the person will understand how the injury has altered sexual functioning, be aware of alternative ways of achieving sexual pleasure and have a positive self-concept and body image.

- Include data about sexuality when obtaining the nursing history and database. *Sexuality is a private matter for most people and the person may not discuss it unless the nurse introduces the topic.*
- Provide accurate information about the effect of the SCI on sexual function. *Accurate information gives the person a realistic picture of how the injury will affect sexuality.*
- Initiate a discussion with the person and partner of alternative means of gaining sexual satisfaction; these include the use of vibrators and oral–genital and manual stimulation. *Alternatives to intercourse can meet sexual needs and help maintain the relationship with a significant other.*
- Refer for sexual counselling, if appropriate, or to local support groups where questions can be answered by others with similar experiences. *Knowing that others have had similar experiences can decrease social isolation and provide a means of learning alternative methods of sexual functioning.*

Low self-esteem

An SCI is often the result of sudden trauma. Within moments, a formerly independent, fully functioning individual is suddenly unable to move and faces enormous adjustments in social, economic and personal roles and relationships. Body image, self-esteem and role performance are all affected by the damage. As a result, the person often demonstrates behaviours that may be difficult for the nurse to handle: depression, denial and anger are seen in the period immediately after the injury. In addition to these responses, the young adult person may act out by making sexually overt statements.

- Encourage talking about all aspects of physical function and care. *Talking provides a safe outlet for fears and frustrations and also increases self-awareness. Acceptance of self facilitates rehabilitation.*
- Encourage self-care and independent decision making. *Participating in self-care can promote positive coping; making decisions decreases feelings of powerlessness.*
- Help identify strategies to increase independence in desired roles; include both short- and long-term goals. Discuss assistive devices (such as hand-operated motor vehicles). *Identifying strategies to increase independence in the future fosters a positive self-concept and motivates the person to achieve rehabilitation goals.*
- Include family members and important others in discussions. *The realisation that others do care and will continue to provide support is important in fostering positive self-regard.*
- Refer the person and family to support groups or for psychological counselling. *Adjustment to change is more likely when the person and family seek peer and professional assistance.*

Community-based care

Rehabilitation of the person with an SCI is an ongoing process that moves from intensive care to intermediate care, to rehabilitation, and then to community-based and home care. Nursing interventions are necessary at all points in the process to prevent the complications of altered physical mobility and body functions, and to teach the person and family measures that promote independence in self-care.

Discharge planning should be addressed even in the initial plan of care while the person is in the critical care setting. Advance planning ensures continuity of care when the person leaves the hospital setting.

The following should be included in teaching the person and family about care at home:

- self-care activities (ADLs, exercises, bowel and bladder programs, skin care)
- mobility (use of assistive devices: wheelchair, crutches, special motor vehicles)
- preparation of the home environment
- if the person is in a wheelchair, will steps, stairs, doors or carpeted floors present physical barriers?
- if a special bed is necessary, have arrangements been made and is it in the home?
- psychological support
- independent activities
- coping skills for the person and caregiver
- referral to a community health agency and physiotherapist for the person who is returning home
- helpful resources:
  - Spinal Cord Injuries Australia: https://scia.org.au 1800 819 775
  - Christopher and Dana Reeve Foundation: https://www.christopherreeve.org
  - Australian Quadriplegic Association (Victoria): https://www.aqavic.org.au/.

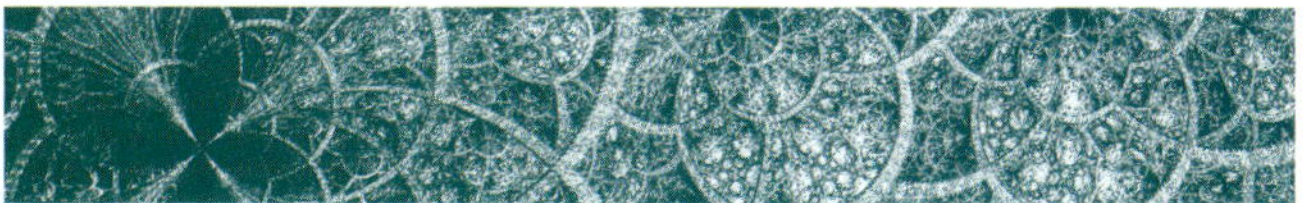

THE PERSON WITH A HERNIATED INTERVERTEBRAL DISC

A herniated intervertebral disc—also called a *ruptured disc, herniated nucleus pulposus* or a *slipped disc*—is a rupture of the cartilage surrounding the intervertebral disc with protrusion of the nucleus pulposus (see Figure 42.10). Perhaps few neuro-orthopaedic disorders are as challenging as those involving the intervertebral discs. The person with herniation (rupture) of a disc has not only excruciating pain but also limited mobility. These problems may in turn cause alterations in role function, coping and the ability to perform ADLs.

Incidence and prevalence

A herniated intervertebral disc may occur at any adult age. However, it is more common as people enter middle age and age-related changes occur. The nucleus pulposus loses fluid

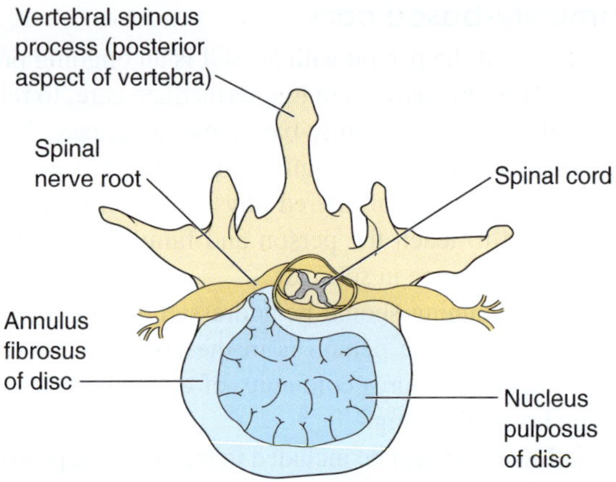

FIGURE 42.10 ***A herniated intervertebral disc. The herniated nucleus pulposus is applying pressure against the nerve root***

content and the discs are less able to absorb shocks. The discs become smaller and slip out of place more easily. Ageing causes degeneration in the annulus fibrosus and the posterior longitudinal ligaments, and the vertebrae and discs are less able to respond to movement and are more easily injured.

FAST FACTS

- A herniated disk refers to a problem with one of the rubbery cushions (disks) that sit between the bones (vertebrae) that stack to make the spine.
- A spinal disk has a soft, jelly-like centre (nucleus) encased in a tougher, rubbery exterior (annulus). Sometimes called a *slipped disk* or a *ruptured disk*, a herniated disk occurs when some of the nucleus pushes out through a tear in the annulus.
- A herniated disk, which can occur in any part of the spine, most often occurs in the lower back (L4 or L5 to S1). Depending on where the herniated disk is, it can result in pain, numbness or weakness in an arm or leg.
- Many people have no symptoms from a herniated disk. For people who do have symptoms, the symptoms tend to improve over time. Surgery is usually not necessary to relieve the problem.

Source: Mayo Clinic (2022). *Herniated disk*. Retrieved from https://www.mayoclinic.org/diseases-conditions/herniated-disk/symptoms-causes/syc-20354095. Used with permission of Mayo Foundation for Medical Education and Research, all rights reserved.

Pathophysiology

The intervertebral discs, located between the vertebral bodies, are made of an inner nucleus pulposus and an outer collar (the annulus fibrosus). The discs allow the spine to absorb compression by acting as shock absorbers. A herniated intervertebral disc occurs when the nucleus pulposus protrudes through a weakened or torn annulus fibrosus of an intervertebral disc (see Figure 42.10). This protrusion may occur anywhere along the vertebral column, but herniation of thoracic discs is uncommon. The protrusion may occur spontaneously or as a result of trauma, with trauma (such as lifting heavy objects or falling) causing about half of all cases. Rupture of the disc allows herniation of the nucleus pulposus in a posterolateral direction, with compression of the associated nerve root. The resulting pressure on adjacent spinal nerves causes characteristic manifestations, which vary with the location and the amount of protruding disc material (see the 'Manifestations' box). Occasionally, the herniation is central rather than posterolateral, with pressure on the spinal cord.

The herniation may be abrupt or gradual. Lifting incorrectly or suddenly twisting the spine can cause rupture with immediate intense pain and muscle spasms. Gradual herniation is the result of degenerative changes, osteoarthritis or ankylosis spondylitis. People with a gradual herniation have a slow onset of pain and neurological deficits.

MANIFESTATIONS A ruptured intervertebral disc

L4 TO L5 LEVEL (AFFECTS FIFTH LUMBAR NERVE ROOT)

- Pain in hip, lower back, posterolateral thigh, anterior leg, dorsal surface of foot, great toe
- Muscle spasms in affected areas
- Paraesthesia over lateral leg and web of great toe
- Foot drop (rare)
- Decreased or absent ankle reflex
- Cauda equina syndrome (with complete nerve root compression): bowel and bladder incontinence, paralysis of lower extremities

L5 TO S1 LEVEL (AFFECTS FIRST SACRAL NERVE ROOT)

- Pain in midgluteal region, posterior thigh, calf to heel, plantar surface of the foot to the fourth and fifth toes
- Paraesthesias in posterior calf and lateral heel, foot and toes
- Difficulty walking on toes

C5 TO C6 LEVEL (AFFECTS SIXTH CERVICAL NERVE ROOT)

- Pain in neck, shoulder, anterior upper arm, radial area of forearm, thumb
- Paraesthesia of forearm, thumb, forefinger and lateral arm
- Decreased biceps and supinator reflex
- Triceps reflex normal to hyperactive

Lumbar disc manifestations

The classic manifestation of a ruptured lumbar disc is recurrent episodes of pain in the lower back. The pain typically radiates across the buttock and down the posterior leg, although it may be experienced only in the leg. **Sciatica** is a term used to describe lumbar back pain that radiates down the posterior leg to the ankle and is increased by sneezing or coughing (the result of pressure on nerve roots L4, L5, S1, S2 or S3, which give rise to the sciatic nerve). Sciatica may be elicited by straight leg raising: the person feels pain when lifting one leg while dorsiflexing the foot of that leg. Sciatica pain varies in intensity, ranging from mildly uncomfortable to excruciating. It is aggravated by a variety of positions and activities, including sitting, straining, coughing, sneezing, climbing stairs, walking and riding in a car.

Other manifestations include postural deformity, motor deficits, sensory deficits and changes in reflexes. In about 60% of people with ruptured lumbar discs, the normal lumbar lordosis is absent. When standing, the person typically has a slight forward tilt to the trunk, scoliosis of the lumbar spine, slight flexion of the hip and knee on the affected side and paravertebral muscle spasms (Hickey, 2019). Motor deficits include weakness and, in some people, problems with sexual function and urinary elimination. Sensory deficits include paraesthesias and numbness. Knee and ankle reflexes are decreased or absent.

Cervical disc manifestations

Cervical discs that herniate laterally cause pain in the shoulder, neck and arm. Other manifestations of lateral cervical herniation include paraesthesias, muscle spasms and stiff neck, and decreased or absent arm reflexes. Central cervical herniations result in mild, intermittent pain; however, the person may also experience lower extremity weakness, unsteady gait, muscle spasms, urinary elimination problems, altered sexual function and hyperactive lower extremity reflexes.

INTERPROFESSIONAL CARE

Considerations for the person with a ruptured intervertebral disc include identifying the location of herniation and determining whether conservative treatment or surgery is indicated. Nursing care is directed towards preparing the person for diagnostic tests and providing teaching and care for the person who has either medical or surgical interventions.

Diagnosis

Diagnostic tests are ordered to differentiate the cause of back pain; for example, back and leg pain is also caused by spinal tumours, degenerative processes or abdominal diseases. Assessing pain is an important part of diagnosis. The tests include x-rays and CT scans of the lumbosacral or cervical area to identify skeletal deformities and narrowing of the disc spaces (see the chapter 'A person-centred approach to assessing the nervous system'). Electromyography (EMG), which measures electrical activity of skeletal muscles at rest and during voluntary contraction, may be conducted to identify specific muscles affected by the pressure of the herniation on the nerve roots.

A myelogram with contrast medium is done to illustrate areas of herniation, although it does not provide the detail found with CT or MRI. However, myelography is diagnostic in 80–90% of all cases and is used both to rule out tumours and locate the herniation. Nursing implications for the care of a person having a myelogram are described in the chapter 'A person-centred approach to assessing the nervous system'.

Medications

The person with a ruptured intervertebral disc is treated with medications to relieve pain and reduce swelling and muscle spasms. Pain is usually managed with NSAIDs (see the chapter 'Nursing care of people in pain'). Muscle spasms are treated with muscle relaxants.

Treatments

A ruptured intervertebral disc may be treated conservatively or with surgery.

CONSERVATIVE TREATMENT A ruptured intervertebral disc is usually managed conservatively unless the person is experiencing severe neurological deficits. The goals of treatment are pain relief and healing of the involved disc by fibrosis. Conservative treatment is usually prescribed for 2 to 6 weeks. If the person continues to have pain after that time, surgery may be considered. The treatment regimen depends on the severity of the manifestations. Decreasing activity level with bed rest is no longer recommended; and in many cases, the person is advised to continue with normal activities while taking prescribed medications for pain, inflammation and muscle spasms.

Medications used to treat back pain include non-narcotic analgesics, anti-inflammatory drugs such as the NSAIDs, muscle relaxants and sedative–tranquillisers.

SURGERY Surgery is indicated for people who do not respond to conservative management or have serious neurological deficits. Several surgical interventions are used to treat a ruptured intervertebral disc. The type of surgery chosen depends on the location of the disc and the stability of the spinal column.

- A **laminectomy**, the type of surgery most often performed, is the removal of a part of the vertebral lamina. The surgery is done to relieve pressure on the nerves. It is often combined with removal of the protruding nucleus pulposus (*nuclectomy*). See the accompanying box for nursing care for the person having a laminectomy. A *discectomy* is the removal of the nucleus pulposus of an intervertebral disc. Discectomy may be performed alone or with a laminectomy.
- Spinal fusion is the insertion of a wedge-shaped piece of bone or bone chips between the vertebrae to stabilise them. The bone is usually taken from a person donor site, such as the iliac crest. A spinal fusion may also be performed through a spinal implant with a device called a BAK (a hollow titanium cylinder with holes), which is packed with grafted bone from a donor site and placed in the space where a disc is removed. Although not appropriate for all people requiring a spinal fusion, this does facilitate a short hospital stay and convalescence.
- Foraminotomy is an enlargement of the opening between the disc and the facet joint to remove bony overgrowth compressing the nerve. The location and size of the incision vary according to the surgeon's preference and the location and size of the ruptured disc. The posterior approach is taken for lumbar surgery. Either the posterior or the anterior approach may be taken for cervical discs.
- Intradiscal electrothermal therapy (IDET) uses thermal energy to treat pain from a bulging spinal disc. A special needle is inserted into the disc and heated to a high temperature. The heat thickens and seals the disc wall and decreases bulging of the disc.
- A *microdiscectomy*, in which microsurgical techniques are used, is performed through a very small incision. This type of surgery decreases the possibility of trauma to surrounding structures during surgery and allows early postoperative mobility and a short hospital stay.

NURSING CARE OF THE PERSON having a posterior laminectomy

PREOPERATIVE TEACHING

- Demonstrate and ask the person to practise log-rolling; explain that it will be done by the nurses for the first day or two and then the person can do it alone. *To ensure healing, the spinal column must remain in alignment when turning and moving.*
- Explain the importance of taking pain medications regularly and of asking for them before the pain is severe. Include information about the possibility of the pain being much the same after surgery. *Pain is easier to control if medications are taken before the pain is severe. Pain may be the same following surgery for a herniated intervertebral disc because oedema due to surgery irritates and compresses the nerve roots.*
- Demonstrate the use of a fracture bedpan and ask the person to practise its use. The person usually must remain flat in bed for a period of time following surgery. *A fracture bedpan is more comfortable for the person who must lie flat.*
- Explain that the person may need to eat while lying flat. *This position prevents flexion of the spine.*
- Demonstrate and ask the person to demonstrate deep breathing, the use of the incentive spirometer and leg exercises. *These measures prevent respiratory and circulatory complications.*

POSTOPERATIVE CARE

- Maintain the person in a position that minimises stress on the surgical wound. For people with cervical laminectomy:
  a. Elevate the head of the bed slightly.
  b. Position a small pillow under the neck.
  c. Maintain the position of the cervical collar.
- For people with lumbar laminectomy:
  a. Keep the bed flat or elevate the head of the bed slightly.
  b. Place a small pillow under the head.
  c. Place a small pillow under the knees or use a pillow to support the upper leg when the person lies on one side.

  These positions minimise stress on the surgical wound and suture line. A cervical collar provides stability and prevents flexing or twisting the neck.
- Turn the person every 2 hours, using the log-rolling technique. Teach the person not to use the side rails to change position. Maintain proper body alignment in all positions. *The person's body is turned as a single unit (usually with a turning sheet) to avoid movement of the operative area. Pulling on the side rails puts stress on the operative area and may also cause misalignment of the vertebral column.*
- Monitor the person for signs of nerve root compression.
  a. Cervical laminectomy: assess hand grips and arm strength, ability to move the fingers and ability to detect touch.
  b. Lumbar laminectomy: assess leg strength, ability to wriggle the toes and ability to detect touch.

  Compare bilateral findings. Report muscle weakness or sensory impairment to the doctor immediately. *Loss of motor and sensory function may indicate nerve root compression.*
- Assess for haematoma formation as manifested by severe incisional pain that is not relieved by analgesics and decreased motor function. Report these findings immediately. *A haematoma may form at the surgical site. If untreated, it may cause irreversible neurological deficits including paraplegia and bowel/bladder dysfunctions (Hickey, 2019).*
- Assess for leakage of cerebrospinal fluid. Assess the dressing for increased moisture. Check the sheets for wetness when the person is lying supine; check for clear liquid running down the back when the person is sitting or standing. Gently palpate the sides of the wound to detect a bulge. Use a Dextrostrix strip to assess any leakage for the presence of glucose, a positive indicator of cerebrospinal fluid. *Although uncommon, leakage of cerebrospinal fluid greatly increases the risk of infection of the wound and of the meninges.*
- Assess for nerve root injury. Assess the person's ability to dorsiflex the foot (lumbar laminectomy) and the person's grip strength (cervical laminectomy). Assess the person who has had a cervical laminectomy for hoarseness. Report hoarseness and further assess the person's ability to swallow. *Nerve root compression may cause permanent damage, resulting in footdrop (in lumbar laminectomy) and hand weakness (in cervical laminectomy). Damage to the laryngeal nerve may cause permanent hoarseness. Impaired ability to swallow puts the person at risk of aspiration.*
- Assess for urinary retention. The person should void within 8 hours after surgery. If the doctor allows, let males stand to void. Compare intake and output for each 8-hour period. *All people who have received a general anaesthetic are at risk of urinary retention. The person who has had a lumbar laminectomy may have even more difficulty voiding as a result of stimulation of sympathetic nerves during surgery.*
- Assess for pain using a scale from 0 (no pain) to 10 (severe pain). Administer prescribed analgesics on a regular basis or teach the person to use patient-controlled analgesia (PCA), if prescribed. Discuss the person's concerns about pain that is unrelieved by surgery. *Compression of the nerve root over time results in oedema and inflammation. Because of surgery-induced oedema, the person is likely to experience either the same pain or perhaps more severe pain in the period immediately after surgery. This pain usually persists for several weeks after surgery. In addition, many people who have had a lumbar laminectomy have muscle spasms in the lower back, abdomen and thighs for the first few days after surgery.*
- Assess for infection by taking and recording vital signs at least every 4 hours; report increased body temperature. Assess the wound and dressing for signs of infection: increased redness, drainage, pain and pus. Use sterile technique to change dressings. *The surgical person is always at risk of infection; the person with a laminectomy is also at risk of arachnoiditis. This inflammation of the arachnoid layer of the spinal meninges results from wound infection or contamination during surgery and may cause the formation of painful adhesions.*

NURSING CARE OF THE PERSON having a posterior laminectomy (continued)

- Encourage deep breathing and the use of the incentive spirometer every 2 hours; coughing may be discouraged. *Anaesthesia and immobility depress respiratory function. Coughing may be discouraged because it can disrupt healing tissues, especially in the person having a cervical laminectomy.*
- Increase mobility as prescribed. (The timeframe for ambulation is prescribed by the doctor; the routine here is representative.) People often sit on the side of the bed and dangle their legs the evening after surgery or the first day thereafter. Many people ambulate the first or second postoperative day. To help the person out of bed, first elevate the head of the bed. Then bring the person's legs over the side of the bed at the same time that the upper body moves into the upright position. *The person should not ambulate without assistance until they are no longer dizzy or weak. Early ambulation increases respiratory and circulatory function and decreases the risk of thrombophlebitis of the lower extremities. The vertebral column should remain in alignment while the person sits and stands. Safety must be considered throughout care.*

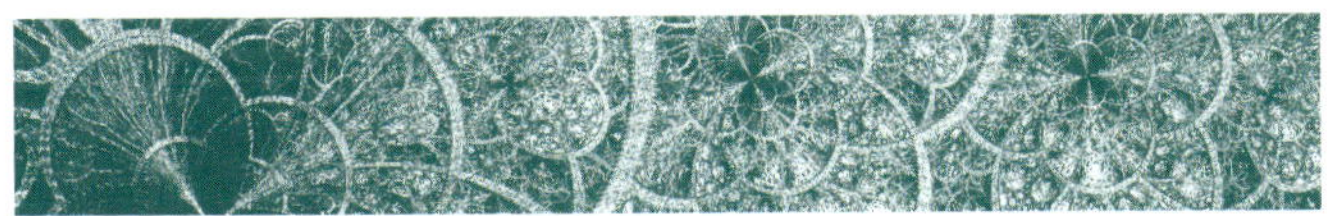

Nursing care

Nursing care for the person with a ruptured intervertebral disc may be provided through information in community and work settings, during conservative treatment and during pre- and postoperative treatment. The pain of the ruptured disc is often discouraging and debilitating and may well affect the person's ability to work.

Health promotion

Proper body mechanics may help prevent the occurrence of a ruptured intervertebral disc. Educating the person about the proper method of lifting and moving heavy objects should begin when children enter school. This information should also be given to all workers (including nurses) who have lifting as part of their responsibilities. The guidelines for proper body mechanics are as follows:

- Begin activities by spreading the feet apart to broaden the base of support.
- Use large muscles of the arms to lift and the legs to push when lifting.
- Work as closely as possible to the object that is to be lifted or moved.
- Slide, roll, push or pull an object rather than lift it.
- When lifting, bend the knees and lift up over your centre of gravity.
- When lifting, use a back support belt.

Assessment

The following data are collected through the health history and physical examination (see the chapter 'A person-centred approach to assessing the nervous system').

- *Health history*: type of employment, risk factors, pain (location, duration, intensity).
- *Physical assessment*: muscle strength and coordination, sensation, reflexes.

Nursing diagnosis and interventions

Nursing care for the person with a herniated intervertebral disc focuses largely on pain management, both during conservative management and after surgery.

Acute pain

People with a ruptured intervertebral disc experience acute back and leg pain. Acute pain may be related to preoperative muscle spasms or nerve root compression. After surgery, the person may have pain at the site of the incision and in the surgical area.

- Assess the degree of pain on a 0 to 10 scale (10 being greatest pain) and identify contributing and relieving factors. *Pain is a subjective experience. The nurse needs to assess it thoroughly before initiating interventions.*
- Use a firm mattress or place a board under the mattress. *A firm bed supports the spinal column and muscles.*
- Educate the person about avoiding turning or twisting the spinal column and to assume positions that decrease stress on the vertebral column (e.g. when in the supine position, flex the hips slightly). A small pillow may be placed under the knees (for the person with a herniated lumbar disc) or under the neck (for the person with a herniated cervical disc). *Correct body positions can decrease intradisc pressure.*
- Provide analgesic medications around the clock. *Intense pain can increase muscle spasms; maintaining serum levels of analgesics often prevents severe pain.*

CONSIDERATION FOR PRACTICE

It is important to maintain a constant level of pain relief. Healthcare providers have the responsibility of relieving pain with adequate medications.

Chronic pain

The person with a ruptured intervertebral disc often has pain for an extended period of time. Despite conservative treatment or previous surgery, pain may be ongoing or intermittent. If previous surgery has not relieved the pain, the person may be depressed or angry. Caring for a person with chronic pain is frustrating and the person is often regarded as difficult.

- Treat the person's reports of pain with respect. *The person is the one experiencing the pain and is thus the expert about it.*
- Do not refer to the person as being addicted to pain medication. *All types of pain medications may be used legitimately to manage pain.*

- Monitor the person carefully for any changes in condition. *Significant changes in the person's condition may go unrecognised when pain is present for a prolonged period of time.*

CONSIDERATION FOR PRACTICE

Although the person may develop tolerance to a narcotic analgesic, tolerance does not imply addiction.

- Maintain written plans of care for pain management that are individualised and ensure continuity of care. *When the person makes several visits (e.g. to an emergency department or a pain clinic), written records help caregivers determine what is effective in managing pain and what is not.*
- Teach the person alternative methods of pain management. *Consider the person's coping style when recommending methods. People who have a passive coping style are often better able to manage pain by depending on others, taking medications and resting. People with an active coping style are probably better able to manage pain by learning self-management methods, taking part in activities and staying busy.*
- Develop effective methods of improving rest and sleep. *Problems with rest and sleep make pain management more difficult. Sleeping poorly at night contributes to decreased motivation, confused thinking, depression and muscle aches.*
- Refer the person to a physiotherapist for an exercise program, if appropriate. *The person needs to know exactly what exercises to do, how many repetitions are recommended, for how long and how often. The person should not exercise to the point of causing increased pain.*
- Assess the need for referrals (and make them, if necessary) for the person who is depressed or anxious. *Anxiety and depression often are a part of long-term chronic pain, making pain management more difficult. Suggest that referrals for help with the frustration (rather than 'depression') may make a significant difference in the person's ability to manage pain.*

Constipation

The person with a ruptured intervertebral disc often has problems with constipation because of reduced mobility. Nursing interventions to alleviate and prevent constipation are important because straining to have a bowel movement can increase intradisc pressure, thus increasing pain.

- Assess the person's usual bowel routine, including diet, fluid intake and the use of laxatives or enemas. *Effective interventions are based on individualised needs.*

CONSIDERATION FOR PRACTICE

People who use laxatives or enemas for long periods of time may be dependent on those methods of having a bowel movement.

- Encourage a fluid intake of 2,500 to 3,000 mL per day unless contraindicated by the presence of renal or cardiac disease. *Adequate fluid intake facilitates the passage of faeces.*
- Increase fibre and bulk in the diet. If the person is unable to tolerate increased fibre, consult with the doctor about the use of stool softeners or bulk-forming agents. *Bulk and fibre promote regularity by retaining water in the large intestine.*

Community-based care

It is the nurse's responsibility to teach the person and family about chronic pain control, including specific interventions to alleviate pain. The nurse's role may be that of advocate and creative problem solver (see the 'Meeting individualised needs' box). The following topics should be addressed:

- Often the goal is to control pain so that the person can perform normal ADLs rather than to reach a pain-free state.
- Non-pharmacological methods of pain management include relaxation techniques, guided imagery,

MEETING INDIVIDUALISED NEEDS Educating the person with a ruptured intervertebral disc

- Sleep on a firm mattress; use a bed board if necessary.
- When lying in the supine position, flex the knees to approximately a 45-degree angle with a small pillow and use a small pillow under the head.
- Avoid any activities that flex the spine, such as bending or lifting, and do not twist the back.
- Follow your diet to maintain body weight or to lose weight if needed.
- Follow the prescribed exercise program—for example:
  a. Lie flat on your back on the floor. Tighten your abdominal and buttock muscles and tilt your pelvis forward so that your lower back is flat on the floor. (This is called a *pelvic tilt.*) Hold the position for 3 seconds and repeat for the prescribed number of times.
  b. Lying on the back on a firm surface, press the feet to the floor, tighten the abdominal muscles and lift the upper half of the body off the floor. Hold the position for 3 seconds and repeat as prescribed.
  c. Lying on your back on a firm surface, bring your knees up to the chest. Put your hands around your knees and raise the buttocks off the floor. Repeat as prescribed.
  d. Sit upright on the floor or a firm surface. Keep one leg straight and bend the other knee. Reach for the toes of the straightened leg. Switch legs. Repeat as prescribed.
  e. Stand upright. Squat down, flexing the hips and knees. Straighten your back. Stand upright by straightening the knees. Repeat as prescribed.
- Wear flat-heeled shoes that provide good support.
- Use proper lifting techniques. For instance, squat and use your thigh muscles to lift an object from the floor and spread your feet to get a wide base of support when you lift while you are standing.

distraction, hypnosis and music. Joining a support group may be an effective intervention in coping with and managing pain.

- The person may be referred to a physiotherapist for education about body mechanics and back-strengthening exercises. Nurses should have the person demonstrate the exercises to reinforce teaching.

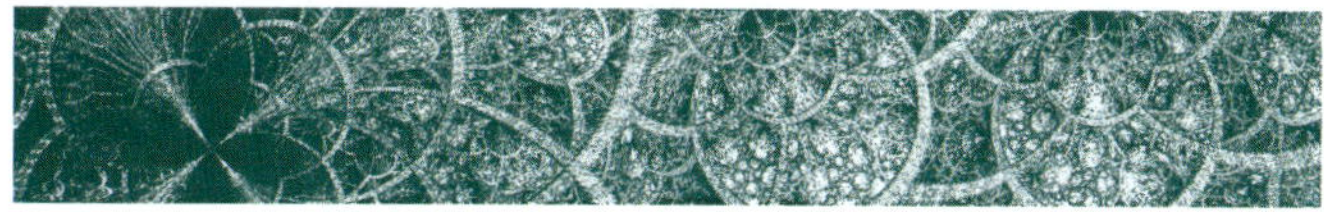

THE PERSON WITH A SPINAL CORD TUMOUR

Spinal cord tumours may be benign or malignant, primary or metastatic. They may arise at any level of the spinal column. Of all spinal cord tumours, 50% are thoracic, 30% are cervical and 20% are lumbosacral. They constitute about 0.5–1% of all tumours (Hickey, 2019). Tumours of the spinal cord are seen equally in men and women, and they most often occur between the ages of 20 and 60. They are rarely seen in the older adult.

Classification

Spinal cord tumours are classified by anatomical location as either intramedullary or extramedullary tumours. Intramedullary tumours, which make up about 10% of spinal tumours, arise from within the neural tissues of the spinal cord; those that occur include astrocytomas, ependymomas, glioblastomas and medulloblastomas (Papadakis et al., 2022). Extramedullary tumours arise from tissues outside the spinal cord, with commonly occurring tumours including neurofibromas, meningiomas, sarcomas, chordomas and vascular tumours.

Extramedullary tumours are further categorised as intradural (arising from the nerve roots or meninges within the subarachnoid space) or extradural (arising from epidural tissue or the vertebrae outside the dura).

Tumours of the spinal cord are also classified as either primary or secondary (metastatic). Primary tumours, arising from the epidural vessels, spinal meninges or glial cells, have an unknown cause. Secondary tumours are metastatic in origin, most commonly the result of malignancies of the lung, breast, prostate, gastrointestinal tract or uterus.

Pathophysiology

Depending on their anatomical location, spinal cord tumours result in pathological changes as a result of compression, invasion or ischaemia secondary to arterial or venous obstruction. Extramedullary tumours (whether benign or malignant) alter normal function through compression of the spinal cord, with destruction of white matter and eventual filling of the space around the spinal cord. Cord compression interferes with normal blood flow and membrane potentials, altering afferent and efferent motor, sensory and reflex impulses. Compression of the spinal cord also causes oedema, which can ascend the cord and cause further neurological deficits. Intramedullary tumours both compress and invade. As the tumour grows within the cord, the cord also enlarges and distorts the white matter.

Manifestations

The manifestations of a spinal cord tumour depend on the anatomical location, level of occurrence, type of tumour and spinal nerves involved. General manifestations of a spinal cord tumour include pain, motor and sensory deficits, changes in bowel and/or bladder elimination, and changes in sexual function. Specific manifestations by anatomical level are outlined in the 'Manifestations' box.

Pain is often the first manifestation of a spinal cord tumour. It is caused by compression of the spinal cord, tension on the spinal nerves or tumour attachment to the proximal dura (the covering of the spinal cord). The pain may be either localised or radicular. Localised pain is felt when pressure is applied over the spinous process of the involved area; this type of pain often accompanies metastatic tumours involving the vertebrae. Radicular pain is felt along the course of a nerve as a result of compression, irritation or tension of a nerve root. The pain is often made worse by any activity that causes intraspinal pressure, such as sneezing or coughing.

Motor manifestations resulting from a spinal cord tumour include paresis and paralysis below the level of the tumour, spasticity and hyperactive reflexes. The Babinski reflex may be positive. These deficits are the result of involvement of the corticospinal tracts.

MANIFESTATIONS Spinal cord tumours

CERVICAL CORD TUMOURS

- Ipsilateral arm motor involvement, followed by ipsilateral and contralateral leg involvement, followed by contralateral arm involvement
- Paresis of the arms and legs
- Stiffness of the neck
- Paraplegia
- Pain in the shoulders and arms
- Hyperactive reflexes

THORACIC CORD TUMOURS

- Paresis and spasticity of one leg, followed by paresis and spasticity of the other leg
- Pain in the back and chest
- Positive Babinski reflex
- Bowel and bladder dysfunction
- Sexual dysfunction

LUMBOSACRAL CORD TUMOURS

- Paresis and spasticity of one leg, followed by paresis and spasticity of the other leg
- Pain in the lower back, radiating to the legs and perineal area
- Loss of sensation in the legs
- Bowel and bladder dysfunction
- Sexual dysfunction
- Decreased or absent ankle and knee reflexes

Many different sensory manifestations may occur, depending on the location and level of the tumour. Lateral tumour growth and compression affect the lateral spinothalamic tracts, causing pain, numbness, tingling and coldness. If the tumour involves the posterior columns, the senses of vibration and proprioception of body parts are affected.

Bladder and bowel elimination and sexual function are often affected. Bowel elimination deficits include constipation that may progress to paralytic ileus. Initial bladder elimination deficits include frequency, urgency and difficulty voiding. The deficits may progress to urinary retention and a neurogenic bladder. In addition, the male person may be impotent.

Syringomyelia is a complication of some spinal cord tumours. In this condition, a fluid-filled cystic cavity forms in the central intramedullary grey matter. This syndrome causes pain, motor weakness and spasticity.

INTERPROFESSIONAL CARE

The medical management of the person with a spinal cord tumour focuses first on diagnosis. Treatment depends on the type of tumour, its location and the person's condition.

Diagnosis

The person with a spinal cord tumour undergoes many of the same diagnostic tests as the person with a ruptured intervertebral disc. The tests used to identify the tumour include x-rays, CT scans, MRI and myelogram (see the chapter 'A person-centred approach to assessing the nervous system'). A lumbar puncture of the person with a spinal cord tumour will demonstrate CSF that is commonly xanthochromic (having a yellow colour), has increased protein, has few to no cells and clots immediately. (This cluster of findings is called Froin's syndrome.)

Medications

The person with a spinal cord tumour is given medications to relieve pain and control oedema. If the pain is severe and the result of a metastatic tumour, narcotic analgesic may be administered via an epidural catheter. Pain management for the person with a spinal cord tumour is provided by narcotic analgesics (see the chapter 'Nursing care of people in pain'). Steroids, such as dexamethasone, are administered to control oedema of the cord.

Surgery

Intramedullary and intradural tumours are surgically excised when possible. Advances in microsurgical techniques and laser surgery have increased the possibility of tumour excision. Metastatic tumours may be partially excised to reduce cord compression; rapidly growing metastatic lesions may require surgical decompression to preserve motor, bowel or bladder function.

The surgical excision is made through a laminectomy. The person with a tumour involving more than two vertebrae often has a spinal fusion and may also have rods inserted to stabilise the spinal column.

Radiation therapy

Radiation therapy is used to treat metastatic spinal cord tumours for several different reasons. It may be used on an emergency basis to treat the person with rapidly progressing neurological deficits. It may be used to reduce pain. Radiation may also be used following surgical excision of as much tumour mass as possible.

Radiation of the spinal cord may cause the development of radiation-induced myelopathy. This complication of radiation exposure occurs over time, with manifestations of *Brown–Séquard syndrome* (weakness or paralysis on one side of the body and loss of sensation on the opposite side) developing 12 to 15 months after therapy. The manifestations may progress to paraplegia, sensory loss and loss of bowel and bladder control (Hickey, 2019).

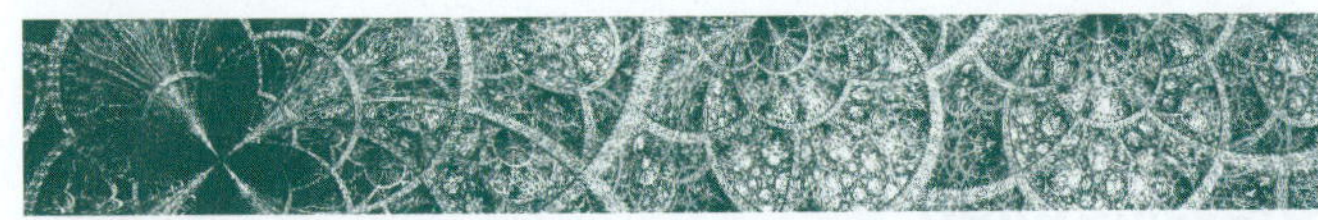

Nursing care

Nursing care for the person with a spinal cord tumour is individualised in accordance with the type of tumour and the type of treatment. The person with a benign tumour that is removed by surgery has different healthcare needs to the person with a metastatic tumour, even though they may have similar neurological deficits. The person with a spinal cord tumour (regardless of type) requires nursing care to monitor for neurological changes, to provide pain management and to manage motor and sensory deficits in order to preserve quality of life.

The assessments and nursing interventions for the person with a spinal cord tumour are similar to those described for the person with an SCI or who is undergoing surgery for a ruptured intervertebral disc. Following surgical treatment, the person may be transferred to a rehabilitation centre or may go home for the recovery period. Referrals for home care, occupational therapy and physiotherapy often help the person regain functional abilities. Teach family members how to move the person in the bed and from the bed to a chair. Also teach them how to provide physiotherapy, care for any appliances (such as an indwelling catheter) and prevent or treat constipation.

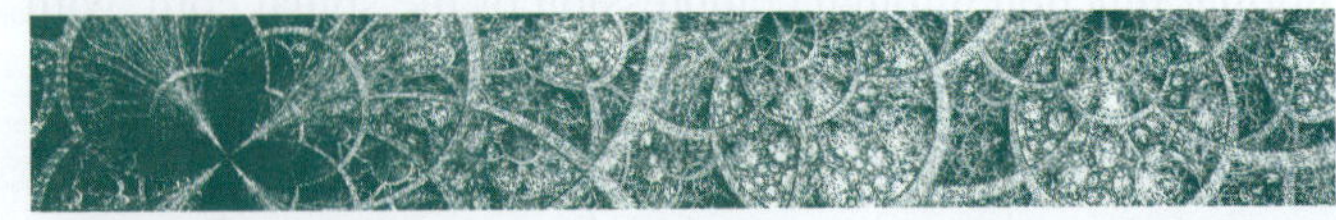

CHAPTER HIGHLIGHTS

- A stroke is a condition in which neurological deficits result from a sudden decrease in blood flow to a localised area of the brain. Strokes may be ischaemic or haemorrhagic. Ischaemic strokes result from a blockage of a cerebral artery by formation of a blood clot or by a clot or foreign substance (such as fat or bacteria) lodging in a blood vessel; they include transient ischaemic attacks, thrombotic strokes and embolic strokes. Haemorrhagic strokes occur when a cerebral blood vessel ruptures.
- Depending on the size and location of cerebral tissue damage, strokes may cause cognitive and behaviour changes, sensory–perceptual deficits, language disorders and motor deficits. Treatment of an ischaemic stroke with fibrinolytic therapy within 3 hours of the onset of manifestations may reverse damage to cerebral neurons.
- Nursing care is directed towards both prevention of a stroke through community-based education programs and interventions to promote recovery and decrease complications.
- Intracerebral haemorrhage may follow rupture of an intracranial aneurysm or arteriovenous malformation. Intracranial aneurysms occur at the site of a weakness in a cerebral blood vessel, while AV malformations are a tangled collection of dilated arteries and veins.
- Spinal cord injuries are almost always the result of trauma, with the main risk factors being age (young adults), gender (male) and alcohol or drug abuse. The causes of injury to the spinal cord include contusion, laceration, transection, haemorrhage and damage to spinal cord blood vessels.
- In a complete SCI, the motor and sensory pathways in the spinal cord are completely interrupted (transected), resulting in total loss of motor and sensory function below the level of the injury. In an incomplete SCI, the motor and sensory pathways are only partially interrupted, resulting in variable loss of function below the level of injury. Injuries of the spinal cord have the potential to affect movement, perception, sensation, sexual function and elimination.
- Spinal shock is the temporary loss of all reflexes (areflexia) below the level of injury. Manifestations of spinal shock include bradycardia, hypotension and flaccid paralysis.
- Autonomic dysreflexia is an exaggerated sympathetic response in the person with an SCI at or above the T6 level. Triggered by noxious stimuli (such as a blocked urinary catheter or a faecal impaction), this condition results in extreme hypertension and, if untreated, may cause seizures, stroke or a myocardial infarction.
- Rehabilitation of the person with an SCI is an ongoing process from intensive care to home care. Nursing interventions are necessary in all settings to promote independence in self-care.
- A herniated intervertebral disc is a rupture of the cartilage surrounding the intervertebral disc with protrusion of the nucleus pulposus. The main manifestation of lumbar discs is lower back and sciatic pain on the affected side. Cervical discs cause pain in the shoulder, neck and arm. A variety of medications, treatments and surgical procedures are available for the person.
- Spinal cord tumours may be benign or malignant, primary or metastatic. Depending on their size and location, they cause pathological changes in spinal cord function through compression, invasion or ischaemia.

CONCEPT CHECK

1 Which of the following manifestations would alert you to the possibility that a person has had a TIA?
1 sudden severe pain over the left eye
2 numbness and tingling in the corner of the mouth
3 complete paralysis of the right arm and leg
4 loss of sensation and reflexes in both legs

2 Although all of the following are risk factors for a stroke, which one is the greatest risk?
1 hypertension
2 heart disease
3 diabetes
4 high cholesterol levels

3 You have been assigned to care for a person who has had an acute ischaemic stroke of a left cerebral vessel. You read the chart and realise the person has contralateral deficits. Indicate what this means?
1 Both sides of the body are involved.
2 The person will have neurological deficits on the left side of the body.
3 The person will have neurological deficits on the right side of the body.
4 Deficits will be present below the level of the stroke.

4 What is the rationale for administration of a tissue plasminogen activator within the first 3 hours of a thrombotic stroke?
1 to reduce the risk of vasospasm
2 to decrease the risk of infection
3 to increase platelet aggregation
4 to cause fibrinolysis of the clot

5 Oxygen is often administered to the person who has had a stroke. Preventing hypoxia and hypercapnia through this treatment will lessen the risk of which complication?
1 fluid accumulation in the lungs
2 pulmonary emboli
3 increased intracranial pressure
4 rebleeding

6 What is the primary pathophysiological process of spinal shock?
1 temporary loss of reflex function below the level of injury
2 loss of control of cardiovascular mechanisms
3 exaggerated sympathetic response
4 damage to the lower motor neurons

7 A person has manifestations of autonomic dysreflexia. Which of these assessments would indicate a possible cause for this condition?
1 extreme hypertension
2 kinked catheter tubing
3 respiratory wheezes and stridor
4 skin breakdown over the coccyx

8 A person is admitted to the emergency department following a motor vehicle accident. An SCI at the cervical level is identified. What will be done to facilitate respirations?
1 No treatments are necessary.
2 Oxygen per nasal prongs will be administered.
3 The person will be placed on a ventilator.
4 The head of the bed will be elevated.

9 **Many different medications may be given to the person with an acute SCI. Which of the following will possibly be administered? (Select all that apply.)**
1 corticosteroids
2 vasopressors
3 antibiotics
4 analgesics
5 antihistamines

10 **You are conducting an educational session at a factory to teach methods to prevent a ruptured intervertebral disc. What should be included in the session? (Choose all that apply.)**
1 Spread the feet apart to broaden the base of support.
2 Bend from the waist to lift articles from the floor.
3 Use large leg muscles to push when lifting.
4 Always lift articles rather than rolling or pushing them.
5 Work as closely as possible to the object to be moved.

BIBLIOGRAPHY

Australian Bureau of Statistics (ABS) (2019). *2018 survey of disability, ageing and carers, customised data report*. Retrieved from https://www.abs.gov.au/statistics/

Australian Bureau of Statistics (ABS) (2020). *Causes of death, Australia*. Retrieved from https://www.abs.gov.au/

Australian Institute of Health and Welfare (AIHW) (2019). *Spinal cord injury, Australia 2015–16*. Injury research and statistics series, no. 122. (Cat. No. INJCAT 202.) Canberra: AIHW.

Australian Institute of Health and Welfare (AIHW) (2021). *Heart, stroke and vascular disease—Australian facts*. Retrieved from https://www.aihw.gov.au/reports/

Brain Aneurysm Foundation (2022). *Unruptured and ruptured aneurysms*. Retrieved from https://www.bafound.org/

Cardiac Research Institute (2022). *Stroke*. Retrieved from https://www.victorchang.edu.au/

Hickey, J. (2019). *The clinical practice of neurological and neurosurgical nursing* (8th ed.). Philadelphia: Lippincott Williams & Wilkins.

Mayo Clinic (2022). *Herniated disk*. Retrieved from https://www.mayoclinic.org/

National Stroke Foundation (2017a). *Clinical guidelines for stroke management 2017*. Retrieved from https://strokefoundation.org.au/.

National Stroke Foundation (2017b). *Facts and figures about strokes*. Retrieved from https://strokefoundation.org.au/

National Stroke Foundation (2018). *More guarantees needed for Australians touched by stroke*. Retrieved from https://strokefoundation.org.au/

National Stroke Foundation (2021). *Our stroke journey*. Retrieved from https://strokefoundation.org.au/

National Stroke Foundation (2022a). *About strokes*. Retrieved from https://strokefoundation.org.au/

National Stroke Foundation (2022b). *About stroke/prevent stroke*. Retrieved from https://strokefoundation.org.au/

National Stroke Foundation (2022c). *Overweight and obesity*. Retrieved from https://strokefoundation.org.au/

National Stroke Foundation (2022d). *Physical inactivity*. Retrieved from https://strokefoundation.org.au/

National Stroke Foundation (2022e). *Treatment for stroke*. Retrieved from https://strokefoundation.org.au/

Norris, T. L. (2018). *Porth's pathophysiology: Concepts of altered health states* (10th ed.). Philadelphia: Lippincott Williams & Wilkins.

Papadakis, M., McPhee, S. & Rabow, M. (2022). *Current medical diagnosis and treatment* (61st ed.). New York: McGraw-Hill Education.

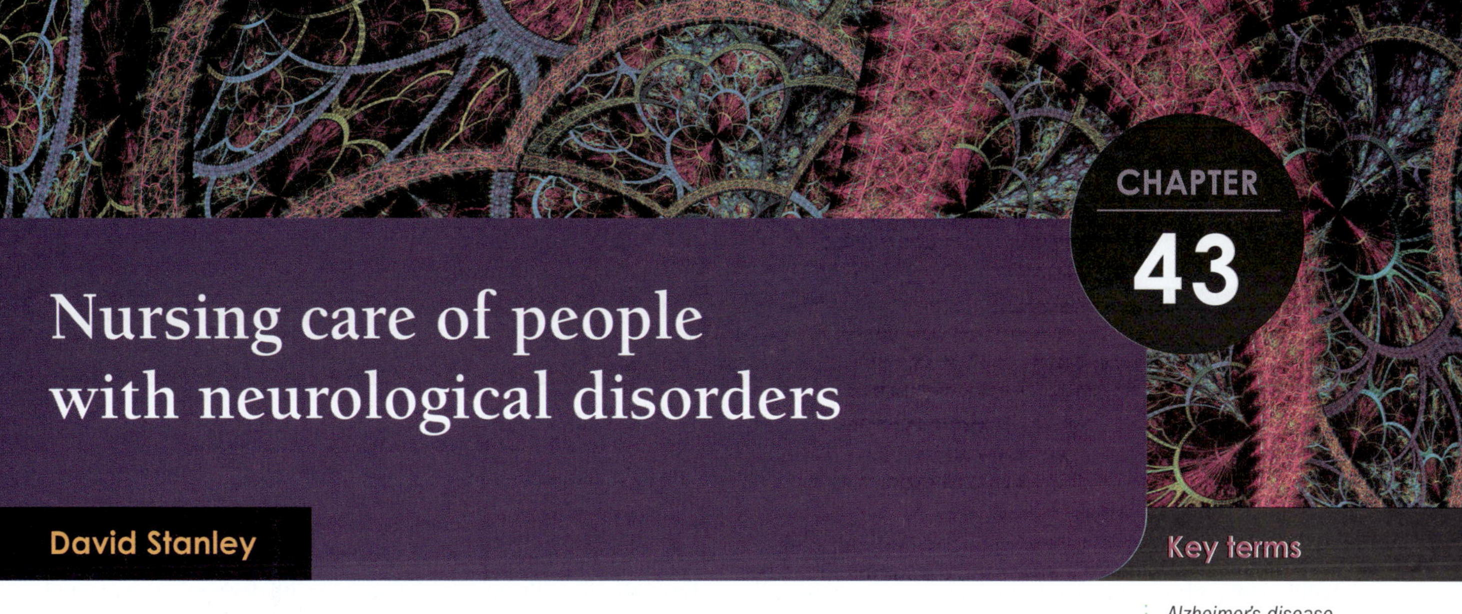

CHAPTER 43

Nursing care of people with neurological disorders

David Stanley

Learning outcomes

- Identify prevalence, incidence and risk factors for degenerative neurological, peripheral nervous system, cranial nerve and infection- and neurotoxin-caused neurological disorders.
- Explain the pathophysiology, manifestations, complications, interprofessional care and nursing care of people with neurological disorders.
- Compare and contrast the manifestations of the progressive stages of Alzheimer's disease.
- Discuss the purposes, nursing implications and health education for the person and their family of medications used to treat Alzheimer's disease, multiple sclerosis, Parkinson's disease, myasthenia gravis and the neurological implications for a person with COVID-19.
- Describe the procedures (thymectomy, percutaneous rhizotomy, plasmapheresis) used to treat selected neurological disorders.

Clinical competencies

- Assess functional status of people with neurological disorders and monitor, document and report abnormal manifestations.
- Use evidence-based research to design nursing interventions specific to the needs of ageing people with multiple sclerosis.
- Determine priority nursing diagnoses, based on assessed data, to select and implement individualised nursing interventions for people with neurological disorders.
- Administer oral and injectable medications used to treat neurological disorders knowledgeably and safely.
- Provide skilled care to people having a thymectomy, percutaneous rhizotomy or plasmapheresis.
- Integrate interprofessional care into the care of people with neurological disorders.
- Provide appropriate teaching to facilitate safety and communication, prevent neurological infections and toxins (rabies, tetanus and botulism) and facilitate community-based acute and chronic self-care for healthcare needs resulting from neurological disorders.
- Revise the plan of care as needed to provide effective interventions to promote, maintain or restore functional health status for people with neurological disorders.

Key terms

Alzheimer's disease (AD) 1595
Bell's palsy 1635
botulism 1641
Creutzfeldt–Jakob disease (CJD) 1636
COVID-19 1638
dementia 1594
Guillain–Barré syndrome (GBS) 1630
Huntington's disease 1619
motor neurone disease (MND) 1622
multiple sclerosis (MS) 1603
myasthenia gravis 1624
Parkinson's disease (PD) 1611
postpoliomyelitis syndrome 1637
rabies 1639
sundowning 1597
tetanus 1640
trigeminal neuralgia 1633

This chapter discusses a variety of neurological disorders. Included are degenerative disorders, peripheral nervous system disorders, cranial nerve disorders and disorders caused by neurotoxins and viruses (including COVID-19). For many of the disorders, nursing care is based on similar nursing diagnoses. To avoid repeating those diagnoses and interventions for each disorder, they have been divided between the nursing care discussions as appropriate.

Degenerative neurological disorders

Degenerative neurological disorders affect the central nervous system and the peripheral nerves. By progressively disrupting cognitive processes or motor functions, disorders such as Alzheimer's disease, Parkinson's disease and multiple sclerosis strike at the core of an individual's sense of personal autonomy and wellbeing and can be psychologically and emotionally devastating to family members and caregivers.

Ongoing medical research into degenerative neurological disorders offers an increasing measure of hope to people and their families. The discovery of genetic or biochemical markers associated with some of these disorders is leading to the development of effective screening and diagnostic methods. In addition, new drugs may make it possible to halt the progression of the disorders in some people, transforming the disorders into manageable conditions. This chapter begins with a discussion of dementia, which is not a specific disease but rather a collection of manifestations caused by a variety of disorders that affect the brain.

DEMENTIA

Dementia affects multiple cortical functions, calculation, learning capacity, language and judgment. Impairments of cognitive function are usually accompanied by deterioration in emotional control, social behaviour and motivation. People with dementia lose their ability to solve problems and may also have personality changes such as agitation and hallucinations. All forms of dementia result from death of neurons and/or the loss of communication between the cells. Although the exact cause is not always known, many forms of dementia are characterised by abnormal structures in the brain called inclusions and there is clearly a genetic component in the development of some kinds of dementia. According to the Australian Bureau of Statistics (ABS, 2020), dementia is the second leading cause of death of Australians and the leading cause of death for women. In 2022, there were an estimated 487,500 Australians living with dementia. Without a medical breakthrough, the number of people with dementia is expected to increase to almost 1.1 million by 2058. In 2022, there were an estimated 28,800 people with younger-onset dementia; this is expected to rise to 29,350 by 2028 and 41,250 by 2058. This can include people in their thirties, forties and fifties. In 2022, it was estimated that almost 1.6 million people in Australia are involved in the care of someone living with dementia. Approximately 70% of people with dementia live in the community and more than two-thirds (68.1%) of aged care residents have moderate to severe cognitive impairment (Dementia Australia, 2022a).

Many different diseases and conditions may cause dementia, including Alzheimer's disease, vascular dementia, Huntington's disease, Creutzfeldt–Jakob disease, medications, metabolic disorders, poisoning and anoxia. Table 43.1 provides an overview of the most common causes of dementia. Doctors do not diagnose dementia unless two or more brain functions (such as memory, language skills, perception, reasoning or judgment) are significantly impaired without loss of consciousness.

Even though the actual cause of all dementias may not be known, factors that increase the risk of developing one or more kinds of dementia have been identified. These risk factors include advancing age, a family history of a disease that causes dementia, smoking and alcohol use, atherosclerosis, high cholesterol and plasma homocysteine levels, diabetes, mild cognitive impairment and Down syndrome.

TABLE 43.1 Common causes of dementia

NAME	CAUSE AND PRIMARY PATHOPHYSIOLOGY
Alzheimer's disease (the most common cause of dementia in people aged 65 and older)	Unknown cause; characterised by two abnormalities in the brain: amyloid plaques and neurofibrillary tangles.
Vascular dementia (the second most common cause of dementia)	Caused by brain damage from cerebrovascular and cardiovascular problems (usually strokes). May also be caused by cerebral blood vessel damage from genetic disorders, endocarditis, myeloid angiopathy, vasculitis and profound hypotension.
Lewy body dementia	Cause usually unknown, although familial cases have been reported. Cells die, and remaining cells in the substantia nigra contain abnormal structures called Lewy bodies.
Frontotemporal dementia	Nerve cells, especially in the frontal and temporal lobes, degenerate. In many people, abnormal tau protein accumulates in neurofibrillary tangles.

Although sometimes confused with dementia, people often experience other conditions that may mimic dementia, including:

- age-related cognitive decline, resulting from slower information processing and mild memory impairment. With ageing, the brain often decreases in volume and some neurons are lost. These changes are normal and are not considered a part of dementia
- mild cognitive impairment, which may progress to dementia but is not severe enough to be initially diagnosed as such
- depression or other emotional problems, causing people to be passive, slow, confused or forgetful
- delirium, characterised by confusion, rapidly altering mental states, disorientation and possible personality changes. Delirium is usually caused by a treatable physical or mental health illness and, when treated, results in a full recovery.

THE PERSON WITH ALZHEIMER'S DISEASE

Alzheimer's disease (AD) (also called *dementia of Alzheimer type* or *senile disease complex*) is a form of dementia characterised by progressive, irreversible deterioration of general intellectual functioning. People with AD live about 8 to 10 years following diagnosis, although some live as long as 20 years. The cause of death is often aspiration pneumonia because of the loss of the ability to swallow late in the disease.

Memory loss is usually the first sign of Alzheimer's disease. Memory deficits are initially subtle and family members and friends may not suspect a problem until the disease progresses and manifestations become more noticeable. Family members and people with AD may also deny the manifestations and hide deficits until the person exhibits unsafe or extremely unusual behaviour. Progression of the disease varies, but the course is one of deteriorating cognition and judgment with eventual physical decline and total inability to perform activities of daily living (ADLs). With the loss of the ability to perform even the most basic ADLs, the burden of meeting the person's needs shifts to the caregiver.

Incidence and prevalence

Alzheimer's disease is the most common degenerative neurological disorder and the most common cause of cognitive impairment in older adults (Norris, 2018). It accounts for up to 70% of cases of dementia in Australia, affecting adults in middle to late life (Dementia Australia, 2022b).

Two types of AD exist: *familial AD* follows an inheritance pattern; *sporadic AD* has no obvious inheritance pattern. AD is further described as early onset (occurring in people younger than 65) and late onset (occurring in people aged 65 and older). Early-onset AD affects people aged 30 to 60, is relatively rare and often progresses more rapidly.

Risk factors and warning signs

As one ages, the risk of developing AD increases. With numbers of older people increasing, the incidence of AD is predicted also to increase. The risk factors for AD are older age, family history and female gender. Warning signs are:

- memory loss that affects job skills
- difficulty performing familiar tasks
- problems with language
- disorientation to time and place
- poor or decreased judgment
- problems with abstract thinking
- misplacing things
- changes in mood or behaviour
- changes in personality
- loss of initiative.

Recognising early manifestations is important because the cause of dementia (such as from depression or hypothyroidism) may be reversible. Dementia from AD is not reversible. Treatment, however, can maximise quality of life and allow the affected person to plan for the future.

FAST FACTS

- From 2011 to 2020, deaths due to dementia, including Alzheimer's disease, increased by 47.8% (4,711 deaths) (ABS, 2020).
- Although usually a disease of later life (generally after the age of 60), it may rarely affect people as young as age 30 (Brain Foundation, 2022).
- AD usually occurs after the age of 65, with the risk increasing with age.
- People who die from dementia have a high median age at death of 89.1 (ABS, 2020).
- Alzheimer's disease affects about 1 in 10 people over 65 years of age and almost 1 in 4 people over 85 years of age (Neuroscience Research Australia, 2022).
- There has been a stabilisation in the rate of deaths due to dementia since 2014 (ABS, 2020).

Pathophysiology

Characteristic findings in the brains of AD people are loss of nerve cells and the presence of *neurofibrillary tangles* and *amyloid plaques* (see Figure 43.1). Neurofibrillary tangles result when *tau*, a kind of protein in the neurons, becomes distorted and twisted. Tau normally holds together the microtubules which guide nutrients and molecules to the end of the axon. In AD, tau changes and twists into pairs of filaments, which then join to form tangles. Because tau no longer maintains the transport system, communication is lost between neurons. Death of neurons may follow, contributing to the development of dementia.

Groups of nerve cells (especially the terminal axons) degenerate and clump around an amyloid core as plaques and are found in the spaces between the neurons of the brain. These plaques, which develop first in areas used for memory and cognition, disrupt transmission of nerve impulses. The plaques consist primarily of insoluble deposits of beta-amyloid, a protein fragment from a larger protein called amyloid precursor protein, mixed with other neurons and non-nerve cells. It is not yet known if plaque formation causes AD or if plaques are a by-product of the AD process.

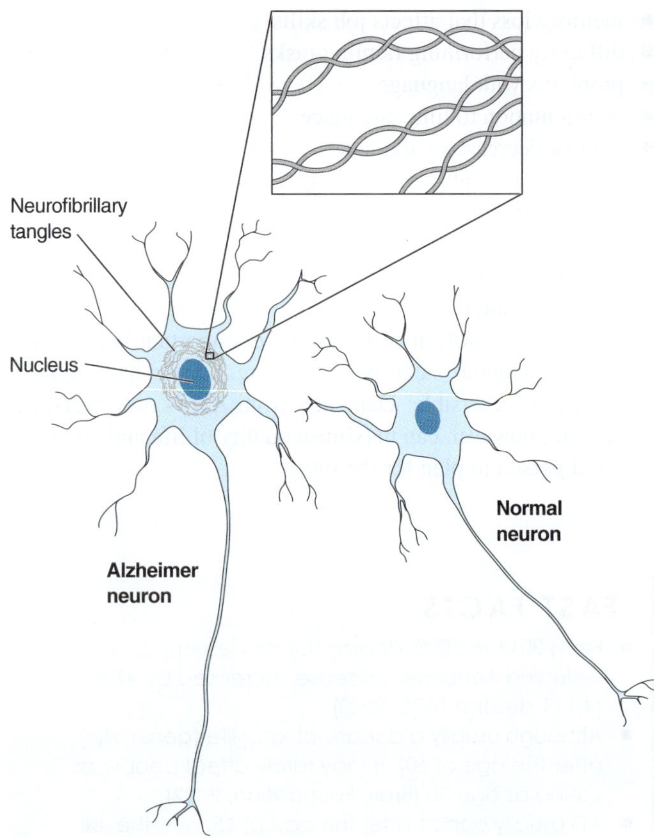

FIGURE 43.1 ***Neuron with neurofibrillary tangles seen in Alzheimer's disease***

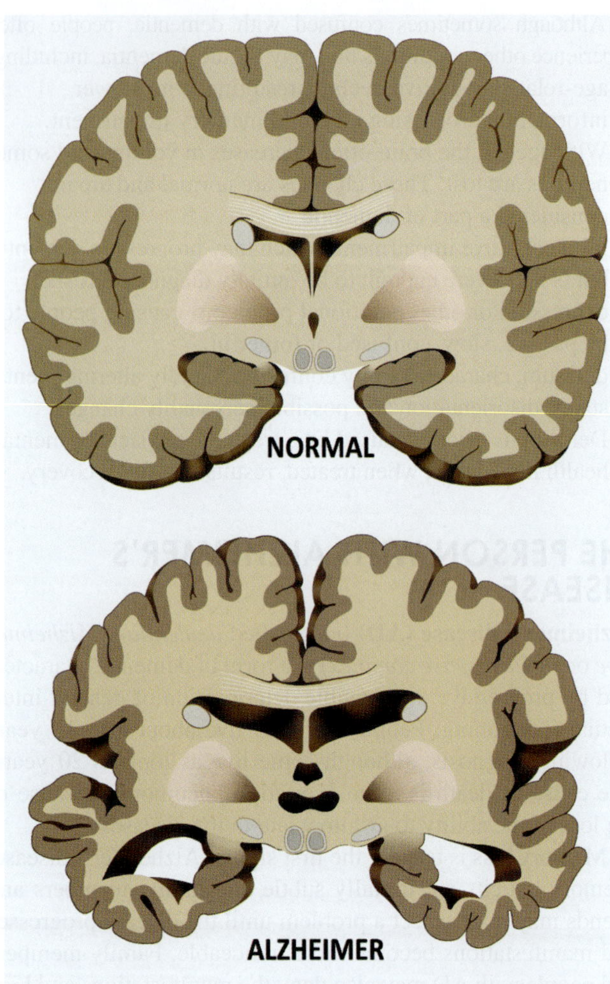

FIGURE 43.2 ***Changes in neuroanatomy associated with Alzheimer's disease. Note areas of cortical atrophy, narrowing of the gyri, enlargement of sulci and ventricular dilation***

Source: ilusmedical/Shutterstock.

Blood flow to the affected areas of the brain is decreased. The brain atrophies and corresponding enlargement of ventricles and sulci is evident (see Figure 43.2). As AD progresses, more areas of the brain are affected, with manifestations correlating to those affected areas of the brain. For example, neuronal and neurotransmitter losses in the parietal lobe result in problems with perception and interpretation of environmental stimuli; deficits in the frontal lobe cause changes in personality and emotional lability.

AD is characterised by atrophy of the cortical area of the brain and loss of neurons, especially in the parietal and temporal lobes. With significant atrophy and loss of brain tissue, the ventricles enlarge (a form of hydrocephalus) (Norris, 2018). Several structural and chemical changes in the brain occur with AD, especially in the hippocampus and the frontal and temporal lobes of the cerebral cortex. As AD destroys neurons in the hippocampus and related structures, short-term memory fails and the ability to perform easy and familiar tasks declines. The effect of AD on neurons in the cerebral cortex is loss of language skills and judgment. Emotional outbursts and behaviour changes (such as wandering and agitation) begin to occur and become more frequent as the disease progresses. Eventually, other areas of the brain are affected; all affected areas begin to atrophy and the person becomes totally helpless and unresponsive.

The exact cause of AD is unknown. Theories include a decrease in choline acetyltransferase activity in the cortex and hippocampus. This enzyme is necessary for the synthesis of acetylcholine, a neurotransmitter associated with memory. The decrease in choline acetyltransferase is about equal to the severity of AD. Other theories include a mutation for encoding amyloid precursor protein and alteration in apolipoprotein E. Other possible causes are gene defects on chromosomes 14, 19 or 21, which may lead to clumping and precipitation of insoluble amyloid as plaques. The role of protein kinase C, the link between AD and aluminium, a viral cause, an autoimmune cause and mitochondrial defects that alter cell metabolism and protein processing are being studied.

Manifestations

Alzheimer's disease is classified into three stages based on the person's manifestations and abilities, as outlined in the 'Manifestations' box. It is important to note that the progression of AD varies for each individual and may not precisely follow the model.

Stage 1 AD

In stage 1, a person typically appears physically healthy and alert, and cognitive deficits can go undetected unless thorough and periodic evaluations are performed. People may seem restless, forgetful or uncoordinated; they may lack spontaneity and be disoriented as to time and date. Usually, family members are the first to notice lapses in memory, subtle changes in personality or problems in doing simple calculations. People with AD and their families may consciously or unconsciously compensate for cognitive deficits by adjusting schedules and routines.

Stage 2 AD

In stage 2, memory deficits are more apparent and the person is less able to behave spontaneously. People may wander and get lost, even in their own homes. Although progression of manifestations continues and orientation to place and time deteriorates, people with AD may still have periods of mental lucidity and engage in time-oriented conversations. Generally, however, people become more confused and lose their sense of time, leading to changes in sleeping patterns, agitation and stress. They may demonstrate repetitive behaviour and eat ravenously. People with AD are less capable of making even simple decisions and adapting to environmental changes and are often unable to carry out ADLs. **Sundowning** is another behavioural change, characterised by increased agitation, time disorientation and wandering behaviours during afternoon and evening hours; it is accelerated on overcast days.

Language deficits are common in stage 2. They include *paraphasia* (using the wrong word), *echolalia* (repetition of words or phrases) and *scanning speech*, in which the person appears to search for words. Eventually, *total aphasia* (absence of speech) may occur. Frustration and depression are common in people with AD as the full extent and implications of the deficits become obvious.

The person with AD slowly loses the ability to perform simple tasks required for hygiene or eating because sequencing of tasks is lost. For example, the person may open a can of soup but not remember to pour it into a pan to heat it. Instead, the person might place the can directly on the burner and leave the heat on high even after a smoke alarm sounds. The person with AD may falsely interpret the smoke alarm as a telephone ringing or an ambulance siren. Thus, safety is a high priority for the person in stage 2.

Sensorimotor deficits in stage 2 include *apraxia*, the inability to perform purposeful movements and use objects correctly; *astereognosis*, the inability to identify objects by touch; and *agraphia*, the inability to write properly. Problems related to malnutrition and decreased fluid intake, such as anaemia and constipation, may be evident. Sleep pattern disturbances are also common and are related to the loss of time orientation, sundowning phenomenon and depression.

Stage 3 AD

Stage 3 brings increasing dependence, with inability to communicate, loss of urinary and faecal continence and progressive loss of cognitive abilities. Common complications include pneumonia, dehydration, malnutrition, falls, depression, delusions, seizures and paranoid reactions. People with AD are indifferent to food and lose weight. They are unable to recognise family or friends, or even themselves. The average life expectancy is 1 to 2 years from the onset of stage 3, although the individual may live as long as 10 years. Most people with AD are institutionalised during this final stage of the disease. Death frequently occurs from pneumonia secondary to aspiration.

INTERPROFESSIONAL CARE

There is no cure for AD and the main objective of care is to provide an environment that matches the person's functional abilities. Nurses, doctors, physical therapists and social workers collaborate with the person's family to provide the least restrictive environment in which the person can safely function.

MANIFESTATIONS Alzheimer's disease

STAGE 1: APPROXIMATELY 2 TO 4 YEARS

- Short-term memory loss: forgets location and names of objects and has difficulty learning new information; long-term memory is unaffected.
- Decreased attention span.
- Subtle personality changes: lacks spontaneity; denial, irritability and depression are possible.
- Mild cognitive deficits: attempts to adjust to and cover up memory loss.
- Visuospatial deficits: some problems with depth perception.

STAGE 2: APPROXIMATELY 2 TO 12 YEARS

- Impaired cognition: obvious memory deficits and confusion; loss of abstract thinking; astereognosis and agraphia; inability to do maths calculations; loss of ability to tell time and time disorientation, manifested as 'sundowning'; wandering behaviour.
- Personality changes: becomes easily agitated and irritable; may have delusions or hallucinations.
- Visuospatial deficits: is unable to dress self; has poor spatial orientation.
- Impaired motor skills: paces and is restless at times; motor apraxia is evident when using familiar objects.
- Impaired judgment: diminished social skills; inability to drive a car; inability to make decisions (e.g. choose clothing).

STAGE 3: APPROXIMATELY 2 TO 4 YEARS OR LONGER

- Cognitive abilities grossly decreased or absent: is usually disoriented to time, place and person.
- Communication skills usually absent: is frequently mute.
- Motor skills grossly impaired or absent: limb rigidity and posture flexion; bowel and bladder incontinence.

Diagnosis

Alzheimer's disease is diagnosed by ruling out causes for the person's manifestations. The only definitive method of diagnosis is postmortem examination of brain tissue. An extensive work-up is especially important because the dementia may be due to a reversible or treatable condition. For example, an older person's misuse of medications can lead to overdosing and resulting confusion. Other categories of conditions that may be considered and ruled out include depression, infection, hypothyroidism, dehydration, heart disease, stroke and chronic obstructive respiratory disease. Mental status is assessed with tests such as the Folstein Mini-Mental State Examination (Folstein, Folstein & McHugh, 1975). This examination assesses areas of function such as the person's orientation to time, ability to repeat a series of words, ability to name objects and ability to follow written instructions.

National policies and practice guidelines for the early recognition and assessment of AD have been established by Dementia Australia. A diagnosis of Alzheimer's disease requires the documented presence of dementia, onset between ages 40 and 90 years (most often after age 65), no loss of consciousness and absence of systemic or brain disorders that could cause mental changes.

Medications

Some medications are effective in slowing the progression of the disease. Tacrine hydrochloride (Cognex) was the first medication specifically approved for the treatment of AD. Donepezil hydrochloride (Aricept) is used to treat mild to moderate AD dementia with some success. Rivastigmine tartrate (Exelon) is also used to treat mild to moderate AD manifestations. It improves the ability to carry out ADLs, decreases agitation and delusions and improves cognitive function. Galantamine hydrobromide (Reminyl) is believed to increase the concentration of acetylcholine in the central nervous system (CNS) and is used as a treatment of mild to moderate AD. Memantine (Ebixa) improves cognitive function in moderate to severe AD and mild to moderate vascular dementia. Memantine acts by blocking receptors for glutamate, resulting in decreased calcium accumulation into neurons (increased calcium accumulation damages neurons). See the 'Medication administration' box for information about selected medications used to treat AD.

Depression often accompanies AD and is treated with the appropriate medication. Antihistamines and tricyclic antidepressants that have high anticholinergic activity are usually avoided because they can increase AD manifestations. Occasionally, people with AD require tranquillisers such as thioridazine (Mellaril) or haloperidol (Serenace) to manage severe agitation. Other therapies under study to prevent or delay the onset of AD include antioxidants such as vitamin E, anti-inflammatory agents and antihypertensive drugs to lower hypertension.

Alternative and complementary therapy

The following types of alternative and complementary therapies may be used in treating the manifestations of AD:

- massage, which decreases agitation
- herbs:
  - ginkgo biloba and vitamin E, which are thought to improve cognition
  - huperzine A, a traditional Chinese medicine, which acts as an acetylcholinesterase inhibitor

MEDICATION ADMINISTRATION The person with Alzheimer's disease

CHOLINERGICS (PARASYMPATHOMIMETICS); CHOLINESTERASE INHIBITORS

Tacrine hydrochloride (Cognex)
Donepezil hydrochloride (Aricept)
Rivastigmine tartrate (Exelon)

In the early stages of AD, the pathological changes in neurons result in a deficiency of acetylcholine (a key neurotransmitter involved in cognitive functioning). Cholinesterase inhibitors slow the breakdown of acetylcholine release by the remaining intact neurons. In addition, rivastigmine tartrate inhibits the G1 form of acetylcholinesterase (found in higher levels in the brain of people with AD), so less acetylcholine is degraded. The drugs are used to improve memory in mild to moderate AD dementia.

Nursing responsibilities

- Administer tacrine hydrochloride 1 hour before meals, if possible.
- Administer donepezil hydrochloride at bedtime.
- Administer rivastigmine tartrate (both capsules and liquid) with food. Liquid form may be administered undiluted or mixed with water, juice or soft drink. Stir to completely dissolve.
- Monitor for jaundice, increased bilirubin levels and other signs of liver involvement, such as rising serum aminotransferase (AST, ALT) levels. Therapy is usually decreased when the enzyme level exceeds four times normal limits and discontinued when the level reaches five times normal.
- Observe for gastrointestinal bleeding and gastric ulcer pain.
- Monitor for cholinergic-related problems: bladder outlet obstruction, seizures and slowed heart rate.
- Assist with ambulation because dizziness is a common side effect.
- Monitor glycaemic control in people with diabetes.
- Assess for improvement in AD symptoms, especially in reasoning, memory and ADLs.

Health education for the person and family

- Notify the healthcare provider promptly if jaundice, seizures, slowed heart rate, GI bleeding or difficulty in urinating occurs.
- Follow directions for times and instructions about administration of specific medication.
- Follow your healthcare provider's recommendation for periodic EEGs, blood tests and urine tests.
- These medications do not cure AD and will at some point become ineffective as the disease progresses.

- coenzyme Q10, an antioxidant that occurs naturally in the body
- supplements, such as zinc, selenium and evening primrose oil
- therapies involving art, music, sound and dance.

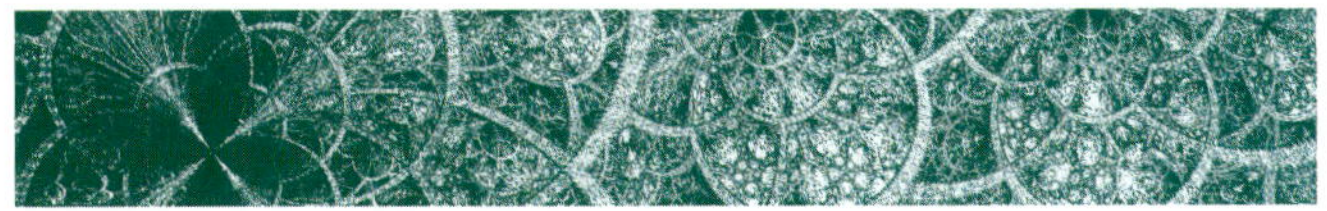

Nursing care

People with AD often require intensive, supportive nursing interventions directed at the physical and psychosocial responses to illness. Equally important, the nurse can facilitate the long-term support of these people by providing teaching and referrals to follow-up care in the community. See the nursing care plan for the person with AD.

Health promotion

Health promotion for the person with AD focuses on maintaining functional abilities and safety. If the person is cared for at home, address safety considerations (see the 'Meeting individualised needs' box) as well as the caregivers' abilities to meet the person's basic needs, such as maintaining hygiene and other ADLs. Adapt nursing interventions and teaching to the person's stage of Alzheimer's disease. Nurses also promote health in the caregiver; information about caregiver support systems and respite care should be provided.

Assessment

Collect the following data through the health history and physical examination (see the chapter 'A person-centred approach to assessing the nervous system'). Further focused assessments are described with nursing interventions below.

NURSING CARE PLAN A person with AD

Arthur and Ruth Joste, both aged 73, have been married for 47 years; he is a retired school teacher and she has been a homemaker. They have four children—two live in the same town and two live out of state. Arthur has noticed that he is having problems remembering friends' names and phone numbers; his wife has been asking him if he is driving in the correct direction when they go shopping.

Mrs Joste has severe osteoarthritis and is unable to lift heavy objects or perform all but light housekeeping tasks. For about 18 months, Mrs Joste has been aware of her husband's progressive cognitive decline, including forgetting current news from last night's TV news; miscalculating bank balances; neglecting his hygiene needs; and confusing their children's and grandchildren's names. The Jostes are referred to a neurologist for evaluation.

ASSESSMENT

Martha Spital, RN, assesses Mr Joste at the neurologist's office. She notes that he is unable to recall his home address without prompting, to name the correct date (although he does know the day of the week), to subtract serial 7s more than twice and to recall two of three objects. He is alert to his surroundings. Mrs Joste states that the problems seem to be getting worse with time and that she has had to 'cover up' mistakes for her husband. Mr Joste seems easily agitated and his wife reports that his sleep habits are 'jumbled'; he has long periods of wakefulness in the night-time hours.

Following a thorough evaluation and diagnostic testing to rule out other possible disorders, the neurologist tells the couple that Mr Joste has probable dementia of the Alzheimer's type. Both have feared this diagnosis; they want to know how they can be sure that Mr Joste has this disease and what they can do to prevent further decline. Both are obviously much saddened and they verbalise their feelings of being overwhelmed. The Jostes intend to remain in their home 'for as long as we can'.

DIAGNOSES

- *Chronic confusion* related to deterioration of brain function and dementia manifested by forgetfulness.
- *Self-care deficits* related to forgetfulness and declining physical abilities, evidenced by poor hygiene.
- *Risk of injury* related to decreased orientation manifested by a decreased awareness of surroundings.
- *Disturbed sleep pattern* related to time disorientation, evidenced by periods of wakefulness.
- *Caregiver role strain* (wife/partner) related to need to care for self and husband manifested by husband's increased need for assistance with ADLs.

PLANNING

Provide education about Alzheimer's disease, evaluate the environment, assess available support and determine needs in order to establish a management plan.

Expected outcomes

- The Joste family becomes aware of the characteristics of Alzheimer's disease and its progression.
- Remain free of injury.
- Navigate home environment with modifications as needed.
- Participate in grooming and hygiene activities with prompting and supervision.
- Obtain a minimum of 7 uninterrupted hours of sleep a night.
- Mrs Joste will participate in a minimum of two out-of-home activities a week.

IMPLEMENTATION

The community nurse, Eric Montane, RN, makes a home visit to evaluate the environment, assess available support and determine needs. He meets two of the Jostes' children, Dawn and Jay, who live in the same community and are willing to participate as much as possible in providing care and modifying the home.

Mr Montane discusses the importance of establishing and maintaining a consistent daily routine. He emphasises the importance of matching activities to Mr Joste's mental abilities to avoid frustration and increased agitation. Mr Montane recommends labelling drawers with their contents, such as Mr Joste's sock drawer. Labelling rooms may be necessary eventually.

(continued)

NURSING CARE PLAN A person with AD (continued)

Because his inability to comprehend and process information distresses and agitates Mr Joste, Mr Montane teaches the family to modify their communications to fit Mr Joste's cognitive ability, such as using simple, direct statements and directions.

Mr Montane recommends that family members keep background noise to a minimum because this may be a source of confusion.

After assessing the home, Mr Montane makes the following recommendations about safety:

- Remove throw rugs from hallways and tack down any remaining carpets.
- Secure the kitchen, bathroom and workshop cabinets, as well as the controls on the oven and stove.
- Modify the doors so that negotiating locks requires a two-step system of unlocking, such as with a deadbolt and a key.
- Provide extra lighting in dark areas, especially a night light in the bathroom.

Mr Montane explains that Mrs Joste will need assistance with housekeeping as Mr Joste continues to decline. Mr Montane provides referrals to community services, including Meals on Wheels, which can supply a daily meal. He also suggests that the Jostes obtain home care services to provide daily hygiene care. Most of the remaining home maintenance needs can be met with the children's help.

Mr and Mrs Joste and the two children attend the weekly local support group meetings for Alzheimer's disease and related disorders for approximately 3 months; thereafter, Mrs Joste attends with her daughter.

EVALUATION

Six months after the initial home visit and family planning session, Mr Joste:

- Has not had a fall, burn or other injury.
- Has periods of confusion when outside his home, but 90% of the time is oriented to place when at home.
- Has attended several support group meetings until 3 months ago. Currently, his wife attends weekly and a daughter occasionally accompanies her. She has continued to participate in their church and maintains contact with a few friends. She is finding it harder to leave her husband unattended for even a few minutes.
- Is able to clean and dress himself with prompting; he is not able to choose his own clothing. If hygiene articles are 'set up' (e.g. if the toothpaste is placed on the toothbrush), he remembers to perform the hygiene activity. The children have been replacing buttons and zippers with Velcro closures on his clothing.
- Sleeps an average of 6 hours a night with a 30-minute nap in the afternoon; this pattern is consistent with his previous sleep pattern.
- Has been more easily agitated for the past month. He wanders from room to room, apparently looking for something. These behaviours are worse in the evening and on cloudy days. Mrs Joste acknowledges her progressive inability to care for her husband.

CRITICAL THINKING IN THE NURSING PROCESS

1. Develop a tool to teach safety needs for the person and the family with Alzheimer's disease.
2. List five interventions to decrease agitation in cognitively impaired older adults; give three additional examples of activities suited to an older adult with AD who has osteoarthritis.

REFLECTION ON THE NURSING PROCESS

1. Outline what you have learned from this case study that you will apply to your future nursing practice.
2. Which education strategies could you use to ensure a person with AD receives adequate nutrition?

MEETING INDIVIDUALISED NEEDS Safety interventions for the person with AD

DECREASING THE RISK OF FALLS

- Assess usual environment for hazards, such as throw rugs, electrical cords and slick floors.
- Observe areas of special concern, such as the bathroom, kitchen and stairs, and modify as needed; for example, provide skid-proof surfaces and mark stairs to show depth.
- Evaluate muscle strength and gait; consult a physiotherapist to plan exercises to increase strength and balance.
- Check shoes for fit and support.
- Enquire about alcohol use and medications that affect balance or cause mobility problems; for example, antihypertensive agents can cause dizziness with position changes.
- Use night lights and increase daytime lighting in dark areas such as hallways.
- Keep traffic areas free from clutter.

DECREASING THE INJURIES RELATED TO COGNITIVE IMPAIRMENTS

- Secure items that may be mistakenly ingested, such as cleaning preparations and house plants.
- Modify potentially unsafe areas, such as unenclosed porches.
- Provide double-lock systems to outside doors and doors to rooms that are off limits.
- Protect from fire hazards; for example, make matches and cigarettes inaccessible.
- Fence the yard with a locked gate to prevent wandering.
- Modify the controls on the oven and stove.
- Adjust the water heater to a safe temperature.

GENERAL SAFETY CONSIDERATIONS

- Plan a calling system for emergencies; have children call at about the same time every day as a check.
- Ensure that the cognitively impaired family member has no access in the home to objects such as knives and guns.

- *Health history*: family member/caregiver support, living arrangements, ability to carry out ADLs, drug use, work history (e.g. exposure to metals), previous history of multiple strokes, brain injury or brain infection, family history of dementia, sleep pattern, changes in cognition and memory, ability to communicate, changes in behaviour.
- *Physical assessment*: height/weight, orientation, abstract reasoning, mental status.

Nursing diagnoses and interventions

During the early stage of AD, nursing care focuses on helping the person make minor adaptations to their environment. As the person becomes progressively unable to manage self-care tasks, more adaptations are required. Equally important, the caregiver needs much support—both physical and psychosocial—as the person becomes increasingly dependent.

Impaired memory

Impaired memory is an appropriate nursing diagnosis in stage 1 AD. At this stage, techniques to help with the memory loss should be included in teaching for both the person and the caregiver.

- Suggest complementary therapies, such as meditation, massage or exercise. *These activities can help reduce stress; stress can aggravate memory loss.*
- Suggest using a calendar, keeping lists of reminders or asking someone else to remind of appointments and events. *Written or verbal reminders are helpful if memory is impaired.*
- Recommend using a medication box labelled with days and times. A *medication box is a good way to remember to take medications.*
- If safety is a concern (such as turning on the stove and forgetting it), suggest using alternatives such as a microwave. Program emergency numbers into the telephone. Ask the person to consider a personal emergency alarm system. *These measures can increase safety.*
- Suggest using cues, such as an alarm on a watch or a mobile phone, to trigger actions at designated times. *Cues are often helpful when memory loss is a problem.*

> **CONSIDERATION FOR PRACTICE**
> **It may be necessary for the caregiver to arrange for the person's medications to be supplied by the pharmacy in a prearranged pack such as a Webster pack.**

Chronic confusion

People with AD often have memory deficits that make functioning in a non-structured environment difficult. Many of the nursing interventions for this diagnosis need to be modified over time as the person continues to lose cognitive function.

- Label rooms, drawers and other items as needed. *Visual cues promote the highest possible degree of independence for the person.*
- Remove potential hazards (such as sharp knives or potentially harmful liquids or chemicals) from the environment. *Ensuring safety is a critical factor in providing care.*
- Keep environmental stimuli to a minimum: decrease noise levels; speak in a calm, low voice; and take an unhurried approach. *Minimising sensory input and maintaining a calm manner may decrease anxiety.*
- Begin each interaction by identifying yourself and calling the person by name. See Box 43.1 for other communication techniques. *These techniques provide information for the person with memory loss.*
- Limit questions to those that require a simple 'yes' or 'no' response. Questions need to be appropriate to the person's ability as decision-making and verbal skills decline.
- Orient to the environment, person and time as able and place large, easy-to-read calendars and clocks in the person's line of vision. Make references to the season or day of the week when conversing with the person. Orient the person according to their own level of ability. *Orienting to precise time may not be possible in the later stages of AD.*
- Provide boundaries by placing red or yellow tape on the floor. *Boundaries help the person stay within safe areas.*

> **CONSIDERATION FOR PRACTICE**
> **Red and yellow are more easily seen by older adults.**

- Provide continuity in nursing staff. *This not only promotes consistency of care for the person but also allows the nurse to determine more accurately changes in the person's condition.*
- Repeat explanations simply and as needed to decrease anxiety. *Loss of short-term memory leads to loss of a point of reference; eventually, people with AD think they are experiencing everything for the first time.*

BOX 43.1 Communicating with the person with AD

- Face the person and talk directly to them; call the person by name.
- When first approaching the person, identify yourself.
- Use simple sentences and words with few syllables.
- Speak in a calm, low voice.
- Ask one question at a time. Use questions that require only a 'yes' or 'no' response.
- Keep non-verbal communication relaxed and parallel to the verbal communication.
- Avoid giving the impression of being in a hurry; try to have a relaxed approach.
- Observe for anxiety—wringing hands, pacing, darting eye movements—and alter your approach to decrease anxiety.
- Avoid arguing with people; do not insist on orienting person to reality; the person's point of reference may not be based in reality.
- Give plenty of time for the person with AD to process what you are trying to say; do not expect people to perform skills beyond their abilities.
- Repeat explanations in simple terms.

Anxiety

Managing the AD person's behaviours associated with anxiety, restlessness and confusion is a major challenge confronting nurses and caregivers. Frequently, people are relatively calm in the morning hours, only to experience increasing periods of agitation in the afternoon and evening hours. The person with AD may even wake from the night's sleep with confusion, fearfulness or panic attacks.

- Monitor for early behaviours of fatigue and agitation. *Early assessment of problems results in prompt intervention to promote rest or to remove the person from the situation causing anxiety.*
- Remove from situations that are causing increased anxiety, such as noisy activities involving large groups. *High-stimulus situations may increase anxious feelings and agitation.*
- Keep daily routine as consistent as possible. *Providing a structured day enhances feelings of familiarity and decreases stress.*
- Schedule rest periods or quiet times throughout the day. *Fatigue contributes to anxiety and lowers the ability to tolerate stress.*
- Provide quiet activities, such as listening to music, in the afternoon or early evening. *Quiet activities may help decrease sundowning.*
- If confusion and agitation persist or escalate, assess for physical causes such as decreased oxygenation, infections, fatigue, constipation and electrolyte imbalance. *Physical factors can increase agitation in people with AD.*
- Use therapeutic touch or gentle hand massage. *These activities induce relaxation and have a calming effect.*

Hopelessness

As the person and their family recognise the effect of AD on their lives, they may feel a sense of hopelessness. They may not have the coping skills to deal effectively with the diagnosis and anticipated problems. The increasingly degenerative, irreversible nature of the disorder tends to diminish hope; only the ability to adapt to the many problems can restore it.

- Assess the person's and family's response to the diagnosis and understanding of AD; encourage expression of feelings. *Understanding the person/family's perspective enables the nurse to dispel myths about AD.*
- Provide realistic information about the disorder; provide information at the person/family's level of understanding. *The person and their family may need to have separate sessions. Factual information provides a foundation for decision making.*
- Avoid criticising or judging expressed feelings. *An environment accepting of the expression of real feelings promotes both further expression of feelings and willingness to discuss other issues.*
- Support positive family bonds and enhance communication between family members; promote mutual positive regard. *Strong family relationships can provide direction for living and convey willingness to share the burden.*
- Encourage the person to make as many decisions as possible. *Self-determination enhances a feeling of control over a situation and may give a sense of hope.*
- Encourage the person and their family to seek spiritual guidance that previously inspired hope. *The person's religious affiliation is a legitimate support system. Belief in a higher being can inspire hope beyond present circumstances.*

Caregiver role strain

Most caregivers of people with AD are spouses or other family members. Because AD is a chronic and eventually debilitating disorder, caregivers may feel overwhelmed by their responsibilities. The caregiving spouse faces not only the responsibility for the person's multiple physical demands but also economic and psychosocial stressors. An area that must be discussed is the ability and safety of the person in driving an automobile. Although it may be necessary, the loss of independence represented by the loss of the ability to drive may further trigger anxiety and anger. Fear of the future, loss of income, loss of companionship and a mate—combined with fatigue—make the caregiver vulnerable. Caregivers may become physically and mentally exhausted and socially isolated because of the overwhelming responsibilities of providing total care to the incapacitated family member.

- Teach the caregivers self-care techniques, such as taking rest periods and avoiding fatigue. *Fatigue adds to stress and potentially leads to poor decision making.*
- Have the caregivers list and regularly take part in physical activities they enjoy, such as walking or swimming. *Regular physical exercise decreases stress.*
- Refer the caregivers to local AD support groups. Suggest books pertinent to the subject. *Explicit suggestions in locating support systems and providing specific information promote coping.*
- Refer the caregivers to Meals on Wheels, home care, respite care and other community services. *Community agencies can relieve some of the daily care burdens, thus providing time for other activities. Programs that support caregivers have been shown to delay nursing home placement.*
- Ensure the family knows that hospice care is available during the end stages of AD. *Hospice services can support the family during this difficult time.*

Community-based care

Teaching for people and families initially centres on explaining the disorder and exploring available support systems. Anticipate the need to re-explain the disorder and its consequences because people and families may be in shock or denial during the initial period of the disease.

In addition, suggest practical solutions to identified problems. It is important to evaluate both the person and caregivers; interventions must be appropriate for the family's situation and resources. Maintaining the least restrictive environment that promotes safety for the person is a major goal of teaching. Using memory cues, such as labelling drawers to indicate the specific types of clothing and labelling rooms, can help orient the person and foster independence. Consistency in the environment and daily routine is an essential part of care. Emphasising realistic expectations means adjusting care and communication techniques to the person's level of ability.

Address the following topics for home care of the person and for the caregiver:

- Support groups and peer counselling are helpful in handling caregiver stress.
- A person with AD who is confused or agitated is not comfortable and is usually frightened.
- Plan care that matches the person's level of coping, using a consistent routine.
- Provide regular rest periods to decrease the person's stress and fatigue (these do not increase night-time wandering).
- Plan care for the caregiver. Periodic adult day care or respite care during the initial stages, with plans for increasing assistance to meet the person's daily needs as the disease progresses, may be sufficient. Referrals to the appropriate agency for long-term care, including skilled nursing facilities, may be indicated. Family members may need help adjusting to the idea of extended care but may be relieved to relinquish the physical care needs.
- Suggest the following resources:
  - Alzheimer's Association: https://www.alz.org/au/dementia-alzheimers-australia.asp
  - National Dementia Helpline: 1800 100 500
  - Dementia Australia: https://www.dementia.org.au
  - Carer Gateway Australia: https://www.carergateway.gov.au or 1800 422 737
  - My Aged Care: https://www.myagedcare.gov.au or 1800 200 422.

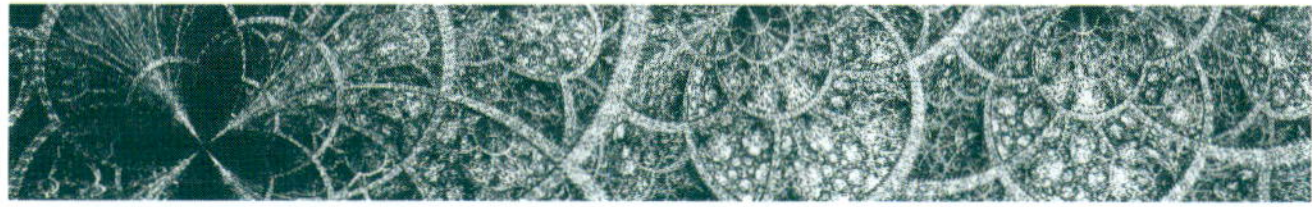

THE PERSON WITH MULTIPLE SCLEROSIS

Multiple sclerosis (MS) is a chronic demyelinating neurological disease of the CNS (brain, optic nerves and spinal cord), associated with an abnormal immune response to an environmental factor. The manifestations of MS vary according to the area of the nervous system affected. The initial onset may be followed by a total remission, making diagnosis difficult. In about 60% of people, MS is characterised by periods of exacerbation, when manifestations are highly pronounced, followed by periods of remission, when manifestations are not obvious. However, the end result is progression of the disease with increasing loss of function.

Incidence and prevalence

The onset of MS is usually between 20 and 40 years of age, with three times as many women as men being diagnosed. MS is the most prevalent CNS demyelinating disorder and is a leading cause of neurological disability in young adults. MS is more common in Caucasians, especially those of northern European ancestry; however, MS does occur in people of African, Asian and Hispanic descent. A definite genetic factor has not been established, but studies suggest that genetic factors may make some individuals more susceptible than others.

Pathophysiology

MS is believed to occur as a result of an autoimmune response to a prior viral infection in a genetically susceptible person. The infection, which is thought to occur early in life, activates T cells. T cells usually move in and out of the CNS across the blood–brain barrier but, for an unknown reason, they remain in the CNS in people with MS. The T cells facilitate infiltration by other leucocytes and an inflammatory process follows. Inflammation destroys myelin and oligodendrocytes (myelin-producing cells), leading to axon dysfunction.

Myelin sheaths are fatty, segmented wrappings that normally protect and insule nerve fibres and increase the speed of transmission of nerve impulses. In multiple sclerosis, these myelin sheaths of the white matter of the spinal cord, brain and optic nerve are destroyed in patches, called *plaques*, along the axon (see the 'Pathophysiology illustrated' feature). The demyelination of nerve fibres slows and distorts the conduction of nerve impulses and sometimes results in the total absence of impulse transmission. The neurons usually affected by MS are located in the spinal cord, brainstem, cerebral and cerebellar areas and the optic nerve.

Both plaques and diffuse lesions form as demyelinating lesions. Plaques typically are scattered through the white matter of the CNS, although they may extend into adjacent grey matter. Early manifestations are the result of inflammatory oedema in and around the plaque and partial demyelination. These manifestations typically disappear within weeks after the initial episode. With progression of the disease, the demyelination and plaque formation result in scarring of glia (*gliosis*) and degeneration of axons. Continued loss of function leads to permanent disability, usually over about 20 years.

FAST FACTS

- Approximately 25,600 people in Australia have MS (0.1% of the population).
- Females are affected three times as often as males, with the incidence highest in young adults under 55 years old.
- The disease affects more young people than any other acquired chronic disease.
- As yet, there is no cure (MS Australia, 2022).

There are four classifications of MS: relapsing–remitting, primary progressive, secondary progressive and progressive–relapsing (see Box 43.2). Most people with MS present with the relapsing–remitting type.

Various stressors have been suggested as triggers for MS. These stressors include febrile states, pregnancy, extreme physical exertion and fatigue. These precipitating factors can also cause a relapse of the manifestations during the course of the disease.

Manifestations

The manifestations of MS vary according to the areas destroyed by demyelination and the affected body system (see 'Multisystem effects of MS'). Fatigue is one of the most

Multiple sclerosis

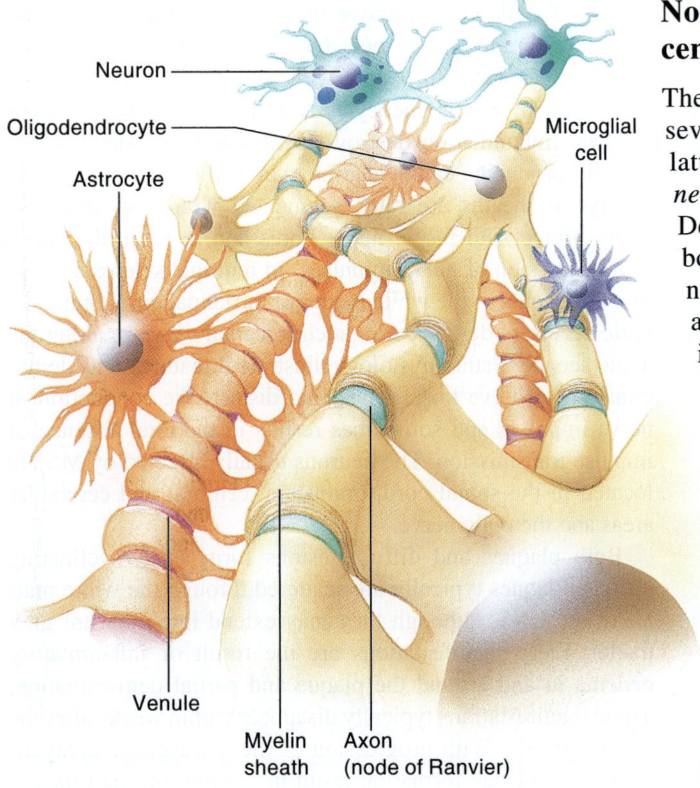

Normal anatomy of the central nervous system

The central nervous system (CNS) is composed of several cell types arranged in a dense, interconnected lattice. The basic functional cell of the CNS is the *neuron*, which transmits electrochemical impulses. Dendrites, thin projections extending from the neuron body, receive impulses that are passed down the neuronal axon for transmission to other cells. Myelin, a lipid-protein substance, surrounds the axons, insulating them and speeding nerve impulse transmission.

Neurons are surrounded by a network of cells:

- *Astrocytes* support neurons and connnect them to surrounding capillaries and venules.
- *Microglia* are motile phagocytic cells.
- *Oligodendrocytes* wrap concentric layers of myelin around nearby axons.

Acute attack

Multiple sclerosis (MS) is a demyelinating disease in which axonal myelin in the central nervous system is eroded, destroyed and replaced by scar tissue.

An autoimmune process apparently triggered by genetic and environmental factors is believed to cause inflammation of venules in the CNS. This disrupts the blood–brain barrier, allowing lymphocytes to enter CNS tissue. These lymphocytes proliferate and produce IgG, an antibody that attacks and damages myelin and causes the release of inflammatory chemicals and oedema. As the inflammation subsides, the myelin regenerates and manifestations of the disease subside.

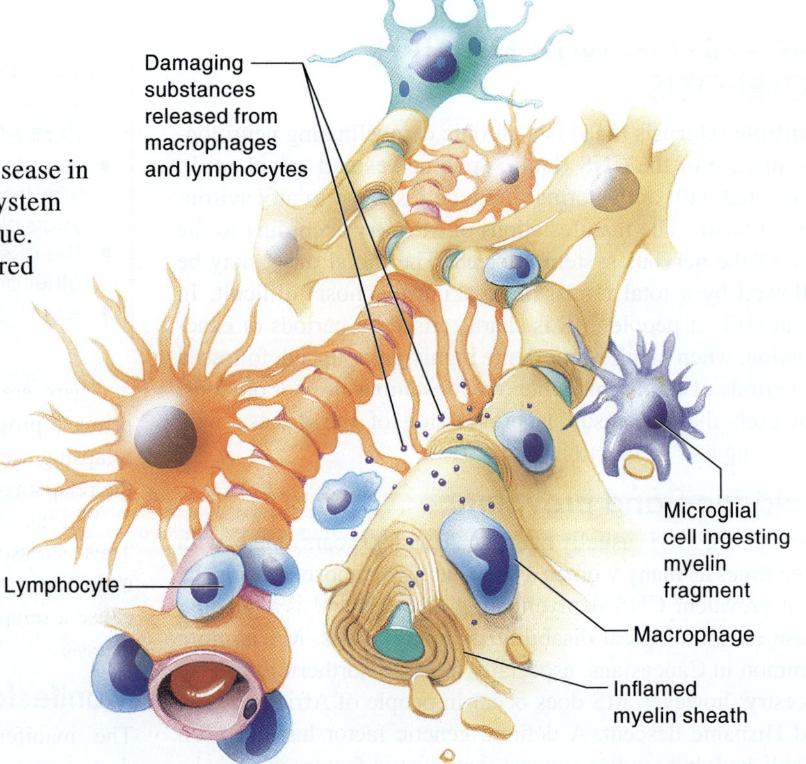

Chronic lesion

After repeated inflammatory attacks, myelin is irreparably damaged. Segments of axons become totally demyelinated and may degenerate. Astrocytes proliferate in damaged regions of the CNS (a process called *gliosis*), forming plaques. The plaques are scattered throughout the CNS, appearing as grey or pinkish lesions. The relapsing-remitting character of MS and the scattered areas of damage within the CNS account for the variable nature of MS manifestations.

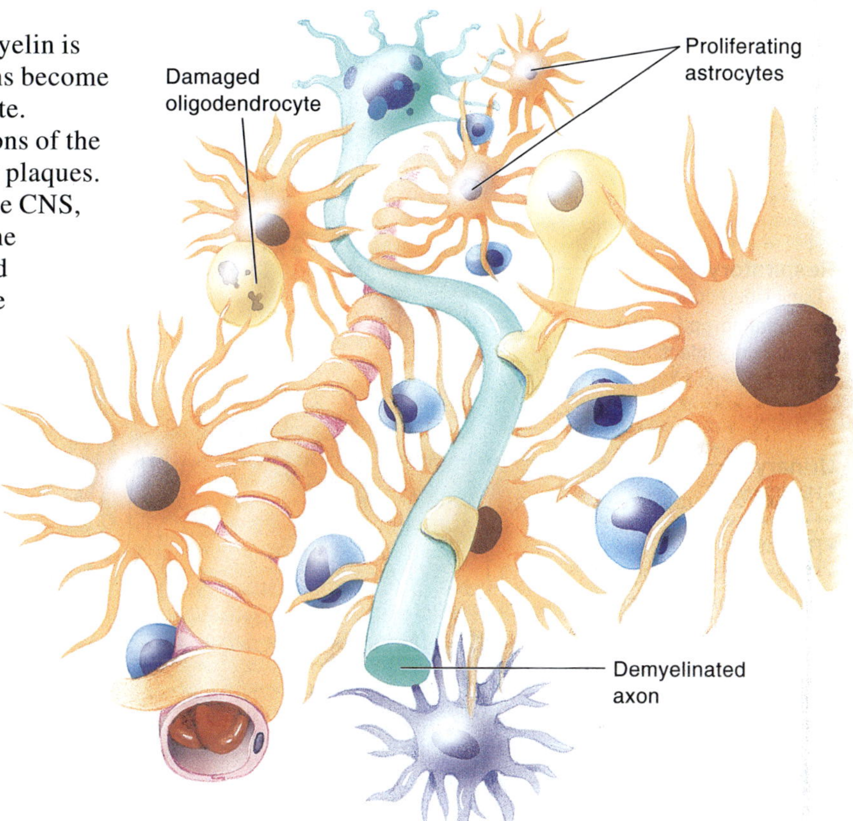

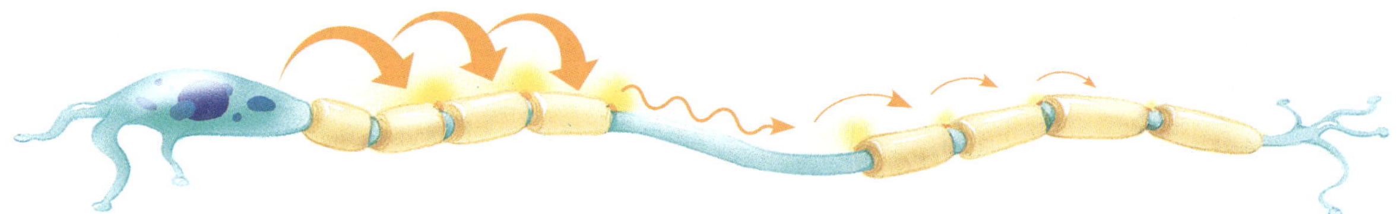

Abnormal nerve impulse transmission

In an undamaged neuron, nerve impulses travel down the axon by 'leaping' from one node of Ranvier to the next, thus greatly increasing the speed of impulse transmission. When nerve impulses travel down an axon damaged by MS, they are significantly slowed and weakened as they pass across the surface of demyelinated areas. Impulses may be blocked entirely when axons degenerate. The weakening or interruption of the transmission of nerve impulses and plaque formation within the CNS cause the manifestations of MS, including extremity weakness, paraesthesias, visual disturbances, bladder dysfunction and vertigo.

Multisystem effects of multiple sclerosis

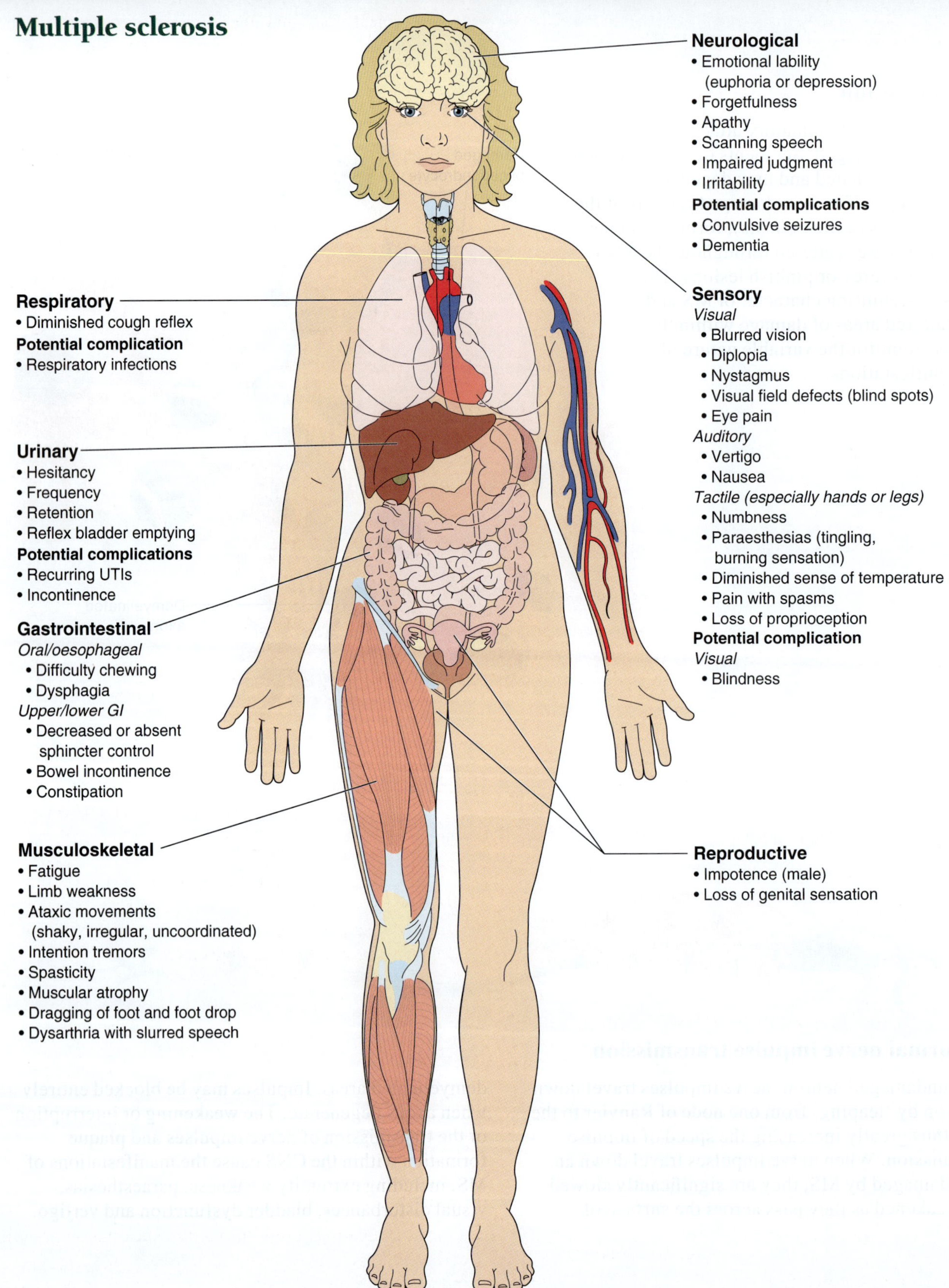

BOX 43.2 classifications of multiple sclerosis

Relapsing–remitting: the most common clinical course of MS, characterised by exacerbations (acute attacks) with either full recovery or partial recovery with disability.

Primary progressive: steady worsening of disease from the onset with occasional minor recovery.

Secondary progressive: begins as with relapsing–remitting, but the disease steadily becomes worse between exacerbations.

Progressive–relapsing: this rare form continues to progress from the onset but also has exacerbations.

disabling manifestations and affects almost all people with MS. The manifestations, categorised by the established syndromes of MS, are listed in the 'Manifestations' box.

Brief attacks of manifestations are described as short lived or paroxysmal. Short-lived attacks of neurological deficits indicate the appearance or worsening of manifestations. Conditions that cause short-lived attacks include: (1) minor increases in body temperature or serum calcium concentrations (both increase the leakage of current through demyelinated neurons), and (2) functional demands that exceed conduction capacity. Paroxysmal attacks are sensory or motor manifestations that occur abruptly and last for only seconds or minutes; the manifestations are paraesthesias, dysarthria and ataxia, and tonic head turning. Paroxysmal attacks, which may occur many times a day, result from the direct transmission of nerve impulses between adjacent demyelinated axons.

MANIFESTATIONS Multiple sclerosis

MIXED OR GENERALISED TYPE (50% OF CASES)

- Visual deficits, with visual blurring, fogginess or haziness; impaired colour perception, decreased central visual acuity, area of diminished vision in the visual fields, acquired colour-vision deficit (especially to red and green) and an altered pupillary reaction to light.
- Brainstem lesions (cranial nerves III to XII) with nystagmus, dysarthria, deafness, vertigo, vomiting, tinnitus, facial weakness, decreased sensation, diplopia and eye pain; and cognitive dysfunctions involving concentration, short-term memory, word finding and planning.
- Mood alterations are manifested as depression more often than euphoria.

SPINAL TYPE (25% OF CASES)

- Weakness and/or numbness in one or both extremities (most often the legs).
- Upper motor neuron involvement is manifested by stiffness, slowness, weakness (spastic paresis).
- Bladder dysfunctions include urgency, hesitancy and incontinence.
- Bowel dysfunction is most often seen as constipation.
- Neurogenic impotence is noted.

CEREBELLAR TYPE (5% OF CASES)

- Manifestations of nystagmus, ataxia and hypotonia.

AMAUROTIC FORM (5% OF CASES)

- Blindness

INTERPROFESSIONAL CARE

Management of the person with MS varies according to the severity of the manifestations. The focus is on retaining the optimal level of functioning possible, given the degree of disability. Rehabilitation—physical, occupational/vocational and psychosocial—is a cornerstone of an interprofessional approach to treatment. During exacerbations, the focus of interventions shifts to controlling manifestations and quickly returning to remission.

Diagnosis

Diagnosis of MS is challenging because the disease does not present uniformly. A diagnosis requires that the person has one of the following: (1) two or more exacerbations separated by 1 month or more and lasting more than 24 hours, followed by recovery, (2) a history of repeated exacerbations and remissions with or without complete recovery, followed by progressively more severe manifestations lasting for 6 months or more, or (3) slowly increasing manifestations for at least 6 months.

Diagnostic tests vary with the presenting complaints. Magnetic resonance imaging (MRI) with findings of lesions is the most definitive test available; however, it is only one of several laboratory and diagnostic tests that may be performed when establishing the diagnosis. Other tests (described in the chapter 'A person-centred approach to assessing the nervous system') include:

- Cerebrospinal fluid (CSF) analysis reveals an increased number of T lymphocytes that are reactive with antigens, indicating the presence of an immune response in the person (but is not specific to MS). Eighty per cent of people with MS have elevated levels of immunoglobulin G (IgG) in the CSF.
- Computed tomography (CT) scan of the brain shows atrophy and white matter lesions. In about 25% of people with MS, enlarged ventricles are visible on CT.
- Positron emission tomography (PET) scan measures brain activity. In people with MS the scan reveals areas with changes in glucose metabolism.
- Evoked response testing of visual, auditory or somatosensory impulses may show delayed conduction.

Medications

Medications slow the progression of MS and decrease the number of attacks. Medications are used for a variety of reasons, including to treat manifestations, modify the course of the disease or interrupt the progression of the disease.

The medications used during an exacerbation are aimed at decreasing inflammation to inhibit manifestations and induce remission. Frequently, a combination of adrenal corticosteroid hormone (ACTH) and glucocorticoids is used to decrease inflammation and suppress the immune system.

MEDICATION ADMINISTRATION The person with multiple sclerosis

IMMUNOMODULATORS

Interferon beta-1a (Avonex)
Interferon beta-1b (Betaferon)
Glatiramer acetate (Copaxone, Copolymer-1)

Interferon beta-1a, interferon beta-1b and glatiramer acetate are administered to people with relapsing–remitting MS to prolong the time of onset to disability. Their use is based on the assumption that MS is an immunologically mediated disease. Interferon beta-1b produces a decrease in the MS lesions in some people. Some people, however, develop a decrease in the absolute neutrophil count and increases in the levels of liver enzymes. Anxiety, confusion and depression with suicidal tendencies also have been reported. Other adverse reactions include pain, inflammation, hypersensitivity at the injection site and generalised flu-like manifestations. Some women experience menstrual disorders. Pregnant women should not take these medications.

Nursing responsibilities

- Assess baseline parameters to evaluate drug side effects: psychological profile, liver function tests and FBC with differential.
- Monitor FBC and liver function tests every 3 months or as prescribed.
- Assess injection site and report ulceration promptly (pain and redness are common reactions).
- Evaluate the person's baseline neurological, sensory and motor function. Monitor changes in condition and function.
- Report if the person is pregnant or breastfeeding.

Health education for the person and family

- These drugs may cause depression and thoughts of suicide; report these feelings immediately to the healthcare provider.
- Administer medication within 3 hours of reconstitution. Rotate injection sites and avoid any areas that are red or show other skin reactions.
- Seek follow-up care to monitor neurological changes, FBC and liver function.
- Avoid prolonged exposure to sunlight.

ADRENAL CORTICOSTEROIDS

Adrenocorticotropic hormone (ACTH) (Acthar)
Prednisone (Deltasone, Meticorten, Predsone, Prednisolone)
Methylprednisolone (Depo-Medrol, Solu-Medrol)

Adrenal corticosteroids are used both to sustain a remission and to treat exacerbations of MS. ACTH is usually given to induce a remission; it is administered intravenously for 1 week and may be followed by oral prednisone therapy. Another protocol involves administering ACTH intravenously for 3 days followed by intramuscular injections every 12 hours for 1 week (Hickey, 2019). The drugs are given to suppress the immune system, which is implicated in the aetiology of MS. If the drug is used long term the usual steroid precautions are indicated, such as monitoring for glucose intolerance, osteoporosis and cataract formation. The drugs are used with caution in pregnant and lactating women.

MUSCLE RELAXANTS

Baclofen (Lioresal)
Dantrolene (Dantrium)
Diazepam (Valium)

Muscle relaxants are given to people with MS to relieve muscle spasms. Baclofen and diazepam act by suppressing CNS reflexes that regulate muscle activity; neither drug affects muscle strength. Baclofen therapy should be discontinued over 1 to 2 weeks; sudden withdrawal may cause seizures and paranoid ideation. In contrast to diazepam and baclofen, dantrolene acts directly on skeletal muscles and may affect muscle strength. Dantrolene may cause hepatotoxicity and should not be administered when hepatitis or cirrhosis is present.

Nursing responsibilities

- Evaluate baseline muscle strength and spasticity, range of movement and dexterity.
- Maintain safety or fall precautions; dizziness and drowsiness are common side effects.
- For the person taking dantrolene, monitor liver function tests (enzymes and bilirubin) for signs of hepatotoxicity.

Health education for the person and family

- These drugs may cause sedative effects. Take appropriate safety measures (e.g. avoid driving).
- Avoid CNS depressants (antihistamines, alcohol); they can increase the sedative effects of the medication.
- Continue follow-up care; if you are taking dantrolene, for example, liver function will need to be monitored.
- If you are taking baclofen, do not suddenly stop the medication.
- Increase fibre and fluids in the diet to prevent constipation.
- Change positions slowly to minimise dizziness and other effects of orthostatic hypotension.

IMMUNOSUPPRESSANTS

Azathioprine (Imuran)
Cyclophosphamide (Endoxan)

Immunosuppressants are given to people with MS because of the autoimmune component of the disease. Both medications can cause bone marrow suppression and increase the risk of cancer. Azathioprine may produce hepatitis. Toxic effects of cyclophosphamide include haemorrhagic cystitis, sterility and stomatitis.

Nursing responsibilities

- Monitor baseline parameters: FBC with platelet count and differential, urinalysis, liver function tests, hepatitis profile.
- Assess for anaemia: fatigue, lethargy, pallor.
- Watch for bleeding.
- Protect against and observe for subtle signs of infection.

Health education for the person and family

- Report infection, bleeding and anaemia immediately.
- Drink at least 2 L of fluid a day and observe urine for blood.
- Report jaundice immediately.
- Check oral cavity daily for changes or ulcers.
- Avoid becoming pregnant while taking these drugs.
- Obtain follow-up care, including frequent blood tests.

Immunosuppressive agents, including azathioprine (Imuran) and cyclophosphamide (Endoxan), are also used. Interferon and glatiramer acetate are used to reduce exacerbations in people with relapsing–remitting MS. Interferon alpha, beta and gamma (Roferon-A, Intron A, Wellferon, Imukin, Avonex or Rebif, Betaferon, Actimmune) enhance immune function, while glatiramer acetate (Copaxone) stimulates parts of the myelin basic protein to reduce the relapse rate of MS. Both drugs are given by injection and are usually well tolerated.

Other medications treat the manifestations of MS. Anticholinergics are administered for bladder spasticity; cholinergics are given if the person has a problem with urinary retention related to flaccid bladder. Depression is treated with antidepressant drugs.

Surgery

Surgery may be indicated for people who experience severe spasticity and deformity. However, physical therapy can prevent most severe problems. Foot drop from severe plantar flexion can be relieved with an Achilles tenotomy, a surgical procedure in which the Achilles tendon is transected.

Nutrition and fluids

Several diets involving manipulation of fats are currently under investigation. People with MS may be overweight because of their inability to ambulate; depression may contribute to the problem because people who are depressed tend to eat more. Ideally, the person should maintain a weight as close as possible to that recommended for the person's height and body type.

As MS progresses, the person's ability to prepare food and eat is compromised. Changes in muscle tone, tremor, weakness and ataxia all contribute to nutritional problems. Dysphagia also is a common problem. The diet must be adapted to accommodate changes in the person's ability to chew and swallow.

Rehabilitation

Physical and rehabilitative therapies are tailored to the person's level of functioning. The long-term goal is to enable the person to retain as much independence as possible. One major intervention is to maintain and increase existing muscle strength.

Spasticity is managed with stretching exercises, gait training and braces, splints or other assistive devices. To maintain balance, the person is encouraged to widen the base of support by standing with the feet slightly further apart. Walkers and canes may be weighted to provide support and balance for the ataxic person.

An interprofessional approach to rehabilitation will provide supportive services: speech therapy for problems with phonation, occupational therapy to maintain strength in the upper extremities and carry out ADLs, and occupational counselling. Referrals to a urologist are indicated for problems with urinary incontinence, urinary tract infections, retention and impotence. Consultation with a physiotherapist may be needed if the person develops chronic respiratory in.ions due to the inability to cough, move secretions or breathe deeply, especially with increased debilitation.

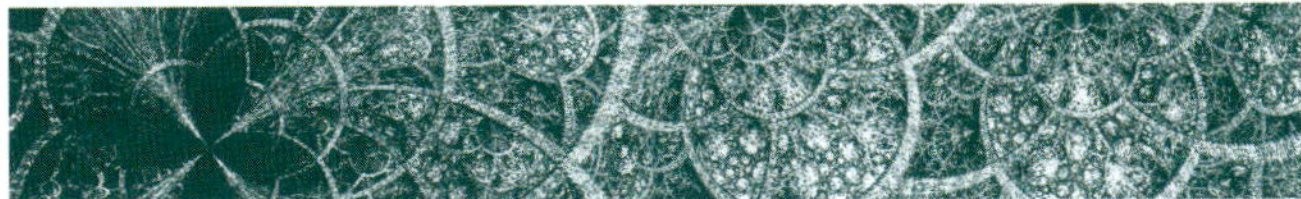

Nursing care

Because the disease most often affects young adults in the prime of life, the psychosocial and economic effect can be devastating. People with MS have to make adjustments to body image changes while simultaneously adapting to the altered relationships and decreased earnings usually encountered with the disease. A once-healthy spouse becomes wheelchair bound; a person once independent may eventually become dependent for even the most basic ADLs. The unpredictable course of MS is a challenge for long-term planning. See the nursing care plan for the person with MS.

- Suggest performing tasks in the morning hours. *People usually have greater energy reserves in the morning hours.*
- Advise to avoid temperature extremes, such as hot showers or exposure to cold. *Maintaining a relatively constant body temperature may avoid exacerbation of the disorder. Heat can delay impulse transmission across demyelinated nerves, which contributes to fatigue.*
- Refer to the appropriate professionals to manage fatigue: stress management groups, support groups, occupational or physical therapist, as indicated. *Support groups and therapy can facilitate self-management and improve coping.*

Health promotion

Following an overview of the disorder, the person needs to understand how to prevent fatigue and exacerbations. Advise the person to avoid stress, extremes of cold and heat, high humidity, physical overexertion and infections. Because pregnancy can exacerbate manifestations, counselling about this risk is indicated. Also, address preventive measures to avoid risk of respiratory and urinary tract infections.

Assessment

Collect the following data through the health history and physical examination (see the chapter 'A person-centred approach to assessing the nervous system'):

- *Health history*: history of childhood viral illnesses, geographical residence when a child, exposure to physical or emotional stressors (pregnancy/delivery, extremes of heat), medications, symptom onset, severity of manifestations.
- *Physical assessment*: affect, mood, speech, eye movements, gait, tremors, vision and hearing, reflexes, muscle strength and movement, sensation.

NURSING CARE PLAN A person with MS

George McMurphy, a 45-year-old from Gosford, NSW, was diagnosed with MS approximately 5 years ago. He states that he probably had mild symptoms as long ago as 10 years. He works as a manager for a large grocery store chain near his home. He lives at home with his wife and two children, aged 12 and 15. Recently, Mr McMurphy has had increasing problems with urinary incontinence, lack of energy, weakness, extreme fatigue and altered mobility from spasticity in his leg muscles. He also has a fever, chest congestion and a cough productive of green sputum. He is admitted to the hospital for evaluation and treatment of pneumonia and exacerbation of his MS.

ASSESSMENT

Denise Miller, RN, is assigned to care for Mr McMurphy. His main complaint is the inability to 'bring up all this sputum; I feel rotten from being so congested. I hate not being able to get to work and for my wife to have to tend to my personal needs'. Vital signs are as follows: BP 134/84, P 94, R 30, T 38.8°C. Mr McMurphy is admitted for an acute exacerbation of the disorder, probably triggered by pneumonia. He will be treated with ACTH and intravenous antibiotics during this admission.

DIAGNOSES

- *Ineffective airway clearance* related to lung infection and thick mucus, evidenced by tachypnoea and a productive cough.
- *Activity intolerance* related to fatigue and spasticity, evidenced by the inability to attend work and attend to own ADLs.
- *Self-care deficit: toileting, feeding and grooming* related to muscle weakness, evidenced by the inability to attend to own ADLs without assistance.

PLANNING

Management of symptoms of pneumonia and implementation of strategies to cope with an exacerbation of MS.

Expected outcomes

- Be able to clear airway.
- Have breath sounds clear to auscultation and pulse oximetry readings above 95%.
- Be able to ambulate using assistive devices, if needed.
- Perform self-care activities without becoming overly fatigued and tired.
- Verbalise methods to adapt daily routine to his level of tolerance.

IMPLEMENTATION

- Initiate pulmonary hygiene measures (e.g. incentive spirometry, turning, deep breathing and coughing, breathing exercises and postural drainage) at least every 2 hours. Assess lung sounds, oxygen saturation and ability to clear airway.
- Teach the importance of maintaining an oral fluid intake of at least 2 L per day to prevent tenacious sputum and urinary tract infections. Teach signs and symptoms of urinary and respiratory infections.
- Encourage participation in decision making about care.
- Assist with ADLs only as needed, based on level of fatigue and muscle weakness.
- Plan self-care activities so that they are performed during periods of peak level of energy; intersperse rest periods throughout the day.
- Refer to an MS support group.
- Refer to physical and occupational therapists for counselling regarding control of spasticity and possible splinting of spastic muscles.
- Consult a urologist for assessment of bladder incontinence; teach intermittent catheterisation. Alternatively, the use of an external condom catheter may be indicated.

EVALUATION

Mr McMurphy is discharged 3 days following admission. He states that he feels stronger; on discharge, he has no problem clearing his airway. Although he continues to pace his activities to avoid fatigue, his muscle strength and 'tiredness' have improved. He is able to complete ADLs unassisted.

Pulmonary function has returned to normal pre-hospitalisation levels: ABGs and pulse oximetry are within normal limits. Both Mr McMurphy and his wife have listed several ways to modify their daily routine to allow more rest and decrease stress. Follow-up visits to Mr McMurphy's primary care provider have been arranged and the McMurphys have been provided with information about the local MS support group.

CRITICAL THINKING IN THE NURSING PROCESS

1. Describe approaches the nurse could take to ensure that Mr McMurphy does not exceed his activity tolerance.
2. Develop a teaching plan for Mr McMurphy to help prevent future respiratory infections.

REFLECTION ON THE NURSING PROCESS

1. Which education and communication strategies could you suggest to reduce the risk of injury related to fatigue, muscle weakness and spasticity?
2. Outline what you have learned from this case study that you will apply to your future nursing practice.

Nursing diagnoses and interventions

Interventions for the person with MS vary with the acuity of exacerbations and the presenting problems. Many nursing diagnoses relate to the inability to perform ADLs—for example, *Self-care deficit* and *Impaired home maintenance*. Others reflect problems with musculoskeletal changes or altered nerve conduction—for example, *Impaired physical mobility*, *Ineffective breathing pattern*, *Constipation* and *Functional urinary incontinence*. The nursing diagnoses discussed in this section are *Fatigue* and *Self-care deficit*.

Fatigue

Fatigue is an overwhelming, sustained sense of exhaustion and decreased capacity for physical and mental work at the usual level. Fatigue affects every aspect of the life of a person with MS: the ability to remain independent and perform self-care, sexual function, mobility, airway clearance and, ultimately, self-concept and coping. A great deal of teaching is needed to help the person and their family understand fatigue and how to adapt. People and their families need assistance managing fatigue in a society in which energy is highly valued.

- Assess degree of fatigue and identify contributing factors. *Fatigue is a subjective experience that needs to be evaluated thoroughly before planning can begin.*
- Arrange daily activities to include rest periods. *Rest is essential to manage feelings of fatigue; periods of relaxation may help replenish energy reserves.*

CONSIDERATION FOR PRACTICE

It is important to remember that the fatigue from chronic illnesses such as MS is very different from being 'tired' and that rest and sleep may not result in improvement.

- Ask the person to consider which activities are really necessary and to set priorities. *Prioritising activities promotes independence and self-control.*

Self-care deficit

People with MS may need assistance with all aspects of their ADLs. The help needed can range from minimal guidance to total dependence. The person's ability to perform self-care activities is the gauge by which family members and caregivers need to adjust assistance. Self-care encompasses both the decisions about care and the provision of care; most people are capable of making decisions even after physical limitations prevent physical self-care. The need to maintain self-determination cannot be overemphasised and must be incorporated into each intervention. As the person with MS ages, there may be even more need for teaching to provide self-care.

- Assess the extent of the person's self-care deficit; refer to other health team members for assessment as appropriate. For example, refer to a speech pathologist to assess swallowing and gag reflex, if indicated. *An accurate assessment is crucial to individualising interventions.*
- Suggest adaptive devices, such as arm or wrist braces, as needed. *Meeting hygiene needs and feeding self are essential for positive self-concept, self-esteem and socialisation.*
- Teach to use assistive devices, such as plate guards; to modify consistency of foods; and to eat when energy level is better. If unable to buy and prepare meals, provide referral to Meals on Wheels. *Proper nutrition is basic to health; adapting utensils and foods can facilitate meeting nutritional needs.*
- Teach interventions related to altered bowel and bladder function: fluid intake of at least 2 L daily, bowel routine as indicated to prevent constipation, self-catheterisation skills as necessary. *Maintaining optimal bowel and bladder function decreases the risk of urinary tract infection and bowel impaction.*

Community-based care

The inconsistent and erratic nature of MS can make teaching for self-care difficult. Initial teaching focuses on a realistic explanation of MS. Referral to a support group early in the course of the disease is indicated. Social support can make a positive difference to a person's ability to cope with MS. Address the following topics in preparing the person for home care:

- various treatment options and their side effects
- information about medications, particularly steroid use, and about possible interactions with prescription or over-the-counter (OTC) medications
- ongoing care from nurses, counsellors and physical, occupational and speech therapists, as well as the doctor and community health nurse
- helpful resources:
  - MS Australia: https://www.msaustralia.org.au
  - National Institute of Neurological Disorders and Stroke (NINDS): https://www.ninds.nih.gov
  - Brain Foundation: https://brainfoundation.org.au/disorders/multiple-sclerosis.

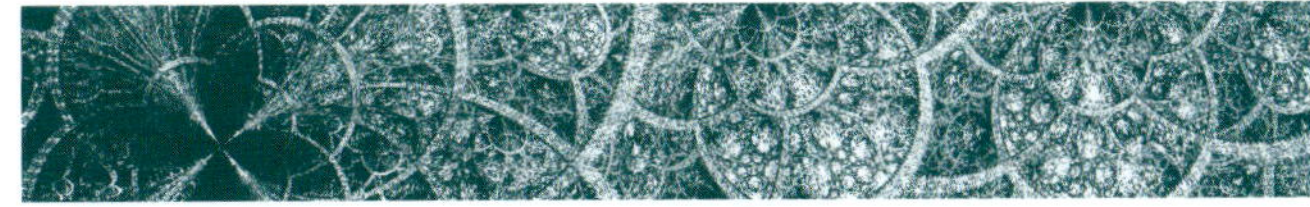

THE PERSON WITH PARKINSON'S DISEASE

Parkinson's disease (PD) is a progressive, degenerative neurological disease characterised by tremor (shaking), muscle rigidity and bradykinesia (slowness of movement) (Norris, 2018). People with PD are faced with multiple problems involving independence in ADLs, emotional wellbeing, financial security and relationships with caregivers.

Incidence and prevalence

PD is one of the most common neurological disorders affecting older adults. It is estimated that there as many as 82,000 (1 in every 308) Australians are currently living with PD; of these, a small majority are male. People who develop PD are three times more likely to do so after the age of 65 (Garvan Institute, 2021). The recent discovery of inherited forms of PD suggests a genetic role in the development of this disease, although this is still being investigated (Garvan Institute, 2021).

Parkinson's-like manifestations, called *secondary Parkinsonism*, may result from other disorders such as trauma, encephalitis, tumours, toxins and drugs. Drug-induced Parkinsonism, which is usually reversible, may occur in people taking neuroleptics, anti-emetics, antihypertensives and illegal designer drugs containing MPTP, a toxic chemical (Norris, 2018). Carbon monoxide or cyanide poisoning can also cause secondary Parkinsonism. This discussion focuses on primary Parkinson's disease, the cause of which is unknown.

Pathophysiology

Coordinated, voluntary body movement is achieved through the actions of neurotransmitters in the basal ganglia of the brain. Some neurotransmitters facilitate the transmission of excitatory nerve impulses, while other neurotransmitters inhibit their transmission. Together, this system allows control of movement. A disturbed balance between excitatory and inhibitory neurotransmitters causes disorders of voluntary motor function, such as PD.

In PD, neurons in the cerebral cortex atrophy and are lost, the dopaminergic nigrostriatal (pigmented) pathway degenerates and the number of specific dopamine receptors in the basal ganglia decreases. These pathological processes cause a decrease in the production of dopamine (a neurotransmitter that helps regulate nerve impulses involved in motor function) from the substantia nigra. The usual balance of dopamine (an inhibitory neurotransmitter) and acetylcholine (an excitatory neurotransmitter) in the brain is disrupted and dopamine no longer inhibits acetylcholine. The failure to inhibit acetylcholine is the underlying basis for the manifestations of the disorder. PD has five stages, outlined in Box 43.3.

Manifestations

Parkinson's disease begins with subtle manifestations. People complain of feeling tired and seem to move more slowly; a slight tremor may accompany the fatigue. Over time, the manifestations progressively increase in severity. The manifestations and complications of PD are presented in the 'Manifestations and complications' box.

Tremor

Tremor at rest is usually the first manifestation experienced, with one of the upper extremities more often affected. Resting tremors of the hand show a 'pill-rolling' motion of the thumb and fingers. (This name reflects the way in which medicinal pills were formed in the early days of medicine.) The tremor may be controlled with purposeful, voluntary movement and is worsened by stress and anxiety. People have progressive impairment in performing skills that require dexterity and fine muscle control, such as writing and eating.

Rigidity and bradykinesia

Manifestations related to motor and postural effects include rigidity, bradykinesia and uncoordinated movements. Rigidity (resulting from involuntary contraction of all skeletal muscles) makes both active and passive movement difficult. It is manifested as increased resistance to passive range of motion. Although the extremity moves, it does so in a jerky motion, called *cogwheel rigidity*. The first manifestation of rigidity may be muscle cramps in the toes or hands, but most often the person describes stiffness, heaviness or aching in muscles.

Bradykinesia, experienced as difficulty in starting, continuing or coordinating movements, is the most common and crippling manifestation. All striated muscles are affected, including those that involve chewing, swallowing and speaking. Slowed or delayed movements affect the eyes, mouth and voice, causing a mask-like face and softened or muffled voice. Disorders of swallowing result in problems with eating and with drooling. People have a staring gaze with minimal change in expression (see Figure 43.3). People describe being 'frozen' in place as voluntary movement is lost and they sit

BOX 43.3 Stages of Parkinson's disease

1. Unilateral involvement only, usually with minimal or no functional impairment.
2. Bilateral or midline involvement, without impairment of balance.
3. First sign of impaired righting reflexes, evidenced as unsteadiness as the person turns or demonstrated when the person is pushed from standing equilibrium with the feet together and eyes closed. Functionally, the person is somewhat restricted in activities but may have some employment potential, depending on the type of employment. People are physically capable of leading independent lives and their disability is mild to moderate.
4. Fully developed, severely disabling disease; the person is still able to walk and stand unassisted but is markedly incapacitated.
5. Person is confined to bed or wheelchair unless aided.

MANIFESTATIONS AND COMPLICATIONS

Parkinson's disease

RELATED TO MOTOR DYSFUNCTION

- Non-intentional tremor
- Bradykinesia or akinesia
  a. Slowed movements; inability to initiate voluntary movements
  b. Slowed speech, low amplitude
  c. Poor articulation
  d. Decreased eye movements (i.e. blinking)
  e. Mask-like, expressionless face
- Rigidity
- Posture and gait disturbances
  a. Trunk tilted forwards
  b. Shuffling gait, propulsive at times
  c. Retropulsion
- Complications: falls, fractures, impaired communication, social isolation

RELATED TO AUTONOMIC SYSTEM DYSFUNCTION

- Skin problems
  a. Seborrhoea
  b. Excess sweating on face and neck, absence of sweating of trunk and extremities
  c. Mottled skin
- Heat intolerance
- Postural hypotension
- Constipation
- Complications: skin breakdown, dizziness, falls, constipation

RELATED TO COGNITIVE AND PSYCHOLOGICAL DYSFUNCTION

- Dementia
  a. Memory loss
  b. Lack of insight and problem-solving ability
  c. Declining intellectual abilities
- Anxiety
- Depression
- Complications: loss of ability to function, social isolation

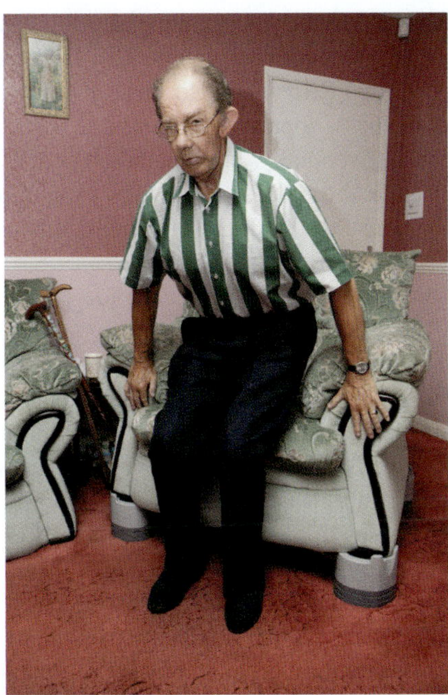

FIGURE 43.3 ***In Parkinson's disease, the person's face lacks expression or animation***

Source: John Birdsall/Alamy Stock Photo.

or lie in one position without movement for long periods of time. Movement is interspersed with freezing, brought about by turning, increasing the effort to move or making visual or touch contacts.

Abnormal posture

The loss of normal postural reflexes results in postural abnormalities, including disorders of postural fixation, equilibrium and righting. Involuntary flexion of the head and shoulders means the person with PD cannot maintain an upright position of the trunk when sitting or standing. This problem of postural fixation results in the characteristic stooped, forwards-leaning position. Disorders of equilibrium follow loss of postural fixation, with an inability to adjust when leaning or falling, increasing the risk of injury from falls. (The person usually falls backwards.) The person takes short, accelerated steps to try to maintain an upright position when walking.

Autonomic and neuroendocrine effects

Many manifestations result from the loss of functions controlled by the autonomic nervous system. Elimination problems include constipation and urinary hesitation or frequency. People may experience problems related to orthostatic hypotension, including dizziness with position change. Eczematous skin changes and seborrhoea are related to the increase in sweat gland activity secondary to increased sebotrophic hormone production.

Mood and cognition

Both depression and dementia are pathologies associated with PD. Depression occurs in half of all people and one-third have dementia. Dementia, resulting from loss of cholinergic cells, loss of neurons, senile plaques, neurofibrillary tangles and amyloid changes in small blood vessels, occurs in 20% of people with PD and develops later in the disease (Norris, 2018). The person has manifestations similar to the person with Alzheimer's disease, including confusion, disorientation, memory loss, distractibility and changes in abstraction and judgment. *Bradyphrenia* may also occur, resulting in slow thinking and a decreased ability to form thoughts, to plan or to make decisions.

Sleep disturbances

People with PD commonly have sleep disturbances, although they may experience decreased manifestations during sleep in the early stages. The ability to fall and stay asleep is affected by acetylcholine. Muscle rigidity may compromise sleep because of the inability to change position. This lack of muscle movement causes the person to awaken and consciously shift position.

Interrelated effects

Some of the manifestations that people with PD experience have multiple contributing factors. For example, constipation is common because of decreased peristalsis. However, decreased peristalsis is not the only cause: immobility, tremors (resulting in being unable to drink from a glass easily) and dietary changes from dysphagia all contribute to the problem of constipation.

Complications

The following complications are associated with PD:

- oculogyric crisis, in which the eyes become fixed with a lateral and upwards gaze
- paranoia and hallucinations, which may accompany dementia
- impaired communication due to changes in speech, handwriting and expressiveness
- falls from balance, posture and motor changes
- infections, such as pneumonia, related to immobility
- malnutrition related to dysphagia and inability to prepare meals
- altered sleep patterns due to loss of dopamine, levodopa side effects (nightmares, dreams) or side effects of anticholinergics (hyperreflexia, muscle twitching) and depression
- skin breakdown and pressure ulcers associated with urinary incontinence, malnutrition and sweat reflex changes
- depression and social isolation.

INTERPROFESSIONAL CARE

Prognosis is poor, owing to the progressive degeneration that ultimately affects multiple physiological systems and their function. Psychosocial effects are equally devastating and the family needs more support as the person's debilitation increases. Total disability is usually seen 10 to 20 years after diagnosis. The leading cause of death is pneumonia.

Diagnosis is based primarily on a thorough history and physical examination and is made based on having two of the following manifestations: tremor at rest, bradykinesia, rigidity and postural instability. Interventions vary with the clinical stage of the disorder and include medication, surgery and rehabilitation to retain the optimal level of functioning possible. An interprofessional approach is essential for people with PD.

Diagnosis

Diagnostic studies may support a potential diagnosis of PD; no test clearly differentiates PD from other neurological disorders (Hickey, 2019). However, a PET scan will show decreased uptake of 6-[18F]-fluorodopa.

Medications

The goal of drug therapy is to control manifestations to the extent possible. Generally, medications vary with the stage of the disease; however, response is individualised and guides the selection of medications. Types of drugs used include monoamine oxidase (MAO) inhibitors, dopaminergics, dopamine agonists and anticholinergics. Information about these drugs is presented in the 'Medication administration' box.

Initially people are treated with selegiline (Carbex, Eldepryl), amantadine (Symmetrel) or anticholinergics. As the disease progresses, levodopa (Dopar, Larodopa) in combination with carbidopa (Lodosyn) is used in a medication named carbidopa–levodopa (Sinemet). Because levodopa eventually loses its effectiveness, dopamine agonists are added to increase its effectiveness. Eventually, pharmacotherapeutic agents lose their efficacy and the disease continues to progress despite treatment. Response to the drugs fluctuates; this phenomenon is called the 'on–off' response.

Bromocriptine (Parlodel) and pergolide (Permax), agents that inhibit the breakdown of dopamine, are used to delay progression of the disease. Catecholamine-O-methyl transferase (COMT) inhibitors (tolcapone (Tasmar) and entacapone (Comtan)) are used in conjunction with carbidopa–levodopa therapy to reduce the metabolism of levodopa, leading to more sustained dopaminergic stimulation of the brain. Selegiline (Eldepryl) increases dopaminergic activity and is used as an adjunctive therapy for people who have fluctuations in response, or become unresponsive, to levodopa.

Other medications may be used to treat problems related to PD. Antidepressants may be prescribed. Propranolol (Inderal) may be used to treat tremors; it should be used cautiously when people have orthostatic hypotension. Botulism toxin injections may be given to treat eyelid spasms and abnormal posturing (dystonia) involving the extremities.

MEDICATION ADMINISTRATION The person with Parkinson's disease

DOPAMINERGICS

Levodopa (Larodopa, Dopar)

Carbidopa–levodopa (Sinemet)

Amantadine (Symmetrel)

These drugs have their main effect on the akinesia of DP, improving mobility while decreasing muscle rigidity and tremor. Levodopa is a metabolic precursor of dopamine, but unlike dopamine it can cross the blood–brain barrier. Levodopa is converted to dopamine in the brain by decarboxylase, a catalytic enzyme, and stimulates dopamine receptors to balance the dopamine/acetylcholine concentrations. Carbidopa prevents decarboxylase from converting levodopa to dopamine in the peripheral tissues; therefore, carbidopa is frequently given in combination with levodopa. Amantadine is used to treat dyskinesia and also elevates mood.

Levodopa is avoided in people with narrow-angle glaucoma, severe angina pectoris, transient ischaemic attacks or melanoma. The 'on–off' phenomenon occurs after the person takes levodopa for several years; this phenomenon is characterised by unexpected dyskinesias and lack of symptom control.

Common side effects are nausea and vomiting; darkening of urine and sweat; dyskinesias, especially in the first few months of therapy; arrhythmias; orthostatic hypotension; and psychological reactions, such as hallucinations and vivid dreams. Older adults are particularly susceptible to psychological disturbances.

Nursing responsibilities

- Establish the person's baseline functional abilities in performing ADLs and administering the medication; assess motor control and coordination.
- To avoid adverse reactions, assess the person's overall health status before initiating therapy.
- Monitor medications known to cause adverse drug interactions: anticholinergics, pyridoxine and antipsychotic agents alter the effectiveness of levodopa; MAO-B inhibitors can cause severe hypertension because of their vasoconstrictive effects.
- Withhold levodopa for 8 hours prior to administering carbidopa–levodopa to avoid potentiating the effects of the circulating levodopa.

Health education for the person and family

- Levodopa may not take effect for several weeks to months.
- Do not alter dosages of medications; taking more of a medication may not result in better symptom control and can cause severe side effects.
- Your protein intake should be divided into equal amounts for the day's meals. Avoid foods high in pyridoxine, such as pork, beef, ham, avocado, beans and oatmeal.
- Levodopa may cause a darker colour of urine; however, this is harmless.
- To prevent side effects:
  - Prevent nausea by taking medication with food.
  - Change position slowly to avoid a drop in blood pressure and risk of falling.
  - Prevent constipation by increasing fluid intake and exercising regularly.
- Notify the healthcare practitioner if you begin to have difficulty making voluntary movements, or cardiac or psychological symptoms develop.

MEDICATION ADMINISTRATION The person with Parkinson's disease (continued)

- Watch for the 'on–off' phenomenon, in which periods of symptom control alternate with periods when the drug fails to control symptoms.

MONOAMINE OXIDASE INHIBITORS

Selegiline (Eldepryl, Carbex)

Selegiline works by selectively inhibiting the enzyme that inactivates dopamine in the brain. It may be administered alone or as an adjunct therapy with levodopa: selegiline inhibits the enzyme system that would otherwise break down and destroy dopamine. This synergistic effect lasts approximately 1 to 2 years. The combination of selegiline and levodopa increases the adverse reactions of dopamine; nurses must be alert for orthostatic hypotension, changes in movement, hallucinations and confusion. These responses can be modified by lowering the dose of levodopa. Because it is highly selective for the MAO-A enzyme, selegiline does not have antidepressant effects like the MAO-B inhibitors. The risk of severe hypertension is low.

Nursing responsibilities

- Establish baseline functional abilities: motor control and movements, position changes, mental status.
- Monitor problems with insomnia.
- Assess for orthostatic hypotension; look for unsteadiness with position change and complaints of dizziness.
- Assess for hypertension, which can occur with higher than usual doses.

Health education for the person and family

- It is very important to take the medication as directed, especially the dose and time of administration.
- Notify the healthcare practitioner if insomnia occurs.
- Report signs of dizziness when changing positions or standing, changes in ability to move or psychological changes.
- Change positions slowly, especially when moving from a sitting to a standing position.
- Keep follow-up appointments for evaluation of the medication's effectiveness.

DOPAMINE AGONISTS

Bromocriptine (Parlodel)
Pergolide (Permax)
Pramipexole (Sifrol)
Ropinirole (Repreve)

Dopamine agonists act by directly activating dopamine receptors in the brain. They are frequently used in combination with levodopa therapy: when dopamine agonists are given with levodopa, they increase the therapeutic effects of levodopa and reduce fluctuations in motor symptoms. Adverse reactions are similar to those of levodopa: nausea, orthostatic hypotension and psychological disturbances are common. Nursing responsibilities and personal and family teaching information are similar to those for the dopaminergics.

COMT INHIBITORS

Tolcapone (Tasmar)
Entacapone (Comtan)

COMT inhibitors inhibit catechol-O-methyltransferase (COMT), which is responsible for metabolising dopamine. The concurrent administration of a COMT inhibitor with levodopa increases the amount of levodopa available to the brain to control Parkinson's disease.

Nursing responsibilities

- Monitor liver function test results and manifestations of liver impairment (dark urine, jaundice).
- Administer with food.
- If given concurrently with warfarin, monitor APTT and INR.

Health education for the person and family

- Avoid using alcohol and sedatives.
- Rise slowly from a sitting or lying position to avoid falling.
- Nausea is common at the beginning of therapy.
- Do not abruptly stop taking the medication.
- Report increased loss of muscle control, yellow skin or eyes, dark urine, hallucinations, severe diarrhoea.

ANTICHOLINERGICS

Benzhexol (Artane)
Benztropine (Cogentin)
Biperiden (Akineton)
Cycrimine (Pagitane)
Procyclidine (Kemadrin)
Chlorphenoxamine (Phenoxene)

Anticholinergics are effective in PD because they block the excitatory action of the neurotransmitter acetylcholine. They are frequently used during the early stages of the disease or when the person can no longer take levodopa. They may be given in combination with carbidopa–levodopa therapy. These medications ease drooling, tremors and rigidity; however, side effects are common and may include blurred vision, dry mouth, constipation, delayed gastric emptying, urinary retention, photophobia and tachycardia. Older adults are especially susceptible to heat stroke and psychological side effects, including confusion, depression, delusions and hallucinations. Anticholinergics should be tapered slowly when discontinued to avoid enhancing Parkinsonian symptoms.

Nursing responsibilities

- Perform baseline assessment for presence of glaucoma, cardiac dysfunction and prostatic hypertrophy.
- Note other medications, including OTC medications that have anticholinergic effects, such as antihistamines and tricyclic antidepressants.
- Monitor for side effects, especially changes in vision, elimination, gastric emptying and mentation.

Health education for the person and family

- Inform your healthcare practitioner if you begin taking any new medications or notice any new symptoms.
- Avoid overexposure to heat and take precautions to avoid heat stroke: drink fluids, keep cool and avoid strenuous activity on hot days.
- Drink adequate amounts of fluid to minimise constipation.
- Practise home safety to prevent falls associated with blurred vision.
- Avoid taking OTC antihistamines or sleeping aids; these have anticholinergic activity.
- Have the eyes examined annually to check for glaucoma; wear dark glasses if photophobia develops.
- Do not suddenly stop taking anticholinergics.

Deep brain stimulation

Activa® tremor control therapy uses an implanted pacemaker-like device to deliver mild electrical stimulation to block the brain impulses that cause tremor, rigidity, stiffness, slowed movement and problems with walking. In this procedure, an insulated wire is surgically placed in the thalamus and connected to an implanted pulse generator (similar to an advanced cardiac pacemaker) near the clavicle. It is used only for people who cannot adequately control manifestations with medications.

Surgery

Pallidotomy is a surgical technique for Parkinson's disease and its results have been helpful for many people. In this procedure, the neurosurgeon locates the affected areas of the globus pallidus and destroys the involved tissue. As a result, people who could not previously ambulate are able to walk and tremors cease. The long-term effects are still being evaluated.

Stereotaxic thalamotomy (an x-ray is taken during neurosurgery to guide the insertion of a needle into a specific area of the brain) has been used only for people who do not respond to medications—generally, younger people with extreme unilateral tremor. The surgeon destroys a small amount of tissue by creating a lesion in the ventrolateral nucleus of the thalamus. This surgery decreases tremors and rigidity in the contralateral extremity.

Fetal tissue transplantation is a controversial surgical procedure limited to a few medical centres. In this procedure, brain cells from aborted fetuses are implanted into the brain in the hope that the new cells will grow and produce enough dopamine to restore some lost mobility.

Rehabilitation

Depending on their individual needs, people frequently benefit from rehabilitation therapy with a physiotherapist, social worker, psychologist and/or speech therapist.

Physiotherapists (PTs) can implement an individual exercise program to improve coordination, balance, gait and transfers. Preventing contractures is an important goal of exercise therapy. It is crucial that family and healthcare personnel permit the person adequate time to perform not only exercise regimens but also ADLs. Activities should not be rushed.

An occupational therapist (OT) helps the person adapt to changing abilities pertinent to work, self-care and recreational activities. Some rehabilitation centres assign OT personnel the responsibility of addressing the person's upper extremity functions while assigning PT personnel to manage lower extremity problems. For example, skills related to cooking and grooming would be supervised by the OT, whereas mobility and posture skills would be supervised by the PT.

Speech therapists frequently address not only the person's speech but also chewing and swallowing. These therapists evaluate people and plan treatment regimens. The challenge with people who have PD is that they have not only vocalisation problems but also dexterity deficits; speech therapists therefore must evaluate the potential benefits of assistive devices, such as a magic slate, voice synthesiser or computer, for each person.

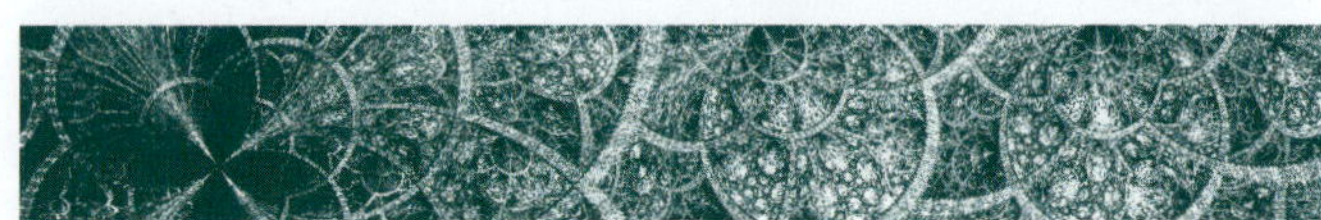

Nursing care

The chronic and eventually debilitating nature of PD poses many challenges to people, families and healthcare professionals. Dependence due to declining physical and mental abilities is of major concern. In the early stages, most people are able to remain at home, with the family support as needed. As the disease progresses and the burden of care increases, the person and their family may prefer placement in a long-term care facility. See the nursing care plan for the person with PD.

Health promotion

Teaching preventive measures is extremely important when caring for people who have PD. Preventing malnutrition, falls and other environmental accidents, constipation, skin breakdown from incontinence or immobility, and joint contracture requires teaching and reinforcement.

NURSING CARE PLAN A person with PD

Walter Avneil, aged 78, was diagnosed with PD at age 64. His wife died 5 years ago and he has no other family living. Mr Avneil worked for more than 40 years as a mechanic in a large factory. He now lives in a residential aged care facility. During his last clinic visit for a review of his medications, the following assessment was made.

ASSESSMENT

Caucasian male with history of PD for the past 14 years. Skin oily and damp. Tremors in both hands and the lips. Gait is slow and shuffling, with a forwards-leaning posture. Speech slow and slurred. Face expressionless. Has lost 5 kg since last visit 3 months ago. Has been on levodopa with carbidopa since diagnosis. States his main problems are 'eating problems, bowel problems, walking problems'.

DIAGNOSIS

- *Constipation* related to lack of exercise, decreased food intake and effects of medications manifested by difficulty opening bowels.
- *Impaired verbal communication* related to lip tremors, slow/slurred speech and facial muscle involvement of PD, evidenced by difficulty communicating needs to others.
- *Poor nutrition* related to difficulty swallowing and chewing, evidenced by weight loss.
- *Impaired physical mobility* related to rigidity and bradykinesia, evidenced by slow, shuffling gait.

PLANNING

- Provide interventions to manage complications of PD.

NURSING CARE PLAN A person with PD (continued)

Expected outcomes

- Have a soft stool at least every other day.
- Practise exercises provided by speech therapist twice a day.
- Increase number of kilojoules, fluids and fibre in diet provided at long-term facility.
- Improve joint mobility and ability to ambulate.

IMPLEMENTATION

- Discuss problems with bowel elimination with staff at long-term facility; suggest increasing fluids to 3 L per day and increasing fibre in the diet with more fruit and high-fibre vegetables at meals.
- Encourage exercises provided by speech therapist to improve speech and swallowing. If these are not effective, make a referral for another evaluation.
- Discuss diet plan with dietitian at the long-term care facility, including consistency of foods and number of kilojoules. Suggest dietitian be part of the swallowing evaluation by the speech therapist.
- Refer for physiotherapy and occupational therapy for a program to improve gait and joint mobility and to decrease risk of falling.

EVALUATION

In a return visit 3 months later, Mr Avneil reports that 'my bowels are working better'. He has gained 3.2 kg and the staff report that this is related to multiple factors, including practising his swallowing exercises, getting more exercise which stimulated his appetite and changing his diet to six small meals a day of soft or puréed foods. The staff are offering him liquids at meals and snack times and he usually drinks all they give him. His speech is not much improved. His posture and gait are somewhat better and he is doing the exercises provided by the physiotherapist and occupational therapist. Mr Avneil's functional abilities have improved so much that the staff are considering training sessions specific to care of residents with PD.

CRITICAL THINKING IN THE NURSING PROCESS

1 Although Mr Avneil did not mention it, the staff report that he is frustrated by not being able to dress himself. Which suggestions could you make to facilitate his independence?
2 Mr Avneil spends most of his time alone, although he enjoys the company of the other residents. List assessments and interventions you might provide to increase his diversional activity.
3 The loss of his wife and the debilitating effects of his disease increase Mr Avneil's risk of the nursing diagnosis of *Chronic sorrow*. What might you suggest the long-term staff do to reduce this risk?

REFLECTION ON THE NURSING PROCESS

1 Which communication and education strategies could you use to assist people with PD who are experiencing speech difficulties?
2 Outline what you have learned from this case study that you will apply to your future nursing practice.

In addition to incorporating information about safety needs, teach ways to prevent orthostatic hypotension when the person changes positions; some people may also benefit from wearing individually fitted compression hose. In addition, address safety considerations about proper administration of medications.

Assessment

Collect the following data through the health history and physical examination (see the chapter 'A person-centred approach to assessing the nervous system'). Further focused assessments are described with nursing interventions. When assessing the older person, be aware of normal changes with ageing, outlined in the chapter 'A person-centred approach to assessing the nervous system'.

- *Health history*: brain trauma, stroke, infection, exposure to heavy metals or carbon monoxide, medication and drug use, incontinence, constipation, weight loss, sweating, sleep problems, muscle pain, mood.
- *Physical assessment*: affect; appearance; speech, scalp, eyelashes and skin; drooling; tremor; coordination; posture; gait; muscle rigidity; mental status.

Nursing diagnoses and interventions

People with PD have complex and, ultimately, multisystem needs. Deficits in mobility and self-care are common. Psychosocial needs may include problems related to *Ineffective coping*, *Powerlessness* and *Disturbed body image*. Refer to the nursing care sections throughout this chapter for discussions of fatigue, self-care deficit, ineffective airway clearance and other pertinent diagnoses. This section focuses on the nursing diagnoses related to *Impaired physical mobility*, *Impaired verbal communication*, *Imbalanced nutrition: less than body requirements* and *Disturbed sleep pattern*.

Impaired physical mobility

People with PD have impaired mobility for several reasons, including tremors, gait-pattern disturbances and alterations in body positioning, such as forwards bending of the trunk. Poor self-esteem may contribute to the person's lack of motivation and willingness to be mobile.

- Suggest referral to a physiotherapist to develop an individualised exercise program. *A program specific to the person supplies motivation as well as helping the person maintain muscle tone, flexibility and mobility.*
- Request the physiotherapist teach caregivers how to do ROM exercises at least twice a day, emphasising the trunk, neck, arms, hips and legs. *Maintaining joint mobility promotes better function and strength, improving gait pattern. Consistent ROM exercises can prevent contractures.*
- Ask caregivers to ambulate the person at least four times a day if possible. *Exercise fosters independence and self-esteem.*
- Recommend assistive devices, such as lift chairs, canes, splints or braces, as indicated. *Adaptive equipment*

improves balance, protects joints and promotes proper anatomical positioning.

- To promote mobility and safety:
  - Slightly elevate the back legs of chairs and raise the toilet seat to help rise from a sitting position to a standing position.
  - Wear shoes with Velcro closures.
  - Remove potential hazards, such as unanchored throw rugs.
  - Install handrails and non-skid surfaces in bathtubs and showers.
  - Ensure adequate lighting throughout the home and in outside areas, especially in areas where transfers are common.

  Safety measures prevent potential complications that may result from falls or other accidents and promote self-esteem through self-care.

CONSIDERATION FOR PRACTICE

Parkinson's disease is a disorder common in older adults, who are at greater risk of falls resulting from orthostatic hypotension, osteoporosis, poor vision and problems causing disorientation and confusion, such as Alzheimer's disease.

Impaired verbal communication

Diminished vocal amplitude and loss of muscular control can impair the person's ability to speak. Both caregivers and family members must remember to give people enough time for self-expression; an unhurried approach is recommended. Seek input from family members when determining alternative methods of communicating with the person.

- Assess current communication abilities in speech, hearing and writing. *Communication involves both sending and receiving messages.*
- Develop methods of communication appropriate to coordination abilities, such as a magic slate, flash cards with common phrases and pointing to objects. *Individualising a method of communication decreases anxiety and isolation.*
- Suggest referral to a speech pathologist to develop oral exercises and interventions that will facilitate speaking. *The muscles of speech and swallowing are affected by the PD process.*
- Remind the person to speak more loudly, if possible. *A low, monotonous voice is characteristic of the person with PD.*

Imbalanced nutrition: less than body requirements

Tremors, altered gait and impaired chewing and swallowing can cause nutritional problems in the person with PD. As the disorder progresses, interventions for ensuring optimal nutrition need to be adapted to the person's functional abilities. Assess the person's swallow reflex before starting any feeding program. During the initial stages of the disorder, some people may have the nursing diagnosis of *Poor nutrition* related to excess intake of kilojoules manifested by kilojoule intake exceeding energy expenditure.

- Assess nutritional status and self-feeding abilities; suggest referral to an occupational or speech therapist, if needed. *An initial assessment of abilities ensures that interventions are personalised to the person's current functional abilities.*
- Teach caregivers how to prepare foods of proper consistency as determined by swallowing function. *The person may aspirate food that is too liquid.*
- Weigh weekly. *Early recognition of weight loss allows for intervention.*
- Teach eating methods to decrease tremors, such as holding a piece of bread in the hand that is not holding an eating utensil. *Non-intentional tremor may be reduced through purposeful activity.*
- Encourage diet that is high in bulk and fluids. *Several anti-Parkinson's medications and inactivity can cause constipation.*

Disturbed sleep pattern

Rigidity and weakness can cause people with PD to lose the ability to move and change positions during sleep. The resulting discomfort causes periods of wakefulness. Medications to treat PD contribute to sleep pattern disturbance; for example, levodopa can cause vivid dreams. Nurses can help in accurately assessing the sleep pattern disturbance and in planning interventions to improve or increase sleep time.

- Assess sleep pattern and existing conditions that may affect sleep, such as depression or pain. *People experiencing anxiety, depression and dementia have a difficult time falling asleep and may wake up more at night.*

CONSIDERATION FOR PRACTICE

Remember to assess pain status; lack of adequate pain control may interfere with sleep.

- Explain the disease process and the effects of decreased dopamine on the sleep–wake cycle. *Depending on the dosage, levodopa causes less REM sleep and deep sleep.*
- Review the person's medication. Bromocriptine and levodopa, especially if used with an anticholinergic, can cause vivid dreams. *Other medications (diuretics, theophylline, hypnotics) also may interfere with sleep.*
- Teach how to modify lifestyle activities that affect sleep:
  - Institute a routine of activities with limited rest periods during the day; avoid napping close to bedtime. Avoid strenuous exercise in the evening. *Daytime sleeping may contribute to decreased night-time sleeping. Vigorous exercise just before bedtime may act as a stimulant.*
  - Incorporate diet modifications, such as limiting caffeine and alcohol intake. *Caffeine is a stimulant and alcohol may cause early morning awakenings, increased daytime sleepiness and nightmares.*
  - Drink a glass of milk before bedtime. *Milk contains l-tryptophan, which produces sedative effects by shortening the time taken to fall asleep (sleep latency).*
  - Adapt the environment to aid sleep (e.g. darken the room and decrease noises). *Reducing environmental stimuli decreases external sleep disturbances.*

Community-based care

It is important for both the person and their family to maintain independence and self-care as long as possible. To maintain function and quality of life, the following topics should be addressed:

- realistic expectations
- equipment suppliers
- home environment conducive to using equipment
- referrals to speech therapist, occupational therapist, physiotherapist and dietitian
- gait training and exercises for improving ambulation, speech, swallowing and self-care
- increased fluid intake of 3 L/day and increased fibre in every meal
- stool softeners or laxatives as needed for bowel elimination
- swallowing during eating and taking medications. Have suction equipment available and know first aid treatment for choking:
  - Encourage the person to relax and breathe deeply.
    - Ask the person to cough.
    - If unsuccessful, bend the person well forwards and give 5 sharp blows between shoulder blades.
    - If still unsuccessful, place the person on their left side on the floor and call 000 for an ambulance.
  - Total blockage:
    - Lie the person on their left side on the floor.
    - Give 5 sharp blows between shoulder blades.
    - If unsuccessful, give 5 quick downward lateral chest thrusts (place one hand in the middle of the person's back for support and heel of other hand in the CPR compression position and give 5 chest thrusts, slower but sharper than compressions).
    - If still unsuccessful, call 000 for an ambulance and continue alternating 5 back blows with 5 chest thrusts until medical aid arrives (St John Ambulance Australia, 2020).
- foods that can be easily swallowed (such as puréed or soft foods) and feed six small meals a day if possible
- helpful resources:
  - Parkinson's Australia: https://www.parkinsons.org.au
  - Brain Foundation: https://brainfoundation.org.au
  - Michael J. Fox Foundation: https://www.michaeljfox.org
  - The National Institute of Neurological Disorders and Stroke: https://www.ninds.nih.gov
  - Parkinson's Alliance: https://www.parkinsonalliance.org.

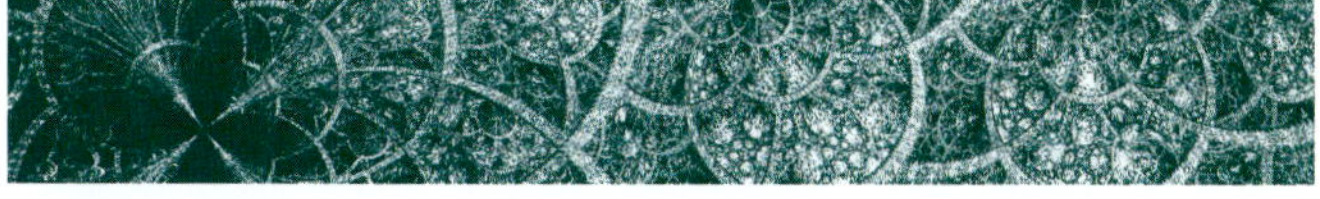

THE PERSON WITH HUNTINGTON'S DISEASE

Huntington's disease (HD) is a progressive, degenerative, inherited neurological disease characterised by increasing dementia and chorea (jerky, rapid, involuntary movements). It is a single-gene autosomal dominant disease that causes localised death of neurons of the basal ganglia (Norris, 2018). The exact cause is unknown, but postmortem studies have demonstrated a decrease in gamma-aminobutyric acid (GABA), an inhibitory neurotransmitter in the basal ganglia. There is also a decrease in acetylcholine levels, suggesting that the manifestations are the result of an imbalance in dopamine and acetylcholine. HD is a familial disease; each child of an HD parent has a 50% chance of inheriting the HD gene and, if they do, will eventually develop the disease (National Institute of Neurological Disorders and Stroke (NINDS), 2022a). There is no cure for the disease. Huntington's disease causes progressive chorea, speech problems and dementia.

Because the person is usually asymptomatic until age 30 to 40, they may already have passed the gene to the next generation. The psychological effect is devastating to people and their families. The family not only experiences guilt from passing the disease from one generation to the next, but also is faced with the overwhelming long-term care needs of those affected. It is common for several family members to have the disease.

Pathophysiology

HD causes destruction of cells in the caudate nucleus and putamen areas of the basal ganglia. Other areas of the brain, such as the frontal lobes, may selectively atrophy. Several neurotransmitters and their receptors are decreased, including GABA and acetylcholine. The neurotransmitter dopamine is not affected in HD, but the decrease in acetylcholine results in a relative excess of dopamine in the basal ganglia. Whereas in PD a deficit of dopamine causes slow movement or lack of movement, in HD the opposite occurs: there is a relative excess of dopamine, causing excessive, uncontrolled movement.

Manifestations

Manifestations and complications primarily involve abnormal movement and progressive dementia (see the 'Manifestations and complications' box). The progression and sequence of manifestations varies somewhat; however, initially the psychological manifestations are more debilitating than the choreiform (rapid and jerky) movements.

Early signs of personality change include severe depression, memory loss with decreased ability to concentrate, emotional lability and impulsiveness. The person experiences frequent mood swings ranging from uncontrollable periods of anger to apathy. Eventually, signs of dementia, including disorientation, confusion and lack of sense of time, become evident and interfere with self-care.

Motor manifestations usually parallel personality and mood changes. The motor manifestations worsen with environmental stimuli and emotional stress but are absent when the person is sleeping. Initially, movement problems are described as 'fidgeting' or restlessness, followed by progressive worsening of abnormal movements. The choreiform movements, which begin in the face and arms and then involve the entire body, are manifested by facial grimaces, tongue protrusion, jerky movement of the distal arms or legs

MANIFESTATIONS AND COMPLICATIONS Huntington's disease

MOTOR EFFECTS

Early

- Restlessness
- 'Fidgety' feeling
- Minor gait changes—unsteady on feet
- Posture and positioning disturbances, frequent falls
- Inability to keep the tongue from protruding
- Slurred speech with poor articulation
- Complications: increasing problem with self-care activities, such as bathing, grooming, eating

Late

- Chorea—severely altered gait with irregular, uncontrollable movement; shoulders shrug arrhythmically
- Facial grimacing—raising of eyebrows, uncontrollable protrusion of the tongue
- Dysphagia
- Unintelligible speech
- Impaired diaphragmatic movement
- Complications: immobility, aspiration, choking and, eventually, total dependence, poor oxygenation, emaciation and cachexia

PSYCHOSOCIAL EFFECTS

Early

- Irritability
- Outbursts of rage alternating with euphoria
- Depression
- Complication: suicide

Late

- Decreasing memory
- Loss of cognitive skills
- Eventual dementia
- Complication: total dependence

and a rhythmic, lurching gait that almost resembles a dance. (The term *chorea* comes from *choreia*, the Greek word meaning 'dance'.) Gait changes cause uncoordinated movements and contribute to frequent falls.

The muscles of swallowing, chewing and speaking are affected, leading to dysphagia and dysarthria and associated problems with communication and nutrition. The person's constant movement and difficulty in swallowing contribute to weight loss and eventual cachexia. Breathing is impaired because the diaphragm is unable to move effectively.

The manifestations slowly progress over approximately 15 to 20 years after initial manifestations appear. Prognosis is poor, with inevitable debilitation and total dependence. Death usually results from aspiration pneumonia or another infectious process.

INTERPROFESSIONAL CARE

Treatment addresses the disease's manifestations, with nurses providing care to people with HD in a variety of community settings. Initially, people and families can manage care needs at home but, as the disease progresses, the person may require constant supervision, such as that provided in day respite facilities or in long-term care facilities. People who develop acute problems may be hospitalised until the crisis is managed. Because of the inevitable total multisystem debilitation of people with Huntington's disease, nurses and other caregivers face many challenges.

Diagnosis

Genetic testing is the only test available to diagnose people suspected of having HD. Both blood and amniotic fluid may be tested for the presence of a gene mutation on chromosome 4 using DNA analysis. The test can predict with 95% accuracy who is a carrier of the disease.

Medications

The following medications are given for the manifestations of HD:

- Antipsychotics, specifically phenothiazines and butyrophenones, are effective in HD because they block dopamine receptors in the brain. The therapeutic goal is to restore the balance between the neurotransmitters.
- Antidepressants are prescribed in the early stage of the disease; however, medications are no substitute for intense follow-up counselling for people and their families.

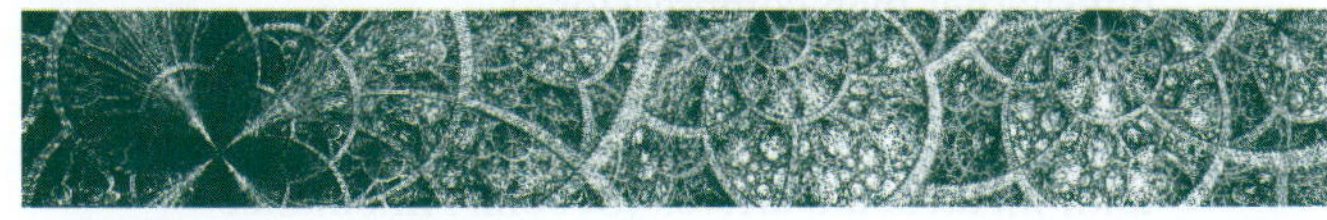

Nursing care

Nurses are faced with a multitude of challenges when caring for families who have Huntington's disease, including physiological, psychosocial and ethical problems. Physiological problems are related to the progressive and eventually debilitating nature of the disease. Psychosocial concerns occur as a result of the person's personality and mental changes, the family's responsibility for providing care and the guilt implicit in a genetically transmitted disease. Ethical difficulties relate to the genetic nature of the disease: DNA testing for the marker on chromosome 4 can determine whether the person is a carrier of the disease before they begin to exhibit manifestations. Children of people with HD are thus faced with the choice of finding out whether they will eventually be affected. If they choose not to be tested, they may pass the disease on to yet another generation; and if a fetus is affected, they may face the decision of whether to undergo an abortion.

Nursing diagnoses and interventions

Initially, much of the nursing care focuses on teaching about the disease, psychological support and genetic counselling.

As manifestations become more severe, nursing considerations centre on problems related not only to immobility and altered nutrition, but also to the increasing self-care deficits. Families and people experiencing HD face many psychosocial issues. Nurses must be prepared to listen actively as well as to provide comfort and encouragement throughout the lengthy illness. There are many possible nursing diagnoses for the person with HD; this section focuses on nursing diagnoses related to aspiration, nutrition, skin integrity and communication.

Risk of aspiration

Uncoordinated movements and swallowing and chewing problems put the person at high risk of aspiration.

- Maintain in an upright position while the person eats; support the head. *Proper positioning may prevent aspiration during meals.*
- Teach the first aid treatment for choking to caregivers and family members (see above). *Aspiration is a real possibility; caregivers must be prepared to re-establish the person's airway.*
- Provide food that is thick enough to manage, such as thick soups, mashed potatoes, stews or casseroles. *These foods are more readily tolerated and manipulated by the tongue than liquids.*
- Make sure food is swallowed before giving another spoonful of food. *The automatic phase of swallowing may be disrupted in the person with HD; providing adequate time and smaller bites may improve the ability to manipulate foods.*
- Provide a calm, relaxing eating environment. *Stress worsens choreiform movements and inappropriate behaviours.*

Poor nutrition

People with HD have unpredictable choreiform movements of the extremities and decreased ability to control muscles involved with chewing and swallowing. Families and caregivers are challenged to provide sufficient kilojoules to maintain the person in positive nitrogen balance.

- Evaluate current weight and nutritional status, including serum prealbumin and transferrin levels. *Establishing a baseline is crucial for meeting individual kilojoule, protein, vitamin and mineral needs.*
- Assess ability to swallow and manipulate eating utensils. *Aspiration is an ever-present danger that must be avoided; utensils may need to be adapted to the person's abilities if the person is able to assist at all.*
- Continue feeding even if the person physically turns away from the meal. *Involuntary choreiform movements should not be interpreted as a refusal to eat.*
- Provide high-kilojoule, nutritious foods and sufficient snacks; request input from a dietitian. *The constant movement of HD increases kilojoule requirements.*
- Avoid milk; provide frequent oral hygiene. *Milk tends to thicken secretions. Decreasing thick secretions may improve ability to swallow and enable the person to ingest more kilojoules.*

Impaired skin integrity

Skin integrity is only one component of the person's general need for protection and avoidance of injury. Several factors increase the risk of impaired skin integrity, including poor nutritional status, eventual total immobility and incontinence.

- Evaluate the skin for actual and potential areas of breakdown. *Establishing a baseline is necessary to modify care and provide prophylactic protection of high-risk pressure areas.*
- Determine nutritional status, especially serum prealbumin level and vitamin, mineral and kilojoule intake. *Optimal nutritional status and positive nitrogen balance help prevent skin breakdown and formation of pressure ulcers.*
- Turn and inspect the skin at least every 2 hours, giving special consideration to areas that are most prone to breakdown, such as heels and coccyx. *Pressure points are particularly susceptible to skin breakdown.*
- Provide ROM exercises on a regular schedule in the daytime. *Movement stimulates circulation, which provides oxygenation and allows nutrients to reach muscles and skin.*
- Keep the skin clean and dry; pay particular attention to the perineal area if incontinent. *Skin in close proximity to the perineal area, such as the sacral area, is highly susceptible to breakdown due to exposure to wet, acidic urine and faecal material.*
- Place on an alternating-pressure mattress with foot board. *Decreasing pressure on bony prominences and preventing shearing forces serve to prevent skin breakdown.*
- Pad side rails and headrests of special chairs; have the person wear a helmet. *The person's violent movements can cause trauma to the head and extremities.*

Impaired verbal communication

The inability to control muscles related to speech, swallowing and facial movement contributes to problems of verbal communication. Because HD affects fine motor movement, especially the distal portion of the extremities, the hands are not effective in communication. As the disease progresses, mental abilities are also compromised, making both receptive and expressive communication impossible.

- Choose alternative methods of communication while the person is able to participate. *Anticipatory planning may facilitate communication and decrease anxiety.*
- Continue to incorporate therapeutic communication techniques, even though the person is not responsive: maintain eye contact, use touch and talk directly to the person rather than to others in the room. *These techniques enhance the individual's dignity and self-worth.*
- Seek input from family about the person's usual preferences and how they are communicated; be alert for subtle cues. *Non-verbal communication techniques may be individualised and more readily recognised by the family member or caregiver who usually provides care.*
- Continue talking to the person, even though there is no apparent response. *Hearing may not be impaired, even though the person cannot speak.*

Community-based care

People with HD and their families may know how devastating the illness is because they may have cared for a parent or other close family member who had the illness. Many families are overwhelmed with just the thought of the physical and psychosocial debilitation that the disease brings. Fear, anxiety and hopelessness leading to depression are common reactions. Teaching ways to cope effectively with the psychosocial and physical changes is an integral part of the nurse's responsibilities. Referrals to appropriate agencies, such as adult day care centres, Huntington's Australia and local support groups or a psychologist, should be considered.

Another aspect of personal teaching concerns the genetic transmission of HD; refer people and family members to a geneticist. Nurses are frequently involved with clarifying information, especially concerning the transmission, course of illness and prognosis. A caring, sensitive approach is crucial. Information about transmission of an autosomal dominant trait is discussed in the chapter 'Genetic implications of adult health nursing'.

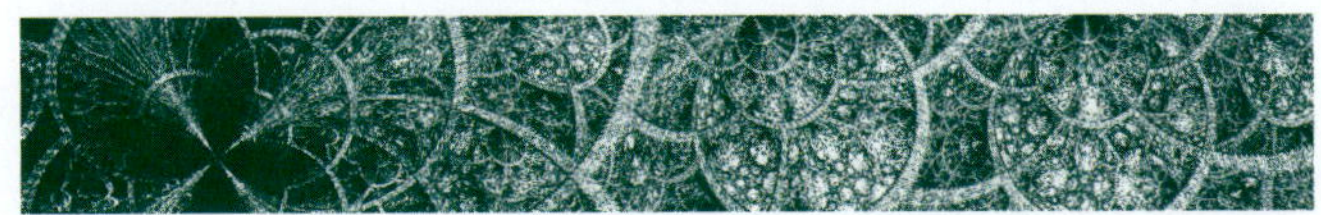

THE PERSON WITH MOTOR NEURONE DISEASE

Motor neurone disease (MND), also known as amyotrophic lateral sclerosis (ALS) or *Lou Gehrig's disease*, is a rapidly progressive and fatal degenerative neurological disease characterised by weakness and wasting of muscles under voluntary control, without any accompanying sensory or cognitive changes. The name is derived from the pathophysiological processes of muscle atrophy (*amyotrophy*), resulting from lower motor neuron involvement, and sclerosis of the corticospinal tract in the lateral column of the spinal cord, resulting from upper motor neuron involvement. Death results in 2 to 5 years after onset of the manifestations (although some people live 10 years or more), usually due to respiratory failure.

It is estimated that in Australia, around 2,100 people are living with MND, with two people diagnosed each day and two people dying from the disease each day. Although the lifetime risk of developing MND is about 1 in 300 by the age of 85, with risk increasing steadily as people get older, many people have not heard of MND before they themselves, or someone they know, has been diagnosed. Slightly more men than women are diagnosed with MND, most commonly in their fifties or sixties. However, MND may be diagnosed in adults at any age. Globally, over 400,000 people are currently living with MND. It affects people from every country and ethnicity in the world (Motor Neurone Disease Australia, 2021). Most of the health problems a person with MND encounters are related to swallowing and managing secretions, communication and dysfunction of the muscles used in respiration.

Pathophysiology

MND results from the degeneration and demyelination of both upper and lower motor neurons in the anterior horn of the spinal cord, brainstem and cerebral cortex. Death of the motor neurons results in axonal degeneration, demyelination, glial proliferation and scarring along the corticospinal tract. In the early stages of the disease, surviving motor neurons sprout new branches to reinnervate affected muscle fibres, preserving muscle strength. However, when more than half of the lower motor neurons are affected, reinnervation fails and weakness is evidenced.

Although the pathogenesis of MND is not clear, abnormal glutamate metabolism and hydrogen peroxide production are being studied. Echovirus RNA has also been isolated in spinal cord tissue in some people with non-familial MND. Environmental factors, excess intracellular calcium and antibodies to calcium channels are also being researched.

Manifestations

The initial manifestations may relate to dysfunction of upper motor neurons, lower motor neurons or both. Dysfunction of upper motor neurons results in spastic, weak muscles with increased deep tendon reflexes. Dysfunction of lower motor neurons results in muscle flaccidity, paresis (weakness), paralysis and atrophy.

Weakness and paresis are common early manifestations. The weakness may initially affect only one muscle group. Manifestations vary according to the particular muscle group involved; *fasciculations* (twitching) of involved muscles are common in the early stage of the disorder. With the loss of muscle innervation, the muscles atrophy and paralysis results. Muscle mass decreases and people complain of progressive fatigue. Typically, the disease first affects the hands, then the shoulders, upper arms and, finally, the legs.

Increasing brainstem involvement causes progressive atrophy of the tongue and facial muscles with eventual dysphagia and dysarthria. Emotional lability and loss of control occur, but dementia is not part of the pathological progression of MND. Vision, hearing, sensation and cognitive ability usually remain intact. A summary of manifestations and complications is presented in the 'Manifestations and complications' box.

INTERPROFESSIONAL CARE

Because many treatable disorders may cause manifestations similar to those that appear in the initial stage of MND, a thorough evaluation is required. Once MND is diagnosed, the primary goal is to support the person and their family in meeting physical and psychosocial needs, particularly as the disease progresses.

Medical and nursing care for people with MND is primarily supportive. Referral for home health management is indicated. Occupational, physical, speech and respiratory (physiotherapy) are major supportive and rehabilitative treatments. As the disorder progresses and swallowing becomes ineffective, a gastrostomy tube may be necessary to provide adequate nutritional intake. Ventilatory assistance should be discussed with people before the need occurs.

MANIFESTATIONS AND COMPLICATIONS MND

MUSCULOSKELETAL SYSTEM
- Weakness and fatigue
- 'Heaviness' of legs
- Fasciculations
- Uncoordinated movements, loss of fine motor control in hands
- Spasticity
- Paresis
- Hyperreflexia
- Atrophy
- Problems with articulation
- Complications: paralysis, loss of ability to perform ADLs, total immobility, aspiration, loss of verbal communication

RESPIRATORY SYSTEM
- Dyspnoea
- Difficulty clearing airway
- Complications: pneumonia, eventual respiratory failure

NUTRITIONAL EFFECTS
- Difficulty chewing
- Dysphagia
- Complication: malnutrition

EMOTIONAL EFFECTS
- Loss of control, lability
- Complication: depression

Diagnosis

There is no specific test to diagnose MND. Rather, diagnosis is made based on manifestations and tests to rule out other diseases. Several disorders may mimic early MND, including hyperthyroidism, hypoglycaemia, compression of the spinal cord, toxic agents, infections and neoplasms.

Medications

Riluzole (Rilutek), an antiglutamate, is the first medication developed to treat MND. It inhibits the presynaptic release of glutamic acid in the CNS and protects neurons against the excitotoxicity of glutamic acid. This oral medication is administered without food at the same time each day. People are regularly monitored for liver function, blood count, blood chemistries and alkaline phosphatase. They should be warned to report any febrile illness to their healthcare provider and to avoid alcohol.

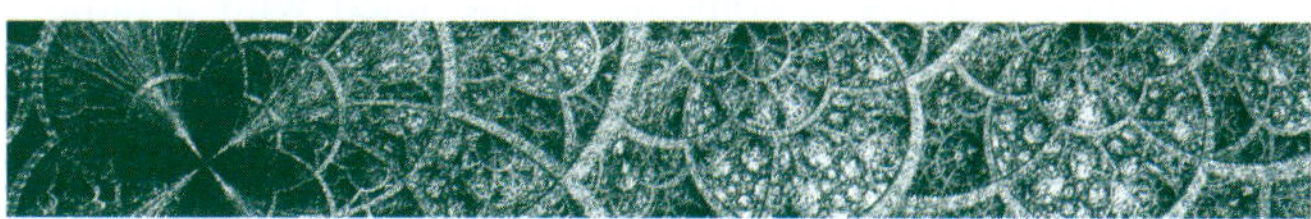

Nursing care

Nursing care focuses on current health problems and on anticipating future difficulties. As with other disorders causing incapacitation and dependence, individualised nursing goals and interventions relate to decreasing complications, especially those associated with loss of muscular function and immobility; promoting independence to the extent possible; initiating referrals, particularly to a support group for both the person and their family; and providing physical and psychosocial support as indicated.

Of special consideration is planning for the person's eventual inability to communicate. Because the person's eye muscles and movements remain intact, signals can be prearranged before the loss of speech.

Nursing diagnoses and interventions

Two nursing diagnoses that frequently apply to people with MND are *Risk of disuse syndrome* and *Ineffective breathing pattern.*

Risk of disuse syndrome

People with MND are at risk of developing problems associated with bed rest not only because they cannot move and reposition themselves, but also because they frequently have altered nutritional and hydration status. Nursing interventions focus on preventing skin breakdown and infections such as urinary tract infections.

- Assess current condition for baseline parameters, particularly skin over bony prominences, lung sounds and vital signs. *Understanding the person's current condition allows accurate future assessment and realistic planning.*
- Assess skin; provide skin care and obtain an alternating-pressure mattress. *Pressure points are at risk of breakdown; early detection is crucial to instituting appropriate care.*
- Institute active ROM exercises, as the person is able. Perform passive ROM exercises every 2 hours, when the person is turned. *Contractures can develop within a week because extensor muscles are weaker than flexor muscles.*
- Maintain positive nitrogen balance and hydration status: monitor prealbumin levels, haemoglobin and haematocrit levels and urine specific gravity. *Adequate protein is required to maintain osmotic pressure and prevent oedema; positive nitrogen balance promotes optimal body functioning.*
- Monitor for manifestations of infection; for example, assess urine, especially if a urinary catheter is present. *Urinary catheters place people at high risk of sepsis; bed rest places the person at greater risk of urinary stasis.*

CONSIDERATION FOR PRACTICE

Urinary tract infection is indicated by cloudy, foul-smelling urine, pain on urination, fever and general malaise.

Ineffective breathing pattern

As the muscle weakness of MND continues, people become less able to breathe. The respiratory muscles are affected and people may eventually require ventilatory assistance. The nurse must initiate measures to support the existing respiratory effort.

- Obtain a baseline assessment of breathing pattern, air movement and oxygen saturation. *Assessments indicating the person's current condition provide data to plan individualised interventions.*
- Turn at least every 2 hours. *Movement enhances the ability to move pulmonary secretions and prevents stasis.*
- Elevate the head of the bed at least 30 degrees, suction as indicated and provide oxygen. *This supports ventilation and enhances lung expansion as the person's condition changes.*
- Monitor temperature and lung sounds routinely; obtain sputum culture as indicated. *Early detection of a possible infectious process leads to prompt treatment.*

CONSIDERATION FOR PRACTICE

A pulmonary infection is indicated by respiratory difficulty, crackles and/or wheezes, cough productive of yellow or green sputum, fever and malaise.

Community-based care

Initial teaching centres on explaining the disease process, expected course and prognosis. Referral to a social worker to determine home care needs and financial assistance is helpful. Counselling and referrals to a home health agency, dietitian, physiotherapist and speech and occupational therapists can help the family meet the person's changing needs and abilities. The realistic anticipation of needs cannot be overemphasised.

As the person becomes more debilitated, family members or other care providers focus on preventing complications. For example, family members need to know how to suction the person and perform the first aid treatment for choking to prevent aspiration. Teaching the family how to prevent problems related to immobility is a primary consideration for the nurse.

Another focus of teaching is basic care needs, such as care required to meet elimination needs. Teach families methods to establish a bowel routine, considerations related to a urinary catheter and the need to promptly report manifestations of an infection.

Throughout the early stage and continued care of the person with MND and their family, much consideration is given to psychosocial concerns. Depression, anger and denial may be initial reactions; refer the person and their family to an MND support group, social worker, psychologist or psychiatrist as indicated.

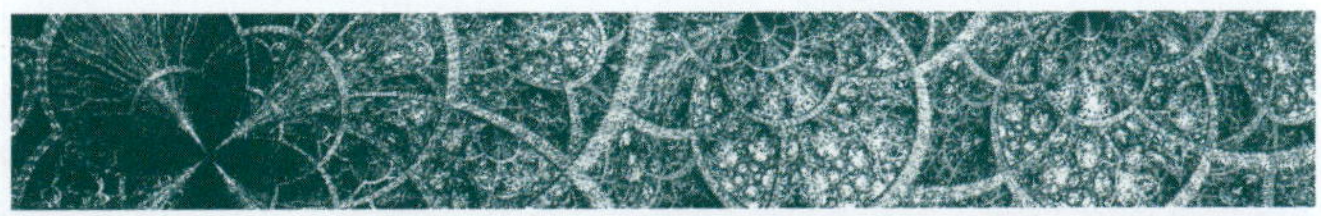

Peripheral nervous system disorders

Many aetiological agents are responsible for peripheral nervous system disorders. Autoimmune disorders, viruses, environmental toxins, such as heavy metals, and nutritional deficiencies can affect the peripheral nervous system.

THE PERSON WITH MYASTHENIA GRAVIS

Myasthenia gravis is a chronic autoimmune neuromuscular disorder characterised by fatigue and severe weakness of skeletal muscles. People experience periods of remission and exacerbation, and mild forms of the disorder exist. Weakness may remain limited to a few muscle groups, especially the ocular muscles, or may become generalised with all muscles eventually becoming weakened.

Women are affected three times more frequently than men. The average age of onset for women is 28 and men is 42. Treatment with anticholinesterase medications has greatly improved the prognosis and symptom management (NINDS, 2022b).

Pathophysiology

The axons of motor neurons divide as they enter skeletal muscles and each axonal ending forms a neuromuscular junction. Although the axonal ending and the muscle fibre are extremely close, they are separated by the synaptic cleft. The transmission of nerve impulses from the nerve to the muscles occurs at the neuromuscular junctions. The neurotransmitter acetylcholine is released from the axonal ending, crosses the synaptic cleft, attaches to acetylcholine receptors on the muscle fibre and stimulates the muscle.

In myasthenia gravis, antibodies destroy or block neuromuscular junction receptor sites, resulting in a decreased number of acetylcholine receptors. Structural changes also result in diminished acetylcholine uptake. The net result is a decrease in the muscle's ability to contract despite a sufficient amount of acetylcholine. A comparison of a normal neuromuscular junction and one affected by myasthenia gravis is shown in Figure 43.4.

In about 75% of people with myasthenia gravis, the thymus gland, which is usually inactive after puberty, continues to produce antibodies because of hyperplasia of the gland or because of tumours. It is believed that the thymus is a source of autoantigen that triggers an autoimmune response in myasthenia gravis. The exact mechanism and reason for the thymus gland's antibody production are unknown.

Myasthenia gravis is sometimes associated with a tumour of the thymus, thyrotoxicosis (hyperthyroidism), rheumatoid arthritis and lupus erythematosus. The disorder is often diagnosed when a person seeks treatment for a coincidental infection that exacerbates manifestations. Exacerbations may also occur before the menstrual period and during or soon after pregnancy.

Manifestations

The manifestations of myasthenia gravis correspond to the muscles involved. Initially, the eye muscles are affected and the person experiences either diplopia (unilateral or bilateral double vision) or ptosis (drooping of the eyelid) (see Figure 43.5). Next, the facial, speech and mastication muscles become weak and people may have periods of dysarthria and dysphagia. Fatigue is evident even when the person tries to eat a meal; the muscles of chewing tire and the person is forced to stop eating momentarily. A smile becomes a snarl or grimace and the voice is weak with a muffled nasal quality. Problems performing fine motor movements of the hands, such as writing, appear early in the disease.

As the disease progresses, the muscles of the neck and extremities are affected. When the muscles of the neck become affected, the head juts forward. Deep tendon reflexes are usually normal, however, even in weak muscles. Fatigue and weakness are exacerbated with stress, fever, overexertion and exposure to heat and are relieved by rest.

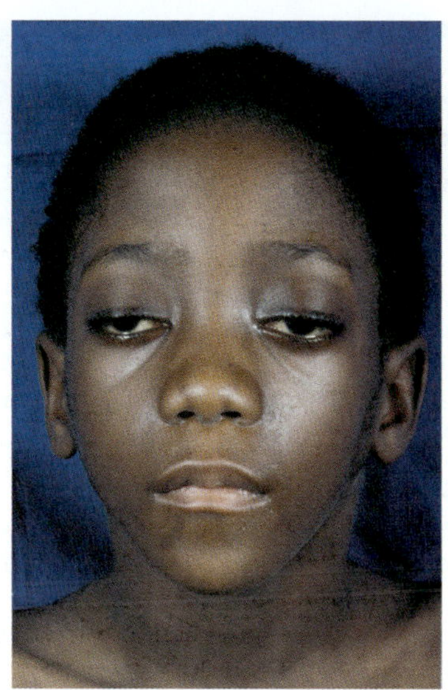

FIGURE 43.5 ***In myasthenia gravis, the person experiences unilateral weakness of the facial muscles***

Source: Dr M. A. Ansary/Science Photo Library/Alamy Stock Photo.

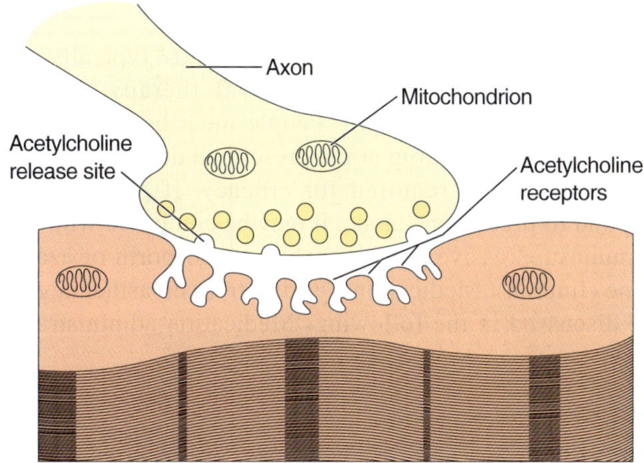

A Normal neuromuscular junction

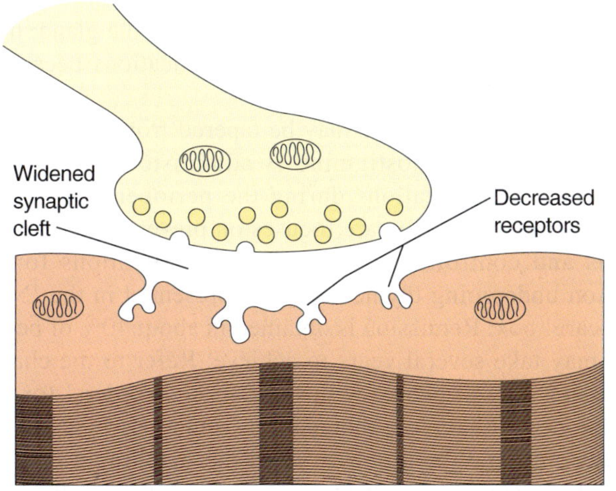

B Myasthenia gravis

FIGURE 43.4 ***A, A normal neuromuscular junction and B, one showing the changes seen in myasthenia gravis. These changes interfere with the transmission of nerve impulses to the muscle***

Manifestations vary each day. Manifestations and complications of myasthenia gravis are listed in the 'Manifestations and complications' box.

Complications

Complications are directly related to the degree of muscle weakness and the specific muscles involved. For example, when the pharyngeal and palatal muscles are affected, the person cannot manage swallowing and may aspirate food or fluids. The person is at increased risk of pneumonia because weakness of the diaphragm and muscles of respiration compromises gas exchange. People with myasthenia gravis can develop life-threatening emergencies, including myasthenic crisis and cholinergic crisis.

Myasthenic crisis

Myasthenic crisis is a sudden exacerbation of motor weakness putting the person at risk of respiratory failure and aspiration. Myasthenic crisis most often is due to undermedication, missed doses of medication or a developing infection. Manifestations of myasthenic crisis include tachycardia, tachypnoea, severe respiratory distress, dysphagia, restlessness, impaired speech and anxiety.

Cholinergic crisis

Cholinergic crisis is the result of overdosage with the anticholinesterase (cholinergic) medications used to treat myasthenia gravis. Gastrointestinal manifestations, severe muscle weakness, vertigo and respiratory distress are signs of cholinergic crisis. Both types of crises are emergency, life-threatening situations; people frequently require ventilatory assistance. Differentiation is based on the person's response to edrophonium chloride (Tensilon). In myasthenic crisis, the test

MANIFESTATIONS AND COMPLICATIONS

Myasthenia gravis

OCULAR AND FACIAL
- Ptosis
- Diplopia
- Facial weakness
- Dysphagia
- Dysarthria
- Complications: difficulty closing eyes, aspiration, impaired communication and nutrition

MUSCULOSKELETAL
- Weakness and fatigue
- Decreased function of hands, arms, legs and neck muscles
- Complications: inability to perform ADLs and self-care activities, complications related to immobility, myasthenic and cholinergic crises

RESPIRATORY
- Weakening of intercostal muscles
- Decrease in diaphragm movement
- Breathlessness and dyspnoea
- Poor gas exchange
- Complications: decreasing ability to walk, eat and perform other ADLs, pneumonia

NUTRITIONAL
- Inability to chew and swallow
- Decreasing ability to move tongue
- Impairment of fine motor movements: inability to feed self
- Complications: weight loss, dehydration, malnutrition, aspiration

is positive; in cholinergic crisis, the test is negative (see the discussion that follows under 'Diagnosis').

INTERPROFESSIONAL CARE

Care of the person with myasthenia gravis focuses on providing appropriate treatment, preventing complications and supporting the person and their family in meeting physical and psychosocial needs, especially as the disease progresses.

Diagnosis

Diagnostic tests are conducted following a thorough history and physical examination, with special attention to the facial, oculomotor, laryngeal and respiratory muscles. Diagnostic tests include the anticholinesterase (Tensilon) test, nerve stimulation studies and an analysis of antiacetylcholine receptor antibodies.

In the Tensilon test, the person is injected with edrophonium chloride, a short-acting anticholinesterase. People with myasthenia gravis show a significant improvement in muscle strength that lasts approximately 5 minutes. This test is also used to differentiate myasthenic crisis (caused by insufficient medication, so the person shows improvement with the drug) from cholinergic crisis (caused by overmedication, so the person does not show improvement).

Single-fibre electromyography can detect delayed or failed neuromuscular transmission in muscle fibres supplied by a single nerve fibre. Serum assay of circulating acetylcholine receptor antibodies, if increased, is diagnostic of myasthenia gravis with a sensitivity of 80–90%.

Medications

The primary group of medications used to treat myasthenia gravis is the anticholinesterases. These drugs act at the neuromuscular junction and allow acetylcholine to concentrate at the receptor sites, thus promoting muscle contraction. Pyridostigmine (Mestinon) is the most commonly used acetylcholinesterase inhibitor for myasthenia gravis. The person's decrease in manifestations guides dosage.

Immunosuppression with glucocorticoids, typically prednisone, is another pharmacological therapy aimed at improving muscle strength. People must be aware of the need to stay on the drug at the prescribed dose to determine the least amount required for efficacy. If people do not respond to prednisone alone, it may be combined with other immunosuppressive agents, such as cyclosporin or azathioprine (Imuran). Medications used to treat myasthenia gravis are discussed in the following 'Medication administration' box.

Surgery

Approximately 75% of people with myasthenia gravis have dysplasia of the thymus gland. Therefore, thymectomy is often recommended for people younger than 60. The two surgical approaches used are the transcervical approach, which is considered less invasive, and the transsternal approach. The latter approach allows a more extensive removal of the gland; however, it also poses more potential complications because it involves splitting the sternum.

Preoperatively, people may be tapered from steroid therapy. Usually, pyridostigmine is administered to prevent muscular manifestations during the perioperative period. Postoperative nursing care focuses on preventing complications and controlling pain. Nursing implications for the person undergoing thymectomy are presented in the 'Nursing care' box. Remission is obtained in about 40% of people but may take several years to achieve. Refer to the chapter 'Nursing care of people with ventilation disorders' for care of the person having a thoracotomy and chest tubes. A tracheostomy may be required when the diaphragm or intercostal muscles are involved.

Plasmapheresis

Plasma exchange in myasthenia gravis may be used in conjunction with other therapies; for example, it may be performed prior to surgical intervention. The goal of therapy is to remove the antiacetylcholine receptor antibodies, thus improving severe

MEDICATION ADMINISTRATION The person with myasthenia gravis

ANTICHOLINESTERASES/CHOLINESTERASE INHIBITORS
Neostigmine (Prostigmin)
Ambenonium (Mytelase Caplets)
Pyridostigmine (Mestinon, Regonol)
For diagnosis: edrophonium chloride (Tensilon)

Cholinesterase inhibitors are used in myasthenia gravis to enhance the effects of acetylcholine at the remaining skeletal muscle receptors. Cholinesterase inhibitors do not cure or change the underlying pathophysiological processes, but they can provide effective, lifelong improvement of symptoms. Because the cholinesterase inhibitors are non-selective, the neuromuscular, muscarinic and ganglionic junctions are each affected.

Adjusting the dose to obtain maximum benefit with minimal side effects is a major consideration when administering cholinesterase inhibitors. Initially, small doses are given, followed by incremental increases until optimal muscle strength is obtained. The dose may need to be adjusted when activities result in symptoms of undermedication, such as increased ptosis. Severe undermedication results in myasthenic crisis. Although a sustained-release form of pyridostigmine is available for bedtime use, it should not be used during the day because of its inconsistent absorption.

Cholinesterase inhibitors should not be administered to people experiencing obstruction of the intestinal or urinary tract. Caution is advised when administering these drugs to people with asthma, hyperthyroidism, bradycardia or peptic ulcer disease. Cholinesterase inhibitors can cross the placenta; reproductive counselling is indicated.

Nursing responsibilities

- Obtain a baseline assessment of muscle strength and abilities, concentrating on swallowing and ptosis.
- Administer the medication parenterally if the person has dysphagia. Check the dose of the medication carefully when changing from oral to parenteral routes.
- Evaluate the effectiveness of the medication and document the response—for example, time when fatigue occurs in relation to activities.
- Promptly recognise and respond to manifestations of excessive stimulation of muscarinic receptors: excess salivation, urinary urgency, bradycardia, gastrointestinal hypermotility, diaphoresis. Atropine can be administered to combat these manifestations. Respiratory depression and failure can occur and require mechanical ventilation.
- Have a muscarinic antagonist (e.g. physostigmine) readily available to treat poisoning.

Health education for the person and family

- Balancing symptom control with dosage is crucial; record time of dose and response in a journal. Note the time of day when fatigued and any adverse effects, such as excess salivation, sweating, slow heartbeat and diarrhoea.
- Take the medication about 30 minutes prior to meals to enhance swallowing and chewing.
- Report manifestations of myasthenic crisis immediately: severe muscle weakness, fast heartbeat, restlessness, difficulty breathing and increasing difficulty swallowing or speaking.
- Report slow heartbeat, increased salivation or sweating, and/or decreased blood pressure immediately.
- Review possible causes of myasthenic crisis: physical or emotional stress, infection or reduction in the medication dosage.
- Wear or carry MedicAlert® identification.

NURSING CARE OF THE PERSON having a thymectomy

PREOPERATIVE CARE

- Reinforce the doctor's explanation of the procedure and prepare the person for chest tubes and tracheostomy. *Realistic preparation of what to expect postoperatively encourages compliance and allays anxiety.*
- Anticipate the need for alternative communication. *The person may have a tracheostomy; preoperative planning facilitates communication after surgery.*
- Allow sufficient time for questions. Thymectomy is a major surgery requiring either a thoracotomy and sternal split, or a transcervical approach. *The person is usually anxious and adequate time must be allocated to preoperative instruction.*

POSTOPERATIVE CARE

- Provide meticulous pulmonary hygiene: turning, deep breathing and coughing at least every 2 hours; use an incentive spirometer. *Regardless of surgical approach, measures are aimed at preventing pulmonary complications of atelectasis and pneumonia.*
- People with a thoracotomy and sternal split procedure will require care of the anterior chest tube. *Observe for complications, such as pneumothorax. Air may enter the thoracic cavity—be alert for sudden chest pain and dyspnoea, decreased breath sounds and early signs of shock, such as restlessness.*
- Manage pain with scheduled analgesic therapy. *Maintaining a therapeutic blood level of analgesic provides better pain control than waiting until the person requests medication, as on a prn basis.*

NURSING CARE OF THE PERSON having plasmapheresis

PRE-PROCEDURE CARE

- Teach about the procedure and what to expect, including what the machine looks like, the need for arterial and venous insertion sites and the length of time of the procedure (2 to 5 hours). *Giving information, answering questions and addressing concerns decrease anxiety.*
- Check with the doctor about withholding medications until after the procedure. *Medications may be removed from the body as an incidental part of the plasmapheresis process.*
- Assess vital signs and weight. *Baseline parameters are necessary to evaluate for fluid imbalances and response to therapy.*
- Assess FBC, platelet count and clotting studies. *People undergoing plasmapheresis are at high risk of anaemia and coagulation problems secondary to haemolysis of cells.*
- Check blood type and cross-match for replacement blood products. *Hypersensitivity reactions can occur and close monitoring is important.*

CARE DURING AND AFTER THE PROCEDURE

- Observe for dizziness or hypotension. *Hypovolaemia is a complication of plasma exchange, especially during the procedure when up to 15% of the person's blood volume is in the cell separator.*
- Apply pressure dressing to access site(s). *Direct pressure helps decrease or prevent bleeding.*
- Monitor for infection and bruises at the intravenous port site. *The site of vascular access is at risk of complications and must be routinely and carefully assessed for signs of infection and bleeding or haematoma formation.*
- Monitor electrolytes and signs of electrolyte loss. Report imbalances and replace electrolytes as ordered. Observe for circumoral tingling, Chvostek's and Trousseau's signs if calcium levels are low, and cardiac arrhythmias and leg cramps if potassium levels are low. *Hypocalcaemia and hypokalaemia may occur. Hypocalcaemia occurs because the anticoagulant citrate dextrose binds with calcium.*
- Re-evaluate pre-procedure laboratory data, especially FBC, platelet count and clotting times. *The cell-separating process can damage cells; anticoagulation is part of the procedure.*

muscle weakness, fatigue and other manifestations. The procedure is frequently performed when respiratory muscle involvement is evident. See the accompanying box for nursing care of the person having plasmapheresis.

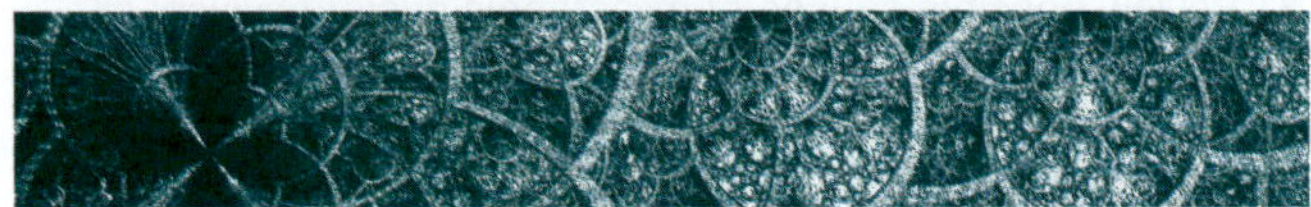

Nursing care

Because avoiding fatigue is a major part of teaching for myasthenia gravis, it is important to incorporate interventions to enhance rest and conserve energy (see Box 43.4). For example, suggest sitting while preparing meals and performing hygiene and grooming. Anticipating problems, such as impaired communication, and developing alternative solutions can be helpful in promoting independence. See the nursing care plan for the person with myasthenia gravis.

Nursing diagnoses and interventions

Nursing care of people with myasthenia gravis focuses not only on present problems but also on anticipated needs. Preventing myasthenic and cholinergic crises and providing psychological support to people and families, are two important aspects of care. Individualised care depends on the specific therapy instituted. This section discusses the nursing diagnoses related to ineffective airway clearance and impaired swallowing; other nursing diagnoses that commonly apply, such as *Fatigue*, are addressed in other sections of this chapter.

BOX 43.4 Personal and family teaching: myasthenia gravis

- **Schedule periods of rest and avoid stress; conserve energy when possible.**
- **Avoid cigarette smoke, alcohol and beverages with quinine (e.g. tonic water).**
- **Take medications as prescribed. If manifestations change, consult the doctor; the dose may need to be adjusted.**
- **Avoid extremes of temperature; an environment that is too hot or too cold may cause an exacerbation of myasthenia gravis.**
- **Avoid people with upper respiratory infections; infections can result in an exacerbation and extreme weakness.**

Ineffective airway clearance

The underlying causes of ineffective airway clearance for the person with myasthenia gravis include poor cough mechanism, decreased rib cage expansion, diminished diaphragm movement and decreased expiratory effort. The following interventions require particular attention if the person undergoes a thymectomy.

- Assist with turning, deep breathing and coughing at least every 2 hours. Teach proper coughing techniques; use an incentive spirometer every 2 hours while the person is awake. *Position changes promote lung expansion; coughing helps clear secretions from the tracheobronchial tree.*
- Place in a semi-Fowler's position. *This position expands the lungs and alleviates pressure from the diaphragm; these are especially important considerations if the person is obese.*
- Maintain hydration status and monitor for dehydration; use a humidifier as needed. If needed, teach family how to perform percussion, postural drainage and suction. *Interventions to*

NURSING CARE PLAN A person with myasthenia gravis

Kirsten Avis, a 44-year-old homemaker and mother of two teenage sons, was diagnosed with myasthenia gravis 2 years ago. She takes an anticholinesterase medication, pyridostigmine (Mestinon), four times a day. Over the past month she has been experimenting with decreasing the dose of her pyridostigmine because she has 'felt so good'. She was prescribed 60 mg of pyridostigmine three times a day before meals and one-half of a long-acting 180 mg pyridostigmine tablet at night.

Three days ago, she began having chills and fever and her myasthenic symptoms became markedly worse. Mrs Avis is easily fatigued and has been experiencing increasing weakness, bilateral ptosis and mild dysphagia in the late afternoon and evenings. She is admitted to the hospital.

ASSESSMENT

Lela Silva, RN, is caring for Mrs Avis. Physical examination of Mrs Avis reveals severe muscle weakness bilaterally in her hands, arms and thorax. Her voice is nasal and she speaks slowly; the longer she speaks, the more difficult it becomes to understand her. She is anxious and dyspnoeic. Her complaints of weakness, dysphagia, dysarthria, problems with mobility and ptosis are more pronounced later in the day. Vital signs are as follows: BP 138/88, P 88, R 28, T 39°C.

Some improvement in muscle weakness is noted following a restful night's sleep; however, the respiratory distress is more evident and Mrs Avis is increasingly restless. She is moved to the critical care unit for advanced monitoring and possible ventilatory assistance. The medical diagnosis is myasthenic crisis secondary to pulmonary infection.

DIAGNOSES

- *Impaired gas exchange* related to ineffective breathing pattern and muscle weakness, evidenced by dyspnoea, restlessness and fatigue.
- *Risk of aspiration* related to dysphagia, manifested by difficulty swallowing.
- *Fatigue* related to increased energy needs from muscular involvement, manifested by limb weakness and mobility difficulties.

PLANNING

- Management of pulmonary infection and exacerbated symptoms of myasthenia gravis.

Expected outcomes

- Pulse oximetry readings will be maintained at 92% or above.
- No aspiration will occur.
- Will verbalise decreasing fatigue when performing ADLs.
- Will state the correct method of medication dosing and demonstrate how she will maintain schedule.

IMPLEMENTATION

Mrs Avis's manifestations improve following administration of edrophonium chloride (Tensilon) to verify myasthenic crisis. She is placed on oxygen by mask and suctioned as needed; equipment for possible intubation and ventilation is made readily available. She is placed in a semi-Fowler's position and vital signs are assessed every 5 minutes during the acute exacerbation. The nurses in the critical care unit remain in constant attendance throughout the crisis period and provide explanations to Mrs Avis in an effort to decrease her stress and to avoid further severity of manifestations.

Three days after the crisis period, Mrs Avis is moved to a progressive nursing care unit. Nurses follow up on teaching her the manifestations of both myasthenic and cholinergic crises. They discuss the need to wear MedicAlert® identification and review medication administration techniques with Mrs Avis. The nurses emphasise in particular that Mrs Avis must not split time-released medications.

Within 5 days, Mrs Avis's condition stabilises and her weakness decreases sufficiently to allow discharge home. Although her temperature has returned to normal and her respiratory status has improved, she still has a productive cough. Oral antibiotics are prescribed for 2 weeks, after which she will have a follow-up visit with her GP. She is instructed to seek treatment promptly if respiratory symptoms or temperature indicate recurrence of infection.

EVALUATION

Mrs Avis is discharged without developing aspiration pneumonia or any symptoms of aspiration. Her airway was maintained throughout the myasthenic crisis and her pulse oximetry readings remained above 92% once oxygen therapy was initiated. On discharge, pulse oximetry is above 95% without oxygen therapy. Mrs Avis states that her fatigue and weakness have significantly improved.

Both Mrs Avis and her husband are able to explain the difference between myasthenic and cholinergic crises and to identify methods to avoid both problems. Mrs Avis correctly relates her proper medication regimen and makes an appointment for a follow-up visit with her doctor.

CRITICAL THINKING IN THE NURSING PROCESS

1. What is the rationale for administering Tensilon to evaluate a myasthenic crisis?
2. Develop a plan to assist Mrs Avis to avoid fatigue when preparing and eating meals.
3. Which factors contributed to Mrs Avis's diagnosis of myasthenic crisis?

REFLECTION ON THE NURSING PROCESS

1. Which communication and education strategies could you use to reduce fatigue related to the performance of ADLs and daily tasks?
2. Outline what you have learned from this case study that you will apply to your future nursing practice.

liquefy secretions, such as ensuring a daily fluid intake of up to 2,500 mL (perhaps via feeding tube or parenteral route), help the person mobilise and expectorate sputum.

- Monitor lung sounds, the rate and character of respirations and pulse oximetry readings at least every 4 hours or as indicated by the person's condition. *Frequent assessments are critical to early identification of ineffective respirations and oxygenation of tissues.*

Impaired swallowing

People with myasthenia gravis have weakness of the laryngeal and pharyngeal muscles involved with swallowing. Alterations in swallowing place the person at risk of poor nutrition as well as possible aspiration. Family members need to be included in teaching, particularly the person who prepares and assists with meals.

- Assess the ability to safely manage various consistencies of foods; consult with a speech therapist for evaluation. *People with dysphagic are at risk of aspiration; matching food consistency to the person's ability to swallow enhances safety.*
- Plan meals to promote medication effectiveness. *Pyridostigmine should be given 30 minutes before the meal to provide optimal muscle strength for swallowing and chewing.*
- Have the person eat slowly, using small bites of food. Schedule meals during periods when the person is adequately rested; develop a daily schedule incorporating rest periods. *Fatigue may add to dysphagia, putting the person at greater risk of aspiration.*
- If necessary, give cues while eating, such as 'Chew your food thoroughly; swallow.' *Keeping the person focused may enhance swallowing.*
- Teach caregivers the first aid treatment for choking and how to suction. *Knowing specific measures to take in case of aspiration decreases both the person's and the family's anxiety and promotes confidence in managing potential problems.*

Community-based care

Teaching for the person and family with myasthenia gravis focuses on prevention and recognition of crisis situations, understanding the disorder and methods for coping with both physical and psychosocial problems. Setting realistic goals with the person and family provides opportunities for self-assessment and promotes active participation in rehabilitation.

Address the following topics:

- the importance of maintaining consistency in medication dosage and management
- realistic expectations
- methods to avoid fatigue and undue stress; specific measures for avoiding upper respiratory infections and exposure to extreme heat or cold
- birth control measures or referral for counselling (Pregnancy can exacerbate manifestations; also, medications used to control myasthenia gravis, such as neostigmine bromide (Prostigmin), cross the placenta.)
- referral to support groups
- helpful resources such as:
  - Myasthenia Alliance Australia: https://myastheniaalliance.org.au
  - National Institute of Neurological Disorders and Stroke (NINDS): https://www.ninds.nih.gov.

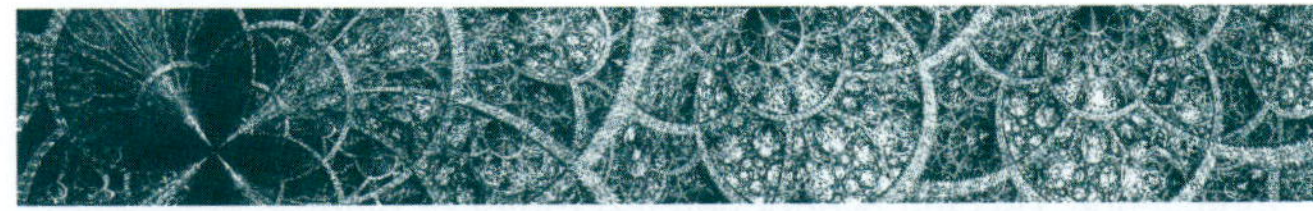

THE PERSON WITH GUILLAIN–BARRÉ SYNDROME

Guillain–Barré syndrome (GBS) is an acute inflammatory demyelinating disorder of the peripheral nervous system characterised by an acute onset of motor paralysis (usually ascending). The classification of Guillain–Barré subtypes includes acute inflammatory demyelinating polyradiculoneuropathy, acute axonal motor neuropathy and acute motor and sensory axonal neuropathy.

GBS is one of the most common peripheral nervous system disorders, affecting about 1 to 2 people per 100,000 in Australia (Guillain–Barré Syndrome Association of NSW, 2018). The cause is unknown, but precipitating events include a respiratory or gastrointestinal viral or bacterial infection 1 to 3 weeks prior to the onset of manifestations, surgery, viral immunisations and other viral illnesses. In 60% of cases, *Campylobacter jejuni* is identified as the cause of the preceding infection. Recently, the Therapeutic Goods Administration (TGA) revealed that two people in Australia died after developing GBS in cases that may be related to vaccination with AstraZeneca's COVID-19 vaccine (Tsirtsakis, 2021). Approximately 90% of people with GBS have a spontaneous recovery with little or no residual disabilities.

The disease is characterised by progressive ascending flaccid paralysis, accompanied by paraesthesias and numbness. About 20% of people have respiratory involvement to the point that ventilatory assistance is required. GBS is often a medical emergency.

Pathophysiology

The primary pathophysiological process in GBS is the destruction of myelin sheaths covering the axons of peripheral nerves. The demyelination is thought to be the result of both a humoral- and a cell-mediated immunological response. The loss of myelin results in poor conduction of nerve impulses, causing sudden muscle weakness and loss of reflex response. Other manifestations occur when nerve conduction to various muscles is interrupted. The stages of GBS and their usual manifestations are presented in Box 43.5.

Manifestations

Muscles, sensory nerves and cranial nerves are commonly affected in people with GBS. Most people experience symmetrical muscle weakness, initially in the lower extremities. The weakness and sensory loss then ascend to the upper extremities,

BOX 43.5 Stages of Guillain-Barré syndrome

I. Acute stage

- Characterised by severe and rapid weakness, especially in the lower extremities; loss of muscle strength progressing to quadriplegia and respiratory failure; decreasing deep tendon reflexes; decreasing vital capacity; paraesthesias, numbness; pain, especially nocturnal; facial muscle involvement (inability to wrinkle forehead or change expressions).
- Involvement of the autonomic nervous system manifested by bradycardia, sweating, fluctuating blood pressure (notably hypotension) which may last for 2 weeks.

II. Stabilising/plateau stage

- Occurs 2 to 3 weeks after initial onset.
- Marks the end of changes in condition; characterised by a 'levelling off' of symptoms.
- Generally, the labile autonomic functions stabilise.

III. Recovery stage

- May take from several months to 2 years.
- Marked by improvement in symptoms.
- Generally, muscle strength and function return in descending order.

torso and cranial nerves. Sensory involvement includes severe pain, paraesthesia and numbness. Cognition and level of consciousness are not affected. Facial nerve involvement results in the inability to change facial expressions and close the eyes. Muscles involved with chewing, swallowing and speaking may be affected.

Paralysis of intercostal and diaphragmatic muscles may alter respiratory function. These people require ventilatory assistance and supportive care. Involvement of the autonomic nervous system is characterised by fluctuating blood pressure, cardiac arrhythmias and tachycardia, paralytic ileus, syndrome of inappropriate antidiuretic hormone secretion and urinary retention.

The weakness usually plateaus or improves by the fourth week. Strength then improves slowly over weeks or months. Women who have had GBS are at increased risk of relapse in the first trimester of pregnancy.

INTERPROFESSIONAL CARE

Interventions during the acute phase (1 to 3 weeks) focus primarily on ensuring oxygenation via ventilatory assistance and preventing complications from immobility. Rehabilitation time to regain muscle strength and function varies; most people return to full pre-syndrome muscle function within 6 months to 2 years.

Care of the person with GBS requires a team approach. From the initial acute phase through rehabilitation, many members of the healthcare team are involved. An accurate and rapid diagnosis is needed to ensure prompt supportive treatment, particularly if there is respiratory involvement combined with widespread paralysis.

Diagnosis

Diagnosis of GBS is made after a thorough history and clinical examination. It must be differentiated from several disorders, among them influenza, heavy metal poisoning, Lyme disease and cranial haemorrhage. Diagnosis is made based on manifestations, history of a recent viral infection, elevated CSF protein levels and electromyography studies reflecting decreased nerve conduction. Although there is no specific test to diagnose this syndrome, several findings support and confirm the diagnosis.

Medications

No medications are available for the specific treatment of GBS. Other medications may be prescribed to provide support or prophylaxis or to combat concurrent problems; for example, antibiotics may be prescribed for urinary tract or respiratory infections. Morphine is commonly administered to control muscle pain. Anticoagulation therapy is usually instituted to prevent thromboembolic complications, such as deep venous thrombosis and pulmonary embolism, which are associated with prolonged bed rest. If hypotension is a problem, vasopressors are prescribed.

Surgery

Tracheostomy is performed if respiratory failure occurs. People who need ventilatory support are usually able to be weaned after 2 to 3 weeks, but the time frame varies greatly. When the person's vital capacity reaches 8 to 10 mL/kg, they may be weaned from the ventilator (Hickey, 2019). Insertion of a temporary pacemaker may be indicated for bradycardia.

Plasmapheresis

Plasma exchange has been beneficial, particularly when performed within the first 2 weeks of the syndrome's development. Antibodies are removed and immunosuppressive agents are administered concurrently. People typically have five exchanges during an 8–10-day period.

Nutrition and fluids

Nutritional support for the person who is immobilised for prolonged periods of time is crucial. Maintaining positive nitrogen balance, ensuring sufficient fluid intake and electrolyte balance and ensuring recommended kilojoule intake are goals of therapy. When swallowing problems occur, total parenteral nutrition may be indicated if feeding via a nasogastric or gastrostomy tube is ineffective.

Physiotherapy and occupational therapy

Long-term physiotherapy and occupational therapy are crucial to recovery. People with GBS usually require prolonged rehabilitation care, which begins during the acute phase and focuses on preventing complications and limiting the effects of immobility. The severe muscle atrophy and loss of muscle tone require that people relearn many functions and skills, such as walking. Compromise in respiratory function may delay physical rehabilitation; people need positive reinforcement when they make even small gains in their progress. Continued attention to pain control is essential because paraesthesia and pain can interfere with physical therapy.

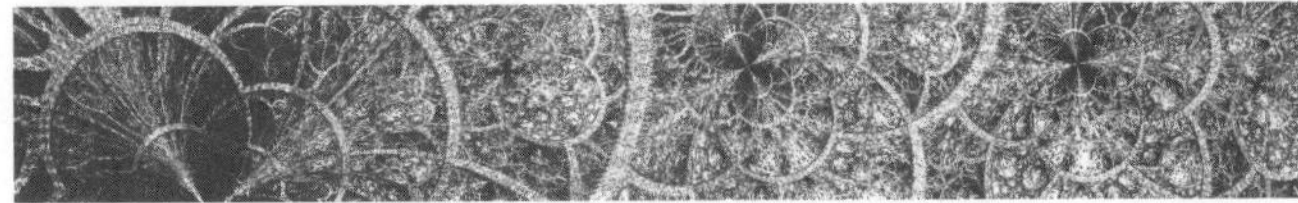

Nursing care

Many of the nursing interventions for people with Guillain–Barré syndrome involve monitoring neurological function, preventing problems of immobility, ensuring adequate hydration and nutrition and promoting respiratory function. Anticipating needs of both the person and their family is an important aspect of care. For example, developing an alternative method of communication before it is necessary may decrease anxiety. It is important that nursing care focuses on preventing complications that may be fatal by following a rigorous predetermined schedule for turning and respiratory care (e.g. coughing, deep breathing, suctioning), using strict aseptic technique and providing continuous psychosocial support.

Nursing diagnoses and interventions

Anxiety and powerlessness are major nursing considerations. The person is almost always admitted to the critical care unit for care and is mentally alert but suddenly mute, ventilator dependent and immobile. Refer to previous nursing care sections in this chapter for interventions related to anxiety, imbalanced nutrition, impaired swallowing, impaired verbal communication and ineffective airway clearance. This section focuses on the nursing diagnoses related to pain and risk of impaired skin integrity.

Acute pain

Pain experienced with GBS varies. Frequently, there is a 'stocking–glove' pattern, with pain in the hands, feet and legs. Pain and tenderness in muscles can be severe; interventions must be individualised to personal needs. The intense pain combined with altered sensations leads to anxiety; nursing interventions can make a difference in breaking the cycle of increasing pain that leads to increased anxiety and in turn causes more pain.

- Listen to the description of pain; determine presence of triggers or a pattern. *Acknowledging the person's perception of pain is a basis for treatment; listening establishes trust.*
- Use a pain scale for determining extent of pain. *Consistent measurement is essential to evaluate degree of pain and effectiveness of intervention.*
- Use complementary therapies to help manage pain:
  - application of heat/cold
  - guided imagery
  - relaxation techniques
  - massage.

  Presenting options for managing pain gives the person control over the situation and helps reduce anxiety. Non-invasive interventions may augment the therapeutic benefit of medications.
- Provide analgesics as indicated; administer on a regular schedule rather than waiting until pain becomes severe. *Anticipating and managing pain before it becomes severe decreases anxiety and averts the cycle of increased anxiety leading to increased pain.*
- Monitor for side effects of analgesics, particularly respiratory depression; assess respirations and lung sounds. Perform routine pulmonary care measures and monitor for aspiration. *People with GBS have weakened thoracic muscles; frequent respiratory monitoring is indicated.*

Risk of impaired skin integrity

During the acute and plateau stages of GBS, people are at risk of problems related to immobility and malnutrition. Impaired skin integrity is one such problem. Preventing areas of skin breakdown is important. Prophylactic interventions will help ensure that ingested protein and kilojoules are used to maintain ideal body weight and other body functions rather than to heal an avoidable problem. Implicit in interventions is maintenance of adequate nutrition.

- Inspect bony prominences and provide skin care at least every 2 hours. Reposition the person and clean, dry and lubricate the skin as needed. *These activities stimulate circulation and ensure even distribution of body weight; baseline observations allow discovery of early signs of altered integrity.*
- Pad bony prominences, such as sacral area, heels and elbows. *This decreases shearing tears on these pressure points.*
- Use an alternating-pressure mattress or water bed. *Relieving pressure stimulates circulation and promotes oxygenation of tissues.*
- Monitor for incontinence and provide thorough skin care following each episode of incontinence. *Urine is caustic to the skin and the moisture promotes skin breakdown.*

Community-based care

People and family members are frequently stunned by the rapid deterioration of function and by fear that the paralysis will be permanent. Regularly reinforce teaching because the person's high anxiety level may interfere with listening and understanding. When possible, include the person and their family in decision making; for example, seek their input when planning a daily schedule of care that incorporates various therapies.

Teaching the rationales for preventive measures reinforces the person's and family's understanding and may promote compliance during the lengthy rehabilitation. For example, because of autonomic nerve involvement, people need to be monitored for cardiac arrhythmias and taught to avoid changing position suddenly to prevent orthostatic hypotension.

Referrals to appropriate therapists are a component of anticipating needs; speech, nutritional, occupational and physical therapists are an integral part of rehabilitation. Another focus of care is teaching both the person and their family; incorporate explanations for interventions aimed at promoting self-care. For further information, refer the person and their family to the Guillain–Barré Syndrome Association in their state.

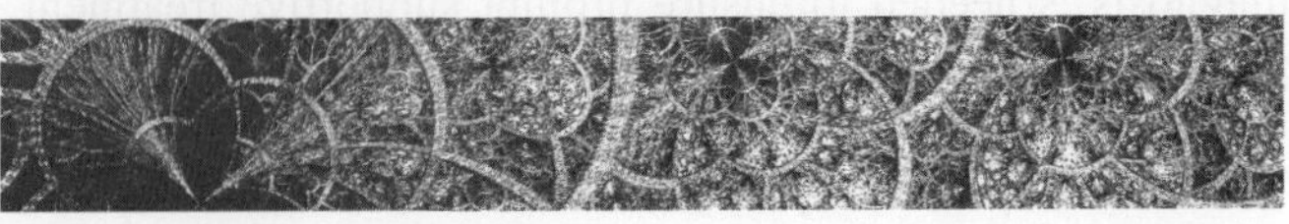

Cranial nerve disorders

Disorders of the cranial nerves may be caused by intracranial trauma or by pathological processes. The pairs of cranial nerves, described in the chapter 'A person-centred approach to assessing the nervous system', are numbered in the order in which they arise in the brain and are named according to their anatomical characteristic or primary function. The most common cranial nerve disorders are those affecting the trigeminal (cranial nerve V) and the facial (cranial nerve VII) nerves. These disorders, discussed in the following sections, result primarily in pain or loss of sensory or motor function.

THE PERSON WITH TRIGEMINAL NEURALGIA

Trigeminal neuralgia, also called *tic douloureux*, is a chronic disease of the trigeminal cranial nerve (V) that causes severe facial pain. The trigeminal nerve has three divisions: the ophthalmic, the maxillary and the mandibular (see Figure 43.6). The ophthalmic division supplies the forehead, eyes, nose, temples, meninges, paranasal sinus and part of the nasal mucosa. The maxillary division supplies the upper jaw, teeth, lip, cheeks, hard palate, maxillary sinus and part of the nasal mucosa. The mandibular division supplies the lower jaw, teeth, lip, buccal mucosa, tongue, part of the external ear and the meninges. Sensory fibres of the nerve conduct impulses for touch, pain and temperature; motor fibres innervate the temporal and masseter muscles used for chewing and lateral movement of the jaw. The maxillary and mandibular divisions are the divisions of the trigeminal nerve affected in almost all cases of this disorder.

Trigeminal neuralgia occurs more commonly in middle-aged and older adults and affects women more often than men.

Pathophysiology

The actual cause of trigeminal neuralgia is unknown; however, contributing factors include irritation from flu-like illnesses, trauma or infection of the teeth or jaw, and pressure on the nerve by an aneurysm, a tumour or arteriosclerotic changes of an artery close to the nerve (Hickey, 2019).

Stimulating specific areas of the face, called *trigger zones*, may initiate the onset of pain. These trigger zones usually parallel the distribution of the nerve and typically follow a track leading from just over the eyebrow to the ridge of the cheekbone, along the nasolabial fold, around the corner of the mouth and down the side of the chin. The episodes of pain are initiated by many factors, including light touch, eating, swallowing, talking, sneezing, shaving, chewing gum, brushing the teeth or washing the face. Other factors that may trigger a pain episode include changes in temperature and exposure to wind. In an attempt to control the pain, people may refuse to wash, shave, eat or talk.

The episodes of pain may recur for several weeks or months. The disease then spontaneously goes into remission and the person is free of pain for periods lasting from days to years. As the person grows older, the remissions tend to become shorter and a dull ache may be present between episodes of acute pain.

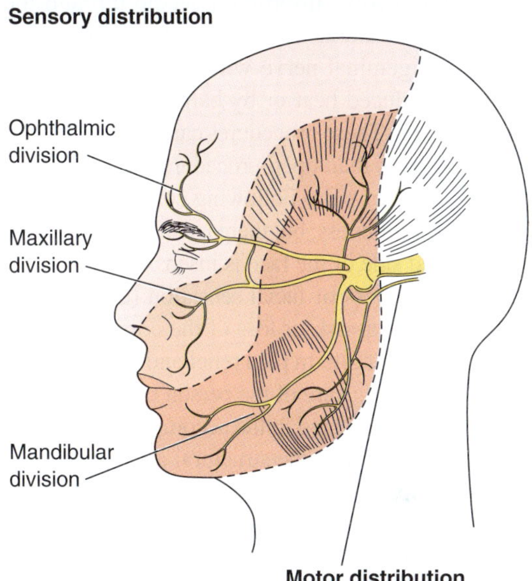

FIGURE 43.6 ***Sensory and motor distribution of the trigeminal nerve. The three sensory divisions are ophthalmic, maxillary and mandibular***

Manifestations

Trigeminal neuralgia is characterised by brief (lasting a few seconds to a few minutes), repetitive episodes of sudden severe (usually unilateral) facial pain. The pain may occur as often as hundreds of times a day to as infrequently as a few times a year. The pain is experienced over the surface of the skin. It most often begins near one side of the mouth and rises towards the ear, eye or nostril on the same side of the face. People describe the pain as stabbing or lightning-like, and often respond to the pain by wincing or grimacing.

INTERPROFESSIONAL CARE

There are no specific diagnostic tests for trigeminal neuralgia. The disorder is diagnosed by the characteristic location and type of pain. The disorder is treated by pharmacological or surgical interventions.

Medications

The drug most useful in controlling the pain is the tricyclic anticonvulsant carbamazepine (Tegretol). If carbamazepine is ineffective, other medications such as the anticonvulsants phenytoin (Dilantin) or gabapentin (Neurontin) or the skeletal muscle relaxant baclofen (Lioresal) may be used. These drugs are administered to decrease paroxysmal afferent impulses and stop the pain. Drugs in this category may cause side effects of dizziness, nausea and drowsiness. Liver function, bone marrow function and blood levels of the medications should be monitored on a regular basis.

Surgery

If medications do not control the pain, surgical procedures may be performed, including various types of *rhizotomy*—the surgical severing of a nerve root. Closed surgical interventions by percutaneous rhizotomy involve inserting a needle through the cheek into the foramen ovale at the base of the brain and partially destroying the trigeminal nerve with glycerol (an alcohol), by radiofrequency-induced heat or by balloon compression of the trigeminal ganglion. These procedures carry less risk and result in shorter hospital stays than open procedures, but there is a possibility of recurrence of pain. Following surgery, the person may have some facial numbness, but there usually is no residual paralysis. The involved side of the face is insensitive to pain. The person will have some loss of facial sensation (e.g. to temperature and/or touch) and is at risk of loss of the corneal reflex. Closed procedures provide long-term pain relief and are well tolerated by the older adult. Nursing care of the person undergoing a percutaneous rhizotomy is presented in the accompanying box.

It has been found that some structural abnormalities (such as an artery or vein compressing the nerve) may cause the neuralgia and, if so, decompression and separation of the blood vessel from the nerve root produce lasting relief of the pain (Papadakis, McPhee & Rabow, 2022). The Jannetta procedure involves locating and lifting the involved vessel and placing a small piece of silicone sponge between the vessel and the nerve. Possible complications of the procedure include headache and facial pain.

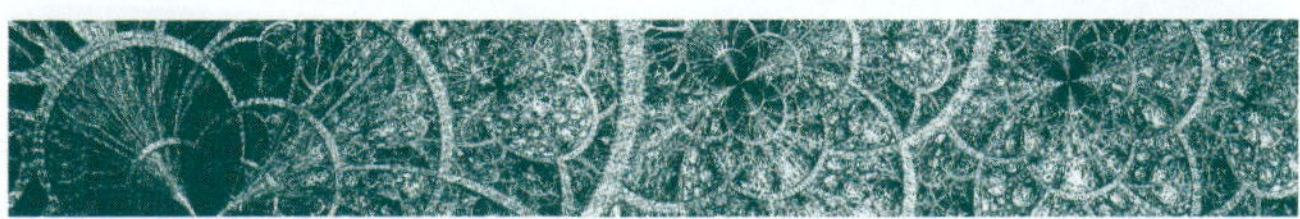

Nursing care

Nursing care for the person with trigeminal neuralgia involves teaching self-management at home after medical or surgical intervention. Primary personal concerns are managing pain, maintaining nutrition and preventing injury.

Nursing diagnoses and interventions

Interventions for managing pain and improving nutritional intake are addressed here; teaching to prevent injury following surgery is discussed in the 'Meeting individualised needs' box.

Acute pain

The person with trigeminal neuralgia has excruciating pain and often avoids ADLs and socialising with others in an attempt to prevent the onset of pain. Pain management is fully discussed in the chapter 'Nursing care of people in pain'. Nursing interventions for pain in people with this disorder focus on strategies for self-management.

- Identify factors that trigger an attack and discuss strategies to avoid these precipitating factors. *Most people can clearly identify trigger zones and triggering factors. Identification is the first step in pain control.*
- Determine usual response to pain. *Sensitivity and reaction to pain are influenced by previous experiences with pain and by age, gender, emotional factors and cultural background.*
- Assess factors that affect the ability to influence pain tolerance, including the knowledge and cause of the pain, the meaning of the pain, the ability to control the pain, cultural background and support systems. *Pain tolerance, which is the duration and intensity of pain a person is willing to endure, differs greatly between individuals and may also vary within particular people in different situations.*
- Monitor the effects of the medication prescribed for the neuralgia. *If the prescribed medication does not provide relief, other medications or methods of treatment may be used to control the pain.*

Risk of altered nutrition: less than body requirements

People often refuse to eat during periods of pain attacks, fearing that the movements of chewing may precipitate the pain. In addition, the chronic nature of the illness often causes depression, which may depress the appetite.

NURSING CARE OF THE PERSON having a percutaneous rhizotomy

POSTOPERATIVE CARE

- Follow routine postoperative interventions for people having surgery(see the chapter 'Nursing care of people having surgery').
- Monitor cranial nerve function every 2 to 4 hours:
  a. Assess the corneal reflex by lightly touching the cornea with a gauze square. If the reflex is intact, the person will blink. *Severing the ophthalmic division of the trigeminal nerve destroys the corneal reflex and leaves the cornea at risk of dryness and injury.*
  b. Assess the facial nerve by asking the person to blow out the cheeks, wrinkle the forehead, frown, wink and close both eyes tightly. Test taste by placing bitter, salty and sweet substances on the anterior portion of the tongue. *Facial weakness is evidenced by changes in movement in the involved side of the face. The facial nerve also innervates the anterior two-thirds of the tongue.*
  c. Assess the function of the oculomotor muscles by asking the person to follow your finger through the cardinal positions of vision (see the chapter 'A person-centred approach to assessing the eye and ear'). *The eyes should move together; alterations in movement indicate an abnormal response.*
  d. Assess the motor portion of the trigeminal nerve by asking the person to clench the teeth while you palpate the tightness of the contracted masseter and temporal muscles. *Loss of motor function is indicated by loss of bulk and tightness of these muscles.*
  e. Apply as prescribed an ice pack to the jaw on the operative site. *Cold decreases bleeding and swelling.*
  f. Teach the person to avoid rubbing the eye on the involved side. *Loss of the corneal reflex removes protection because the person no longer has the sensation of pain in the involved eye. Rubbing the eye could cause corneal abrasions.*

MEETING INDIVIDUALISED NEEDS **Teaching for home care of trigeminal neuralgia**

EYE CARE

- Do not rub the eyes; use artificial tears four times a day if the eyes are dry or irritated.
- Wear an eye patch at night.
- Wear protective sunglasses or goggles when outside, working in dusty areas, mowing the lawn and using any type of spray material (e.g. hair spray, cleaning materials, paint, insecticides).
- Remember to blink frequently.
- Check your eyes for redness or swelling each day.
- Schedule regular eye examinations.

FACE AND MOUTH CARE

- Chew on the unaffected side of the mouth.
- Avoid eating hot foods or drinking hot liquids.
- After every meal, brush your teeth and inspect the inside of your mouth for food that may collect between the gums and cheek.
- Have regular dental examinations; you will not be able to feel pain associated with gum infection or tooth decay.
- Use an electric razor to shave the face.
- Protect your face from very cold or windy conditions.

- Monitor dietary intake and weight at each visit and ask the person to keep a weekly weight record. *Ongoing assessments are necessary for early detection of nutritional deficiencies.*
- Discuss the temperature and consistency of foods eaten and suggest referral to a dietitian if necessary. *Hot or cold foods may trigger an attack; soft, warm or cool foods are less likely to act as triggers.*
- Suggest chewing on the unaffected side of the mouth. *Chewing on the unaffected side is less likely to trigger an attack of pain and so facilitate food intake.*
- If unable to tolerate oral food, tube feedings may be necessary. *Adequate kilojoules and nutrients for metabolic processes are essential.*

Community-based care

The person with trigeminal neuralgia who is receiving medical treatment and providing self-care at home requires teaching about the disease process, medication(s) being taken and ways to reduce the incidence of attacks or pain. Diet teaching and assistance with self-management of pain are also important. For example, if the home setting is draughty and attacks of pain are triggered by wind blowing across the face, it may be necessary to encourage the person to put weather stripping around windows and doors. To prevent injury to affected areas, the topics in the 'Meeting individualised needs: teaching for home care of trigeminal neuralgia' box should be addressed.

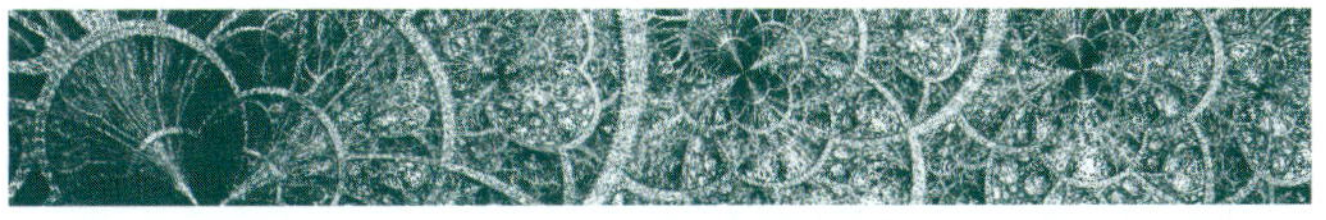

THE PERSON WITH BELL'S PALSY

Bell's palsy, also called *facial paralysis*, is a disorder of the seventh cranial (facial) nerve, characterised by unilateral paralysis of the facial muscles. The facial nerve is primarily a motor nerve that supplies all the muscles associated with expression on one side of the face. The sensory component innervates the anterior two-thirds of one side of the tongue.

This disorder can occur at any age but is seen most often in people aged between 15 and 60. The incidence is equal in men and women. The majority of people recover completely within 2 weeks to 6 months, and most recover without any treatment. Of those remaining, many recover some function but have some permanent facial paralysis; these people are usually older, have diabetes mellitus or have more severe manifestations, such as vertigo, a sensitivity to noise and deep head pain (NINDS, 2022c).

Pathophysiology

The exact cause of the disorder is unknown, although inflammation of the nerve and a relationship to the herpes simplex virus have been suggested (Papadakis et al., 2022).

Manifestations

The onset of Bell's palsy is usually sudden and almost always involves one side of the face. Pain behind the ear or along the jaw may precede the paralysis. The person initially notices numbness or stiffness of one side of the face that distorts the appearance. As the disease progresses, the distortion becomes more obvious and the face appears asymmetrical. The facial paralysis causes the entire side of the face to droop and the person cannot wrinkle the forehead, close the eye or pucker the lips on the affected side (see Figure 43.7). When the person attempts to smile, the lower facial muscles are pulled to the opposite side of the face. Some people have only mild manifestations, whereas others have complete facial paralysis. People often believe they have had a stroke. Manifestations of Bell's palsy are listed in the 'Manifestations' box.

MANIFESTATIONS **Bell's palsy**

- Paralysis of the facial muscles on one side of the face
- Paralysis of the upper eyelid with loss of the corneal reflex on the affected side
- Loss or impairment of taste over the anterior portion of the tongue on the affected side
- Increased tearing from the lacrimal gland on the affected side

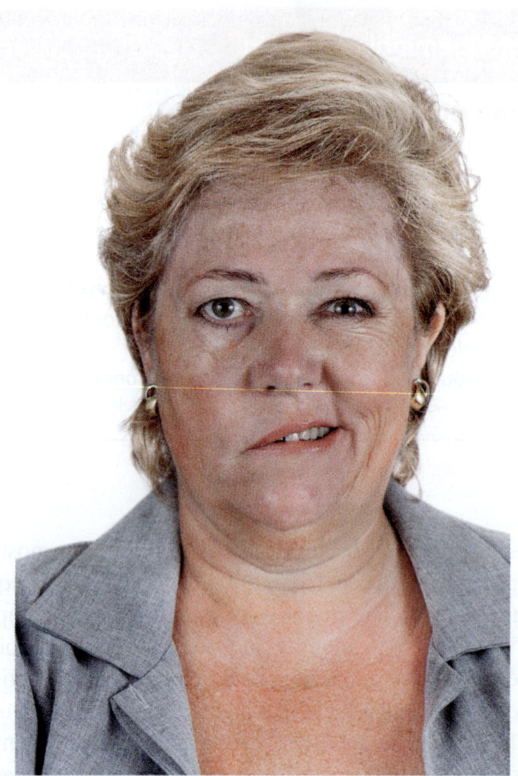

FIGURE 43.7 ***The person with Bell's palsy shows the typical drooping of one side of the face***

Source: Jo Ann Snover/Shutterstock.

INTERPROFESSIONAL CARE

There are no definitive laboratory or diagnostic tests for Bell's palsy, nor are there any specific treatments. Treatment includes medications and physiotherapy. Antiviral drugs such as aciclovir combined with an anti-inflammatory drug such as prednisone may be effective by limiting damage to the nerve. Physiotherapy to stimulate the facial nerve and help maintain muscle tone may help prevent permanent contractures before recovery takes place. Moist heat applied to the affected side of the face may decrease pain.

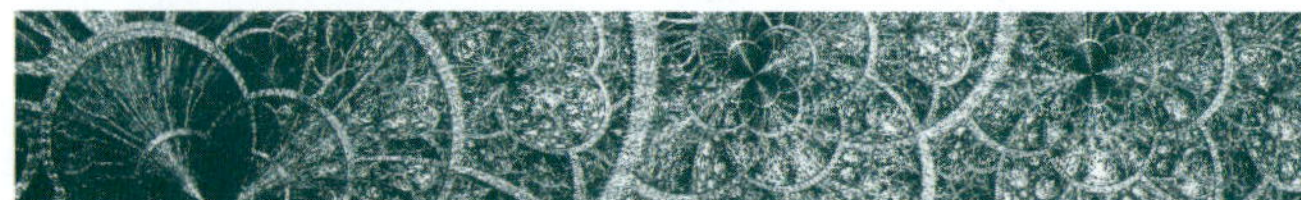

Nursing care

Although people provide self-care at home, the nurse plays a key role in teaching the person and their family about Bell's palsy and how to prevent injury and maintain nutrition. The person is often anxious about their appearance and may require counselling if any deficits in facial expression become permanent. The following topics should be addressed:

- Use artificial tears four times a day to lubricate the eye; wear an eye patch or tape the eye shut at night. Wear sunglasses or goggles when outside, working in dusty conditions and using any type of spray.
- Massage combined with warm, moist heat often is effective in relieving the pain.
- A soft diet that does not require chewing and six small meals a day are helpful. Chew slowly on the unaffected side and avoid hot foods. Clean the mouth and carefully inspect the area between the gums and cheek for food after each meal.
- As function returns, practise wrinkling the forehead, closing the eyes, blowing air out of the puckered mouth and whistling for 5 minutes three or four times a day.

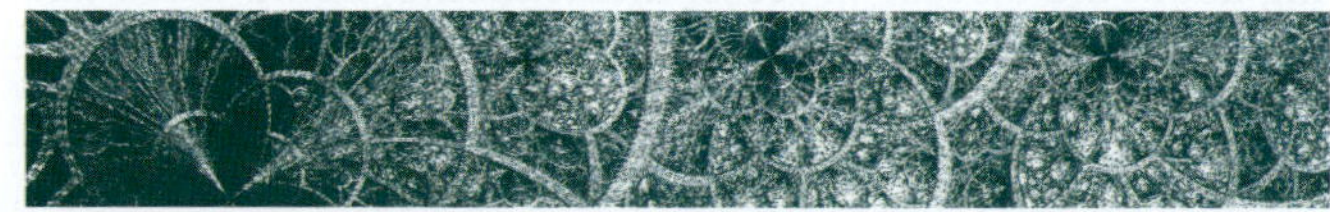

Disorders resulting from infections and neurotoxins

A variety of disorders of the nervous system may have infectious or toxic causes. Although these disorders are not common, those included here require significant nursing care when they do occur.

THE PERSON WITH CREUTZFELDT–JAKOB DISEASE

Creutzfeldt–Jakob disease (CJD) (also called *spongiform encephalopathy*) is a rapidly progressive, degenerative, neurological disease that causes brain degeneration without inflammation. The disease is transmissible and progressively fatal. The causative agent is believed to be an abnormal form of a cellular glycoprotein known as the prion protein. Transmission of the agent is by direct contamination with infected neural tissue, such as during eye and brain surgery. The injection of contaminated human growth hormone from cadaveric pituitaries has also been implicated.

A different form of the disease, called *variant CJD (vCJD)* is also a rare, degenerative, fatal brain disorder, but is not the same as the classic form of CJD. New variant CJD, referred to as 'mad cow disease', is believed to result from consumption of cattle products contaminated with bovine spongiform encephalopathy (BSE). This form primarily affects young adults. Because the illness is fatal and is associated with infected cattle, severe restrictions have been placed on the importation of cattle, sheep and goats, and on products from these animals, from countries in which BSE is known to exist.

Both forms of CJD occur worldwide, but clusters occur in several areas, more often in England, Chile and Italy. The incidence is approximately one case per 1 million Australians every year (NSW Health, 2019). Classic CJD affects adults over the age of 50; vCJD affects younger adults. The median age of death for people with classic CJD is 68 years. In contrast, the median age of death with vCJD is 28 years. No cases of vCJD have been identified in Australia to date. Australian cattle remain free of BSE (NSW Health, 2019).

Pathophysiology

Creutzfeldt–Jakob disease is characterised by degeneration of the grey matter of the brain. The spongiform degeneration (involving the formation of tiny holes and resembling a sponge) produces severe dementia, myoclonus (muscle contractions) and characteristic changes in brain waves. On autopsy or biopsy of brain tissue, the brain shows loss of neurons and a proliferation of astrocytes (indicating destruction of nearby neurons).

Manifestations

The disease has characteristic stages and manifestations. The onset is characterised by memory changes, an exaggerated startle reflex, sleep disturbances and nervousness. The person then experiences rapid deterioration in motor, sensory and language function. Tremors, hyperreflexia, rigidity and a positive Babinski reflex are often present, and confusion progresses to dementia in almost all cases. People in the terminal state are comatose and exhibit decorticate and decerebrate posturing. The median duration of illness for CJD is 4 to 5 months and the median duration of illness for vCJD is 13 to 14 months, although the vast majority of CJD patients usually die within 1 year of illness onset (Centers for Disease Control and Prevention, 2022).

INTERPROFESSIONAL CARE

No specific treatment is available to stop or slow the progression of CJD. Collaborative interventions focus on the disease's manifestations. The disease is diagnosed by a thorough neurological examination, specific EEG changes and a CT scan. However, the final diagnosis of CJD can be made only by postmortem examination. It is often difficult to differentiate this disease from Alzheimer's disease, especially in the early stages.

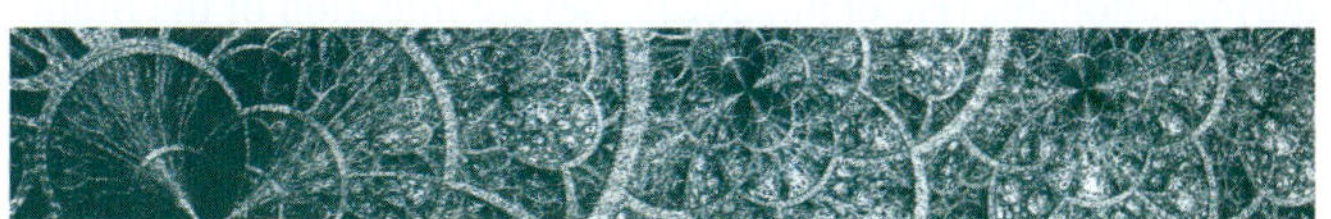

Nursing care

The nurse may identify the manifestations of CJD when conducting a health history and total physical assessment. Include questions about familial history, cultural and geographical risk, and high-risk occupations or procedures in the history. Assessment of mental function, reflexes and cranial nerve function may provide information to assist in diagnosis.

Nursing care focuses on maximising comfort, preventing injury, preventing transmission and providing support. The following guidelines are useful in designing the plan of care:

- Although comfort is difficult to assess in people with impaired cognitive function, interventions that provide a quiet environment and analgesia are important.
- Communication is essential, even if the person is unable to respond.
- Institute seizure precautions and pad side rails.
- Provide skin care, changes in position and pressure-relief mattresses to decrease the risk of pressure ulcers, venous stasis and pneumonia.
- Use standard precautions for blood and body fluids when providing care. Disinfect surfaces with a solution of 5% bleach. Sterilise contaminated equipment by autoclave or soak in 5% bleach solution for 1 hour. Label all specimens as biohazardous. Teach staff members and family members guidelines for care, including careful handwashing. However, it is not necessary to place the person in isolation.
- Provide time for family members to verbalise grief and loss, which may be manifested as anger and frustration with the healthcare system.
- Provide information to family members about all procedures and the plan of care.
- Refer family members to sources of support, such as social services and the appropriate clergy.

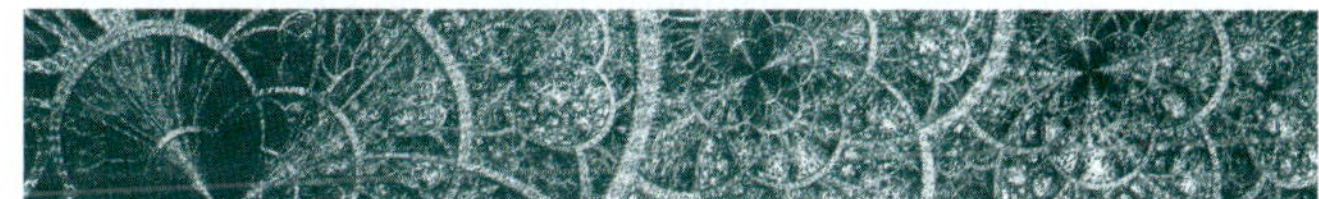

THE PERSON WITH POSTPOLIOMYELITIS SYNDROME

Postpoliomyelitis syndrome is a complication of a previous infection by the poliomyelitis virus. Polio (also called *poliomyelitis* or *infantile paralysis*) is a viral infection that was common in the Western world until the early 1960s. Most cases of polio developed only mild symptoms but others were more severe and progressed to a paralytic form. In Australia, there were major polio epidemics in the late 1930s, early 1940s and the 1950s. The last epidemic was in 1956. Polio vaccines were introduced in Australia in 1956 (Salk) and 1966 (Sabin) and were followed by mass immunisation programs. With the continuing immunisation of children, the disease was all but eradicated in Australia as well as in other parts of the Western world (Polio NSW, 2022). Although, in the wake of antivaccination propaganda following COVID-19, it may be re-emerging (NPR, 2022). It is estimated that a minimum of 20,000 to 40,000 people had paralytic polio in Australia between the 1930s and the 1960s. Actual figures for the number of people infected with the virus are up to a hundred times greater: 2 million to 4 million Australians. Polio no longer threatens Australian society; however, it is not forgotten (Polio NSW, 2022).

People with polio have struggled for years to rehabilitate themselves and lead productive lives. Now, as they reach retirement age, they are again experiencing manifestations which may be physically and psychologically incapacitating.

The poliomyelitis virus destroys some of the motor cells of the anterior horn cells of the spinal cord, causing neuromuscular effects that range from mild to severe flaccid paralysis and atrophy. The primary cause of death is respiratory arrest (Papadakis et al., 2022).

Manifestations of motor neuron degeneration and weakness may emerge 10 to 40 years after the initial infection. Most people with postpoliomyelitis syndrome initially had a more severe case of polio and required hospitalisation, contracted the disease after the age of 10, required ventilator assistance for respiration and had paralysis in all four extremities. The incidence is slightly higher in women. As the population ages, it is projected that the number of older adults with postpoliomyelitis syndrome will increase.

Pathophysiology

The pathophysiological process in postpoliomyelitis syndrome is not known.

Manifestations

The manifestations of postpoliomyelitis syndrome include fatigue, muscle and joint weakness, loss of muscle mass, respiratory difficulties and pain. The manifestations are most often seen in muscles affected by the initial infection, but new muscle groups may also be affected. In addition to neuromuscular manifestations, the person may experience cold intolerance, dizziness, headaches, urinary incontinence and sleep disorders.

INTERPROFESSIONAL CARE

Postpoliomyelitis syndrome is diagnosed by a previous history of polio and the current manifestations. Diagnostic studies of nerve conduction, muscle strength and pulmonary function determine current physical status. Treatment addresses the manifestations and often involves physical physiotherapy and pulmonary rehabilitation programs.

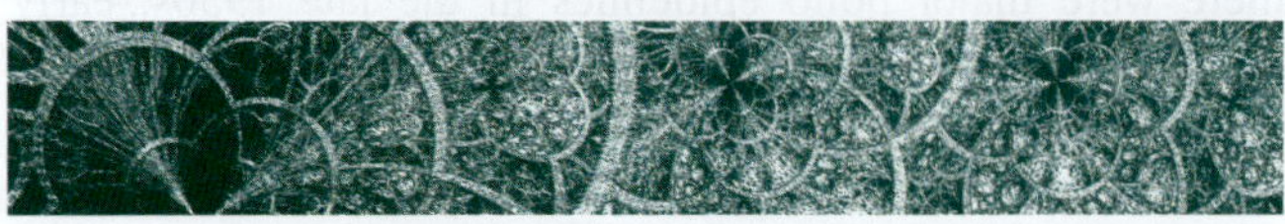

Nursing care

The person with postpoliomyelitis syndrome faces the challenge of unexpected physical changes. People are often anxious about how others will react or what the future holds. Respiratory dysfunction may result in the need for oxygen. Muscular weakness and decreased pulmonary function may make walking difficult, if not impossible. ADLs, independent self-care and careers are threatened.

Many people have not fully recovered psychologically from having polio and may respond to a recurrence of manifestations with denial and disbelief. Older people may not know they had polio as children. Nurses are responsible for assessing and identifying the manifestations of postpoliomyelitis syndrome. It is essential to question middle to older adults about a past history of polio when conducting the health history and to ask specific questions about manifestations the person may be experiencing.

The nurse individualises teaching to meet the physical and psychosocial needs of the person and their family. The nurse should provide candid explanations and teach the person how to prevent fatigue, promote optimal respiratory function, meet self-care needs, modify ADLs and maintain safety. Follow-up care with nurses, doctors, physiotherapists, respiratory therapists and counsellors is indicated. Referral to a support group can make a positive difference in the person's and family's ability to cope with the disorder.

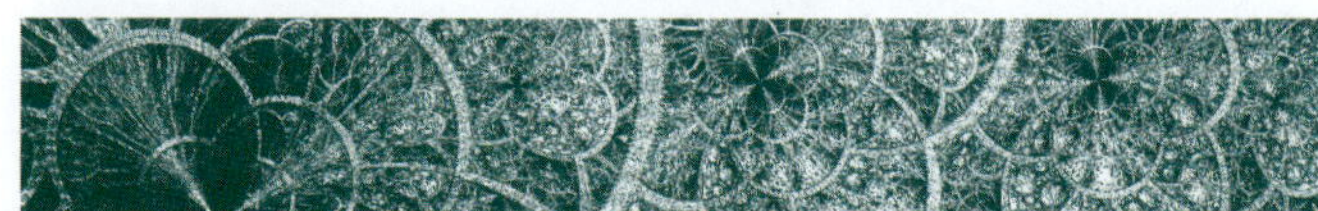

THE PERSON WITH COVID-19

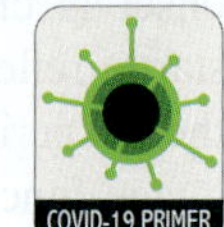

Nervous system consequences of COVID-19

Severe acute respiratory syndrome coronavirus 2 (SARS-CoV-12), or **COVID-19**, and its variants are a common cause of usually mild to moderate upper respiratory tract infection or illness with a range of symptoms. The condition can also present with a range of neurological complications including confusion, stroke and neuromuscular disorders (Spudich & Nath, 2022), as well as other conditions such as impaired concentration, headache, sensory disturbances, nausea and vomiting (He et al., 2021). Depression and even psychosis may remain for months after the infection as part of a constellation of symptoms called *long COVID* (Spudich & Nath, 2022). (See the COVID-19 Primer.)

Pathophysiology

Novel coronaviruses have the potential to be neuroinvasive and can cause adverse effects to neurological function. The novel coronavirus can enter the CNS via haematogenous or retrograde neuronal pathways or, in severe cases, via the olfactory nerve in the nasal cavity (Kissler et al., 2020). Researchers have found evidence of the virus in cerebrospinal fluids and brain tissue during autopsies (He et al., 2021). Severe infection of the brainstem with COVID-19 has been reported in the brains of both human patients and experimental animals. Coronaviruses have viral synapses similar to neuronal synapses and these contribute to rapid infection and the escape of viruses to the nerves (Desforges et al., 2019). Therefore, COVID-19 has the potential for direct nerve infection, retention, cross-neuronal transmission and latency. This means that even when the host has been treated and has recovered from an acute infection, the virus may remain in the neurons for a long time, suggesting that viruses from previously infected neurons can persist (Wu et al., 2020).

Manifestations

Human COVID-19 sufferers show clinical manifestations that include myalgia and fatigue (He et al., 2021). Asadi-Pooya and Simani (2020) suggested that 25% of people with COVID-19 infections (especially with a severe infection) develop CNS manifestations. Mao et al. (2020) analysed data from 214 laboratory-confirmed COVID-19 patients and observed neurological clinical manifestations in 78 of them (approximately 37%). Most showed CNS symptoms including vertigo, headache, impaired consciousness, irritability, delirium, psychosis, acute cerebrovascular disease, stroke, ataxia, encephalitis and epilepsy. A minority displayed peripheral nervous system (PNS) symptoms including taste disturbance, olfactory disturbance, visual disturbance and neuralgia. Following an acute infection with COVID-19, long-term symptoms included fatigue, muscle weakness, sleep difficulties, anxiety and depression (Cheng et al., 2020). Other data suggests that Kawasaki syndrome has also been reported in patients with COVID-19 (Divani et al., 2020). Therefore, neurological manifestation should be monitored in patients with (particularly) severe COVID-19 infections.

INTERPROFESSIONAL CARE

Data on the incidence of COVID-19 infection and its impact on the neurological system and neurological manifestations have not been fully studied (He et al., 2021). However, it is clear from recent information that people with COVID-19 and corresponding neurological involvement have a poor prognosis and medical and nursing teams should pay close attention to neurological manifestations (Ahmed et al., 2020) in order to initiate rapid interventions.

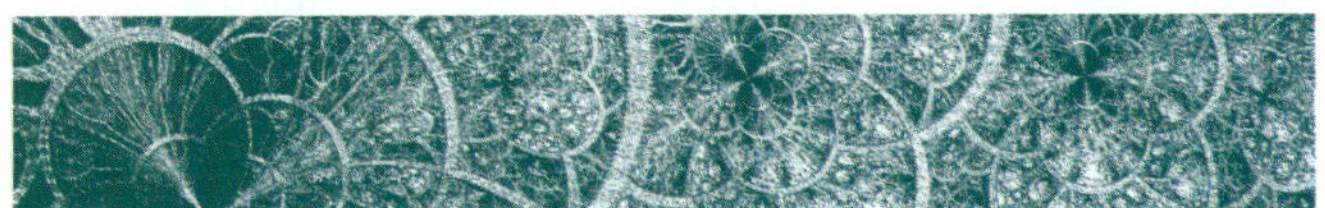

Nursing care

Nursing care will depend on the clinical manifestations evident and on the stage of infection. The first stage of care involves recognition of and understanding the potential range of neurological disorders associated with COVID-19 infection or long COVID. Patients should be reassured and provided with care for acute respiratory support and relevant medication therapy. It should be noted that many patients requiring neurological care have comorbidities that increase their risk of developing severe COVID-19 disease or more serious complications (Zubair et al., 2020). People with pre-existing neurological conditions such as multiple sclerosis, neuromuscular disorders and epilepsy may have increased risk of developing severe COVID-19 illness (Zubair et al., 2020).

Health promotion

Personal and family teaching should focus on the additional risks of the impact of COVID-19 for people with pre-existing neurological conditions, when to seek immediate medical attention and how to avoid contracting COVID-19 with up-to-date vaccination (if possible), social distancing, the use of face masks in public spaces and excellent personal hygiene and hand hygiene.

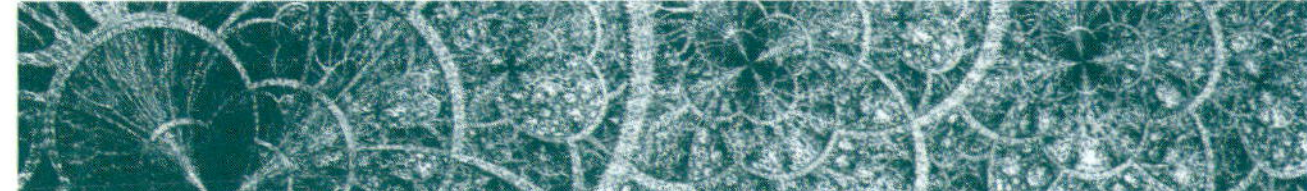

THE PERSON WITH RABIES

Rabies is a rhabdovirus infection of the central nervous system transmitted by infected saliva that enters the human body through a bite or an open wound. It is a fatal viral encephalitis that causes tens of thousands of deaths worldwide each year, with more than 15 million people worldwide receiving post-exposure vaccination. Rabies is estimated to cause 59,000 human deaths annually in over 150 countries, with 95% of cases occurring in Africa and Asia. Due to underreporting and uncertain estimates, this number is likely a gross underestimate. The burden of disease is disproportionally borne by rural poor populations, with approximately half of cases attributable to children under 15 years of age (World Health Organization (WHO), 2021).

Rabies does not currently occur in Australia, but a rabies-like virus, called the lyssavirus (which is lethal to humans), is carried by Australian animals such as bats and flying foxes; therefore, understanding the effects remains important to Australians. Australian health authorities suggest lyssavirus poses a low public health risk. However, they strongly recommend that anyone scratched or bitten by a bat should immediately wash the affected area with soap and water and contact their local doctor (CSIRO, 2021).

Rabies is a critical illness that almost always causes death if untreated. The rabies virus is carried by both wild and domestic animals, including bats, skunks, foxes, raccoons, cats and dogs. Dogs make up the largest single vector across the world (WHO, 2021). After an incubation period that may last from 10 days to many years (the norm is 3 to 7 weeks), the virus travels to the brain of the infected animal via the nerves. It multiplies and migrates to the salivary glands.

Pathophysiology

The person with rabies usually has a history of an animal bite but may also become infected through an abrasion or open wound that is exposed to the infected saliva. The virus spreads from the wound to local muscle cells and then invades the peripheral nerves. It eventually travels to the central nervous system. The incubation period in humans varies according to the severity and location of the bite. For example, bites on the face may result in manifestations in 10 days to a few weeks, whereas bites on the lower extremities may incubate for as long as 1 year.

Manifestations

The manifestations occur in stages. During the initial—or prodromal—stage, the site of the wound is painful and then exhibits various paraesthesias. The infected person is anxious, irritable and depressed. General manifestations of infection (such as headache, loss of appetite and sore throat) may appear. The person may also have increased sensitivity to light and sounds, and the skin is especially sensitive to changes in temperature.

The prodromal stage is followed by an excitement stage. The infected person has periods of excitement that alternate with periods of quiet. Attempts to drink cause such painful laryngospasms that the person refuses to drink (a phenomenon called *hydrophobia*). Large amounts of thick, tenacious mucus are present. The person experiences convulsions, muscle spasms and periods of apnoea. If untreated, death occurs approximately 7 days from the onset of manifestations and is usually due to respiratory failure.

INTERPROFESSIONAL CARE

Sick animals should be euthanised and their brains examined for presence of the rabies virus, which is detected by fluorescent antibody testing. The blood of an infected person can also be tested with the same diagnostic study to demonstrate the presence of rabies antibodies.

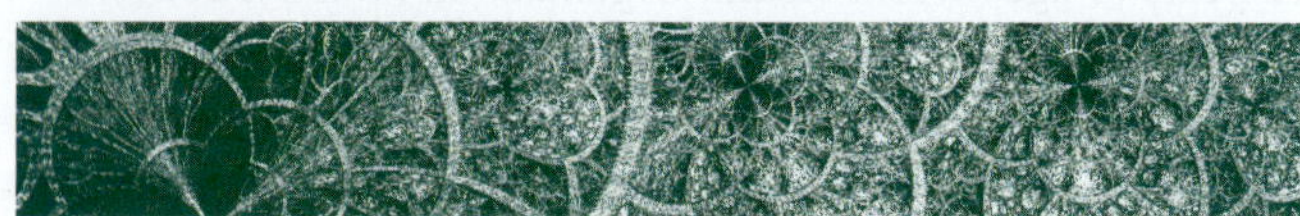

Nursing care

Nursing care for people with rabies is provided in a critical care unit, with the person in a quiet, darkened room to decrease stimulation as much as possible. The person requires interventions to maintain the airway, maintain oxygenation and control seizures. Standard precautions are essential, because the rabies virus is present in the saliva of the person. If an open wound of a healthcare provider is contaminated with infected saliva, the provider must receive post-exposure immunisations.

Health promotion

Personal and family teaching focuses on the importance of providing proper care of wounds, seeking immediate medical attention for animal bites and obtaining treatment after any suspicious bite.

Because the untreated disease is almost always fatal, the best intervention is prevention. Preventive activities include:

- Immunisation of those at risk of injury from bats (i.e. bat handlers, vets and wildlife officers).
- Local treatment of animal bites and scratches:
  - Carefully and thoroughly clean and flush wounds with soap and water to remove the saliva and dilute the viral exposure.
  - Immediately take the person with the bite for emergency treatment.
- Post-exposure care: post-exposure prophylaxis (PEP) is the immediate treatment of a bite victim after rabies exposure. This prevents virus entry into the central nervous system, which results in imminent death. PEP consists of:
  - Extensive washing and local treatment of the bite wound or scratch as soon as possible after a suspected exposure (WHO, 2021).
  - Human rabies immunoglobulin (RIG) is administered for passive immunisation. A dose of 20 units/kg of the immunoglobulin is infiltrated around the wound and the rest is administered intramuscularly. At the same time, an inactivated human diploid cell vaccine (HDCV) is administered intramuscularly, with 1 mL given on the day of exposure and on days 3, 7, 14 and 28 after exposure (WHO, 2021).
  - HRIG and HDCV should never be given in the same syringe or at the same site. Local and mild systemic reactions include itching, tenderness, headaches, muscle aches and nausea.
  - If RIG is not available, equine rabies antiserum may be administered after testing the person for horse serum sensitivity.

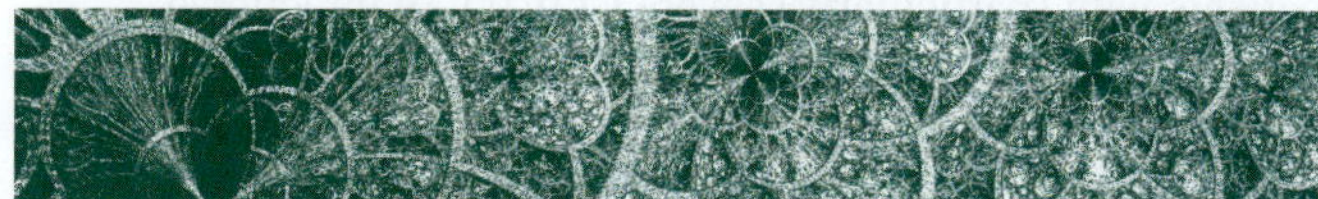

THE PERSON WITH TETANUS

Tetanus is a disorder of the nervous system caused by a neurotoxin elaborated by *Clostridium tetani*. This anaerobic bacillus lives in the soil. Spores of the bacillus enter the body through open wounds contaminated with dirt, street dust or faeces (animal or human). The wounds may result from punctures, scratches or abrasions, bee stings, abortions, surgery, trauma, burns or intravenous drug use. Incidence is highest in people who have never been immunised, the very young who are not fully immunised and older adults whose immunity has been lost. Tetanus causes severe muscle spasms, especially in the neck and jaw (called *lockjaw*). Tetanus has a high mortality rate, with around 1 in 10 people who contract the disease dying from it (Department of Health and Aged Care, 2022). Contaminated lesions of the head and face are more dangerous than those in other parts of the body.

Pathophysiology

When the spores of *C. tetani* enter the open wound, they germinate and produce a toxin called tetanospasmin. The incubation period averages 8 to 12 days but can range from 5 days to 15 weeks (Papadakis et al., 2022). The toxins are absorbed by the peripheral nerves and carried to the spinal cord, where they block the action of inhibitory enzymes at spinal synapses and interfere with transmission of neuromuscular impulses. As a result, even minor stimuli cause uncontrolled muscle spasms.

Manifestations

The manifestations begin with pain at the site of the infection. The infected person has stiffness of the jaw and neck, and dysphagia. There is often profuse perspiration and drooling from increased salivation. As the infection progresses, the person experiences hyperreflexia, spasms of the jaw muscles (*trismus*) or facial muscles, and rigidity and spasms of the abdominal, neck and back muscles. Generalised tonic seizures are caused by even minor stimuli and the person assumes a typical opisthotonic position during the seizures: the head is retracted, the back is arched and the feet are extended. The muscle spasms are painful. The person may be unable to breathe from spasms of the glottis and respiratory muscles. Despite these physical effects, the person has no change in mental status.

The complications of tetanus include urinary retention and airway obstruction from the spasms. Cardiac and respiratory failure are late, life-threatening complications.

INTERPROFESSIONAL CARE

There are no specific diagnostic tests for tetanus; diagnosis is based on manifestations. Tetanus is completely preventable by active immunisation. Immunisation for children includes tetanus toxoid, administered as part of the diphtheria-pertussis-tetanus (DPT) immunisation series. In adults, immunisation is obtained by administering tetanus toxoid as two doses 4 to 6 weeks apart, with a third dose in 6 to 12 months. All individuals should have a booster dose every 10 years throughout life or at the time of a major injury if the last booster dose was given more than 5 years prior to the injury.

If a wound is contaminated, or if the person's immunisation status is uncertain, passive immunisation with tetanus immune globulin is administered. Active immunisation with tetanus toxoid is begun at the same time. The wound is carefully and thoroughly debrided and antibiotics are administered.

The person with tetanus requires intensive care in an area of minimal stimulation. Penicillin is administered to help destroy the toxin-producing organism. Muscle spasms and seizures are controlled by chlorpromazine (Largactil) or diazepam (Valium), often combined with a sedative. Anticoagulants may be prescribed to prevent venous thrombosis. In severe cases, seizures and spasms are controlled with paralysis by a curare-like medication and airway obstruction is managed by mechanical ventilation.

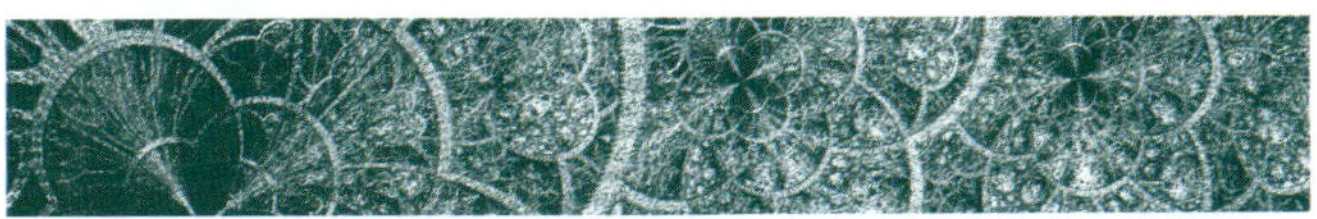

Nursing care

Nursing care for the person with tetanus is intensive and focuses on assessments and interventions to promote safety, prevent injury, maintain nutrition and maintain pulmonary and cardiovascular function. The person usually requires in-hospital care for 2 to 5 weeks. The nursing care plan commonly includes the following:

- Place in a quiet, darkened room to decrease stimuli that cause muscle spasms and seizures.
- Provide only necessary physical care and do so during periods of maximal sedation to decrease tactile stimulation that causes muscle spasms.
- Maintain oxygenation through mechanical ventilator and frequent suctioning of secretions.
- Maintain intravenous access for the administration of fluids and medications.
- Administer prescribed antibiotics, anticonvulsants and sedatives. In the case of cardiovascular complications, administer prescribed beta-adrenergic blocking agents such as propranolol (Inderal).
- Provide adequate nutrition through prescribed nutritional support, such as total parenteral nutrition.
- Monitor respiratory and cardiovascular status and provide immediate interventions for respiratory or cardiovascular failure.
- Monitor fluid and electrolyte status. Ensure adequate fluid intake to maintain hydration and urinary output.
- Monitor urinary output, which should be maintained at 1.5 to 2 L per day.
- Monitor for the hazards of immobility, including constipation, pneumonia, deep venous thrombosis and pressure ulcers.

Health promotion

Tetanus is a preventable disorder and nurses have a major role in promoting immunisations for all children and for educating adults about the need for booster doses. The older population is especially at risk of never having been immunised or for letting immunisations lapse. Information for this age group can be provided through activities such as community health fairs and programs at senior citizen groups.

It is also necessary to teach the proper care of wounds. All wounds, no matter how small, should be thoroughly washed with soap and water. All foreign material should be carefully flushed out or removed from a wound and medical care should be sought for wounds that are more extensive or contaminated.

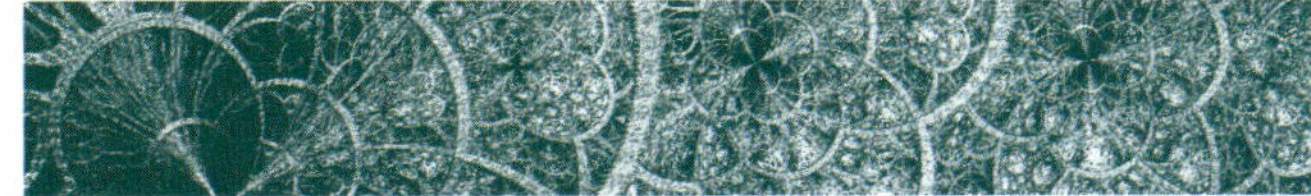

THE PERSON WITH BOTULISM

Botulism is food poisoning caused by ingestion of food contaminated with a toxin produced by the bacillus *Clostridium botulinum*. This anaerobic spore-forming bacillus is found in the soil. Most cases of botulism occur from eating improperly canned or cooked foods, especially home-canned vegetables and fruits, smoked meats and vacuum-packed fish. The mortality rate is high if the disease is untreated.

Pathophysiology

The toxins liberated by *C. botulinum* are absorbed by the gastrointestinal tract and bound to nerve tissues. They block the release of acetylcholine from nerve endings and thus cause respiratory paralysis due to paralysis of skeletal muscles.

Manifestations

Manifestations appear 12 to 36 hours after ingestion of the contaminated food. They usually begin with visual disturbances such as diplopia, loss of accommodation and fixed, dilated pupils. Ptosis is often present. Gastrointestinal manifestations include nausea and vomiting, diarrhoea, dysphagia and dry mouth. Involvement of the larynx is manifested by dystonia (impaired muscle tone). Paralysis of all muscle groups progresses throughout the body, with respiratory paralysis causing death if the person is not placed on a mechanical ventilator. There is no effect on mental status.

INTERPROFESSIONAL CARE

Infection with the *Clostridium* toxin is verified by laboratory analysis of the serum and stool and of suspected food, if possible. If botulism is suspected, the local Public Health Unit should be notified for assistance with laboratory assays and procuring botulism antitoxin. All people who may have eaten the contaminated food must be located and observed.

Any toxins in the gastrointestinal system are removed by cathartics, enemas and gastric lavage. The person with respiratory paralysis is placed on a mechanical ventilator and may require a tracheostomy. Botulism antitoxin is administered to eradicate toxins in the circulation. Nutritional support is often provided with total parenteral nutrition. Intravenous fluids are administered to prevent dehydration and renal failure. If ventilation can be maintained, the person often recovers without further neurological deficits.

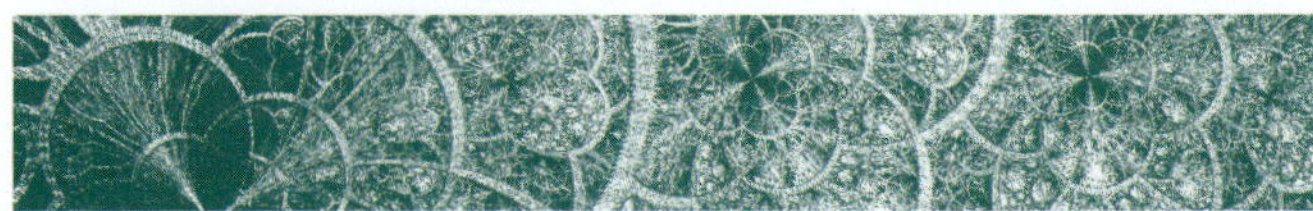

Nursing care

The person with botulism is hospitalised and interventions focus on monitoring for respiratory failure and providing ventilatory assistance if necessary. Ongoing assessments are also made for manifestations of paralytic ileus and urinary retention. The person will be nil by mouth until able to swallow and breathe; therefore, hydration and nutritional status are monitored. Teach the person and their family that fatigue and weakness may persist for up to a year. During this time, the person may need to modify ADLs and take rest periods throughout the day.

Health promotion

Education of the public to prevent botulism is important. Address the following topics at health fairs and community programs:

- Home-canned foods must be processed in a pressure cooker rather than in boiling water because the organism is difficult to kill.
- Do not eat home-processed foods that have a change in colour, are soft, contain gas bubbles or have a bad odour.
- Always heat both home-processed and commercial foods at temperatures over 120°C or boil for 10 minutes before tasting or eating them.
- Discard home-processed or commercially canned or bottled foods with defective seals.
- Discard commercially prepared canned foods that are damaged or have bulging sides or leaking contents.

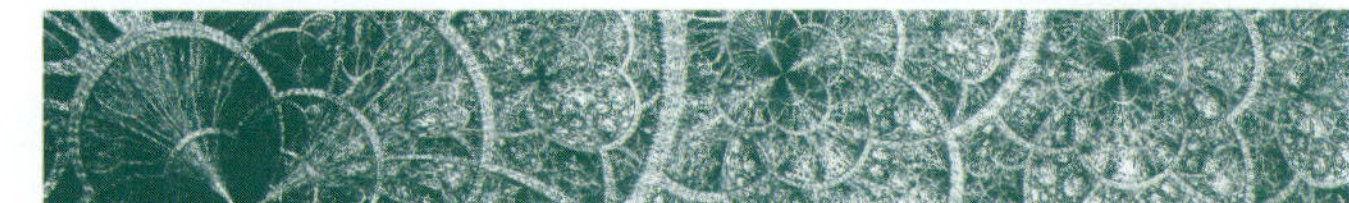

CHAPTER HIGHLIGHTS

- **Alzheimer's disease (AD) is a form of dementia (a disease of the brain) of older adults with progressive irreversible deterioration of general intellectual functioning. The disease is characterised by atrophy of brain tissue, loss of neurons, neurofibrillary tangles and amyloid plaques. AD finally leaves the person unable to communicate, maintain continence and recognise self or others. Caregivers need much teaching and support not only to provide care but also to avoid caregiver burden.**
- **Multiple sclerosis (MS) is a chronic demyelinating neurological disease of the CNS (brain, optic nerves and spinal cord). Occurring in young to middle-aged adults, it is believed to be due to an autoimmune response to a prior viral infection. The loss of myelin leads to axon dysfunction, which slows and distorts nerve impulses. Medications (ACTH, immunosuppressive agents, interferon and glatiramer acetate) are used to slow the progression of the disease, decrease the number of exacerbations and treat manifestations.**
- **Parkinson's disease (PD) is a progressive degenerative neurological disease characterised by tremor, muscle rigidity and bradykinesia. The loss of voluntary motor control is the result of pathological processes resulting in a decrease of dopamine (an inhibitory neurotransmitter) so that it can no longer inhibit acetylcholine (an excitatory neurotransmitter). Medications are used to treat manifestations and include MAO inhibitors, dopaminergics, dopamine agonists and anticholinergics. Other treatments include deep brain stimulation and surgery.**
- **Huntington's disease (HD) (chorea) is a progressive, degenerative, inherited neurological disease characterised**
- **by increasing dementia and chorea. There is an excess of dopamine, causing excessive, uncontrolled movement.**
- **Motor neurone disease (MND) is a rapidly progressive and fatal degenerative disease characterised by weakness and wasting of voluntary control muscles, but without sensory or cognitive changes. The person eventually loses the ability to communicate**

and breathe. Riluzole, antiglutamate medication, is used to treat (but not cure) manifestations.

- Myasthenia gravis (MG) is a chronic autoimmune peripheral nervous system disorder characterised by fatigue and severe skeletal muscle weakness. It results from a decreased number of acetylcholine receptors at the neuromuscular junction, so muscles are unable to contract. Life-threatening emergencies include myasthenic crisis (sudden increase in motor weakness) and cholinergic crisis (from an overdose of the anticholinesterase medications used to treat MG).
- Guillain–Barré syndrome (GBS) is an acute inflammatory demyelinating disease of the peripheral nervous system characterised by an acute onset of flaccid motor paralysis that begins in the lower extremities and ascends to involve the upper extremities, torso and cranial nerves. Paralysis of intercostal and diaphragmatic muscles often necessitates ventilatory assistance. The acute phase lasts from 1 to 3 weeks, followed by recovery, which takes from 6 months to 2 years.
- Cranial nerve disorders include trigeminal neuralgia (tic douloureux) and Bell's palsy. Trigeminal neuralgia is a chronic disorder of cranial nerve V and causes severe facial pain. Bell's palsy is an acute disorder of cranial nerve VII, characterised by unilateral paralysis of the facial muscles. People provide self-care at home and require teaching to help prevent complications.
- Neurological disorders resulting from neurotoxins or viruses include Creutzfeldt–Jakob disease, postpoliomyelitis syndrome, rabies, tetanus, botulism and complications from COVID-19 and its variants. Community-based health education can not only provide information but can also prevent illness in the case of rabies, tetanus and botulism.

CONCEPT CHECK

1 Which of the following statements is true of dementia? (Choose all that apply.)
1 Dementia is a general term used to describe manifestations of damage or death of neurons.
2 Dementia is the term used to describe the cognitive and behavioural manifestations of AD.
3 Dementia is an acute disorder resulting from an injury to the brain.
4 Dementia is the primary manifestation of Guillain–Barré syndrome.

2 Which manifestation is usually the first indication of the onset of AD?
1 inability to perform ADLs
2 sundowning at night
3 subtle memory deficits
4 inability to communicate

3 Which of the following nursing diagnoses is appropriate for people with MS, regardless of type or severity?
1 *Fatigue*
2 *Risk of aspiration*
3 *Acute pain*
4 *Impaired gas exchange*

4 You are preparing information to teach a person about medications for MS. Which drugs would you expect to be used?
1 antibiotics
2 antihistamines
3 interferon
4 levodopa

5 Which of the following topics is important when teaching a young adult with MS?
1 how to prevent sexually transmitted infections
2 how pregnancy can improve manifestations
3 what can be done to cure the disease
4 why it is important to avoid extremes of heat and cold

6 The manifestations of Parkinson's disease are the result of:
1 autoimmune responses to a viral infection
2 the failure of dopamine to inhibit acetylcholine
3 effects of a neurotoxin
4 a genetic defect

7 When teaching care at home for the person with PD, what would be a major area to discuss with caregivers?
1 preventing an overdose of medications
2 avoiding daily baths and showers
3 preventing falling
4 increasing appetite

8 Which drug classification is the medication used to treat MND?
1 dopamine agonist
2 anticholinergic
3 anti-inflammatory
4 antiglutamate

9 You are preparing a teaching plan for a person with Bell's palsy. What information would you include?
1 'You will experience severe facial pain during attacks.'
2 'The disease affects your muscles so you can't walk.'
3 'One side of your face will not move normally.'
4 'Be sure to boil all home-canned foods before eating them.'

10 How can the nurse prevent tetanus?
1 Teach safe food preparation techniques.
2 Promote immunisation for adults and children.
3 Demonstrate proper disposal of soiled dressings.
4 Promote immunisation of household pets.

BIBLIOGRAPHY

Ahmed, W., Khan, A., Sundar, W. H. et al. (2020). Neurological diseases caused by coronavirus infection of the respiratory airways. *Brain Science Advances*, 6(4), 324–343.

Asadi-Pooya, A. A. & Simani, L. (2020). Central nervous system manifestations of COVID-19: A systematic review. *Journal of Neurological Sciences*, *413*, 116832.

Australian Bureau of Statistics (ABS) (2020). *Causes of death, Australia*. Retrieved from https://www.abs.gov.au/

Brain Foundation (2022). *Disorders—Alzheimer's disease*. Retrieved from https://brainfoundation.org.au/

Centers for Disease Control and Prevention (2022). *CJD (Creutzfeldt–Jakob disease, classic)*. Retrieved from https://www.cdc.gov/

Cheng, K. B., Wie, M., Shen, H. et al. (2020). Clinical characteristics of 463 patients with common and severe type coronavirus disease (in Chinese). *Shanghai Medical Journal*, *43*(4), 224–232.

CSIRO (2021). *Australian bat lyssavirus*. Retrieved from https://www.csiro.au/

Dementia Australia (2022a). *Statistics*. Retrieved from https://www.dementia.org.au/

Dementia Australia (2022b). *Alzheimer's disease*. Retrieved from https://www.dementia.org.au/

Department of Health and Aged Care (2022). *Tetanus*. Retrieved from https://www.health.gov.au/

Desforges, M., Le Coupanec, A., Dubeau, P. et al. (2019). Human coronaviruses and other respiratory viruses: Understanding opportunistic pathogens of the central nervous system. *Viruses*, *12*(1), E14.

Divani, A. A., Andalib, S., Biller, J. et al. (2020). Central nervous system manifestations associated with COVID-19. *Current Neurological and Neuroscience Reports, 20*(12), 60. doi: 10.1007/s11910-020-01079-7

Folstein, M. F., Folstein, S. E. & McHugh, P. R. (1975). Mini-Mental State: A practical method for grading the cognitive state of patients for the clinician. *Journal of Psychiatric Research, 12*, 189–198.

Garvan Institute (2021). *Parkinson's disease*. Retrieved from https://www.garvan.org.au/

Guillain–Barré Syndrome Association of NSW (2018). *What is GBS?* Retrieved from http://www.gbs-cidp-nsw.org.au/

He, C., He, L., Chen, L. & Wang, W. (2021). Advances in the study of nervous system infections in COVID-19. *Brain Science Advances, 7*(3), 163–171.

Hickey, J. V. (2019). *The clinical practice of neurological and neurosurgical nursing* (8th ed.). Philadelphia: Lippincott Williams & Wilkins.

Kissler, S. M., Tadijanto, C., Goldstein, E. et al. (2020). Projecting the transmission dynamics of SARS-CoV-2 through the post pandemic period. *Science, 368*(6493), 860–868.

Mao, L., Jin, H. J., Wang, M. D. et al. (2020). Neurologic manifestations of hospitalized patients with coronavirus disease 2019 in Wuhan, China. *JAMA Neurology, 77*, 683–690.

Motor Neurone Disease Australia (2021). *What is MND?* Retrieved from https://www.mndaustralia.org.au/

MS Australia (2022). *What is multiple sclerosis?* Retrieved from https://www.msaustralia.org.au/

National Institute of Neurological Disorders and Stroke (NINDS) (2022a). *Huntington's disease*. Retrieved from https://www.ninds.nih.gov/

National Institute of Neurological Disorders and Stroke (NINDS) (2022b). *Myasthenia gravis*. Retrieved from https://www.ninds.nih.gov/

National Institute of Neurological Disorders and Stroke (NINDS) (2022c). *Bell's palsy*. Retrieved from https://www.ninds.nih.gov/

Neuroscience Research Australia (2022). *Alzheimer's disease*. Retrieved from https://www.neura.edu.au/

Norris, T. L. (2018). *Porth's pathophysiology: Concepts of altered health states* (10th ed.). Philadelphia: Lippincott Williams & Wilkins.

NPR (2022). *Vaccine-derived polio is on the rise. A new vaccine aims to stop the spread*. Retrieved from https://www.npr.org/

NSW Health (2019). *Creutzfeldt–Jakob disease (CJD) fact sheet*. Retrieved from https://www.health.nsw.gov.au/

Papadakis, M., McPhee, S. & Rabow, M. (2022). *Current medical diagnosis and treatment* (61st ed.). New York: McGraw-Hill Education.

Polio NSW (2022). *Polio*. Retrieved from https://www.polionsw.org.au/

Spudich, S. & Nath, A. (2022). Nervous system consequences of COVID-19. *Science, 375*(6578), 267–269.

St John Ambulance Australia (2020). *Fact sheet: CPR*. Retrieved from https://stjohn.org.au/

Tsirtsakis, A. (2021). Guillain-Barré Syndrome deaths 'likely linked' to COVID vaccine. *newsGP*. Retrieved from https://www1.racgp.org.au/

World Health Organization (WHO) (2021). *Rabies fact sheet*. Retrieved from https://www.who.int/

Wu, Y. S., Xu, X. L., Chen, Z. J. et al. (2020). Nervous system involvement after infection with COVID-19 and other coronaviruses. *Brain Behavior, and Immunity, 87*, 18–22.

Zubair, A. S., McAlpine, L. S., Gardin, T. et al. (2020). Neuropathogenesis and neurologic manifestations of the coronavirus in the age of coronavirus disease 2019. *JAMA Neurology. Clinical Review and Education, 77*(8), 1018–1027.

UNIT 11 BUILDING CLINICAL COMPETENCE

Responses to altered neurological function

Clinical scenario

- You have been assigned to work with the following people on a neurological hospital unit. Significant data obtained during report are as follows:
- Sam Kwon is a 74-year-old male who was admitted from the emergency department to the neurology ward last night. Mr Kwon was found by family in his home. He was unable to speak or move the right side of his body and continues to experience paralysis on the right side in both his arm and his leg. He is aphasic with facial drooping but is able to nod his head to communicate. Mr Kwon has a known history of hypertension, CHF and type 2 diabetes controlled by oral hypoglycaemic medications. He has smoked a packet of cigarettes a day for 40 years. BP is now 140/105, P 98, R 24. Lungs reported to have crackles in the bases. He is receiving 2 L of oxygen via nasal prongs. A swallowing evaluation has been ordered to be done today.
- Jane Thomas is a 56-year-old female. She was admitted 4 days ago and underwent a lumbar laminectomy. She was able to ambulate with assistance on day 2 after surgery and now reports no dizziness on ambulation. Her leg strength has progressively increased since surgery. She has equal sensation and is able to wriggle her toes on both feet. Pain is controlled at her desired level of 2 to 3 on a scale of 1 to 10 with oral medications.
- Cesar Phillips is a 39-year-old male, admitted 4 days ago after experiencing paralysis and severe headache at work. He has been diagnosed with stroke following an MRI. He has a history of smoking one packet of cigarettes per day and hypertension. His wife reported that he had stopped taking his blood pressure medication due to the side effects of impotence. Mr Phillips is awake and alert but has exhibited impulsive behaviour and agnosia. He also has a difficult time remembering words and neglects the left side of his body in ADLs. BP had been 130/85 at the beginning of last shift but has increased to 170/110. He received an additional prn blood pressure medication 1.5 hours ago.
- Tonya Walton is a 29-year-old female. She was involved in a car crash 12 hours before her admission 5 days earlier. She developed a headache, drowsiness, confusion and pupil enlargement several hours after the crash. Following an MRI, Ms Walton underwent intracranial surgery to evacuate a subdural haematoma. She has been complaining of a headache that has increased in intensity from a 2 to a 6 on a scale of 1 to 10 on the previous shift. She received two Nurofen ES tabs 1 hour ago. BP was 140–150 systolic and 90–100 diastolic for most of the shift. Her BP at the time of the Nurofen administration was 175/115. She has not experienced any changes in her neuro assessment except for the increasing headache and blood pressure elevation.

Critical-thinking questions

1 In what order would you visit these people after report?

1.
2.
3.
4.

2 Which two top-priority nursing diagnoses would you choose for each of the people presented above? Can you explain, if asked, the rationale for your choices?

	Priority Nursing Diagnosis #1	Priority Nursing Diagnosis #2
Sam Kwon		
Jane Thomas		
Cesar Phillips		
Tonya Walton		

3 After completing Mr Kwon's beginning-of-shift baseline assessment, which assessment would be your next priority?

1. rhythm strip interpretation
2. intake and output
3. heart sounds
4. level of pain

4 You are completing the beginning-of-shift assessment for Mr Phillips. Which changes would best indicate that the plan initiated by the previous shift was effective?

1. Mr Phillips no longer has a craving for cigarettes.
2. Mr Phillips's respiratory rate is 18–20.
3. Mr Phillips's pain score is now 1–2.
4. Mr Phillips's blood pressure has decreased to 145/90.

5 What are the top two education priorities for Jane Thomas as you plan for discharge? (Select all that apply.)

1. appropriate exercise
2. pain management
3. weight control
4. incision care
5. importance of rest

6 You review the lab reports for Jane Thomas. You are most interested in the results for which of the following studies? (Select all that apply.)

1. white blood cell count
2. red blood cell indices
3. serum sodium
4. haemoglobin
5. haematocrit
6. osteocalcin
7. prealbumin

7 You are completing the beginning-of-shift assessment for Ms Walton. Which changes would best indicate that the plan initiated by the previous shift was effective?

1. Ms Walton has no neurological changes or deterioration.
2. Ms Walton's BP is 142/94.
3. Ms Walton's pain score is now 1–2.
4. Ms Walton's dressing is dry and intact.

8 If you re-evaluated Ms Walton and her headache pain had not decreased, what should be your next priority?

1. Reposition Ms Walton on her left side with the head of the bed flat.
2. Call the doctor about Ms Walton's report of increasing headache.
3. Decrease stimuli in the room by darkening the room and limiting noise.
4. Check the prn orders to evaluate if a stronger pain medication has been ordered.

9 If you were planning an effective team meeting with all disciplines that should be collaborating to provide care and a discharge plan for Mr Phillips, which six disciplines should be represented and why?

1. ____________________
2. ____________________
3. ____________________
4. ____________________
5. ____________________
6. ____________________

10 Review the five steps of the abbreviated neurological assessment as outlined in the text. What are three findings you would expect when conducting a neuro check with Mr Kwon?

1. ____________________
2. ____________________
3. ____________________

Case study

Shirley Tayler is a 54-year-old Indigenous Australian female. She was admitted 2 days earlier after being diagnosed with a stroke. She lives with her husband of 34 years and her 14-year-old grandson. Her grandson found her lying on the kitchen floor when he got home from school. When he asked her what had happened, she was unable to say words that were clear or understandable. He tried to help her stand up but was unable to because she was extremely weak in her left side. He called 000 and an ambulance transported her to the emergency department. Her blood pressure when the ambulance arrived was 220/125, P 105, R 24, and she was very anxious and spoke garbled words loudly at the paramedics. She was diagnosed with acute stroke after evaluation at the hospital and was admitted for treatment. Mrs Tayler has a history of hypertension and type 2 diabetes. She recently stopped taking her blood pressure medication because it made her feel 'tired'.

The pathophysiology of a stroke is dependent on location of the causative factor, size of tissue affected and time of loss of cellular perfusion and oxygenation. Time is critical when it involves compromised perfusion to any organ and the brain is no exception. Cerebral neuron cellular metabolism is severely affected within 4 to 5 minutes of compromised perfusion. Compromised cellular metabolism leads to glucose, glycogen and adenosine triphosphate depletion and sodium–potassium pump failure. Wherever sodium goes, water follows. When the sodium–potassium pump fails, the sodium in the cell draws water into the cell, resulting in oedema. Additionally, cerebral vessel walls also swell, further compromising blood and oxygen supply. Severe or prolonged ischaemia leads to cellular death. The manifestations of a stroke include, but are not limited to, motor deficits, elimination disorders, sensory–perceptual deficits, communication disorders and behavioural changes. The manifestations are always sudden in onset, focal and usually unilateral. Typically, a stroke is manifested by weakness of the face, arm and leg; loss of vision in one eye; speech and swallowing problems; and difficulties with balance. There are many different complications of a stroke, including increased intracranial pressure, coma, death, chronic long-term confusion and intellectual changes.

The nursing diagnosis of *Ineffective cerebral tissue perfusion* is appropriate for implementing care for Mrs Tayler.

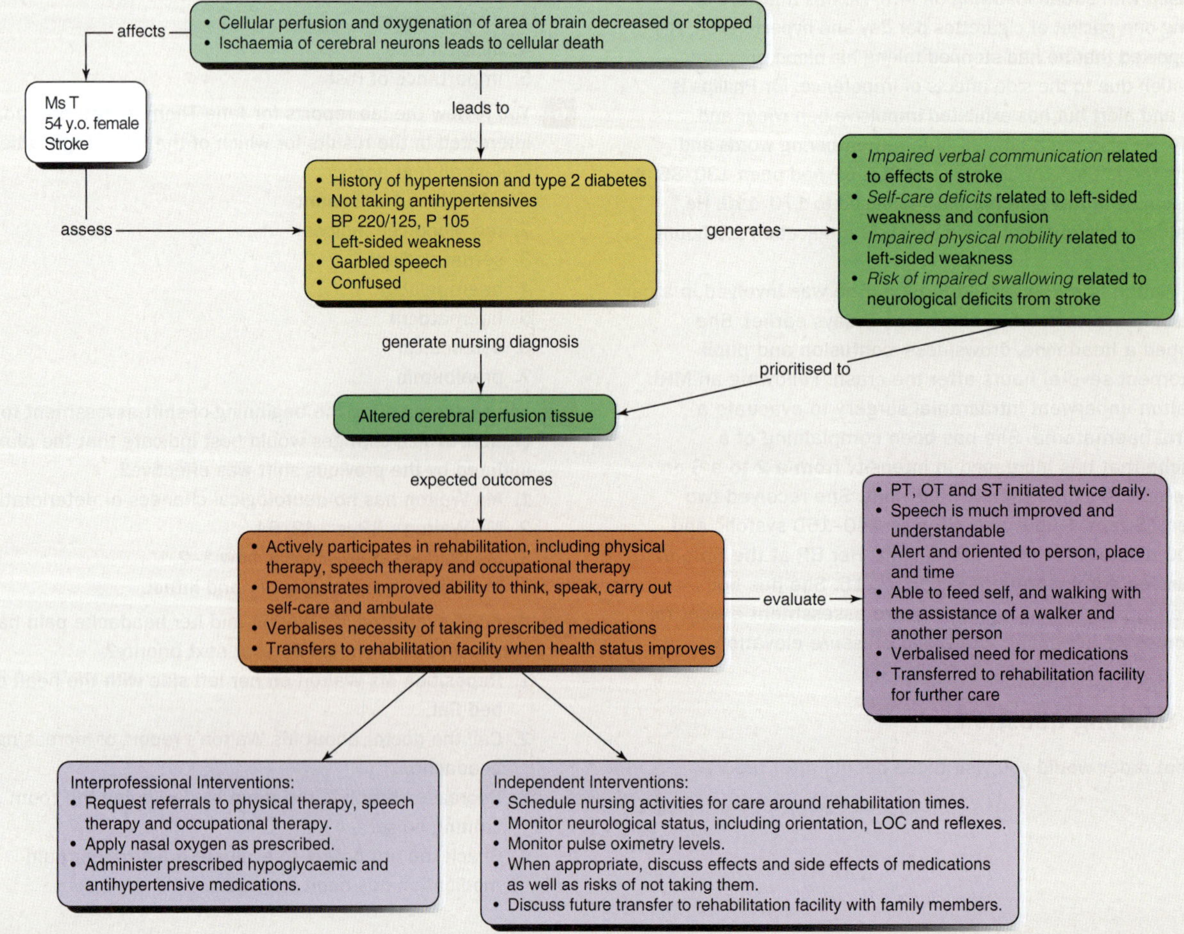

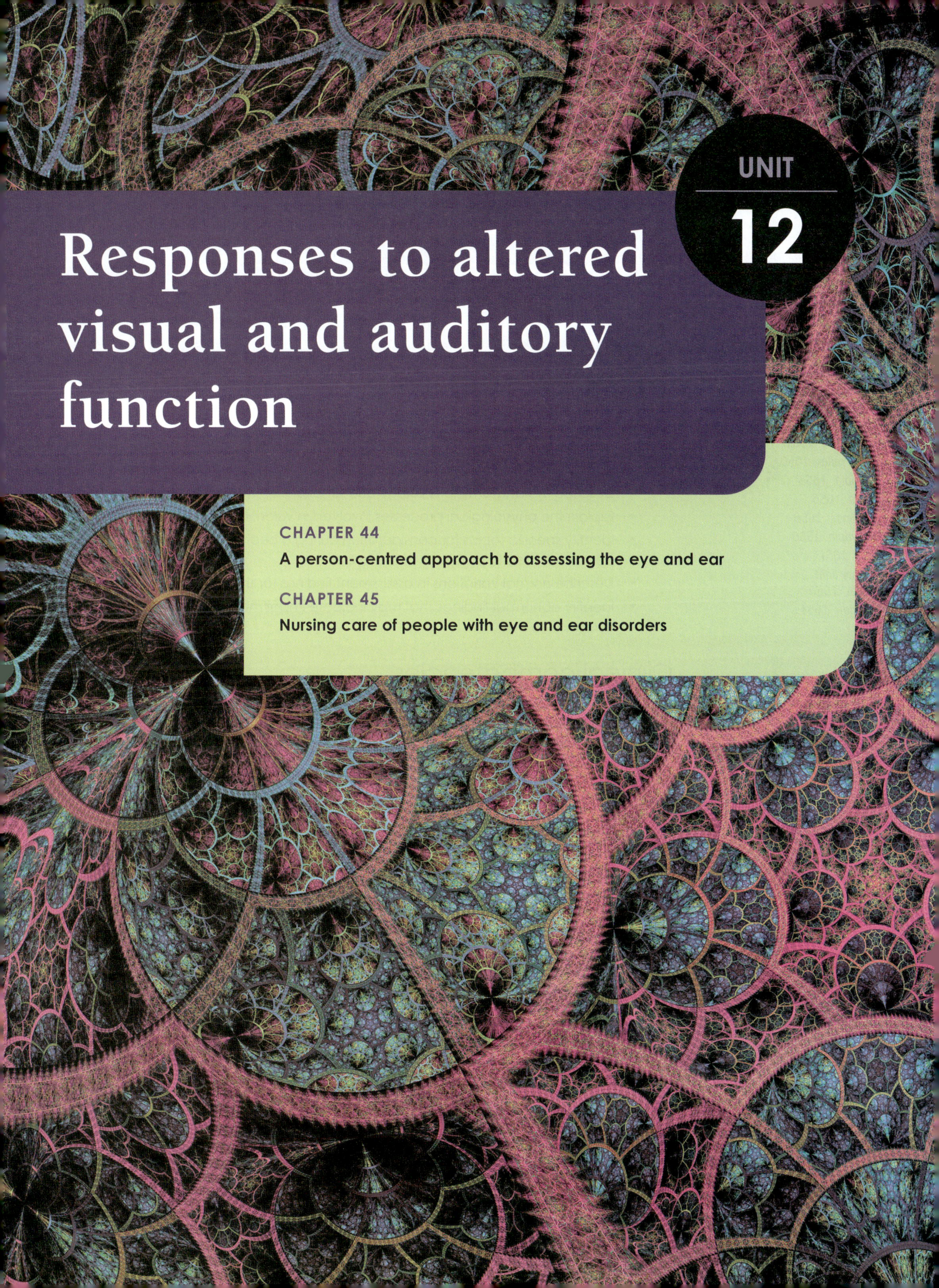

UNIT 12

Responses to altered visual and auditory function

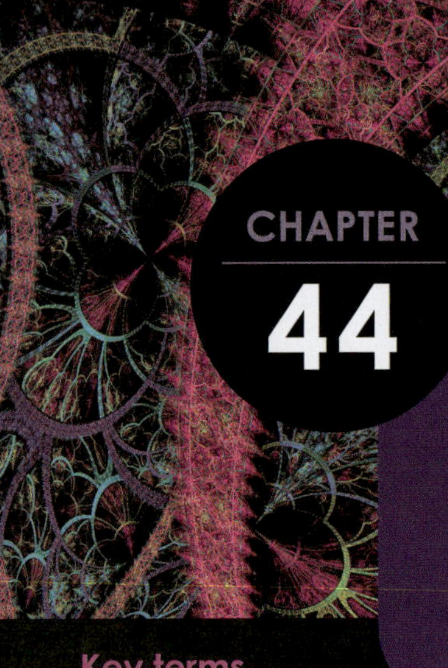

CHAPTER 44

A person-centred approach to assessing the eye and ear

Kamaree Houlis-Berry

Key terms

accommodation 1652
cerumen 1660
convergence 1652
corneal reflex 1650
hyperopia 1656
myopia 1656
nystagmus 1656
presbyopia 1656
ptosis 1657
pupillary light reflex 1650
refraction 1651

Learning outcomes

- Describe the anatomy, physiology and functions of the eye and ear.
- Explain the physiological processes involved in vision, hearing and equilibrium.
- Identify specific topics for consideration during a health history interview of the person with health problems of the eye or ear.
- Describe normal variations in assessment findings for the older adult.
- Identify abnormal findings that may indicate impairment in the function of the eye and the ear.

Clinical competencies

- Conduct and document a health history for people having or at risk of alterations in the structure or functions of the eye and ear.
- Monitor the results of diagnostic tests and report abnormal findings.
- Conduct and document a physical assessment of the structure and/or functions of the eye and ear.

Equipment needed

- Visual acuity charts
- Opaque eye cover
- Pen
- Penlight
- Cotton-tipped applicator
- Ophthalmoscope
- Otoscope
- Tuning fork

Vision and hearing allow us to experience the world in which we live. The eyes and ears provide pathways for visual and auditory stimuli to reach the brain, while specialised structures within the ear help maintain position sense and equilibrium. Deficits in vision and hearing may limit self-care, mobility, safety, independence, communication and relationships with others.

Anatomy, physiology and functions of the eyes

The eyes are complex structures that contain 70% of the sensory receptors of the body.

Each eye is a sphere measuring about 2.5 cm in diameter, surrounded and protected by a bony orbit and cushions of fat. The primary functions of the eye are to encode the patterns of light from the environment through photoreceptors and to carry the coded information from the eyes to the brain. The brain gives meaning to the coded information, allowing us to make sense of what we see. Both extraocular and intraocular structures are considered parts of the eye.

Extraocular structures

Although the extraocular structures of the eye are outside the eyeball, they are vital to its protection. These structures are the eyebrows, eyelids, eyelashes, conjunctiva, lacrimal apparatus and extrinsic eye muscles (see Figure 44.1).

The eyebrows shade the eyes and keep perspiration away from them. The eyelids are thin, loose folds of skin covering the anterior eye; they protect the eyes from foreign bodies, regulate the entry of light into the eye and distribute tears by blinking. The eyelashes are short hairs that project from the top and bottom borders of the eyelids. An unexpected touch to the eyelashes initiates the blinking reflex to protect the eyes from foreign objects.

The conjunctiva is a thin, transparent membrane that lines the inner surfaces of the eyelids and folds over the anterior surface of the eyeball. The palpebral conjunctiva lines the upper and lower eyelids, whereas the bulbar conjunctiva loosely covers the anterior sclera (the white part of the eye). The conjunctiva is a mucous membrane that lubricates the eyes. The lacrimal apparatus is composed of the lacrimal gland, the puncta, the lacrimal sac and the nasolacrimal duct. Together, these structures secrete, distribute and drain tears to cleanse and moisten the eye's surface.

The six extrinsic eye muscles control movement of the eye, allowing it to follow a moving object and move precisely. The muscles also help maintain the shape of the eyeball. The cranial nerves control the extrinsic muscles (see Figure 44.2).

Intraocular structures

The intraocular structures transmit visual images and maintain homeostasis of the inner eye. Those in the anterior portion of each eyeball are the sclera and the cornea (forming the outermost coat of the eye, known as the fibrous tunic), the iris, the pupil and the anterior cavity (see Figure 44.3).

Sclera and cornea

The white sclera lines the outside of the eyeball it protects and provides its shape. The sclera gives way to the cornea over the iris and pupil, which is transparent, avascular and sensitive to touch. The cornea forms a window that allows light to enter the eye

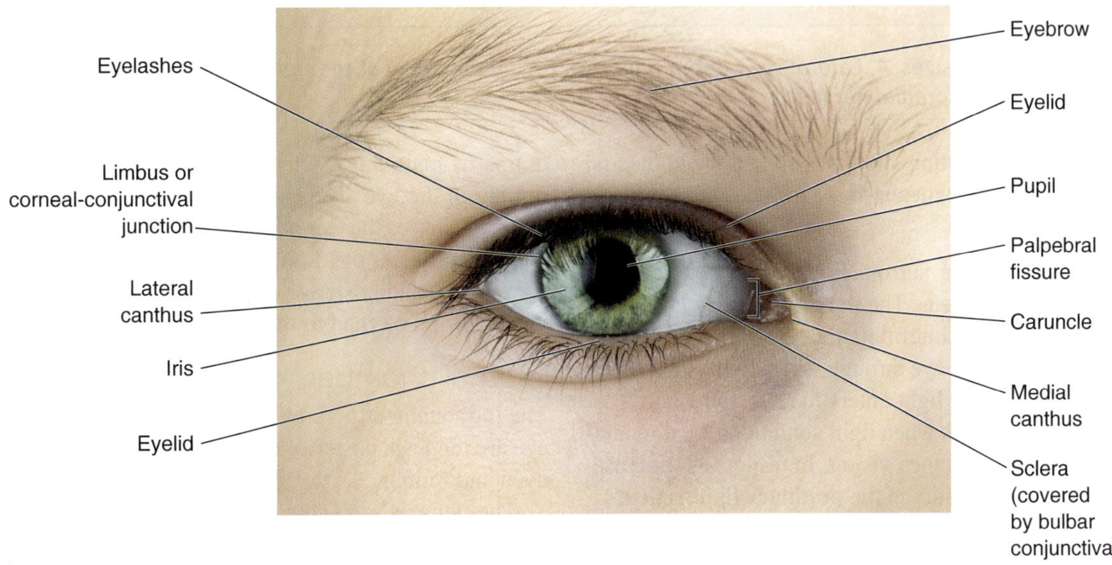

FIGURE 44.1 ***Accessory and external structures of the eye***

Source: Bo Valentino/Shutterstock.

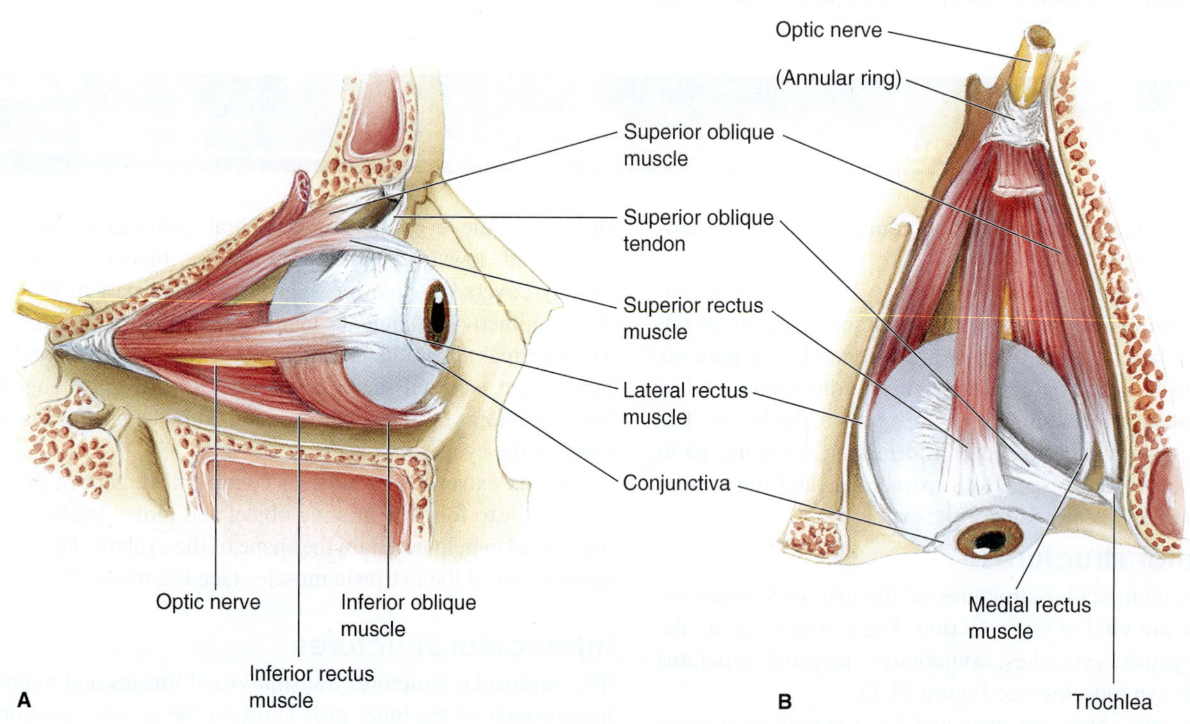

Name	Controlling cranial nerve	Action
Lateral rectus	VI (abducens)	Moves eye laterally
Medial rectus	III (oculomotor)	Moves eye medially
Superior rectus	III (oculomotor)	Elevates eye or rolls it superiorly
Inferior rectus	III (oculomotor)	Depresses eye or rolls it inferiorly
Inferior oblique	III (oculomotor)	Elevates eye and turns it laterally
Superior oblique	IV (trochlear)	Depresses eye and turns it laterally

C

FIGURE 44.2 ***Extraocular muscles. A, Lateral view of the right eye. B, Superior view of the right eye. C, Innervation of the extraocular muscles by the cranial nerves***

and is a part of its light-bending apparatus. When the cornea is touched, the eyelids blink (**corneal reflex**) and tears are secreted.

Iris

The iris is a disc of muscle surrounding the pupil and lying between the cornea and the lens. The iris gives the eye its colour and regulates light entry by controlling the size of the pupil. The pupil is the dark centre of the eye through which light enters. The pupil constricts when bright light enters the eye and when it is used for near vision; it dilates when light conditions are dim and when the eye is used for distance vision. In response to intense light, the pupil constricts rapidly in the **pupillary light reflex**.

Aqueous fluid

The anterior cavity is made of the anterior chamber (the space between the cornea and the iris) and the posterior chamber (the space between the iris and the lens). The anterior cavity is filled with aqueous humour, a clear fluid which constantly forms and drains to maintain a relatively constant pressure of 15 to 20 mmHg in the eye. The canal of Schlemm, a network of channels that circles the eye in the angle at the junction of the sclera and the cornea, is the drainage system for fluid moving between the anterior and posterior chambers. Aqueous humour provides nutrients and oxygen to the cornea and the lens.

Internal chamber

The intraocular structures that lie in the internal chamber of the eye are the lens, posterior cavity, vitreous humour, ciliary body, uvea and retina.

The lens is a biconvex, avascular, transparent structure located directly behind the pupil. It can change shape to focus and refract light onto the retina. The posterior cavity lies behind the lens. It is filled with a clear gelatinous substance, the vitreous humour, which supports the posterior surface of the lens, maintains the position of the retina and transmits light. The

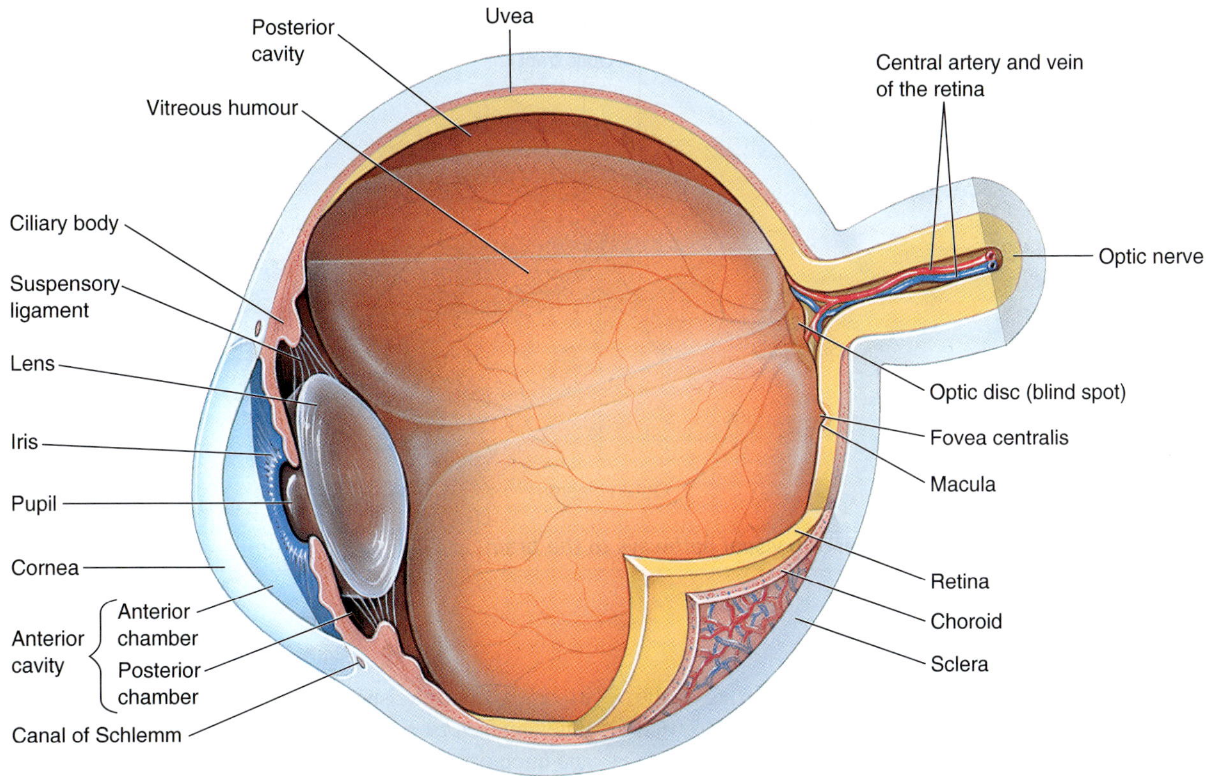

FIGURE 44.3 *Internal structures of the eye*

uvea, also called the vascular tunic, is the middle layer of the eyeball. This pigmented layer has three components: the iris, ciliary body and choroid. The ciliary body encircles the lens and, along with the iris, regulates the amount of light reaching the retina by controlling the shape of the lens. Most of the uvea is made up of the choroid, which is pigmented and vascular. Blood vessels of the choroid nourish the layers of the eyeball and its pigmented areas absorb light, preventing it from scattering within the eyeball.

The retina is the innermost lining of the eyeball. It has an outer pigmented layer and an inner neural layer. The outer layer, next to the choroid, serves as the link between visual stimuli and the brain. The transparent inner layer is made up of millions of light receptors in structures called rods and cones. Rods enable vision in dim light as well as peripheral vision and cones enable vision in bright light and the perception of colour. The optic disc, a cream-coloured round or oval area within the retina, is the point at which the optic nerve enters the eye. The slight depression in the centre of the optic disc is called the physiological cup. Located laterally to the optic disc is the macula, a darker area with no visible blood vessels and which contains primarily cones. The fovea centralis is a slight depression in the centre of the macula that contains only cones and is a main receptor of detailed colour vision.

The visual pathway

The optic nerves are cranial nerves formed of the axons of ganglion cells. The two optic nerves meet at the optic chiasma, just anterior to the pituitary gland in the brain. At the optic chiasma, axons from the medial half of each retina cross to the opposite side to form pairs of axons from each eye. These pairs continue as the left and right optic tracts (see Figure 44.4). The crossing of the axons results in each optic tract carrying information from both eyes. The left optic tract carries visual information from the lateral half of the retina of the left eye and the medial half of the retina of the right eye, whereas the right optic tract carries visual information from the lateral half of the retina of the right eye and the medial half of the retina of the left eye.

The ganglion cell axons in the optic tracts travel to the thalamus and synapse with neurons, forming pathways called optic radiations. The optic radiations terminate in the visual cortex of the occipital lobe and the nerve impulses that originated in the retina are interpreted here.

The visual fields of each eye overlap considerably and each eye sees a slightly different view. Because of this overlap and the crossing of the axons, information from both eyes reaches each side of the visual cortex, which then fuses the information into one image. This fusion of images accounts for the ability to perceive depth; however, depth perception depends on visual input from two eyes that focus well.

Refraction

Refraction is the bending of light rays as they pass from one medium to another of different optical density. As light rays pass through the eye, they are refracted at several points: as they enter the cornea; as they leave the cornea and enter the aqueous humour; as they enter the lens; and as they leave the lens and enter the vitreous humour. At the lens, the light is bent so that

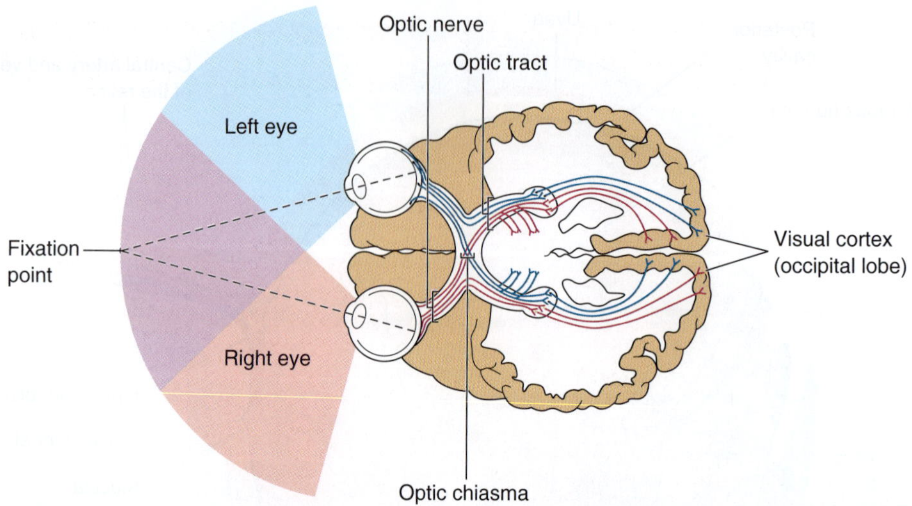

FIGURE 44.4 *The visual fields of the eye and the visual pathways to the brain*

it converges at a single point on the retina. The focusing of the image is called **accommodation**. Because the lens is convex, the image projected on to the retina (the real image) is upside down and reversed from left to right. This real image is coded as electric signals that are sent to the brain; the brain then decodes the image so that the person perceives it as it occurs in space.

The eyes are best adapted to see distant objects. Both eyes fix on the same distant image and do not require any change in accommodation. For people with emmetropic (normal) vision, the distance from the viewed object at which the eyes require no accommodation is 6 metres. This point is called the far point of vision. To focus for near vision, the eyes must instantly accommodate the lens, constrict the pupils and converge the eyeballs. Accommodation is accomplished by contraction of the ciliary muscles. This contraction reduces the tension on the lens capsule so that it bulges outwards to increase the curvature. This change in shape also achieves a shorter focal length, another requirement for focusing close images on the retina. The closest point on which a person can focus is called the near point of vision; in young adults with normal vision this is usually 20 to 25 cm. Pupillary constriction helps eliminate most of the divergent light rays and sharpens focus. **Convergence** (the medial rotation of the eyeballs so that each is directed towards the viewed object) allows the focusing of the image on the retinal fovea of each eye.

ASSESSING THE EYES

Structures and functions of the eyes are assessed by findings from a health assessment interview to collect subjective data, a physical assessment to collect objective data and diagnostic tests.

Health assessment interview

To determine problems with the eyes and vision, a health assessment interview may be conducted during a health screening. It may focus on a chief complaint, such as blurred vision or an eye infection, or may be part of a complete health assessment. If the person has a health problem involving one or both eyes, analyse its onset, characteristics and course, severity, precipitating and relieving factors, and any associated symptoms, noting the timing and circumstances. For example, ask the person:

- Describe the type of pain you experience in your eyes. When did it begin? How long does it last?
- Have you noticed rings of colour around streetlights at night?
- When did you first notice having difficulty reading the paper?

Throughout the interview, be alert to non-verbal behaviours, such as squinting and/or abnormal eye movements, that may suggest problems with eye function. Explore problems such as watery, irritated eyes or changes in vision. Assess the person's use of corrective eyewear and care of eyeglasses or contact lenses. If the person uses eye medications, ask about the type, purpose, frequency, dose and duration of use. When taking the history, find out about eye trauma, surgery or infections, as well as the date and results of the last eye examination. In addition, ask the person about a medical history of diabetes, hypertension, thyroid disorders, glaucoma, cataracts and eye infections. Include questions about a family history of myopia (nearsightedness) or presbyopia (farsightedness), cancer of the retina, colour blindness and any other eye or vision disorders.

Collect information about environmental and/or work exposure to irritating chemicals, sport participation or hobbies that pose the risk of eye injury and the use of protective eyewear during dangerous activities such as sawing wood or using a lawn trimmer.

Interview questions categorised by functional health patterns are listed in the 'Functional health pattern interview' table.

Physical assessment of the eyes and vision

Physical assessment of the eyes and of visual acuity may be performed as part of a total assessment or separately for people with known or suspected eye problems. The eyes and vision are primarily assessed through inspection of external structures

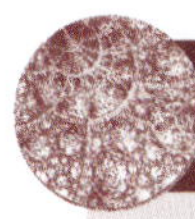

FUNCTIONAL HEALTH PATTERN INTERVIEW The eye

FUNCTIONAL HEALTH PATTERN	INTERVIEW QUESTIONS AND LEADING STATEMENTS
Health perception–Health management	▪ Describe your vision. Rate it on a scale of 1 to 10, with 10 being excellent vision. Is it the same in both eyes? If not, which eye is better?
	▪ Describe your current vision problems. How have these been treated?
	▪ What eye medications do you use? What type and how often?
	▪ Have you ever had eye surgery? Provide details.
	▪ Describe the type of corrective lens that you wear. Are you satisfied with this appliance? How do you care for it?
	▪ Describe how you care for your eyes each day.
	▪ Do you wear sunglasses when you are outside?
	▪ When was your last eye examination? Have you been tested for glaucoma?
Nutritional–Metabolic	▪ Do you have any redness, swelling, watering or dryness of your eyes?
Activity–Exercise	▪ Does your vision problem interfere with your usual activities of daily living? Provide details.
	▪ Do you wear protective goggles when you take part in activities that increase the risk of injury to your eyes (such as at work or when operating machinery at home)?
Sleep–Rest	▪ Does your eye problem interfere with your ability to rest or sleep (e.g. pain)? If so, what do you do?
Cognitive–Perceptual	▪ Do you have any difficulty focusing on objects? If so, do you have more difficulty with near objects or distant objects?
	▪ Is your vision blurry? Do you see halos around lights? Do you see flashes of light or 'floaters'? Do you see double?
	▪ Do you have pain in or around your eyes? If so, describe its location, intensity, what makes it worse and how long it lasts. How do you treat it?
Self-perception–Self-concept	▪ Has this problem with your eyes affected how you feel about yourself?
Role–Relationships	▪ How has having this condition affected your relationships with others?
	▪ Has having this condition interfered with your ability to work? Provide details.
	▪ Has anyone in your family had problems with eye disease? Provide details.
Sexuality–Reproductive	▪ Has this condition interfered with your usual sexual activity?
Coping–Stress–Tolerance	▪ Has having this condition created stress for you? If so, does your health problem seem to be more difficult when you are stressed?
	▪ Have you experienced any kind of stress that makes the condition worse? Provide details.
	▪ Describe what you do when you feel stressed.
Value–Belief	▪ Describe how specific relationships or activities help you cope with this problem.
	▪ Describe specific cultural beliefs or practices that affect how you care for and feel about this problem.
	▪ Are there any specific treatments that you would not use to treat this problem?

and assessment of visual fields and visual acuity, extraocular muscle function and internal structures. Palpation—for example, of a blocked lacrimal duct—may be used if a problem is identified. Prior to the examination, explain the techniques to the person to decrease anxiety. The person may sit or stand during the assessment. Normal age-related findings for the older adult are summarised in Table 44.1.

Assessing visual fields

Visual fields are tested to assess the functioning of the macula and peripheral vision. The visual fields of the examiner (which must be normal to perform this assessment) are used as the standard. To measure visual fields, sit directly opposite the person at a distance of 45 to 60 cm. Ask the person to cover

PATIENT SAFETY COMPETENCY FRAMEWORK

5 Clinical reasoning

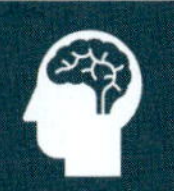

The Patient Safety Competency Framework indicates that nursing students must demonstrate clinical reasoning through the ability to accurately assess, interpret and respond to individual patient data in a systematic and timely way (Levett-Jones et al., 2017).

TABLE 44.1 Age-related changes in the eye

AGE-RELATED CHANGE	SIGNIFICANCE
The lens: • ↓ elasticity, decreasing focus and accommodation for near vision (presbyopia). • ↑ density and size, making lens more stiff and opaque. • Yellowing of the lens and changes in the retina affect colour perception.	Most older adults require corrective lenses to accommodate close and detailed work. Increased opacity leads to the development of cataracts. As cataracts develop, they increase sensitivity to glare and interfere with night vision.
The cornea: • Fat may be deposited around the periphery and throughout the cornea.	A partial or complete white circle may form around the cornea (arcus senilis). Lipid deposits in the cornea cause vision to be blurred.
• ↓ corneal sensitivity.	Decreased sensitivity increases the risk of injury to the eye.
The pupil: • ↓ size and responsiveness to light pupil; sphincter hardens.	Increased light perception threshold and difficulty seeing in dim light or at night means increased light is needed to see adequately.
The retina and visual pathways: • Visual fields narrow. • Photoreceptor cells are lost. • Rods work less effectively. • Macular degeneration is a risk. • Depth perception is distorted. • Adaptation to dark and light takes longer.	Peripheral vision is decreased and central vision may be lost from macular degeneration. Increased risk of falls as a result of changes in depth perception and adaptation to changes in light. Vision progressively declines with age.
The lacrimal apparatus: • ↓ reabsorption of intraocular fluid. • ↓ production of tears.	Increased risk of developing glaucoma and eyes feel and look dry.
The posterior cavity: • Debris and condensation become visible. • Vitreous body may pull away from the retina.	Vision is blurred and distorted and 'floaters' are often seen by the older adult.

one eye with the opaque cover while you cover your own eye opposite to the person (e.g. if the person covers the right eye, you cover your left eye). Ask the person to look directly at you. Move the penlight from the periphery towards the centre from right to left, above and below, and from the middle of each of these directions. Both you and the person should see the penlight enter the field of vision at the same time, if the examiner has normal peripheral vision.

The central visual field may be assessed with an Amsler grid (see Figure 44.5). The most basic form has black lines on a white grid, forming squares (boxes) that measure 5 mm with a black dot in the centre of the grid. The Amsler grid is useful for identifying early changes in vision from macular degeneration and diabetes mellitus. To use the Amlser grid, ask the person to hold the grid at normal reading distance (about 30 to 35 cm), cover one eye and stare at the centre dot. Ask the person if any of the lines look crooked or bent, if any of the boxes are different in size or shape, and if any of the lines are wavy, missing, blurry or discoloured. Repeat with the other eye. The test should be conducted before the pupils are dilated and the person should be wearing their best correction lenses.

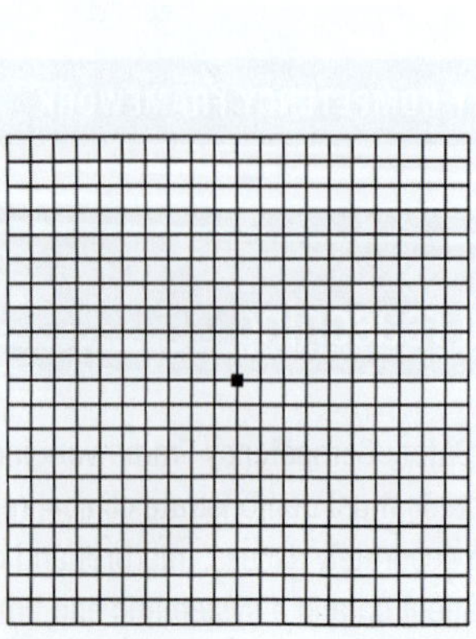

FIGURE 44.5 *The Amsler grid*

Diagnostic tests

The results of diagnostic tests of the structure and functions of the eyes are used to support the diagnosis of a specific injury, disease or vision problem; to provide information to identify and/or modify the appropriate medications or assistive devices used to treat the disease or problem; and to help nurses monitor the person's responses to treatment and nursing care interventions. Diagnostic tests of the eye, especially for vision testing, are most often conducted in a healthcare provider's office. Diagnostic tests to assess the structure and functions of the eyes are described in the 'Diagnostic tests' box and summarised in the following list. More information is included in the discussion of specific injuries or diseases in the chapter 'Nursing care of people with eye and ear disorders'.

- Refractive errors (with prescription for corrective lenses) are evaluated by retinoscopy and/or refractometry. Pupils must be dilated for accurate diagnosis.
- Tonometry is used to identify and evaluate increased intraocular pressure, characteristic of glaucoma.
- A CT scan may be used to identify foreign objects or tumours of the eye.
- Fluorescein angiography is used to evaluate blood vessels in the eye in conditions such as diabetes, macular degeneration or vessel occlusion.

DIAGNOSTIC TESTS Eye disorders

NAME OF TEST Refraction, retinoscopy, refractometry

PURPOSE AND DESCRIPTION Used to measure refractive error. Either a hand-held retinoscope or an instrument with multiple lenses is used; with the latter method, the person chooses lenses that provide the best vision.

RELATED NURSING CARE No special preparation is needed; advise the person that pupils will be dilated with medication and may be enlarged for several hours.

NAME OF TEST Tonometry

PURPOSE AND DESCRIPTION Used to diagnose increased intraocular pressure in glaucoma. A variety of methods are used, ranging from a hand-held instrument (tonometer) to a computerised component of the device used to evaluate refraction. The cornea is anaesthetised prior to being touched with the device.

NORMAL VALUE: 10–22 mmHg.

RELATED NURSING CARE No special preparation is needed.

NAME OF TEST Computed tomography (CT) scan of the eye

PURPOSE AND DESCRIPTION Radiological examination used to identify foreign objects or tumours within the eyeball or orbit.

RELATED NURSING CARE No special preparation is needed.

NAME OF TEST Fluorescein angiography

PURPOSE AND DESCRIPTION Fluorescein solution is injected IV to evaluate blood vessels in the eye in conditions such as diabetes, macular degeneration or vessel occlusion.

RELATED NURSING CARE Informed consent is required for this test. Note current medications and notify the doctor if the person is pregnant. Inform the person that a hot flush and transient nausea may be experienced when the dye is injected. Monitor for anaphylactic hypersensitivity responses that may occur. Fluorescent yellow urine and a yellow skin colour may be noted for 1–2 days after the procedure; these are not considered harmful.

Regardless of the type of diagnostic test, the nurse may be responsible for explaining the procedure and any special preparation needed, assessing any medication use that might affect the outcome of the tests, supporting the person during the examination as necessary, documenting the procedures as appropriate and monitoring the results of the tests.

Genetic considerations

When conducting a health assessment interview and a physical assessment, it is important for the nurse to consider genetic influences on the health of the adult, as several diseases of the eyes have a genetic component. During the health assessment interview, ask about a family history of glaucoma and/or blindness.

During the physical assessment, assess for any manifestations that might indicate a genetic disorder (see the accompanying 'Genetic considerations' box). If the data are found to indicate genetic risk factors or alterations, ask about genetic testing and refer for appropriate genetic counselling and evaluation. The chapter 'Genetic implications of adult health nursing' provides further information about genetics in medical–surgical nursing.

GENETIC CONSIDERATIONS Eye disorders

- *Glaucoma* is a term used for a group of diseases that damage the optic nerve and cause blindness. Approximately 300,000 people in Australia may suffer from glaucoma, with nearly half of them not being aware that they suffer from this disease (Centre for Eye Research in Australia, 2022).
- Gyrate atrophy of the choroid and retina is a genetic disorder resulting in a progressive vision loss, with total blindness occurring between ages 40 and 60.
- Best disease is a familial disorder found most often in Caucasians who originated in Europe. It leads to gradual loss of vision, beginning during the teenage years.
- Retinitis pigmentosa may be transmitted in an autosomal recessive, dominant or X-linked pattern. It results in progressive night blindness, with loss of visual acuity and peripheral vision.

EYE AND VISION ASSESSMENTS

Vision assessment

Visual acuity is assessed with an eye chart, such as the Snellen or the E chart for testing distance vision and the Rosenbaum chart for testing near vision. The Snellen chart contains rows of letters in various sizes, with standardised numbers at the end of each row. The number at the end of the row indicates the visual acuity of a person who can read the row at a distance of 6 metres. If the person is unable to read or does not read English, use the E chart to test visual acuity. The top number at the end of the row is always 6, representing the distance between the person and the chart. The bottom number is the distance (in metres) at which a person with normal vision can read the line. A person with normal vision can read the row marked 6/6. To conduct the assessment, ask the person to stand 6 metres from the chart in a well-lit area. Ask the person to cover one eye with an opaque cover or with the palm of their hand (see Figure 44.6). Then ask the person to read each row of letters, moving from largest letters to the smallest ones that the person can see. Measure visual acuity in the other eye the same way and then assess visual acuity while the person has both eyes uncovered. You may test the person who wears corrective lenses with and without the lenses.

The Rosenbaum chart is held at a distance of from 30 to 35 cm from the eyes, with visual acuity measured in the same manner as with the Snellen chart (see Figure 44.7). A gross estimate of near vision may also be assessed by asking the person to read from a magazine or newspaper.

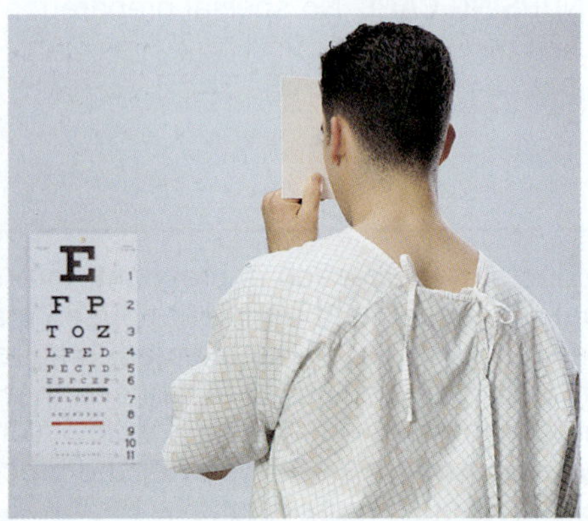

FIGURE 44.6 *Testing distant vision using the Snellen eye chart*

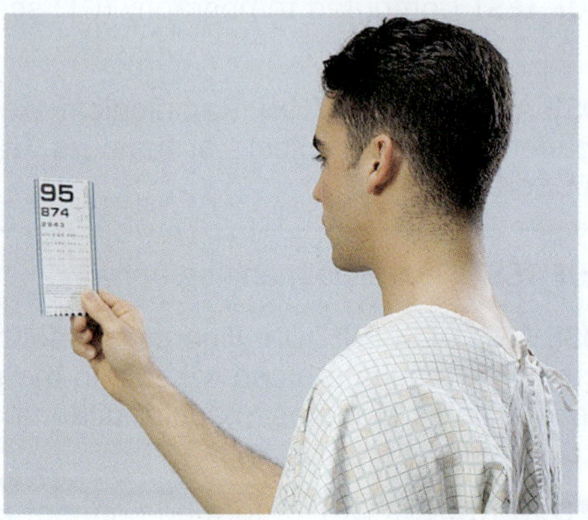

FIGURE 44.7 *Testing near vision using Rosenbaum eye chart*

Technique/normal findings	Abnormal findings
Vision	
Assess distant vision using the Snellen or E chart. *When standing 6 metres from the chart, the person can read the smallest line of letters with or without corrective lenses (recorded as 6/6).*	▪ Changes in distant vision are most commonly the result of **myopia** (nearsightedness). For example, a reading of 6/9 indicates impaired distance vision. A person has to stand 6 metres from the chart to read a line that a person with normal vision could read 9 metres from the chart.
Assess near vision, using a Rosenbaum chart or a card with newsprint held 30 to 35 cm from the person's eyes. *Normal near visual acuity is 35/35 with or without corrective lenses.*	▪ Changes in near vision, especially in people over age 45, can indicate **presbyopia**, impaired near vision resulting from a loss of elasticity of the lens related to ageing. In younger people, this condition is referred to as **hyperopia** (farsightedness).
Eye movement assessment	
Assess the cardinal fields of vision to gain information about extraocular eye movements. Ask the person to follow a pen or your finger while keeping the head stationary. Move the pen or your finger through the 6 fields one at a time, returning to the central starting point before proceeding to the next field (see Figure 44.8). *The eyes should move through each field without involuntary movements.*	▪ Failure of one or both eyes to follow the object in any given direction may indicate extraocular muscle weakness or cranial nerve dysfunction. ▪ An involuntary rhythmic movement of the eyes, **nystagmus**, is associated with neurological disorders and the use of some medications.

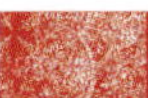

EYE AND VISION ASSESSMENTS (continued)

Technique/normal findings	Abnormal findings
The cover–uncover test is a test for strabismus, a weakening of a muscle that causes one eye to deviate from the other when the person is focusing on an object. To conduct the test, hold a pen or your finger about 300 cm from the eyes and ask the person to focus on that object. Cover one of the person's eyes and note any movement in the uncovered eye; as you remove the cover, assess for movement in the eye that was just uncovered. Repeat the procedure with the other eye. *The uncovered eye should remain fixed straight ahead. The covered eye should remain fixed straight ahead after being uncovered.*	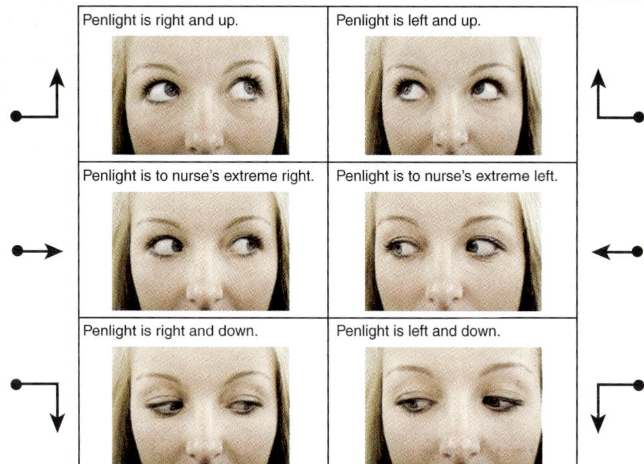 **FIGURE 44.8** ***The six cardinal fields of vision*** *Source*: Michael Heron/Pearson Education, Inc.
Assess convergence. Ask the person to follow an object as you move it towards the person's eyes. *Normally both eyes converge towards the centre.*	■ Failure of the eyes to converge equally on an approaching object may indicate a neuromuscular disorder or improper eye alignment.
Assess the corneal light reflex. Direct a light source onto the bridge of the nose from 30 to 40 cm. *Observe for equal reflection of the light from each eye.*	■ Reflections of the light from different sites on the eyes reveal improper alignment.
Pupils	
Observe pupil size and equality. *Pupils should be of equal size, 3 to 5 mm.*	■ Pupils that are unequal in size may indicate a severe neurological problem, such as increased intracranial pressure.
Assess direct and consensual pupil response. Ask the person to look straight ahead. Shine a light obliquely into one eye at a time. Observe for constriction of the pupil in the illuminated eye. Test both eyes. To test consensual pupil response, again shine a light obliquely into one eye at a time as the person looks straight ahead. Observe constriction of the pupil in the opposite eye. *The normal direct and consensual pupillary response is constriction.*	■ Failure of the pupils to respond to light may indicate degeneration of the retina or destruction of the optic nerve. ■ A person who has one dilated and unresponsive pupil may have paralysis of the oculomotor nerve. ■ Some eye medications may cause unequal dilation, constriction or inequality of pupil size. Morphine and narcotic drugs may cause small, unresponsive pupils and anticholinergic drugs such as atropine may cause dilated, unresponsive pupils.
Test for accommodation. Hold an object at a distance of approximately 600 cm from the person. The pupils should dilate. Ask the person to follow the object as you bring it to within a few centimetres of the person's nose. *The pupils should constrict and converge as they change focus to follow the object.*	■ Failure of accommodation along with lack of pupil response to light may signal a neurological problem. ■ Lack of response to light with appropriate response to accommodation is often seen in people with diabetes.
External eye	
Inspect the eyelids. *Eyelids should be the colour of the person's facial skin, without redness, discharge or drooping. The sclera should not be visible.*	■ Unusual redness or discharge may indicate an inflammatory state due to trauma, allergies or infection. ■ Drooping of one eyelid, called **ptosis**, may be the result of a stroke, indicate a neuromuscular disorder or be congenital (see Figure 44.9).

(continued)

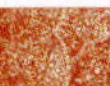

EYE AND VISION ASSESSMENTS (continued)

Technique/normal findings	Abnormal findings
	■ Unusual widening of the lids may be due to exophthalmos (protrusion of the eyeball). Exophthalmos is often associated with hyperthyroid conditions (see the chapter 'Nursing care of people with endocrine disorders'). ■ Yellow plaques noted on or near the lid margins are referred to as xanthelasma and may indicate high lipid levels. ■ An acute localised inflammation of a hair follicle is known as a *hordeolum* (sty) and is generally caused by staphylococcal organisms. ■ A *chalazion* is an infection or retention cyst of the meibomian glands.
Inspect the puncta. *The puncta should be free of redness or discharge.*	■ Unusual redness or discharge from the puncta may indicate an inflammation due to trauma, infection or allergies.
Inspect the bulbar and palpebral conjunctiva. *The conjunctiva should be clear, moist and smooth. The upper and lower palpebral conjunctiva should be clear, without redness or swelling.*	■ Increased erythema or the presence of exudate may indicate acute conjunctivitis. ■ A cobblestone appearance is often associated with allergies. ■ A fold in the conjunctiva, called a *pterygium*, may be seen as a clouded area that extends over the cornea. This is an abnormal growth of the bulbar conjunctiva, usually seen on the nasal side of the cornea. It may interfere with vision if it covers the pupil.
Inspect the sclera. *The sclera is white in Caucasians; people with darker skin normally have yellow sclera.*	■ Unusual redness may indicate an inflammatory state as a result of trauma, allergies or infection. ■ Yellow discolouration of the sclera in people with fair skin may be seen in conditions involving the liver, such as hepatitis. ■ Bright red areas in the sclera are often subconjunctival haemorrhages and may indicate trauma or bleeding disorders. They may also occur spontaneously.
Inspect the cornea. *The cornea is normally transparent.*	■ Dullness, opacities or irregularities of the cornea may be abnormal. ■ *Corneal arcus* is a thin, greyish-white arc seen towards the edge of the cornea. It is normal in older adults.
Assess corneal sensitivity. Lightly touch a wisp of cotton to the person's cornea. *This action should cause a corneal reflex (blinking the eye).*	■ Failure of the corneal reflex may indicate a neurological disorder.
Inspect the iris. *The iris is normally round, flat and evenly coloured.*	■ Lack of clarity of the iris may indicate a cloudiness of the cornea. ■ Constriction of the pupil accompanied by pain and circumcorneal redness indicates acute iritis.
Internal eye	
Assess internal structures of the eye by using the ophthalmoscope, an instrument that allows visualisation of the lens, the vitreous humour and the retina. Box 44.1 provides guidelines for using the ophthalmoscope.	
Inspect for the red reflex. *The red reflex should be clearly visible.*	■ Absence of a red reflex often indicates improper position of the ophthalmoscope, but also may indicate total opacity of the pupil by a cataract or a haemorrhage into the vitreous humour.

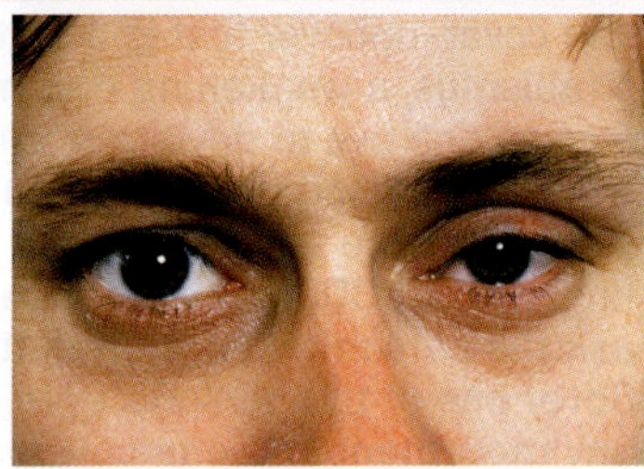

FIGURE 44.9 ***Ptosis***

Source: © Mediscan/Alamy Stock Photo.

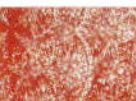

EYE AND VISION ASSESSMENTS (continued)

Technique/normal findings	Abnormal findings
Inspect the lens and vitreous body. *The lens should be clear.*	■ A cataract is an opacity of the lens, often seen as a dark shadow on ophthalmoscopic examination. It may be due to ageing, trauma, diabetes or a congenital defect.
Inspect the retina. *There should be no visible haemorrhages, exudate or white patches.*	■ Areas of haemorrhage, exudate and white patches may be a result of diabetes or long-standing hypertension.
Inspect the optic disc. *The optic disc should be round to oval in shape with clear, well-defined borders.*	■ Loss of definition of the optic disc, as well as an increase in the size of the physiological cup, is seen in papilloedema from increased intracranial pressure.
Inspect the blood vessels of the retina. *The retinal blood vessels should be distinct.*	■ Glaucoma often results in displacement of blood vessels from the centre of the optic disc due to increased intraocular pressure. ■ Hypertension may cause a narrowing of the vein where an arteriole crosses over. ■ Engorged veins may occur with diabetes, atherosclerosis and blood disorders.
Inspect the retinal background. *The retina should be a consistent red-orange colour, becoming lighter around the optic disc.*	■ Variations in colour or a pale colour overall may indicate disease.
Inspect the macula. *The macula should be visible on the temporal side of the optic disc.*	■ Absence of the fovea centralis is common in older adults. It may indicate macular degeneration, a cause of loss of central vision.
Palpate over the lacrimal glands, puncta and nasolacrimal duct. *There should be no tenderness, drainage or excessive tearing.*	■ Tenderness over any of these areas or drainage from the puncta may indicate an infectious process. (Wear gloves if you see any drainage.) ■ Excessive tearing may indicate a blockage of the nasolacrimal duct.

BOX 44.1 Guidelines for using the ophthalmoscope

The ophthalmoscope has a head and a handle (see figure). The head contains a focus wheel (also called a lens selector dial) located on the side, lenses of varying magnification and an opening through which the eye structures are visualised. The focus wheel adjusts the lens refraction, which is measured in diopters. The diopter measurements range from 0 to +40 when the lens is rotated clockwise and from 0 to −25 when the lens is rotated anticlockwise. By moving the focus wheel, the examiner can converge or diverge light rays to visualise the retina. The handle usually contains batteries that can be recharged.

Before the examination, explain the procedure to the person. Assemble the ophthalmoscope. Wash hands and wear disposable gloves if the person has any drainage from the eyes. Darken the room (to allow the pupils of the person to dilate) and ask the person to look straight ahead, focusing on a fixed point such as an object on the wall. Hold the ophthalmoscope in one hand, resting the index finger on the focus wheel (see the figure).

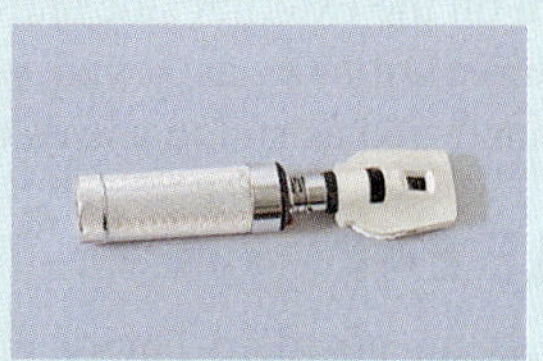

An ophthalmoscope

Source: Pearson Education.

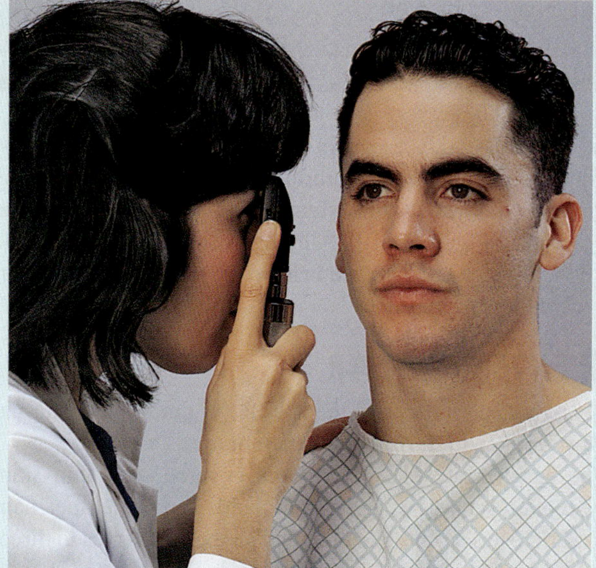

Technique for holding an ophthalmoscope

Source: Pearson Education.

(continued)

BOX 44.1 Guidelines for using the ophthalmoscope (continued)

1. Turn on the ophthalmoscope light and set focus wheel to 0 diopters. Hold the ophthalmoscope in your right hand with your index finger on the focus wheel. Standing in front of the person, position yourself at a 15-degree angle to the person's line of vision.
2. Hold the opening of the ophthalmoscope up to your right eye and direct the light towards the person's right eye from a distance of about 30 cm.
3. As the beam of light falls on the person's pupil, observe for the red reflex which appears as a sharply outlined orange glow from within the pupil. This glow is the reflection of the light from the retina.
4. Move closer to the person, turning the focus wheel clockwise towards the positive numbers as needed to maintain clear focus.
5. Examine the lens and the vitreous body; both should be clear.
6. Gradually rotate the focus wheel anticlockwise towards the negative numbers as needed, focusing on a structure of the retina (such as the disc or a blood vessel). Turn the focus wheel until the image is clear. Examine the structures of the retina as follows:
   a. The optic disc (see the figure). Assess for size, shape, colour, distinct margins and the physiological cup. The disc is round to slightly oval and about 1.5 mm in diameter. It has a yellow to pink colour that is lighter than the retina itself. The margins should be sharp and clear. The physiological cup is a small depression that occupies about one-third of the optic disc, lying temporal to the centre of the disc.
   b. The vessels of the retina. Assess for colour, arteriolar light reflex, ratio of arterioles to veins and arteriovenous crossings. The arterioles are red, brighter than the veins and about one-quarter smaller. The arterioles normally have a narrow light reflex from the centre of each vessel; veins do not have this light reflex. The ratio of arterioles to veins is usually 2:3 or 4:5. The vessels normally cross and become smaller towards the periphery.
   c. The retinal background. Assess colour and changes in colour. The retina is normally reddish orange and regular in colour.
   d. The macula. Assess size and colour. To assess the macula, ask the person to look directly into the ophthalmoscope light. The macula is temporal to the optic disc, appears slightly darker than the retina and has no visible vessels. The fovea centralis may be seen as a bright spot of light. Because looking directly into the light causes some discomfort, conduct this portion of the examination last. The macula is often difficult to visualise.
7. Using the same technique, examine the left eye.

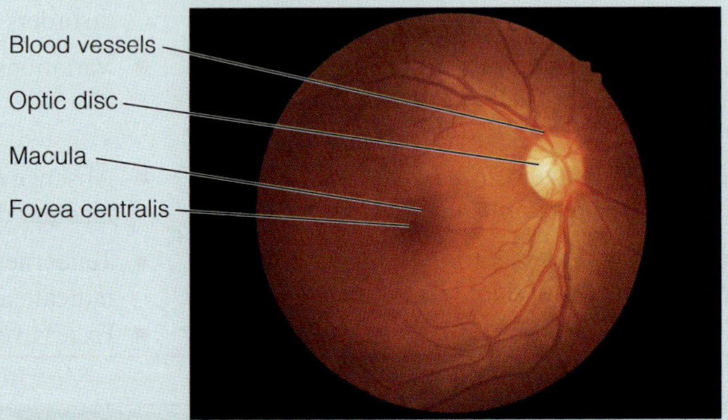

The optic disc as seen through an ophthalmoscope

Source: memorisz/Shutterstock.

Anatomy, physiology and functions of the ears

As a sensory organ, the ears have two primary functions: hearing and maintaining equilibrium. Anatomically, each ear is divided into three areas: the external ear, the middle ear and the inner ear (see Figure 44.10). Although each area has a unique function, all three are involved in hearing, but only the inner ear is involved in equilibrium.

THE EXTERNAL EAR

The external ear consists of the auricle (or pinna), the external auditory canal and the tympanic membrane.

The auricles are elastic cartilage covered with thin skin. They contain sebaceous and sweat glands and sometimes hair. Each auricle has a rim (the helix) and a lobe that serves to direct sound waves into the ear.

The external auditory canal, which is about 2.5 cm long, extends from the auricle to the tympanic membrane. The canal is lined with skin that contains hair, sebaceous and ceruminous glands. The external auditory canal serves as a resonator for the range of sound waves typical of human speech and increases the pressure that sound waves in this frequency range place on the tympanic membrane. The canal's ceruminous glands (modified apocrine glands) secrete a yellow to brown waxy substance called **cerumen** (earwax). Cerumen traps foreign bodies; it also has bacteriostatic properties, protecting the tympanic membrane and the middle ear from infections.

The tympanic membrane lies between the external ear and the middle ear. It is a thin, semi-transparent, fibrous structure covered with skin on the external side and mucosa on the inner side. The membrane vibrates as sound waves strike it; these vibrations are transferred as sound waves to the middle ear.

THE MIDDLE EAR

The middle ear is an air-filled cavity in the temporal bone and contains three auditory ossicles: the malleus, the incus and the stapes. These bones extend across the middle ear. The medial side of the middle ear is a bony wall containing two membrane-covered openings: the oval window and the round window. The posterior wall of the middle ear contains the

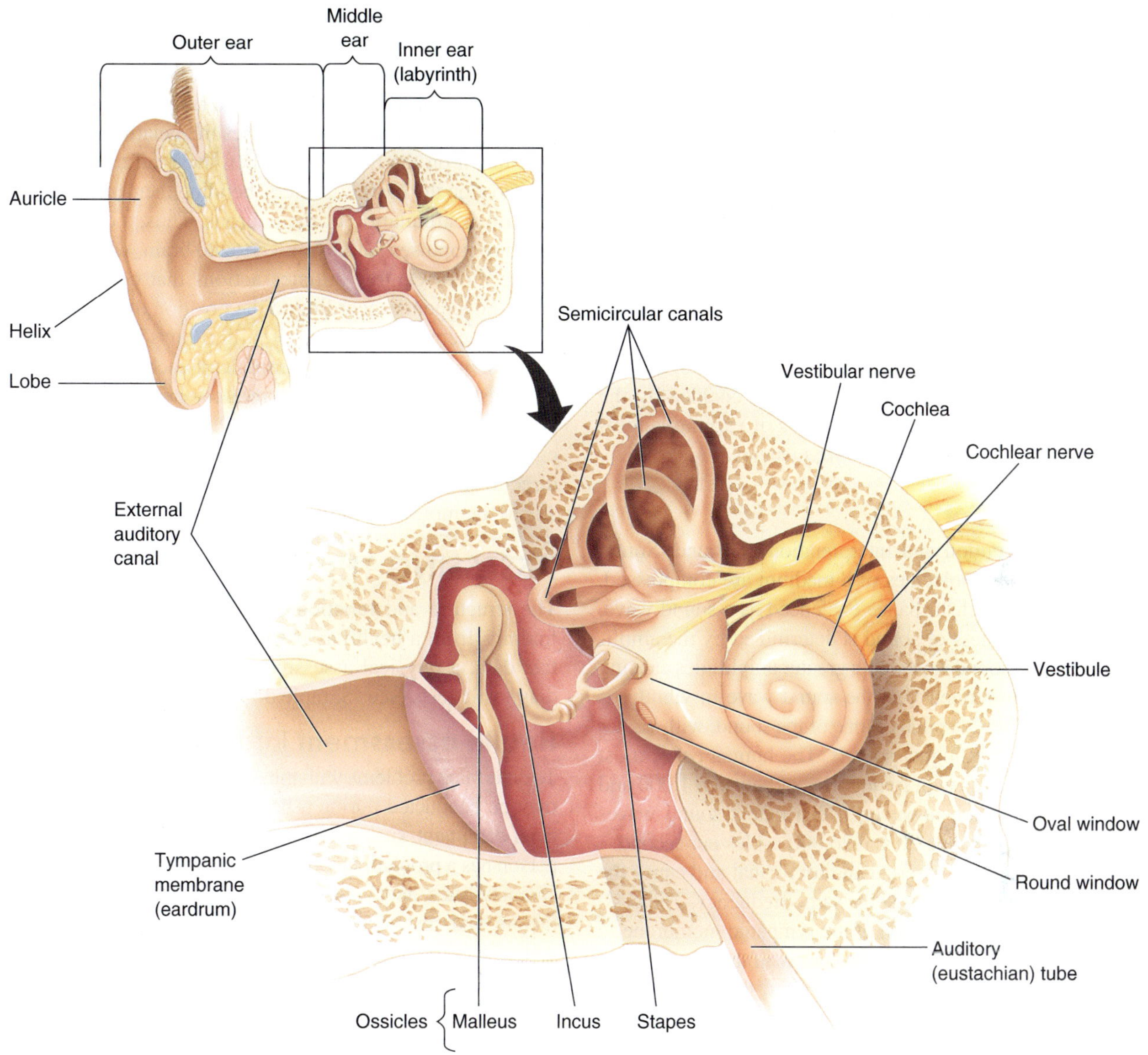

FIGURE 44.10 ***Structures of the external ear, middle ear and inner ear***

Source: © Todd Buck, Pearson Education.

mastoid antrum. This cavity communicates with the mastoid sinuses, which help the middle ear adjust to changes in pressure. It also opens into the eustachian tube, which connects with the nasopharynx. The eustachian tube helps to equalise the air pressure in the middle ear by opening briefly in response to differences between the pressure in the middle ear and atmospheric pressure. This action also ensures that vibrations of the tympanic membrane remain adequate. The mucous membrane lining the middle ear is continuous with the mucous membranes lining the throat.

The malleus attaches to the tympanic membrane and articulates with the incus, which in turn articulates with the stapes. The stapes fits into the oval window. When the tympanic membrane vibrates, the vibrations are conducted across the middle ear to the oval window by the ossicles. The vibrations then set in motion the fluids of the inner ear, which in turn stimulate the hearing receptors. Two small muscles attached to the ossicles contract reflexively in response to sudden loud noises, decreasing the vibrations and protecting the inner ear.

THE INNER EAR

The inner ear, also called the labyrinth, is a maze of bony chambers located deep within the temporal bone, just behind the eye socket. The labyrinth is further divided into two parts: the bony labyrinth, a system of open channels that houses the second part, the membranous labyrinth. The bony labyrinth is filled with a fluid (similar to cerebrospinal fluid) called perilymph, which bathes the membranous labyrinth. Within the chambers of the membranous labyrinth is a fluid called endolymph.

The bony labyrinth has three regions: the vestibule, the semicircular canals and the cochlea. The vestibule is the central portion of the inner ear, one side of which is a bony wall containing the oval window. Two sacs within the vestibule (the saccule and the utricle) join the vestibule with the cochlea and the semicircular canals. The saccule and the utricle contain receptors for equilibrium that respond to changes in gravity and changes in position of the head. The three semicircular canals each project into a different plane (anterior, posterior and lateral). Each canal contains a semicircular duct that communicates with the utricle of the vestibule. Each duct has an enlarged area at one end containing an equilibrium receptor that responds to angular movements of the head.

The cochlea is a tiny bony chamber that houses the organ of Corti, the receptor organ for hearing. The organ of Corti is a series of sensory hair cells, arranged in a single row of inner hair cells and three rows of outer hair cells. The hair cells are innervated by sensory fibres from the VIII (acoustic) cranial nerve. The organ of Corti is supported in the cochlea by the flexible basilar membrane, which has fibres of varying lengths that respond to different sound wave frequencies.

Sound conduction

Hearing is the perception and interpretation of sound. Sound is produced when the molecules of a medium are compressed, resulting in a pressure disturbance evidenced as a sound wave. The intensity or loudness of sound is determined by the amplitude (height) of the sound wave, with greater amplitudes causing louder sounds. The frequency of the sound wave in vibrations per second determines the pitch or tone of the sound, with higher frequencies resulting in higher sounds. The human ear is most sensitive to sound waves with frequencies of between 1,000 and 4,000 cycles per second; however, it can detect sound waves with frequencies of between 20 and 20,000 cycles per second.

Sound waves enter the external auditory canal and cause the tympanic membrane to vibrate at the same frequency. The ossicles not only transmit the motion of the tympanic membrane to the oval window, but also amplify the energy of the sound wave. As the stapes moves against the oval window, the perilymph in the vestibule is set in motion. The increased pressure of the perilymph is transmitted to fibres of the basilar membrane and then to the organ of Corti (directly above the basilar membrane). The up-and-down movements of the fibres of the basilar membrane pull the hair cells in the organ of Corti, which in turn generates action potentials that are transmitted to the VIII (acoustic) cranial nerve and then to the brain for interpretation.

Several brainstem auditory nuclei transmit impulses to the cerebral cortex. Fibres from each ear cross, with each auditory cortex receiving impulses from both ears. Auditory processing is so finely tuned that a wide variety of sounds of different pitch and loudness can be heard at any one time. In addition, the source of the sound can be localised.

Equilibrium

The inner ear also provides information about the position of the head. This information is used to coordinate body movements so that equilibrium and balance are maintained. The types of equilibrium are static balance (affected by changes in the position of the head) and dynamic balance (affected by the movement of the head).

Receptors called maculae in the utricle and the saccule of the vestibule detect changes in the position of the head. Maculae are groups of hair cells that have protrusions covered with a gelatinous substance. Embedded in this gelatinous substance are tiny particles of calcium carbonate called otoliths (ear stones), which make the gelatin heavier than the endolymph that fills the membranous labyrinth. As a result, when the head is in the upright position, gravity causes the gelatinous substance to bear down on the hair cells. When the head changes position, the force on the hair cells alters, bending them and changing the pattern of stimulation of the neurons. Thus, a different pattern of nerve impulses is transmitted to the brain, where stimulation of the motor centres initiates actions that coordinate various body movements according to the position of the head.

The receptor for dynamic equilibrium is in the crista, a crest in the membrane lining the ampulla of each semicircular canal. The cristae are stimulated by rotatory head movement (acceleration and deceleration) as a result of changes in the flow of endolymph and of movement of hair cells in the maculae. The direction of endolymph and hair cell movement is always opposite to the motion of the body.

ASSESSING THE EARS

The structure and functions of the ears are assessed through findings from a health assessment interview to collect subjective data, a physical assessment to collect objective data and diagnostic tests (see 'Sample documentation').

Health assessment interview

To determine problems with the ear, a health assessment interview may be conducted during a health screening. It may focus on a chief complaint, such as hearing problems or pain in the ear. If the person has a problem involving one or both ears, analyse its onset, characteristics and course, severity, precipitating and relieving factors, and any associated symptoms, noting the timing and circumstances. For example, the following questions may be asked:

- Have you noticed any difficulty hearing high-pitched sounds, low-pitched sounds, or both?
- When did you first notice the ringing in your ears?
- Is your workplace very noisy? If so, do you wear protective ear equipment at work?

SAMPLE DOCUMENTATION

Assessment of the ear

25/9/2023 NURS 0930 hrs	22-year-old male complaining of 'having some problems hearing these days'. States he often listens to music in his car 'as loud as it will go' and uses ear phones at home so as not to bother other family members. Ears are placed bilaterally; skin smooth without lesions. Small amount of dark brown cerumen present in both ear canals. Tympanic membranes grey and shiny. No bulging or retraction noted. Whisper test: unable to repeat back words spoken by examiner. Weber's test: sound lateralised to left ear. Rinne test: BC $\geq$ AC. No tenderness noted when mastoids palpated. Referred to ear clinic for further evaluation. ________________ O Fehon (OLIVIA FEHON, RN)

Throughout the examination, be alert to non-verbal behaviours, such as inappropriate answers or requests to repeat statements that may suggest problems with ear function. Explore changes in hearing, ringing in the ears (*tinnitus*), ear pain and drainage from the ears or the use of hearing aids. When taking a medical history, ask about trauma, surgery or infections of the ear, as well as the date of the last ear examination. In addition, ask the person about a history of infectious diseases, such as meningitis or mumps, as well as the use of medications that may affect hearing. Because ear problems tend to run in families, ask about a family history of hearing loss, ear problems or diseases. If the person has a hearing aid, ascertain the type and assess measures for its care.

Interview questions categorised by functional health patterns are found in the 'Functional health pattern interview' table.

Physical assessment of the ears and hearing

Physical assessment of the ears and hearing may be performed as part of a total health assessment or separately for people with known or suspected problems with the ears. The ears and hearing are assessed primarily through inspection of external structures through palpation, the external auditory canal and the tympanic membrane. Disorders of the middle ear may be identified with tympanometry and hearing acuity is assessed by

FUNCTIONAL HEALTH PATTERN INTERVIEW The ear

FUNCTIONAL HEALTH PATTERN	INTERVIEW QUESTIONS AND LEADING STATEMENTS
Health perception–Health management	■ Describe your hearing. Rate it on a scale of 1 to 10, with 10 being excellent hearing. Is it the same in both ears? If not, which ear is better?
	■ Describe any current hearing problems. How have these been treated?
	■ Do you use ear medications? What type, dosage and how often?
	■ Have you ever had ear surgery? Provide details.
	■ Describe the type of hearing aid that you use. Are you satisfied with this appliance? How do you care for it?
	■ Describe how you care for your ears each day.
	■ Have you ever had your hearing tested? When was your last ear examination?
	■ Do you listen to loud music? Do you use ear phones when you listen to loud music?
Nutritional–Metabolic	■ Do you have any swelling or tenderness in the ears or drainage from the ears?
Activity–Exercise	■ Does your hearing problem interfere with your usual activities of daily living? Provide details.
	■ Do you wear protective earplugs when you take part in activities that increase the risk of injury to your ears (such as at work or when operating machinery)?
Sleep–Rest	■ Does your ear problem interfere with your ability to rest or sleep (e.g. pain)? If so, what do you do?
Cognitive–Perceptual	■ Do you have pain in or around your ears? Have you ever had ringing in your ears? If so, describe its location, intensity, what makes it worse and how long it lasts. How do you treat it?
	■ Do you have difficulty hearing conversations, either in person or on the telephone? Do you have trouble hearing the television? Do you have difficulty hearing when you are in crowds or there is background noise?
	■ Have you noticed your hearing is different in each ear?
	■ Do you have buzzing, ringing or crackling noises in one or both ears? Provide details.
	■ Do you ever feel dizzy?
Self-perception–Self-concept	■ Has this problem with your ears affected how you feel about yourself?
Role–Relationships	■ How has having this condition affected your relationships with others?
	■ Has having this condition interfered with your ability to work? Provide details.
	■ Has anyone in your family had problems with ear disease? Provide details.
Sexuality–Reproductive	■ Has this condition interfered with your usual sexual activity?
Coping–Stress–Tolerance	■ Has having this condition created stress for you? If so, does your health problem seem to be more difficult when you are stressed?
	■ Have you experienced any kind of stress that makes the condition worse? Provide details.
	■ Describe what you do when you feel stressed.
Value–Belief	■ Describe how specific relationships or activities help you cope with this problem.
	■ Describe specific cultural beliefs or practices that affect how you care for and feel about this problem.
	■ Are there any specific treatments that you would not use to treat this problem?

TABLE 44.2 Age-related changes in the ear

AGE-RELATED CHANGE	SIGNIFICANCE
The inner ear:	
• Loss of hair cells, ↓ blood supply, less flexible basilar membrane, degeneration of spiral ganglion cells and ↓ production of endolymph result in progressive hearing loss with age (presbycusis). • High-frequency sounds are lost; middle- and low-frequency sounds may also be lost or decreased. • Vestibular structures degenerate, organ of Corti and cochlea atrophy.	Older adults may require hearing aids to hear well. With loss of high-frequency sounds, speech may be distorted, contributing to a risk of problems with communication. Degeneration and atrophy of inner ear structures concerned with balance and equilibrium increase the risk of falls.
The middle ear:	
• Muscles and ligaments weaken and stiffen, decreasing the acoustic reflex.	Own speech and sounds are louder and may further interfere with hearing, speech and communications.
The external ear:	
• Increased cerumen in the ear canal is due to its high keratin content.	Accumulated cerumen may impair hearing.

voice and tuning fork tests. Normal age-related findings for the older adult are summarised in Table 44.2.

Prior to the assessment, collect all necessary equipment and explain the techniques to the person to decrease anxiety. During the assessment, the person should be sitting and the examiner's head should be level with the head of the person. The auditory canal and tympanic membrane are inspected with the otoscope. Guidelines for use of the otoscope are listed in Box 44.2.

BOX 44.2 Guidelines for using the otoscope

The otoscope has a handle that contains batteries for the light and various specula that fit on to the handle (see figure). It is used to inspect the auditory canal and the tympanic membrane. A pneumatic otoscope is used to determine the mobility of the tympanic membrane. It has an attached rubber bulb that can be squeezed to inject air into the auditory canal, causing a normal tympanic membrane to move in and out.

Before the examination, explain the procedure. Assemble the otoscope using the largest speculum that will fit into the person's auditory canal without discomfort. Wash your hands; wear disposable gloves if the person has any drainage from the ears. Turn on the otoscope light. Ask the person to tip the head slightly towards the shoulder opposite the ear being examined. When they are in this position, the auditory canal is aligned with the speculum.

1. Hold the handle of the otoscope in your dominant hand. If the person is restless, hold the otoscope handle upward, resting the hand against the person's head. If the person is cooperative, hold the handle downward.
2. For adults, grasp the superior portion of the auricle and pull up, out and back to straighten the auditory canal (see figure).
3. Insert the speculum into the ear and advance it gently. Assess the walls of the auditory canal while advancing the speculum, inspecting for colour, obstructions, hair growth and cerumen. Old cerumen is very dark and may obstruct visualisation of part or all of the tympanic membrane.
4. Move the otoscope so that you can see the tympanic membrane. You may need to realign the auditory canal by gently continuing to pull up and back on the auricle. A normal membrane is semi-transparent, allowing visualisation of a

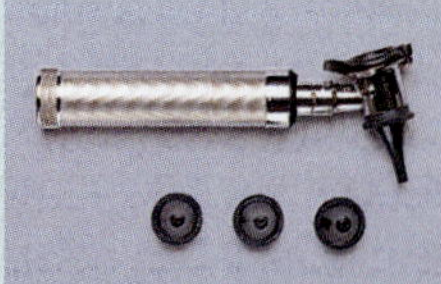

An otoscope

Source: Pearson Education.

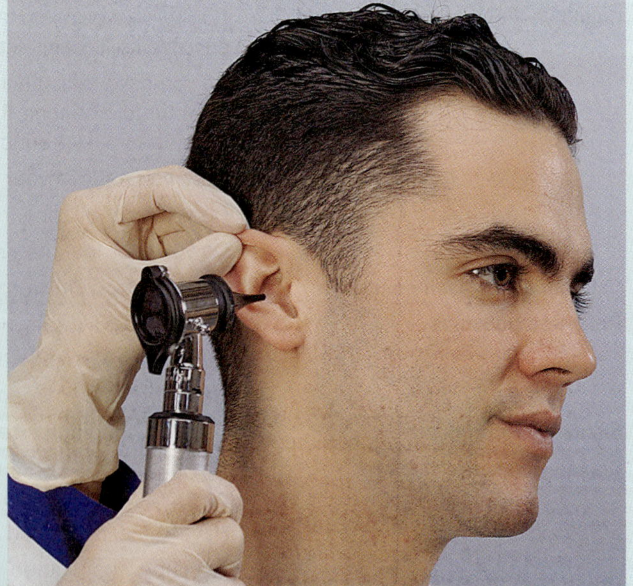

Technique for using an otoscope

BOX 44.2 Guidelines for using the otoscope (continued)

portion of the auditory ossicles. The concave nature of the tympanic membrane and its oblique position in the auditory canal account for the triangular light reflex (cone of light) seen on otoscopic examination.

5. Note the colour and surface of the membrane. The normal tympanic membrane is pearly grey, shiny and semi-transparent. The surface should be continuous, intact and either flat or concave.
6. Identify the landmarks on the tympanic membrane (see figure):
   a. the cone of light, located over the anteroinferior quadrant
   b. the malleus, pars tensa, annulus, pars flaccida and malleolar folds.
7. Assess movement of the tympanic membrane. If the auditory tube is patent, the membrane moves in and out when air is injected or when the person performs the Valsalva manoeuvre.
8. Gently withdraw the speculum. If the speculum is soiled with drainage or cerumen, use a clean speculum for the other ear.
9. Using the same technique, examine the other ear.

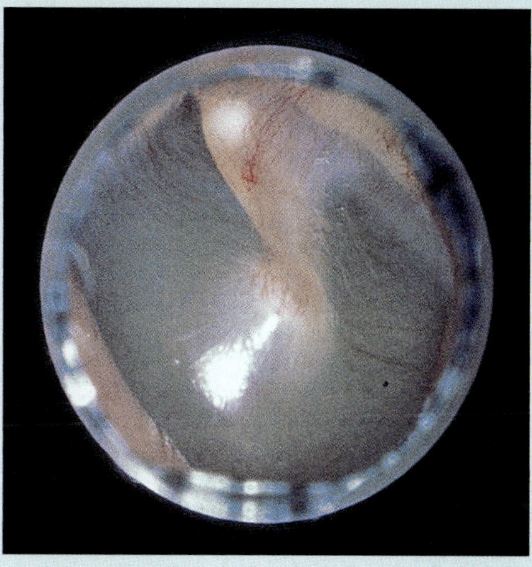

The tympanic membrane as it appears through the otoscope

Source: Pearson Education.

PATIENT SAFETY COMPETENCY FRAMEWORK

5 Clinical reasoning

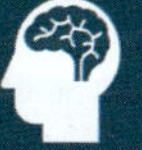

The Patient Safety Competency Framework indicates that nursing students must demonstrate clinical reasoning through the ability to accurately assess, interpret and respond to individual patient data in a systematic and timely way (Levett-Jones et al., 2017).

Diagnostic tests

The results of diagnostic tests of the structure and functions of the ears are used to support the diagnosis of a specific injury, disease or hearing problem; provide information to identify and/or modify the appropriate medications or assistive devices used to treat the disease or problem; and help nurses monitor the person's responses to treatment and nursing care interventions. Diagnostic tests of the ear, especially for hearing, are most often conducted in a healthcare provider's office. Diagnostic tests to assess the structure and functions of the ears are described in the 'Diagnostic tests' table and summarised in the following list. More information is included in the discussion of specific injuries or diseases in the chapter 'Nursing care of people with eye and ear disorders'.

- Audiometry is used to evaluate and diagnose conductive and sensorineural hearing loss.
- Electrical activity of the auditory nerve may be evaluated by using an auditory evoked potential (AEP) or an auditory brainstem response (ABR).
- Vestibular system function is evaluated with a caloric test. If no nystagmus occurs during the test, further testing for brain lesions is conducted.

Regardless of the type of diagnostic test, the nurse may be responsible for explaining the procedure and any special preparation needed, assessing for any medication use that might affect the outcome of the tests, supporting the person during the examination as necessary, documenting the procedures as appropriate and monitoring the results of the tests.

Genetic considerations

When conducting a health assessment interview and a physical assessment, it is important for the nurse to consider genetic influences on the health of the adult as several diseases of the ears have a genetic component. During the health assessment interview, ask about a family history of congenital deafness or deafness associated with a thyroid goitre or with tumours of the auditory nerve.

During the physical assessment, assess for any manifestations that might indicate a genetic disorder (see the 'Genetic considerations' box). If data are found to indicate genetic risk factors or alterations, ask about genetic testing and refer for appropriate genetic counselling and evaluation. The chapter 'Genetic implications of adult health nursing' provides further information about genetics in medical–surgical nursing.

DIAGNOSTIC TESTS Ear disorders

NAME OF TEST Audiometry

PURPOSE AND DESCRIPTION Used to evaluate and diagnose conductive and sensorineural hearing loss. Person sits in soundproof room and responds by raising a hand or pressing a button when sounds are heard.

RELATED NURSING CARE No special preparation is needed.

NAME OF TEST Auditory evoked potential (AEP)

PURPOSE AND DESCRIPTION Used to identify electrical activity of the auditory nerve. Electrodes are placed on various areas of the ear and on the forehead, and a graphic recording is made.

RELATED NURSING CARE No special preparation is needed.

NAME OF TEST Auditory brainstem response (ABR)

PURPOSE AND DESCRIPTION Measures electrical activity of the auditory pathway from inner ear to brain to diagnose brainstem pathology, stroke and acoustic neuroma.

RELATED NURSING CARE No special preparation is needed.

NAME OF TEST Caloric test

PURPOSE AND DESCRIPTION Used to assess vestibular system function. Cold or warm water is used to irrigate the ear canals one at a time and the person is observed for nystagmus (repeated abnormal movements of the eyes). Normally, the nystagmus occurs in the eye opposite to the ear being irrigated. If no nystagmus occurs, the person needs further testing for brain lesions.

RELATED NURSING CARE Assess person for use of alcohol, central nervous system depressants and barbiturates. These chemicals may alter the test results.

GENETIC CONSIDERATIONS Ear disorders

- Deafness (hearing loss) is a common disorder that is seen from newborns to those of old age. About 1 in 1,000 infants have a profound hearing loss, with about half being genetic in origin (National Center for Biotechnology Information, 2022). Early diagnosis is important to facilitate language and social skill development in adults.
- Penred syndrome is an inherited disorder that accounts for as much as 10% of hereditary deafness. The deafness is usually accompanied by a thyroid goitre.
- Neurofibromatosis, a rare inherited disorder, is characterised by the development of acoustic neuromas (benign tumours of the auditory nerve) and malignant central nervous system tumours.

EAR AND HEARING ASSESSMENTS

Hearing assessment

Tuning forks are used to determine whether hearing loss is conductive or perceptive (sensorineural). Hold the tuning fork at the base and make it ring softly by stroking the prongs or by lightly tapping them on the heel of the opposite hand. The vibrating tuning fork emits sound waves of a particular frequency, measured in hertz (Hz). Tuning forks with a frequency of 512 to 1024 Hz are preferred for auditory evaluation because that range corresponds to the range of normal speech.

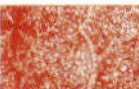

EAR AND HEARING ASSESSMENTS (continued)

Technique/normal findings	Abnormal findings
Perform the Weber test. Place the base of a vibrating tuning fork on the midline vertex of the person's head (see Figure 44.11). Ask whether the person hears the sound equally in both ears or better in one than the other. *Sound is normally heard equally in both ears.*	■ Sound heard in, or lateralised to, one ear indicates either a conductive loss in that ear or a sensorineural loss in the other ear. The sound will be louder on the impaired side with conductive hearing loss. Conductive losses may be due to a build up of cerumen, an infection such as otitis media or perforation of the eardrum. The sound will be softer on the impaired side, suggesting sensorineural hearing loss. 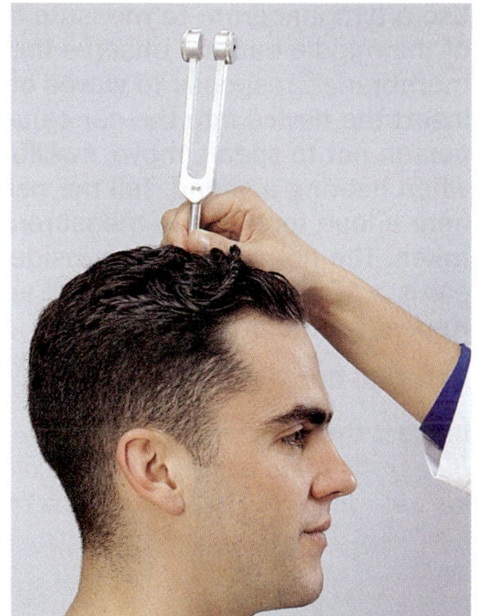 **FIGURE 44.11** ***Performing the Weber test with a tuning fork*** *Source*: Pearson Education.
Perform the Rinne test. Place the base of a vibrating tuning fork on the person's mastoid bone. Ask the person to indicate when the sound is no longer heard. When the person does so, quickly reposition the tuning fork in front of the person's ear close to the ear canal. Ask whether the person can hear the sound. If the person says yes, ask the person to indicate when the sound is no longer heard. Repeat over the opposite mastoid bone (see Figure 44.12). *The person with no conductive hearing loss will hear the sound twice as long by air conduction as by bone conduction.*	■ Bone conduction is greater than air conduction in the ear with a conductive loss. The normal pattern is air conduction greater than bone conduction (AC > BC). 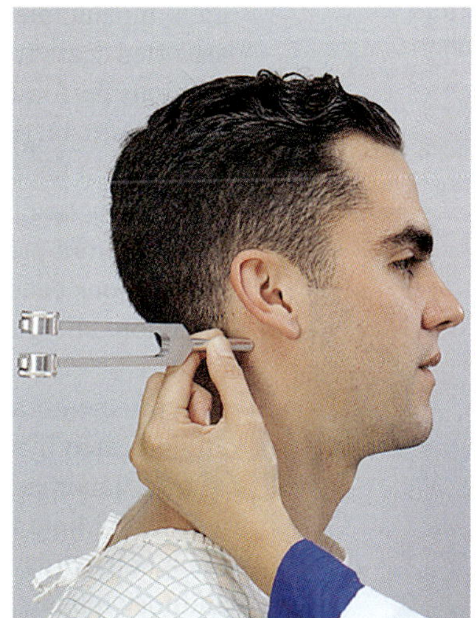 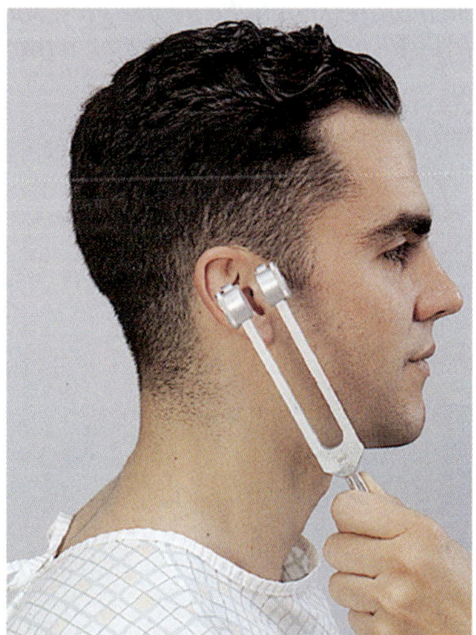 **FIGURE 44.12** ***Performing the Rinne test with a tuning fork*** *Source*: Pearson Education.
Perform the whisper test. Ask the person to occlude one ear with a finger. Stand 30–60 cm away from the person, on the side of the opposite ear. Softly whisper numbers and ask the person to repeat them. Repeat the procedure, having the person occlude the other ear. Note whether you need to raise your voice or to stand closer to make the person hear you.	■ This test provides a rough estimate of hearing loss.

(continued)

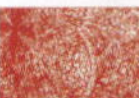

EAR AND HEARING ASSESSMENTS (continued)

Technique/normal findings	Abnormal findings
Use a tympanogram to measure the pressure of the middle ear and observe the tympanic membrane's response to waves of pressure. Insert the device into the ear canal. Ask the person not to speak, move, swallow or jump when hearing a sound. Tell the person they will hear a loud tone as the measurements are taken. The normal pressure inside the middle ear is a 100 daPa (a very small amount). Repeat for the other ear.	■ Abnormal findings may include fluid in the middle ear, a perforated eardrum, impacted earwax or a tumour of the middle ear.
External ear	
Inspect the auricle. *External ears are normally bilaterally equal in size, of equal colour with the person's face, and without redness or lesions.*	■ Unusual redness or drainage may indicate an inflammatory response to infection or trauma. ■ Scales or skin lesions around the rim of the auricle may indicate skin cancer. ■ Small, raised lesions on the rim of the ear are known as tophi and indicate gout.
Inspect the external auditory canal with the otoscope. *Canal walls should be pink and smooth without lesions. Cerumen is normally present in small, odourless amounts.*	■ Unusual redness, lesions or purulent drainage may indicate an infection. ■ Cerumen varies in colour and texture, but hardened, dry or foul-smelling cerumen may indicate an infection or an impaction of cerumen that requires removal. People with darker skin tend to have darker cerumen.
Inspect the tympanic membrane. *The tympanic membrane should be pearly grey, shiny and translucent without bulging or retraction.*	■ White, opaque areas on the tympanic membrane are often scars from previous perforations (see Figure 44.13). ■ Inconsistent texture and colour may be due to scarring from previous perforations caused by infection, allergies or trauma. ■ Bulging membranes are indicated by a loss of bony landmarks and a distorted light reflex. Such bulges may be the result of otitis media or malfunctioning auditory tubes. ■ Retracted tympanic membranes are indicated by accentuated bony landmarks and a distorted light reflex. Such retraction is often due to an obstructed auditory tube.
Palpate the auricles and over each mastoid process. *There should be no pain or swelling on palpation.*	■ Tenderness, swelling or nodules may indicate inflammation of the external auditory canal or mastoiditis.

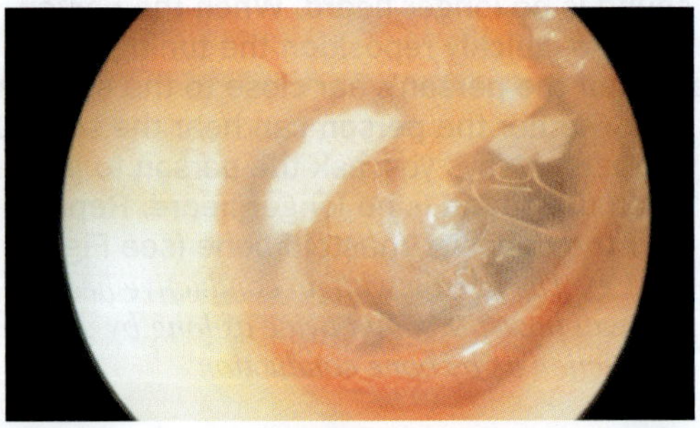

FIGURE 44.13 ***Scarring of the tympanic membrane***

Source: Professor Tony Wright/Inst. of Laryngology & Otology/Science Photo Library/Alamy Stock Photo.

CONCEPT CHECK

1 During an eye assessment, you touch the part of the eye covering the iris and pupil. What normal response would you expect?
1 excess tearing
2 blinking of eyelids
3 bilateral nystagmus
4 pupil dilates

2 Which of the following statements would indicate a person has presbyopia?
1 'I am having so much trouble hearing music.'
2 'I can't seem to remember anything these days.'
3 'I think I have a lot of earwax in my ears.'
4 'My arms don't seem long enough for reading.'

3 What equipment would be necessary to test sound conduction during an assessment of the ear?
1 ophthalmoscope
2 tuning fork
3 otoscope
4 penlight

4 What occurs when light enters the lens of the eye?
1 accommodation
2 convergence
3 pupillary reflex
4 hyperopia

5 What would you tell a person before a test of refraction is done?
1 'This test is uncomfortable, but it doesn't take long.'
2 'You will be blindfolded during the test.'
3 'Are you allergic to seafood?'
4 'Your pupils will be dilated for several hours.'

6 Which function, in addition to hearing, is provided by the inner ear?
1 Coordinates visual pathways.
2 Integrates efferent neuron messages.
3 Provides information about head position.
4 Maintains middle ear structure and function.

7 Why is the Snellen eye chart used during vision assessment?
1 to test distant vision
2 to test near vision
3 to determine visual fields
4 to examine convergence

8 Of the following ear assessments, which one is a rough estimate of the ability to hear?
1 whisper test
2 Rinne test
3 Weber test
4 audiometry

9 What is a high-priority risk for the older adult with age-related changes in the vestibular structures of the ear?
1 infection
2 falls
3 medication errors
4 food intolerance

10 Which criterion is important to accurately assess visual fields?
1 Person must wear corrective lenses.
2 Person must have no less than 6/9 vision.
3 Examiner must not wear glasses.
4 Examiner must have normal visual field.

BIBLIOGRAPHY

Centre for Eye Research in Australia (2022). *Glaucoma*. Retrieved from https://www.cera.org.au/

Levett-Jones, T., Dwyer, T., Reid-Searl, K., Heaton, L., Flenady, T., Applegarth, J., Guinea, S. & Andersen, P. (2017). *Patient Safety Competency Framework (PSCF) for Nursing Students*. Sydney. Retrieved from http://psframework.wpengine.com/

National Center for Biotechnology Information (2022). *Genes and disease*. National Center for Biotechnology Information (US). Retrieved from https://www.ncbi.nlm.nih.gov/

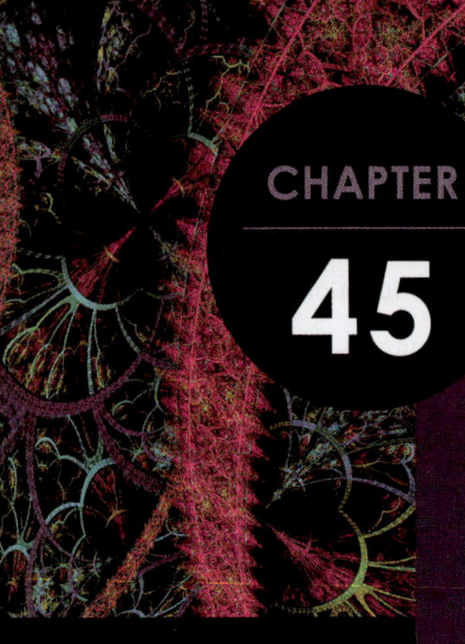

CHAPTER 45

Nursing care of people with eye and ear disorders

Kamaree Houlis-Berry

Key terms

acoustic neuroma 1709
astigmatism 1675
cataract 1683
chalazion 1680
conjunctivitis 1672
corneal ulcer 1675
diabetic retinopathy 1694
enophthalmos 1681
enucleation 1697
glaucoma 1685
hordeolum (sty) 1679
hyperopia 1675
hyphaema 1681
keratitis 1675
labyrinthitis 1706
macular degeneration 1693
mastoiditis 1703
Ménière's disease 1706
myringotomy 1702
otitis externa 1698
otitis media 1701
otosclerosis 1705
presbycusis 1710
retinal detachment 1695
tinnitus 1698
trachoma 1673
tympanoplasty 1704
vertigo 1701

Learning outcomes

- Relate knowledge of normal anatomy, physiology and sensory functions of the eye and ear to the effects of disorders of these organs on the cognitive/perceptual functional health pattern.
- Describe the pathophysiology of commonly occurring disorders of the eyes and ears, relating their manifestations to the pathophysiological process.
- Explain the risk factors for selected disorders of the eyes and ears, identifying the nursing implications for these risk factors.
- Identify diagnostic tests used for specific eye and ear disorders.
- Discuss the effects of and nursing implications for medications prescribed to treat eye and ear disorders.
- Describe surgical and other invasive procedures used to treat eye and ear disorders, identifying their implications for nursing care.
- Discuss the nurse's role in caring for a person with impaired vision or hearing loss.

Clinical competencies

- Assess vision, hearing and functional health of people with eye and ear disorders.
- Using assessed data, determine priority nursing interventions and care for people with eye and ear disorders.
- Collaborate with other members of the healthcare team to provide effective care for people with eye and ear disorders.
- Plan and implement appropriate and individualised evidence-based nursing interventions and education for the person with an eye or ear disorder.
- Safely and effectively administer eye and ear medications and prescribed treatments.
- Provide appropriate care and education for the person having eye or ear surgery.
- Evaluate the effectiveness of nursing care provided for people with eye and ear disorders and revise the plan of care as indicated.

Vision and hearing provide the primary means of input for much of what we know about the world. The ability to receive and organise information orients us to our surroundings. These senses allow us to communicate easily, gain access to information and derive pleasure from the sights and sounds of the world around us.

This chapter discusses conditions affecting vision and hearing as the result of eye and ear disorders. Nursing care focuses on people with vision and hearing deficits that can result from the disorders presented.

Eye disorders

Any portion of the eye and its protective structures may be affected by an acute or a chronic condition. While many disorders of the eye are minor and have little or no effect on vision, others can and often do result in permanent vision impairment. Disorders and diseases of the outer, visible portion of the eye often cause discomfort and may have cosmetic effects. Vision impairment can often be prevented or reversed with appropriate treatment.

Disorders affecting the internal structures or the function of the eye are more likely to have adverse effects on vision (e.g. disorders of the cornea present the greatest risk to vision in this group) and are more likely to affect adults over the age of 40 and the older adult. The person who has had eye surgery or minor trauma may experience either temporary or permanent vision impairment.

Although disorders that commonly affect vision cannot often be prevented or cured, some can be controlled with vision corrected to normal or near normal. Regardless of the real threat a disorder poses to vision, the person may experience anxiety related to a perceived threat. The nursing care box discusses major causes of significantly impaired vision and nursing care for the person who is blind. These principles of nursing care may apply to people with many of the disorders discussed in this chapter.

PATIENT SAFETY COMPETENCY FRAMEWORK

5 Clinical reasoning

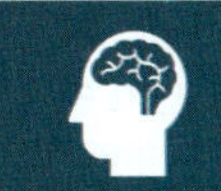

The Patient Safety Competency Framework indicates that nursing students must demonstrate clinical reasoning through the ability to accurately assess, interpret and respond to individual patient data in a systematic and timely way (Levett-Jones et al., 2017).

NURSING CARE OF THE PERSON who is blind

Vision impairment exists on a continuum from blindness to decreased visual acuity that can be corrected with refractive lenses, to normal or near normal vision. *Vision impairment* is defined as 6/12 vision in the better eye, even with corrective lenses. The legal definition of *blindness* is visual acuity no better than 6/60 in the better eye with optimal correction or a visual field of less than 20 degrees in diameter (compared to the normal of 180 degrees) (Vision Australia, 2022). Total blindness usually indicates that the person has no light perception at all. In practical terms, a person with a visual deficit sufficient to need assistive devices or aid from other people for normal activities of daily living is considered blind.

According to the World Health Organization (2021), there are 2.2 billion people worldwide with vision impairment. Although blindness often can be prevented or cured, it remains a significant problem worldwide because of lack of access to care, fear of surgery or treatment, poor sanitation and nutrition, and ignorance of need. In Australia, cataracts, age-related macular degeneration, glaucoma and diabetic retinopathy remain significant causes of blindness in adults.

NURSING CARE

Blind people need to cope not only with the loss of a major sense but often also with societal attitudes that may make them feel inferior, helpless and inadequate. The idea of losing the ability to see is uniformly feared, leaving sighted people often unable to understand the magnitude and impact of the loss in those who have experienced it. Because of this fear and confusion, sighted people are unsure of what the blind expect from them.

The adjustment of the person who is born blind and raised to become an independent member of society differs from that of the person who has been sighted and becomes blind. The person who has been blind from birth has developed numerous adaptive strategies that the newly blind person has yet to learn.

Although adaptation may be easier for the person who experiences a gradual loss of vision than for someone with an abrupt loss, both grieve the lost sense. The blind person needs to grieve the lost body part as well as the loss of mobility, self-sufficiency, perhaps economic security and, to a certain extent, contact with reality as it has previously been perceived. The person's self-concept and self-esteem are threatened. Anger, denial, remorse and self-pity are not uncommon in the initial period following loss of sight. Interpersonal relationships and roles are affected and communication patterns change with the loss of the ability to perceive many non-verbal cues. In addition, expressions of sexuality may be impaired.

(continued)

NURSING CARE OF THE PERSON who is blind (continued)

Acceptance of the change from sighted to blind is characterised by releasing the hope that vision will be regained. Self-esteem increases as the person attempts and masters activities of self-sufficiency such as completing ADLs, cooking and becoming mobile outside the known home environment.

Health professionals often confuse the blind person with someone helpless, dependent and lacking in personal identity and control. Although nurses need to take blindness into account in planning care and maintaining the person's safety, it is vital to give the blind person the same respect and decision-making control and power that all people deserve. Nurses who have dealt with their own emotions and responses to vision loss are better prepared to help the person adapt.

Nurses can foster independence in the hospitalised person with a significant vision deficit by carrying out the following:

- Orientation to the environment verbally and physically. Describe the room using a central point such as the bed, then lead the person around the room, identifying chairs, sink, bathroom and other landmarks. Be sure that objects such as chairs, personal items and clothing remain in the same place unless moved by the person. Leave doors either fully open or closed as the person requests but preserve safety by not leaving doors partially open. Keep the room and hallways free of clutter.
- Use verbal communication freely. Introduce yourself as you enter the room and let the person know when you are leaving, and describe activities going on around the person.
- Provide other sensory stimuli such as radio and television, as desired by the person.
- Orient to food trays by using the face of a clock to describe the position of food items on the plate and tray (unless the person has always been blind and cannot visualise a clock face).
- When assisting with ambulation, allow the person to hold your arm as you walk slightly ahead. Do not hold the person's arm. Verbally describe the environment; for example: 'There will be two steps up 1.5 metres ahead.'
- Do not hesitate to ask what assistance the person desires.

For the person with a new loss of sight, refer to available services. Counselling can help the person cope with and eventually adapt to the loss of sight. People who are blind can receive mobility training, assistance with relearning self-care activities, education in the use of Braille to communicate and vocational and other forms of rehabilitation. Local, state and national agencies such as the Association for the Blind, state and territory guide dog associations, Seeing Eye Dogs Australia, Australian Braille Authority, Vision Australia, Blind Welfare Association and Blind Citizens Australia coordinate services for the blind. They provide many assistive devices, including guide dogs, computer services, talking books and tape players, and low-vision aids.

FAST FACTS

- In 2016, more than 453,000 Australians were blind or vision impaired (Vision 2020 Australia, 2018). As the population in Australia ages, the number of people who are blind or have vision loss is expected to be over 800,000 by 2020 (Vision Initiative, 2020).
- The economic impact of vision impairment in Australia has been estimated at $9.85 billion. Vision disorder direct spending costs are more than the combined costs associated with stroke, arthritis and depression (Australian Institute of Health and Welfare (AIHW), 2020).
- Over the past 4 years, the Australian Government has committed $58 billion to deal with chronic ear and eye conditions in Indigenous Australians. The prevalence of blindness and vision impairment is three times higher in Indigenous Australians than in the general population (AIHW, 2021) (see Table 45.1).

TABLE 45.1 Eye conditions causing vision impairment in the Australian population

CONDITION	NON-INDIGENOUS	INDIGENOUS
Aged-related macular degeneration	9%	1%
Diabetic retinopathy	1.5%	5.5%
Glaucoma	1.5%	0.5%
Cataract	14%	20%
Uncorrected refractive error	62%	63%
Other	12%	10%

THE PERSON WITH CONJUNCTIVITIS

The conjunctiva—the thin, transparent membrane that covers the anterior surface of the eye and lines the inner surfaces of the eyelids—is vulnerable to inflammation and infection because of its constant exposure to the environment. **Conjunctivitis**, inflammation of the conjunctiva, is the most common eye disease caused by a bacterial or viral infection. These infections can be transmitted to the eye by direct contact (e.g. hands, tissues, towels). Allergens, chemical irritants and exposure to radiant energy such as ultraviolet light from the sun or tanning devices can also lead to this common condition. Its severity can range from mild irritation with redness and tearing to conjunctival oedema, haemorrhage or a severe necrotising process with tissue destruction.

Pathophysiology and manifestations

Acute conjunctivitis

Infectious conjunctivitis may be bacterial, viral or fungal in origin. Bacterial conjunctivitis, also known as 'pink eye', is highly contagious and often is caused by *Staphylococcus* and *Haemophilus*. Adenovirus infection is the leading cause of conjunctivitis in adults. Systemic infections that may affect the eyes include herpes simplex and other viral infections. Contact with genital secretions infected with *Gonococcus* can cause gonococcal conjunctivitis, a medical emergency that can lead to corneal perforation.

Redness and itching of the affected eye are common manifestations of acute conjunctivitis (see Figure 45.1). The person may also complain of a scratchy, burning or gritty sensation.

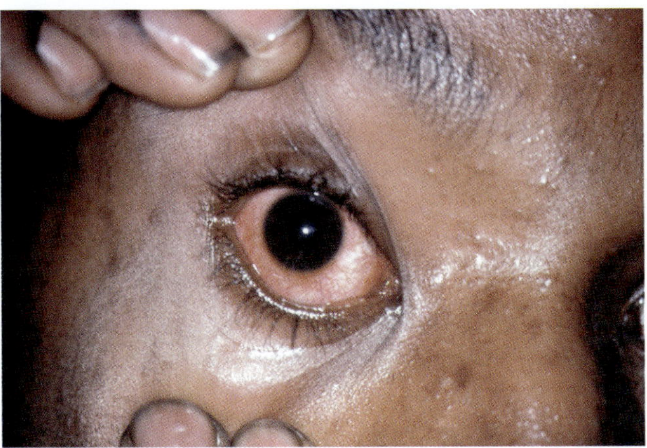

FIGURE 45.1 ***The appearance of an eye with conjunctivitis***

Source: CDC/Joe Miller, VD.

Pain is not common; however, photophobia may occur. Tearing and discharge accompany the inflammatory process. The discharge may be watery, purulent or mucoid, depending on the cause of conjunctivitis. The person may have associated manifestations such as pharyngitis, fever, malaise and swollen pre-auricular lymph nodes.

Trachoma

Trachoma, a chronic conjunctivitis caused by *Chlamydia trachomatis*, is a significant preventable cause of blindness worldwide. Trachoma is endemic in sub-Saharan Africa, the Middle East and parts of Asia. Australia is the only developed country with endemic trachoma, with extremely high incidence in the Indigenous population. Trachoma is contagious, transmitted primarily by close personal contact (eye to eye, hand to eye) or by fomites such as towels, handkerchiefs and flies (Loscalzo et al., 2022). Certain forms of trachoma are transmitted during delivery when the newborn is exposed to contaminated genital secretions of the mother (Loscalzo et al., 2022).

Early manifestations of trachoma include redness, eyelid oedema, tearing and photophobia. Small conjunctival follicles develop on the upper lids. The inflammation also causes superficial corneal vascularisation and infiltration with granulation tissue. Scarring of the conjunctival lining of the lid causes entropion (see Figure 45.2). The lashes then abrade the cornea, eventually causing ulceration and scarring. The scarred cornea is opaque, resulting in loss of vision.

INTERPROFESSIONAL CARE

Management of the person with conjunctivitis focuses on establishing an accurate diagnosis and prompt treatment.

Diagnosis

Diagnosis is especially important because of other potentially vision-threatening conditions, such as acute uveitis or acute angle-closure glaucoma, which can also cause acute red eye (see Table 45.2). Diagnostic procedures may include:

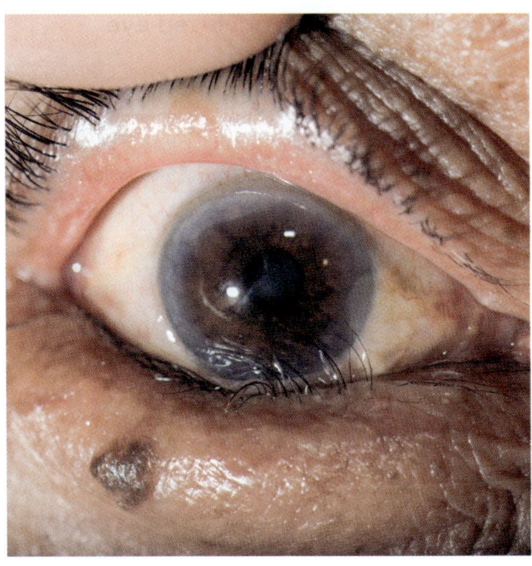

FIGURE 45.2 ***Entropion***

Source: PHUCHONG CHOKSAMAI/123RF.

- *culture and sensitivity* of exudates to determine presence of an infection and identify the infecting organism
- *fluorescein stain* with slit-lamp examination to identify possible corneal ulcerations or abrasions, which appear green with staining
- *conjunctival scrapings* that are examined microscopically or cultured to identify the organisms.

Additional laboratory testing such as blood counts or antibody titres may be used to identify underlying infectious or autoimmune processes.

Medications

Conjunctivitis is treated with antibiotic, antiviral or anti-inflammatory drugs as appropriate. Topical antibiotic eye drops or ointments are usually prescribed with severe cases of conjunctivitis. Trachoma is usually treated with a single dose of oral azithromycin (Knights et al., 2022). Antihistamines are used to minimise symptoms of conjunctivitis when an allergic response underlies the inflammatory process.

Complementary therapies

Frequent eye irrigations may be ordered to remove the copious purulent discharge associated with conjunctivitis. Soaking the lids with warm saline compresses prior to cleansing promotes comfort and facilitates the removal of crusts and exudate in conjunctivitis.

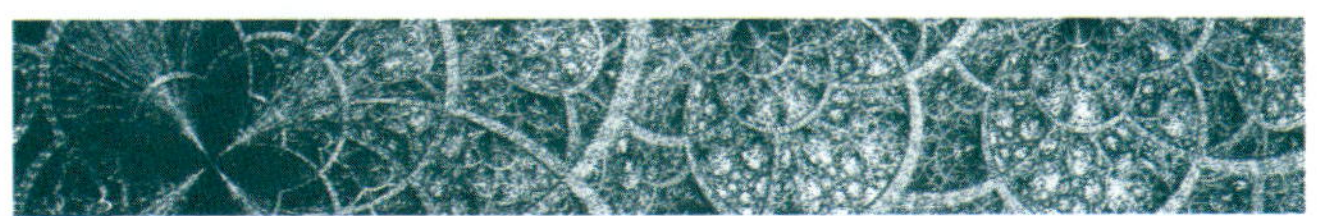

Nursing care

The nursing role in treating conjunctivitis is primarily education to prevent the disorder and its spread when it does occur.

TABLE 45.2 Possible causes of acute red eye

	ACUTE CONJUNCTIVITIS	CORNEAL TRAUMA OR INFECTION	ACUTE UVEITIS	ACUTE ANGLE-CLOSURE GLAUCOMA
Incidence	Very common	Common	Common	Rare
Pain	Mild	Moderate to severe	Moderate	Severe
Vision	Normal	Blurred	Blurred	Markedly blurred
Discharge	May be copious	Watery, may be purulent	None	None
Conjunctival erythema	Diffuse	Primarily around cornea	Primarily around cornea	Primarily around cornea
Cornea	Clear	Depends on cause	Usually clear	Cloudy
Pupils	Normal size, response to light	Normal size, response to light	Small, minimal response to light	Moderately dilated, fixed

Health promotion

Education is a vital strategy for preventing conjunctivitis. Teach all people about proper eye care, including the importance of not sharing towels, make-up or contact lenses, and avoiding rubbing or scratching the eyes. Instruct to avoid using old eye make-up, which can cause eye infections. Educate contact lens users about appropriate care (see Box 45.1). Emphasise the need to follow precise cleaning instructions to avoid bacterial contamination of lenses. If the eyes become red, irritated or develop discharge, instruct the person to avoid wearing contact lenses until the inflammatory process has cleared.

Assessment

- *Health history*: presence of redness, discomfort, tearing, photophobia and drainage; symptom onset; care measures; use of contact lenses; exposure to 'pink eye' or recent travel; allergies; previous history of conjunctivitis; presence of any chronic diseases.
- *Physical assessment*: visual acuity; inspect eyelids, conjunctiva, sclera and cornea; vital signs (temperature, heart rate, respirations, blood pressure).

Nursing diagnoses and interventions

Nursing care focuses primarily on preventing complications from the disorder. The priority nursing diagnoses include risk of infection and altered vision.

BOX 45.1 Contact lens care

- **Wash hands thoroughly before handling contact lenses.**
- **Keep storage case clean.**
- **Remove lenses before sleep, cleaning and storing as recommended by the manufacturer, or dispose of if single-use only.**
- **Use cleaning and wetting solutions recommended by the eye care professional or lens manufacturer. Do not use water or home-made solutions for wetting or cleaning lenses.**
- **If eye redness, tearing, vision loss or pain occurs, remove lenses and contact eye care professional as soon as possible.**
- **Do not share contact lenses with another person.**

Risk of infection

Acute conjunctivitis is highly contagious. While most people experience discomfort from the disease, the infection carries a risk of scarring and damage to the delicate cornea. Preventing the spread of this infection is a vital nursing role.

- Educate to wash hands thoroughly before instilling eye medications. Instruct to avoid touching or rubbing the eyes. Advise to use a new, clean cotton-tipped swab or cotton ball for cleaning each eye. *Handwashing is the single most important measure to prevent transmission of infection to the eye. Touching or rubbing the eyes increases the risk of infection and corneal trauma. Using a new swab or cotton ball prevents cross-contamination between eyes.*
- Educate person to instil prescribed eye drops as ordered. *Prescribed medications reduce inflammation and eliminate infection.*
- Discuss the importance of avoiding contact lens use until the infectious process has cleared, and of completing the prescribed treatment. *Use of contact lenses in the inflamed eyes can lead to further damage and impair healing.*

Risk of disturbed visual perception

Conjunctivitis can potentially disrupt the integrity or clarity of the cornea. Because of its vital role in focusing light on the retina, corneal damage can impair visual acuity.

- Assess vision with and without corrective lenses. *Assessment provides a baseline to evaluate possible changes in vision resulting from the infection.*
- Instruct to avoid activities requiring high visual acuity until the infection has cleared. *The inflammatory process, oedema of the conjunctiva and local antibiotic applications can decrease visual acuity and cloud vision.*
- Instruct to use dark sunglasses with appropriate UV protection when outdoors, even on cloudy days. *Photophobia, a common manifestation of conjunctivitis, causes eye pain with increased light intensity.*

Community-based care

People with conjunctivitis are typically managed in the community, reinforcing the need for effective education for home care. Emphasise to the individual and family ways to prevent transmission of infection. If the person is unable to administer eye medications, involve and educate the family in the following:

- safety and medical asepsis when cleansing the eye
- instillation of prescribed eye drops and ointments
- comfort measures such as reducing lighting intensity and wearing sunglasses
- avoiding activities such as excessive reading while the eye is inflamed.

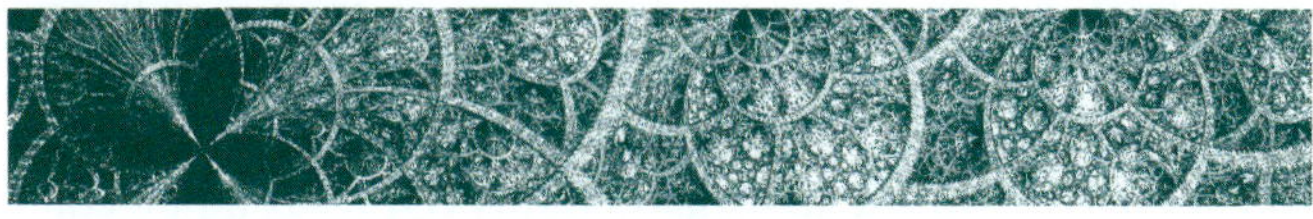

THE PERSON WITH A CORNEAL DISORDER

The clear cornea allows light rays to enter the eye and transmits images onto the retina. It helps to focus light on the retina and protects the internal eye structures. The cornea can be affected by a variety of disorders, including infection and trauma. While the cornea heals quickly after minor injuries or abrasions, injury to its deeper layers can delay healing or result in scarring.

Physiology review

The cornea has three main layers: the outermost epithelium, which consists of five or six layers of cells that are constantly being renewed; the stroma, which makes up 90% of corneal tissue; and the single-cell-thickness endothelium adjacent to the aqueous humour of the anterior chamber. The cornea is avascular tissue; the central cornea is dependent on atmospheric oxygen to meet its metabolic needs. Because there is no blood supply, immune defences have difficulty fending off infections of the cornea.

Pathophysiology and manifestations

When light enters the eye through the normally clear curved cornea, it is bent or *refracted* onto the lens, which then focuses the light on the sensory cells of the retina. A change in the curvature of the cornea or in its clarity affects the ability of the eye to clearly focus; as a result, vision is distorted or blurred. Refractive errors such as myopia, hyperopia and astigmatism are common. Corneal scarring or ulceration are two main causes of blindness worldwide.

Refractive errors

Refractive errors are the most common problems affecting visual acuity; they result from an abnormal curvature of the cornea or an altered shape of the eyeball. People with *emmetropia* (normal vision) can see near and far objects clearly because light rays focus directly on the retina. In myopia (nearsightedness) the curvature of the cornea is excessive or the eyeball is elongated, causing the image to focus in front of the retina instead of on it. Objects in close range are seen clearly and those at a distance are blurred. The eyeball is too short in **hyperopia** (farsightedness), causing the image to focus behind the retina. People with this condition see objects at a distance more clearly than they see those close to them.

Astigmatism develops due to an irregular or abnormal curvature of the cornea. Instead of the round, even curvature, it curves more in one direction than the other, resembling the back of a spoon. As a result, light rays focus on more than one area of the retina, distorting both near and distance vision.

Keratitis

Keratitis is inflammation of the cornea. (When the inflammatory process involves both the conjunctiva and the cornea, the term *keratoconjunctivitis* may be used.) Keratitis may be caused by infection, hypersensitivity reactions, ischaemia, tearing defects, trauma and impaired innervation of the cornea. Scarring that occurs as a result of keratitis is a leading cause of blindness worldwide (Norris, 2018).

Keratitis is described as either non-ulcerative or ulcerative. In *non-ulcerative keratitis*, all layers of corneal epithelium are affected, but remain intact. Viral infections, tuberculosis and autoimmune disorders such as lupus erythematosus may cause non-ulcerative keratitis. *Ulcerative keratitis*, in contrast, affects the epithelium and stroma of the cornea, leading to tissue destruction and ulceration. Bacterial conjunctivitis (e.g. *Staphylococcus*, *S. pneumoniae*, *Chlamydia*) may lead to ulcerative keratitis.

Keratitis commonly causes tearing, discomfort ranging from a gritty sensation in the eye to severe pain, decreased visual acuity and *blepharospasm* (spasm of the eyelid and inability to open the eye). A discharge may be present, especially if the conjunctiva is also inflamed. Corneal ulceration may be visible on direct examination.

Corneal ulcer

A **corneal ulcer**, local necrosis of the cornea, may be caused by infection, exposure trauma or the misuse/overuse of contact lenses. Herpes viruses (e.g. herpes simplex and herpes zoster) are a leading cause of ulcerative corneal disease. Corneal ulcers may also complicate bacterial conjunctivitis, trachoma, gonorrhoea and other acute infections. People who are immunosuppressed because of disease or drug therapy are at particular risk of developing corneal ulcers due to infection.

In corneal ulceration, a portion of the epithelium and/or stroma is destroyed. Ulcers may be superficial or deep, penetrating underlying layers and posing a risk of perforation. Fibrous tissue may form during healing, resulting in scarring and opacity of the cornea. Perforation can lead to infection of deeper eye structures or extrusion of eye contents. Partial or total vision loss may result.

Corneal dystrophies

A corneal dystrophy is accumulation of cloudy material in part or parts of the normally clear cornea, potentially affecting visual acuity. Corneal dystrophies are typically inherited disorders that progress gradually and affect both eyes. *Keratoconus*, progressive thinning of the cornea, is the most common corneal dystrophy. It typically affects teenagers and young adults. In keratoconus, the centre of the cornea thins and bulges outwards, affecting its shape and ability to focus light on the lens of the eye. In most cases, the thinning stabilises over time. In Australia, there is a 98.1% success rate in reconstructive surgery for this condition in which corneal transplantation and the sclera are used.

INTERPROFESSIONAL CARE

Management of the person with a disorder of the cornea focuses on establishing an accurate diagnosis and prompt treatment to reduce the risk of permanent vision deficit. The person's history and physical assessment are key in diagnosing these disorders.

Although many eye disorders can be treated in the community, the person with a severe corneal infection or ulcer may require hospitalisation. Corneal ulcers are medical emergencies that require prompt referral to an ophthalmologist for treatment. Pressure dressings may be applied to both eyes for comfort in order to reduce the risk of perforation and possible loss of eye contents.

Diagnosis

Visual acuity is tested on all people presenting with refractory or corneal disorders. See the chapter 'A person-centred approach to assessing the eye and ear' for more information about testing visual acuity. The following tests may be ordered to identify the cause and extent of eye infections or inflammations:

- *Fluorescein stain* with slit-lamp examination allows visualisation of any corneal ulcerations or abrasions, which appear green with staining.
- *Conjunctival* or *ulcer scrapings* are examined microscopically or cultured to identify the organisms.

Additional laboratory testing such as blood counts or antibody titres may be used to identify any underlying infectious or autoimmune disease processes.

Medication

Infectious processes are treated with antibiotic or antiviral therapy as appropriate. The only topical antiviral available in Australia is acyclovir (Knights et al., 2022). Corticosteroids may be prescribed for keratitis related to systemic inflammatory disorders or trauma; however, it is important to avoid their use with local infections to avoid suppressing the immune and inflammatory responses.

Corrective lenses

Corrective lenses, either in the form of eyeglasses or contact lenses, generally are prescribed to restore visual acuity for people with refractive errors such as myopia, hyperopia and astigmatism. Specially fitted contact lenses to reduce vision distortion are ordered for people with keratoconus. Because contact lenses are a risk factor for corneal infection and ulcers, providing appropriate education regarding lens care is vital (see Box 45.1).

Surgery

LASER EYE SURGERY Laser eye surgery is commonly performed to correct refractive errors such as myopia, hyperopia and astigmatism. A laser is used to permanently change the shape of the cornea, and in most cases the need to use corrective lenses is reduced or eliminated. Several surgical procedures are now available:

- laser in situ keratomileusis (LASIK)
- photorefractive keratectomy (PRK)
- laser epithelial keratomileusis (LASEK)
- laser thermokeratoplasty (LTK).

These procedures reshape the cornea using laser technology to remove a thin layer of epithelial cells or to shrink and reshape the cornea. Candidates for laser vision-correction surgery should be in good health and must have adequate corneal thickness to ensure that the risk of perforation does not occur.

Following surgery, people may experience a temporary loss of contrast sharpness (images do not appear crisp as with corrective lenses), over- or under-correction of visual acuity, dry eyes or temporarily decreased night vision with halos, glare and starbursts. Diffuse lamellar keratitis (DLK) is a rare complication of surgery that, while treatable, can lead to vision impairment if not identified and treated early.

Phototherapeutic keratectomy (PTK) provides an alternative to corneal transplant in treating corneal dystrophies, scars and some infections. In this procedure, diseased corneal tissue is vaporised and surface irregularities are corrected with little trauma to surrounding tissue; healing occurs rapidly.

CORNEAL TRANSPLANT Once the cornea has become scarred and opaque, no treatment can restore its clarity. The first successful corneal transplant (*keratoplasty*), replacement of diseased cornea by healthy corneal tissue from a donor, was performed in 1906. Current corneal transplant procedures have a success rate of approximately 90% in Australia. Data collected from the Australian Corneal Graft Registry (2018), one of the world's largest registries, show that 91.2% of such transplants in Australia survive for approximately 1 year.

Corneas are harvested from the cadavers of uninfected adults who were under the age of 65 and who died as a result of acute trauma or illness. After harvesting, the cornea can be stored in a tissue-culture medium for up to 4 weeks before being used as a graft. Corneal transplantation is usually an elective surgery, although emergency transplantation may be required for perforation of the cornea.

Corneal transplant may be either lamellar or penetrating. In a lamellar keratoplasty, the superficial layer of cornea is removed and replaced with a graft. The anterior chamber remains intact. In a penetrating keratoplasty, a button or full thickness of cornea is removed and replaced by donor tissue (see Figure 45.3). The graft is then sutured in place using suture finer than human hair and a continuous or interrupted stitch. Because the cornea is avascular, these sutures remain in place for up to a year to ensure healing.

Most corneal transplants do not require hospitalisation. The eye is patched for 24 hours following surgery. Narcotic analgesia may be required initially because the cornea is extremely sensitive. Corticosteroid eye drops are ordered to reduce the inflammatory response and prevent oedema of the graft, and antibiotic drops may be prescribed to prevent infection.

The risk of transplant rejection is low as the cornea is avascular and there is little exposure of the transplanted corneal tissue to the host's immune defences (Norris, 2018). Research suggests that matching of blood type (not tissue type, as is required for major organ transplants) between the donor and the transplant recipient may reduce the risk of transplant rejection (Gurnani et al., 2022). When rejection does occur, it occurs within 3 weeks of the transplant, beginning with inflammation at the edge of the grafted tissue and spreading to involve the entire graft. In many

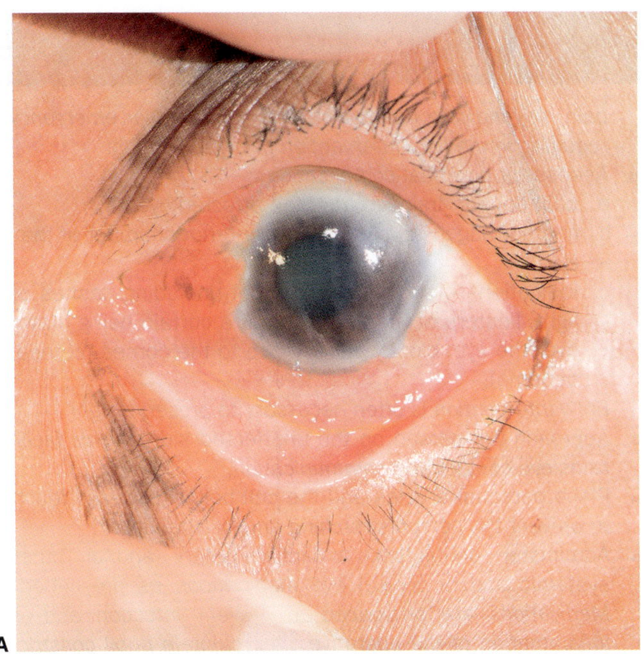
A

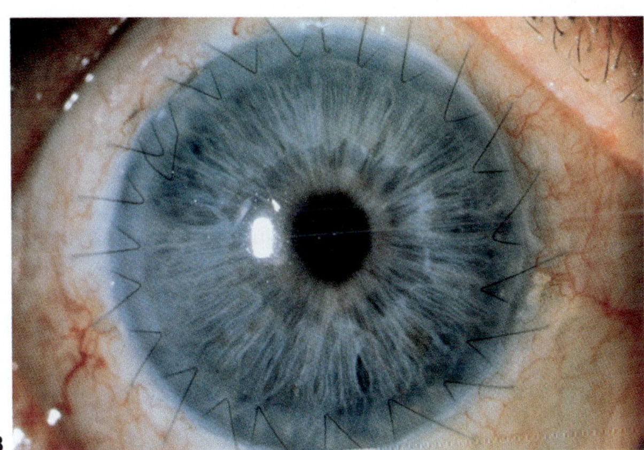
B

FIGURE 45.3 ***Corneal transplant. A, The diseased, opaque cornea. B, The diseased cornea is removed and a corneal graft is sutured in place using material finer than a human hair***

Sources: A, ARZTSAMUI/Shutterstock; B, Mediscan/Alamy Stock Photo.

cases, rejection can be successfully treated using corticosteroid therapy, preserving the graft. (See the accompanying box for nursing care of the person undergoing eye surgery.)

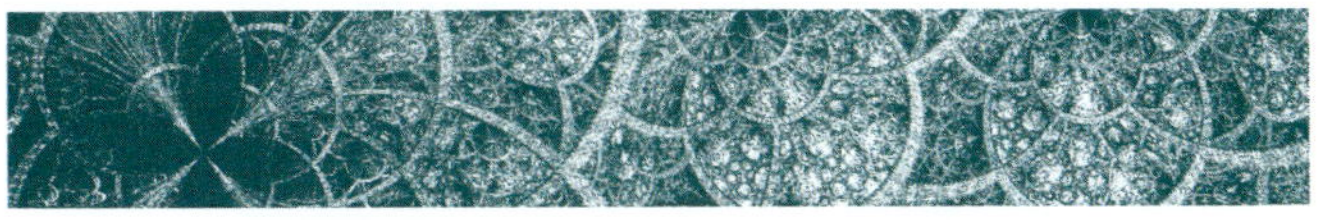

Nursing care

Nurses working in clinics and outpatient surgical settings care for people undergoing corneal transplant and surgeries to correct refractive errors. The nursing role in caring for people with corneal disorders may involve direct care; however, the focus is on prevention and education.

Health promotion

Education is a vital strategy for preventing many corneal disorders. Educate all involved about proper eye care, including the importance of not sharing towels and make-up, and avoiding rubbing or scratching the eyes, as well as preventing trauma and infection. Teach contact lens users appropriate care and cleaning techniques. Stress the importance of periodic removal of lenses, even extended-wear or single-use lenses. In general, lenses should be removed at night, even though manufacturers may claim it is safe to wear them while sleeping. Emphasise the need to follow cleaning instructions (as per the manufacturer's instructions) to avoid bacterial contamination of lenses and possible corneal infection. If the person experiences a corneal abrasion or keratitis, instruct the person to avoid wearing contact lenses until the cornea has healed completely.

Assessment

Collect the following data through a health history and physical examination (see the chapter 'A person-centred approach to assessing the eye and ear'). Additional focused assessments are described with the interventions below:

- *Health history*: risk factors; presence of redness, discomfort, tearing, photophobia, oedema and drainage; symptom onset; presence of pain, effect on vision.
- *Physical assessment*: visual acuity; inspect external eye, including conjunctiva, sclera and cornea; extraocular movements.

Nursing diagnoses and interventions

Nursing care focuses primarily on preventing complications and promoting healing. The priority nursing diagnosis for people with corneal disorders includes risk of altered vision, pain and injury.

Risk of disturbed visual perception

Disorders affecting the cornea may disrupt its integrity and/or clarity as the cornea plays a vital role in focusing light on the retina. Any corneal damage can affect vision, impairing visual acuity and even causing legal blindness.

- Assess vision with and without corrective lenses. *Assessment provides a baseline to evaluate possible vision changes resulting from the disorder and/or treatment.*
- Educate the person about thorough handwashing before inserting or removing contact lenses or instilling any eye medications, and about avoiding touching or rubbing the eyes. Instruct to use a new, clean cotton-tipped swab or cotton ball for cleaning each eye. *Handwashing is the single most important measure to prevent transmission of infection to the eye. Touching or rubbing the eyes increases the risk of infection and possible corneal trauma. Using a new swab or cotton ball prevents cross-contamination between eyes.*
- Emphasise the importance of proper care of contact lenses specific to the type of lens used. *People who wear hard contact lenses must remove them daily, as the central cornea requires exposure to atmospheric oxygen. Although soft and extended-wear lenses allow the cornea to 'breathe', improper cleaning carries a major risk of infection.*

NURSING CARE OF THE PERSON having eye surgery

PREOPERATIVE CARE

- Review the chapter 'Nursing care of people having surgery' for routine preoperative care.
- Assess visual acuity of the affected eye prior to surgery. *The person with limited vision in the affected eye may need additional attention and ADL assistance postoperatively to ensure safety.*
- Assess the person's support systems and the possible effect of impaired vision on lifestyle and ability to perform ADLs in the postoperative period. *Safety measures such as installing handrails and removing throw rugs from the home can help promote mobility and safety, especially if the person has limited vision in the unaffected eye.*
- Educate the person regarding measures to prevent eye injury postoperatively, such as avoiding possible vomiting, straining with stool movement, coughing, sneezing, lifting more than 2 kg and bending over at the waist. *These activities can temporarily increase intraocular pressure and may lead to postoperative complications.*
- Remove all eye make-up and contact lenses or glasses prior to surgery. Store corrective lenses and eyeglasses in a safe place and make them readily available to the person on return from surgery. *Maintaining visual acuity in the unaffected eye helps reduce fear and maintains safety.*
- Administer preoperative medications and eye drops and/or ointments as prescribed. *Mydriatic (pupil-dilating) or cycloplegic (ciliary-paralytic) drops, and/or drops to lower intraocular pressure, may be prescribed preoperatively.*

POSTOPERATIVE CARE

- Review the chapter 'Nursing care of people having surgery' for routine postoperative care.
- Assess eye dressing for bleeding and/or drainage following surgery *as it may indicate a surgical complication.*
- Maintain the eye patch or shield in place *to prevent inadvertent injury to the operative site.*
- Place in semi-Fowler's or Fowler's position on the unaffected side. *Elevating the head of the bed and lying on the unaffected side reduces intraocular pressure in the affected eye.*
- Remind the person to avoid coughing, sneezing and/or straining, *as these activities can increase intraocular pressure.*
- Assess and medicate as necessary for complaints of pain, aching and/or a scratchy sensation in affected eye. *Complaints of sudden sharp eye pain must be reported to the doctor immediately. An abrupt increase in or onset of eye pain may indicate haemorrhage or other ocular emergency requiring immediate intervention to preserve sight.*
- Assess for potential complications:
  a. pain and/or drainage from the affected eye
  b. haemorrhage with blood in the anterior chamber of the eye
  c. indications of retinal detachment, including flashes of light, floaters or the sensation of a curtain being drawn over the eye; cloudy appearance to the cornea (corneal oedema).

  Early intervention is often necessary to preserve sight.
- Approach the person on the unaffected side *as this facilitates eye contact and communication.*
- Place personal articles and the call bell within easy reach *to prevent the person stretching and/or straining.*
- Administer antibiotics, anti-inflammatory and/or other systemic and/or topical eye medications as prescribed. *Medications are prescribed to prevent infection and/or inflammation of the operative site, maintain pupil constriction and control intraocular pressure.*
- Administer anti-emetic medication as required. *It is important to prevent vomiting, in order to maintain normal intraocular pressures.*

HEALTH EDUCATION FOR THE PERSON AND FAMILY

- Educate the person and family about home care:
  a. how to instil eye drops
  b. the name, dosage, schedule, duration, purpose and side effects of medications
  c. how and when to use the eye patch and eye shield
  d. the importance of avoiding scratching, rubbing, touching or squeezing the affected eye
  e. measures to avoid constipation and straining
  f. activity limitations, if ordered
  g. reporting of symptoms including eye pain or pressure, redness or cloudiness, drainage, decreased vision, floaters, or flashes of light or halos around bright objects
  h. the need to wear sunglasses with side shields when outdoors to reduce photophobia
- Remind the person that vision may not stabilise for several weeks following eye surgery. If new corrective lenses are required, they will not be prescribed until vision has stabilised. *A person may be alarmed that vision seems worse after surgery and need reassurance that visual acuity usually improves with time and healing of the affected eye.*
- Emphasise the importance of keeping follow-up appointments. Provide referral to a community service for assistance with home care after discharge as required.

- Emphasise the importance of using eye protection when engaging in potentially dangerous activities. *Trauma can increase the risk of infection and scarring of the cornea.*
- If corneal perforation is suspected, place the person in the supine position, close the eye and cover it with a dry, sterile dressing. Notify the doctor immediately. *Corneal perforation may occur without warning in people with corneal ulcers. It places the person at risk of loss of eye contents. Emergency measures are taken to reduce intraocular pressure and maintain eye integrity to preserve vision.*

> **CONSIDERATION FOR PRACTICE**
> **Suspect corneal perforation with complaints of sudden, severe eye pain and photophobia.**

Acute pain

The cornea of the eye is extremely sensitive; therefore, corneal disorders frequently cause significant pain. This in turn increases the stress response and interferes with rest, potentially impairing healing.

- Assess pain, using verbal and non-verbal cues. *Pain is a subjective experience and can be evaluated only by the person's response and in terms of its effect on the person.*
- Administer prescribed analgesia routinely in the first 12 to 24 hours after corneal surgery. *Routine administration of analgesics prevents pain from reaching a level of severity at which it becomes difficult to relieve.*
- Patch both eyes if necessary. *Patching both eyes reduces eye movement and irritation of the affected eye.*
- Instruct to apply warm compresses to reduce inflammation and pain. *Warm compresses for 15 minutes, three to four times a day, promote comfort for people with keratitis or corneal injury.*
- Instruct to use dark sunglasses with appropriate UV protection when outdoors, even on cloudy days. *True photophobia, often associated with corneal disorders, causes eye pain with increased light intensity.*
- Instruct how to instil prescribed eye drops/ointment as ordered. *Prescribed medications may reduce inflammation and eliminate infection, reducing discomfort.*

Risk of injury

The person who has undergone corneal transplantation has an increased risk of injury for several reasons. The eye on which surgery was performed is patched for 24 hours after surgery, changing depth perception and increasing the risk of falls. Increased intraocular pressure or trauma to the eye may damage the graft, resulting in graft rejection.

- Instruct to call for help before getting up or ambulating after surgery. Ensure access to the call bell. It may take time for the person to adjust to changes in depth perception caused by the eye patch. *Assistance helps prevent falls that may not only injure the person but also traumatise the operative site.*
- Encourage deep breathing and use the incentive spirometer to promote lung expansion. *These important postoperative measures help prevent pulmonary complications. Coughing is avoided because it increases intraocular pressure.*
- Educate the person on how to apply an eye shield at night after the eye patch is removed. *An eye shield may be recommended at night to prevent inadvertent rubbing or trauma to the eye during sleep.*
- Encourage the person not to rub or scratch the eye. *Rubbing or scratching may disrupt suture lines or damage the grafted tissue.*
- Reinforce the importance of using eye protection during hazardous activities. *Following a corneal transplant, the person has the same risk of eye injury as other people who perform hazardous activities.*

> **CONSIDERATION FOR PRACTICE**
> **Administer prescribed anti-emetics and stool softeners postoperatively to prevent vomiting and straining at stool—activities that increase intraocular pressure and can damage suture lines.**

Community-based care

Following treatment, educate the person to manage these conditions at home. Emphasise to the person and family ways to prevent transmission of infection. If the person is unable to administer eye medications or to perform other eye care required, involve the family in the education session. The following topics should be included:

- safety and medical asepsis when cleansing the eye
- instillation of prescribed eye drops and ointments
- application of an eye patch/shield and where to obtain supplies
- avoidance of activities such as excessive reading while eye is inflamed
- follow-up appointments after corneal transplant surgery
- signs and symptoms of graft rejection
- avoidance of activities that increase intraocular pressure, such as straining, coughing, sneezing, bending over, lifting heavy objects
- helpful resources:
  - Lions Eye Institute: https://www.lei.org.au
  - state organ and tissue agencies.

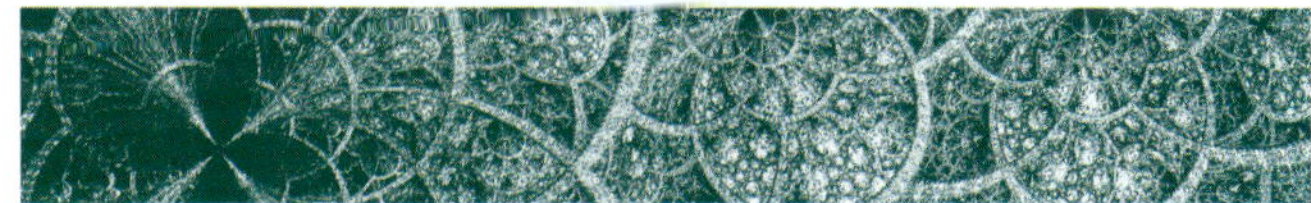

DISORDERS AFFECTING THE EYELIDS

The eyelids and eyelashes are constantly exposed to the environment as they protect the eye from damage. When these structures are inflamed, deformed or their function is impaired, this affects both appearance and their protective functions.

Pathophysiology and manifestations

The most common disorder affecting the eyelids is *marginal blepharitis*, an inflammation of the glands and lash follicles on the margins of the eyelids. This inflammatory disorder can be caused by a staphylococcal infection, or it may be seborrhoeic in origin; commonly, both types are present. Seborrhoeic blepharitis is usually associated with seborrhoea (dandruff) of the scalp or eyebrows. Irritation, burning and itching of eyelid margins are common manifestations of blepharitis. The eye appears red rimmed with mucus discharge and there is crusting or scaling of lid margins. Lid margins may ulcerate, resulting in a loss of eyelashes.

Infection of one or more of the sebaceous glands of the eyelid may cause a **hordeolum (sty)**. Hordeolum is a staphylococcal abscess that may occur on either the external or internal margin of the lid (see Figure 45.4). An external hordeolum is characterised initially by acute pain at the lid margin with redness, and a small tender raised area is visible. The person may also experience photophobia, tearing and the sensation of a foreign body in the affected eye. Internal hordeola are seen on the conjunctival side of the lid and may have more severe manifestations.

Chronic inflammation of a meibomian gland may lead to formation of a **chalazion**, a granulomatous cyst or nodule of the lid (see Figure 45.5). It presents as a hard swelling on the lid, and the surrounding conjunctival tissue is red and inflamed. Chalazion may also follow a hordeolum that was inadequately treated. Unlike a hordeolum, a chalazion is painless; however, it may slowly increase in size and eventually require removal, although most resolve within several months.

Entropion, the inversion of the lid margin (see Figure 45.2), may be associated with the normal ageing process (senile entropion) or result from an infectious process such as trachoma. Entropion can lead to corneal irritation and, potentially, scarring as the lashes rub on the conjunctiva and cornea during blinking and sleep. *Ectropion*, or eversion of the lid margin, occurs primarily as an effect of ageing (see Figure 45.6). Other conditions may also lead to ectropion, including facial nerve paralysis or palsy (Bell's palsy), scarring or infection. Here the eye does not close effectively, increasing the risk of drying and damage to the conjunctival membrane and cornea. Both entropion and ectropion have cosmetic effects as they alter the appearance of the eyes and face.

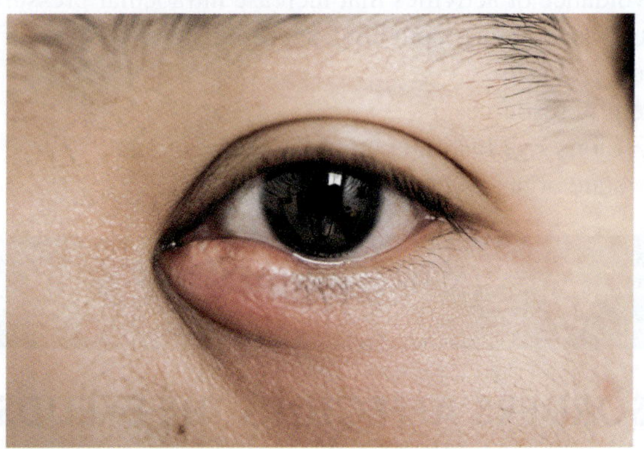

FIGURE 45.4 ***Hordeolum***

Source: Sorapop Udomsri/123RF.

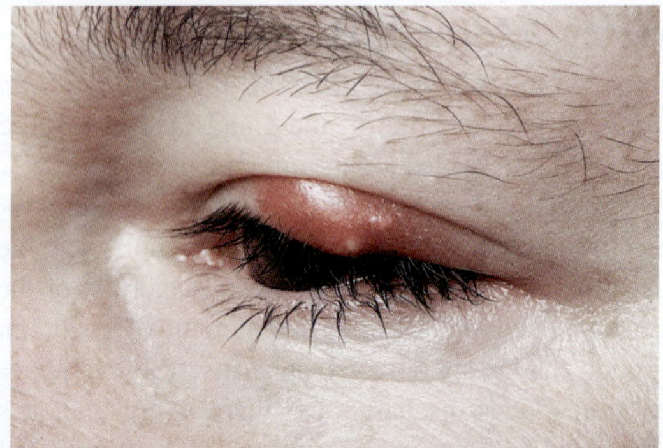

FIGURE 45.5 ***Chalazion***

Source: Gromovataya/Shutterstock.

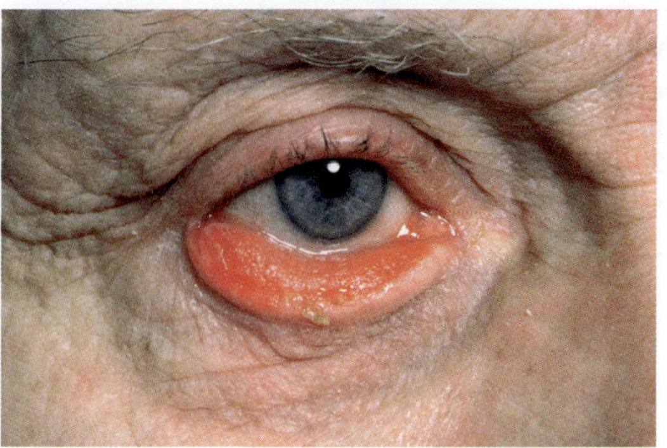

FIGURE 45.6 ***Ectropion***

Source: Mediscan/Alamy Stock Photo.

INTERPROFESSIONAL CARE

Disorders affecting the eyelids typically are managed in the community. Diagnosis is typically made through the person's history and physical examination. Diagnostic tests are rarely required except to identify corneal or conjunctival damage resulting from the condition.

Topical antibiotics (eye drops or ointments) may be prescribed for the person with hordeolum and to treat infection resulting from irritation of the eye by a deformed lid. Careful cleansing of the lid margins using a 'no-tears' baby shampoo is often recommended for marginal blepharitis. Soaking the lids with warm saline compresses prior to cleansing facilitates the removal of crusts and exudate in blepharitis. Local heat applications may be used to treat hordeolum or chalazion; excision and drainage may be required if this is not effective. In entropion or ectropion, surgery may be performed to correct the defect, reduce the risk of damage to the eye and improve cosmetic appearance.

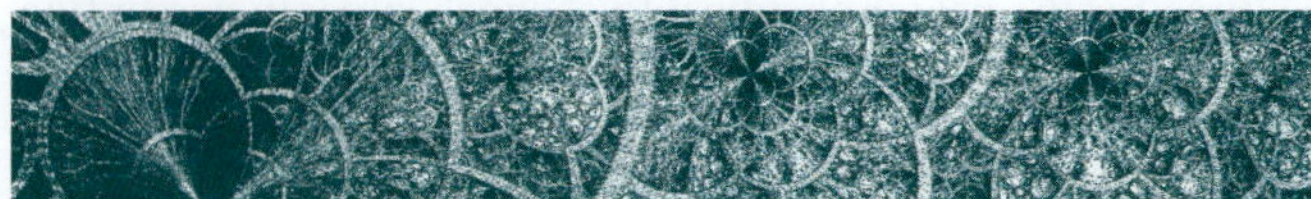

Nursing care

The nursing role focuses on education and comfort measures. Educate people about appropriate eye care, including avoiding rubbing or scratching the eyes. Discuss the importance of not using old eye make-up, which can cause lid infections. Instruct to wash hands well before cleansing the eyelids or instilling any eye medications. Instruct to use a new, clean cotton-tipped swab or cotton ball for cleaning each eye. Instruct to instil prescribed eye drops and apply ointments as ordered. If the person is unable to administer eye medications, involve the family. Instruct to apply warm compresses to reduce inflammation and discomfort.

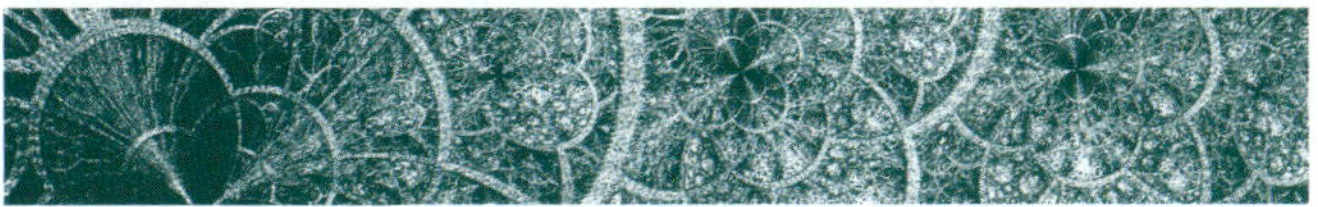

THE PERSON WITH EYE TRAUMA

Most eye injuries are minor but, without timely and appropriate intervention, even a minor injury can threaten a person's vision. Therefore, all eye injuries should be considered medical emergencies requiring immediate evaluation and intervention.

Pathophysiology and manifestations

Any part of the eye, especially the exposed parts, may be affected by trauma. Foreign bodies, abrasions and lacerations are the most common types of eye injury, along with traumatic injuries such as burns, penetrating objects and/or blunt force.

Corneal abrasion

Corneal abrasion is the disruption of the superficial epithelium of the cornea. Objects commonly causing corneal abrasion include contact lenses, eyelashes, small foreign bodies (dust, dirt and fingernails), drying of the eye surface and chemical irritants.

Superficial abrasions of the cornea are extremely painful but generally heal rapidly without complications or scarring. Photophobia and tearing are commonly present. When the stroma is damaged by a deep abrasion or laceration, there is an increased risk of infection, healing is slowed and scar formation occurs.

Burns

The outer surface of the eye may be subjected to burns caused by heat, radiation or explosion; however, chemical burns are the most common. Acid or alkaline substances may burn the eye. Ammonia, products that contain lye (such as oven and drain cleaners) and acids from car batteries or other sources are often implicated in eye injuries. Burns caused by alkaline substances are particularly serious as tiny particles of the chemical may remain in the conjunctival sac, causing progressive damage. Acid causes rapid damage to the eye; however, in general it causes less serious burns than alkaline substances.

Explosions and flash burn injuries pose the greatest risk of thermal burns of the eye. UV rays can also cause corneal damage ranging from mild to extensive. Depending on the source of the ultraviolet light, these burns may be known by various names such as snow blindness, welder's arc burn or flash burn.

In addition to giving a history of the face and eye contact with a caustic substance or other burning agent, the person complains of eye pain and decreased vision, and eyelids are often swollen. Burns may also affect the face or lids, and the appearance of the eye may vary, depending on the type of burn. The conjunctiva is reddened and oedematous; sloughing may be seen, particularly with chemical burns. The cornea often appears cloudy or hazy, and ulcerations may be evident.

Penetrating trauma

Perforation of the eye occurs from a variety of causes including metal flakes or other particles produced by high-speed drilling or grinding, glass shards or other substances. In a *perforating* injury, the layers of the eye do not spontaneously reapproximate, resulting in rupture of the globe and potential loss of ocular contents.

In a *penetrating* injury, the layers of the eye spontaneously reapproximate after entry of a sharp-pointed object or small missile into the globe (e.g. knives, arrows and gunshot). These injuries may not be readily apparent through inspection of the eye. Penetrating injuries may be hidden or missed due to tissue swelling or when the person has other significant injuries that command attention. When the eyelid is lacerated or has a puncture wound, inspection of the underlying eye tissue for possible damage is vital. Eye perforations/penetrations cause pain, partial or complete loss of vision, and possible bleeding or extrusion of eye contents.

Blunt trauma

Sports injuries are a common cause of blunt trauma to the eye; for example, being struck with a ball or injured in contact sports. Other causes include injury from a motor vehicle accident, falls and physical assault.

Blunt trauma may lead to a minor eye injury such as lid ecchymosis (black eye) or subconjunctival haemorrhage caused by rupture of a blood vessel in the conjunctiva. A well-defined bright area of erythema appears under the conjunctiva; however, no pain or discomfort is associated with the haemorrhage and no treatment is necessary. The blood typically reabsorbs within 2 to 3 weeks.

Hyphaema, bleeding into the anterior chamber of the eye, is a potential result of blunt eye trauma. When the highly vascular uveal tract of the eye is disrupted by blunt force, haemorrhage may result, filling the anterior chamber. The person complains of eye pain, decreased visual acuity and seeing a reddish tint. Blood is visible in the anterior chamber.

An orbital blowout fracture is another potential result of blunt eye trauma. Although any part of the eye orbit may be fractured, the ethmoid bone on the orbital floor is the most likely site. Orbital contents, including fat, muscles and the eye itself, may herniate through the fracture into the underlying maxillary sinus. The person complains of diplopia (double vision), pain with upward movement of the affected eye and decreased sensation on the affected cheek. The eye appears sunken (**enophthalmos**) and has limited movement on examination.

INTERPROFESSIONAL CARE

When trauma to the eye is known or suspected, a thorough examination is conducted to determine the type and extent of the injury. Unless immediate treatment is indicated, as with a chemical burn, vision is evaluated initially. If the person normally wears corrective lenses, vision assessment is performed while glasses are worn. Eye movement is evaluated unless a penetrating object is present, and the lid and eye are inspected for lacerations. Inspection is performed using strong light and magnification with a headband loupe or slit lamp. Topical anaesthesia may be used prior to inspection if eye pain and photophobia make eye opening difficult. Fluorescein staining can help identify foreign bodies and abrasions. Any conjunctival or anterior chamber haemorrhage is noted, as is the presence or absence of the red reflex. Ophthalmoscopic examination is used to detect haemorrhage or trauma to the interior chamber. Facial x-rays and computed tomography (CT) scans are used to identify orbital fractures or foreign bodies within the globe. Ultrasonography may be employed to detect a detached retina or vitreous haemorrhage.

Foreign bodies are removed using irrigation, a sterile cotton-tipped applicator or a sterile needle or other instrument. Antibiotic ointments can be applied once objects have been removed. In a person with corneal abrasion and large foreign bodies, an eye patch is applied firmly after the antibiotic application to keep the eye closed for approximately 24 hours.

The immediate priority of care for people with chemical burns is flushing the affected eye with copious amounts of fluid. Normal saline is preferred; however, water may be used if saline is not available. A special contact lens irrigating unit (Morgan lens), normal saline eye bath or bag of irrigation with intravenous tubing held to flush all eye surfaces may be useful. The eyelid is everted to identify and remove material from the conjunctival sac. A topical anaesthetic helps relieve pain, making inspection and irrigation easier. During irrigation, fluid is directed from the inner canthus of the eye to the outer. Tipping the person's head slightly to the affected side prevents contamination of the unaffected eye. Irrigation is continued until the pH of the eye is normal (in the range 7.2 to 7.4). Following irrigation, a topical antibiotic ointment may be applied.

Penetrating wounds of the eye generally require surgical intervention by an ophthalmic surgeon. Immediate care focuses on relieving pain and protecting the eye from further injury. To prevent loss of intraocular contents, pressure should not be placed directly on the eye, but gently cover with a sterile gauze or an eye pad. If a foreign body is embedded in or sticking out of the eye, no attempt should be made to remove it. The object should be immobilised and the eye protected with a metal eye shield until the surgeon can review it. A paper cup or other protective device may be used if the object is too large to use an eye shield. Patching the unaffected eye decreases ocular movement. Pain is managed using narcotic analgesics such as morphine. The person may also require sedation (e.g. diazepam), anti-emetic medications to prevent vomiting and antibiotics to prevent infection.

Interventions for the person with blunt trauma to the eye include placing the person on bed rest in semi-Fowler's position and protecting the eye from further injury with an eye shield. The unaffected eye is also patched to minimise eye movement. A carbonic anhydrase inhibitor may be prescribed to reduce intraocular pressure.

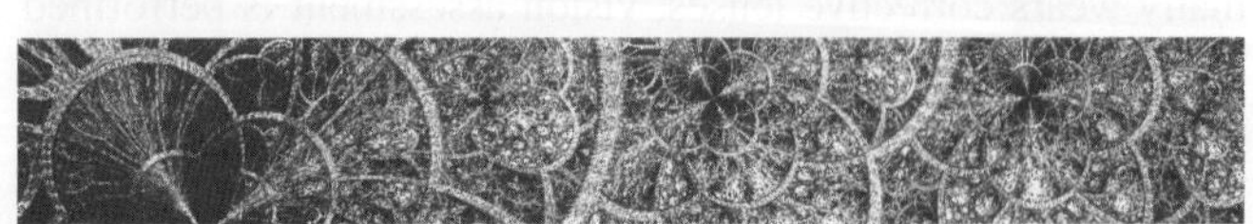

Nursing care

The nursing role involves educating people about prevention and providing direct care regarding eye injuries.

Health promotion

Educating individuals and groups about how to prevent eye injuries, the use of protective devices and first aid measures is an important nursing role, especially for people involved in hazardous occupations and high-risk sports. Emphasise the importance of using seat belts and air bags to prevent eye injury in motor vehicle accidents. Instruct people to immediately flush the eye with copious amounts of water if a chemical splash occurs. Loose, visible foreign bodies can be removed using a clean, moistened cotton-tipped swab. If an abrasion, penetrating or blunt injury is suspected, the eye should be covered loosely with sterile gauze and medical attention sought immediately; people should not try to remove objects.

Nursing diagnoses and interventions

Ocular injuries require immediate interventions simultaneously with assessment and accurate history collection, including pre-existing vision problems. The time, type and extent of injury, and the circumstances under which it occurred, must be determined.

Impaired ocular tissue integrity

All types of eye trauma pose the risk of violating the integrity of the eye and threatening vision. The goals of nursing care are to preserve vision and the integrity of the eye and prevent further damage.

- Assess vision in each eye followed by both eyes together, with and without corrective lenses, on entry into the emergency department or primary care setting. *An initial assessment provides valuable information about the effect of the injury on the person's vision and a baseline for future comparisons.*
- Inspect eye(s) carefully for evidence of foreign bodies, burns, penetrating injury or blunt trauma. Note if lacerations, burns or other trauma are evident in tissues surrounding the eye. *Eye trauma may be hidden by other injuries and, as a result, remain untreated.*
- If a burn or foreign body is present, anaesthetic drops may be instilled and the eye irrigated either before or after the doctor evaluates the person. *Blepharism and eye pain may impair assessment of the injured eye. Irrigation to remove the chemical is of higher priority than assessment of the eye.*
- Loose foreign bodies may be removed using a moist, sterile cotton-tipped applicator. *Prompt removal of foreign bodies may prevent corneal abrasion.*
- For a severe or penetrating injury, promote rest and stabilise the injured eye by applying an eye pad or gauze dressing loosely over both the affected and unaffected eye. Stabilise any penetrating object if possible. *These measures reduce eye movement and can help preserve the person's vision.*
- Following treatment, apply eye drops or ointment as prescribed and apply an eye pad or shield as required. *An eye pad is applied to the affected eye to reduce pain and photophobia and to promote healing.*

Community-based care

Following an injury, discuss the following topics with the person and family:

- prescribed medications and possible adverse effects
- strategies to prevent further trauma
- application of the eye pad or shield
- avoidance of activities that increase intraocular pressure
- importance of restricting activities.

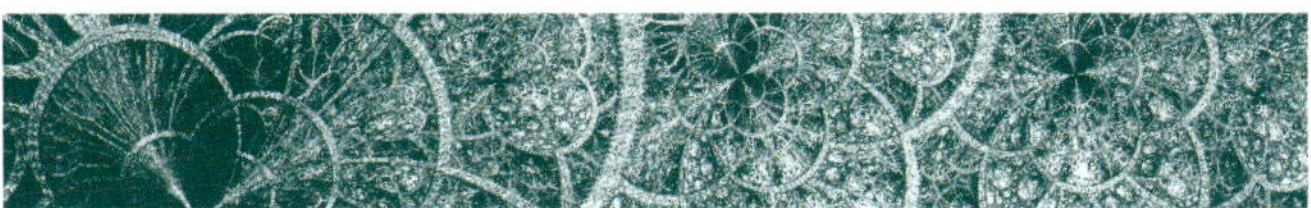

THE PERSON WITH UVEITIS

The middle vascular layer of the eye, including the choroid, the ciliary body and the iris, is known as the uvea and uveal tract. *Uveitis* is inflammation of all or part of this vascular layer; *iritis*, inflammation of the iris, occurs more commonly than uveitis.

Uveitis is a disease limited to the eye; it may be idiopathic or caused by an autoimmune process, infection, parasitic disease or trauma. Many cases can be linked to a systemic disease, often an arthritic or autoimmune disorder such as ankylosing spondylitis, Reiter's syndrome, rheumatoid arthritis or sarcoidosis (see the chapter 'Nursing care of people with musculoskeletal disorders'). Uveitis has also been linked with tuberculosis and syphilis. Manifestations of uveitis include pupillary constriction and erythema around the limbus, severe eye pain and photophobia and blurred vision.

Immunosuppressive therapy may be used to suppress the inflammatory response in people with severe uveitis. Atropine may also be prescribed for associated inflammation of the iris. The person may require analgesics for pain management. Nursing care is supportive, focusing on promotion of comfort and education regarding the disorder and its management.

THE PERSON WITH CATARACTS

A **cataract** is an opacification (clouding) of the lens of the eye which can significantly interfere with light transmission to the retina and the ability to perceive images clearly.

Incidence and risk factors

Age is the greatest single risk factor for cataract; however, genetics may contribute to the risk, although the link is unclear. Environmental and lifestyle factors also play a role, such as long-term exposure to sunlight (UVB rays); cigarette smoking and heavy alcohol consumption are associated with earlier cataract development. Although senile cataracts are by far the most common, cataracts may also be congenital or acquired in origin. Eye trauma, including injury to the lens capsule by a foreign body, blunt trauma or exposure to heat or radiation, can precipitate cataract formation. Diabetes mellitus is associated with earlier development of cataracts, especially when the blood glucose level is not carefully controlled at or near normal levels. Certain drugs such as systemic or inhaled corticosteroids also prompt the formation of cataracts.

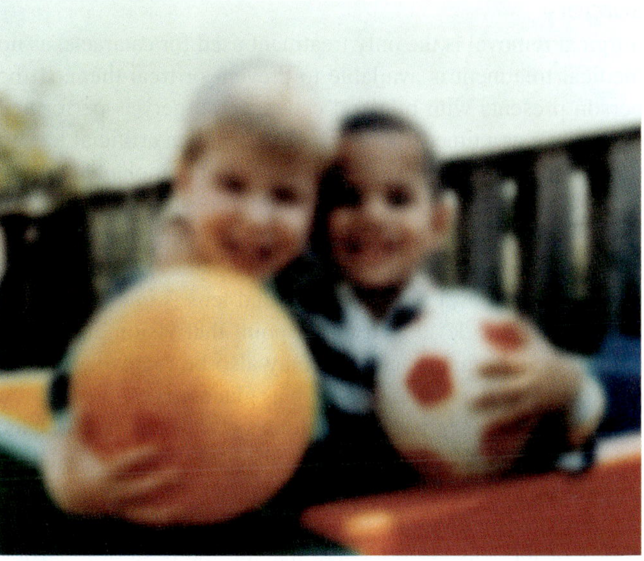

FIGURE 45.7 ***A scene as viewed by a person with cataracts***

Source: Courtesy of National Eye Institute, National Institutes of Health (NEI/NIH).

Pathophysiology

The majority of cataracts are known as senile and are formed as a result of the ageing process. As the lens ages, its fibres and proteins change and degenerate. In addition, the proteins clump, clouding the lens and reducing light transmission to the retina. This process generally begins at the periphery of the lens, gradually spreading to involve the central portion. As the cataract continues to develop, the entire lens may become opaque. An immature cataract occurs when only a portion of the lens is affected; however, a mature cataract affects the entire lens. In addition to clouding, the lens may discolour over time, affecting the ability to accurately discriminate colours.

Manifestations

Cataracts tend to occur bilaterally unless they are related to eye trauma. Fortunately, they tend to develop at different rates and one cataract generally matures more rapidly than the other. As a cataract interferes with light transmission through the lens, visual acuity decreases, affecting both close and distance vision (see Figure 45.7). Light rays are scattered as they pass through the lens, causing complaints of glare, which affects the ability to adjust between light and dark environments. Colour discrimination is impaired, particularly in the blue to purple range. When the cataract is mature, the pupil may appear cloudy grey or white, rather than black.

INTERPROFESSIONAL CARE

The diagnosis of a cataract is made based on the person's history and eye examination. Ophthalmoscopic examination confirms the diagnosis by identifying the location and extent of a cataract. As the cataract matures, ophthalmoscopy reveals a dark area instead of the red reflex.

Surgery

Surgical removal is the only treatment used for cataracts, as no medical treatment is available to prevent or treat them. If the person presents with bilateral cataracts, surgery is performed on one eye at a time. If an intraocular lens (an artificial lens to replace the diseased lens of the eye) is to be implanted during surgery, the corneal curvature and anteroposterior diameter of the eye are measured prior to surgery to determine the lens power needed for the intraocular lens implant.

Surgical removal of the cataract and lens is indicated when the cataract has developed to the point that vision and ADLs are affected. A mature cataract may also be removed when it causes a secondary condition such as glaucoma or uveitis.

Cataract surgery is usually done on a day surgery basis, using local anaesthesia. If general anaesthesia and/or sedation is required, the person may be hospitalised overnight. Extracapsular extraction, in which the anterior capsule, nucleus and cortex of the lens are removed, leaving the posterior capsule intact, is the procedure of choice (see Figure 45.8). Using an operating microscope, the surgeon makes a small incision at the edge of the cornea and extracts the lens intact or via emulsification and aspiration. In the latter technique, ultrasound vibrations are used to break the lens material into fragments (phacoemulsification), which are then suctioned out of the eye. The remaining capsule supports the lens implant and protects the retina.

After removal of the lens, the eye can no longer focus light on the retina and vision is seriously affected. Usually a polymethylmethacrylate (PMMA or Plexiglas) intraocular lens is implanted at the time of surgery. This implant rapidly restores binocular vision and depth perception. Following extracapsular lens removal, the intraocular lens is positioned in the posterior capsule behind the iris (see Figure 45.8).

If an intraocular lens cannot be implanted, convex corrective glasses or contact lenses may be used to correct vision after cataract removal. Although contact lenses can provide excellent vision correction following cataract surgery, they may be difficult for some people to adapt to or manipulate. The person with a pre-existing refractive error may continue to require corrective lenses and often needs a prescriptive change even after surgery.

Complications of cataract surgery are unusual and occur in less than 1% of the surgeries. Loss of vitreous humour, corneal oedema, increased intraocular pressure, haemorrhage, inflammation or infection, retinal detachment and displacement of the implanted lens are considered potential complications. Up to 35% of people who undergo extracapsular extraction may develop opacification of the remaining posterior capsule. Vision can be restored using laser capsulotomy (creating an opening for light to pass through the opacified capsule) or surgical incision into the posterior capsule to allow light to reach the retina (Rothrock, 2022).

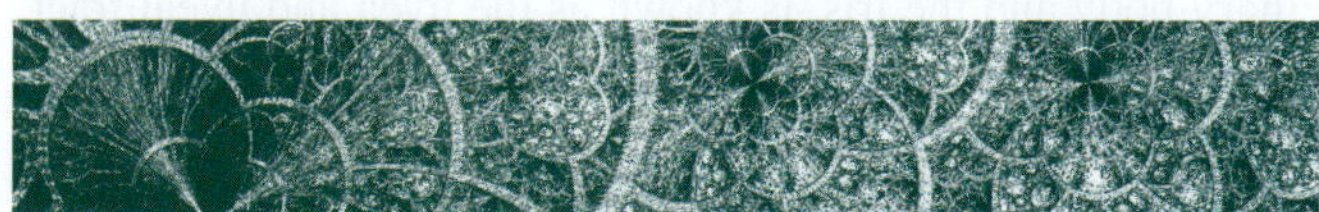

Nursing care

Health promotion

Advise all people about the importance of protecting the eyes from UVB rays by wearing eye protection during activities such as welding and when outdoors. Discuss the link between heavy smoking and cataract development and provide necessary education and resources to young people regarding the additional effects of smoking.

Assessment

- *Health history*: effect of vision changes on lifestyle and activities (e.g. ability to read, watch television, participate

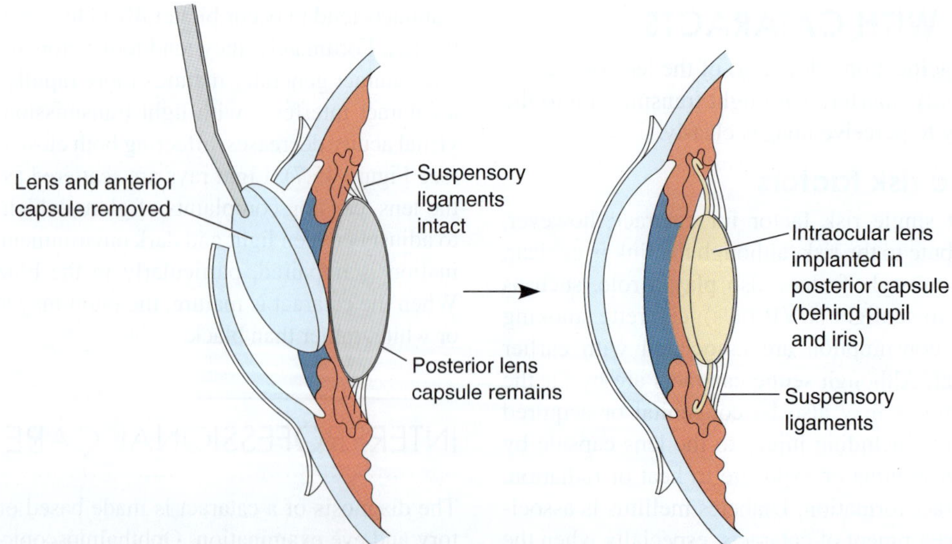

FIGURE 45.8 ***Extracapsular cataract extraction with removal of the lens and anterior capsule, leaving the posterior capsule intact. The intraocular lens is implanted within the posterior capsule***

in work and recreational activities); history of smoking, diabetes, use of prescription drugs associated with increased risk of cataract.
- *Physical examination*: general health; visual acuity (using corrective lenses and Snellen chart) in each eye; presence of red reflex.

Nursing diagnoses and interventions

The person with cataracts has few physical care nursing requirements. Patient advocacy, psychological and emotional support, and education are typically of higher priority for these people. (See 'Nursing care of the person having eye surgery' in the earlier box.)

Decisional conflict: cataract removal

With the initial diagnosis of a cataract, the nurse often becomes an important information resource for the person.

- Explain the non-emergent nature of the condition and help the person determine the extent to which the cataract is affecting daily life. *Providing information about cataracts and their surgical removal assists with decision making and helps the person decide whether to proceed with the surgery.*
- Attend to verbalised concerns about surgery and its outcome. Address questions factually and completely. Fear of blindness is second only to fear of cancer for many people. *Careful listening, education and a caring, understanding attitude can help the person deal with possible fear prior to surgery.*

Risk of ineffective therapeutic regimen management

- Assess for factors that may interfere with the person's ability to be self-caring in the postoperative phase. *A chronic condition such as arthritis may affect the ability to administer eye drops and may indicate the need to include the education and support of a family member.*
- Assess for additional care needs that may be necessitated by vision changes in the early postoperative period. *Additional needs, such as insulin injections, may suggest the requirement for additional home or nursing care postoperatively.*

Community-based care

Following the initial diagnosis, the focus is on education, indications for surgery and vision restoration following cataract removal. Provide adaptive strategies to deal with effects of the cataract on vision and depth perception. When surgery is scheduled, provide pre- and postoperative education and include a significant other in the sessions. Reinforce the following information with written instructions:

- limitations such as avoiding reading, lifting, strenuous activity and sleeping on operative side
- importance of not disturbing the eye dressing
- importance of not rubbing or scratching the eye
- prescribed medications and side effects
- importance of follow-up appointments
- manifestations of postoperative complications such as eye pain, decreased visual acuity or other change in vision, headache, nausea or itching and redness of the affected eye
- instillation of eye drops and application of eye patch or shield
- care, insertion and removal of contact lenses as appropriate
- visual changes associated with thick-lensed eyeglasses as appropriate.

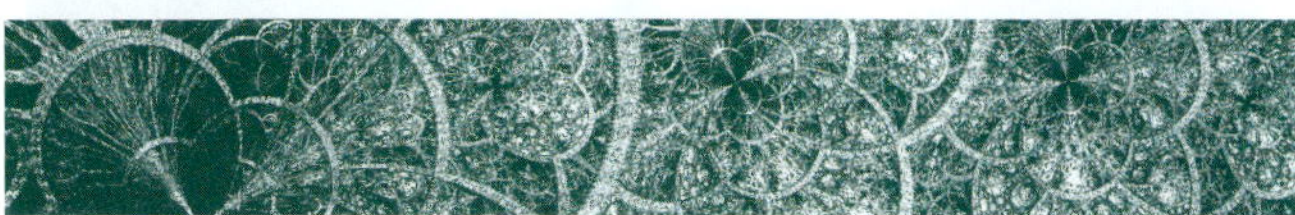

THE PERSON WITH GLAUCOMA

Glaucoma is a condition characterised by optic neuropathy with gradual loss of peripheral vision and, usually, increased intraocular pressure. Glaucoma is a silent thief of vision in that the person typically experiences no manifestations other than narrowing of the visual field, which occurs so gradually that it often goes unnoticed until late in the disease process.

Incidence and risk factors

Glaucoma affects over 300,000 Australians aged over 60 (this number is expected to grow to around 400,000 by 2025 due to the ageing population) and is the leading cause of blindness worldwide. The limited data available to date highlight the prevalence of glaucoma in the older generation of Indigenous Australians (Vision Australia, 2017).

Glaucoma is usually a primary condition without an identified cause. Primary glaucoma is most common in adults over the age of 60; however, it may be a congenital condition in infants and children. Secondary glaucoma can develop as a result of infection or inflammation of the eye, cataract, tumour, haemorrhage or eye trauma.

Pathophysiology

The aqueous humour occupies both the anterior and posterior chambers of the eye. The normal intraocular pressure of approximately 10 to 20 mmHg is maintained by a balance between the production of aqueous humour in the ciliary body, its flow through the pupil from the posterior to the anterior chamber of the eye and its outflow or absorption through the trabecular meshwork and canal of Schlemm (see Figure 44.3). If the balance is disrupted, due to a decrease in the outflow or absorption of aqueous humour, the intraocular pressure increases. Although the exact relationship is unclear, it appears that increased intraocular pressure injures the optic nerve. Axons in the periphery of the optic disc are damaged first. As optic fibres are destroyed, the rim of the optic disc shrinks and the normal depression in its centre (the *optic cup*) becomes larger and deeper (called optic 'cupping'). These changes to the optic disc are visible before visual field changes can be detected. As the disease progresses, there is a painless, progressive narrowing of the visual field (see Figure 45.9) and eventual blindness. Vision loss is often significant before the person seeks treatment and glaucoma is diagnosed.

Primary glaucoma in adults has two main forms: open-angle and angle-closure glaucoma. Both terms refer to the angle formed at the point where the iris meets the cornea in the eye's anterior chamber (see Figure 45.10). Forms of primary glaucoma are compared in Table 45.3.

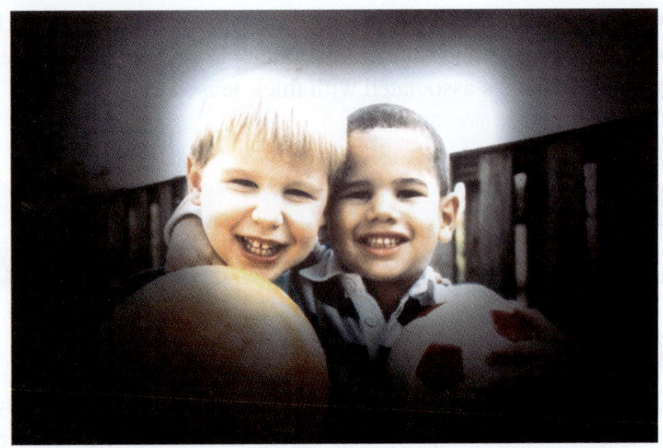

FIGURE 45.9 ***Narrowing of visual fields typical of untreated glaucoma***

Source: Courtesy of National Eye Institute, National Institutes of Health (NEI/NIH).

Open-angle glaucoma

Open-angle glaucoma, often called chronic simple glaucoma, is the most common form of glaucoma in adults, accounting for approximately 90% of all glaucoma. Its cause is unknown; it is thought to have a hereditary component, but no clear inheritance pattern can be identified.

In open-angle glaucoma, the anterior chamber angle between the iris and cornea is normal (see Figure 45.10A); hence the term *open angle*. However, the flow of aqueous humour through the trabecular meshwork and into the scleral venous sinus is relatively obstructed: the cause of this obstruction is unknown. Restricted outflow leads to an increased amount of fluid in the eye and increased intraocular pressure. Open-angle glaucoma tends to be a chronic, gradually progressive disease. The trabecular meshwork increasingly inhibits the outflow of aqueous humour and the intraocular pressure gradually increases. The result is neuronal ischaemia and optic nerve degeneration, leading to gradual loss of vision.

Open-angle glaucoma typically affects both eyes, although the pressures and progression may not be symmetrical.

MANIFESTATIONS Open-angle glaucoma is painless, with gradual loss of visual fields. The loss of peripheral vision generally is so gradual that the person is often unaware of it until it is detected through a comprehensive vision examination. Intraocular pressure is usually, but not always, elevated (Loscalzo et al., 2022).

Angle-closure glaucoma

Acute angle-closure (also called narrow-angle or closed-angle) glaucoma is a less common form of primary glaucoma in adults. It accounts for approximately 5–10% of all cases of glaucoma (Norris, 2018). Approximately 1% of people over the age of 40 have narrowed anterior chamber angles; the incidence is higher in older adults and in people of Far Eastern, Asian or Inuit ancestry (Papadakis, McPhee & Rabow, 2022).

Narrowing of the anterior chamber angle (see Figure 45.10A for an illustration of the normal anterior chamber angle) occurs because of corneal flattening or bulging of the iris into the anterior chamber. When the lens thickens during accommodation, or the iris thickens during pupil dilation, this angle can close completely. Closure of the angle blocks the outflow of aqueous humour through the trabecular meshwork and scleral venous sinus, and the intraocular pressure rises abruptly (see Figure 45.10B). This abrupt increase in intraocular pressure

TABLE 45.3 A comparison of open-angle and angle-closure glaucoma

	OPEN-ANGLE GLAUCOMA	ANGLE-CLOSURE GLAUCOMA
Incidence	• Common • Accounts for 90% of all cases of glaucoma	• Uncommon
Risk factors	• Over age 40 • Genetic link	• Narrow anterior chamber angle • Ageing • Far Eastern, Asian or Inuit ancestry
Pathophysiology	• Impaired aqueous outflow through the scleral venous sinus • Damage to axons of retinal ganglion cells with optic nerve atrophy • Gradual, consistent increase in intraocular pressure • Usually bilateral	• Pupil dilation or lens accommodation causes already narrowed angle to close, blocking aqueous outflow • Rapid rise in intraocular pressure • Usually unilateral
Manifestations	• No initial manifestations • Frequent lens changes in glasses • Impaired dark adaptation • Halos around lights • Gradual reduction of visual fields with preservation of central vision until late in the disease • Mild to severe increased intraocular pressure	• Abrupt onset of eye pain, headache • Decreased visual acuity • Nausea and vomiting • Reddened conjunctiva • Cloudy cornea • Fixed pupil • Rapid, significant increase in intraocular pressure
Management	• Topical medications such as miotics, beta-blockers, prostaglandin analogues • Carbonic anhydrase inhibitors • Laser trabeculoplasty, trabeculectomy	• Topical miotics or beta-blockers • Systemic osmotic agents, carbonic anhydrase inhibitors • Laser iridotomy or peripheral iridectomy

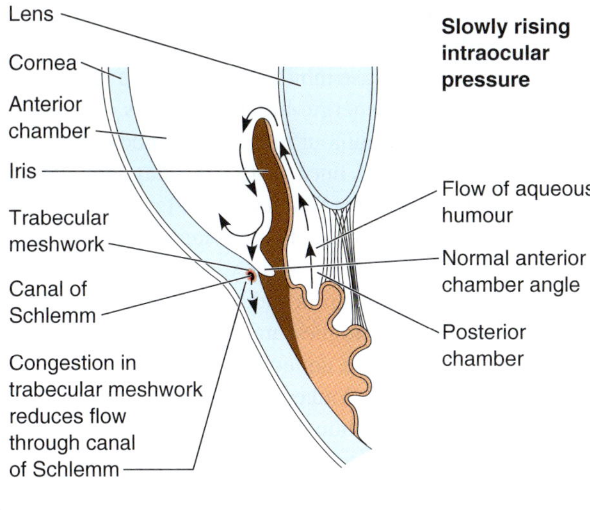

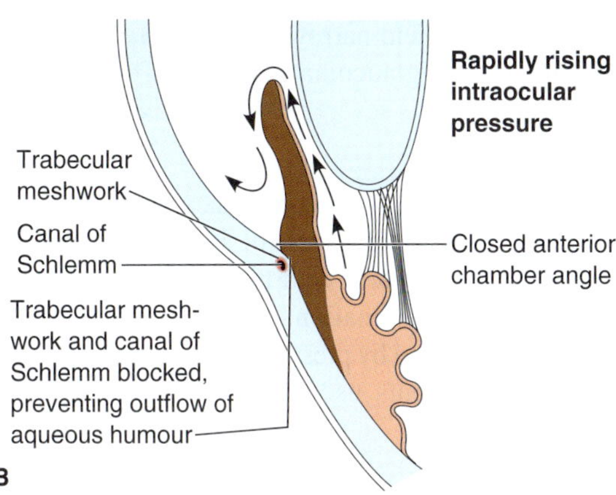

FIGURE 45.10 *Forms of primary adult glaucoma. A, In chronic open-angle glaucoma, the anterior chamber angle remains open, but drainage of aqueous humour through the canal of Schlemm is impaired. B, In acute angle-closure glaucoma, the angle of the iris and anterior chamber narrows, obstructing the outflow of aqueous humour*

damages the neurons of the retina and the optic nerve, leading to a rapid and permanent loss of vision if not treated promptly.

Episodes of angle-closure glaucoma are typically unilateral. However, a history of angle-closure glaucoma of one eye increases the risk that it will occur in the other eye.

Because of the effect of pupil dilation on aqueous outflow in angle-closure glaucoma, episodes often occur in association with darkness, emotional upset/stress or other factors that cause the pupil to dilate. People may have intermittent episodes lasting several hours before having a more typically prolonged attack of angle-closure glaucoma. For people with a history of the condition, it is vital to avoid medications such as atropine and other anticholinergics, which have a mydriatic or pupil-dilating effect.

MANIFESTATIONS Symptoms such as severe eye and face pain, general malaise, nausea and vomiting, seeing coloured halos around lights and an abrupt decrease in visual acuity are associated with acute episodes of angle-closure glaucoma. The conjunctiva of the affected eye may be reddened and the cornea clouded with corneal oedema, and the pupil may be fixed (non-reactive to light) at midpoint. Some people may experience periodic mild attacks, usually in the evening, with eye discomfort, impaired vision and coloured rings around lights.

INTERPROFESSIONAL CARE

Although glaucoma cannot be predicted, prevented or cured, in most cases it can be controlled and vision can be preserved if diagnosed early. Because open-angle glaucoma, the most prevalent type of glaucoma, has few symptoms, routine eye examinations are recommended for early detection. Measurement of intraocular pressure, fundoscopy to assess the optic disc and visual field testing are used for diagnosis and monitoring of treatment effectiveness.

Diagnosis

The following diagnostic studies are used to detect and evaluate for the presence, severity, type and effects of glaucoma:

- *Tonometry* indirectly measures intraocular pressure (see Figure 45.11). Contact or non-contact tonometry may be used. Routine tonometry screening is recommended for all people over the age of 60. A single elevated pressure reading does not warrant a diagnosis of glaucoma; variations in intraocular pressure occur throughout the day. See the chapter 'A person-centred approach to assessing the eye and ear' for more information about tonometry.
- *Fundoscopy* (visual inspection of the optic fundus using an ophthalmoscope) identifies pallor and an increase in the size and depth of the optic cup on the optic disc. These changes are significant for diagnosing glaucoma.

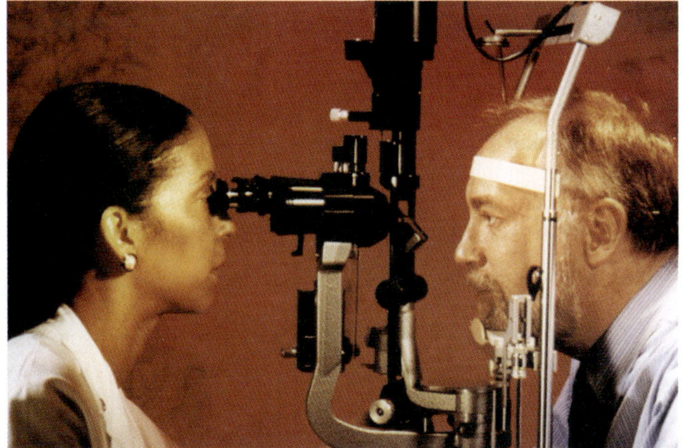

FIGURE 45.11 *An eye professional uses a tonometer to indirectly measure the intraocular pressure of a person's eye*

Source: Courtesy of National Eye Institute, National Institutes of Health (NEI/NIH).

- *Gonioscopy* uses a gonioscope to measure the depth of the anterior chamber. This test differentiates open-angle from angle-closure glaucoma.
- *Visual field testing* (see Figure 45.12) identifies the degree of central visual field narrowing and peripheral vision loss. The person with glaucoma may retain 6/6 central vision even though there is severe peripheral vision loss.

Medications

Although medications cannot cure glaucoma, many people with open-angle glaucoma can control intraocular pressure and preserve vision indefinitely with medications. Medications are used alone or in combination, with the timing and dosage individually determined by pressure measurements. The primary pharmacological agents used to treat glaucoma are topical beta-adrenergic blocking agents, adrenergics (mydriatics), prostaglandin analogues or carbonic anhydrase inhibitors. An oral carbonic anhydrase inhibitor also may be used.

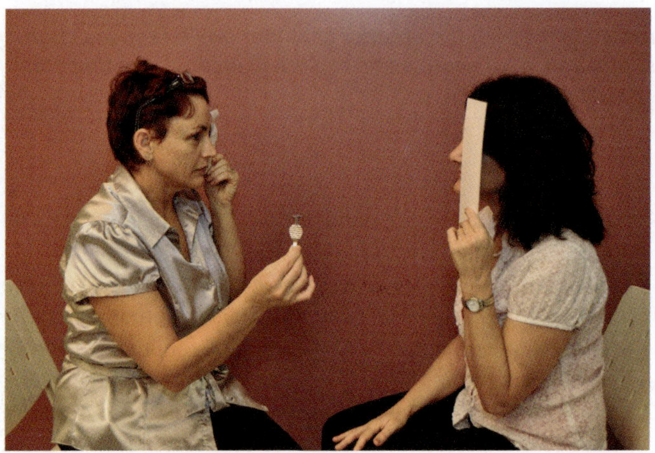

FIGURE 45.12 ***Visual field testing. Peripheral vision or visual fields are assessed by testing the person's ability to detect an object brought into the line of vision from the periphery. The person's peripheral vision is compared to that of the nurse examiner. Each eye is tested separately***

Topical beta-adrenergic blocking agents decrease the production of aqueous humour in the ciliary body. Beta-adrenergic blockers can be used once or twice a day, depending on the drug and dosage form. When administering beta-blockers or teaching about their use, it is important to remember that ophthalmic preparations can produce systemic effects, including bronchospasm, bradycardia and heart failure.

Prostaglandin analogues are a newer class of ophthalmics prescribed to increase aqueous outflow. They are similar to beta-blockers in their longer duration of action, thus requiring only a daily dose. Although they have fewer systemic effects, these drugs may cause conjunctival hyperaemia and permanent changes in the colour of the iris and eyebrows.

An adrenergic agonist may be prescribed along with a beta-blocker, or, if beta-blockers are contraindicated (e.g. in a person with heart failure, asthma or chronic obstructive pulmonary disease (COPD)), another adrenergic agonist may be prescribed when other drugs do not sufficiently reduce intraocular pressure, but adverse effects make it inappropriate for long-term use (Papadakis et al., 2022).

A carbonic anhydrase inhibitor decreases the production of aqueous humour and reduces intraocular pressure. It is used with other drugs to control pressures and in people for whom beta-blockers are contraindicated because of heart failure or reactive airway disease. A systemic carbonic anhydrase inhibitor also may be used for some people.

Nursing implications for medications used to control chronic glaucoma are outlined in the 'Medication administration' box.

In acute angle-closure glaucoma, diuretics may be administered intravenously to achieve a rapid decrease in intraocular pressure prior to surgical intervention. Carbonic anhydrase inhibitors and osmotic diuretics are used. Fast-acting miotic drops, such as acetylcholine, are also administered to constrict the pupil and draw the iris away from the angle and the scleral venous sinus.

MEDICATION ADMINISTRATION The person with glaucoma

ADRENERGIC AGONISTS (MYDRIATICS)

Brimonidine

Apraclonidine

Adrenergic agonists dilate the pupil, reduce the production of aqueous humour and increase its absorption, effectively reducing intraocular pressure in open-angle glaucoma.

Nursing responsibilities

- Assess the person for contraindications and adverse reactions to adrenergic agonists, including acute angle-closure glaucoma, hypertension, cardiac arrhythmias and coronary heart disease.
- Assess for central nervous system side effects of anxiety, nervousness and muscle tremors. If these side effects are severe, notify the doctor.
- Assess for a hypersensitivity reaction, including itching, lid oedema and discharge from the eyes. Notify the doctor if you notice these signs.

Health education for the person and family

- Report any change in visual acuity or eye pain. (Eye pain may indicate an attack of angle-closure glaucoma and must be reported to the doctor immediately.)
- Avoid over-the-counter sinus and cold medications containing pseudoephedrine and phenylephrine, as they may accentuate the side effects of this drug.

BETA-ADRENERGIC BLOCKERS

Betaxolol

Carteolol

Levobunolol

Metipranolol

Timolol

Selected beta-adrenergic blockers reduce intraocular pressure by decreasing the production of aqueous humour. Because beta-blockers do not affect pupil size and lens accommodation, they do not have the adverse effects on

MEDICATION ADMINISTRATION **The person with glaucoma (continued)**

visual acuity that adrenergic agonists do. Their systemic effects, however, may limit their usefulness for certain people.

Nursing responsibilities

- Assess the person for allergies or contraindications to beta-blocker therapy, including asthma, COPD, heart block and heart failure.
- Maintain pressure over the lacrimal sac after administration to prevent systemic absorption.
- Assess for side effects such as bradycardia, hypotension and depression.
- Educate about the drug, its dose, administration and desired and side effects.

Health education for the person and family

- After instilling the eye drops, put pressure on the lacrimal sac, at the corner of the eye near the bridge of the nose, to keep the drug from entering your system.
- Your vision may be blurred during the initial period of therapy, but it will improve as you continue to use the drug.
- Report adverse effects, including worsening vision, difficulty breathing, reduced exercise tolerance and sweating or flushing, to the doctor.

CARBONIC ANHYDRASE INHIBITORS

Dorzolamide
Brinzolamide
Acetazolamide (most common)

The carbonic anhydrate inhibitors lower intraocular pressure and are used primarily as adjunctive therapy. Dorzolamide and brinzolamide are administered as eye drops; acetazolamide may be given PO, IM or IV in glaucoma emergencies.

Nursing responsibilities

- Assess for allergies or other contraindications to the use of carbonic anhydrase inhibitors, including known allergy to sulfur or severe kidney or hepatic disease.
- Monitor for increased drug interactions of amphetamines, procainamide, quinidine, tricyclic antidepressants, and ephedrine and pseudoephedrine.
- Assess daily weight, intake and output, serum electrolytes and vital signs in people taking oral or parenteral carbonic anhydrase inhibitors.
- Administer PO in the morning to prevent sleep disruption because of the diuretic effect.
- If used with another topical ophthalmic, administer 10 minutes apart.
- Educate the person about the drug, its dose, administration and desired and side effects.

Health education for the person and family

- For oral medications, maintain a fluid intake of 2 to 3 L per day and rise slowly from lying or sitting positions because you may feel dizzy when you first stand (orthostatic hypotension).
- For topical medications, notify the doctor if you have prolonged eye irritation.

PROSTAGLANDIN ANALOGUES

Bimatoprost
Latanoprost
Travoprost

The prostaglandin analogue drugs relax the ciliary muscle, improving the outflow of aqueous humour and reducing intraocular pressure. These drugs have the advantage of requiring only a single daily dose; however, they do have some adverse effects such as blurred vision and stinging and, when used long term, cause permanent darkening of the iris of the eye and eyebrows, increased growth of eyelashes and conjunctival hyperaemia (redness).

Nursing responsibilities

- Assess and note eye colour, presence of inflammation, exudates or pain.
- Note vital signs and most recent liver function test results because these may be altered by the drug.

Health education for the person and family

- Use once daily at bedtime as directed. This drug may blur vision; use at bedtime minimises associated safety risks.
- Remove contact lenses before administering this drug.
- Minor eye discomfort, including burning and tearing, may occur with this drug. Notify your doctor if adverse effects are severe or intolerable.
- This drug may cause darkening of your iris, the skin around the eyes and the eyebrows, as well as increased growth of the eyelashes. These colour changes are permanent and will not progress if the drug is discontinued by your doctor.

Surgery

Surgical intervention is indicated for people with acute angle-closure and chronic open-angle glaucoma that is not effectively controlled by medication.

Surgical management of chronic open-angle glaucoma involves improving the drainage of the aqueous humour from the anterior chamber of the eye. Trabeculoplasty and trabeculectomy filtration surgery are the most commonly used procedures.

In a *laser trabeculoplasty*, an argon laser is aimed through a gonioscope to create multiple laser burns spaced evenly around the trabecular meshwork. As the burns heal, the scars they create cause tension, stretching and opening the meshwork. This non-invasive technique is the treatment of choice because it requires no incision and can be performed as an outpatient procedure.

Trabeculectomy is a type of filtration surgery in which a permanent fistula is created to drain aqueous humour from the anterior chamber of the eye. A portion of trabecular meshwork is removed and a flap of sclera is left unsutured to create a channel or fistula between the anterior chamber and the subconjunctival space. Aqueous humour is able to drain into the space under the conjunctiva, where it can be absorbed into the systemic circulation. A trabeculectomy is usually performed under general anaesthesia and requires hospitalisation.

If these procedures are not fully effective, either photocoagulation using an argon laser (heat) or cyclocryotherapy using a probe to freeze tissue may be employed to destroy portions of the ciliary body. This tissue destruction reduces the production of aqueous humour, subsequently reducing intraocular pressure. Another surgical procedure involves insertion of a glaucoma drainage device that regulates the outflow of aqueous humour.

Surgical procedures used in the treatment of acute angle-closure glaucoma include gonioplasty, laser iridotomy and peripheral iridectomy. Because of the high risk of a future attack of angle-closure glaucoma in the unaffected eye, these procedures are often performed prophylactically.

In *gonioplasty*, the healing and scarring of microscopic lesions created at the periphery of the iris draws the iris away from the cornea, widening the anterior chamber, increases the angle and opens drainage channels for the aqueous humour.

Laser iridotomy is a non-invasive procedure using a laser to create multiple small perforations in the iris of the eye. These perforations allow aqueous humour to drain from the posterior chamber to the anterior chamber, and out through the trabecular meshwork and the scleral venous sinus. During an *iridectomy*, a small segment of the iris is removed to facilitate the flow of aqueous humour between the posterior and anterior chambers and to open the anterior chamber angle.

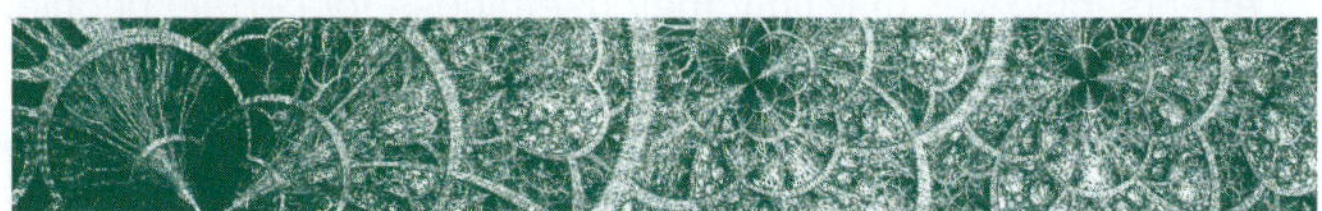

Nursing care

When planning and providing nursing care for the person with glaucoma, both the specific form of the disease and its actual or potential effects on the person's vision, lifestyle, safety and psychosocial wellbeing must be considered. In the hospitalised person, glaucoma is typically a concurrent diagnosis rather than the primary reason for seeking care, unless the diagnosis is acute angle-closure glaucoma. For additional nursing activities for the person with glaucoma, see the accompanying nursing care plan.

NURSING CARE PLAN A person with glaucoma and cataracts

Lila Rainey is an 80-year-old widow who lives alone in the house she and her late husband built 50 years ago. She has worn glasses for myopia since she was a young girl and now wears bifocals to correct her near vision as well. She was diagnosed 4 years ago with chronic open-angle glaucoma, for which she takes timolol maleate 0.5%—one drop in each eye twice a day. Recently she has noticed difficulty reading and watching television despite a new lens prescription. She has stopped driving at night because the glare of oncoming headlights makes it difficult for her to see. Mrs Rainey's ophthalmologist has told her that she has cataracts but that they do not need to come out until they bother her. Although her glaucoma is still controlled by the medication, her intraocular pressure measurements have been gradually increasing. Mrs Rainey has taken 325 mg of aspirin daily since a transient ischaemic attack 8 years ago. She is being admitted to the outpatient surgery unit for a cataract removal and intraocular lens implant in her right eye.

ASSESSMENT

Mrs Rainey is admitted to the eye surgery unit by Susan Schafer, RN. In her assessment, Ms Schafer finds Mrs Rainey to be alert and oriented, though apprehensive about her upcoming surgery. Assessment findings include BP 134/72, P 86 and R 18. Mrs Rainey's neurological, respiratory, cardiovascular and abdominal assessments are essentially normal. Her pupils are round, equal and react briskly to light and accommodation. Her conjunctiva are pink; sclera and corneas, clear. Using the ophthalmoscope, Ms Schafer notes that the red reflex in Mrs Rainey's right eye is diminished. Ophthalmic examination shows visual acuity of 6/45 OD (right eye) and 6/15 OS (left eye) with corrective lenses. Her intraocular pressures are 21 mmHg OD and 17 mmHg OS. On fundoscopic exam, no disease of the blood vessels, retina, macula or disc is found. Ms Schafer reviews the operative procedure with Mrs Rainey, answering her questions and advising what to expect after surgery. Following preoperative protocols, Mrs Rainey is prepared and transported to surgery.

NURSING DIAGNOSIS

- *Risk of disturbed visual perception* related to myopia and lens extraction.
- *Risk of anxiety* related to anticipated surgery.
- *Risk of knowledge deficit* related to lack of information regarding postoperative care.
- *Risk of impaired home maintenance* related to activity restrictions and impaired vision.

PLANNING

- Provide a safe environment, placing the call bell and personal care items within easy reach.
- Encourage Mrs Rainey to express her fears about surgery and its potential effect on vision.
- Explain all procedures related to surgery and recovery.

Expected outcomes

- To regain sufficient visual acuity to maintain ADLs, including reading and watching television for enjoyment.
- Demonstrate the procedure for instilling eye drops postoperatively.
- Demonstrate knowledge of the home care she will require after surgery, signs of complications and actions to take if complications occur.
- Use appropriate resources to assist with home maintenance until vision stabilises and activity restrictions are lifted.
- Demonstrate a reduced level of anxiety.

IMPLEMENTATION

- Instruct her to avoid shutting her eyelids tightly, sneezing, coughing, laughing, bending over, lifting or straining to have a bowel movement. Educate her to wear glasses during the day and an eye shield at night to prevent injury to the surgical site.
- Explain and demonstrate the procedure for administering eye drops.
- Provide verbal and written instructions about postoperative care, including a schedule of follow-up examinations, potential complications and actions to take in response.

NURSING CARE PLAN **A person with glaucoma and cataracts (continued)**

- Refer Mrs Rainey to a discharge planner or social worker to help establish a plan for home maintenance as required.

EVALUATION

Mrs Rainey is discharged the morning after her surgery. She is visibly relieved when the eye patch is removed because her vision in the operated eye is better than before surgery, even without her glasses. She is able to relate the recommended activity restrictions. Mrs Rainey administers her own eye drops before discharge and relates an understanding of the prescribed postoperative care and safety precautions. Mrs Rainey's daughter plans to visit her mother two to three times a week to help with laundry and vacuuming until she is able to resume all her household activities. Mrs Rainey says that she will not 'be so scared when I need my other eye done'. She understands the chronic nature of her glaucoma and states that her vision is too important for her to neglect her timolol drops and routine eye exams.

CRITICAL THINKING IN THE NURSING PROCESS

1 Why did it become more difficult to control Mrs Rainey's intraocular pressure as her cataract matured?
2 Identify medications that are commonly prescribed following cataract surgery. What are the risks of interactions between these medications and Mrs Rainey's timolol drops?
3 Develop a care plan for the nursing diagnosis *Self-care deficit: dressing/grooming*, related to vision impairment and restricted bending.

REFLECTION ON THE NURSING PROCESS

1 Outline what you have learned from the case study and how this applies to your future practice.
2 What communication strategies could you use when caring for a person experiencing issues with their vision?

Health promotion

Although glaucoma cannot be prevented, its severity and potentially deleterious permanent effects can be limited with early visual screening. The nurse assumes an important role in educating the public about the risk factors for glaucoma, such as increased age and the higher incidence in certain cultures. All people over the age of 40 are encouraged to receive an eye examination every 2 to 4 years, including tonometry screening. Those with a predominant family history should be evaluated more frequently, every 1 to 2 years. After the age of 65, yearly ophthalmological examinations are recommended.

Assessment

- Collect the following data through a health history and physical examination (see the chapter 'A person-centred approach to assessing the eye and ear').
- *Health history*: family history; presence of altered vision, halos and excessive tearing; sudden, severe eye pain; use of corrective lenses; most recent eye examination.
- *Physical examination*: distant and near vision, peripheral fields and retina for optic nerve cupping.

Nursing diagnoses and interventions

Nursing care planning focuses on problems associated with the temporary or permanent vision impairment, the resultant increased risk of injury and the psychosocial problems of anxiety and coping.

Disturbed visual perception

Whether glaucoma and resulting impaired vision is the person's primary problem or a pre-existing condition in a person with another disorder, it must be a primary consideration in nursing care planning.

- Establish rapport with the person. Orient to time, place, person and situation as indicated. State the purpose of your visit. *The person with impaired vision must rely on input from the other senses. A lack of visual cues increases the importance of verbal ones. For example, the person with impaired vision cannot see the nurse checking an intravenous infusion and needs a verbal explanation of who is in the room and why. When the person's normal daily routine is disrupted by illness or hospitalisation, additional sensory input such as a radio or television, and explanations of the routine and activities, are useful to maintain the person's orientation.*
- Provide any visual aids that are routinely used. Keep them close, making sure that the person knows where they are and can reach them easily. *Easy access encourages the person to use these items and enhances the ability to provide self-care.*
- Orientate the person to the environment. Explain the location of the call bell, personal items and the furniture in the room. If able, tour the person's room, including the bathroom and sink. *People with vision impairments are usually very capable of providing self-care in a known environment.*
- Provide other tools or items that can help compensate for diminished vision:
  a. bright, non-glare lighting
  b. books, magazines and instructions in large print
  c. books on tape, CD or MP3 player
  d. telephones with oversized pushbuttons
  e. a clock with numbers and hands that can be felt.
- Assist with meals by:
  a. reading menu selections and marking choices
  b. describing the position of foods on a meal tray according to the clock system—for example, 'On the plate, the peas are at 9 o'clock, the mashed potatoes at 1 o'clock and the chicken breast at 6 o'clock. The water glass is at 2 o'clock on the tray above the plate and coffee is at 11 o'clock'
  c. placing the utensils in a readily accessible position
  d. removing lids from containers, buttering bread and cutting meat, as needed
  e. if the vision impairment is new or temporary, the person may need feeding or continued assistance during the meal.

Providing assistance during meals is important to maintain the person's nutritional status. The person may be ashamed of needing help or embarrassed to request it, and may respond by not eating or by claiming not to be hungry.

- Assist with mobility and ambulation as needed:
  a. Have the person hold your arm or elbow and walk slightly ahead as a guide. Do not hold the person's arm or elbow.
  b. Describe the surroundings and progress as you proceed. Warn in advance of potential hazards, turns and steps.
  c. Educate on how to feel the chair, bed or commode with the hands and the back of the legs before sitting.

  These measures help ensure the person's safety while providing for mobility and helping prevent complications associated with immobility.
- If the vision loss is unilateral and recent, provide instructions related to this loss and change in depth perception:
  a. Caution about the loss of depth perception and educate about safety precautions, such as reaching slowly for objects and using visual cues for distance, especially when driving.
  b. Educate the person to scan their environment, turning the head fully towards the affected side to identify potential hazards and looking up and down to compensate for the loss of depth perception.

  The person with a unilateral vision loss is often unaware of its effects on peripheral vision and depth perception.

Risk of injury

Whether the person is experiencing a sudden loss of vision due to acute angle-closure glaucoma or significant vision impairment due to inadequately managed chronic glaucoma, both are at an increased risk of injury. People who have had surgical interventions for glaucoma are at even greater risk.

- Assess ability to perform ADLs. People may be reluctant to request assistance, believing that they should be able to perform these familiar tasks. *Careful assessment and provision of needed assistance help prevent injury and maintain the person's self-esteem and confidence.*
- Notify all staff and place a sign on the person's door to alert all personnel not to change the arrangement of the person's room. *The person with impaired vision is at high risk of falling when in an unfamiliar environment. It is important to maintain a safe, familiar room when the person is hospitalised.*
- Raise the person's side rails on their bed. *Raised rails remind people to ask for assistance before ambulating in an unfamiliar environment.*
- Discuss possible adaptations in the home to help the person remain as independent as possible and prevent falls or other injuries. *Often minor changes in the home environment, such as removing scatter rugs and small items of furniture, allow the person to navigate safely in this already familiar environment.*

CONSIDERATION FOR PRACTICE

Keep traffic areas free of clutter to reduce the risk of injury in people with impaired vision.

Anxiety

The actual or potential loss of sight threatens the person's self-concept, role functioning, patterns of interaction and, potentially, environment. The person with impaired vision who functions well in a familiar environment will feel anxious in the unfamiliar setting of a hospital or care facility.

- Assess for verbal and non-verbal indications of anxiety levels and for normal coping mechanisms. Repeated expressions of concern or denial that the vision change will affect the person's life indicate anxiety. Non-verbal indicators include tension, difficulty concentrating or thinking, restlessness, poor eye contact and changes in vocalisation (rapid speech, voice quivering). Physical indicators include tachycardia, dilated pupils, cool and clammy skin, and tremors. *The person may not recognise this feeling as anxiety. Identifying and acknowledging the anxiety state can help the person recognise and deal with it.*
- Encourage to verbalise fears, anger and feelings of anxiety. *Verbalising helps externalise the anxiety and allows fears to be addressed.*
- Discuss perception of the eye condition and its effects on lifestyle and roles. *Discussion provides an opportunity to correct misperceptions and introduce alternative activities and assistive devices for people with vision impairments.*
- Establish rapport with the person by explaining all procedures fully before and as they are being performed, and use touch to convey proximity and caring. *The person with impaired vision must rely on the other senses to make up for the loss of sight. Because the person cannot see what you are doing, complete explanations of even simple tasks such as refilling a water glass help to relieve anxiety.*
- Identify coping strategies that have been useful in the past and adapt these strategies to the present situation. *Previously successful coping strategies may be employed to increase the person's sense of control.*

Community-based care

People with glaucoma require education about lifetime strategies for managing the disease at home. They need to understand the importance of lifetime therapy to control the disease and prevent blindness. If a permanent vision impairment has resulted, the person needs information on achieving the maximum possible independence while maintaining safety. The following topics should be discussed with the person and family:

- prescribed medications, including proper way to instil eye drops
- importance of not taking certain prescription and over-the-counter medications without consulting a doctor
- periodic eye examinations with intraocular pressure measurement
- risks, warning signs and management of acute angle-closure glaucoma
- possible surgical options
- available state and territory community resources.

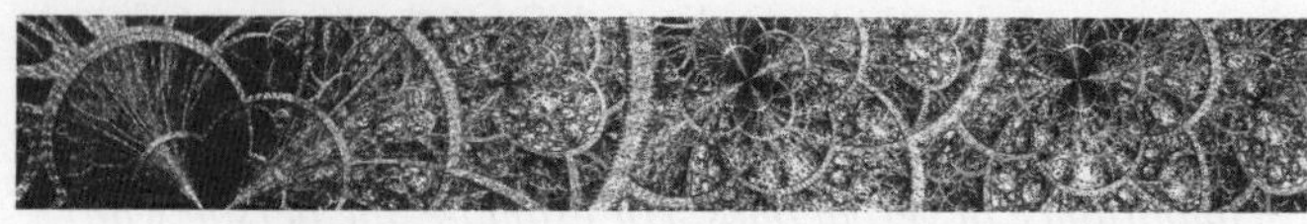

THE PERSON WITH AGE-RELATED MACULAR DEGENERATION

In Australia, age-related **macular degeneration** (AMD) is the second most common eye disease that causes vision impairment after cataracts.

FAST FACT

The total cost of vision loss associated with AMD in Australia was estimated at $5 billion in 2010. In 2021, there were approximately 1.29 million Australians with AMD, equivalent to 1 in 7 people over the age of 50. This could reach almost 2 million by 2030 (Department of Health, 2020).

Although the exact cause of AMD is unknown, factors associated with it include ageing, smoking, race and, possibly, genetic factors and cultural background. The destructive changes in the macula occur most often as a response to the ageing process. AMD affects males and females equally. Recent evidence suggests that inflammation plays a role in the development of AMD (Loscalzo et al., 2022), as does the interaction of certain genes with the immune system (NEI, 2018). Evidence suggests that the risk of developing AMD may be reduced by consumption of omega-3 fatty acids in fish, and vegetables high in lutein and zeaxanthin (carotenoids found in vegetables such as spinach, kale and broccoli).

Pathophysiology

The macula is the area of the retina that provides sharp central vision, receiving light from the centre of the visual field. Two forms of AMD identified are non-exudative (dry) and exudative (wet). Although both are progressive disorders, their manifestations and management differ.

Non-exudative or *dry macular degeneration* is the more common form of AMD. It is a gradual process that begins with accumulation of deposits called *drusen* beneath the pigment epithelium of the retina. Over time, these deposits enlarge and become more numerous. The pigment epithelium detaches in small areas and becomes atrophic, interfering with sensory function of the macula. Vision loss typically is not significant and the disorder progresses slowly. There is, however, a risk that the disorder will progress to the exudative stage of the disease.

Exudative macular degeneration is characterised by the formation of new, weak blood vessels in the potential space between the choroid (vascular layer of the eye) and the retina (neurosensory layer). These new vessels are prone to leak, elevating the retina from the choroid and distorting vision. Although exudative macular degeneration typically is a gradual process, bleeding can lead to acute vision loss in some cases. With significant or repeated bleeding episodes, scar tissue forms and central vision is permanently lost (Loscalzo et al., 2022).

Manifestations

When the macula is damaged, central vision becomes blurred and distorted, but peripheral vision remains intact. Distortion of vision in one eye is a common initial manifestation; straight lines appear wavy or distorted. With the loss of central vision, activities that require close central vision, such as reading and sewing, are particularly affected (see Figure 45.13).

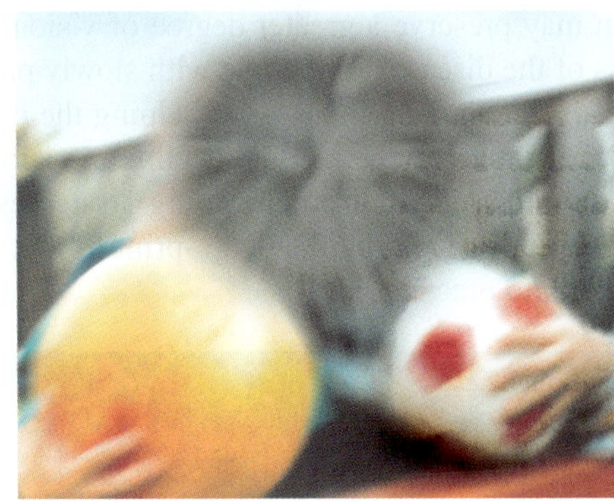

FIGURE 45.13 ***Loss of central vision with advanced age-related macular degeneration***

Source: Courtesy of National Eye Institute, National Institutes of Health (NEI/NIH).

INTERPROFESSIONAL CARE

Age-related macular degeneration is diagnosed through vision and retinal examination. The Amsler grid (see Figure 44.5) may be used to identify distortion of central vision caused by AMD. If treatment for wet AMD is planned, a *fluorescein angiogram* may be done. Pictures are taken as the dye passes through the blood vessels of the retina, allowing detection of leaks.

In its early or intermediate stages, the progress of dry AMD can be slowed through the use of high-dose antioxidants and zinc. Research demonstrated a benefit when vitamins C and E, beta-carotene (vitamin A), zinc and copper were administered daily.

Wet AMD is treated with laser surgery or photodynamic therapy. Although these treatments do not cure the disease, they may slow the rate of vision loss. In laser surgery, fragile blood vessels are destroyed, preventing bleeding. There is a risk, however, of damage to surrounding healthy tissue, some vision loss and continued growth of new vessels. In photodynamic therapy, verteporfin, a drug that tends to adhere to the surface of new blood vessels, is injected systemically. Light is then shined into the affected eye, activating the drug and destroying new blood vessels. This treatment is relatively fast and painless but does require avoidance of exposure to direct sunlight or bright indoor light for 5 days following treatment (NEI, 2021).

Large-print books and magazines, the use of a magnifying glass and high-intensity lighting can help the person to cope with the reduced vision of macular degeneration.

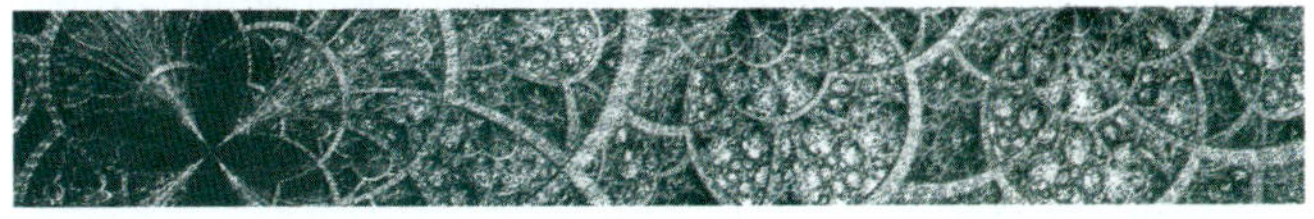

Nursing care

Nurses should be alert for people demonstrating new and rapid onset manifestations of macular degeneration and promptly refer these people for ophthalmological evaluation. Early intervention may preserve a greater degree of vision and slow the progress of the disease. For people with slowly progressive manifestations, the nursing focus is on helping the person and family members adapt to the gradual decline in vision by recommending visual aids and other coping strategies. Person education materials should be in a large-print format. See also the 'Translation to practice' box.

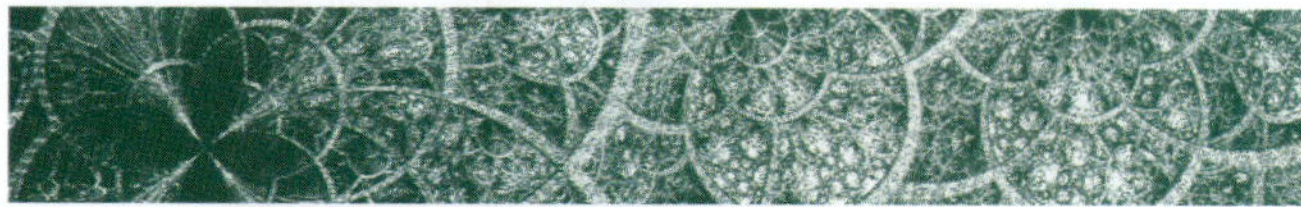

THE PERSON WITH DIABETIC RETINOPATHY

Diabetic retinopathy is a vascular disorder affecting the capillaries of the retina. The capillaries become sclerotic and lose their ability to transport sufficient oxygen and nutrients to the retina.

The risk of developing diabetic retinopathy is related to the duration of the diabetes and the degree of glycaemic control. Hypertension also is a risk factor (Loscalzo et al., 2022). Retinopathy is seen in both type 1 and type 2 diabetes. Nursing care of the person with diabetes is discussed in the chapter 'Nursing care of people with diabetes mellitus'.

FAST FACTS

- In Australia, diabetic retinopathy is the third most common eye disease that causes vision impairment after cataracts and age-related macular degeneration.
- People with diabetes are 25 times more likely to become legally blind than people unaffected by the disease (Loscalzo et al., 2022).

Pathophysiology and manifestations

Diabetic retinopathy progresses through four stages: (1) mild *non-proliferative* or background retinopathy, (2) moderate non-proliferative retinopathy, (3) severe non-proliferative retinopathy, and (4) *proliferative* retinopathy (NEI, 2022). Non-proliferative retinopathy is typically the initial form seen. The venous capillaries of the eye dilate and develop microaneurysms that may then leak, causing retinal oedema; or they may rupture, causing small haemorrhages into the retina. On ophthalmoscopic examination, yellow exudates, cotton-wool patches indicative of retinal ischaemia and red-dot haemorrhages are observed (see Figure 45.14). When the peripheral retina is involved, the person may experience few symptoms other than light glare. Oedema of the macula or a large haemorrhage may cause vision loss.

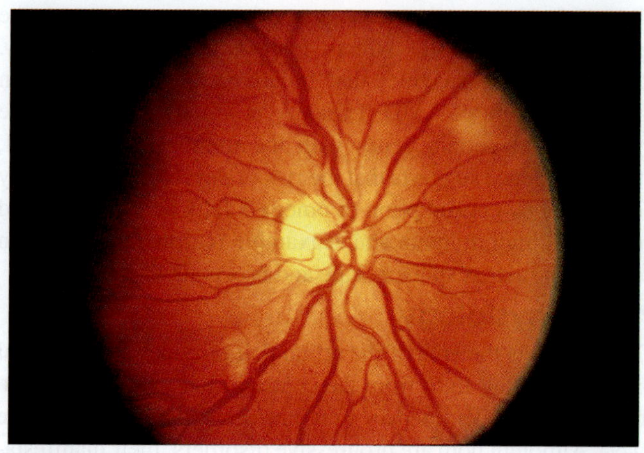

FIGURE 45.14 ***Appearance of the ocular fundus in diabetic retinopathy***

Source: Courtesy of National Eye Institute, National Institutes of Health (NEI/NIH).

TRANSLATION TO PRACTICE Evidence-based practice: the person with impaired vision

Age-related macular degeneration is the leading cause of significant vision impairment among older adults. Research is ongoing in relation to the effect of vision impairment on the lives of older adults, spanning both social and physical impacts including depression, social isolation, loneliness, balance, dementia, cognitive decline and supports required to be put into place for positive lifestyle outcomes.

IMPLICATIONS FOR NURSING

Older adults with significant vision deficit continue to cherish their independence and focus on their remaining abilities (as opposed to their disabilities). While it is important to present clear, accurate and realistic information to people with irreversible vision impairment, maintenance of hope and optimism also is important to the older adult. Many people faced with impaired vision make conscious choices to maintain a positive attitude and lifestyle, developing strategies that allow them to continue with activities that are important to them or provide pleasure. The nurse can help support and encourage these choices and selection of positive behaviours to maintain independence and self-worth.

CRITICAL THINKING IN PERSON-CENTRED CARE

1. Discuss ideas to suggest for a person with impaired vision to continue to engage in activities such as shopping, attending cultural events and playing golf or participating in other sports.
2. Men participating in one study expressed more scepticism about their diagnosis and prognosis and criticism of their treatment than did older women with AMD who had participated in an earlier study. What factors might account for this difference? What implications could this difference have for nursing assessment and care?
3. Develop a teaching plan for a person with newly diagnosed AMD using the nursing diagnosis of *Deficient diversional activity* related to recent change in visual acuity.

Diabetic retinopathy may progress to the proliferative form. This disease is marked by large areas of retinal ischaemia and the formation of new blood vessels (neovascularisation) spreading over the inner surface of the retina and into the vitreous body. These vessels are fine and fragile, making them permeable and easily ruptured. Blood and blood protein leakage contribute to retinal oedema, and haemorrhage into the vitreous body may occur. The vessels gradually become fibrous and firmly attached to the vitreous body, increasing the risk of retinal detachment.

INTERPROFESSIONAL CARE

People with diabetes should be examined yearly by an ophthalmologist. The development of any new visual manifestations is an additional indication for prompt ophthalmological examination and possibly retinal angiography.

Laser photocoagulation is used to treat both the non-proliferative and proliferative forms of diabetic retinopathy. Leaking microaneurysms are sealed and proliferating vessels destroyed, reducing the risk of haemorrhage, retinal oedema and retinal detachment. This treatment also slows the progress of aneurysms and new vessel formation; however, it does not cure the disorder. People with severe proliferative retinopathy may undergo vitrectomy to remove vitreous haemorrhage or treat associated retinal detachments (Papadakis et al., 2022). Although conclusive research is lacking, the diabetic person with retinopathy may be advised to avoid physical activity associated with the Valsalva manoeuvre (e.g. weight training) (Loscalzo et al., 2022).

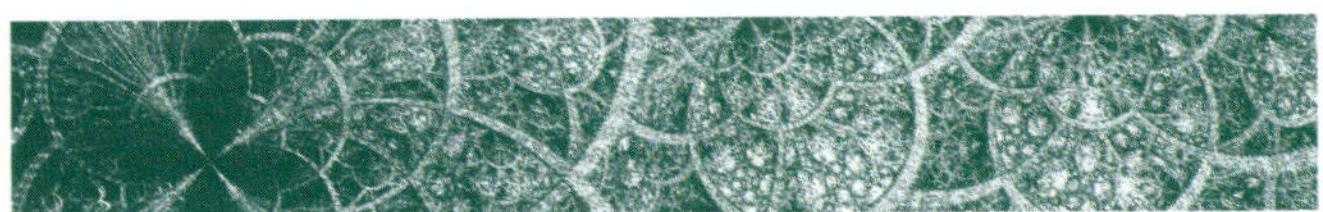

Nursing care

As with many other eye disorders, the nursing care focus for diabetic retinopathy is primarily educational. The newly diagnosed diabetic person needs to understand the importance of regular eye examinations, beginning approximately 5 years after the onset of type 1 diabetes and at the time of onset of type 2 diabetes. Changes of diabetic retinopathy may already be present when type 2 diabetes is diagnosed.

Educate the person to report promptly any new visual manifestation, including blurred vision; black spots (floaters), cobwebs or flashing lights in the visual field; or a sudden loss of vision in one or both eyes. Emphasise to the person that careful blood glucose control may help prevent diabetic retinopathy from developing; it may also slow its progress. The person's blood pressure should also be maintained within normal limits to prevent further damage to retinal vessels. Although diabetic retinopathy cannot be halted or cured, its progress can be slowed with aggressive management. Much of the burden for this management falls on the person, increasing the importance of good teaching.

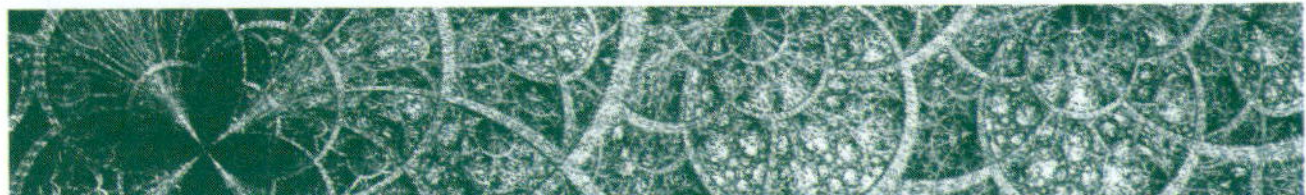

THE PERSON WITH A RETINAL DETACHMENT

The retina contains the photoreceptors of the eye, which allow the perception of light and initial processing of images and stimuli for transmission to the optic centre of the brain. Disruption of this neural layer of the eye by trauma or disease interferes with light perception and image transmission, potentially resulting in blindness.

Both primary eye conditions and systemic diseases can affect the retina and interfere with vision.

Pathophysiology and manifestations

Separation of the retina or sensory portion of the eye from the choroid, the pigmented vascular layer, is known as a **retinal detachment**. Although retinal detachment may be precipitated by trauma, it usually occurs spontaneously. The vitreous humour normally adheres to the retina at the optic disc, the macula and the periphery of the eye. With ageing, the vitreous humour shrinks and may pull the retina away from the choroid. Ageing therefore is a common risk factor, as are myopia and aphakia—absence of the lens (e.g. following lens removal for cataracts) (Norris, 2018; Papadakis et al., 2022).

The retina may actually tear and fold back on itself or may remain intact but no longer adhere to the choroid. A break or tear in the retina allows fluid from the vitreous cavity to enter the defect. This, along with fluid that escapes from choroid vessels, the pull of gravity and traction exerted by the vitreous humour, separates the retina from the choroid. The detached area may rapidly increase in size, increasing loss of vision. Unless contact between the retina and choroid is re-established, the neurons of the retina become ischaemic and die, causing permanent vision loss. For this reason, retinal detachment is a true medical emergency, requiring prompt ophthalmological referral and treatment.

The person experiences floaters, 'spots', lines or flashes in the visual field when the retina detaches. Often the person describes the sensation of having a curtain drawn across the vision, much like a curtain being drawn over a window. The area of the visual field affected is directly related to the area of detachment. For example, because light rays cross as they pass through the lens, a retinal tear in the superior portion of the eye results in a deficit in the lower part of the visual field. The person feels no pain and the eye appears normal to visual inspection. Common manifestations of retinal detachment are listed in the 'Manifestations' box.

MANIFESTATIONS Retinal detachment

- Floaters: irregular dark lines or spots in the field of vision.
- Flashes of light.
- Blurred vision.
- Progressive deterioration of vision.
- Sensation of a curtain or veil being drawn across the field of vision.
- If the macula is involved, loss of central vision.

INTERPROFESSIONAL CARE

Retinal detachment is a medical emergency; prompt treatment is necessary to preserve vision. The manifestations and examination of the ocular fundus by ophthalmoscopy establish the diagnosis of retinal detachment, as early diagnosis and intervention are vital. If the condition is left untreated, the detached portion will become necrotic because of separation from the vascular supply of the choroid. The result is permanent blindness in that portion of the eye. If an ophthalmologist is not readily available, the person's head is positioned so that gravity pulls the detached portion of the retina into closer contact with the choroid.

Interventions are directed towards bringing the retina and choroid back into contact and re-establishing the blood and nutrient supply to the retina. Either cryotherapy, using a super-cooled probe, or laser photocoagulation may be used to create an area of inflammation and adhesion to 'weld' the layers together.

A surgical procedure called *scleral buckling* also may be used. In this procedure, an indentation or fold is created in the sclera, bringing the choroid into contact with the retina. Contact is maintained with a local implant on the sclera or an encircling strap or 'buckle'. Air may also be injected into the vitreous cavity, a procedure called pneumatic retinopexy. The person is positioned so that the air bubble pushes the detached portion of the retina into contact with the choroid.

With a retinal tear, it may be necessary to use surgical instruments to manipulate the detached section of retina into place. Air or a liquid is then injected into the vitreous to maintain retinal contact with the choroid or laser therapy is used to create a bond.

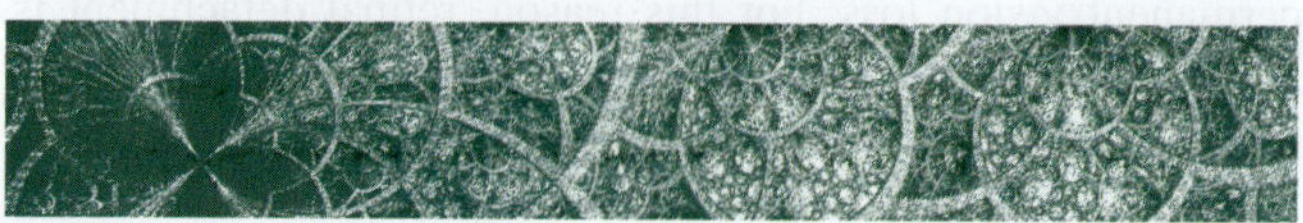

Nursing care

The nursing focus for the person with a detached retina is on early identification and treatment. Because early intervention is vital to preserve the person's sight, nurses must recognise early manifestations of retinal detachment and intervene appropriately to obtain definitive treatment for the person. Retinal detachment can be successfully treated on an outpatient basis, often in an ophthalmologist's office. For these people, the nursing focus is on education.

Nursing diagnoses and interventions

Ineffective retinal tissue perfusion

Restoring contact between the retina and choroid is a priority of nursing and medical care for the person with retinal detachment. Vitreous humour may leak through a retinal tear and fluid exudate may collect behind the tear, causing further detachment. If the macula is detached, central vision is lost and the prognosis for full vision restoration is poorer.

CONSIDERATION FOR PRACTICE

Carefully assess anyone who complains of a sudden rapid loss of vision because this often signals a medical emergency.

- Assess for other manifestations of eye disease. Retinal detachment is painless and has no outward manifestations. *The person with a red eye or cloudy cornea may be experiencing acute angle-closure glaucoma rather than retinal detachment.*
- Notify the doctor and ophthalmologist immediately. *Immediate medical intervention is required in people with retinal detachment to preserve vision.*
- Position so the area of detachment is inferior. For instance, for a superior temporal retinal detachment of the right eye (with corresponding vision loss in the inferior medial visual field of that eye), place supine with the head turned to the right. *Correct positioning allows the contents of the posterior portion of the eye to place pressure on the detached area, bringing the retina in closer contact with the choroid.*

Anxiety

Retinal detachment causes a rapid decline in vision in the affected eye, often occurring spontaneously and without pain. Unless previous episodes have occurred, the person usually does not know what is causing the problem. Anxiety and fear of complete vision loss are common, expected reactions.

- Maintain a calm, confident attitude while carrying out priority interventions. *Administering care in a calm, although urgent, manner helps reassure the person that the problem is treatable and that appropriate measures are being taken.*
- Reassure that most retinal detachments are successfully treated, usually on an outpatient basis. *Reassurance can help allay the person's fear of permanent vision loss.*
- For spontaneous detachments, assure the person that they did not cause the detachment to occur. *The person may believe that the detachment is related to a specific activity and feel guilty for 'causing' this loss of vision.*
- Explain all procedures fully, including the reason for positioning. *Explanations facilitate understanding and help relieve anxiety in unfamiliar settings.*
- Allow supportive family members or friends to remain with the person as much as possible. *Additional support helps lower the person's anxiety level.*

Community-based care

Teaching for the person undergoing surgical repair of retinal detachment is similar to that for people experiencing other types of eye surgery. If the retina remains detached, provide instructions about the change in peripheral vision or other visual fields, and changes in depth perception.

Discuss the following topics with the person and family to prepare for home care:

- limitations on positioning the head before or following repair
- activity restrictions such as no bending or straining at stool movement
- use of eye shield
- early manifestations and the importance of seeking immediate treatment
- follow-up treatment with the ophthalmologist.

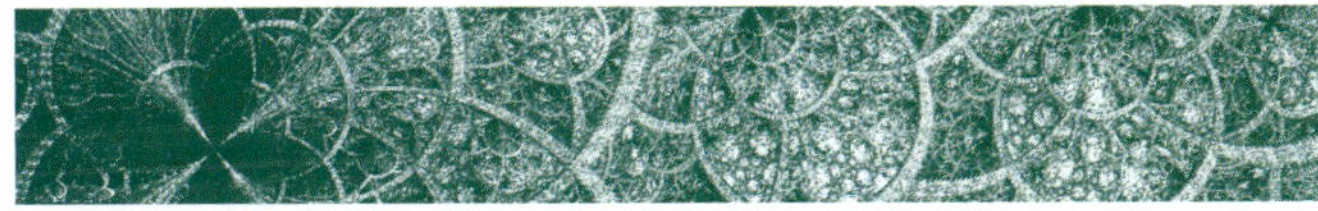

THE PERSON WITH RETINITIS PIGMENTOSA

Retinitis pigmentosa is a hereditary degenerative disease characterised by retinal atrophy and loss of retinal function progressing from the periphery to the central region of the retina. It is inherited as an autosomal dominant, autosomal recessive or X-linked trait, and may be associated with other genetic defects (Loscalzo et al., 2022; Norris, 2018).

In retinitis pigmentosa, the genetic defect appears to cause production of an unstable form of rhodopsin, the receptor protein of rod cells in the retina. Rod cells degenerate, initially at the periphery of the retina. The areas of degeneration and cell death slowly expand, causing vision to narrow. Central vision is finally lost as well.

The initial manifestation of retinitis pigmentosa, difficulty with night vision, is often noted during childhood. As the disease progresses, there is slow loss of visual fields, photophobia and disrupted colour vision. The progression to tunnel vision and blindness is gradual; the person may be totally blind by age 40.

Currently, there is no effective treatment for retinitis pigmentosa. Research into defective rhodopsin holds future promise for the development of therapy that may at least slow its progress.

People with retinitis pigmentosa may benefit from low-vision aids, much like those for the person with macular degeneration. Additionally, information about the disease and its progress is vital so the person can plan for the eventual total loss of sight. People should be referred for genetic counselling prior to starting a family to determine the risk of transmitting the disease to their children.

THE PERSON WITH HIV INFECTION

More than 50% of people infected with the human immunodeficiency virus (HIV) develop an infectious or non-infectious ocular condition, generally as a late manifestation of the disease (Loscalzo et al., 2022).

HIV retinopathy, seen as cotton-wool spots around the optic nerve, is the most common non-infectious ophthalmic lesion in AIDS. Cotton-wool spots indicate areas of retinal ischaemia. Microaneurysms and dot-, blot- or flame-shaped haemorrhages may also be seen in HIV retinopathy.

Neoplasms common in the person with AIDS can also affect the eye. Kaposi's sarcoma may affect the external surface or anterior segment of the eye or the eyelids. Kaposi's lesions vary in colour (red, brown or purple) and in size, shape and location. Conjunctival lesions resemble a benign subconjunctival haemorrhage. Kaposi's lesions of the lid may cause ptosis (drooping of the lid) and abnormal lid function. Vision or eye position and movement may be affected by the tumour or by the effect of increased intracranial pressure on the cranial nerves.

The most serious and frequent opportunistic eye infection associated with HIV infection is cytomegalovirus (CMV) retinitis. CMV retinitis generally develops when CD4 cell counts drop below 50 mL. Initially unilateral, CMV retinitis commonly progresses to become bilateral because of the systemic nature of the infection. CMV invades the retina of the eye directly, producing exudate and cotton-wool spots, haemorrhage, cell death and necrosis. Visual field deficits develop and can progress to eventual blindness.

Corneal ulcers from opportunistic bacterial, fungal, protozoal or viral infections are also associated with HIV infection. Toxoplasmic and fungal retinal infections may occur.

The person with an HIV-associated eye disorder may complain of a change in visual acuity, blurring, floaters or gaps in the field of vision. Extensive retinal damage may cause retinal detachment and symptoms of flashing lights, multiple floaters and a loss of vision. Because the observed changes in the retina are non-specific, it is important for the examining healthcare provider to know that the person is HIV positive in order to make an accurate diagnosis.

In addition to the general treatment of HIV infection with retroviral medications, specific therapies may be directed towards the ocular manifestations of the disease. CMV retinitis is commonly treated with the antivirals ganciclovir and foscarnet sodium.

Although treatment of ocular Kaposi's sarcoma is usually not indicated, conjunctival lesions may be excised for comfort or cosmetic reasons. Lid lesions may be treated with radiation or intralesional chemotherapy.

THE PERSON WITH AN ENUCLEATION

Occasionally, surgical removal of an eye is necessary because of trauma, infection, glaucoma, intractable pain or malignancy. This procedure is known as **enucleation**.

Enucleation is performed under local or general anaesthesia. After the globe is removed, the conjunctiva and eye muscles are sutured to a round implant inserted into the orbit to maintain its shape. A pressure dressing is left in place for 24 to 48 hours. The person is permitted out of bed on the day of surgery. Haemorrhage and infection are the most commonly seen complications.

Postoperative nursing care includes education, psychological support and observation for potential complications. The person may be instructed to apply warm compresses and instil antibiotic ointment or drops postoperatively.

Within 1 week, a temporary prosthesis called a conformer is fitted into the empty socket. The permanent prosthesis is individually designed to closely resemble the person's other eye. The prosthesis can be fitted 1 to 2 months after surgery. Often it is difficult to discern which eye is functional and which is the prosthesis. Procedure 45.1 outlines the proper way to remove and reinsert an eye prosthesis when the person is unable to do so.

PROCEDURE 45.1 Removing and reinserting a prosthetic eye

GATHER SUPPLIES

- Gloves
- Clean basin or plastic denture cup
- Sterile normal saline or soap and water for cleaning the prosthesis
- Gauze squares or cotton cloth for cleaning the socket
- A bulb syringe for irrigation if necessary

BEFORE THE PROCEDURE

Most people who have an artificial eye provide self-care and require little assistance. However, it may be necessary for the nurse to remove an eye prosthesis from the unconscious or debilitated person. If the person is conscious, explain the procedure and provide for privacy.

PROCEDURE

- Follow standard precautions.
- Wash the hands and put on clean exam gloves.
- To remove the prosthesis, do one of the following:
  - Pull down the lower lid and gently exert outward and upward pressure on the lower edge of the prosthesis. This pressure usually causes the prosthesis to slip out.
  - Pull down the lower lid and apply a moistened suction cup to the prosthesis by squeezing the device. Twist gently to remove the prosthesis from the socket.
- Wash the prosthesis using mild soap and water or normal saline. Rinse thoroughly. Do not use abrasives or chemicals for cleaning.
- If the prosthesis is not immediately replaced in the eye socket, store it in a clearly labelled plastic container lined with a soft cloth or gauze squares. Avoid scratching or damaging the prosthesis. Store it in a safe place to prevent loss.
- If irrigation of the eye socket is ordered, have the person lean over a sink or basin if possible or position on the affected side with a clean emesis basin to hold the irrigant as it flows out of the socket. Gently hold the lids open and irrigate the socket using a bulb syringe and clean warm water.
- Reinsert the prosthesis.
  a. Moisten the prosthesis with warm normal saline or water.
  b. Gently hold the lids open. Insert the upper edge of the prosthesis under the upper lid first, then the lower edge under the lower lid using slight pressure.
  c. If a suction device is used, attach it to the cleaned prosthesis over the pupil. Holding the lids open, insert the prosthesis using the above procedure, then remove the suction cup by squeezing it gently and exerting slight pressure on the edge of the cup with the lower lid.

AFTER THE PROCEDURE

Ensure that the person is comfortable. Chart the procedure and any abnormal findings, such as drainage or inflammation.

Ear disorders

For a person to hear, sound waves must enter the external auditory meatus and travel through the ear canal to vibrate the tympanic membrane and bony structures of the middle ear, which in turn activate the receptors of the cochlea. Trauma or disease involving any portion of this pathway can affect hearing. **Tinnitus**, the perception of sound such as ringing, buzzing or roaring in the ears, is another potential result of problems affecting the auditory system.

Disorders of the external ear, including the auricle, auditory meatus and ear canal, can affect the conduction of sound waves and hearing. Obstruction of the external auditory canal or damage to the tympanic membrane, which separates the outer from the middle ear, may lead to conductive hearing loss. Infection or inflammation, trauma and obstruction of the ear canal with cerumen (wax) or a foreign body are the most common conditions affecting the external ear.

Disorders of the middle ear may be either acute or chronic. Unless these disorders are treated promptly and effectively, damage and scarring of middle ear structures can result in a permanent conductive hearing loss. Infectious or inflammatory disorders such as otitis media and mastoiditis are the most common conditions affecting the middle ear. Otosclerosis, a genetic condition, may also affect the structures of the middle ear.

THE PERSON WITH OTITIS EXTERNA

Otitis externa is inflammation of the ear canal. Commonly known as *swimmer's ear*, it is most prevalent in people who spend significant time in the water. Competitive athletes, including swimmers, divers and surfers, are particularly prone to otitis externa. Wearing a hearing aid or ear plugs, which hold moisture in the ear canal, is an additional risk factor. Although *Pseudomonas aeruginosa* or other bacterial infection is the most common cause, external otitis may also be due to fungal infection, mechanical trauma (such as cleaning the ear with a toothpick) or a local hypersensitivity reaction.

Pathophysiology and manifestations

Disruption of the normal environment within the external auditory canal typically precedes the inflammatory process. Retained moisture, cleaning or drying of the ear canal removes the protective layer of cerumen, an acidic, water-repellent substance with antimicrobial properties. Its removal leaves the skin of the ear canal vulnerable to invasion and infection. For surfers, the presence of *exostoses*, bony growths in the ear canals resulting from prolonged exposure to cold, predisposes to impaction and retained moisture within the canal.

The person with otitis externa often complains of a feeling of fullness in the ear. Ear pain typically is present and may be severe. The pain of otitis externa can be differentiated from that associated with otitis media by manipulation of the auricle. In external otitis, this manoeuvre increases the pain, whereas the person with otitis media experiences no change in pain perception. Odourless watery or purulent drainage may be present. The ear canal appears inflamed and oedematous on examination.

INTERPROFESSIONAL CARE

Management of the person with an external ear disorder focuses on restoring the normal balance of the external ear and canal and teaching the person how to prevent future problems.

For otitis externa, the following steps are recommended in treatment:

- thorough cleansing of the ear canal, particularly if drainage or debris is present
- treatment of the infection with local antibiotics; if cellulitis is present, systemic antibiotics may be necessary
- medication to relieve the pain and itching
- education on the prevention of future episodes of swimmer's ear.

Topical antimicrobials used to treat otitis externa include chloramphenicol, framycetin, neomycin, gramicidin, ciprofloxacin and bacitracin. Nystatin, an antifungal agent, is also used (Knights et al., 2022).

A topical antibiotic is often prescribed for the treatment of otitis externa. A topical corticosteroid may be ordered in combination with the antibiotic to provide immediate relief of the pain, swelling and itching. Chloramphenicol ear drops (broad-spectrum antibiotic) are effective against *Pseudomonas*, *Staphylococcus aureus* and *Enterobacter*. Other ear drop preparations include aminoglycoside antibiotics (framycetin and neomycin); however, it is important to identify known sensitivity to any of the drugs in this preparation prior to initiating therapy. People who are sensitive to neomycin may develop dermatitis, in which case the drug must be stopped.

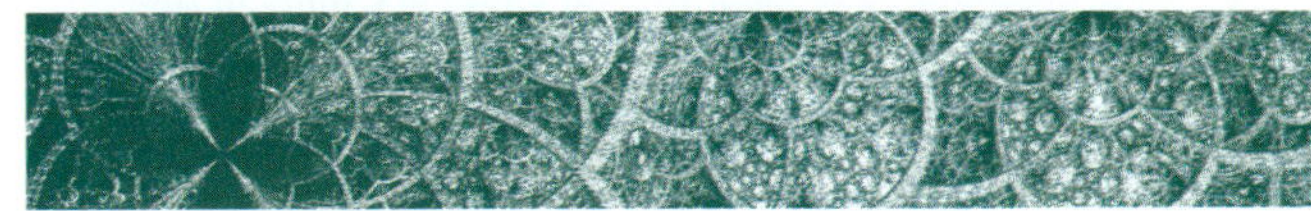

Nursing care

External otitis can cause severe pain and discomfort. Although the disorder is rarely serious enough to require hospitalisation, the nurse teaches the person about the disorder, comfort measures and prevention of future episodes.

Nursing diagnoses and interventions

Impaired tissue integrity

External otitis may result from attempts to clean the ear canal with a toothpick, cotton-tipped applicator or other implement that damages the skin, allowing an infectious organism to invade the tissue. Even if the canal is not damaged by attempts to clean it, the cleaning process often interrupts normal mechanisms, causing cerumen and debris to collect in the canal. The collected debris, in turn, tends to trap water within the canal, causing maceration of the skin.

- Inform that ear canals rarely need cleansing beyond washing of the external meatus with soap and water. Educate people of all ages not to clean ear canals with any implement. *'Cleaning' increases the risk of tissue damage and impairs the normal mechanism that clears the canal of accumulated cerumen and debris.*
- Educate person (and, if necessary, a family member) about how to instil prescribed ear drops:
  a. Wash hands.
  b. Warm the medication briefly by holding the container in the hand or placing it in a pocket for approximately 5 minutes before instilling the drops. *Warming the medication promotes comfort.*
  c. Lie on the unaffected side; if sitting, tilt the head towards the unaffected side. *This position allows gravity to assist in moving the medication to the inner portion of the ear canal.*
  d. Partially fill the ear dropper with medication.
  e. Using the non-dominant hand, straighten the ear canal by pulling the pinna of the ear up and back. *Straightening helps the medication travel along the length of the canal.*
  f. Administer the prescribed number of drops into the ear canal. *It is important that the full amount of prescribed medication be administered to penetrate the length of the canal and achieve full effectiveness.*
  g. Remain in the side-lying position for approximately 5 minutes after the instillation of drops. *This position allows the medication to penetrate into deeper portions*

BOX 45.2 Teaching to prevent otitis externa

- Stay out of the water until the acute inflammatory process is completely resolved. Ideally, allow 7 to 10 days before resuming water activities.
- Take precautions to keep the ear canal dry while in the water:
  a. Use silicone ear plugs, which can keep water out of the ear without reducing hearing significantly.
  b. Wear a tight-fitting swim cap or wetsuit hood, especially in cold ocean water. Although these do not prevent water from entering the ear, they protect the ear from the cold and possibly slow the formation of bony growths in the ears. They also protect the ear from sand and other water debris.
- Immediately after swimming, dry the ear canal. Allow water to drain by tilting the head and jumping to shake water out of the ear. Dry the outer ear with a towel, then use a hair dryer on the lowest setting several centimetres from the ear to dry the canal.
- Do not insert cotton swabs or other objects into the ear canal to dry it. This removes the protective layer of cerumen and may damage the skin of the canal, increasing the risk of bacterial infection. In addition, if debris such as sand is present, the swab may actually push debris further into the canal, forming an impacted mass.
- Consult primary care provider about using a drying agent in the ear canal after swimming. A 2% acetic acid solution or 2% boric acid in ethyl alcohol is effective in drying the canal and restoring its normal acidic environment.
- If it is necessary to remove impacted debris from the ear canal, irrigate the ear with warm tap water. A bulb syringe available over the counter or a 20 mL syringe attached to a short Teflon intravenous catheter (with the needle removed) is effective. With the head tilted towards the affected side, direct a stream of warm water towards the upper wall of the ear canal, allowing the water to run out into a bowl or sink. Repeated instillations may be necessary to break up and flush out impacted wax and debris.
- Follow manufacturer's directions for cleaning and disinfecting pools and spas (hot tubs). Use a pool test kit to check for adequate disinfectant and pH levels before entering.

of the canal and prevents it from running out when the head is moved upright.

h. Loosely place a small piece of cotton in the auditory meatus for 15 to 20 minutes. *The cotton helps keep the medication in the canal.*

- Educate to avoid getting water in the affected ear until it is fully healed. Cotton balls may be used while showering to prevent water from entering the ear canal. *The person should refrain from water sports and activities until approved by the primary care provider. Retained moisture in the ear canal can further impair skin integrity, increasing inflammation.*

Community-based care

The person is ultimately responsible for carrying out the prescribed treatment regimen in external otitis and for implementing measures to prevent future episodes. Education is vital. Provide verbal and written instructions on use of the prescribed medications. Educating the person about care measures to prevent recurrent episodes is especially important in swimmers, divers and surfers (see Box 45.2).

Cellulitis of the surrounding tissue is a possible complication of external otitis. Instruct the person to report to the primary care provider any increase in pain, swelling or redness of surrounding tissues; fever; or other manifestations of infection such as malaise or increased fatigue.

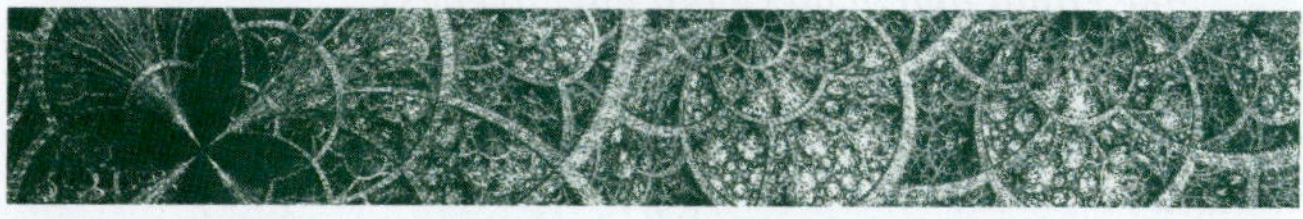

THE PERSON WITH IMPACTED CERUMEN OR A FOREIGN BODY

The external auditory canal can be obstructed by cerumen or foreign bodies. The curved shape and narrow lumen of the canal make it particularly vulnerable to obstruction.

Pathophysiology and manifestations

As cerumen dries, it moves down and out of the ear canal. In some individuals it tends to accumulate, narrowing the canal. Ageing is a risk factor for impaction because less cerumen is produced and it is harder and drier. The accumulation of cerumen is often aggravated by attempting to remove it using cotton-tipped swabs or hair pins, which pack it more deeply into the ear canal.

A variety of objects become foreign bodies in the ear canal. In adults, implements used to clean the ear canal may break and become lodged. Insects also may enter the ear canal and be unable to exit.

When the ear canal becomes occluded with either cerumen or a foreign body, the person experiences a conductive hearing loss in the affected ear. Manifestations include a sensation of fullness, along with tinnitus and coughing due to stimulation of the vagal nerve. The foreign body or impacted cerumen may be visualised on otoscopy. Impacted cerumen appears as a yellow, brown or black mass in the canal.

INTERPROFESSIONAL CARE

Treatment focuses on clearing the canal. If there is no evidence of tympanic membrane perforation, irrigation of the canal is often the initial therapy.

Impacted wax, objects or insects may require physical removal using an ear curette, forceps or right-angle hook inserted via an otoscope and ear speculum. Mineral oil or topical lignocaine drops are used to immobilise or kill insects prior to their removal from the ear. When an organic foreign body such as a bean or an insect is suspected, water should not be instilled into the ear canal because it may cause the object to swell, making its removal more difficult. Smooth, round objects present the biggest challenge to remove from the ear canal. Suction applied using a piece of soft intravenous tubing may be effective.

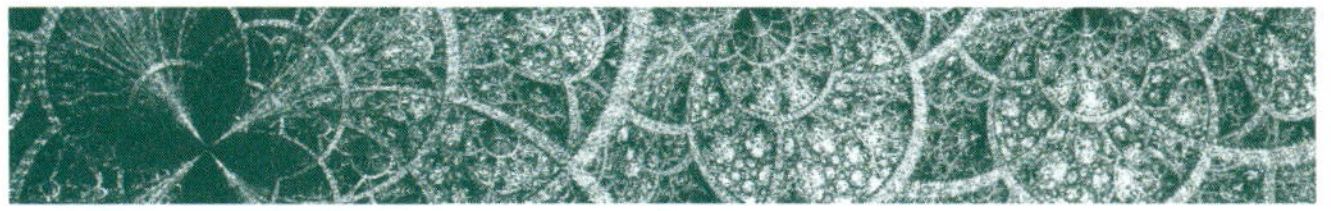

Nursing care

Nurses are often involved in identifying and relieving obstructions of the ear canal, especially in outpatient and community settings. Any person with evidence of a new conductive hearing loss or complaints of discomfort and fullness in one ear should be evaluated for possible obstruction. Inability to visualise the tympanic membrane or observation of a dark, shiny mass obstructing the canal may indicate a need for irrigation or other procedure to clear the canal. It is important to determine that the tympanic membrane is intact before irrigating; assessment by a doctor or advanced practitioner may be necessary if a ruptured membrane is suspected.

Because obstruction of the ear canal with cerumen or a foreign body is generally preventable, education is a key component of nursing care. People need to know appropriate care measures for the external ear. Although the ear canal rarely needs cleaning, the person prone to cerumen impaction requires education regarding the use of mineral oil or commercial products to soften wax, and irrigation to remove it. All people should understand the importance of not inserting anything smaller than a finger wrapped with a washcloth into the ear canal to avoid trauma to the canal or eardrum. Stress the risk of impacting cerumen against the tympanic membrane when using cotton-tipped swabs to clean the ear canal. Additionally, the swab may break and lodge in the canal. If ear drops have been prescribed, educate the person and a family member about how to instil them.

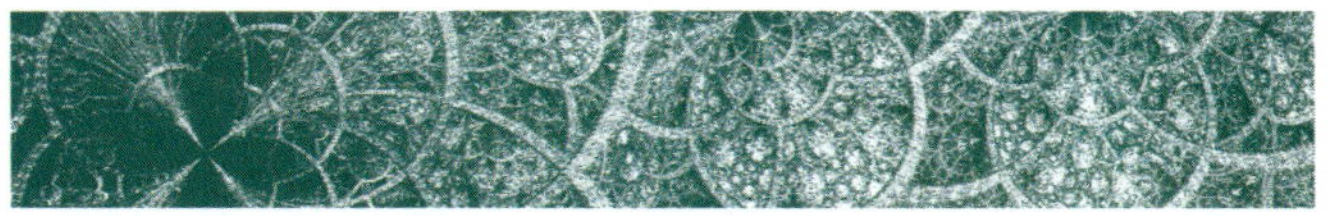

THE PERSON WITH OTITIS MEDIA

Otitis media, inflammation or infection of the middle ear, primarily affects infants and young children but may also occur in adults. It can persist from infancy through adolescence and adulthood. The tympanic membrane, which separates the middle ear from the external auditory canal, protects the middle ear from the external environment. The eustachian (auditory) tube connects the middle ear with the nasopharynx to help equalise the pressure in the middle ear with the atmospheric pressure. Unfortunately, this connecting tube also provides a route by which infectious organisms enter the middle ear from the nose and throat, causing otitis media, the most common disease of the middle ear. This is the most common cause of hearing loss in the Australian Indigenous population.

Pathophysiology

There are two primary forms of otitis media: (1) serous, and (2) acute or suppurative. Both forms are associated with upper respiratory infection and eustachian tube dysfunction. The eustachian tube is narrow and flat, normally opening only during yawning and swallowing. Allergies or upper respiratory tract infections can cause oedema of the tube lining, impairing its function. Air within the middle ear is trapped and gradually absorbed, creating negative pressure in this space.

Serous otitis media

Serous otitis media (also called *otitis media with effusion*) occurs when the eustachian tube is obstructed for a prolonged time, impairing equalisation of air pressure in the middle ear. Air within the middle ear space is gradually absorbed; the tube obstruction prevents more air from entering the middle ear. The resulting negative pressure in the middle ear causes sterile serous fluid to move from the capillaries into the space, forming a sterile effusion of the middle ear.

Upper respiratory infections or allergies such as hay fever predispose the person to serous otitis media. In addition, people with narrowed or oedematous eustachian tubes may also be subject to barotrauma or barotitis media. In these people, the middle ear cannot adapt to rapid changes in barometric pressure such as those that occur during air travel or underwater diving. Barotrauma tends to occur during descent in an aeroplane because negative pressure within the middle ear causes the eustachian tube to collapse and lock. However, underwater diving places even greater stress on the eustachian tube and middle ear.

MANIFESTATIONS Typical manifestations of serous otitis media include decreased hearing in the affected ear and complaints of 'snapping' or 'popping' in the ear. On examination, the tympanic membrane demonstrates decreased mobility and may appear retracted or bulging. Fluid or air bubbles are often visible behind the drum. Severe pressure differences such as those occurring with barotrauma may cause acute pain, haemorrhage into the middle ear, rupture of the tympanic membrane or even rupture of the round window with sensory hearing loss and severe **vertigo** (a sensation of whirling or rotation). *Haemotympanum*, bleeding into or behind the tympanic membrane, may be observed on otoscopic examination.

Acute otitis media

The eustachian tube also provides a route for the entry of pathogens into the normally sterile middle ear, resulting in acute or suppurative otitis media. Acute otitis media typically follows an upper respiratory infection. Oedema of the eustachian tube impairs drainage of the middle ear, causing mucus and serous fluid to accumulate. This fluid is an excellent environment for the growth of bacteria, which may enter from the oronasopharynx via the eustachian tube. Although a viral upper respiratory infection may predispose the person to a middle ear infection, the bacteria *Streptococcus pneumoniae*, *Haemophilus influenza* and *Streptococcus pyogenes* account for most cases of otitis media in adults. Invasion and colonisation of the middle ear by bacteria and the resultant migration of white blood cells cause pus formation. Accumulated pus can increase middle ear pressure sufficiently to rupture the tympanic membrane. The bacterial infection may also migrate internally, causing mastoiditis, brain abscess or bacterial meningitis. A more common complication of otitis media is a persistent conductive hearing loss, which typically resolves when the middle ear effusion clears.

MANIFESTATIONS The person with acute otitis media experiences mild to severe pain in the affected ear. The person's temperature is often elevated. Diminished hearing, dizziness, vertigo and tinnitus are common associated complaints. Pus within the mastoid air cells often causes mastoid tenderness in acute otitis media. On otoscopic examination, the tympanic membrane appears red and inflamed or dull and bulging (see Figure 45.15). Decreased movement of the membrane is demonstrated by tympanometry or air insufflation. Spontaneous rupture of the tympanic membrane releases a purulent discharge. **Myringotomy** (an incision of the tympanic membrane) may be performed to relieve the pressure.

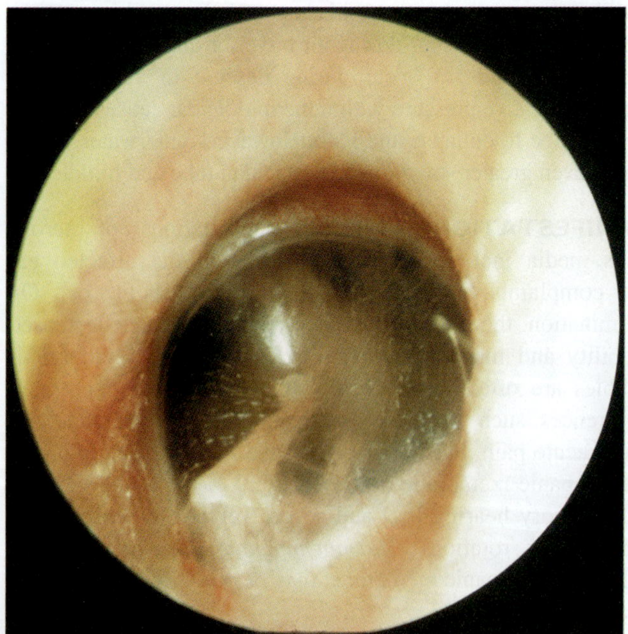

FIGURE 45.15 ***A red, bulging tympanic membrane of otitis media***

Source: Mediscan/Alamy Stock Photo.

INTERPROFESSIONAL CARE

The diagnosis of otitis media is usually based on the person's history and the physical examination. The tympanic membrane can be visualised and its mobility evaluated using a pneumatic otoscope that allows a puff of air to be instilled into the ear canal. Generally, the tympanic membrane moves slightly when air is instilled or the person performs the Valsalva manoeuvre. Less movement is seen in people with eustachian tube dysfunction and acute otitis media with effusion.

Diagnosis

- *Impedance audiometry*, also known as tympanometry, is an accurate diagnostic test for otitis media with effusion. A continuous tone is delivered to the tympanic membrane by an audiometer with a sealed probe tip. Compliance of the tympanic membrane and middle ear is measured by recording energy reflected from the membrane surface. With middle ear effusion, compliance is reduced.
- A *full blood count (FBC)* may be done to assess for an elevated WBC count and increased numbers of immature cells indicative of acute bacterial infection.
- If the tympanic membrane has ruptured or a tympanocentesis or myringotomy is performed, drainage is cultured to determine the infecting organism.

Medications

When eustachian tube dysfunction and serous otitis media do not spontaneously resolve or lead to hearing loss, a short course of an anti-inflammatory drug (e.g. oral prednisone for 7 days) is prescribed to reduce mucosal oedema of the tube and improve its patency.

Although a decongestant or antihistamine may be used, there is little evidence of their effectiveness in treating serous otitis media. Antibiotic/corticosteroid ear drops or ointments can be prescribed. See the chapter 'Nursing care of people with altered immunity' for the nursing implications of corticosteroid medications.

The person with auditory tube dysfunction may be taught to auto-inflate the middle ear by performing the Valsalva manoeuvre or by forcefully exhaling against closed nostrils. Additionally, the person is advised to avoid air travel and underwater diving.

Acute otitis media usually is treated with antibiotic therapy, especially amoxicillin, trimethoprim-sulfamethoxazole, cefaclor or azithromycin for 5 to 10 days. This course of treatment is long enough to ensure eradication of the infective organism, yet short enough to reduce the incidence of bacterial resistance. (See the chapter 'Nursing care of people with infections' for further discussion of antibiotics.) Symptomatic relief may be provided by analgesics, antipyretics, antihistamines and local application of heat.

Surgery

A myringotomy or tympanocentesis may be performed to relieve excess pressure in the middle ear and prevent spontaneous rupture of the eardrum. To perform a tympanocentesis, the doctor inserts a 20-gauge spinal needle through the inferior portion of the tympanic membrane, allowing aspiration of fluid and pus from the middle ear to relieve pressure and, if necessary, obtain a specimen for culture. Myringotomy may be performed to relieve severe pain or when complications of acute otitis media, such as mastoiditis, are present. As soon as the pressure is released, pain subsides and hearing improves.

People who do not respond to antibiotic therapy may require myringotomy with insertion of ventilation (tympanostomy) tubes. Small tubes are inserted into the inferior portion of the tympanic membrane, providing for ventilation and drainage of the middle ear during healing. The tube is eventually extruded from the ear and the tympanic membrane heals. While the tube is in place, it is important to avoid getting any water in the ear canal because it may then enter the middle ear space.

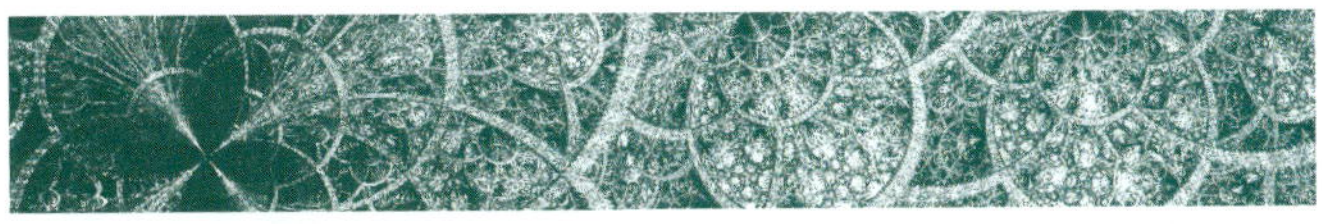

Nursing care

People with otitis media are commonly treated in outpatient and community settings. The nursing role is primarily one of support and education. A comprehensive intersectoral and multidisciplinary approach specifically addressing prevention and early intervention will assist in improving awareness in the Australian Indigenous population, to reduce the incidence of this condition.

Health promotion

Health promotion for otitis media focuses on educating people about the importance of seeking medical care for prolonged, severe ear pain with or without drainage combined with an upper respiratory tract infection. Untreated or repeated attacks of otitis media can progress to a chronic form of otitis media, acute mastoiditis or eardrum perforation.

Assessment

Collect assessment data through a health history and physical examination (see the chapter 'A person-centred approach to assessing the eye and ear').

- *Health history*: recent upper respiratory infection; presence, intensity and nature of pain in affected ear; sense of fullness or pressure in the ear; change in hearing; snapping or popping sensation in the affected ear; presence of vertigo.
- *Physical examination*: temperature; hearing test; inspect tympanic membrane.

Nursing diagnoses and interventions

Pain can be a significant problem for people with otitis media, as can the risk of damage to delicate tissues of the middle ear by the infectious and inflammatory processes.

Pain

Tissue oedema, effusion of the middle ear and the inflammatory response can affect the pain-sensitive tissues of the middle ear in otitis media, causing acute discomfort. This discomfort is increased by pressure changes, such as those that occur during air travel or underwater diving.

- Assess pain for severity, quality and location. A thorough assessment is important to determine the source of the pain. *Unlike that of external otitis, the pain of otitis media is not aggravated by movement of the external ear.*
- Encourage the use of mild analgesics such as aspirin or paracetamol every 4 hours as needed to relieve pain and fever. *These non-prescription medications are effective in reducing the perception of pain. Aspirin also has anti-inflammatory properties that may help relieve the inflammation of the ear.*
- Advise to apply heat to the affected side unless contraindicated. *Heat dilates blood vessels, promoting the reabsorption of fluid and reducing swelling.*
- Instruct to avoid air travel, rapid changes in elevation or diving. *A rapid change in barometric pressure can increase the person's pain significantly.*
- Instruct to report promptly an abrupt relief of pain to the primary care provider. *Pain that subsides abruptly may indicate spontaneous perforation of the tympanic membrane with relief of pressure within the middle ear.*

Community-based care

The person who has otitis media needs educating regarding the disorder, its causes and prevention, and any specific treatment recommended or prescribed. Discuss the following topics with the person and family:

- antibiotic therapy and potential side effects
- importance of completing all ordered doses
- follow-up examinations in 2 to 4 weeks
- avoiding swimming, diving or submerging the head while bathing if ventilation tubes are in place.

If surgical intervention is necessary, educate the person and family members about the surgery and postoperative care. Provide instructions regarding any special postoperative precautions, such as avoiding water in the ear canals or avoiding sudden changes in air pressure.

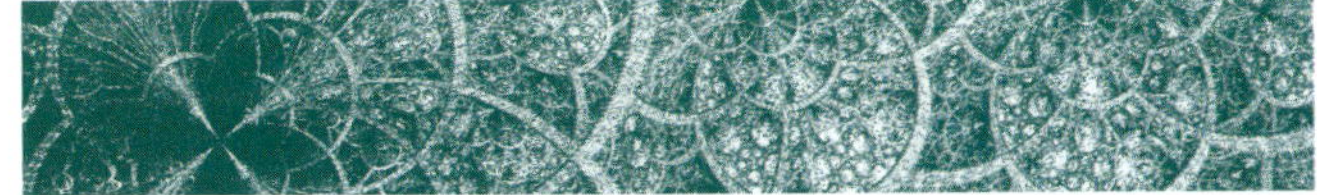

THE PERSON WITH ACUTE MASTOIDITIS

The mastoid process is a portion of the temporal bone of the skull lying adjacent to the middle ear. It is full of air cavities called mastoid air cells or mastoid sinuses. The infection of acute otitis media generally extends into the mastoid air cells; effective treatment of acute otitis media eliminates the infection from the mastoid cells as well. When treatment is ineffective, pus remains in the mastoid air cells and acute **mastoiditis**, bacterial infection of the mastoid process, may develop.

The incidence of acute mastoiditis is low in countries where the prescription and use of antibiotics to treat acute otitis media is widespread. Its incidence is higher in countries where antibiotics are less likely to be prescribed.

Pathophysiology and complications

In acute mastoiditis, the bony septa between mastoid air cells are destroyed and cells coalesce to form large spaces. Portions of the mastoid process are eroded. With chronic infection, an abscess may form or bony sclerosis of the mastoid may result. Acute mastoiditis increases the risk of meningitis because only a very thin bony plate separates mastoid air cells from the brain. Fortunately, this complication is rare since the advent of effective antibiotic therapy for treating otitis media.

Manifestations

Manifestations of acute mastoiditis usually develop approximately 2 to 3 weeks after an episode of acute otitis media and include recurrent earache and hearing loss on the affected side. The pain is persistent and throbbing; tenderness is present over the mastoid process (behind the ear). It may also be red and inflamed. Swelling of the process can cause the auricle of the ear to protrude more than normal. Fever may be accompanied by tinnitus and headache, and profuse drainage from the affected ear may be noted.

INTERPROFESSIONAL CARE

In addition to the manifestations of acute mastoiditis, loss of septa between mastoid air cells may be noted on radiological examination. Acute mastoiditis is treated aggressively with antibiotic therapy tailored to the infecting organism. Antibiotics are continued for at least 14 days. Infections that do not respond to medical therapy or that pose a high risk of spreading to the brain may necessitate a *mastoidectomy*, the surgical removal of the infected mastoid air cells, bone and pus, and inspection of the underlying dura for possible abscess. The extent of tissue destruction determines the extent of surgery required. In a modified mastoidectomy, as much tissue is preserved as possible to avoid disruption of hearing. A radical mastoidectomy involves removal of middle ear structures, including the incus and malleus, as well as the diseased portions of the mastoid process. Unless reconstruction is performed at the time of surgery, this surgery results in conductive hearing loss. **Tympanoplasty**, surgical reconstruction of the middle ear, can restore or preserve hearing.

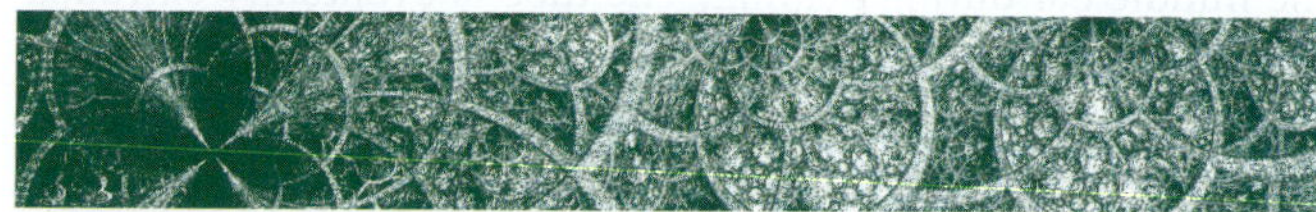

Nursing care

Prevention is the primary focus of collaborative and nursing care related to mastoiditis. Adequate, effective antibiotic treatment of acute otitis media prevents mastoiditis in nearly all instances.

Following surgical intervention, carefully assess the wound and drainage for evidence of infection or other complications. The person's hearing may be temporarily or permanently affected, depending on the extent of the surgery. If the person has impaired hearing in the unaffected ear as well, develop a means of communication with the person prior to surgery. If the hearing is preserved in the unaffected ear, position the person with that ear towards the door. Speak slowly and clearly; do not shout or speak unusually loudly. Be sure that family and staff know about the person's hearing loss and use appropriate communication techniques. Assist the person with ambulation initially because dizziness and vertigo are not unusual following surgery. Nursing care of the person having ear surgery is discussed in the accompanying box.

NURSING CARE OF THE PERSON having ear surgery

PREOPERATIVE CARE

- Review the chapter 'Nursing care of people having surgery' for routine preoperative care.
- Assess hearing and/or verify documentation of preoperative hearing assessment. *This data is important in evaluating the results of the surgical procedure.*
- Establish a means of communication to be used after surgery, *when hearing may be impaired.*
- Explain that blowing of the nose, coughing and sneezing need to be restricted postoperatively to prevent pressure changes in the middle ear and potential disruption of the surgical site. *Keeping the mouth open during a cough or sneeze minimises pressure changes in the middle ear. Providing education and the opportunity to practise before surgery promotes cooperation in the postoperative period.*

POSTOPERATIVE CARE

- Review the chapter 'Nursing care of people having surgery' for routine postoperative care.
- Assess for bleeding and/or drainage from the affected ear. *Infection and haemorrhage are possible complications.*
- Administer anti-emetics as ordered to prevent vomiting. *Vomiting may increase the pressure in the middle ear, disrupting the surgical site.*
- Elevate the head of the bed and position the person on the unaffected side. *This position minimises the pressure in the middle ear.*
- Assess for vertigo or dizziness, especially with ambulation or movement in bed. Avoid unnecessary movements such as turning. *Take measures to ensure safety during ambulation. Surgery on the ear may disrupt equilibrium, increasing the risk of falling.*
- Assess hearing postoperatively. Stand on the unaffected side to communicate and use other measures such as written messages as needed for effective communication with the person with impaired hearing. Reassure the person that decreased hearing acuity immediately after surgery

NURSING CARE OF THE PERSON **having ear surgery (continued)**

is expected. *Hearing improvement is an expected result of the ear surgery and typically does not occur until ear plugs are removed and oedema and drainage at the operative site have resolved. If no reconstruction of the middle ear is carried out or the cochlea is involved, permanent hearing loss in the affected ear may be an expected result.*

- Remind to avoid coughing, sneezing or blowing the nose. *These increase pressure in the middle ear.*

HEALTH EDUCATION FOR THE PERSON AND FAMILY

- Provide education and instructions for home care:
  a. To prevent contamination of the ear canal, avoid showers, shampooing and immersing the head until the doctor says you can do so.
  b. Keep the outer earplug clean and dry, changing it as needed. Do not remove inner ear dressing until instructed to do so by the doctor.
  c. Avoid blowing the nose; if you need to cough or sneeze, keep the mouth open.
  d. Do not swim or dive without doctor approval. Check with your doctor regarding air travel.
  e. Meclizine hydrochloride or other anti-emetic and/or antihistamine medication may be necessary for up to 1 month following surgery.
  f. Fever, bleeding, increased drainage, increased dizziness or decreased hearing after discharge may indicate a complication. Notify the doctor if any of these occur.

Community-based care

When educating about acute mastoiditis, stress the importance of complying with the prescribed antibiotic therapy and recommendations for follow up. Instruct the person and family to report any adverse reactions to the primary care provider so that therapy can be adjusted. Educate the person and family about how to change the surgical dressing using aseptic technique. Provide referrals to appropriate community agencies for the person with a new hearing loss resulting from mastoiditis or its treatment.

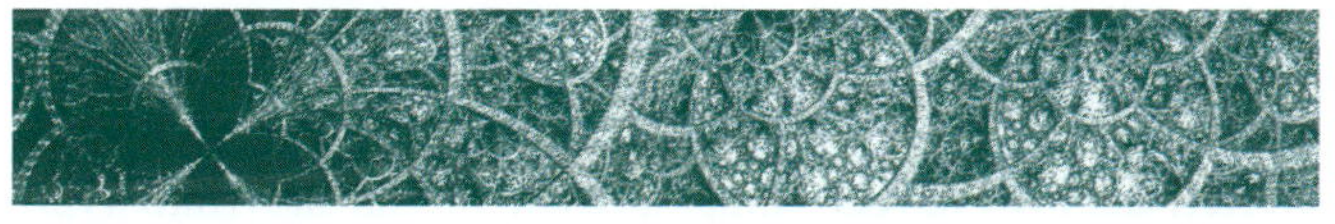

THE PERSON WITH CHRONIC OTITIS MEDIA

Chronic otitis media involves permanent perforation of the tympanic membrane, with or without recurrent pus formation. Changes in the mucosa and bony structures (ossicles) of the middle ear often accompany chronic otitis media. It usually is the result of recurrent acute otitis media and eustachian tube dysfunction but may also result from trauma or other diseases.

Marginal perforations, which usually occur in the posterior–superior portion of the tympanic membrane, are associated with more complications than central perforations. With marginal perforations, squamous epithelium may migrate from the ear canal into the middle ear, where it begins to desquamate and accumulate, forming a *cholesteatoma* (a cyst or mass filled with epithelial cell debris). Its incidence is highest in children and young adults. The desquamating epithelium continues to accumulate and remains infected, producing collagenases (enzymes) that destroy adjacent bone. The inflammatory process impairs the blood supply to the stapes, causing its destruction and conductive hearing loss. Cholesteatomas are benign and slow-growing tumours which can enlarge to fill the entire middle ear. Untreated, the cholesteatoma can progressively destroy the ossicles and erode into the inner ear, causing profound hearing loss.

Systemic antibiotics are prescribed for exacerbations of purulent otitis media. Tympanic membrane perforation is repaired with a tympanoplasty to restore sound conduction and the integrity of the middle ear. A cholesteatoma may require delicate surgery for its removal. If at all possible, radical mastoidectomy with removal of the tympanic membrane, ossicles and tumour is avoided.

As with other complications of acute otitis media, a priority of nursing care is prevention of chronic otitis media and cholesteatoma. People with chronic otitis media need to understand various treatment options and their risks and benefits, as well as the long-term risk of not treating a perforated tympanic membrane. They are also educated on how to instil ear drops, to clean the external auditory meatus and to not irrigate the ear when the tympanic membrane is perforated or if they think it might be.

If surgical treatment of chronic otitis media will affect the person's hearing, include this information in preoperative teaching. Teach the person and family how to use alternative means of communication if this will be necessary postoperatively. When an assistive device is ordered, teach the person and a family member about its use.

THE PERSON WITH OTOSCLEROSIS

Otosclerosis is a common cause of conductive hearing loss. Abnormal bone formation in the osseous labyrinth of the temporal bone causes the footplate of the stapes to become fixed or immobile in the oval window. The result is a conductive hearing loss.

Otosclerosis is a hereditary disorder with an autosomal dominant pattern of inheritance. It occurs most commonly in Caucasians and females. The progressive hearing loss typically begins in adolescence or early adulthood and seems to be accelerated by pregnancy. Although both ears are affected, the rate of hearing loss is asymmetrical. Because bone conduction of sound is retained, the person may be able to use the telephone but have difficulty conversing in person. Tinnitus may also be associated with this condition.

On examination, a reddish or pinkish-orange tympanic membrane may be noted because of increased vascularity of the middle ear. The Rinne test (the chapter 'A person-centred approach to assessing the eye and ear') shows bone sound conduction to be equal to or greater than air conduction, an abnormal finding.

People with otosclerosis may choose conservative treatment, relying on a hearing aid to improve their ability to hear and interact with others. Sodium fluoride may be prescribed to slow bone reabsorption and overgrowth. Surgical treatment involves a stapedectomy and middle ear reconstruction, or a stapedotomy. A *stapedectomy* is a microsurgical technique for removing the diseased stapes. A metallic prosthesis is then inserted, with one end connected to the incus and the other inserted into the oval window. *Stapedotomy* involves creation of a small hole in the footplate of the stapes and insertion of a wire or platinum ribbon prosthesis. An argon, KTP or CO_2 laser may be used for surgery. Surgery usually restores hearing for the person with otosclerosis.

Education and referral of the person to appropriate community agencies are important nursing care priorities for the person with otosclerosis. For the person who chooses surgical treatment, nursing care is similar to that for other people undergoing ear surgery. The following may be appropriate:

- *Risk of injury* related to hearing loss or postoperative vertigo.
- *Risk of disturbed auditory perception* related to bony sclerosis of the stapes.
- *Risk of impaired verbal communication* related to hearing loss.
- *Risk of anxiety* related to concern about transmission of a genetic disorder to children.

THE PERSON WITH AN INNER EAR DISORDER

Disorders affecting the inner ear are much less common than disorders of the outer or middle ear. Inner ear disorders affect equilibrium and may also affect sensorineural hearing, the perception of sound. Labyrinthitis and Ménière's disease are the most common diseases of the inner ear. Vertigo may be a disorder of the inner ear itself or a manifestation of other disorders.

Pathophysiology and manifestations

The labyrinth (the inner ear) contains the cochlea and the semicircular canals. The hair cells and neurons that allow sound perception and transmission to the auditory centre of the brain are in the cochlea. The semicircular canals filled with endolymph are the primary organs involved in maintaining equilibrium. Disruption of this portion of the ear by an inflammatory process or excess endolymph not only affects balance but may also result in permanent hearing loss.

Vertigo

Normally, the integration of input from the labyrinths, eyes, muscles, joints and neural centres maintains balance and posture. This input and integration can be affected by disorders of the labyrinth, vestibular nerve or nuclei, eyes, cerebellum, brainstem or cerebral cortex, causing vertigo. Vertigo, the sensation of movement when there is none, is a disorder of equilibrium. The sensation of whirling, rotation or movement is described as either subjective or objective.

People with subjective vertigo report the sensation of being in motion in a stable environment. This is not always a sense of spinning; the person may have a sense of tumbling or falling forwards or backwards. The sensation is reversed in objective vertigo; people report a sensation of stability in a moving environment. This motion may be perceived as the room spinning around the person or the ground rocking beneath the person's feet. Dizziness, which may be mistaken for vertigo, is a sensation of unsteadiness, lack of balance, light-headedness or movement within the head. The person who is dizzy does not have the rotational sensation felt with vertigo.

Vertigo may be disabling, resulting in falls, injury and difficulty walking. Attacks of vertigo are often accompanied by nausea and vomiting, nystagmus and autonomic symptoms such as pallor, sweating, hypotension and salivation.

Labyrinthitis

Labyrinthitis, also called otitis interna, is inflammation of the inner ear. It is an uncommon disorder because the bony protection of the membranous labyrinth makes it difficult for organisms to enter the inner ear. However, bacteria, viruses and other organisms may enter and infect the inner ear through the oval window during acute otitis media, the cochlear aqueduct during meningitis, or the blood. Viral labyrinthitis is suspected when the person has a sudden onset of symptoms after an upper respiratory infection or when there is no evidence of concurrent otitis media. Labyrinthitis also may result from an autoimmune process of unknown aetiology.

MANIFESTATIONS Inflammation of the labyrinth typically causes vertigo, sensorineural hearing deficit and nystagmus (rapid involuntary eye movements).

Vertigo is the hallmark manifestation of inner ear disorders. The vertigo of labyrinthitis is severe and often accompanied by nausea and vomiting. Any movement can aggravate the vertigo and falling is a significant risk if the person attempts to stand. Vertigo lasts days to weeks in labyrinthitis, making education a vital component of care.

Hearing loss in the ear affected by labyrinthitis may be temporary or permanent. If inflammation destroys tissue of the membranous labyrinth, the hearing loss may be complete and permanent.

The involuntary rhythmic eye movements of nystagmus may not be present in all people with labyrinthitis. When present, the eye movement is typically horizontal. Applying positive or negative pressure to the tympanic membrane of the affected ear may stimulate nystagmus, as will caloric testing (irrigating the ear canal with warm or cool water). Although nystagmus may also be a symptom of brainstem or cerebellar dysfunction, vertigo and hearing loss are not typically associated with those disorders.

Ménière's disease

Ménière's disease, also known as endolymphatic hydrops, is a chronic disorder characterised by recurrent attacks of vertigo with tinnitus and a progressive unilateral hearing loss. This disorder affects men and women equally, with adults between the ages of 35 and 60 at highest risk. The cause of Ménière's disease is unclear, although the most common form of the disease is thought to result from viral injury to the fluid transport system of the inner ear. Other factors that may increase the risk of Ménière's disease include trauma, bacterial infections such as syphilis, autoimmune processes, vascular disorders, selected drugs and toxins (Norris, 2018). A family history of the disease increases risk, suggesting a possible genetic link in some people.

Ménière's disease results from an excess of endolymph, the fluid in the membranous labyrinth of the inner ear. Although the precise pathophysiological mechanism leading to accumulation of endolymph is unclear, it is thought to result from impaired filtration and excretion of the fluid by the endolymphatic sac (Norris, 2018). Excessive pressure resulting from the increased fluid volume causes neural organs of the cochlea to degenerate.

COURSE AND MANIFESTATIONS The onset of Ménière's disease may be gradual or sudden. It is characterised by recurrent attacks of vertigo, gradual loss of hearing and tinnitus. Attacks may be preceded by a feeling of fullness in the ears and a roaring or ringing sensation. The sensorineural hearing loss and tinnitus are usually unilateral but can become bilateral. Attacks of severe rotary vertigo occur abruptly and often unpredictably, lasting from minutes to hours. An attack may be linked to increased sodium intake, stress, allergies, vasoconstriction or premenstrual fluid retention. As the disease continues, hearing loss progresses and the vertigo can be severe enough to cause immobility, nausea and vomiting. Attacks are often accompanied by hypotension, sweating and nystagmus.

INTERPROFESSIONAL CARE

The manifestations associated with inner ear disorders are similar, making testing necessary to establish a diagnosis. Once the diagnosis is determined, collaborative care is directed towards managing symptoms and preventing permanent hearing loss. People with labyrinthitis or an acute attack of Ménière's disease may require hospitalisation to manage the vertigo and its effects.

Diagnosis

The following diagnostic studies may be ordered:

- *Caloric testing (electronystagmography)* evaluates the vestibulo-ocular reflex by identifying eye movements (nystagmus) in response to caloric testing. In people with impaired vestibular function, the normal nystagmus response is blunted or absent. This portion of the test is contraindicated in people who have a perforated tympanic membrane.
- *Rinne* and *Weber tests* of hearing (the chapter 'A person-centred approach to assessing the eye and ear') show decreased air and bone conduction on the affected side if a sensorineural hearing loss is present. In Ménière's disease, audiology shows sensorineural hearing loss involving the low tones.
- *X-rays* and *CT scans* of the petrous bones are used to evaluate the internal auditory canal. In people with Ménière's disease, the vestibular aqueducts may be shorter and straighter than normal.
- *Glycerol test* is conducted by giving the person oral glycerol to decrease fluid pressure in the inner ear. An acute temporary hearing improvement is considered diagnostic for Ménière's disease.

Medications

A scopolamine patch may be used for people with recurrent vertigo, although adverse effects such as dry mouth, blurred vision and urinary retention may limit its use. In Ménière's disease, a diuretic such as hydrochlorothiazide may be prescribed to reduce endolymphatic pressure. A central nervous system depressant such as diazepam or lorazepam may halt an attack of vertigo. Parenteral droperidol provides both a sedative and an anti-emetic effect, making it a useful drug for acute attacks. Anti-vertigo/anti-emetic medications such as meclizine, prochlorperazine or hydroxyzine hydrochloride are prescribed to reduce the whirling sensation and nausea. If the nausea and vomiting are severe, intravenous fluids may be necessary to maintain fluid and electrolyte balance.

Treatments

Bed rest in a quiet, darkened room with minimal sensory stimuli and minimal movement provides the most comfort for the person experiencing an acute attack of vertigo.

Between acute attacks, management of the person with Ménière's disease is directed at preventing future attacks and preserving hearing. A low-sodium diet helps reduce labyrinthine pressure. The Furstenberg diet, a salt-free neutral ash diet, may be prescribed if moderate sodium restriction is ineffective in controlling attacks. People should avoid tobacco, which causes vasoconstriction and can precipitate an attack, along with alcohol and caffeine.

Surgery

When episodes of vertigo are not controlled through medical interventions, surgery may be necessary. Surgical *endolymphatic decompression* relieves the excess pressure in the labyrinth; a shunt is then inserted between the membranous labyrinth and the subarachnoid space to drain excess fluid away from the labyrinths and maintain lower pressure. This procedure preserves hearing for most people. Vertigo is relieved in approximately 70% of people, but about half of people undergoing this procedure continue to experience sensations of fullness and tinnitus.

Destruction of a portion of the acoustic nerve is an alternative to shunting procedures. In a *vestibular neurectomy*, the portion of cranial nerve VIII that controls balance and sensations of vertigo is severed. This procedure relieves vertigo for up to 90% of people. Although there is a risk of damage to the cochlear portion of the nerve and resultant hearing loss, for most people hearing loss stabilises after neurectomy, even improving for some.

The surgery of last resort for Ménière's disease is a *labyrinthectomy*. The labyrinth is completely removed, destroying cochlear function. This procedure is used only when hearing loss is nearly complete and vertigo is persistent. Although labyrinthectomy relieves vertigo in nearly all cases, the person may remain unsteady and have continued problems with balance.

After surgery on the inner ear, the person is positioned to minimise ear pressure and vertigo. Movement is restricted and assistance is provided when the person gets up. Anti-emetics and anti-vertigo medications are used to manage symptoms resulting from disruption of the inner ear. Complications include infection and leakage of cerebrospinal fluid.

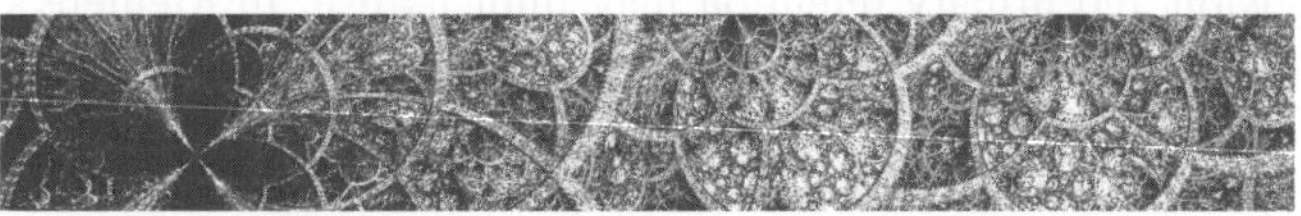

Nursing care

The person with an inner ear disorder has multiple nursing care needs related to the manifestations of the disorder.

Health promotion

Health promotion focuses on identifying people with potential inner ear disorders. Persistent episodes of dizziness, ringing in the ears, balance problems or loss of hearing should be reported to a healthcare provider. People diagnosed early may have a lower risk of injury and can be taught strategies for maintaining, as near normal as possible, their work and social life.

Assessment

In addition to the following, assess the older person for other medical causes of imbalance and dizziness, such as neurological dysfunction, musculoskeletal and cardiovascular disorders, and endocrine problems.

- *Health history*: medication use; presence of vertigo, tinnitus, nausea and vomiting and hearing loss; balance problems; frequency and duration of symptoms; precipitating factors for an attack.
- *Physical examination*: vital signs, general health; hearing, nystagmus, balance.

Nursing diagnoses and interventions

The risk of trauma in people with inner ear disorders is great. Attacks of vertigo may occur without warning and can be so severe that the person is unable to remain upright. If frequent attacks are accompanied by nausea, nutrition may be compromised. Constant or intermittent tinnitus can interfere with sleep and rest. Finally, because nearly all inner ear disorders are associated with some degree of hearing loss, which may be progressive, the person has significant psychosocial needs.

Risk of trauma

Because of the unpredictable nature of attacks, the person with vertigo due to an inner ear disorder needs to learn strategies for dealing with an acute episode. Because vertigo tends to be chronic except in acute labyrinthitis, the emphasis is on helping the person develop strategies to reduce the frequency of attacks and the risk of injury.

- Monitor for vertigo, nystagmus, nausea, vomiting and hearing loss. *Monitoring is important to determine the severity of impairment, the duration of attacks and the person's ability to predict an impending attack.*
- Instruct to not get up without assistance during episodes of vertigo. *During attacks of vertigo, assistance reduces the risk of falling.*

> **CONSIDERATION FOR PRACTICE**
> **During an acute attack of vertigo, keep on bed rest with the side rails raised and the call bell readily accessible.**

- Educate to avoid sudden head movements or position changes. *Sudden movement may precipitate an attack of vertigo.*
- Administer prescribed medications as ordered, including anti-emetics, diuretics and sedatives. *These medications may reduce the frequency, severity and duration of vertigo attacks.*
- Instruct to take the prescribed medication and lie down in a quiet, darkened room when an impending attack is sensed. *These measures help protect the person from injury and may shorten the duration and reduce the severity of the attack.*
- Advise to pull to the side of the road and wait for the symptoms to subside if an attack occurs while driving. *Perception and judgment necessary for safe driving may be impaired during an acute attack; pulling off the road is vital to protect the safety of the person and others.*
- Discuss the effect of unilateral hearing loss on the ability to identify the direction of sounds. To ensure safety, encourage the person to use other senses (e.g. when crossing the street). *Sound perception and differentiation of direction change when hearing is lost unilaterally, just as depth perception changes when vision is lost in one eye.*

Disturbed sleep pattern

The tinnitus often associated with inner ear disorders may be loud and continuous, interfering with the person's ability to concentrate, relax and sleep. It may be perceived as a continuous high-pitched whine, buzzing, ringing or humming sound. In some people, it may have a pulsatile quality.

- Refer for a complete hearing and ear examination if one has not been done. *Although most tinnitus is associated with hearing loss, often due to noise exposure, it may also be associated with treatable conditions such as impacted cerumen, hypertension, cerebrovascular disorders and other conditions.*
- Discuss options for masking tinnitus to promote concentration and sleep:
  a. ambient noise from a radio or sound system
  b. masking device or white-noise machine
  c. hearing aid that produces a tone to mask the tinnitus
  d. hearing aid that amplifies ambient sound.
  These techniques or devices help mask the subjective perception of tinnitus, allowing the person to focus on something other than the sound.
- Discuss the possible risks and benefits of medications to treat tinnitus. *Many medications have been used to treat tinnitus; oral antidepressants such as nortriptyline taken at bedtime have been shown to be most effective.*

Community-based care

Because disorders of the inner ear disrupt balance, safety is a primary focus of education. Assist the person to identify possible hazards in the home environment. Discuss the following points during the teaching session:

- Change positions slowly, especially when ambulating.
- Turn the whole body rather than just the head.
- Sit down immediately with the onset of vertigo and lie down if possible.
- Take prescribed anti-emetic and anti-vertigo medications.
- Wear MedicAlert® identification.
- If appropriate, discuss the surgical procedure, the immediate postoperative period and the long-term effects of the surgery.
- Discuss alternative communication techniques and associated community resources as needed.

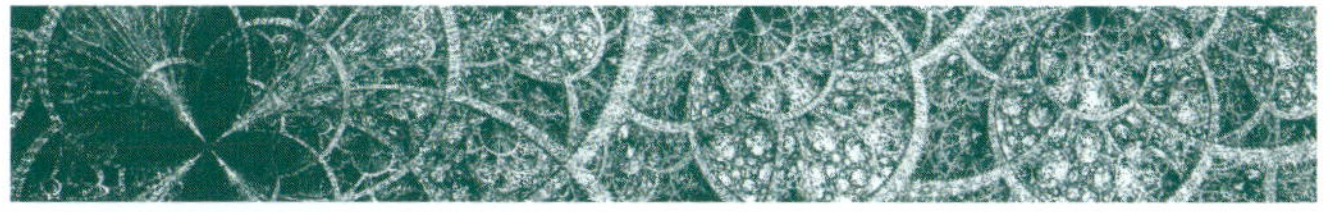

THE PERSON WITH AN ACOUSTIC NEUROMA

An **acoustic neuroma**, or schwannoma, is a benign tumour of cranial nerve VIII. It typically occurs in adults between the ages of 40 and 50. They are common and account for about 9% of primary brain tumours. Although usually unilateral, people with neurofibromatosis type 2, a genetic disorder, frequently develop bilateral schwannomas (Loscalzo et al., 2022).

These tumours usually occur in the internal auditory meatus, compressing the auditory nerve where it exits the skull to the inner ear. Both the vestibular and the cochlear branches are affected; however, the tumour arises from the vestibular division of the auditory nerve twice as often. If allowed to grow, the tumour eventually destroys the labyrinth, including the cochlea and vestibular apparatus. As the tumour expands, it erodes the wall of the internal auditory meatus. The tumour may eventually impinge on the inferior cerebellar artery, which provides blood to the lateral pons and medulla, the brainstem and the cerebellum. An obstructive hydrocephalus can also occur. Cranial nerves VII (facial) and V (trigeminal) are often affected by the expanding tumour; the tumour frequently wraps around the facial nerve.

Early manifestations of an acoustic neuroma are those associated with disorders of the inner ear: tinnitus, unilateral hearing loss and nystagmus. Dizziness or vertigo may occur. As the tumour expands and occupies increasing amounts of space in the closed cranium, the person experiences neurological signs related to the area of the brain affected.

The presence of the tumour can generally be identified on CT or MRI scans. X-ray films of the petrous pyramid of the temporal bone may show erosion caused by the tumour. The treatment of choice for an acoustic neuroma is surgical excision. In surgery, every effort is made to preserve this nerve and its function as well as other cranial nerves that may be affected.

Postoperative nursing care focuses on preserving cerebral function. Position the person to minimise cerebral oedema and monitor frequently for signs of increased intracranial pressure. Because the gag reflex may be affected, assess the person carefully before food and fluids are allowed by mouth. Speech therapy is often prescribed for the person after surgery. Because deficits may not resolve for a long time after surgery, education and support are vital components of nursing care for the person. (See the chapter 'Nursing care of people with intracranial disorders' for care of the person undergoing craniotomy.)

THE PERSON WITH HEARING LOSS

One in 6 people in Australia is reported to be affected by hearing loss. This is expected to increase to 1 in 4 by 2050. In 2019, 3.6 million 14.5% Australians had at least one long-term hearing disorder, the most common being complete or partial deafness, followed by tinnitus (ringing in the ears) (Department of Health, 2019). In 2018–2019, around 1 in 10 Aboriginal and Torres Strait Islander people reported having diseases of the ear and mastoid, and/or hearing problems. The proportion of Aboriginal and Torres Strait Islander people with ear/hearing problems was higher for people living in remote areas (59%) than non-remote areas (39%) (Australian Bureau of Statistics, 2019; AIHW, 2020).

Hearing loss impairs the ability to communicate in a world filled with sound and hearing individuals. A hearing deficit can be partial or total, congenital or acquired. It may affect one or both ears. In some types of hearing loss, the ability to perceive sound at specific frequencies is lost. In others, hearing is diminished across all frequencies.

People with a hearing loss often display signs that caregivers can recognise. The voice volume of the person with impaired hearing frequently increases and the person positions the head with the better ear towards the speaker. The person frequently may ask people to repeat what they have said or respond inappropriately to questions or statements. A question may elicit a blank look if the person has not heard or understood its content.

Pathophysiology and manifestations

Lesions in the outer ear, middle ear, inner ear or central auditory pathways can result in hearing loss. The process of ageing also can affect the structures of the ear and hearing. Hearing loss is classified as conductive, sensorineural or mixed, depending on which portion of the auditory system is affected. Profound deafness is often a congenital condition.

Conductive hearing loss

Anything that disrupts the transmission of sound from the external auditory meatus to the inner ear results in a conductive hearing loss. The most common cause of conductive hearing loss is obstruction of the external ear canal. Impacted cerumen, oedema of the canal lining, stenosis and neoplasms all may lead to canal obstruction. Other causes of conductive loss include a perforated tympanic membrane, disruption or fixation of the ossicles of the middle ear, fluid, scarring or tumours of the middle ear.

With conductive hearing loss, there is an equal loss of hearing at all sound frequencies. If the level of sound is greater than the threshold for hearing, speech discrimination is good. Because of this, the person with a conductive hearing loss benefits from amplification by a hearing aid.

Sensorineural hearing loss

Disorders that affect the inner ear, the auditory nerve or the auditory pathways of the brain may lead to a sensorineural hearing loss. In this type of hearing loss, sound waves are effectively transmitted to the inner ear. In the inner ear, however, lost or damaged receptor cells, changes in the cochlear apparatus or auditory nerve abnormalities decrease or distort the ability to receive and interpret stimuli.

A significant cause of sensorineural hearing deficit is damage to the hair cells of the organ of Corti. Damage may result from either loud impulse noise (e.g. an explosion) or loud continuous noise (e.g. machinery). Exposure to a high level of noise (e.g. standing close to the stage or speakers at a rock concert) on an intermittent or continuing basis damages the hair and supporting cells of the organ of Corti. Ototoxic drugs also damage the hair cells; when combined with high noise levels, the damage is greater and resultant hearing loss more profound. Ototoxic drugs include aspirin, furosemide, aminoglycosides, streptomycin, vancomycin, antimalarial drugs and chemotherapy such as cisplatin. Other potential causes of sensory hearing loss include prenatal exposure to rubella, viral infections, meningitis, trauma, Ménière's disease and ageing.

Tumours such as acoustic neuromas, vascular disorders, demyelinating or degenerative diseases, infections (bacterial meningitis, in particular) or trauma may affect the central auditory pathways and produce a neural hearing loss.

Sensorineural hearing losses typically affect the ability to hear high-frequency tones more than low-frequency tones. This loss makes speech discrimination difficult, especially in a noisy environment. Hearing aids are often not useful because they amplify both speech and background noise. The increased sound intensity may actually cause discomfort for the person.

Presbycusis

With ageing, the hair cells of the cochlea degenerate, producing a progressive sensorineural hearing loss. In **presbycusis**, gradual hearing loss associated with ageing, hearing acuity begins to decrease in early adulthood and progresses as long as the individual lives. Higher-pitched tones and conversational speech are lost initially. Hearing aids and other amplification devices are useful for most people with presbycusis.

Because the hearing loss of presbycusis is gradual, the person and family may not realise the extent of the deficit. The individual with a hearing impairment may be described as unsociable or paranoid. The family may worry that the person is becoming increasingly forgetful, absentminded or perhaps 'senile'. Depression, confusion, inattentiveness, tension and negative attitudes and/or behaviours have been noted in older adults with hearing impairments. Functional problems such as poor general health, reduced mobility and impaired interpersonal communication are also associated with hearing loss. Caregivers need to be alert for signs of impaired hearing such as cupping an ear, difficulty understanding verbal communication when the person cannot see the speaker's face, difficulty following conversation in a large group and withdrawal from social activities.

Tinnitus

Tinnitus is the perception of sound or noise in the ears without stimulus from the environment. The sound may be steady, intermittent or pulsatile and is often described as a buzzing, roaring or ringing.

Tinnitus is usually associated with hearing loss (conductive or sensorineural); however, the mechanism producing the sound is poorly understood. It is often an early symptom of noise-induced hearing damage and drug-related ototoxicity. Tinnitus is especially associated with salicylate, quinine or quinidine toxicity. Other aetiologies include obstruction of the auditory meatus, presbycusis, middle or inner ear inflammations and infections, otosclerosis and Ménière's disease. Most tinnitus, however, is chronic and has no pathological importance.

Tinnitus that is intermittent or slight enough to be masked by environmental sounds is often well tolerated. When it is loud, continuous and not responsive to treatment, tinnitus can be a significant stressor. It can interfere with activities of daily living, sleep and rest.

INTERPROFESSIONAL CARE

The best treatment for hearing loss is prevention. People need to know the risk of hearing damage and how to prevent it. Awareness of the effects of noise exposure, especially when combined with the ototoxic effects of aspirin or other drugs, is important to prevent sensorineural hearing loss.

Diagnosis

Hearing evaluation includes gross tests of hearing (such as the whisper test), the Rinne and Weber tests, and audiometry.

- *Rinne* and *Weber tests* compare air and bone sound conduction. When bone conduction of sound is better than air conduction, the hearing deficit is a conductive loss. The Rinne test can identify even mild conductive hearing losses. If both air and bone conduction are impaired, a sensorineural loss is indicated (see the chapter 'A person-centred approach to assessing the eye and ear').
- *Audiometry* identifies the type and pattern of hearing loss. Specific sound frequencies are presented to each ear by either air or bone conduction.
- *Speech audiometry* identifies the intensity at which speech can be recognised and interpreted. *Speech discrimination* evaluates the ability to discriminate between various speech sounds.
- *Tympanometry* is an indirect measurement of the compliance and impedance of the middle ear to sound transmission. The external auditory meatus is subjected to neutral, positive and negative air pressure while the resultant sound energy flow is monitored.
- *Acoustic reflex testing* uses a tone presented at various intensities to evaluate movement of the structures of the middle ear.

Amplification

A hearing aid or other amplification device can help many people with hearing deficits. These assistive devices do nothing to prevent, minimise or treat the hearing loss itself. They amplify the sound presented to the hearing apparatus of the ear, which may bring the level of sound above the hearing threshold, allowing more accurate perception and interpretation of its meaning. When sound perception is distorted, a hearing aid may be less helpful because it simply amplifies the distorted sound.

Unfortunately, fewer than one-fifth of older people with a hearing deficit have and/or use a hearing aid. Denial of the deficit, other health problems, poor visual acuity, decreased manual dexterity and cost all contribute to this low usage. Hearing aids must be individually prescribed by an audiologist. Proper design, proper fit and regular maintenance are necessary for their effectiveness.

All hearing aids include a microphone, amplifier, speaker, earpiece and volume control. Most allow volume control, reduce background noise and can be adjusted for the person's pattern of hearing loss. Behind-ear and in-ear aids often include a telecoil, which amplifies sound from the telephone without feedback. The models also may allow direct audio input (e.g. MP3 player) or include Bluetooth capability for hands-free telephone use. Hearing aids are available in a variety of styles, each with advantages and disadvantages:

- Canal hearing aids (in-the-canal and completely-in-canal) are the least noticeable style, fitting in the ear canal. They are appropriate for mild to moderately severe hearing loss. These small and unobtrusive devices allow use of the telephone and can be worn during exercise. Because of their small size, the person must have good manual dexterity to insert, clean and change the batteries on canal hearing aids. For this reason, older people or people with impaired dexterity may be unable to use them.
- The in-ear style of hearing aid fits into the external ear and is used for mild to severe hearing loss (see Figure 45.16). Its larger size makes manipulation somewhat easier, although it still may be difficult for less dexterous individuals. A greater degree of amplification is possible with the in-ear aid. Many have a toggle switch for telephone usage.
- The behind-ear hearing aid allows finer adjustment of the level of amplification and is easier for the person to manipulate (see Figure 45.17). It can be used by people with mild to profound hearing loss. For the person who wears glasses, this style can be modified, with all components fitting into the temple of the eyeglasses.
- People with profound hearing loss may require a body hearing aid. The microphone and amplifier of this aid are contained in a pocket-sized case that the person clips on to clothing, slips into a pocket or carries in a harness. The receiver is attached by a cord to the case and clips on to the ear mould, which delivers the sound to the ear canal.

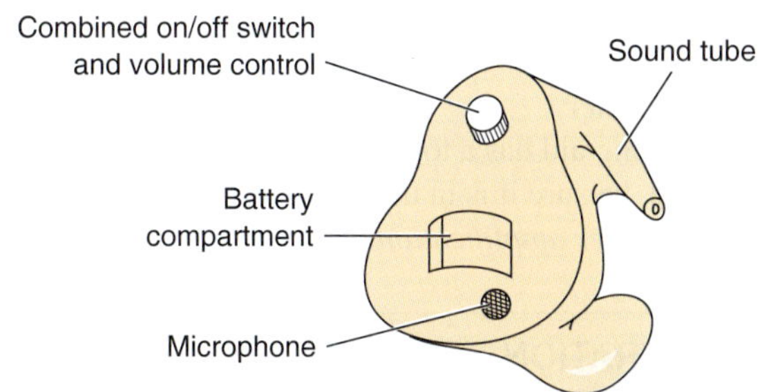

FIGURE 45.16 ***An in-ear hearing aid***

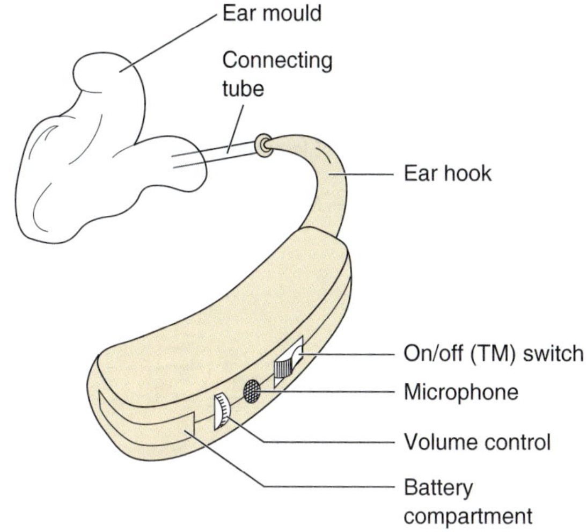

FIGURE 45.17 ***A behind-ear hearing aid***

With both the in-canal and in-ear style, cleaning is important. Small portals may become plugged with cerumen, interfering with sound transmission.

For the person who does not have a hearing aid, an *assistive listening device* or 'pocket talker', with a microphone and ear buds, is useful. Pocket talkers are available over the counter or through an audiologist and are relatively inexpensive. The earpiece requires no special fitting and the external microphone allows the person to focus on the desired sound rather than simply amplifying all sounds. Assistive listening devices may also be used in conjunction with a hearing aid.

People with tinnitus may find a white-noise masking device helpful to promote concentration and rest. These devices conduct a pleasant sound to the affected ear, allowing the person to block out the abnormal sound.

Surgery

Reconstructive surgeries of the middle ear, such as a stapedectomy or tympanoplasty, may help restore hearing with a conductive hearing loss. Stapedectomy is the removal and replacement of the stapes. This procedure is used to treat hearing loss related to otosclerosis.

In a tympanoplasty, the structures of the middle ear are reconstructed to improve conductive hearing deficits. Chronic otitis media with necrosis and scarring of the middle ear is a common indication for this type of surgery.

For the person with a sensorineural hearing loss, a *cochlear implant* may be the only hope for restoring sound perception. The cochlear implant consists of a microphone, speech processor, transmitter and receiver/stimulator, and electrodes (see Figure 45.18). Its function is more similar to the way the ear normally receives and processes sounds than it is to a hearing aid. The microphone picks up sounds, sending them to the speech processor, which selects and processes useful sounds.

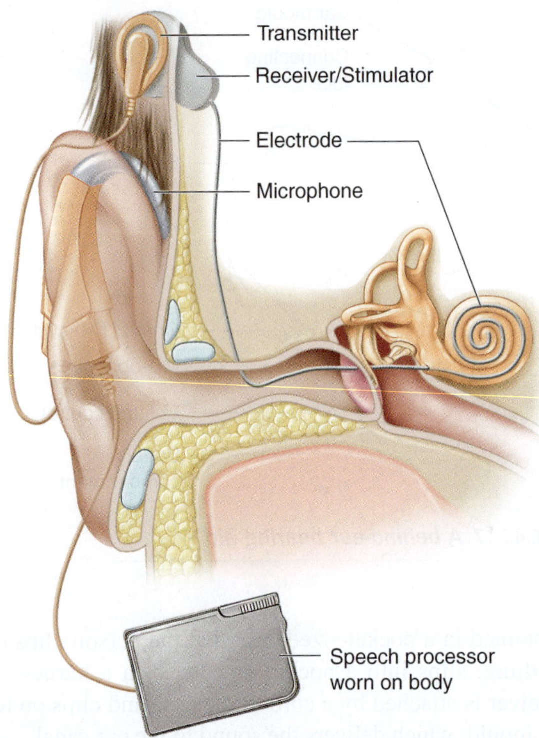

FIGURE 45.18 ***A cochlear implant for hearing loss***

The transmitter and receiver/stimulator receive signals from the speech processor, convert them to electrical impulses and send these impulses to the electrodes for transmission to the brain.

Cochlear implants provide sound perception but not normal hearing. The person is able to recognise warning sounds such as cars, sirens, telephones and doors opening or closing. They also receive stimuli to alert them to incoming communication so they can focus on the person speaking. Many people learn to interpret perceived sounds as words, especially when the hearing loss is acquired as an adult.

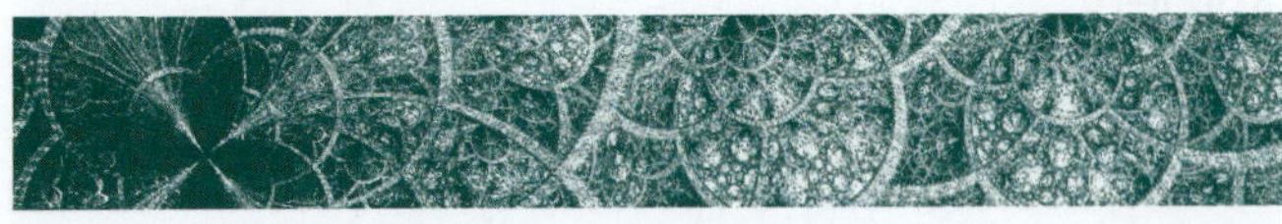

Nursing care

In planning and implementing nursing care for the person with a hearing deficit, the type and extent of hearing loss, the person's adaptation to the loss and the availability of assistive hearing devices are considered, as well as the person's ability and willingness to use assistive devices.

Health promotion

Healthcare personnel can be instrumental in preventing hearing loss through education. It is important to promote environmental noise control and the use of ear protection. Workplace Health and Safety legislation requires ear protection for work environments that consistently exceed 85 decibels. Education for primary prevention focuses on the following:

- care of the ears and ear canals, including cleaning and treatment of infection
- not placing hard objects into the ear canal
- use of plugs to protect the ears during swimming or diving
- avoiding intermittent or frequent exposure to loud noise
- monitoring for side effects with ototoxic medications
- hearing evaluation when hearing difficulty is present.

Assessment

- *Health history*: perceived ability to hear; effect of hearing loss on function and lifestyle; risk factors such as use of ototoxic medications; upper respiratory tract or frequent ear infection; noise exposure; presence of vertigo, tinnitus, unsteadiness or imbalance.
- *Physical examination*: apparent perception of normal speech; inspection of external ear, tympanic membrane; whisper, Rinne and Weber tests; tests of balance and cranial nerve function.

Nursing diagnoses and interventions

This section focuses on the problems of having a hearing deficit, impaired communication and social isolation for the person who is hearing impaired.

Disturbed auditory perception

Whether the person's hearing deficit is partial or total, impaired sound perception is the primary problem. The person needs to understand what causes the deficit and what to expect for the future. Nursing interventions focus on maximising available hearing and preventing further deterioration to the extent possible.

- Encourage the person to talk about the hearing loss and its effect on activities of daily living. *Hearing loss affects each individual in a different way. The person may be denying the extent of the deficit or grieving the loss. Listening and providing support encourage the person to develop coping strategies.*
- Provide information about the type of hearing loss. Refer the person to an audiologist for evaluation of the hearing loss and possible exploration of amplification devices. *With improved understanding of the deficit, the person can plan ways to compensate.*
- Replace batteries in hearing aids regularly and as needed. *Hearing aid batteries last approximately 1 week. If a battery is old or has been improperly stored, the life may be reduced further.*
- If the hearing aid has a toggle switch for microphone/telephone, be sure it is in the appropriate position. *This ensures proper amplification with the hearing aid.*

> **CONSIDERATION FOR PRACTICE**
> **Check hearing aids for patency, cleaning out cerumen as necessary.**

Impaired verbal communication

A hearing deficit impairs the person's ability to receive and interpret verbal communication. A hearing loss affects the person's ability to follow conversations, use the telephone and enjoy television or other forms of entertainment.

- Use the following techniques to improve communication:
  a. Wave the hand or tap the shoulder before beginning to speak.
  b. If the person wears corrective lenses, ensure that they are clean and encourage the person to wear them.
  c. When speaking, face the person and keep your hands away from your face.
  d. Keep your face in full light.
  e. Reduce the noise in the environment before speaking.
  f. Use a low voice pitch with normal loudness.
  g. Use short sentences and pause at the end of each sentence.
  h. Speak at a normal rate and do not overarticulate.
  i. Use facial expressions or gestures.
  j. Provide a magic slate for written communication.
  Individuals with hearing impairments often lip read, making good visibility of the speaker's face necessary. Excessive environmental noise interferes with the ability to perceive the message. Higher tones are typically lost with presbycusis and other types of hearing loss. Using short sentences and pausing give the person time to interpret the message. Overarticulating makes it more difficult to follow the flow and to lip read. Non-verbal cues and written messages enhance the person's understanding.
- Be sure the hearing aid is properly placed, is turned on and has fresh batteries. *The person may not be aware that the hearing aid is not functioning well.*
- Do not place intravenous catheters in the dominant hand. *The person may need to use that hand to write in order to communicate.*
- Rephrase sentences when there is difficulty understanding. *Hearing losses may affect different sound tones, making some words more difficult to comprehend. Using alternative words and phrases may increase the person's ability to perceive the message.*
- Repeat important information. *The nurse makes sure that the person understands the information.*
- Inform other staff about the person's hearing deficit and effective strategies for communication. *Consistent use of effective strategies for communication decreases the person's frustration.*

Social isolation

The person with impaired hearing often becomes socially isolated. This isolation may be self-imposed because of difficulty communicating, especially in a group. Often, however, the isolation comes about gradually and without intention. The person finds social settings such as family dinners or community gatherings increasingly difficult. Friends and family become frustrated trying to communicate with someone who has a hearing impairment and invitations to participate in social activities dwindle.

- Identify the extent and cause of the social isolation. Help to differentiate the reality of the isolation and its cause from the person's perception of isolation. *People with impaired hearing may be unaware that they are isolated. Identifying factors that contribute to isolation may provide the needed impetus to remedy the hearing loss. People may also experience paranoid thinking as a result of impaired communication and believe that friends and family have purposely begun to avoid interactions.*
- Encourage the person to interact with friends and family on a one-to-one basis in quiet settings. *People with impaired hearing are more successful in understanding conversations that take place in small groups and quiet settings.*
- Treat the person with dignity and remind friends and family that a hearing deficit does not indicate loss of mental faculties. *Inappropriate responses due to a hearing deficit can cause others to perceive the person as 'stupid' or demented.*
- Involve the person in activities that do not require acute hearing, such as draughts and chess. *The person has an opportunity to interact socially without the stress of straining to hear.*
- Obtain a pocket talker or encourage the person and family to do so.
- Refer the person to an audiologist for evaluation and possible hearing-aid fitting.
- Refer the person to resources such as support groups and senior citizen centres. *These groups provide new social outlets.*

Community-based care

Educating for home and community-based care for the person with hearing loss and family focuses on managing the deficit and developing coping strategies. Referral to an audiologist for evaluation of the deficit and the usefulness of a hearing aid may be appropriate. In addition, discuss the following topics as appropriate for each person:

- use, care and maintenance of a hearing aid
- strategies for coping with the hearing deficit
- voicing a preference for individual visits and small-group interactions rather than large social functions
- highlighting relevant resources available within the state and/or territory.

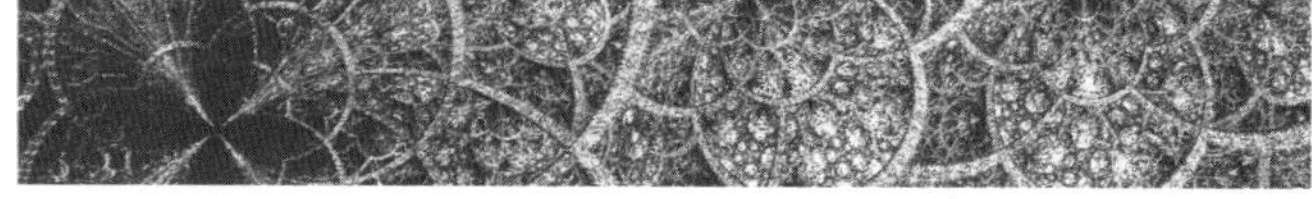

CHAPTER HIGHLIGHTS

- Structures of the external eye are vulnerable to trauma and infection. While usually minor, these problems can cause significant pain, scarring and clouding of the cornea, and loss or impairment of vision.
- Cataracts, glaucoma, age-related macular degeneration and diabetic retinopathy are leading causes of vision impairment in Australia. While these conditions cannot, in most cases, be prevented, they often can be treated or their progress slowed, preserving vision.
- Age, smoking, diabetes and long-term use of certain drugs are risk factors for cataract development. Removal of the clouded lens with insertion of an intraocular lens is the treatment of choice for cataracts. Surgery is elective, performed only when the cataract significantly impairs the ability to maintain ADLs and recreational activities.
- Glaucoma is progressive loss of visual fields associated with increased intraocular pressure and impaired aqueous humour drainage. Open-angle glaucoma, the predominant form of the disorder, can be controlled using medications and, as needed, laser surgery to promote aqueous humour drainage.
- Angle-closure glaucoma is a medical emergency requiring immediate treatment to lower intraocular pressure to preserve vision. Angle-closure glaucoma usually affects only one eye; however, the person is at risk of future attacks affecting the other eye.
- Age-related macular degeneration, a leading cause of blindness, cannot be effectively treated, although its progress may be slowed or halted through use of high-dose antioxidant vitamins and zinc if it is identified early. Macular degeneration affects the macula, the area of high-acuity central vision.
- Diabetic retinopathy eventually affects nearly all people with diabetes. It is a disease of the small blood vessels of the retina, leading to formation of aneurysms, retinal ischaemia and growth of fragile new vessels (neovascularisation) that easily rupture leading to haemorrhage. It is treated with laser surgery to seal fragile vessels.
- Otitis media is related to eustachian tube dysfunction, with impaired pressure equalisation of the middle ear. Otitis media may be either serous (sterile) or infectious (suppurative). Both cause acute discomfort with diminished hearing, snapping, popping and possible vertigo and systemic symptoms. The risk of complications, including rupture of the tympanic membrane, damage to structures of the middle ear and spread of infection to surrounding tissues, is greater with acute suppurative otitis media.
- Potential complications of acute otitis media include mastoiditis, chronic otitis media with tympanic membrane perforation and cholesteatoma formation. Hearing loss in the affected ear is a possibility with these disorders. The primary treatment is prevention through adequate treatment of acute otitis media.
- The primary manifestations of disorders of the inner ear are vertigo and possible hearing loss. Severe vertigo can interfere with safety, nutrition and the person's ability to maintain ADLs and life roles.
- The two main types of hearing loss are conductive and sensorineural. Presbycusis, hearing loss associated with ageing, is a type of sensorineural hearing loss. Hearing loss may be accompanied by tinnitus, the perception of sound without an environmental stimulus. Amplification devices (hearing aids) are the primary treatment for hearing loss.

CONCEPT CHECK

1 A nurse is working with a group of residents in a long-term care facility. All of the residents have moderate to severe hearing or vision impairment. Which of the following does the nurse identify as the highest priority of care?

1 preventing sensory deprivation
2 encouraging social interaction
3 promoting family relationships
4 maintaining resident safety

2 The nurse teaching a person with newly diagnosed glaucoma emphasises which of the following instructions?

1 turning the head side to side to compensate for impaired peripheral vision
2 using the prescribed eye drops as directed on a continuing basis
3 contacting the doctor if further decline in vision is noticed
4 avoiding coughing, sneezing or straining to have a bowel movement

3 A person with glaucoma has a history of heart failure. Which medication should the nurse discuss with the doctor before administering it?

1 brimonidine
2 dorzolamide
3 timolol
4 latanoprost

4 A person with Ménière's disease experiences frequent attacks of vertigo and tinnitus. Of the following teaching points, which one has the highest priority for this person?

1 Follow a low-sodium diet.
2 Stop smoking.
3 Take prescribed anti-emetic medications.
4 Sit down when an attack develops.

5 On a person's return from cataract surgery, the nurse in the ambulatory surgery recovery unit places the person:

1 in semi-Fowler's position
2 on the affected side
3 in a private room
4 in proximity to the nurses' station

6 A person calls her primary care provider's office with complaints of bright flashing lights to the side of her vision. The appropriate response by the nurse is to:

1 recommend that she lie down until the sensation has passed
2 advise her to make an appointment to have her blood pressure checked
3 initiate immediate referral to an ophthalmologist
4 reassure her that this is not unusual and should resolve without treatment

7 A person presents at the urgent care clinic with complaints of right ear pain. Which of the following should be included in physical assessment of this person? (Select all that apply.)

1 vital signs with temperature
2 inspection of the oral pharynx
3 manipulation of the ear pinna
4 palpation of cervical lymph nodes
5 inspection of the ear canal and tympanic membrane

8 An elderly resident in an assisted living facility complains to the nurse that his head 'feels stuffy' and he has ringing in his ears. The appropriate response by the nurse would be to:

1 make an appointment with the resident's primary care provider
2 refer the person for evaluation by a local audiologist
3 provide non-prescription ear drops for daily use
4 inspect the ear canals for patency

9 The nurse caring for a person with a severe hearing deficit identifies which of the following as an appropriate goal towards improving the person's social interactions?

1 Will plan to have dinner with one or two friends weekly.
2 Will participate in senior centre communal lunches at least twice per week.
3 Will engage in activities such as card tournaments and dancing.
4 Will attend religious services of choice.

10 When assessing a person, the nurse notes absence of the red reflex in the person's right eye. On questioning, the person responds: 'Oh yes, my doctor told me I have cataracts. When do you think I should have them removed?' How should the nurse respond?

1 'It appears that the right eye is due for surgery.'
2 'Are you having difficulty reading or doing activities you enjoy?'
3 'Are you starting to experience pain in your right eye or frequent headaches?'
4 'Cataracts can be removed any time that it is convenient for you.'

BIBLIOGRAPHY

Australian Bureau of Statistics (2019). *Australian Aboriginal and Torres Strait Islander health survey: Ear diseases and hearing problems*. Retrieved from http://www.abs.gov.au

Australian Corneal Graft Registry (2018). *2018 report*. Retrieved from https://www.flinders.edu.au/

Australian Institute of Health and Welfare (AIHW) (2020). *Australia's health 2020*. Retrieved from https://www.aihw.gov.au

Australian Institute of Health and Welfare (AIHW) (2021). *Indigenous eye health measures 2021*. Retrieved from https://www.aihw.gov.au

Department of Health (2019). *Roadmap for hearing health*. Canberra: Australian Government.

Department of Health (2020). *National strategic action plan for macular disease*. Retrieved from https://www.health.gov.au/

Gurnani, B., Czyz, C. N., Mahabadi, N. & Havens, S. J. (2022). *Corneal graft rejection*. Retrieved from https://www.ncbi.nlm.nih.gov/

Knights, K., Rowland, A., Darroch, S. & Bushell, M. (2022). *Pharmacology for health professionals* (6th ed.). Sydney: Elsevier.

Levett-Jones, T., Dwyer, T., Reid-Searl, K., Heaton, L., Flenady, T., Applegarth, J., Guinea, S. & Andersen, P. (2017). *Patient Safety Competency Framework (PSCF) for Nursing Students*. Sydney. Retrieved from http://psframework.wpengine.com/

Loscalzo, J., Fauci, A. S., Kasper, D. L., Hauser, S. L. & Longo, D. (2022). *Harrison's principles of internal medicine* (21st ed.). New York: McGraw Hill Medical.

National Eye Institute (NEI) (2018). *Immune cells in the retina can spontaneously regenerate*. Retrieved from https://nei.nih.gov/

National Eye Institute (NEI) (2021). *Aged-related macular degeneration* (AMD). Retrieved from https://nei.nih.gov/

National Eye Institute (NEI) (2022). *Diabetic retinopathy*. Retrieved from https://nei.nih.gov/

Norris, T. L. (2018). *Porth's pathophysiology: Concepts of altered health states* (10th ed.). Philadelphia: Lippincott Williams & Wilkins.

Papadakis, M., McPhee, S. & Rabow, M. (2022). *Current medical diagnosis and treatment* (61st ed.). New York: McGraw-Hill Education.

Rothrock, J. C. (2022). *Alexander's care of the patient in surgery* (17th ed.). St Louis, MO: Elsevier.

Vision Australia (2017). *Glaucoma. The silent thief of sight*. Retrieved from https://www.visionaustralia.org/

Vision Australia (2022). *Blindness and vision loss*. Retrieved from https://www.visionaustralia.org/

Vision Initiative (2020). *Eye health Australia*. Retrieved from http://www.visioninitiative.org.au/

Vision 2020 Australia (2018). Retrieved from https://www.v2020.org

World Health Organization (2021). *Visual impairment and blindness*. Retrieved http://www.who.int/

UNIT 12 BUILDING CLINICAL COMPETENCE

Responses to altered visual and auditory function

Clinical scenario

You have been assigned to work with the following four people for the 0700 shift on a medical–surgical unit. Significant data obtained during report are as follows:

- Andrew Hardy, a 50-year-old type 1 diabetic with hypertension, is a new admission during the night shift with blood glucose of 33.4 mmol/L. On assessment, the person reveals that he has been seeing black spot floaters and flashing lights at times. He is now complaining of blurred vision.
- Gladys Harvey is an 84-year-old who had right eye cataract surgery yesterday. Her vital signs have been stable since surgery. She has begun complaining of itching and slight discomfort in the right eye.
- Georgia Stanley is a 45-year-old admitted with complaints of feeling like she is spinning or falling, and has ringing and a fullness feeling in her left ear. Her vital signs are T 37°C, P 78, R 16, BP 102/68. She is diaphoretic and complains of nausea. She is scheduled for x-rays and a CT scan of her head at 0800.
- Kenneth Koch, a 30-year-old, is a postoperative person who had a right ear tympanoplasty yesterday because of hearing loss due to chronic otitis media. Vital signs are T 37.6°C, P 90, R 20, BP 136/86. The person is requesting medication for ear pain. Pain scale is 9 out of 10 on a scale of 10 being the highest.

Critical-thinking questions

1 In what order would you visit these people after handover?
1.
2.
3.
4.

2 Which top two priority assessments would you choose for each of the people presented above? Can you explain, if asked, the rationale for your choices?

	Priority Assessment #1	Priority Assessment #2
Andrew Hardy		
Gladys Harvey		
Georgia Stanley		
Kenneth Koch		

3 Which is the correct treatment for a person such as Mr Hardy who has symptoms of diabetic retinopathy?
1. scleral buckling
2. enucleation
3. photorefractive keratectomy
4. laser photocoagulation

4 After cataract surgery, Ms Harvey is placed in which position to reduce intraocular pressure?
1. Sims' position on the unaffected side
2. semi-Fowler's position on the unaffected side
3. supine with the head elevated 10 degrees
4. prone position on the affected side

5 A low-sodium diet is ordered for Ms Stanley, who has Ménière's disease. Ms Stanley understands this diet when she picks which meal plan?
1. hot dog on a roll with tomato sauce and mustard
2. ham and cheese sandwich with potato salad
3. grilled chicken sandwich with lettuce and tomato
4. hamburger on a roll with potato chips

6 Which assessment data would be most indicative of hyphema, a potential result of blunt eye trauma?
1. eye pain, decreased visual acuity, seeing a reddish tint
2. hypertension, headache, facial pain
3. white eye reflex, pressure and blindness in affected eye
4. double vision, sunken eye, limited eye movement

7 Which techniques may improve communication with the person who has a hearing impairment? (Select all that apply.)
1. Speak loudly to enhance hearing.
2. Speak at a normal rate and avoid overarticulating.
3. Stand in front of a window so person can see the face.
4. Face the person to enhance lip reading.
5. Turn down the television or radio.
6. Use short sentences and pause frequently.

8 A prescription for gentamicin is ordered for a person with conjunctivitis. The nurse understands that a serious adverse effect of aminoglycosides is which effect?
1. damage to the eighth cranial nerve resulting in hearing loss
2. vasodilation leading to migraine headaches
3. leg pain caused by thromboembolism
4. stomach irritation leading to gastric ulcers

9 When evaluating for Ménière's disease, which diagnostic studies would you expect to be ordered? (Select all that apply.)
1. caloric testing
2. Rinne and Weber tests
3. troponins
4. complete blood cell count
5. glycerol test
6. blood glucose test

10 After eye surgery, which measures does the nurse instruct the person in?
1. Avoid lifting more than 7 kg.
2. Avoid coughing or sneezing.
3. Lie on the affected side.
4. Remove the eye patch when sleeping.

11 Which is the correct way to instil ear drops in the adult person with otitis media?
1. Have person hang head over side of bed, pull pinna of the ear straight up, instil ear drops and have person turn to instil drops to other ear.
2. Have person tilt head towards unaffected side, pull pinna of the ear down and back, instil ear drops and have person remain still for 3 minutes.

3. Have person lie on unaffected side, pull the pinna of the ear up and back, instil ear drops and have person remain still for 5 minutes.
4. Have person lie in Sims' position on unaffected side, pull the pinna of the ear back, instil ear drops and have the person turn to other side after 1 minute.

12 Which is the appropriate primary prevention to teach Mr Koch to prevent hearing loss?

1. Cleanse the ear with ear swabs to prevent earwax build-up.
2. Avoid getting water in the ears when showering.
3. Monitor for ringing in the ears when taking paracetamol.
4. Wear ear protectors when exposed to loud noises.

Case study

George Panzarin is a 65-year-old Greek–Australian male who is seen in the eye clinic for a routine eye examination. He states he has not had any recent eye infections or eye injuries. He denies pain in the eyes. Vital signs are T 37.1°C, P 84, R 16, BP 168/88. His height is 172 cm and weight is 90 kg. His medical history indicates that he has hypertension and type 2 diabetes. He is taking hydrochlorothiazide, captopril and glyburide. He states that he is on an 8,400 kilojoule diabetic diet but he is often non-compliant with the diet. He sees his medical doctor about once a year but has not had an eye exam in about 10 years. He is married with five grown children and six grandchildren. Mr Panzarin states he does not know if there is any family history of glaucoma because his father died of a heart attack at age 50 and his mother died of cancer at age 60.

The ophthalmologist performs a tonometry, which indicates an increase in intraocular pressure. A fundoscopic examination indicates pallor and increase in the size and depth of the optic cup on the optic disc. Visual field testing indicates significant peripheral vision loss. The results of these tests indicate a diagnosis of glaucoma.

Based on the medical diagnosis of open-angle glaucoma and the person's decreased peripheral vision, the nursing assessment *Risk of disturbed visual perception* is appropriate for planning care for Mr Panzarin.

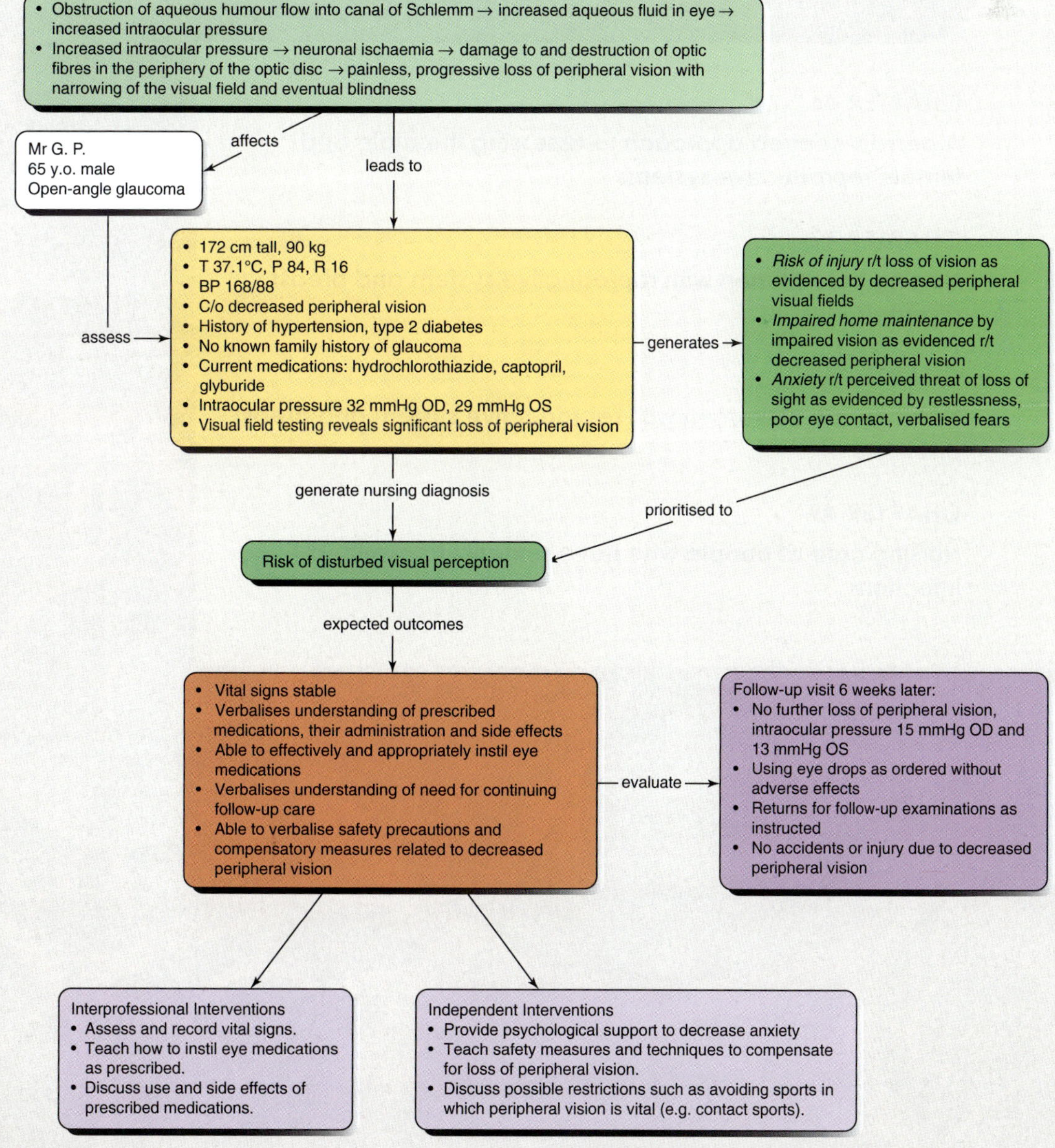

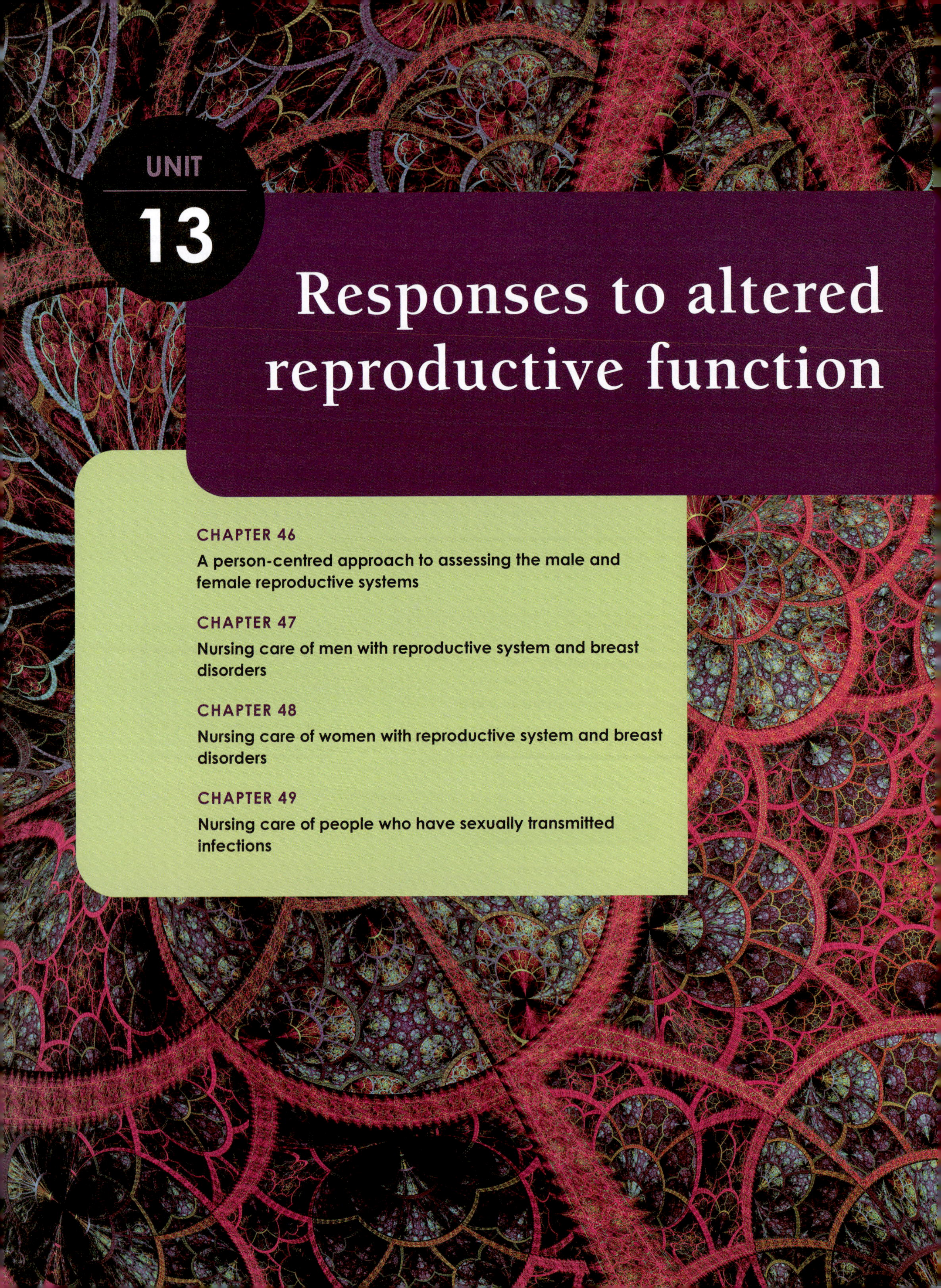

UNIT 13

Responses to altered reproductive function

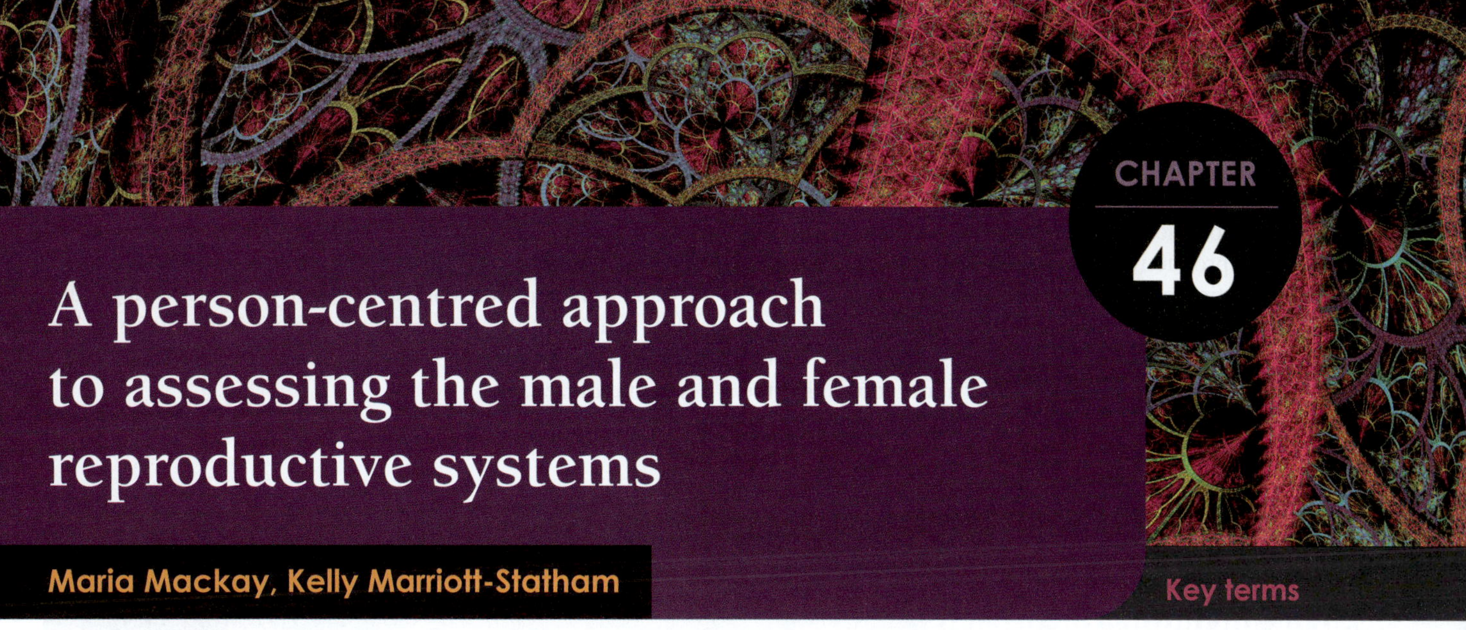

CHAPTER 46

A person-centred approach to assessing the male and female reproductive systems

Maria Mackay, Kelly Marriott-Statham

Key terms

Learning outcomes

- Describe the anatomy, physiology and functions of the male and female reproductive systems and the breasts.
- Explain the functions of the male and female sex hormones.
- Identify specific topics for consideration during a health history interview and person-centred assessment of a person's reproductive system and breast structures and/or functions.
- Describe variations in assessment findings for the older person.
- Identify signs of impairment in the male and female reproductive system and breast structure or function.

Clinical competencies

- Conduct a health history with a person relevant to male and female reproductive systems and functions and the breasts.
- Conduct a person-centred physical assessment of male and female reproductive system structures and functions and the breasts.
- Monitor and interpret findings from diagnostic tests in conjunction with health history and physical assessment and report abnormal findings.

Although the male and female reproductive organs are very different, they share common functions: enabling sexual pleasure and reproduction. The reproductive organs, in conjunction with the neuroendocrine system, produce hormones important in biological development and sexual behaviour. Parts of the reproductive organs also enclose and are integral to the function of the urinary system. Assessment of the reproductive and urinary systems is often difficult for both the nurse and the individual and requires sensitivity on the part of the nurse when asking questions about topics that the person may be hesitant to talk about. Given the high incidence of physical and sexual violence experienced within the community, nurses need to exercise skill and sensitivity in language used and in the conducting of a physical person-centred assessment. Consideration of pronouns and gendered language is vitally important to ensure the consideration of how people choose to identify (or not) with gender. Skill and sensitivity in conducting a person-centred physical examination of an area of the body usually considered private is also required.

Anatomy, physiology and functions of the male reproductive system, including the breasts

The male reproductive system comprises the paired testes, scrotum, ducts, glands and penis (see Figure 46.1). This chapter also includes the breasts as part of the reproductive system. The location and functions of the male reproductive organs are summarised in Table 46.1.

The breasts

The male breast is comprised primarily of an areola (circular pigmented area) and a nipple. These lie over a thin disk of undeveloped breast tissue that may not be overtly different from surrounding tissue. Approximately 1 in 3 people have a firm area of breast tissue 2 cm or larger; the limits of the normal size of this area have not been established (Sencha et al., 2015).

The penis

The penis is the genital organ that encloses the urethra (see Figure 46.1). It is homologous to the clitoris of the female. The penis is composed of a shaft and a tip called the glans, which is covered by the foreskin or prepuce (when uncircumcised). The shaft contains three columns of erectile tissue: the two lateral columns are called the corpora cavernosa and the central mass is called the corpus spongiosum.

Erection occurs when the penile masses become filled with blood in response to a reflex that triggers the parasympathetic nervous system to stimulate arteriolar vasodilation. The erection reflex may be initiated by touch, pressure, sights, sounds, smells or thoughts of a sexual encounter. After ejaculation, the arterioles vasoconstrict and the penis returns to a flaccid state.

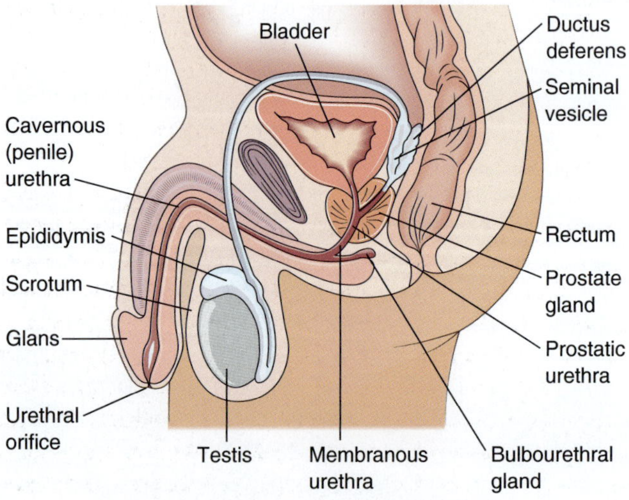

FIGURE 46.1 *The male reproductive system*

The scrotum

The scrotum is a sac or pouch made of two layers. The outer layer is continuous with the skin of the perineum and thighs. The inner layer is made of muscle and fascia. The scrotum hangs at the base of the penis, anterior to the anus, and regulates the temperature of the testes. The optimum temperature for sperm production is about 2 to 3°C below body temperature. When the testicular temperature is too low, the scrotum contracts to bring the testes up against the body. When the testicular temperature is too high, the scrotum relaxes to allow the testes to lie further away from the body.

The testes

The testes develop in the abdominal cavity of the fetus and then descend through the inguinal canal into the scrotum. Approximately one-third of premature boys are born with at least one undescended testicle, compared with 2–8% of full-term infant boys (Niedzielski, Oszukowska & Slowikowska-Hilczer, 2016), a condition that usually corrects itself within 1 year. This is cryptorchidism (the absence of one or both testes from the scrotum) and is distinct from monorchism (the condition of having one testicle). The testes are homologous to the female's ovaries. These paired organs are each about 4 cm long and 2.5 cm in diameter. They are suspended in the scrotum by the spermatic cord. Each is surrounded by two coverings: an outer tunica vaginalis and an inner tunica albuginea. Each testis is divided into 250 to 300 lobules, with each lobule containing one to four seminiferous tubules. The testes produce sperm and testosterone.

The seminiferous tubules are responsible for sperm production. Leydig's (or interstitial) cells lie in the connective tissue surrounding the seminiferous tubules and produce testosterone.

TABLE 46.1 Location and function of the male reproductive organs

MALE REPRODUCTIVE ORGAN	LOCATION	FUNCTION
Penis	Attached to front and sides of the pubic arch. Proximal, ventral surface is directly continuous with the scrotum.	Excretes semen and urine. Deposits sperm.
Scrotum	Hangs from body at the base of penis.	Contains testes, epididymis and portions of the vas (ductus) deferens.
Testes	In the scrotal sac.	Produces sperm and testosterone.
Epididymis	Posterolateral to upper aspect of each testis.	Stores sperm. Promotes sperm maturation. Transports sperm to vas deferens.
Vas deferens (ductus deferens)	Between the epididymis and the seminal vesicle forming the ejaculatory duct.	Stores sperm. Transports sperm.
Urethra	Begins at bladder and passes through prostate and penis.	Serves as passageway for urine or semen.
Prostate gland	Encircles the urethra at the neck of the bladder.	Contributes to ejaculatory volume. Enhances sperm motility and fertility.
Seminal vesicles	Lie on posterior bladder wall.	Contribute to ejaculatory volume. Contain nutrients to sustain sperm and prostaglandins to facilitate sperm motility.
Bulbourethral (Cowper's) glands	Inferior to the prostate.	Secrete mucus into urethra. Neutralise traces of acidic urine in urethra.

The ducts and semen

The seminiferous tubules lead into the efferent ducts and become the rete testis. From the rete testis, 10,000 to 20,000 efferent ducts join the epididymis, a long, coiled tube that lies over the outer surface of each testis. The epididymis is the final area for the storage and maturation of sperm. When sexual excitement occurs, the epididymis contracts to propel the sperm through the vas deferens to the ampulla, where the sperm are stored until ejaculation.

The seminal vesicles at the base of the bladder produce about 60% of the volume of seminal fluid. Seminal fluid is also made of secretions from the accessory sex organs, the epididymis, the prostate gland and Cowper's glands. Seminal fluid nourishes the sperm, provides bulk and increases its alkalinity (an alkaline pH is essential to mobilise the sperm and ensure fertilisation of the ova). Sperm mixed with this fluid is called **semen**. Each seminal vesicle joins its corresponding vas deferens to form an ejaculatory duct, which enters the prostatic urethra. During ejaculation, seminal fluid mixes with sperm at the ejaculatory duct and enters the urethra for expulsion.

The total amount of semen ejaculated is 2 to 4 mL, although the amount varies. The total ejaculate usually contains from 100 to 400 million sperm.

The prostate gland

The prostate gland is about the size of a walnut. It encircles the urethra just below the urinary bladder (see Figure 46.1). It is made of 20 to 30 tubuloalveolar glands surrounded by smooth muscle. Secretions of the prostate gland make up about one-third of the volume of the semen. These secretions enter the urethra through several ducts during ejaculation.

Spermatogenesis

Spermatogenesis is the series of physiological events that generate sperm in the seminiferous tubules. This process begins with puberty and continues throughout life, with several hundred million sperm produced each day.

The inner layer of the seminiferous tubules consists of sustentacular cells (or Sertoli's cells), which contain the spermatocytes and sperm in different stages of development. Sertoli's cells secrete a nourishing fluid for the developing sperm, as well as enzymes that help convert spermatocytes to sperm. The events in spermatogenesis, which take 64 to 72 days, are as follows:

1. The spermatogonia (sperm stem cells) undergo rapid mitotic division. As these cells multiply, the more mature spermatogonia divide into two daughter cells. These daughter cells grow and become the primary spermatocytes (and eventually become sperm).
2. Primary spermatocytes divide by meiosis to form two smaller secondary spermatocytes, which in turn divide to form two spermatids. This process occurs over several weeks.
3. The spermatids elongate into a mature sperm cell with a head and a tail. The head contains enzymes essential to the penetration and fertilisation of the ova. The flagellar motion of the tail allows the sperm to move. The sperm cells then move to the epididymis to mature further and develop motility.

Functions of the male sex hormones

The male sex hormones are called **androgens**. Most androgens are produced in the testes, although the adrenal cortex also produces a small amount. **Testosterone**, the primary androgen produced by the testes, is essential for the development and maintenance of sexual organs and secondary sex characteristics (such as pubic hair or facial hair) and for spermatogenesis. It also promotes metabolism, growth of muscles and bone, and libido (sexual desire).

ASSESSING THE MALE REPRODUCTIVE SYSTEM

The structures and functions of the male reproductive system are assessed by findings from a comprehensive person-centred assessment, which includes both a health assessment interview to collect subjective data and a physical assessment to collect objective data. In addition, a number of diagnostic tests may provide further information. All health assessments should be in partnership with the person, which will contribute to engagement with treatment and feeling empowered.

Health assessment interview

A health assessment interview to determine health issues with the male reproductive system may be conducted for varying reasons; for example:

- during a health screening
- as part of a comprehensive health assessment
- during a focused assessment for a specific health problem (such as a discharge from the penis).

The person having and/or the nurse undertaking the assessment may experience feelings of discomfort when engaging in discussion about reproductive health. It is important to be open and engage in conversations that enable the person to feel safe to share important personal information. The nurse needs to be aware of and consider the psychological, social and cultural factors that affect sexuality and sexual activity. It is important to use words that the person can understand and not to be embarrassed or offended by words that the person may use. The person may perceive the interview as less threatening if the discussion begins with more general questions and then progresses to specific questions. Ask questions in a way that enables the description of changes or concerns. For example, rather than asking if there is difficulty achieving or maintaining an erection, ask them to describe any changes noticed in erections. If there is a health problem identified by the person, the nurse needs to analyse its onset, characteristics and course, severity, precipitating and relieving factors and any associated symptoms, noting the timing and circumstances. For example, you may ask:

- When did you first notice that you were having difficulty urinating?
- Did you use a different brand of condoms before you noticed the rash on your penis?
- Describe the changes that occurred in your ability to have an erection after you started taking medicine for high blood pressure.

When questioning about a person's past medical history, ask about chronic illnesses such as diabetes, chronic kidney failure, cardiovascular disease, multiple sclerosis, spinal cord tumours or trauma, or thyroid disease. The effects of these illnesses, as well as the treatment of the illnesses, may cause impotence (inability to achieve or maintain an erection). The following drugs have the potential to cause sexual function problems: antihypertensives, antidepressants, antispasmodics, tranquillisers, sedatives, antipsychotics and histamine$_2$-receptor antagonists. Psychosocial stressors also may contribute to impotence.

If the person has a maternal history of being treated during pregnancy with diethylstilbestrol (DES) (a drug prescribed in the 1940s to the early 1970s to prevent miscarriage), they may have congenital deformities of the urinary tract as well as decreased semen levels. If they had mumps as a child, fertility issues are possible. Testicular cancer is a rare cancer, but it is one of the most common cancers for people aged 20 to 39, and the rate of diagnosis has grown by more than 50% in the past 30 years in Australia (Australian Institute of Health and Welfare (AIHW), 2021). The incidence is predicted to continue to rise. There are two kinds of testicular cancer: testicular teratoma or non-seminoma, and seminoma. Non-seminoma is a cancer of the mature germ cells, mostly affecting younger people in their late teens or early 20s. Seminoma develops in the immature germ cells, primarily affecting those slightly older between the ages of 25 and 45. Both kinds of testicular cancer can be treated successfully, with the chance of surviving more than 5 years being 97%, especially if detected early. The risk of testicular cancer is greatest in those who have a history of an undescended testicle, an inguinal hernia, testicular swelling with mumps, a history of maternal use of DES or oral contraceptives and a family history of testicular cancer.

In a person-centred assessment, you should explore the gender identification, lifestyle, social history and use of alcohol, cigarettes or illicit drugs. Unprotected sexual intercourse increases the potential for sexually transmitted infections, including hepatitis B and HIV infection. Ask about sexual preference. Unprotected sexual intercourse with same-sex partners further increases the risk of hepatitis B and HIV infection. Other questions about sexual activity may include number of sexual partners, history of premature ejaculation, impotence, any history of sexual trauma, use of condoms or other contraceptives, and current level of sexual satisfaction.

Interview questions categorised by functional health patterns are listed in the 'Functional health pattern interview' table.

Links to National Patient Safety Standards

NSQHS: Partnering with Consumers Standard

The intention of this standard is to 'create an organisation in which there are mutually valuable outcomes by having consumers as partners in planning, design, delivery, measurement and evaluation of systems and services' and 'patients as partners in their own care, to the extent that they choose' (Australian Commission on Safety and Quality in Health Care (ACSQHC), 2021, p. 14).

Partnering with consumers supports the active participation of all groups in the evaluation and improvement of an organisation, especially those groups who may not always participate in providing feedback.

Source: ACSQHC (2021). *National Safety and Quality Health Service Standards* (2nd ed.). Sydney: ACSQHC.

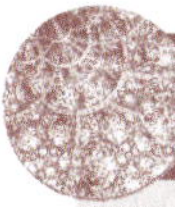

FUNCTIONAL HEALTH PATTERN INTERVIEW The male reproductive system

FUNCTIONAL HEALTH PATTERN	INTERVIEW QUESTIONS AND LEADING STATEMENTS
Health perception–Health management	■ Have you ever had problems or issues with your reproductive organs (penis, testicles, prostate gland)? Can you explain and tell me how was the problem treated?
	■ Have you ever had surgery on your reproductive organs? If so, what type, when, and what was the outcome?
	■ Have you ever noticed any pain or swelling in your breasts? Can you explain the symptoms?
	■ Do you practise testicular self-examination? How often?
	■ Have you ever noticed any pain or swelling in your testicles? Can you explain what you have noticed?
	■ Do you smoke? If so, how much and for how long have you smoked?
Nutritional–Metabolic	■ Describe your usual intake of food and fluids in a 24-hour period.
Elimination	■ Do you now or have you ever had a discharge from your penis? If so, can you describe the colour, odour, consistency, amount and frequency?
	■ Have you ever had any bleeding from your penis? Can you explain when this was, how much blood was present and if there was any associated pain?
	■ Have you noticed any change in your urination, such as burning, frequency, urgency, difficulty starting the stream, size of the stream, dribbling or getting up frequently at night? Can you explain this further?
Activity–Exercise	■ Describe your usual activity in a 24-hour period.
	■ Do you participate in sports or heavy lifting? If so, do you wear a protective cup or athletic support?
Sleep–Rest	■ Describe the quality of your rest and sleep.
Cognitive–Perceptual	■ Describe any pain you have had in the groin area, testicles, penis or scrotum. Where is it? Do you experience it in other parts of your body? How long does it last? What makes it worse or relieves it?
	■ Has there been a change in the condition or colour of the skin on your scrotum or penis? Can you explain the changes?
Self-perception–Self-concept	■ Has this current problem/issue affected how you feel about yourself?
	■ Do you feel that your needs for intimacy and affection are being met?
Role–Relationships	■ Has having this condition affected your relationship with others?
	■ Has having this condition interfered with your ability to work? Can you explain how?
	■ Has anyone in your family had prostate cancer? Can you explain their relationship to you?
Sexuality–Reproductive	■ Are you currently in a sexual relationship? If so, has this condition interfered with your usual sexual activity?
	■ How long have you been with your current partner? Have you had any other partners during this time?
	■ What is your sexual preference?
	■ Has having this problem affected your relationship with your spouse or sexual partner?
	■ Are you satisfied with your current level of sexual functioning?
	■ Have you ever had any problem with achieving or maintaining an erection or ejaculation?
	■ Do you use any medications to facilitate your sexual ability? Can you describe what they are?
	■ Do you use condoms every time you have sexual contact?
Coping–Stress–Tolerance	■ Has having this condition created stress for you? If so, does your health problem seem to be more difficult when you are stressed?
	■ Have you experienced any kind of stress that makes the condition worse? Can you explain this?
	■ Describe what you do when you feel stressed.
Value–Belief	■ Describe how specific relationships or activities help you cope with this problem.
	■ Describe specific cultural beliefs or practices that affect how you care for and feel about this problem.
	■ Are there any specific treatments or interventions that you would not use to treat this problem?

Physical assessment

Physical assessment of the male reproductive system may be performed as part of a comprehensive assessment or separately for those with identified sexual health problems. If conducted as part of a total physical assessment, this is usually the final 'system' to be assessed. Problems of the male reproductive system may involve the urinary system, making an assessment of both systems important. (See the chapter 'A person-centred approach to assessing the renal system' for assessment of the urinary system.) Normal age-related findings are summarised in Table 46.2.

The reproductive system is assessed by history taking, inspection and palpation. It is important for the person to feel safe and comfortable with the healthcare practitioner performing the person-centred assessment; consideration needs to be given to this when describing the assessment (e.g. gender of the healthcare practitioner). The procedures for the physical examination should always be explained using simple language, but thoroughly and in a matter-of-fact way to decrease anxiety and embarrassment. If the person is unfamiliar with internal genitalia, charts may be used to illustrate the parts that will be examined. Ask to empty their bladder (to be more comfortable during the examination), remove clothing and put on a gown. The assessment may be done sitting or standing. Only expose body parts being examined to preserve modesty. Ensure that the examining room is warm and private. Put on gloves before beginning and wear them throughout the examination to prevent infection, in line with the standard outlined in the 'Links to National Patient Safety Standards' box.

Diagnostic tests

The results of diagnostic tests of the structures and functions of the male reproductive system are used to support the diagnosis of a specific sexual problem, injury or disease. Test results also provide information to identify or modify appropriate medications or treatments used to treat the condition and to help nurses monitor responses to treatment and nursing care interventions. Diagnostic tests used to assess the male reproductive system are described in the 'Diagnostic tests' table and summarised in the bulleted list that follows. More information is included in the discussion of specific health problems or diseases in the chapter 'Nursing care of men with reproductive system and breast disorders'.

- Hormone changes and syphilis are diagnosed with blood tests, discussed in the chapters 'Nursing care of men with reproductive system and breast disorders' and 'Nursing care of people who have sexually transmitted infections'. Gonorrhoea, as well as other sexually transmitted infections, is diagnosed by cultures and smears of discharge or mucous membranes.
- Prostate cancer may be diagnosed following a raised prostate-specific antigen (PSA) reading. PSA is a glycoprotein secreted by the cells of the prostatic ductal epithelium. PSA is present in people with a prostate and this level of antigen increases with age (regardless of malignancy).
- The prostate may be examined by ultrasound to identify testicular torsion or masses, by digital rectal examination and by a prostate biopsy to accurately diagnose cancer or benign hypertrophy of the prostate.
- Semen analysis is done to evaluate semen volume, sperm count and motility, and percentage of abnormal sperm.

TABLE 46.2 Age-related changes in the male reproductive system

AGE-RELATED CHANGE	SIGNIFICANCE
Prostate gland • Ageing causes a large proportion of older people have some degree of benign prostatic hyperplasia.	Although ageing does not cause prostate cancer, its incidence does increase with age, with 1 in 6 developing prostate cancer before they turn 85 and 63% of prostate cancers being diagnosed in people over the age of 65 (AIHW, 2021).
Penis, testes and scrotum • Epithelial tissue and mucosa of seminal vesicles are thinner and have reduced capacity to hold fluid. • Sclerosis of penile arteries and veins may occur.	Sperm count can be reduced. Changes in the vascular system of the penis may mean that it takes longer to achieve an erection and ejaculation.

Links to National Patient Safety Standards

NSQHS: Preventing and Controlling Infections Standard

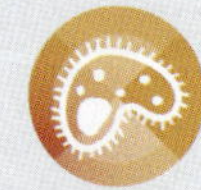

The intent of this standard is to reduce the risk of the person 'acquiring preventable infections; effectively manage infections, if they occur; prevent and contain antimicrobial resistance; promote appropriate prescribing and use of antimicrobials as part of antimicrobial stewardship; and promote appropriate and sustainable use of infection prevention and control resources' (ACSQHC, 2021, p. 22).

Source: ACSQHC (2021). *National Safety and Quality Health Service Standards* (2nd ed.). Sydney: ACSQHC. © Australian Commission on Safety and Quality in Health Care.

DIAGNOSTIC TESTS The male reproductive system

NAME OF TEST Prostate specific antigen (PSA)

PURPOSE AND DESCRIPTION The PSA level is raised in prostate disease, including prostate carcinoma and benign prostatic hypertrophy, and is also elevated following prostate examination. PSA is a protein made in the prostate gland. Low levels of PSA are found usually; however, they tend to rise with age as the prostate grows. PSA is used to monitor recurrence of prostate cancer. PSA as a screening test for cancer is non-specific; it indicates change is occurring in the prostate generally unrelated to cancer. PSA for screening is not recommended for individuals over the age of 70. It is important to note that there are high numbers of false positives and sometimes false negative results.

Normal value: There is no specific normal level for PSA—the 'normal' value for total PSA is age dependent. However, total PSA levels above 10 micrograms/L may indicate a higher probability of prostate cancer. When PSA levels are between 4 and 10 micrograms/L, they will be monitored more closely.

RELATED NURSING CARE No special physical preparation is needed but psychological care is always a consideration, particularly because of the potential implications of a raised PSA result.

NAME OF TEST Prostate ultrasound

PURPOSE AND DESCRIPTION Conducted to identify testicular torsion or masses and to evaluate prostate enlargement. Uses high-frequency sound waves, passed through tissues of various densities, to produce a visual graphic of tissue being examined.

RELATED NURSING CARE A full bladder may be required for the study. Note that if there is urinary frequency, urgency or incontinence, they may be quite anxious about this requirement.

NAME OF TEST Prostate biopsy

- Transrectal biopsy
- Transurethral biopsy
- Transperineal biopsy

PURPOSE AND DESCRIPTION Conducted to diagnose prostate cancer. A transrectal ultrasound (TRUS) is often used to guide the placement of the needle during the procedure.

- A transrectal biopsy is performed with a spring-loaded needle, inserted through the rectal wall and into the prostate gland to remove multiple small tissue samples. This method has a small but significant risk of infection.
- A transurethral biopsy is performed by inserting a cystoscope through the urethra and using a cutting loop to remove small samples of prostate tissue.
- A transperineal biopsy is done under general anaesthetic and is obtained through the skin between the scrotum and anus. An ultrasound probe into the rectum enables visualisation of the prostate. This method allows access to all aspects of the gland, which is not always achieved using the other two methods (Australian Urology Associates, 2016).

RELATED NURSING CARE Prior to the procedure, medications with anticoagulant properties—for example, warfarin, heparin, aspirin, Cartia—should be ceased and antibiotics may be prescribed to commence up to 3 days prior to the procedure for transrectal biopsy. The transrectal and transurethral procedures take 15 to 20 minutes and may be performed either under a local anaesthetic or with sedation. The transperineal biopsy occurs under general anaesthetic and requires preoperative preparation. Advise the person to avoid strenuous activity for 4 hours post procedure and to avoid heavy lifting and sexual activity for the following 24 hours. Explain that there may be some discomfort in the biopsy area for 1 to 2 days, there may be some blood in the urine or from the rectum, and semen may appear dark. Following a transurethral biopsy, a urinary catheter may remain in place for a few hours after the procedure and antibiotics will be prescribed. Excess bleeding, pain or signs of infection should be reported.

NAME OF TEST Gonorrhoea culture

PURPOSE AND DESCRIPTION A culture is performed to evaluate for gonorrhoea. A swab is used to collect a sample of discharge from the infected area (urethra, penis, anus or throat), smeared on a slide and a Gram stain is conducted to identify the organism (*Neisseria gonorrhoeae*). A urine sample is used in some tests.

RELATED NURSING CARE No special physical preparation is needed but psychological care is required. If the test is positive, request the names of all sexual partners and emphasise the need for treatment to eradicate the infection.

(continued)

DIAGNOSTIC TESTS **The male reproductive system (continued)**

NAME OF TEST Venereal disease research laboratory (VDRL); Rapid plasma reagin (RPR); Fluorescent treponemal antibody absorption (FTA-ABS)

PURPOSE AND DESCRIPTION These blood tests are conducted to screen for syphilis. Positive findings can be made within 1 to 2 weeks after the primary lesion appears or 1 to 4 months after the initial infection. The FTA-ABS test is used to detect antibodies to the syphilis-causing bacteria *Treponema pallidum.* It is considered the most accurate and is often used if findings from the VDRL or RPR are questionable, but it remains positive after treatment and so cannot be used to monitor treatment efficacy.

RELATED NURSING CARE No special physical preparation is needed but psychological care is required. If the test is positive, request the names of all sexual partners and emphasise the need for treatment to eradicate the infection.

NAME OF TEST Semen analysis

PURPOSE AND DESCRIPTION Evaluates volume; liquefaction time; sperm count, morphology and motility; pH; white blood cell count and fructose level. Antisperm antibody testing may also be performed.

Normal values:
Volume: > 2.0
pH: ≥ 7.2–7.8
Sperm count (concentration): > 15–25×10^6/mL
Motility: $> 42\%$ motile in a forwards direction
% normal sperm: 30% with normal morphology
WBC: $< 1 \times 10^6$/mL
Sperm antibodies: less than 50% antibodies detected
(World Health Organization, 2021)

RELATED NURSING CARE Ask them to bring in a fresh specimen of semen within 1 hour of ejaculation and following 4–5 days of abstinence.

MALE REPRODUCTIVE SYSTEM ASSESSMENTS

Technique/normal findings	Abnormal findings
Breast and lymph nodes	
Inspect and palpate both breasts, including areola and nipple. *Breast tissue should not be swollen, tender or enlarged (although soft, fatty and enlarged breast tissue does occur with obesity).*	■ A smooth, firm, mobile, tender disc of breast tissue behind the areola indicates gynaecomastia (overdevelopment of breast tissue). Gynaecomastia requires additional investigation to determine the cause but is generally caused by an alteration in the testosterone/oestrogen ratio precipitated by high levels of sex-hormone-binding globulin (SHBG). There are a number of health conditions and also medications that may cause gynaecomastia. ■ A hard, irregular nodule in the nipple area suggests cancer.
Palpate the axillary and supraclavicular lymph nodes. *Lymph nodes should not be palpable.*	■ Enlarged axillary nodes are common with infections of the hand or arm but may be caused by cancer. ■ Enlarged supraclavicular nodes may indicate breast cancer or lymphoma.
External genitalia	
Inspect and palpate the inguinal and femoral area for bulges. Ask the person to cough or strain as you palpate (see Figure 46.2). *There should be no bulging with coughing or straining.*	■ A bulge that increases with coughing or straining suggests a hernia.

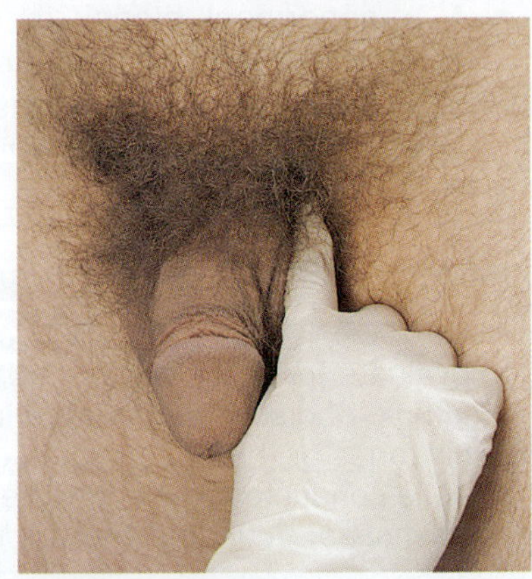

FIGURE 46.2 ***Palpating the male inguinal area for bulges***

Source: Pearson Education.

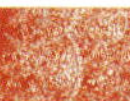

MALE REPRODUCTIVE SYSTEM ASSESSMENTS (continued)

Technique/normal findings	Abnormal findings
Inspect the penis. If the penis is uncircumcised, ask the person to retract the foreskin; help if required. When non-erect, the penis is normally soft, flaccid and non-tender. *The foreskin should be without lesions, the same colour as the penis and should retract easily. The glans is normally free of lesions.*	■ Priapism is the presence of a prolonged, painful erection of the penis that is not related to sexual stimulation. It is a urological emergency as it may lead to necrosis and/or erectile dysfunction if untreated. It may be idiopathic in origin or associated with health conditions such as leukaemia, sickle cell disease, pelvic tumours, spinal cord injury or some medications. ■ Phimosis (tightness of prepuce that prevents retraction of foreskin) may be congenital or due to recurrent balanoposthitis (generalised infection of glans penis and prepuce). ■ Narrow or inflamed foreskin can cause paraphimosis, retraction of the foreskin that causes painful swelling of the glans. ■ Balanitis (inflammation of the glans) is associated with bacterial or fungal infections. ■ Ulcers, vesicles or warts suggest a sexually transmitted infection. ■ Nodules or sores seen on an uncircumcised penis may be cancer.
Inspect the external urinary meatus. Press the glans between the thumb and forefinger (see Figure 46.3). Replace the foreskin if appropriate. *The external urinary meatus is normally in the centre of the glans, without redness or discharge.*	■ Erythema or discharge indicates inflammatory disease or infection. Further assessment is required.
Inspect the skin on the shaft of the penis. *The skin on the shaft of the penis should be free of redness or lesions.*	■ Excoriation or inflammation suggests lice or scabies.
Palpate the shaft of the penis. *The shaft of the penis should not be tender.*	■ Hardening with tenderness along the ventral surface suggests urethritis or urethral stricture with inflammation.
Inspect the scrotum. Further assess any swelling in the scrotum using transillumination: darken the room and place a lit flashlight against the skin of the scrotum. *The normal scrotum and epididymis appear as dark masses with regular borders.*	■ A unilateral or bilateral poorly developed scrotum suggests cryptorchidism (failure of one or both testes to descend into the scrotum). ■ Swelling of the scrotum may indicate indirect inguinal hernia, hydrocoele (accumulation of fluid in the scrotum) or scrotal oedema. Swellings containing serous fluid will transilluminate. Swellings containing blood or tissue will not transilluminate.
Palpate each testis and epididymis. *The testes should not be tender or swollen.*	■ Tender, painful scrotal swelling occurs in acute epididymitis, acute orchitis, torsion of the spermatic cord and strangulated hernia. ■ A painless nodule in the testis is associated with testicular cancer.
Prostate The prostate gland is assessed by digital rectal examination (DRE). (See Figure 20.20 for the technique used to palpate the prostate through the rectal wall.)	
With a gloved index finger, palpate the posterior rectal wall for the rounded, two-lobed structure of the posterior prostate. *The prostate is normally non-tender, with two lateral lobes that are divided, smooth and about 2.5 cm long.*	■ Enlargement (1 cm protrusion into the rectum) with obliteration of the median sulcus suggests benign prostatic hypertrophy. ■ Enlargement with asymmetry and tenderness suggests prostatitis. ■ A hard irregular nodule is suspicious of carcinoma.

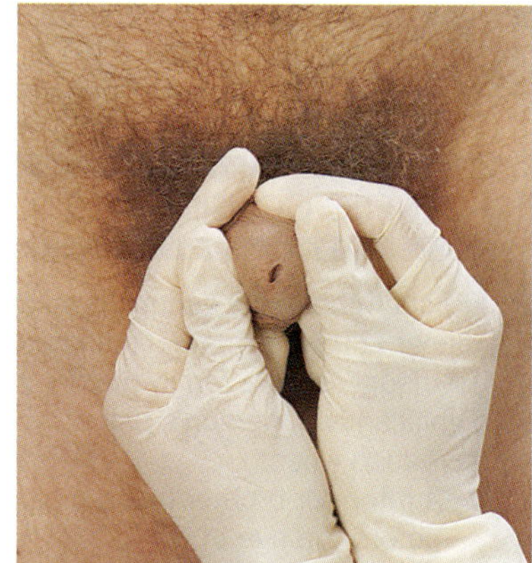

FIGURE 46.3 ***Inspecting the external urinary meatus of the male***

Source: Pearson Education.

Regardless of the type of diagnostic test, and after the person gives informed consent, the nurse is responsible for fully explaining the procedure and any special preparation needed, assessing for any medication use that might affect the outcome of the tests, support during the examination as necessary, documenting the procedures as appropriate and monitoring the results of the tests.

Genetic considerations

When conducting a health assessment interview and a physical assessment, it is important for the nurse to consider genetic influences on the health of an adult. Several diseases of the male reproductive system have a genetic component. During the health assessment interview, it is especially important to ask about a family history of testicular or prostate cancer. During the physical assessment, assess for any signs that might indicate a genetic disorder (see the 'Genetic considerations' box). If data are found to indicate genetic risk factors or alterations, ask about genetic testing and refer for appropriate genetic counselling and evaluation. The chapter 'Genetic implications of adult health nursing' provides further information about genetics in medical–surgical nursing.

GENETIC CONSIDERATIONS Male reproductive system disorders

- Although the exact genetic predisposition for prostate cancer is unknown, the findings of a number of studies have suggested a family history increases a person's risk significantly. A person's risk of prostate cancer is increased when:
  - a father or brother has a diagnosis of prostate cancer before the age of 60
  - there is a family history of prostate, breast or ovarian cancer, especially BRCA1 and BRCA2 gene mutations.
- A family history of testicular cancer is a risk factor for cancer of the testes.
- Two XX chromosomes (instead of XY) often result in altered testicular development because they are missing a gene called the sex-determining region Y gene (SRY), which is responsible for the development of secondary sex characteristics.

Anatomy, physiology and functions of the female reproductive system, including the breasts

The female reproductive system consists of the external genitalia (mons pubis, labia, clitoris, vaginal and urethral openings, and glands) and the internal organs (vagina, cervix, uterus, fallopian tubes and ovaries). This chapter also includes the breasts as part of the reproductive organs. The urethra and urinary meatus are separated from the reproductive organs; however, they are so close to each other that a health problem with one often affects the other. The location and function of the female reproductive organs are summarised in Table 46.3.

The breasts

The breasts (or mammary glands) are located between the third and seventh ribs on the anterior chest wall. They are supported by the pectoral muscles and are richly supplied with nerves, blood and lymph (see Figure 46.4). A pigmented area called the areola is located slightly below the centre of each breast and contains sebaceous glands and a nipple. The nipple is usually protrusive and becomes erect in response to cold and stimulation.

The breasts are made of adipose tissue, fibrous connective tissue and glandular tissue. Cooper's ligaments support the breast and extend from the outer breast tissue to the nipple, dividing the breast into 15 to 25 lobes. Each lobe is made of alveolar glands connected by ducts that open to the nipple.

The external genitalia

The external genitalia collectively are called the vulva. They include the mons pubis, the labia, the clitoris, the vaginal and urethral openings, and glands (see Figure 46.5).

The mons pubis is a pad of adipose (fat) tissue covered with skin. It lies anterior to the symphysis pubis. After puberty, the mons is covered with hair.

The labia are divided into two structures. The *labia majora* are folds of skin and adipose tissue covered with hair following puberty. The labia majora are outermost and begin at the base of the mons pubis and end at the anus. The *labia minora*, located between the clitoris and the base of the vagina, are enclosed by the labia majora. They are made of skin, adipose

TABLE 46.3 Location and function of the female reproductive organs

FEMALE REPRODUCTIVE ORGAN	LOCATION	FUNCTION
Mons pubis (mons veneris)	Anterior and superior to the pubis.	Enhances sexual sensations. Protects and cushions pubic symphysis during intercourse.
Labia majora	Extend from mons pubis to perineum.	Protect labia minora, urethral and vaginal openings. Enhance sexual arousal.
Labia minora	Enclosed by the labia majora.	Protect clitoris. Inferiorly, merge to form posterior ring of vaginal introitus (fourchette). Lubricate vulva. Enhance sexual arousal.
Vestibule	Area enclosed by labia minora.	Contains openings for urethra, vagina, Bartholin's glands and Skene's glands.
Bartholin's (greater vestibular) glands	Posterior on each side of the vaginal orifice. Open onto the sides of the vestibule in the groove between the labia minora and hymen.	Secrete clear, viscid mucus during intercourse.
Skene's (lesser vestibular, paraurethral) glands	Open onto the vestibule on each side of the urethra.	Drain urethral glands. Produce lubricating mucus.
Clitoris	Small bud of erectile tissue just below the superior joining of the labia minora.	Stimulates and elevates levels of sexual arousal.
Perineum	Skin-covered muscular area between vaginal opening and anus.	Provides support for pelvic organs.
Mammary glands	Contained within breasts. Anterior to pectoral muscles of thorax.	Produce human milk. Play a role in sexual arousal.
Ovaries	Lie on each side of the uterus below and behind the uterine tubes.	Produce and secrete ova. Produce the hormones oestrogen and progesterone.
Fallopian tubes (uterine tubes, oviducts)	One tube extends medially from the area of each ovary and empties into the upper portion (fundus) of the uterus.	Transport ova.
Uterus (adnexa of the uterus are composed of the uterine tubes and ovaries)	Anterior to the rectum and posterior/superior to the bladder.	Receives, retains and nourishes the fertilised ovum. Contracts rhythmically to expel infant. Cyclically sheds lining when ovum is not fertilised.
Cervix	Lower portion of uterus extending into the vagina.	Connects uterine cavity with vagina. Opens to allow passage of menstrual flow and infant.
Vagina	Extends from the external orifice in the vestibule to the cervix.	Receives penetration and semen during intercourse. Passageway for menstrual flow and expulsion of infan

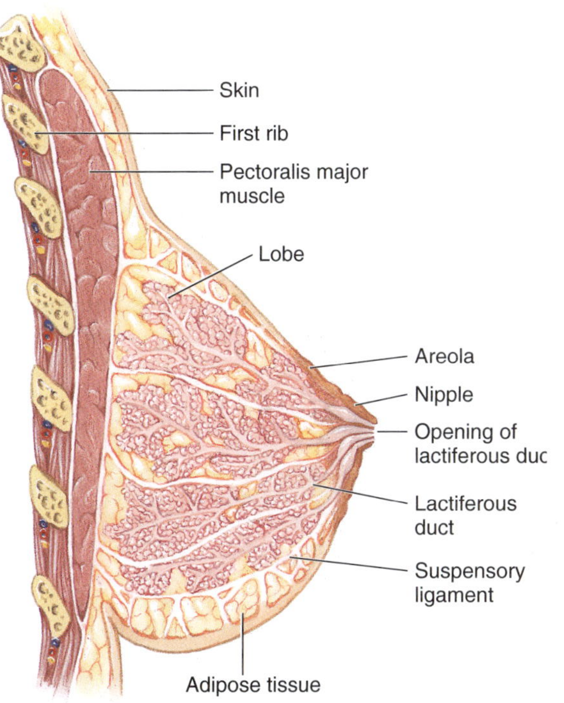

FIGURE 46.4 ***Structure of the female breast***

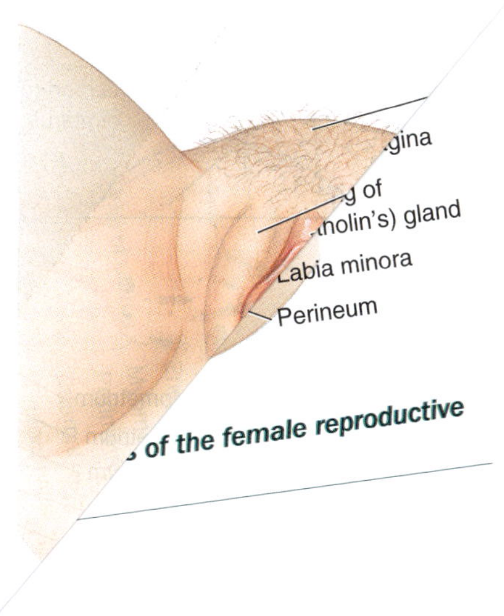

tissue and some erectile tissues. They are usually light pink and hairless.

The area between the labia is called the vestibule and contains the openings for the vagina and the urethra as well as the Bartholin's glands. Skene's glands open on to the vestibule on each side of the urethra. Bartholin's and Skene's glands secrete lubricating fluid during the sexual response cycle prior to menopause.

The clitoris is an erectile organ analogous to the penis in the male. It is formed by the joining of the labia minora. Like the penis, it is highly sensitive and distends during sexual arousal.

The vaginal opening, called the introitus, is the opening between the internal and the external genitals. Prior to rupture from intercourse or trauma, the introitus is surrounded by a connective tissue membrane called the hymen.

The internal organs

The vagina, cervix, uterus, fallopian tubes and ovaries are the internal organs of the female reproductive system (see Figure 46.6). The ovaries are the primary reproductive organs and produce female sex hormones. The vagina, uterus and fallopian tubes serve as accessory ducts for the ovaries and a developing fetus.

fibromuscular tube about 8 to 10 cm in length
to the bladder and urethra, and anterior
walls of the vagina are membranes that
ae. These membranes are composed
atified squamous epithelial cells.
te for the excretion of secretions,
organ of sexual response; and
f an infant.
ually moist and maintain a
H is bacteriostatic and is

maintained by the action of oestrogen and normal vaginal flora. **Oestrogen** stimulates the growth of vaginal mucosal cells so that they thicken and have increased glycogen content. The glycogen is fermented to lactic acid by Döderlein's bacilli (lactobacilli that normally inhabit the vagina), slightly acidifying the vaginal fluid. The upper end of the vagina contains the uterine cervix in an area called the fornix.

The cervix

The cervix is essentially the 'neck of the uterus' and is the lower, narrow part of the uterus, which is cylindrical in shape and protrudes through the upper anterior vaginal wall forming a conduit between the uterus and the vagina. The cervix is a firm structure, protected by mucus that changes consistency and quantity during the menstrual cycle and during pregnancy. The uterine opening of the cervix is called the internal os; the vaginal opening is called the external os. The space between these openings is the endocervical canal. It serves as a route for the discharge of menstrual fluid, the entrance for sperm and delivery of the infant during birth.

The uterus

The uterus is a hollow, pear-shaped muscular organ with thick walls located between the bladder and the rectum. It has three parts: the fundus, the body and the cervix. It is supported in the abdominal cavity by the broad ligaments, the round ligaments, the uterosacral ligaments and the transverse cervical ligaments. The uterus receives the fertilised ovum and provides a site for growth and development of the fetus.

The uterine wall has three layers. The perimetrium is the outer serous layer that merges with the peritoneum. The myometrium is the middle layer and makes up most of the uterine wall. This layer has muscle fibres that run in various directions, allowing contractions during **menstruation** (the periodic shedding of the uterine lining) or childbirth and expansion as the

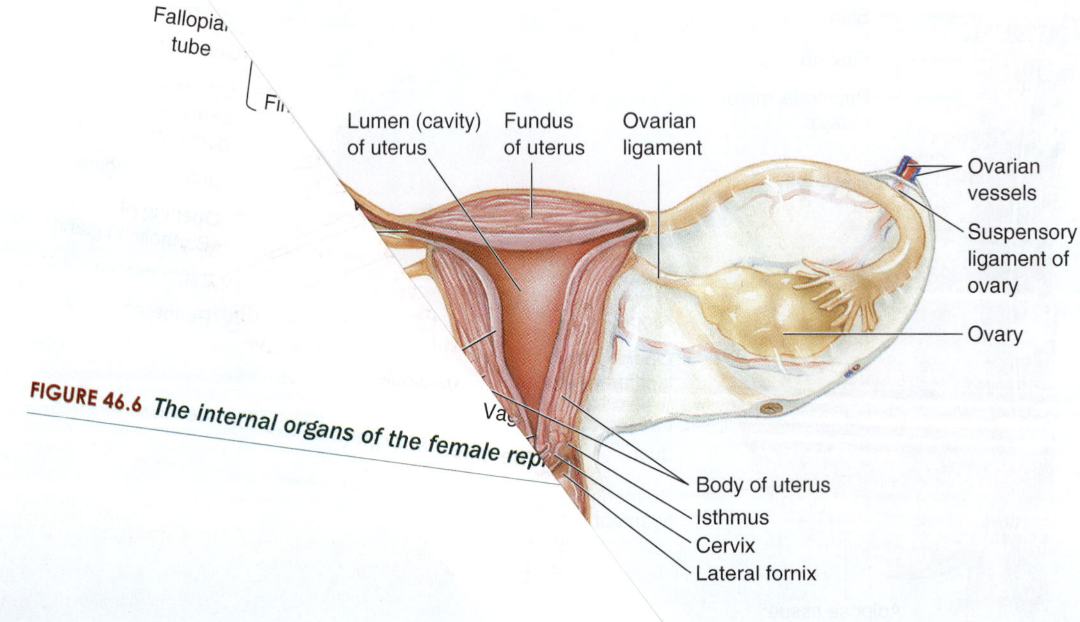

FIGURE 46.6 *The internal organs of the female rep*

fetus grows. The endometrium lines the uterus; its outermost layer is shed during menstruation.

The fallopian tubes

The fallopian tubes are thin cylindrical structures about 10 cm long and 1 cm in diameter. They are attached to the uterus on one end and are supported by the broad ligaments. The lateral ends of the fallopian tubes are open and made of projections called fimbriae that drape over the ovary. The fimbriae pick up the ovum after it is discharged from the ovary.

The fallopian tubes are made of smooth muscle and are lined with ciliated, mucus-producing epithelial cells. The movement of the cilia and contractions of the smooth muscle move the ovum through the tubes towards the uterus. Fertilisation of the ovum by the sperm usually occurs in the outer portion of a fallopian tube.

The ovaries

The ovaries in the adult are flat, almond-shaped structures located on either side of the uterus below the ends of the fallopian tubes. They are homologous to the man's testes. They are attached to the uterus by a ligament and are also attached to the broad ligament. The ovaries store the female germ cells and produce the female hormones oestrogen and progesterone. The formation and development of a female reproductive cell ovum occurs during gestation. The total number of ova is present at birth as oogenesis.

Each ovary contains many small structures called ovarian follicles. Each follicle contains an immature ovum, called an oocyte. Each month, several follicles are stimulated by follicle-stimulating hormone (FSH) and luteinising hormone (LH) to mature. The developing follicles are surrounded by layers of follicle cells, with the mature follicles called graafian follicles. The graafian follicles produce oestrogen, which stimulates the development of endometrium. Each month during menstruation, one or two of the mature follicles eject an oocyte in a process called ovulation. The ruptured follicle then becomes a structure called the corpus luteum. The corpus luteum produces both oestrogen and progesterone to support the endometrium until conception occurs or the cycle begins again. The corpus luteum slowly degenerates, leaving a scar on the surface of the ovary.

Functions of the female sex hormones

The ovaries produce oestrogens, progesterone and androgens in a cyclical pattern. Oestrogens are steroid hormones that occur naturally in three forms: oestrone (E1), oestradiol (E2) and oestriol (E3). Oestradiol is the most potent and is the form secreted in greatest amount by the ovaries. Although oestrogens are secreted throughout the menstrual cycle, they are at a higher level during certain phases of the cycle.

Oestrogens are essential for the development and maintenance of secondary sex characteristics. In conjunction with other hormones, they stimulate the female reproductive organs to prepare for growth of a fetus. Oestrogens are responsible for the normal structure of skin and blood vessels. They also decrease the rate of bone resorption, promote increased high-density lipoproteins, reduce cholesterol levels and enhance the clotting of blood. Oestrogens also promote the retention of sodium and water.

Menopause, a normal physiological process, occurs as a result of the gradual decrease and final cessation of oestrogen production by the ovaries. Menstruation ceases and the tissues that had been supported by oestrogen change. Long-term effects of oestrogen deprivation increase the risk of osteoporosis and cardiovascular disease. Menopause is discussed in the chapter 'Nursing care of women with reproductive system and breast disorders'.

Progesterone primarily affects the development of breast glandular tissue and the endometrium. During pregnancy, progesterone relaxes smooth muscle to decrease uterine contractions. It also increases body temperature.

Androgens are responsible for normal hair growth patterns at puberty and may also have metabolic effects.

Oogenesis and the ovarian cycle

Oogenesis is the process of maturation of oocytes. It begins before birth and is completed after puberty, continuing until menopause. During prenatal oogenesis, the total number of ova develop and are present as primary oocytes in ovarian follicles. Each month from puberty until menopause, the remaining events of oogenesis, known as postnatal oogenesis, occur. Collectively, these events are known as the **ovarian cycle**.

The ovarian cycle has three consecutive phases that occur cyclically, typically every 28 days (although the cycle may vary in length for individuals), as follows:

- The follicular phase lasts from the 1st to the 10th day of the cycle.
- The ovulatory phase lasts from the 11th to the 14th day of the cycle and ends with ovulation.
- The luteal phase lasts from the 14th to the 28th day.

During the follicular phase, the follicle develops and the oocyte matures. These processes are controlled by the interaction of FSH and LH. On day 1 of the cycle, gonadotropin-releasing hormone (GnRH) from the hypothalamus increases and stimulates increased production of FSH and LH by the anterior pituitary. FSH and LH stimulate follicular growth and the oocyte increases in size. The structure, now called the primary follicle, becomes a multicellular mass surrounded by a fibrous capsule, the theca folliculi. As the follicle continues to increase in size, oestrogen is produced and a fluid-filled space (the antrum) forms within the follicle. The oocyte is enclosed by a membrane, the zona pellucida. By about day 10, the follicle is a mature graafian follicle and bulges out from the surface of the ovary. There are always follicles at different stages of development in each ovary, but usually only one follicle becomes dominant and matures to ovulation, while the others degenerate.

The ovulatory phase begins when oestrogen levels reach a level high enough to stimulate the anterior pituitary and a surge of LH is produced. The LH stimulates meiosis in the developing oocyte and its first meiotic division occurs. The LH also stimulates enzymes that act on the bulging ovarian wall, causing it to rupture and discharge the antrum fluid and the oocyte. The oocyte is expelled from the mature ovarian follicle in the process called ovulation.

During the luteal phase, the surge in LH also stimulates the ruptured follicle to change into a corpus luteum and then stimulates the corpus luteum to begin immediately producing progesterone and oestrogen. The increase of progesterone and oestrogen in the blood has a negative feedback effect on the production of LH, inhibiting the further growth and development of other follicles.

If pregnancy does not occur, the corpus luteum begins to degenerate and its hormone production ceases. The declining production of progesterone and oestrogen at the end of the cycle allows the secretion of LH and FSH to increase and a new cycle begins. The ovarian cycle is compared with the menstrual cycle in Figure 46.7.

The menstrual cycle

The endometrium of the uterus responds to changes in oestrogen and progesterone during the ovarian cycle to prepare for implantation of the embryo. The endometrium is receptive to implantation of the embryo for only a brief period each month, coinciding with the time when the embryo would normally reach the uterus from the uterine tube (usually 7 days).

The **menstrual cycle** begins with the *menstrual phase*, lasting from days 1 to 5. The inner endometrial (functionalis) layer detaches and is expelled as menstrual fluid (fluid and blood) for 3 to 5 days. As the maturing follicle begins to produce oestrogen (days 6 to 14), the proliferative phase begins. In response, the functionalis layer is repaired and thickens, while spiral arteries increase in number and tubular glands form. Cervical mucus changes to a thin, crystalline substance, forming channels to help the sperm move up into the uterus.

The final phase, lasting from days 14 to 28, is the secretory phase. As the corpus luteum produces progesterone, the rising levels act on the endometrium, causing increased vascularity, changing the inner layer to secretory mucosa, stimulating the secretion of glycogen into the uterine cavity and causing the cervical mucus again to become thick and block the internal os. If fertilisation does not occur, hormone levels fall. Spasm of the spiral arteries causes hypoxia of the endometrial cells, which begin to degenerate and shed. As with the ovarian cycle, the process begins again with the shedding of the functionalis layer.

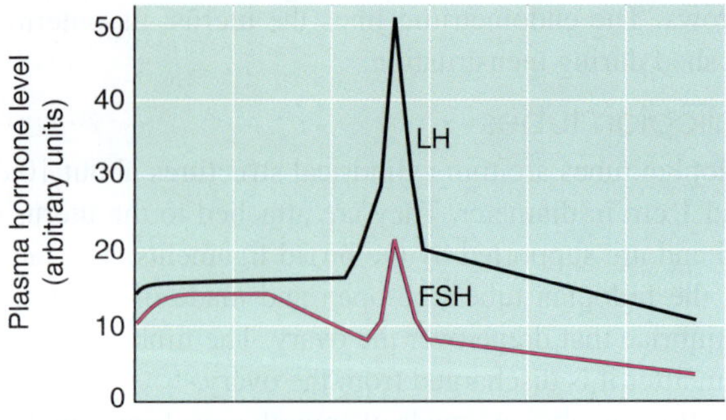

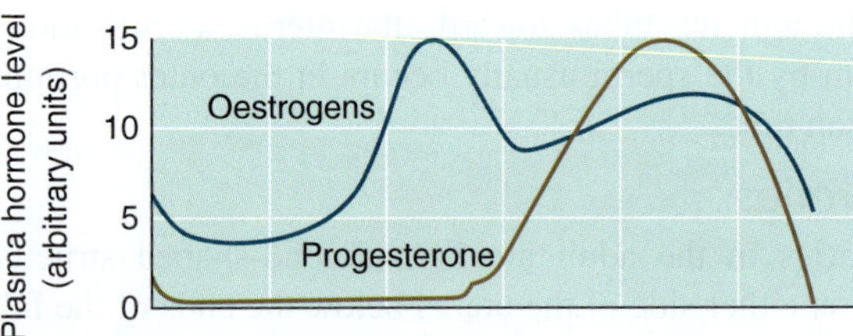

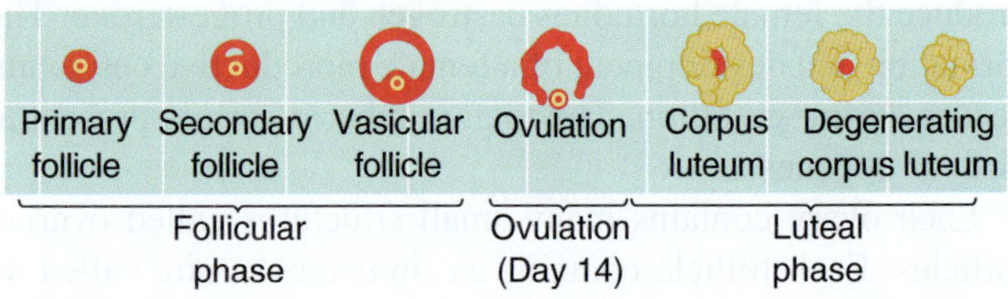

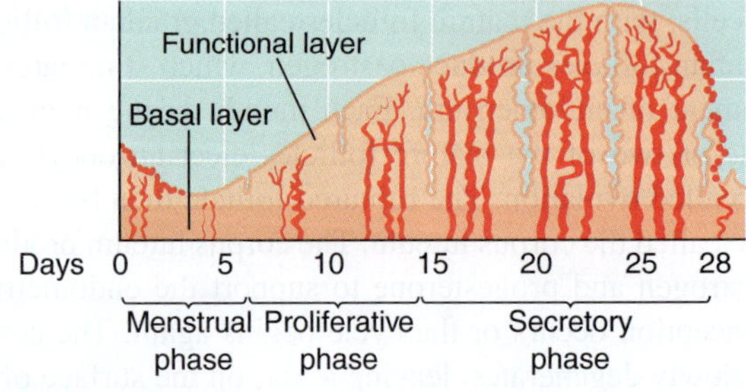

FIGURE 46.7 ***Comparison of the ovarian and menstrual cycles. A, Fluctuating levels of follicle-stimulating hormone (FSH) and luteinising hormone (LH), the pituitary gonadotropins regulating the ovarian cycle. B, Fluctuating levels of ovarian hormones that cause endometrial changes during the menstrual cycle. C, Changes in the ovarian follicles during the 28-day menstrual cycle. D, Corresponding changes in the endometrium during the menstrual cycle***

ASSESSING THE FEMALE REPRODUCTIVE SYSTEM

The structures and functions of the female reproductive system are assessed by findings from a comprehensive person-centred assessment, including both a health assessment interview to collect subjective data and a physical assessment to collect objective data. Diagnostic tests may provide further information.

Information from the health assessment interview is used to individualise the questions that are asked; for example, a person who is postmenopausal would not be asked specific questions about their menstrual cycle, but it would be important to ask about vaginal dryness.

Health assessment interview

A health assessment interview to determine abnormalities or complications with the female reproductive system may be conducted for different reasons, for example:

- during a health screening
- as part of a comprehensive health assessment
- during a focused assessment for a specific health problem (such as severe menstrual cramping).

The nurse needs to be aware of and consider the psychological, gender identification, social and cultural factors that affect sexuality and sexual activity. Use words that can be easily understood. A person may perceive the interview as less threatening if the discussion begins with more general questions and then progresses to specific questions. A safe environment is established when questions are asked in a way that enables the description of changes or concerns. For example, ask about menstrual and childbirth histories before asking questions about sexually transmitted infections.

The focused interview for the female reproductive system is usually extensive. However, the questions may in many instances be tailored to a specific health problem. As with the assessment of other body systems, analyse and document the onset of the problem; the duration, frequency, precipitating and relieving factors; any associated symptoms; treatment; self-care; and outcome. For example, ask:

- Have you noticed vaginal bleeding after intercourse that isn't related to menstruation?
- Does anything relieve the vaginal itching and discharge?
- Have you had any fever or abdominal pain with this vaginal infection?

Ask about menstrual history, obstetric history, use of contraceptives, sexual history, use of medications and reproductive system examinations. Establish when their last menstrual period was. Ask about the use of condoms during intercourse because unprotected sexual intercourse increases the risk of sexually transmitted infections, including hepatitis B and HIV infection. Also ask about smoking because a history of smoking increases the risk of circulatory problems in a person taking oral contraceptives and increases the risk of cancer of the cervix (Allen et al., 2019).

Chronic conditions may affect the function of the female reproductive system. Diabetes increases the risk of vaginal infections and vaginal dryness, both of which interfere with sexual pleasure. Chronic heavy menstrual flow may result in anaemia. Thyroid and adrenal conditions may affect secondary sex characteristics, the menstrual cycle and the ability to become pregnant.

Obtaining any family history of cancer is important. The risk of endometrial cancer is higher in those with a family history of endometrial, breast or colon cancer; the risk of ovarian cancer is higher for those with a family history of ovarian or breast cancer; and the risk of breast cancer is higher in those with a family history of breast cancer. Exposure to DES (diethylstilbestrol, a synthetic form of oestrogen prescribed to prevent miscarriage from the 1940s to the early 1970s) in utero increases the risk of a rare adenocarcinoma cancer of the cervix and vagina (Cancer Australia, 2018). Exposure to asbestos poses a risk of cancer of the ovary (Slomovitz et al., 2021). The risk of breast cancer is also greater if the person has a history of fibrocystic disease.

Carefully explore any history of vaginal bleeding and vaginal discharge. Ask about the onset of vaginal bleeding, any related factors, the colour (pink, red, dark red, brown), the character (thin, watery, presence of mucus, size and number of clots), the amount (spotting, how many pads or tampons in a specific amount of time) and relationship to their menstrual cycle. Ask about the onset of any vaginal discharge; the colour (white, green, grey), character (thin, thick, curd-like), odour, itching and if a rash is present.

Questions about sexual activity may include sexual preference, number of sexual partners, use of condoms, femidoms or other contraceptives, and current level of sexual satisfaction. Ask about any experiences or history of **anorgasmia** (absence of orgasm), **dyspareunia** (painful intercourse) or other problems with intercourse, and any history of sexual trauma.

Interview questions categorised by functional health patterns are listed in the 'Functional health pattern interview' table.

Physical assessment

Physical assessment of the female reproductive system may be performed as part of a comprehensive assessment or separately for a person with identified sexual health problems. If conducted as part of a total physical assessment, this is usually the final system to be assessed. The female reproductive system is assessed by inspection and palpation. The person should empty their bladder before having the examination. Prior to the examination, collect all necessary equipment and explain the procedure fully to decrease anxiety. Put on disposable gloves, in line with the National Safety and Quality Health Service Preventing and Controlling Infections Standard (ACSQHC, 2021), before beginning the examination and wear them throughout the examination. Ask the person to remove clothing and put on a gown. Ensure the examining room is private and warm.

Explain the procedures for the examination thoroughly, sensitively and in a matter-of-fact way to decrease anxiety and embarrassment. If the person is unfamiliar with their reproductive organs, charts may be used to illustrate the parts that will be examined. Carefully explain the procedure for the examination

Links to National Patient Safety Standards

NSQHS: Communicating for Safety Standard

The intent of this standard is to 'ensure timely, purpose-driven and effective communication and documentation that support continuous, coordinated and safe care for patients' (ACSQHC, 2021, p. 54).

Source: ACSQHC (2021). *National Safety and Quality Health Service Standards* (2nd ed.). Sydney: ACSQHC.

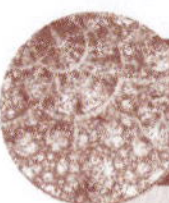

FUNCTIONAL HEALTH PATTERN INTERVIEW The female reproductive system

FUNCTIONAL HEALTH PATTERN	INTERVIEW QUESTIONS AND LEADING STATEMENTS
Health perception–Health management	■ Have you ever had problems or issues with your reproductive organs (ovaries, tubes, uterus, vagina) or with menstruation or menopause? Can you explain them? If so, how was this problem/issue treated?
	■ Do you routinely take any prescribed or herbal medications for symptoms of menopause? If so, what and when do you take it?
	■ Have you ever taken hormone replacement therapy for menopausal symptoms?
	■ Do you practise breast self-examination? When and how often do you do this?
	■ Have you noticed any lumps in your breasts or discharge from your nipples? If so, can you describe the symptoms?
	■ Have you ever had a breast examination or mammogram? When was your last one? How often do you have these?
	■ When was your last gynaecological examination? When was your last cervical screening test? How often do you have these done?
	■ Do you use birth control? If so, what do you use?
	■ What do you do to provide self-care if you have mood swings or menstrual cramps?
	■ Have you ever had a sexually transmitted infection or an infection of the reproductive organs? What was it? How was it treated?
	■ Do you use douches or vaginal sprays? If so, what type and how often?
	■ Do you smoke? If so, how much and for how long have you smoked?
Nutritional–Metabolic	■ Have you noticed a change in your appetite right before your menstrual period?
	■ Have you gained weight recently? If so, why do think this happened?
	■ Describe your usual food intake for a 24-hour period.
Elimination	■ When was your last menstrual period?
	■ At what age did you start/end having menstrual periods?
	■ Describe the length, amount of flow and clotting with your menstrual periods.
	■ Do you ever have bleeding between your menstrual periods? If so, describe the type and amount.
	■ Describe any unusual vaginal discharge you have had (colour, consistency, odour, itching or rash). How long did the discharge occur for?
	■ Have you noticed any changes in urination (frequency, urgency, burning)?
	■ Have you noticed changes in bowel elimination during your menstrual periods?
Activity–Exercise	■ Describe your usual activities in a normal day.
	■ Have you noticed any change in activity or energy levels during your menstrual period?
	■ Have you noticed any change in activity or energy levels since menopause (if applicable)? If so, how?
Sleep–Rest	■ How long do you sleep at night? Is your sleep restful?
	■ Do night sweats wake you?
	■ Do menstrual cramps ever wake you at night?
Cognitive–Perceptual	■ Do you have pain or other symptoms (such as headache, mood swings, irritability, bloating, constipation, diarrhoea and/or breast tenderness) before your menstrual period? Can you describe these and what you do to manage them?
	■ Do you have cramping before or during your menstrual period? Describe the type of cramping, how long it lasts and what you do to be more comfortable.
	■ Do you ever have vaginal itching, pain, burning or dryness? If so, is it affected by sexual intercourse? Does dryness interfere with intercourse?

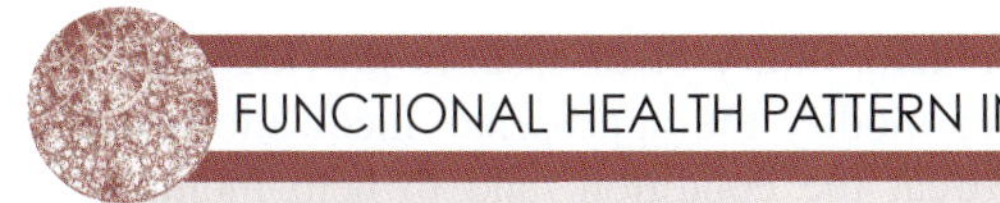

FUNCTIONAL HEALTH PATTERN INTERVIEW The female reproductive system (continued)

FUNCTIONAL HEALTH PATTERN	INTERVIEW QUESTIONS AND LEADING STATEMENTS
Self-Perception–Self-Concept	■ Has this problem affected how you feel about yourself?
	■ Do you believe your needs for intimacy and affection are being met?
Role–Relationships	■ Has having this condition affected your relationship with others?
	■ Has having this condition interfered with your ability to work? In what way?
	■ Has anyone in your family had problems with breast or ovarian cancer? Can you give more information about this?
Sexuality–Reproductive	■ Are you currently in a sexual relationship? If so, has this condition interfered with your usual sexual activity?
	■ How long have you been with your current partner? Have you had any other partners during this time?
	■ What is your sexual preference?
	■ Has having this problem affected your relationship with your spouse or sexual partner?
	■ Have you ever been pregnant? How many times? Have you ever had a miscarriage? Have you ever had a termination of pregnancy?
	■ Do you practise birth control? If so, what do you use?
	■ Do you use a condom every time you have intercourse?
	■ Do you use a vaginal condom?
Coping–Stress–Tolerance	■ Has having this condition created stress for you? If so, does your health problem seem to be more difficult when you are stressed?
	■ Have you experienced any kind of stress that makes the condition worse? Can you provide more details about this?
	■ Describe what you do when you feel stressed.
Value–Belief	■ Describe how specific relationships or activities help you to cope with this problem.
	■ Describe specific cultural beliefs or practices that affect how you care for and feel about this problem.
	■ Are there any specific treatments that you would not use to treat this problem?

and show the speculum. The assessment may be done with the person in the sitting or supine position to examine the breasts and in the lithotomy position to assess the external genitalia and internal organs. Expose only those body parts being examined to preserve modesty. Normal age-related findings are summarised in Table 46.4.

TABLE 46.4 Age-related changes in the female reproductive system

AGE-RELATED CHANGE	SIGNIFICANCE
Breasts	
• Atrophy, with sagging of breast tissue. • Linear strands may appear from shrinkage and fibrotic changes.	Although ageing does not cause breast cancer, the incidence rises with age; age-related changes may make finding tumours more difficult.
Genitalia	
• Labia flatten and vulvar adipose tissue and hair decreases. • Collagen and adipose tissues in the vaginal canal decrease, resulting in loss of rugae, shortening and narrowing of vaginal canal. • Vaginal lubrication decreases, epithelium becomes thinner and avascular. • More alkaline pH of vagina. • Cervix becomes smaller.	Vagina is more easily irritated, increasing the risk of vaginal infections. Greater risk of yeast infections. Lubricants may be used during intercourse.
Internal organs	
• Uterus shrinks. • Fallopian tubes shrink and shorten. • Ovaries are smaller and thicker. • With menopause, hormone production of oestrogen decreases. • Loss of oestrogen may cause pelvic floor muscles to weaken. • Loss of oestrogen causes changes throughout the body, including loss of skin tone and growth of facial hair.	With the completion of menopause, the menstrual cycle ends. Weakening of the pelvic floor muscles may contribute to incontinence with increased intra-abdominal pressure (as with coughing and sneezing). Skin becomes more dry and thinner.

The examination usually begins with examination of the breasts, with the person in the sitting and supine positions. Assist the person to move to the lithotomy position on the examining table, ensuring they are lying on their back with hips and knees flexed and the thighs apart. This position may induce feelings of vulnerability and anxiety related to past experiences. Some people may not be able to tolerate this position. In this case, the examination could occur in the supine position. Although the entire examination is described here, the internal examination is conducted only by a nurse who is accredited to perform the procedure. However, nurses are often asked to assist with the examination and should be able to explain the examination, answer questions about the procedure and provide emotional support.

Diagnostic tests

The results of diagnostic tests of the structures and functions of the female reproductive system are used to monitor the health of female reproductive structures; to support the diagnosis of a specific sexual problem, injury or disease; to provide information to identify or modify the appropriate medications or treatments used to treat the condition; and to help monitor the responses to treatment and nursing care interventions. Diagnostic tests to assess the female reproductive system are described in the 'Diagnostic tests' table and summarised in the following bulleted list. More information is included in the discussion of specific health problems or diseases in the chapter 'Nursing care of women with reproductive system and breast disorders'.

- Blood tests are used to diagnose a variety of hormone changes and sexually transmitted infections. These tests are discussed in the chapters 'Nursing care of women with reproductive system and breast disorders' and 'Nursing care of people who have sexually transmitted infections'.
- Sexually transmitted infections are often diagnosed with cultures and smears of a discharge or mucous membranes.

DIAGNOSTIC TESTS The female reproductive system

SCREENING TESTS, SMEARS AND CULTURES

NAME OF TEST Cervical screening test

PURPOSE AND DESCRIPTION The cervical screening test detects infection with human papillomavirus (HPV) and can detect multiple types of the virus. This screening test replaced the Papanicolaou smear (Pap test) in 2017. HPV is a common virus causing most cervical cancers. Screening should begin at the age of 25 and be repeated every 5 years until an 'exit test' between 70 and 74 years of age. Testing is also indicated if symptoms of cervical cancer are experienced, despite regular testing. Testing can be offered by means of self-collection (the person takes their own sample using a vaginal swab) or by the healthcare provider. Both are accurate and safe.

Self-collection: a self-collected sample is from the vagina (not the cervix). It can only be tested for HPV and not for cytology (cervical cell abnormalities). If a sample is positive for HPV, further testing is required by speculum examination or colposcopy.

Collection by a healthcare provider: a sample of cells is collected from the cervix using a speculum and cotton swab or brush.

RELATED NURSING CARE Nurses need to discuss the options for cervical screening (self-collection or by a healthcare provider) and what option is best for the person's situation. Explain that the best time to have the test is in the middle of the menstrual cycle (a few days after menstruation and a week before it is due again). Provide reassurance and explain the procedure, what to expect and how and when results are provided. Follow the National Cervical Screening Program Guidelines.

NAME OF TEST Chlamydia culture

PURPOSE AND DESCRIPTION Performed to screen for or diagnose chlamydial infections. A swab of cells from the infected area is taken and either smeared on a slide and analysed or cultured. Although usually taken from the urethra, vagina or cervix, cultures may also be taken from the throat and rectum.

RELATED NURSING CARE Assess for pregnancy or enlargement of inguinal lymph nodes. Withhold antibiotics (if prescribed) until after obtaining the specimen. Instruct not to douche before the examination. If the test is positive, request the names of all sexual partners and emphasise need for treatment to eradicate the infection. Provide emotional support.

NAME OF TEST Gonorrhoea culture

PURPOSE AND DESCRIPTION A culture is performed to evaluate for gonorrhoea. A swab is used to collect a sample of discharge from the infected area (cervix, urethra, anus or throat), smeared on a slide and a Gram stain is conducted to identify the organism (*N. gonorrhoeae*). A urine sample is used in some tests.

RELATED NURSING CARE No special physical preparation is needed but psychological care is required. Instruct not to douche before the examination. If the test is positive, request the names of all sexual partners and emphasise the need for treatment to eradicate the infection. Provide emotional support.

DIAGNOSTIC TESTS The female reproductive system (continued)

NAME OF TEST Trichomonas, bacteria, candidae (yeast)

PURPOSE AND DESCRIPTION A culture is performed to identify vaginal organisms or blood cells. A specimen of vaginal discharge is obtained with a swab, placed in solution and examined under the microscope immediately after it is collected (referred to as a wet mount).

RELATED NURSING CARE Request not to douche before the examination.

NAME OF TEST Venereal disease research laboratory (VDRL); Rapid plasma reagin (RPR); Fluorescent treponemal antibody absorption (FTA-ABS)

PURPOSE AND DESCRIPTION These blood tests are conducted to screen for syphilis. Positive findings can be made within 1 to 2 weeks after primary lesion appears or 1 to 4 months after the initial infection. The FTA-ABS test is used to detect antibodies to the syphilis-causing bacteria *Treponema pallidum.* It is considered the most accurate and is often used if findings from the VDRL or RPR are questionable, but it remains positive after treatment and so cannot be used to monitor treatment efficacy.

RELATED NURSING CARE No special physical preparation is needed but psychological care and support is required. If the test is positive, request the names of all sexual partners and emphasise the need for treatment to eradicate the infection.

NAME OF TEST Syphilis (dark-field examination)

PURPOSE AND DESCRIPTION A specimen is obtained from a lesion believed to be caused by syphilis (*T. pallidum*) and examined under the microscope.

RELATED NURSING CARE No special physical preparation is needed but psychological care is required. If the test is positive, request the names of all sexual partners and emphasise the need for treatment to eradicate the infection.

BREAST EXAMINATIONS

NAME OF TEST Mammogram

PURPOSE AND DESCRIPTION Used to detect tumours in the breast. Breasts are flattened in the mammography machine and low-dose x-rays are taken.

RELATED NURSING CARE Explain not to apply body powder or underarm deodorant prior to the test.

NAME OF TEST Breast ultrasound

PURPOSE AND DESCRIPTION This examination uses high-frequency sound waves passing through tissues to detect masses in the breast. May be performed if lesions are identified in a mammogram.

RELATED NURSING CARE No special physical preparation is needed but psychological care is required.

NAME OF TEST Breast biopsy

- Fine-needle aspiration (also known as fine-needle aspiration biopsy, FNA or FNAB)
- Core biopsy (also referred to as core-needle biopsy or CNB)
- Vacuum-assisted core biopsy (VACB or mammotome)
- Large-core surgical biopsy
- Open surgical biopsy

PURPOSE AND DESCRIPTION

- A fine-needle aspiration is simple and quick, taking a few minutes to perform. It is conducted to withdraw fluid from cysts and may be used to sample cells from masses in the breast. A 22- to 25-gauge needle is used to collect 5 to 6 samples of fluid or cells.
- A core biopsy is conducted to obtain a sample of tissue from a solid mass or calcium deposits in the breast. A specialised biopsy needle is used to collect 5 to 6 tissue samples for examination by a pathologist. The test is always done under local anaesthetic.
- A vacuum-assisted core biopsy is primarily used to evaluate calcifications. A specialised biopsy needle with suction is inserted through a small (6 mm) incision and 8 to 10 samples are removed.
- A large-core surgical biopsy is performed to evaluate breast masses or calcification identified with a mammogram, but that are non-palpable. An incision is made and a 5 to 20 mm cylinder of breast tissue (about the size of a wine cork) is removed.
- An open surgical biopsy is performed to evaluate breast masses, hard-to-reach lesions, multiple lesions and masses with calcifications. A 3.8 to 5 cm incision is made and a golf ball size (or larger) area of tissue is removed.

RELATED NURSING CARE For all types of tests, wearing a well-fitted, comfortable bra (preferably with no underwire), applying ice packs and mild analgesics decrease discomfort post procedure.

(continued)

DIAGNOSTIC TESTS **The female reproductive system (continued)**

- Explain that, depending on the medical officer, some procedures may be performed with or without a local anaesthetic.
- Explain that for a core biopsy or a vacuum-assisted core biopsy, a local anaesthetic is used, but no stitches are required.
- Explain that for a large-core biopsy, a local anaesthetic will be administered and stitches will be used to close the incision.
- Explain that for an open surgical biopsy, a general anaesthetic is usually used and the incision will require stitches and leave a scar.

TESTS OF THE INTERNAL REPRODUCTIVE SYSTEM

NAME OF TEST Ultrasound (abdominal, vaginal)

PURPOSE AND DESCRIPTION Used to detect the presence of space-occupying lesions, such as fibroid tumours, cysts, abscesses and neoplasms. The abdomen is coated with transducing gel and a graphical visualisation is made. For a vaginal ultrasound, a transducer is covered with a condom or vinyl glove coated with transducer gel and then introduced into the vagina.

RELATED NURSING CARE Explain the need to increase fluid intake and ask not to void until the test is completed to ensure a full bladder for the abdominal ultrasound. A full bladder lifts the pelvic organs higher in the abdomen and improves visualisation. An empty bladder is required for the vaginal ultrasound.

NAME OF TEST Hysterosalpingogram

PURPOSE AND DESCRIPTION Used to diagnose causes of infertility and abnormalities of the uterus or fallopian tubes. A contrast medium is instilled through the cervix and its passage through the uterus and the fallopian tubes is monitored using serial x-rays.

RELATED NURSING CARE Assess for allergy to seafood (iodine) or previous contrast media. Explain that the procedure is briefly painful.

NAME OF TEST Colposcopy

PURPOSE AND DESCRIPTION Conducted to further study abnormal cervical screening tests and as screening for those exposed to intrauterine DES. A binocular microscope is used to directly visualise the cervix.

RELATED NURSING CARE No special physical preparation is needed but psychological care is required.

NAME OF TEST Conisation, Loop electrosurgical excision of transformation zone (LEETZ), Loop electrosurgical excision procedure (LEEP)

PURPOSE AND DESCRIPTION A conisation, LEETZ or LEEP is performed to remove cervical tissue for evaluation (most often for cervical cancer). A cone-shaped area of tissue surrounding the cervical os is removed.

RELATED NURSING CARE Explain that the procedure requires general anaesthesia; however, local anaesthesia may also be used for the procedure. Postoperative self-care includes rest for 2 to 3 days. Explain that minor vaginal bleeding and discharge are expected for several days after the procedures; perineal pads (not tampons) should be used. Sexual intercourse should be avoided until discharge stops. Notify the health practitioner if increased bleeding or signs of infection (pain, offensive discharge, fever) occur.

NAME OF TEST Endometrial biopsy

PURPOSE AND DESCRIPTION This is performed to identify endometrial hyperplasia or endometrial cancer. The cervix is cleaned and tissue is obtained transcervically from the endometrium, either by curettage or vacuum aspiration.

RELATED NURSING CARE Explain that the procedure is briefly painful and causes vaginal bleeding. Advise to use perineal pads and avoid tampons and sexual intercourse while bleeding continues.

DIAGNOSTIC TESTS **The female reproductive system (continued)**

NAME OF TEST Cervical biopsy

PURPOSE AND DESCRIPTION Performed when cervical screening test results indicate possible cervical cancer or cervical intraepithelial neoplasia (CIN), and for screening of those at high risk of vaginal and cervical cancers from intrauterine exposure to DES. Cervix is cleaned and a sample of tissue is taken for analysis.

RELATED NURSING CARE Explain that minor vaginal bleeding and discharge are expected for several days after the procedures; perineal pads (not tampons) should be used. Sexual intercourse should be avoided until discharge stops. The person should monitor and notify the healthcare provider if increased bleeding or signs of infection (pain, offensive discharge, fever) occur. Provide emotional support.

NAME OF TEST Laparoscopy

PURPOSE AND DESCRIPTION This examination is conducted to visualise the organs in the peritoneal cavity (uterus, fallopian tubes, ovaries); to withdraw fluid for analysis; and to perform a tubal ligation. A fibre-optic scope is inserted through small abdominal incisions and carbon dioxide is inserted into the peritoneal cavity for better visualisation.

RELATED NURSING CARE Ask the person to void prior to the examination and explain that a general anaesthetic will be used. Explain that shoulder pain is common after the procedure (referred pain from the retained carbon dioxide gas); that some vaginal bleeding may occur and a perineal pad should be used; and to report excess bleeding, pain or signs of infection to the healthcare provider.

- A mammogram is used to detect breast tumours, often followed by an ultrasound and breast biopsy for a definitive diagnosis. The type of biopsy conducted depends on many factors, including the size, location, appearance and characteristics of the breast abnormality.
- The cervical screening test detects infection with human papillomavirus (HPV) and can detect multiple types of the virus.
- Space-occupying lesions and abnormalities of the vagina, cervix or uterus may be evaluated with ultrasound, a hysterosalpingogram, a colposcopy, a cervical biopsy, a laparoscopy and/or an endometrial biopsy.

Regardless of the type of diagnostic test, the nurse is responsible for explaining the procedure and any special preparation needed, assessing for any medication use that might impact on findings of the tests, providing support during the examination, documenting the procedures as appropriate and following up with regard to the results of the tests.

Genetic considerations

When conducting a health assessment interview and a person-centred physical assessment, it is important for the nurse to consider genetic influences on the health of an individual. Several conditions affecting the female reproductive system have a genetic component. During the health assessment interview, it is especially important to ask about a family history of ovarian or breast cancer. During the physical assessment, assess for any signs that might indicate a genetic disorder (see the 'Genetic considerations' box). If findings indicate genetic risk factors or conditions, discuss genetic testing and refer for appropriate genetic counselling and evaluation. The chapter 'Genetic implications of adult health nursing' provides further information about genetics in medical–surgical nursing.

GENETIC CONSIDERATIONS **Female reproductive system disorders**

- There is a clear genetic link in some types of breast and ovarian cancers. Two breast-cancer-susceptibility genes have been identified: BRCA1 and BRCA2. If any of these genes are present, there is an increased risk of having breast or ovarian cancer (Davies et al., 2017; Kuchenbaecker et al., 2017).
- A family history of endometrial, colon or breast cancer increases the risk of endometrial cancer.
- Turner's syndrome is a disorder caused by complete or partial absence of one of the two X chromosomes. The disorder is characterised by short stature and the lack of sexual development at puberty. Other physical effects include a webbed neck, heart defects and kidney abnormalities.

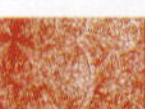

FEMALE REPRODUCTIVE SYSTEM ASSESSMENTS

Technique/normal findings	Abnormal findings
Breasts	
Inspect both breasts simultaneously with the person seated in the following positions: arms at sides, arms overhead, hands pressed on hips, leaning forwards. Inspect breast size, symmetry, contour, skin colour, texture, venous patterns and lesions. Lift the breasts and inspect the lower and lateral aspects. *Breasts normally vary in size and shape and one breast may be larger than the other. Colour should be consistent with the skin tone and texture smooth. There should be no redness, swelling, prominent veins or lesions.*	▪ Retractions, dimpling and abnormal contours suggest benign lesions, but may also suggest malignancy. ▪ Thickened, dimpled skin with enlarged pores (called peau d'orange, orange peel or pig skin) and unilateral venous patterns are also associated with malignancy. ▪ Redness may be seen with infection or cancer
Inspect the areolae and nipples. *The colour of the areolae should be consistent with bodily skin colour (ranging from dark pink to dark brown) and Montgomery tubercles may be present. The nipples should be equal bilaterally in size, centrally located in each breast and free of lesions or discharge. Nipples are usually everted but can be inverted or flat.*	▪ Peau d'orange may be noted first in the areola. ▪ Recent unilateral inversion of the nipple or asymmetry in the directions in which the nipples point may suggest cancer.
Palpate both breasts, axillae and supraclavicular areas. Figure 46.8 illustrates a possible pattern for breast palpation. Various palpation patterns may be used if every part of each breast is palpated, including the axillary tail (also called tail of Spence), which is the breast tissue that extends from the upper outer quadrant towards and into the axillae.	▪ Tenderness may be related to premenstrual fullness, fibrocystic disease or inflammation. Tenderness may also indicate cancer. ▪ Nodules in the tail of the breast may be enlarged lymph nodes. ▪ Hard, irregular, fixed unilateral masses that are poorly delineated suggest cancer. ▪ Bilateral, single or multiple, round, mobile, well-delineated masses are consistent with fibrocystic breast disease or fibroadenoma. ▪ Swelling, tenderness, erythema and heat may be seen with mastitis.
Ask the person to assume a supine position with a small pillow under the shoulder and the arm over the head, and repeat the systematic palpation sequence. Describe identified masses by location, size, shape, consistency, tenderness, mobility and delineation of borders. *Breasts should feel smooth, firm and elastic, without palpable masses. Prior to the menstrual cycle, there may be increased nodularity and tenderness.*	
Palpate the nipple, then compress it between the thumb and index finger. Note the colour of any discharge. *Nipples should be firm and elastic, normally without discharge (although some people normally have a discharge).*	▪ Loss of nipple elasticity is seen in cancer. ▪ Bloody or serous discharge is associated with intraductal papilloma. ▪ Milky discharge not due to prior pregnancy and found on both sides suggests galactorrhoea (lactation not associated with pregnancy or breastfeeding), which is sometimes associated with a pituitary tumour. ▪ Unilateral discharge from one or two ducts can be seen in fibrocystic breast disease, intraductal papilloma or carcinoma.

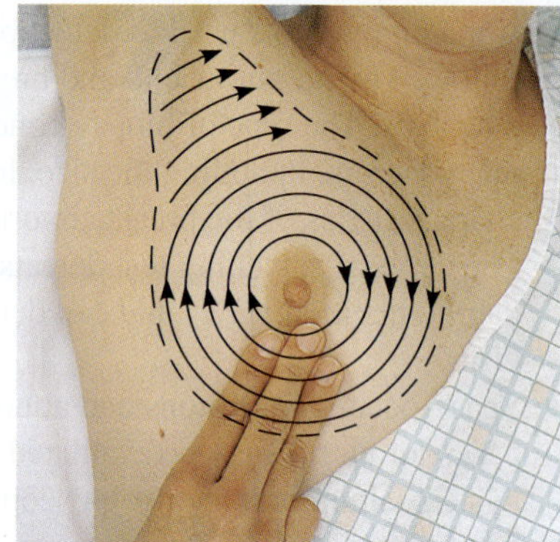

FIGURE 46.8 ***Possible pattern for palpation of the breast***

Source: Pearson Education.

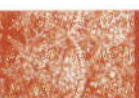

FEMALE REPRODUCTIVE SYSTEM ASSESSMENTS (continued)

Technique/normal findings	Abnormal findings
Axillae	
Inspect the skin of the axillae. *There should be no redness, irritation, lesions or enlarged lymph nodes on palpation.*	■ Rash may be due to allergy or other causes. ■ Signs of inflammation and infection may be due to infection of the sweat glands. ■ Palpate all sections of both axillae for palpable nodes (see Figure 46.9). ■ Enlarged axillary nodes are most often due to infection of the hand or arm but can be caused by malignancy. ■ Enlarged supraclavicular nodes are associated with lymphatic metastases from abdominal or thoracic cancer.
External genitalia	
Help the person to the lithotomy position with the knees flexed and separated.	
Inspect and palpate the labia majora. *The labia majora should be equal in size and free of lesions or bulging.*	■ Excoriation, rashes or lesions suggest inflammatory or infective processes. ■ Bulging of the labia that increases with straining suggests a hernia. ■ Varicosities may be present on the labia.
Inspect the labia minora. Separate the labia majora for better visualisation. *The labia minora should be symmetrical, dark pink and moist, without redness or lesions.*	■ Inflammation, irritation, excoriation or caking of discharge in tissue folds suggests vaginal infection or poor hygiene. ■ Ulcers or vesicles may be symptoms of sexually transmitted infection.
Palpate the inside of the labia minora between thumb and forefinger. *There should be no nodules, ulcers or lesions.*	■ Small, firm, round cystic nodules in labia suggest sebaceous cysts. ■ Wart-like lesions suggest condylomata acuminata (genital warts). ■ Firm, painless ulcers suggest chancre of primary syphilis. ■ Shallow, painful ulcers suggest herpes infection. ■ Ulcerated or red raised lesions suggest vulvar cancer.
Inspect the clitoris. *The clitoris is normally not enlarged.*	■ Enlargement may be a symptom of a masculinising condition.
Inspect the vaginal opening. *There should be no swelling, discolouration, lacerations, discharge or lesions visible in the vaginal opening.*	■ Swelling, discolouration or lacerations may be caused by trauma. ■ Discharge or lesions may be symptoms of infection. ■ Fissures or fistulas may be related to injury, infection, spreading of a malignancy or trauma.
Palpate Skene's glands. Using the index finger, 'milk' Skene's glands on both sides and over the urethra and inspect for possible discharge (see Figure 46.10). *There should be no discharge or tenderness present.*	■ Discharge from Skene's glands and/or tenderness suggests infection.

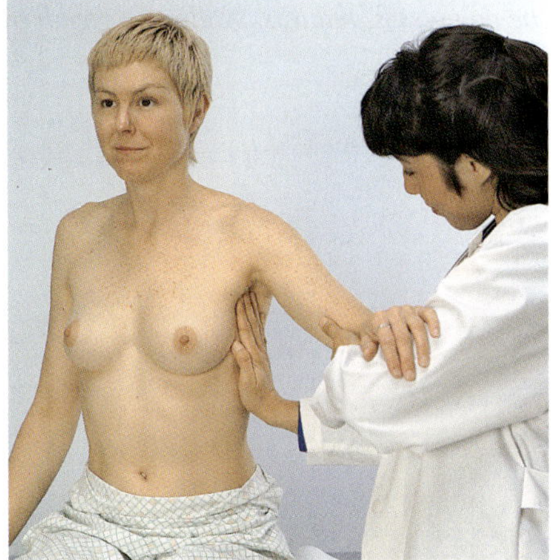

FIGURE 46.9 *Palpating the axillary lymph nodes*

Source: Pearson Education.

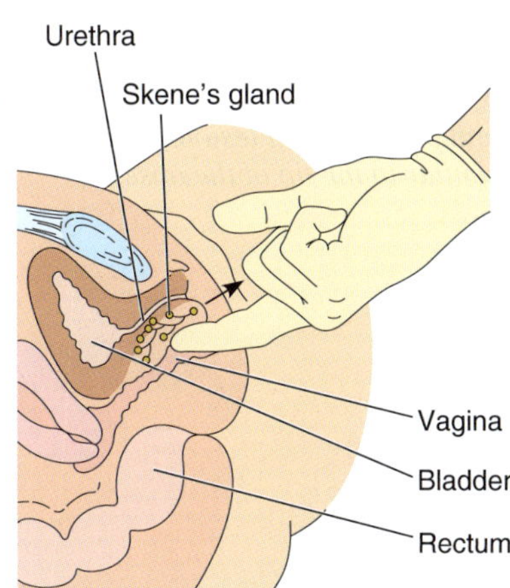

FIGURE 46.10 *Palpating Skene's glands*

(continued)

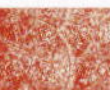

FEMALE REPRODUCTIVE SYSTEM ASSESSMENTS (continued)

Technique/normal findings	Abnormal findings
Palpate Bartholin's glands at the posterior labia majora (see Figure 46.11). *There should be no masses, redness, swelling or tenderness on palpation.*	■ A non-tender mass in the posterolateral portion of the labia majora is indicative of a Bartholin's cyst. ■ Swelling, redness or tenderness, especially if unilateral, may indicate abscess of Bartholin's glands.
Inspect the vaginal orifice for bulging and urinary incontinence. Ask the person to cough or strain. *No bulging should be visible with straining.*	■ Bulging of the anterior vaginal wall and urinary incontinence suggest a cystocele. ■ Bulging of the posterior wall suggests a rectocele. ■ Protrusion of the cervix or uterus into the vagina indicates uterine prolapse.
Inspect and palpate the perineum. The perineum should be free of redness or lesions. *Episiotomy scars are a normal finding.*	■ Inflammation, lesions and growths may be seen in infections or cancer. ■ Fistulas may be the result of injury, trauma, infection or spreading of a malignancy.
Vagina and cervix	
Use a vaginal speculum to inspect the vaginal walls and cervix. See the guidelines in Box 46.1. *The vaginal opening varies, depending on age, experience of sexual penetration and length of the vagina. Vaginal mucosa is normally pink and moist, without discharge or odour. There should be no bulging or loss of urine. The cervix is normally smooth and pink, without lesions, and has a consistency similar to the tip of the nose.*	■ Bluish colour of the cervix and vaginal mucosa may be a sign of pregnancy. ■ A pale cervix is associated with anaemia. ■ A cervix to the right or left of the midline may indicate a pelvic mass, uterine adhesions or pregnancy. ■ Projection of the cervix more than 3 cm into the vaginal canal may indicate a pelvic or uterine mass. ■ Transverse or star-shaped cervical lacerations reflect trauma causing tearing of the cervix. ■ An enlarged cervix is associated with infection. ■ Nabothian cysts (small, white or yellow raised, round areas on the cervix) are considered normal but may become infected. ■ Cervical polyps may be cervical or endometrial in origin.

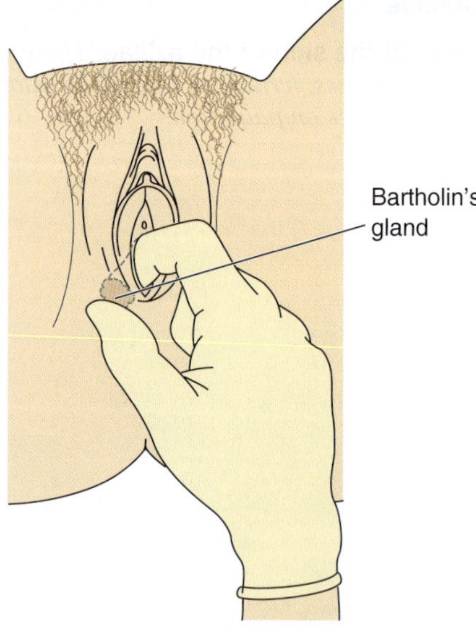

FIGURE 46.11 ***Palpating Bartholin's glands***

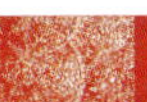

FEMALE REPRODUCTIVE SYSTEM ASSESSMENTS (continued)

Technique/normal findings	Abnormal findings
Palpate the cervix, uterus and ovaries. See the guidelines in Box 46.2. *The cervix can be moved slightly without discomfort. The uterus is normally at the level of the pubis, moves freely and is non-tender. The ovaries (about the size of a walnut) are firm, smooth, mobile and slightly tender on palpation. The ovaries are not usually palpable 3 to 5 years after menopause. A small amount of clear drainage is normal.*	▪ The uterus may be retroverted (tilted backwards) or retroflexed (angled backwards). ▪ Pain on movement of the cervix during manual examination suggests pelvic inflammatory disease (PID). ▪ Softening of the uterine isthmus (Hegar's sign), softening of the cervix (Goodell's sign) and uterine enlargement may be objective signs of pregnancy. ▪ Firm, irregular nodules that vary greatly with size and are continuous with the uterine surface are likely to be myomas (fibroids). ▪ Unilateral or bilateral smooth, compressible adnexal masses are found in ovarian tumours. ▪ Profuse menstrual bleeding is seen with endometrial polyps, dysfunctional uterine bleeding (DUB) and use of an intrauterine device. ▪ Irregular bleeding may be associated with endometrial polyps, DUB, uterine or cervical carcinoma, or oral contraceptives. ▪ Postmenopausal bleeding is seen with endometrial hyperplasia, oestrogen therapy and endometrial cancer.

BOX 46.1 Guidelines for intravaginal assessment and use of the vaginal speculum

The choice of speculum used for an internal examination of the female reproductive system depends on age, experience of sexual penetration and the length of the vagina. There are many types of specula available for use including include Bivalves, paediatric, Huffman, Pederson and Graves. A two-bladed, bivalved speculum is the most commonly used for examinations of adults. It is available in various lengths and widths. The Pederson speculum, which is narrower, may be used to examine adolescents or adults who have not experienced vaginal penetration, have never had a baby or have vaginal atrophy. The speculum should be warm. If cultures or smears are to be obtained, neither water nor gel should be used to warm or to lubricate the speculum.

If cultures or cytological studies are to be taken, the person should avoid sexual activity that includes penetration to the vagina, douching or use of vaginal medications before the examination. Finally, the examination is usually deferred during menstruation or vaginal infection.

The general procedure is as follows:

1. Explain the procedure in full and allow time for a conversation and questions regarding the examination. Ask the person to get undressed from the waist down (ensure privacy) and cover with a sheet or privacy garment.
2. Ask the person to lie on their back with their feet together as close to their buttocks as possible, legs bent and knees falling to the sides.
3. Perform hand hygiene, don gloves and reassure of infection control procedures in place.
4. Perform visual inspection of external genitalia (assessing skin for lesions, warts or erythema, noticing any discharge—including colour and consistency—and observe for any swelling or bleeding of the vulva). Ask the person to cough or strain to observe for any incontinence or prolapse. Discuss any findings and note any changes from pre-existing examinations.
5. Reiterate to the person you are about to undertake an invasive procedure and about to insert the speculum. Lubricate the speculum (if cultures or smears are to be obtained, neither water nor gel should be used to warm or to lubricate the speculum).
6. Use your non-dominant hand to part the labia and your dominant hand to insert the speculum with the blades vertical. During the insertion, rotate the speculum to a horizontal position (see the accompanying figure).
7. Continue to insert the speculum until it reaches the end of the vagina. Open the blades according to manufacturer's instructions. If the cervix is not in full view, try closing the blades, withdrawing the speculum about halfway and inserting it again at a more downward angle. Alternatively,

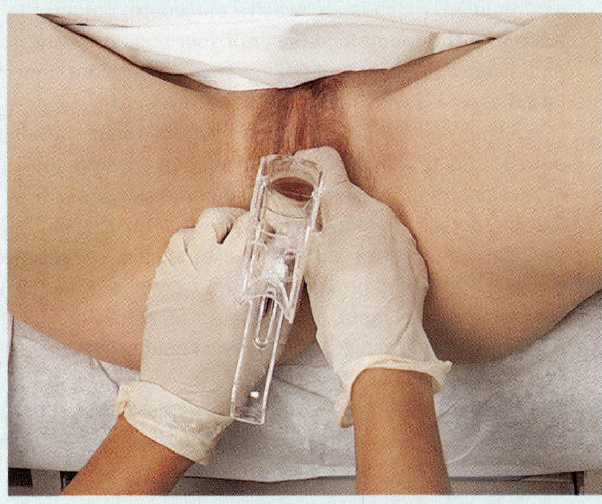

Inserting the vaginal speculum

Source: Pearson Education.

(continued)

BOX 46.1 Guidelines for intravaginal assessment and use of the vaginal speculum (continued)

you can ask the person to make their hands into a fist and place underneath their lower back. When the cervix is in full view, fix the blades to an open position.

8. Inspect the cervix. The normal cervix is pink and midline. Assess colour, position, size, projection into the vagina, surface and shape, and any discharge. If cultures or cytological studies are to be taken, ensure you follow policy and procedure regarding pathology collection and manufacturer instructions.
9. Advise that the examination is over and you will be withdrawing the speculum. Close the speculum blades and rotate slowly while withdrawing the speculum.
10. Offer a tissue or towel for removal of excess lubricant. Ask the person to get dressed (leave the room or provide privacy to do this). Once they are dressed, check in with them about the experience and answer any questions or concerns.

BOX 46.2 Guidelines for bimanual pelvic examination

The bimanual pelvic examination is done to palpate the cervix, uterus and ovaries. The examiner's gloved hand will be inserted intravaginally with the index and middle fingers extended, the thumb abducted and the fourth and fifth fingers folded on the palm of the hand. The extended fingers are lubricated.

The general procedure is as follows:

1. Explain the procedure in full and allow time for a conversation and questions regarding the examination. Ask the person to get undressed from the waist down (ensure privacy) and cover with a sheet or privacy garment.
2. Ask the person to lie on their back with their feet together as close to their buttocks as possible, legs bent and knees falling to the sides.
3. Perform hand hygiene, don gloves and reassure of infection control procedures in place.
4. Perform visual inspection of external genitalia (assessing skin for lesions, warts or erythema, noticing any discharge—including colour and consistency—and observe for any swelling or bleeding of the vulva). Ask the person to cough or strain to observe for any incontinence or prolapse. Discuss any findings and note any changes from pre-existing examinations.
5. Reiterate that you are about to undertake a vaginal examination, which is an invasive procedure. Spread the labia with the thumb and finger of your non-dominant hand and insert two lubricated fingers of your dominant hand into the vagina with your palm upwards.
6. Place your non-dominant hand on the abdomen, pressing down gently to move the internal genitals towards the intravaginal fingers (see the accompanying figure).
7. Ask the person to take deep breaths to relax the abdominal wall. Explain that this part of the examination will be more uncomfortable and provide reassurance. Palpate the cervix, assessing size, contour, position, surface, consistency, tenderness and mobility. The cervix should be freely movable and non-tender.
8. Palpate the uterus by pressing downwards on the abdomen while placing the intravaginal fingers in the anterior fornix and gently lifting against the abdominal hand. Assess the size, shape, surface, consistency, position, mobility and tenderness of the uterus. The normal uterus is freely movable and non-tender.
9. Palpate the adnexal areas, which surround the uterus and contain the fallopian tubes and ovaries. Because these structures are small, palpation may not be possible. If the ovaries are palpable, they should be smooth and firm. The normal ovary is sensitive to touch, firm and highly movable.
10. Advise that the examination is over and you will be withdrawing your fingers. Withdraw your fingers slowly. Offer a tissue or towel for removal of excess lubricant. Ask the person to get dressed (leave the room or provide privacy to do this). Once dressed, check in with them about their experience and answer any questions or concerns.

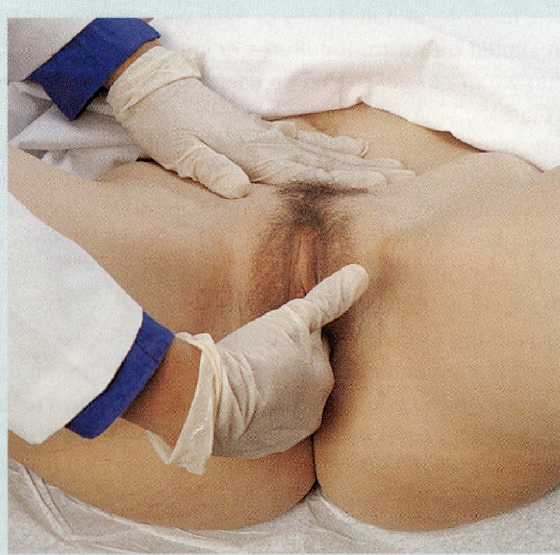

Bimanual pelvic examination

Source: Pearson Education.

CONCEPT CHECK

1 In the male, sex hormones are called:
1 androgens
2 steroids
3 prostaglandins
4 testerones

2 When assessing the breasts of a male who is living with obesity, the nurse may notice what physical change?
1 phimosis
2 gynaecomastia
3 enlarged axillary nodes
4 absent areola

3 You are assessing an 82-year-old person who identifies as a female and uses the pronouns she/her. She tells you that she is suddenly having menstrual bleeding. What should you tell her?
1 'This is normal, and sometimes happens even at your age.'
2 'Do you have menstrual cramps with the bleeding?'
3 'You need to see a doctor because you should not be bleeding.'
4 'Are you sexually active?'

4 Which blood test may be used to monitor prostate cancer?
1 PSA
2 VDRL
3 CBC
4 WBC

5 Atrophy and sagging of breast tissue is associated with:
1 poor nutrition
2 smoking
3 normal ageing
4 breast cancer

6 Oogenesis is the process of oocyte development and continues until which biological event?
1 birth
2 adolescence
3 menopause
4 death

7 Cessation of menstruation in younger person is a normal response to which biological event?
1 implantation of an embryo
2 onset of menopause
3 onset of puberty
4 beginning spermatogenesis

8 Which of the following diagnostic tests may be used to detect HPV?
1 colposcopy
2 mammogram
3 culture
4 cervical screening

9 Which assessment technique is primarily used to determine abnormalities of the breast?
1 inspection
2 auscultation
3 palpation
4 percussion

10 At which anatomical location would you palpate Bartholin's glands?
1 above the clitoris
2 posterior to the labia majora
3 inferior to the urinary meatus
4 internal vaginal wall

BIBLIOGRAPHY

Allen, A. A., Weinberger, A. H., Wetherill, R. R., Howe, C. L. & McKee, S. A. (2019). Oral contraceptives and cigarette smoking: A review of the literature and future directions. *Nicotine & Tobacco Research*, *21*(5), 592–601. https://doi.org/10.1093/ntr/ntx258

Australian Commission on Safety and Quality in Health Care (ACSQHC) (2021). *National Safety and Quality Health Service Standards* (2nd ed.). Sydney: ACSQHC.

Australian Institute of Health and Welfare (AIHW) (2021). *Cancer in Australia, 2021*. Retrieved from https://www.aihw.gov.au/

Australian Urology Associates (2016). *Transperineal prostate biopsy*. Retrieved from https://aua.com.au/

Cancer Australia (2018). *Diethylstilbestrol (DES)*. Retrieved from https://canceraustralia.gov.au/

Davies, H., Glodzik, D., Morganella, S. et al. (2017). HRDetect is a predictor of BRCA1 and BRCA2 deficiency based on mutational signatures. *Nature Medicine*, *23*, 517–525.

Kuchenbaecker, K. B., McGuffog, L., Barrowdale, D. et al. (2017). Evaluation of polygenic risk scores for breast and ovarian cancer risk prediction in BRCA1 and BRCA2 mutation carriers. *JNCI: Journal of the National Cancer Institute*, *109*(7), 1–15.

Niedzielski, J. Z., Oszukowska, E. & Slowikowska-Hilczer, J. (2016). Undescended testis—Current trends and guidelines: A review of the literature. *Archives of Medical Science*, *12*(3), 667–677.

Sencha, A. N., Evseeva, E. V., Ozerskaya, I. A., Fisenko, E. P., Patrunove, Y. N., Mogutov, M. S., Sergeeva, E. D. & Kashmanova, A. V. (2015). Anatomy, physiology, and development of the male breast. In A. Sencha (ed.), *Imaging of male breast cancer*. Cham: Springer.

Slomovitz, B., de Haydu, C., Taub, M., Coleman, R. L. & Monk, B. J. (2021). Asbestos and ovarian cancer: Examining the historical evidence. *International Journal of Gynecological Cancer*, *31*, 122–128.

World Health Organization (2021). *WHO laboratory manual for the examination and processing of human semen* (6th ed.). Geneva: World Health Organization.

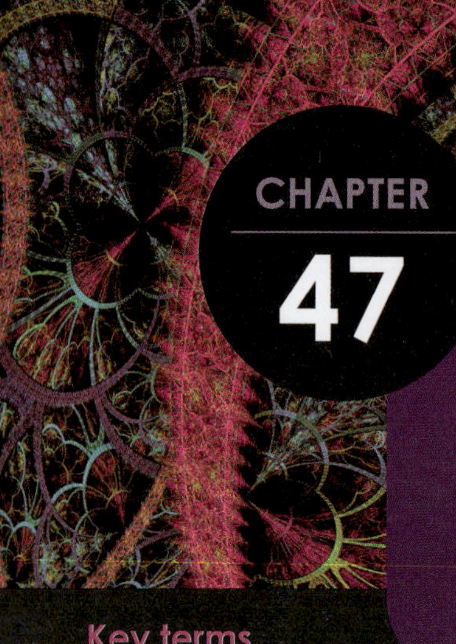

CHAPTER 47

Nursing care of men with reproductive system and breast disorders

Suzi Russell, Peter Thomas

Key terms

benign prostatic hyperplasia (BPH) 1757
epididymitis 1753
erectile dysfunction (ED) 1747
gynaecomastia 1771
hydrocoele 1752
impotence 1747
libido 1747
orchitis 1754
phimosis 1751
priapism 1751
prostatitis 1756
retrograde ejaculation 1750
spermatocoele 1752
testicular torsion 1754
varicocoele 1752

Learning outcomes

- Explain the pathophysiology, manifestations, complications, interprofessional and nursing care of men with disorders of the male reproductive system. Compare and contrast risk factors for cancer of the penis, testes and prostate gland.
- Discuss the purposes, nursing implications and person-centred education required for medications and treatments used to treat disorders of sexual function, the penis, the testes and scrotum, the prostate gland and the breast.
- Describe surgical procedures used to treat men with disorders of the male reproductive system.

Clinical competencies

- Assess functional health status of men with reproductive system and breast disorders, and monitor, document and report abnormal manifestations.
- Use evidence-based research to provide information and education to men having a radical prostatectomy.
- Determine nursing priorities, based on assessed data, to select and implement individualised nursing interventions for men with disorders of the reproductive system and breast.
- Administer or teach men how to knowledgeably and safely administer topical, oral and injectable medications used to treat disorders of the male reproductive system.
- Provide skilled care to men undergoing prostate surgery.
- Revise care plans as needed to provide effective interventions to promote, maintain or restore functional health status to men with disorders of the reproductive system and breast.

Men are subject to disorders of the penis, scrotum and testes, prostate gland and breast. These disorders may be inflammatory, structural, benign or malignant. Young men are at increased risk of testicular cancer (Akers, 2018). As men age, both benign and malignant conditions of the prostate gland become common. Many of the disorders pose significant risk to the man's fertility and sexual and urinary function, and some are life threatening. This chapter discusses disorders of the male reproductive system, including disorders of sexual expression and the male breast. Because many of the treatments and disorders of the male reproductive system have the potential to affect erection and ejaculation, these problems are discussed first.

Disorders of male sexual function

THE MAN WITH ERECTILE DYSFUNCTION

Erectile dysfunction (ED) is the inability of the male to attain and maintain an erection sufficient to permit satisfactory sexual intercourse. **Impotence**, a term often used synonymously with erectile dysfunction, may involve a total inability to achieve erection, an inconsistent ability to achieve erection or the ability to sustain only brief erections. ED has many possible causes (see Table 47.1) and may or may not be associated with a loss of **libido** (sexual desire).

Erectile dysfunction is a common problem. In Australia, 1 in 5 men over the age of 40 experience significant erectile problems and about 1 in 10 men are completely unable to have erections (Healthy Male, 2021a). The incidence of the problem increases with age. Most problems with erection are the result of a disease, injury or chemical substance (such as prescribed medications, alcohol, nicotine, vaping, cocaine, barbiturates, amphetamines, methadone, opiates or marijuana) that decreases blood flow in the penis (WebMD, 2021). Because this is a problem primarily of ageing men, the discussion of pathophysiology focuses on this age group.

TABLE 47.1 Causes of erectile dysfunction

MAJOR PATHOLOGICAL CAUSES		MAJOR IATROGENIC CAUSES	
		MEDICATIONS	PROCEDURES AND INFECTIONS
Neurogenic: Spinal cord injury Stroke Parkinson's disease Multiple sclerosis Epilepsy Alzheimer's disease Guillain-Barré syndrome Endocrinological: Diabetes mellitus Hypogonadism Hypothyroidism Inflammatory Prostatitis Cystitis Activity intolerance: Pulmonary problems Anaemias Myocardial infarction Congestive heart failure Hepatic diseases Kidney failure Substance dependency Alcohol Marijuana Narcotics Sedatives Tobacco	Arterial: Atherosclerosis Hypertension Aortic aneurysm Sickle cell anaemia Mechanical: Decreased penile distensibility Congenital disorders Morbid obesity Hydrocoele Hip or pelvic fractures Psychogenic: Depression Stress Fatigue Fear of failure Compulsive food disorders: Compulsive overeating Anorexia nervosa Bulimia	Antihypertensives: Hydrochlorothiazide Spironolactone Methyldopa Clonidine Prazosin Propranolol Psychotropic agents: Phenothiazines Butyrophenones Tricyclic antidepressants MAO inhibitors Diazepam Endocrinological agents: LHRH agonists Oestrogen compounds Progesterone Other: Antiparkinsonian agents Anticholinergic agents Immunosuppressive agents Antihistamines Non-steroidal anti-inflammatory drugs	Surgery: Coronary artery bypass Pelvic lymphadenectomy Radical prostatectomy Radical cystectomy Abdominal perineal resection Sympathectomy Aortic aneurysm repair Transplant surgeries Spinal surgery Other: Severe healthcare-associated infection Radiation therapy to pelvis

Pathophysiology

Age-related changes in sexual function involve cellular and tissue changes in the penis, decreased sensory activity, hypogonadism and the effects of chronic illness. In the penis, a change from elastic collagen to a more rigid collagen results in decreased distensibility (a less rigid erection). This, in turn, interferes with the veno-occlusive mechanism, which prevents blood from 'leaking' out of the penis into the general vasculature prematurely. Problems with this mechanism result in incomplete erections. Vibrotactile sensation over the skin of the penis declines with age. This decline may explain why some older men require longer stimulation to achieve an erection. Hypogonadism, common in ageing men, results in decreased testosterone levels. There may be a relationship between lower androgen levels and erectile function.

Many illnesses affect erectile function. Damage to arteries, smooth muscles and fibrous tissues are the most common causes of impotence. Diseases such as diabetes, kidney disease, chronic alcohol misuse, liver disease, atherosclerosis, hypertension and vascular disease are responsible for organic ED. Innervation and blood flow to the penis may be damaged during surgery—prostate surgery, in particular, but also by surgery to the bladder, lower bowel and/or spine. Given the effects of ageing on the vasculature of the penis, the increased incidence of chronic illness and the multiple medications and treatments required to manage those illnesses, it is not surprising that many older men have problems with ED.

INTERPROFESSIONAL CARE

The management of men with ED is growing in importance and scale. Because the population as a whole is ageing, so the incidence is increasing proportionately. Another factor is the gradual change in the willingness of men and their partners to discuss sexual concerns. Although sexuality is still a very sensitive and private area for most people, the knowledge that help is available is causing men to seek answers. Many older men are coming to believe that loss of erectile function is not an inevitable part of ageing.

Diagnosis

The diagnostic tests that may be ordered for the man include blood studies, penile monitoring and penile blood flow.

Blood chemistry, testosterone, prolactin, thyroxin and prostate-specific antigen (PSA) levels are measured to identify metabolic and endocrine problems that may be causing the dysfunction. Nocturnal penile tumescence and rigidity (NPTR) monitoring helps differentiate between psychogenic and organic causes. These tests can be performed in a sleep laboratory, although home testing with portable devices is an alternative. The number and quality of erections occurring during REM sleep can be determined. A non-invasive Doppler ultrasound is able to detect poor blood flow in the penis. Cavernosometry and cavernosography of the corpora are invasive techniques to evaluate arterial inflow and venous outflow of blood in the penis.

Medications

- *Oral medications*: oral medications used to treat ED include sildenafil citrate (Viagra), vardenafil hydrochloride (Levitra) or tadalafil (Cialis). Viagra and Levitra are taken an hour before sexual activity; they enhance the effects of nitrous oxide to facilitate relaxation of the smooth muscle in the penis during sexual stimulation to increase blood flow. Both drugs should be taken no more than once a day and should not be taken by men who are also taking nitrate-based drugs (for health problems) or alpha-blockers (used to treat hypertension and prostate enlargement). Cialis is a selective phosphodiesterase type-5 inhibitor that allows smooth muscle relaxation to facilitate inflow of blood into the penis. Its action lasts for 36 hours, but an erection only occurs with sexual stimulation. Cialis should not be taken if the man is also taking nitrates, alpha-blockers, erythromycin or rifampicin (antibiotics), ketoconazole or itraconazole (antifungals) or protease inhibitors (for HIV).
- *Injectable medications*: hormone replacement therapy with testosterone injections (250 mg IM every 3 weeks) or topical patches (Testogel) may be used for men with documented androgen deficiency and who do not have prostate cancer. Injectable medications, including papaverine and prostaglandin E injections (Alprostadil/Caverject), may be used. When injected directly into the penis, papaverine relaxes the arterioles and smooth muscles of the

Links to National Patient Safety Standards

NSQHS: Medication Safety Standard

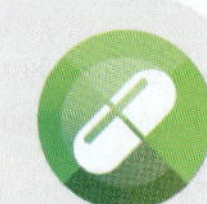

The intention of this standard is to 'ensure clinicians are competent to safely prescribe, dispense and administer appropriate medicines and to monitor medicine use' and that 'consumers are informed about medicines and understand their individual medicine needs and risks' (Australian Commission on Safety and Quality in Health Care (ACSQHC), 2021, p. 36).

Many medications that men take for reproductive system and breast disorders are highly toxic; for these reasons, medications need to be ordered, administered and monitored effectively. ED can be treated with medications taken orally, injected directly into the penis or inserted into the urethra at the tip of the penis.

Source: ACSQHC (2021). *National Safety and Quality Health Service Standards* (2nd ed.). Sydney: ACSQHC. © Australian Commission on Safety and Quality in Health Care.

cavernosum, thus inducing tumescence (swelling). An erection usually develops that lasts from 30 minutes to 4 hours. Prostaglandin E functions much as papaverine does but has fewer side effects. One problem with this treatment is its mode of delivery. There is a high attrition rate and men report dissatisfaction with lack of spontaneity, loss of interest in sex, physical limitations, cost and, occasionally, pain.

Mechanical devices

A frequently prescribed mechanical device for ED is the vacuum constriction device (VCD) (vacuum pump). The VCD draws blood into the penis with a vacuum, trapping it there with a constricting band at the base of the penis. After the device is removed for intercourse, a single small band, often called an O-ring, is left at the base of the penis to maintain the erection. If the man can attain an erection but cannot maintain it, an O-ring alone can be used.

Surgery

Surgical treatment for ED involves either revascularisation procedures or implantation of prosthetic devices. Venous or arterial procedures are generally not successful. The result is often temporary because the underlying cause of the vascular insufficiency is usually not corrected. Implantation of penile prostheses is now common (see Figure 47.1). Men are generally satisfied with their prostheses and they rank the inflatable type highest. Partners are also more likely to report satisfaction with the penile implant, although not to the same degree as men. Some partners report that the implanted penis is harder than a normal erect penis and therefore causes pain. Also, the man can have intercourse for a prolonged period of time and some partners do not find prolonged penetration enjoyable. Education for both the man and their partner is mandatory. Counselling by a sex therapist may be needed to facilitate adaptation to the implant.

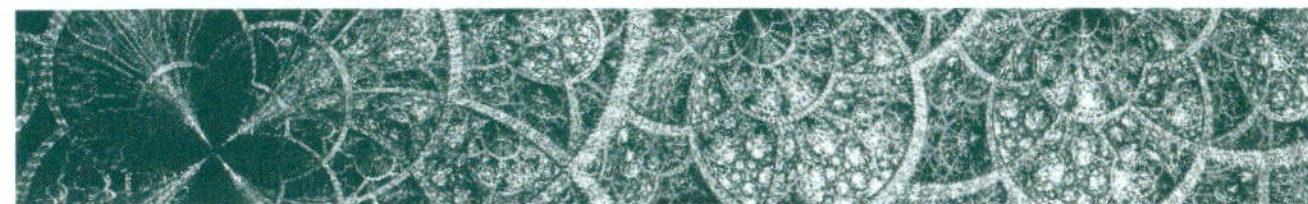

Nursing care

Nurses in any healthcare setting may encounter men with ED, either through routine examinations or through careful assessment of men's conditions and treatments that may incidentally cause ED. Nurses employed in clinics, operating rooms and surgical units with urological services commonly encounter men being treated for ED. Nurses in a variety of settings, including long-term and residential care, encounter men who have had surgical interventions, such as penile implants.

Nursing interventions

Because nurses often complete the man's health history, they are most likely to discover problems of ED. (See the 'Functional health pattern interview' in the chapter 'A person-centred approach to assessing the male and female reproductive systems' for appropriate questions to elicit information.) Once a problem is known, nurses are involved in giving information, providing emotional support and referring men to doctors or counsellors. Although there are many possible nursing interventions, this section focuses on nursing care related to sexual dysfunction and self-esteem.

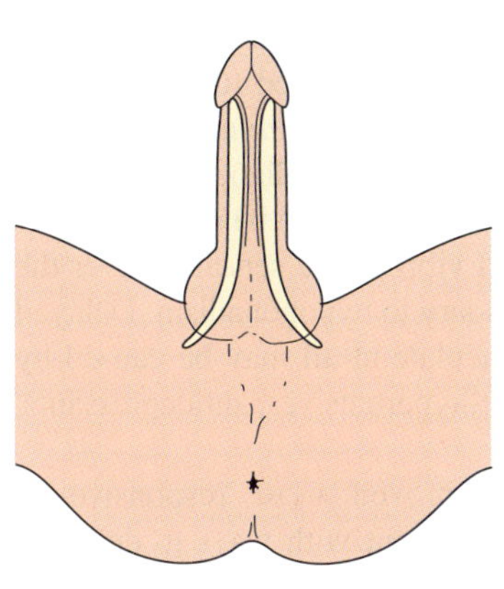

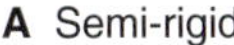

A Semi-rigid

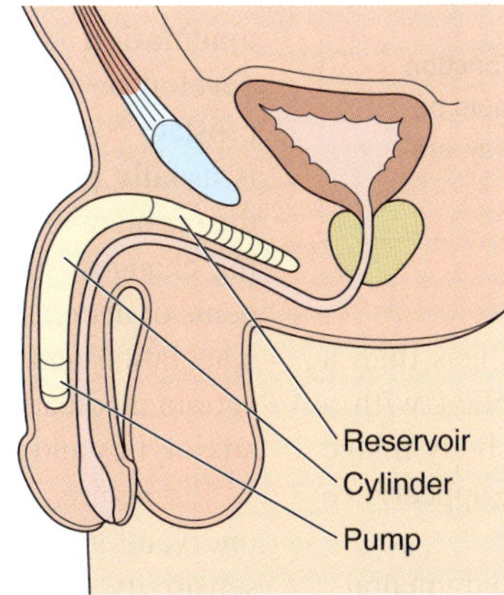

B Self-contained

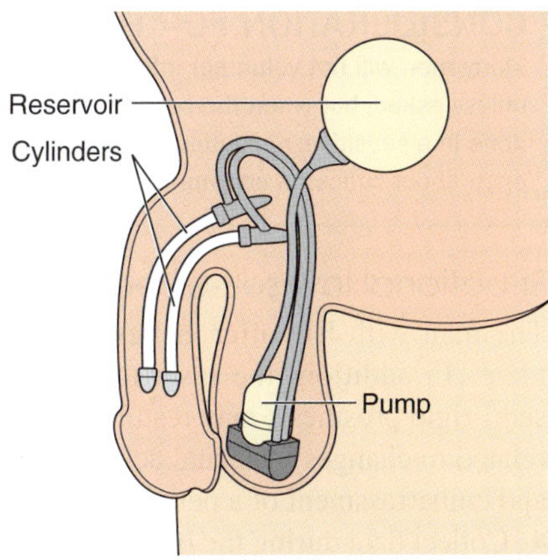

C Inflatable

FIGURE 47.1 *Types of penile implants. A, With semi-rigid rods implanted in the corpora cavernosa, the penis is always in a state of semi-erection, which may not be acceptable to the man. B, With a self-contained penile implant, the penis remains flaccid until the man compresses a pump at the head of the penis, which transfers fluid from a reservoir to a cylinder within the penis to achieve an erection. The man presses a release valve to return the fluid to the reservoir. C, With an inflatable penile implant, the penis remains flaccid until the man compresses a pump in the scrotum, which transfers fluid from an abdominal reservoir to cylinders in the corpora cavernosa to achieve an erection. Pressing a release valve returns the fluid to the reservoir*

Sexual dysfunction

Many men who lose erectile function are not aware of the cause. Often the man blames the loss on unrelated factors, such as age, a medication for an illness, a dangerous illness or his sexual partner. Not knowing causes anxiety, which may disrupt the relationship with his partner or lead him to discontinue an important medication.

- Assess for risk factors for ED. Be especially alert to men who have recently begun medications or had recent surgery that could cause ED. *Awareness of risk factors helps the nurse to prioritise care, although nurses must remember that almost all ageing men have at least one risk factor for ED.*
- Assess for sexual dysfunction. Men have shown greater willingness and comfort to discuss sexual concerns and expect nurses to be aware of the physiological effects of their disease and side effects of treatment on all aspects of their health. *If a problem exists, information obtained in a sexual assessment guides the nurse in deciding if the next step should be health education, referral or both.*
- Perform a detailed assessment of current sexual practices. *It is essential for healthcare providers to understand the man and his partner's sexual pattern in order to provide appropriate, individualised care.*
- Discuss previous methods of coping with ED. *Awareness of coping strategies can provide insight for the nurse and guide health education.*
- Provide information about treatment options. *The man needs to know the details of the intervention, the chances for success and the possible complications. Advice about treatment options should involve patients as partners in their own care, as outlined in the National Safety and Quality Health Service Partnering with Consumers Standard (ACSQHC, 2021).*

CONSIDERATION FOR PRACTICE

Many men will not volunteer information about sexual function unless asked, but when the concept is raised, which should be done in a sensitive, non-judgmental but matter-of-fact way, are open about concerns and appreciate being asked.

Situational low self-esteem

The man with ED often believes himself to be 'less than a man'. In addition, the insertion of a penile implant with a semi-rigid prosthesis may result in disturbances in body image related to changes in sexual activity, as well as the appearance and embarrassment of a permanent semi-erection.

- Collect data during the health history, in a non-judgmental manner, about physiological function, other chronic illnesses and feelings about sexual inadequacy. *This information is necessary to establish the database for individualised interventions.*
- If the man has had a penile implant, teach him and his partner how to use the pump, including how to inflate and deflate the device. Suggest he practise inflation and deflation during the postoperative period. Suggest wearing snug-fitting underwear with the penis placed in an upright position on the abdomen, and loose trousers. Provide information about length of healing and that sexual activity may resume within 6 to 8 weeks post surgery. *Practising using the pump will maintain the pump position and promote tissue growth around the implant. The type of clothing worn can improve the ability to conceal a semi-rigid prosthesis and decrease embarrassment. Recovery from surgery is necessary before resuming sexual activity.*

Community-based care

Many nurses find that men with ED and their partners have lived in isolation with the problem for many years. The partner may even be unaware of the problem. The partner may believe that the man is seeing someone else or that he has lost his attraction to the partner. The man may have kept his problem a secret because an intense feeling of shame makes him unable to admit that he cannot perform sexually. Many men greet the information about the high incidence of ED with a sense of relief that they are not alone in having this problem. All men and their partners need to be aware of support services available to them. Referral sources include:

- Health Male: https://healthymale.org.au
- The Fertility Society of Australia: https://www.fertilitysociety.com.au/anzica/.

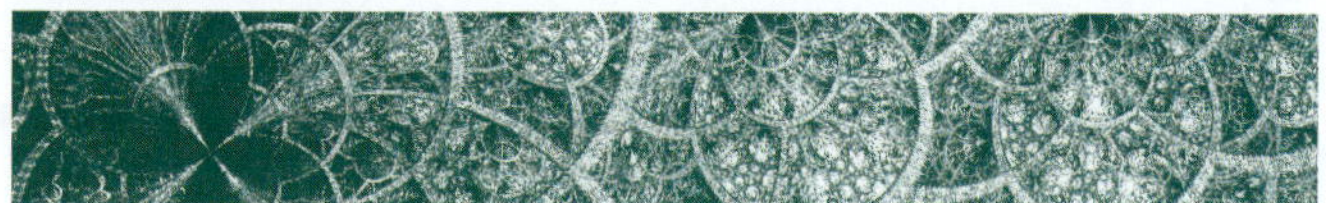

THE MAN WITH EJACULATORY DYSFUNCTION

There are many types of ejaculatory dysfunction. **Retrograde ejaculation** (seminal fluid discharged into the bladder) may develop in ageing men but is usually related to treatment of prostate conditions or testicular cancer. *Premature ejaculation* is usually psychogenic in origin, although diabetes can cause the problem as well. *Delayed ejaculation* can be related to ageing changes, such as decreased vibrotactile sensation over the penis or decreased libido secondary to hypogonadism. Delayed ejaculation and inability to ejaculate at all may be caused by certain medications, such as antihypertensives, antidepressants, anxiolytics and narcotics.

Premature ejaculation has proved most responsive to intervention. The man can experiment with ways to decrease sensitivity (such as wearing condoms). Using relaxation and guided imagery can delay orgasm. Mechanical devices, such as constrictive rings around the base of the penis, can help the man delay ejaculation and sustain an erection.

Nursing care focuses on assessment of the problem and health education for all types of ejaculatory dysfunction. The man's partner can be taught how to avoid excessive stimulation that would result in premature ejaculation. If the problem persists, the man should be referred to a specialist.

Disorders of the penis

THE MAN WITH PHIMOSIS OR PRIAPISM

Two less common disorders of the penis are phimosis and priapism. Although uncommon, these disorders can cause problems with urination and sexual activity. In some cases, they are considered a medical emergency because decreased blood flow to the penis may result in tissue ischaemia and necrosis.

Pathophysiology

Phimosis is constriction of the foreskin in uncircumcised men so that it cannot be retracted over the glans penis. Phimosis may be congenital or it may be related to chronic infections under the foreskin that lead to adhesions. The main problem with this condition is that it prevents adequate hygiene, which may lead to malignant changes of the penis. It also may interfere with urinary elimination and intercourse. In a related disorder, called *paraphimosis*, the foreskin is tight and constricted and is not able to cover the glans penis. The glans becomes engorged and oedematous and is painful. Paraphimosis may result from long-term retraction of the foreskin, such as occurs in placement of an indwelling catheter in the uncircumcised male (Norris, 2018). The tight foreskin can result in ischaemia of the glans.

Priapism is an involuntary, sustained, painful erection that is not associated with sexual arousal. The prolonged erection may result in ischaemia and fibrosis of the erectile tissue with high risk of subsequent impotence (Norris, 2018). The disorder, classified as either primary or secondary, is caused by impaired blood flow in the corpora cavernosa. Primary priapism results from conditions such as tumours, infection or trauma. Secondary priapism is caused by blood disorders (e.g. leukaemia, thalassaemia and thrombocytopenia), neurological disorders (e.g. spinal cord injury or stroke), kidney failure and some medications (see Box 47.1). Men who use intracavernous injection therapy or Cialis for ED are at risk of priapism.

BOX 47.1 Factors implicated in the aetiology of priapism

Illnesses/conditions
- Thalassaemia
- Metastatic cancer
- Leukaemia
- Spinal cord trauma

Drugs
- Papaverine
- Alcohol
- Psychotropic drugs
- Marijuana
- Warfarin
- Cocaine

INTERPROFESSIONAL CARE

Severe phimosis or paraphimosis may require surgical circumcision. If infection is present, the appropriate antibiotic is administered.

Treatment of priapism includes iced saline enemas, intravenous ketamine (Ketalar) administration to induce anaesthesia and spinal anaesthesia. Blood may be aspirated from the corpus through the dorsal glans, followed by catheterisation and pressure dressings to maintain decompression. If necessary, more aggressive surgery to create vascular shunts to maintain blood flow is performed. When priapism is prolonged, it increases the risk of subsequent ED.

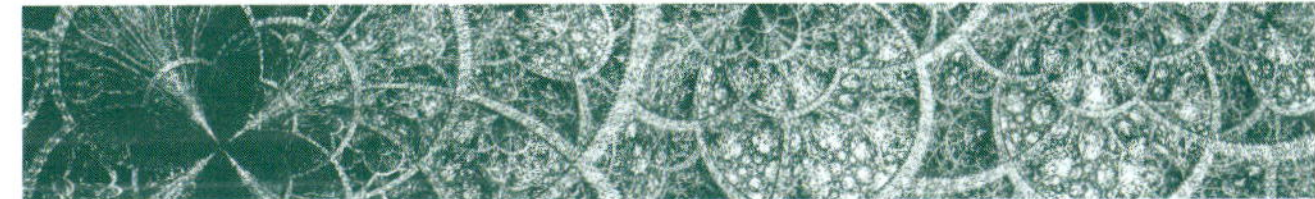

Nursing care

Nursing care for men with priapism focuses on assessing the penis, monitoring urinary output and providing pain management. Assessment of the penis includes inspection for degree of erection and changes in colour due to ischaemia and palpation of the penis for firmness and degree of rigidity. Monitor urine output, assessing for oliguria or signs of acute urinary retention. Pain is treated with analgesics.

The man usually has moderate to severe anxiety related to pain, the treatment and the threat to his sexual function. The treatment may sound bizarre and painful, especially since the area is already extremely sensitive. The man may be acutely embarrassed by the erection and needs reassurance that the nurse understands that the erection is not within his control.

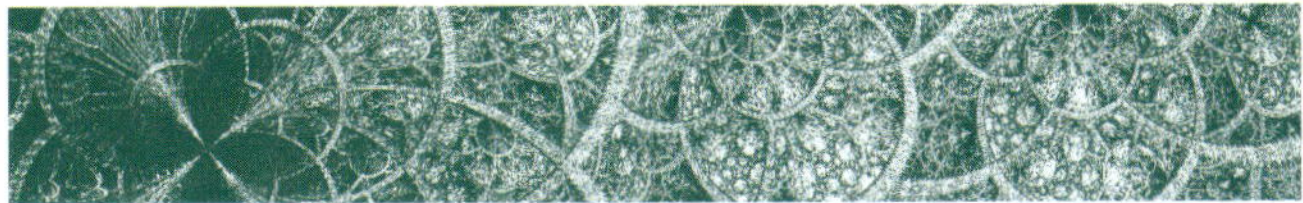

THE MAN WITH CANCER OF THE PENIS

Cancer of the penis is a rare cancer in Australia. It most commonly affects men between the ages of 45 and 60. The cause is unknown. Penile cancer is rare in Jewish and Muslim men, populations in which routine circumcision is practised, although the correlation between circumcision and this cancer is unclear. Phimosis and poor genital hygiene are risk factors, as are human papillomavirus (HPV) and HIV infection. Sunlight and ultraviolet light exposure (such as that used to treat psoriasis) also may play a role (Norris, 2018).

Pathophysiology

Squamous cell carcinoma accounts for 95% of all penile cancers (Healthy Male, 2021b). The tumour usually develops as a nodular or wart-like growth or a red velvety lesion on the glans or foreskin. The tumours tend to grow slowly. Penile cancer spreads to the superficial or deep inguinal nodes and very late in the disease may spread to the bone, liver or lungs. If the lesion is treated before inguinal node involvement, chances for a cure are good. Most of these lesions are painless but there may be significant ulceration and bleeding. Purulent, foul-smelling discharge may be evident under the foreskin. Occasionally, men with penile cancer may present with enlarged inguinal lymph nodes.

INTERPROFESSIONAL CARE

Cancer of the penis is diagnosed by a biopsy of the lesion, including any suspicious inguinal lymph nodes. The cancer is staged according to the size of the tumour, extent of invasion, status of inguinal lymph nodes and the presence or absence of distant metastasis. Small, localised lesions may be treated with fluorouracil cream, external-beam radiation, laser therapy or surgical excision. Larger lesions with superficial or deep infiltration of penile structures require partial or total amputation of the penis. Chemotherapy (discussed in the chapter 'Nursing care of people with cancer') may be administered to men with distant metastasis.

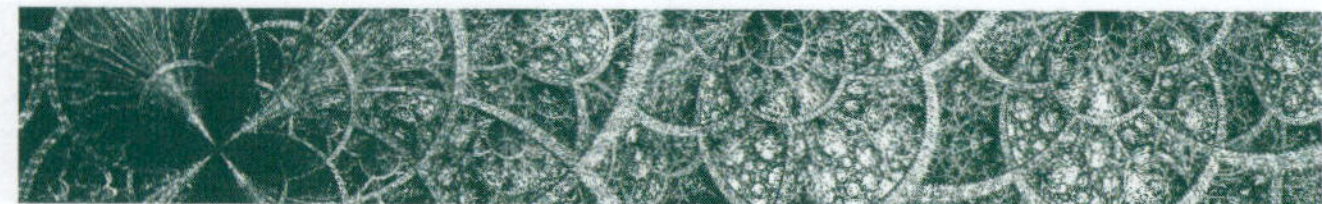

Nursing care

Health education can help prevent this disease or provide early detection and intervention. Teach men about genital hygiene (including retraction of the foreskin if uncircumcised and washing the glans penis while bathing or showering) and the risks of unprotected sex, and encourage condom use. Encourage men to shield their genitals when having ultraviolet light therapy. Discuss the importance of seeking prompt treatment for any lesion or abnormal drainage noted on the penis.

If the man has a penile amputation (*penectomy*), nurses help cope with challenges associated with a shortened or absent penis, including the potentially devastating effect on body image and self-concept. If a total penectomy is performed, the surgeon creates a perineal urethrostomy, preserving urinary continence. However, the man must void in the sitting position, reinforcing the feeling of loss. Dribbling of urine after voiding may be a problem for a few weeks. The man should be taught to perform careful perineal hygiene following surgery, using mild soap and water. Sitz baths may be helpful to relieve pain and to promote healing. Patient teaching about cleanliness should be in line with the National Safety and Quality Health Service Preventing and Controlling Infections Standard (ACSQHC, 2021). If an inguinal lymph node dissection is performed, the man may experience persistent lymphoedema of the lower extremities.

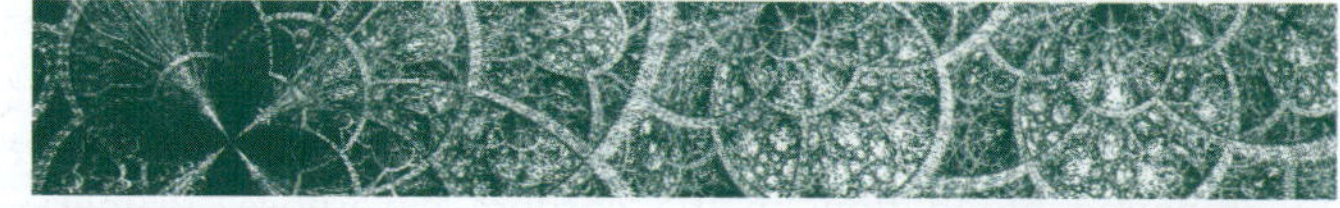

Disorders of the testis and scrotum

THE MAN WITH A BENIGN SCROTAL MASS

Most scrotal masses are benign and can be managed in a manner that is satisfactory to the man. The most common are hydrocoeles, spermatocoeles and varicocoeles (see Figure 47.2).

Pathophysiology

A **hydrocoele**, the most common cause of scrotal swelling, is a collection of fluid within the tunica vaginalis. The swelling ranges from slightly larger than the testicle to larger than a grapefruit. The cause of chronic hydrocoele in men over the age of 40 years is an imbalance between production and reabsorption of fluid within the layers of the scrotum. Hydrocoeles also may occur secondary to trauma, infection or a tumour. A hydrocoele may be differentiated from a solid mass by transillumination or ultrasound of the scrotum. If the hydrocoele becomes large enough to cause embarrassment or significant pain, the fluid is aspirated and an agent is injected into the scrotal sac to sclerose the tunica vaginalis. Hydrocoeles are not associated with infertility.

A **spermatocoele** is a mobile, usually painless mass that forms when efferent ducts in the epididymis dilate and form a cyst. It is thought to result from leakage of sperm due to trauma or infection. Treatment is usually not necessary. Spermatocoeles are not associated with infertility.

A **varicocoele** is an abnormal dilation of a vein within the spermatic cord. It is caused by incompetent or congenitally missing valves that allow blood to pool in the spermatic cord veins. The dilated vein forms a soft mass that may be painful. Most varicocoeles occur on the left side after puberty. A major concern with this condition is that it can decrease blood flow through the testis, interfere with spermatogenesis and cause infertility. Varicocoeles can be felt by scrotal palpation. Scrotal ultrasound is frequently used for diagnosis. If infertility is a concern, the spermatic vein may be ligated or occluded

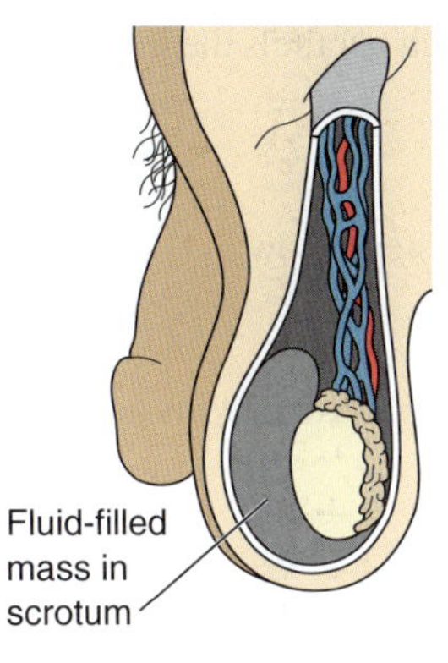

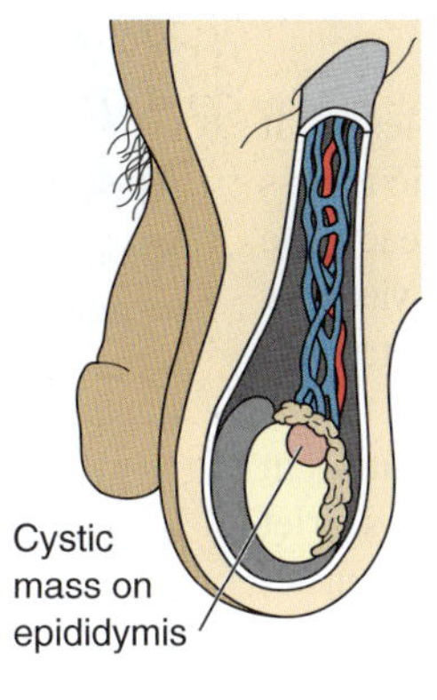

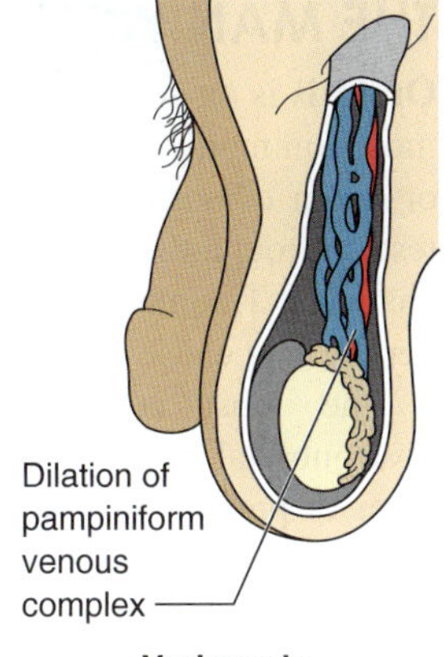

FIGURE 47.2 *Common disorders of the scrotum. Hydrocoeles and spermatocoeles do not usually require treatment unless they become large and cause pain. Varicocoeles are usually treated to prevent infertility*

with a sclerosing agent or balloon catheter. If the varicocoele is small and infertility is not a concern, a scrotal support is recommended.

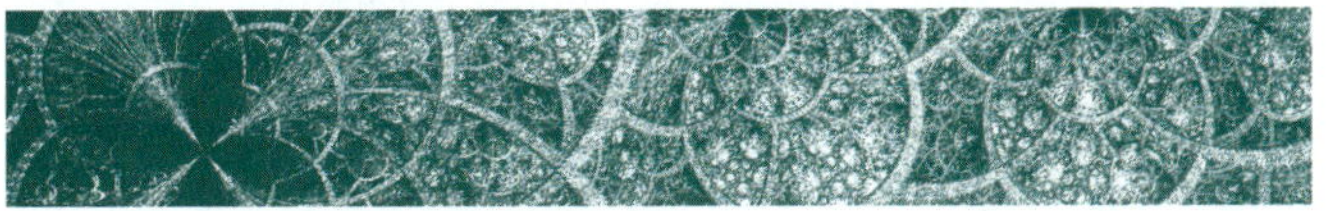

Nursing care

Nursing care focuses on reducing anxiety and providing health education about comfort measures. Almost all men are aware of the possible pain associated with scrotal manipulation. They need information and reassurance about pain management if surgical treatment is necessary. External bleeding is minimal after surgery; however, some men do develop scrotal haematomas, manifested by scrotal oedema and a purple discolouration.

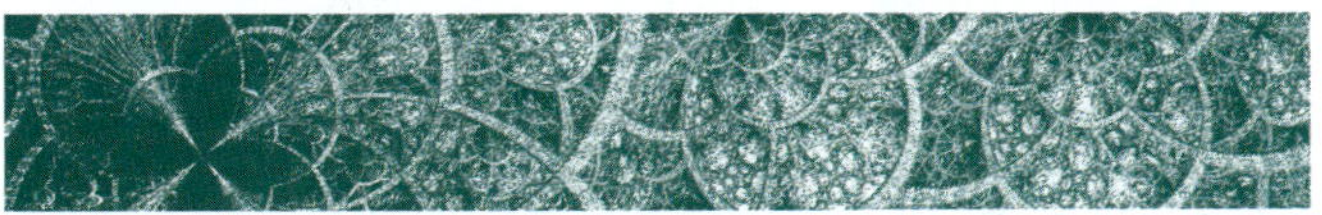

THE MAN WITH EPIDIDYMITIS

Epididymitis is an infection or inflammation of the epididymis, the structure that lies along the posterior border of the testis. This disorder is more often seen in sexually active men who are less than 40 years of age (Rupp & Leslie, 2021).

Sexually transmitted urethritis caused by *Chlamydia trachomatis* or *Neisseria gonorrhoeae* is the usual precipitating factor for epididymitis in younger men. Men who practise unprotected anal intercourse may acquire sexually transmitted epididymitis from *Escherichia coli, Haemophilus influenzae, Cryptococcus* or tuberculosis. In men older than age 35, epididymitis is usually associated with a urinary tract infection or prostatitis. Chemical epididymitis is associated with an inflammatory response to the reflux of urine into the ejaculatory ducts from urethral strictures, congenital structural anomalies or increased abdominal pressure from excessive heavy lifting. This type is usually self-limiting and does not require treatment.

Infectious epididymitis spreads by ascending the vas deferens from an already infected urethra or bladder. Early manifestations include pain and local oedema, which can progress to erythema and oedema of the entire scrotum, especially on the side of the involved epididymis. Complications include abscess formation, infarction of the testis and infertility.

INTERPROFESSIONAL CARE

The infection is diagnosed with a specimen culture from a urethral swab or epididymal aspiration. Severe epididymitis may be treated with intravenous antibiotics and hospitalisation. Less acute forms of the disease are treated with antibiotic therapy. The man's sexual partner should also be treated with antibiotics if the causative organism is sexually transmitted.

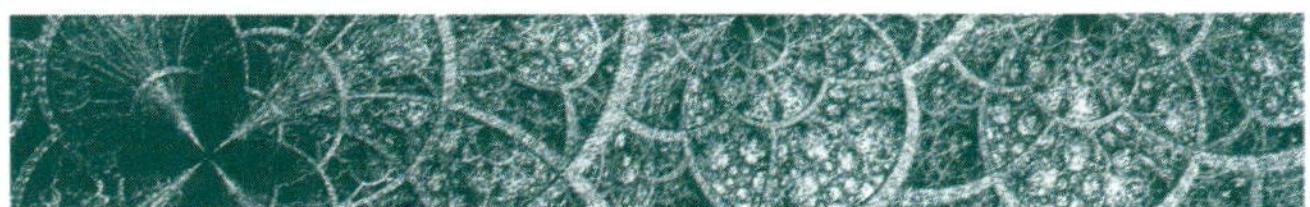

Nursing care

Nursing care involves symptomatic relief and health education. Ice packs and a scrotal support may be applied to the scrotum to relieve pain. Ensure the man knows that complete resolution of the infection may take weeks to months and that treatment should continue until the infection is gone. Provide information about the possibility of infertility because the man may wish to seek evaluation for this problem at a later date.

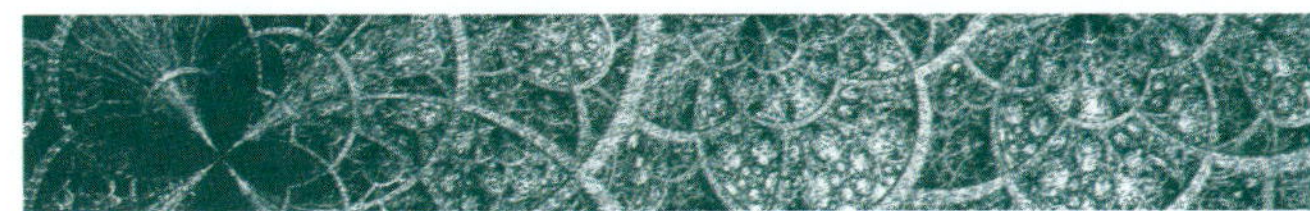

THE MAN WITH ORCHITIS

Orchitis is an acute inflammation or infection of the testes. It most commonly occurs as a complication of a systemic illness or as an extension of epididymitis. Infection may reach the testes through the vas deferens and the lymphatic and vascular channels. Trauma, including vasectomy and other scrotal surgeries, may cause inflammation of the testes.

The most common infectious cause of orchitis in post-pubertal men is mumps. Other causes include scarlet fever or pneumonia. The manifestations have a sudden onset, usually within 3 to 4 days after the swelling of the parotid glands. Manifestations include a high fever, increased WBCs and unilateral or bilateral scrotal redness, swelling and pain. If both testes are involved, permanent sterility may result, but this is rare (Norris, 2018).

INTERPROFESSIONAL CARE

Treatment is supportive and symptomatic, including antibiotic therapy if urine cultures are positive. Bed rest, scrotal support and elevation, hot or cold compresses, and analgesics for pain are prescribed. If a hydrocoele occurs, it is aspirated. Nursing care is similar to that of the man with epididymitis and other scrotal disorders.

THE MAN WITH TESTICULAR TORSION

Testicular torsion, twisting of the spermatic cord with scrotal swelling and pain, is a potential medical emergency. The condition occurs most often in males between birth and age 20 but can occur at any age. Testicular torsion may occur spontaneously or it may follow trauma or physical exertion. The torsion of the arteries and veins decreases or stops testicular circulation, with resultant vascular engorgement and ischaemia.

Testicular torsion is usually diagnosed by history and physical examination. Testicular scanning may be used to determine if blood flow to the testicle is reduced, or a prostate ultrasound may be done to identify masses or torsion. Surgical treatment, which involves detorsion of the testicle and fixation to the scrotum, must begin as quickly as possible. If the testicle is necrotic or has sustained significant damage, an *orchidectomy* (surgical removal of a testis) is performed.

THE MAN WITH TESTICULAR CANCER

Testicular cancer accounts for only 1% of all cancers in men and it most commonly affects men between 15 and 50 years of age (Cancer Council South Australia, 2020). In 2021, an estimated 980 men in Australia were diagnosed with this cancer (Australian Institute of Health and Welfare (AIHW), 2021). Survival from testicular cancer has improved dramatically as a result of treatment with effective combination chemotherapy.

The cause of testicular cancer is unknown, but both congenital and acquired factors have been associated with tumour development. About 5% of cases develop in a man with a history of undescended testicle (*cryptorchidism*). Testicular cancer is more common on the right side, which parallels the incidence of cryptorchidism (Akers, 2018).

Risk factors

Risk factors for testicular cancer are listed below:

- age
- cryptorchidism
- genetic predisposition, especially in identical twins and brothers
- Klinefelter's syndrome
- cancer of the other testicle
- other risk factors under investigation, including occupational risks, presence of multiple atypical naevi, HIV infection, cancer in situ, body size and maternal hormone use (Dreyer, Macfarlane & Hendry, 2018).

Pathophysiology

Approximately 95% of testicular malignancies are germ-cell tumours (Norris, 2018). Germ-cell tumours are classified, depending on their origin and ability to differentiate, as seminomas and non-seminomas. Seminomas are the most common type and are believed to arise from the seminiferous epithelium of the testes. Non-seminomas contain more than one cell type; they include embryonal carcinoma, teratoma, choriocarcinoma and yolk cell carcinoma. The most common type in men ages 20 to 30 is embryonal carcinomas. Testicular cancer may also arise from specialised cells of the gonadal stroma. These tumours are named for the cells from which they originate: Leydig cell, Sertoli cell, granulosa cell and theca cell tumours.

Manifestations

The first sign of testicular cancer may be a slight enlargement of one testicle with some discomfort. The man may also have an abdominal ache and a feeling of heaviness in the scrotum. Local spread of the cancer to the epididymis or spermatic cord is inhibited by the outer covering of the testicles, the tunica albuginea. Therefore, spread by lymphatic and vascular channels to other organs often causes distant disease before large masses develop in the scrotum. Lymphatic dissemination usually leads to disease in retroperitoneal lymph nodes, whereas vascular dissemination can lead to metastasis in the lungs, bone or liver. Bilateral presentation of testicular cancer is unusual. Manifestations of testicular cancer are summarised in the 'Manifestations' box. Manifestations of metastasis include lower extremity oedema, back pain, cough, haemoptysis or dizziness. Human chorionic gonadotropin (hGC)-producing tumours may cause breast enlargement (*gynaecomastia*).

INTERPROFESSIONAL CARE

Care focuses on diagnosis, elimination of the cancer and prevention or treatment of metastasis. Once testicular cancer is suspected, the man undergoes a number of screening tests to help identify the disease and its stage. If the disease is confined

MANIFESTATIONS **Testicular cancer**

COMMON
- Painless swelling on one testicle

OCCASIONAL
- Dull ache in pelvis or scrotum
- Painless nodule on one testicle

UNCOMMON
- Acute pain in scrotum

RARE
- Infertility
- Gynaecomastia

METASTATIC SYMPTOMS
- Neck mass
- Respiratory symptoms
- Gastrointestinal disturbance
- Lumbar back pain

to the testicle, it is classified as stage I. Stage II disease is limited to the testicle and regional lymph nodes. Stage III disease involves metastasis above the diaphragm or extensive visceral involvement. Often, the man does not undergo biopsy before the beginning of treatment, but instead receives a definitive diagnosis after orchidectomy. Most men treated for testicular cancer will live a normal lifespan.

Diagnosis

Diagnosis may be made by various laboratory tests. Serum studies are done to identify tumour markers. Germ-cell tumours produce biochemical markers such as beta-hCG and alpha-fetoprotein (AFP) that can be measured using radioimmunoassay techniques. Elevated levels provide strong evidence of testicular cancer. These markers are also measured after surgery to help determine the presence of residual disease that remains undetected by other means. Persistent elevation may indicate the need for further therapy. Serum lactic acid dehydrogenase (LDH) levels are elevated in testicular cancer and may be significantly elevated when metastatic disease is present. LDH is a less specific indicator of testicular cancer than beta-hCG and AFP.

Medications

Progress in chemotherapy to treat testicular cancer is one of the chief reasons why most men survive the disease. The man who has an advanced disease receives platinum-based combination chemotherapy. Two frequently used combinations are: (1) cisplatin, bleomycin and etoposide (BEP); and (2) etoposide plus cisplatin (EP). Toxicity from the BEP regimen can be significant, with nausea, vomiting, hair loss, bone marrow suppression, nephrotoxicity, ototoxicity and peripheral neuropathy. Decreasing the number of BEP cycles to three (rather than four) or using the EP regimen reduces both the mortality and morbidity associated with chemotherapy. Chemotherapy is discussed in the chapter 'Nursing care of people with cancer'.

Surgery

Radical orchidectomy is the treatment used in all forms and stages of testicular cancer. A modified retroperitoneal lymph node dissection that preserves the nerves necessary for ejaculation often is performed at the same time.

Radiation therapy

Radiation therapy is used for stage I seminoma to treat cancer in the retroperitoneal lymph nodes, the most frequent site for distant metastasis. The man may experience temporary diarrhoea, nausea or a decline in bone marrow function, such as thrombocytopenia or leucopenia. These problems are usually mild and respond well to symptomatic treatment or time. Damage to the contralateral testicle is minimised by careful shielding. Pre-treatment and post-treatment analysis of sperm number and function is necessary. The most common long-term complication is dyspepsia or ulcer disease. Radiation therapy is discussed in the chapter 'Nursing care of people with cancer'.

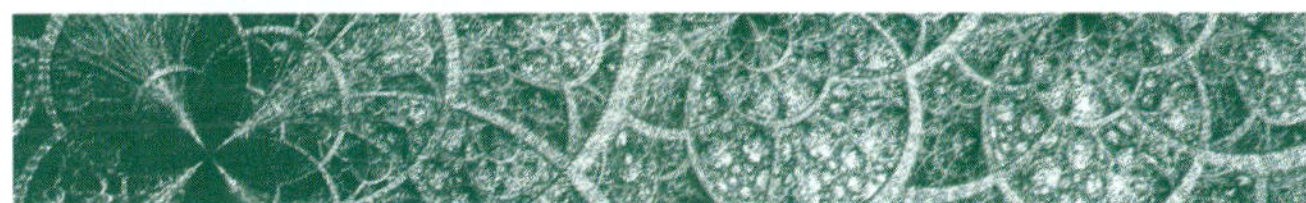

Nursing care

Health promotion

Unfortunately, most men who develop testicular cancer do not have overt risk factors. Therefore, beginning at about the age of 15, all men should perform monthly testicular self-examination, as described in Box 47.2.

Nursing interventions

Nursing care of the man with testicular cancer is complex. The nurse must consider the reactions to the diagnosis, the change in body image accompanying treatment and sexual and reproductive issues. Although chances of a cure are excellent, the

BOX 47.2 Testicular self-examination

- Examine your testicles when you are taking a warm shower or bath, or just after if you prefer to use a mirror to compare size.
- The scrotum, testicles and hands should be soapy to allow easy manipulation of the tissue.
- Gently roll each testicle between the thumb and fingers of each hand. If one testicle is substantially larger than the other or if you feel any hard lumps, consult your doctor immediately.
- Normal scrotal contents may be confusing. Just above and behind the testicle is the epididymis. It feels soft and tender overall, although parts of it may be rather firm. This is normal. The spermatic cord, a small, round, movable tube, extends up from the epididymis. It feels firm and smooth. Of greatest concern is any hard lump felt directly on the testicle, even if it is painless.
- Choose a day out of each month on which to examine yourself. Most men choose an easy day to remember, such as the first or last day of the month. Note this day on your calendar to help you remember.
- Start examinations young so that you become aware of what your testicles normally feel like. This way you will detect changes more readily.

long-term effect on quality of life may be extensive, requiring a change in life goals.

Deficient knowledge

The nurse often initiates and reinforces health education about what to expect after radical orchidectomy. The man's knowledge about surgery is assessed and postoperative routines such as early ambulation are explained (see the chapter 'Nursing care of people having surgery').

- Explain pain management methods. In addition to the usual analgesics used to control postoperative incisional pain, ice bags may be applied to the scrotum. A scrotal support provides relief, especially when the man ambulates. *Surgery results in incisional pain and the scrotum is tender and slightly swollen.*
- Educate the man about the manifestations of complications. The incision is closed with Steri-Strips™ or staples, and, although rare, wound dehiscence is possible. If the incision gapes open or if there is bleeding beyond slight oozing after 24 hours, the man should contact the surgeon. Another rare complication is a haematoma in the scrotum caused by bleeding from the spermatic cord stump. *Rapid onset of scrotal oedema is a sign of this problem. Because the man is usually discharged early, complications may not become apparent until he is at home.*

Ineffective sexuality patterns

The effect of testicular cancer and its treatment on sexual and reproductive function is varied. If the man has a retroperitoneal lymph node dissection, severing of the sympathetic plexus may result in retrograde ejaculation or failure to ejaculate. Infertility may be caused by ejaculation disorders, surgery, chemotherapy or radiation therapy.

- Assess the man's pre-diagnosis sexual function. To assess this, the nurse must establish an atmosphere of trust, openness and permission to discuss sexual concerns. After the initial shock of the diagnosis, men report intense concern about sexual and reproductive issues, which can be relieved only by information. *Knowledge of the man's usual sexual function can guide health education.*
- Discuss the possibility of preserving sperm in a bank prior to treatment. *This option may help relieve the man's fears about his ability to father children in the future, but must be completed prior to initiating treatment with surgery, chemotherapy or radiation therapy.*
- Help coping with feelings about altered sexual function and appearance. Explain that testicular implants can be inserted to preserve appearance. *Many men, regardless of whether they are in a significant relationship, deeply grieve the loss of the ability to father children. It is important to maintain body image despite disfiguring surgery.*

Community-based care

Families need to be included in health education for a variety of reasons. If the man is of reproductive age, his partner will have significant anxiety and will also require information. For the teenager, parents need information about the effect on sexual function and are often very involved in postoperative care. The man needs the support of the people he loves, and knowledgeable loved ones can give effective support.

Provide health education and reinforcement of the need for follow up, especially if the retroperitoneal lymph nodes were not surgically explored. For men with a risk of recurrence, surveillance with periodic physical examinations, chest x-ray films, tumour markers and computed tomography (CT) scans of the retroperitoneal nodes could continue for a minimum of 5 years, and possibly 10 years, after orchidectomy.

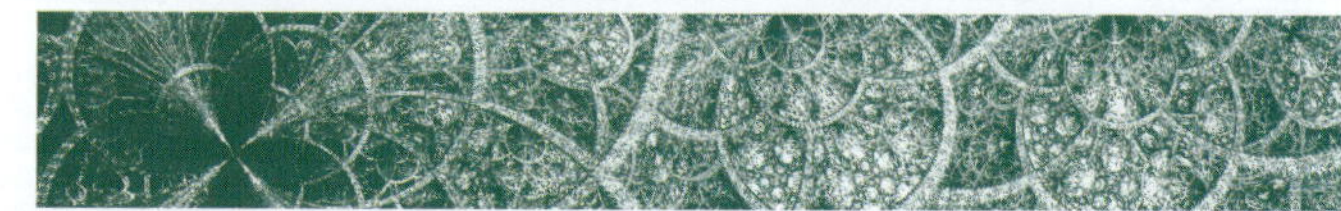

Disorders of the prostate gland

THE MAN WITH PROSTATITIS

Prostatitis refers to different types of inflammatory disorders of the prostate gland. *Prostatodynia* is a condition where the man experiences the symptoms of prostatitis but shows no evidence of inflammation or infection. Manifestations of prostatitis and prostatodynia are summarised in the 'Manifestations' box.

Pathophysiology and manifestations

The National Institutes of Health in the United States has defined four types of prostatitis. To gain a consistent approach to classification, Australia and New Zealand have adopted these definitions. The types are known as: acute bacterial prostatitis, chronic bacterial prostatitis, chronic prostatitis/pelvic pain syndrome and asymptomatic inflammatory prostatitis. Men with asymptomatic inflammatory prostatitis have no subjective symptoms but are diagnosed when a biopsy or prostatic fluid examination is conducted.

Acute bacterial prostatitis

Acute bacterial prostatitis is most often caused by an ascending infection from the urethra or reflux of infected urine into the ducts of the prostate gland. *E. coli* is the most common causative organism; other causative organisms include *Pseudomonas, Klebsiella* and *Chlamydia*.

Symptoms of acute bacterial prostatitis include fever, malaise, muscle and joint pain, urinary frequency and urgency, dysuria and urethral discharge. The man often experiences dull, aching pain in the perineum, rectum or lower back. On rectal examination, the prostate is enlarged and painful.

Chronic bacterial prostatitis

Men with chronic bacterial prostatitis often present with a history of recurrent urinary tract infections. The causative organisms are most often *E. coli, Proteus* or *Klebsiella*. Calculi may form in the prostate and contribute to the chronicity of the problem.

MANIFESTATIONS **Prostatitis and prostatodynia**

ACUTE BACTERIAL PROSTATITIS

- Onset (may be abrupt): obstruction, irritation or pain upon voiding; frequency; and urgency
- Positive cultures of infectious organism
- Non-urinary symptoms: chills, fever, low back and pelvic floor pain

CHRONIC BACTERIAL PROSTATITIS

- Urinary symptoms sometimes similar to those of the acute form, except less sudden, less dramatic or even absent
- Positive cultures of causative organism not always obtainable

CHRONIC PROSTATITIS

- Perineal, suprapubic, lower back or genital pain
- Irritation upon voiding
- Post-ejaculatory pain
- Negative cultures of organisms

PROSTATODYNIA

- Pelvic, lower back or perineal pain
- Irritation or obstruction upon voiding
- No evidence of inflammation in the prostate
- No urinary tract infection
- Normal prostatic secretions

The manifestations of chronic bacterial prostatitis include urinary frequency and urgency, dysuria, lower back pain and perineal discomfort. Epididymitis may be associated with the prostatitis.

Chronic prostatitis/chronic pelvic pain syndrome

This type of prostatitis is both the most common and the least understood of the syndromes (Lotti & Maggi, 2018). The two types (inflammatory and non-inflammatory) are based on the presence of white blood cells in the prostatic fluid.

- *Inflammatory prostatitis* is believed to be an autoimmune disorder, but the actual cause is unknown. Men with this type of prostatitis have lower back pain; urinary manifestations; pain in the penis, testicles, scrotum, lower back and rectum; decreased libido; and painful ejaculations. They do not have bacteria in their urine, but have leukocytes in the urine and abnormal inflammatory cells in prostatic secretions.
- *Non-inflammatory prostatitis* (prostatodynia) has manifestations that imitate those of inflammatory prostatitis, but no evidence of urinary or prostatic infection or inflammation can be found. The cause is not known but is believed to be the result of a problem outside the prostate gland, such as obstruction of the bladder neck. Treatment is mainly symptomatic.

Asymptomatic inflammatory prostatitis

This type of prostatitis is generally diagnosed during investigation of other genitourinary complaints. No symptoms are evident in the man. Leukocytes are found in the seminal fluid from the prostate.

INTERPROFESSIONAL CARE

Diagnosis

It is often difficult to diagnose prostatitis. Urine and prostatic secretion examination and cultures are obtained to determine the presence and type of blood cells and/or bacteria. X-ray studies and ultrasound may be useful to visualise pelvic structures.

Medications

Bacterial prostatitis is treated with antibiotics appropriate for the causative organism. Oral antibiotics are usually administered up to 4 weeks for acute bacterial prostatitis, but men with the chronic form must take antibiotics for a much longer period. This can be up to 4 months, and they may still relapse as soon as the antibiotic is discontinued. Non-bacterial prostatitis does not usually respond satisfactorily to drug therapy, although relief from symptoms is possible. Non-steroidal anti-inflammatory drugs are often useful for pain, but it can be difficult to manage pain in chronic prostatitis where moderate relief may be obtained only. At times opioid analgesia may be necessary to control chronic pain, but careful monitoring and evaluation is needed. Anticholinergics may assist in reducing voiding symptoms. Prostatodynia is treated symptomatically to relieve muscle tension, usually with alpha-adrenergic blocking agents or muscle relaxants.

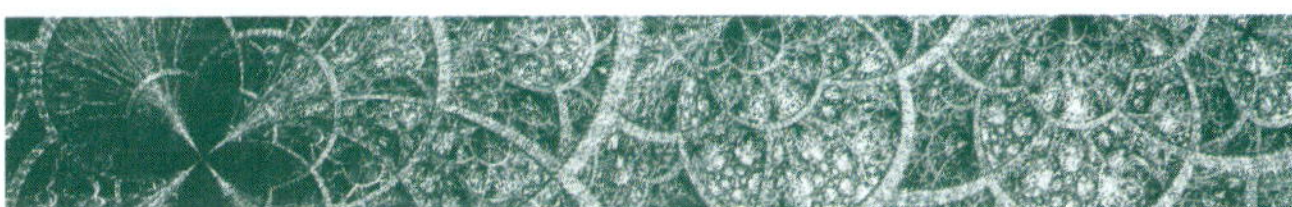

Nursing care

Educating men with prostatitis focuses on symptom management. Men with acute and chronic bacterial prostatitis should be taught to increase fluid intake to approximately 3 L daily and to void every few hours. These measures help decrease irritation when voiding and assist in minimising the effects of increased fluid loss due to fever and infection. Management of fever is important in reducing fluid loss and minimising discomfort. Regular bowel movements help ease potential pain associated with defecation. It is important to educate the man on the need to complete the course of antibiotic therapy. Men with chronic prostatitis/chronic pelvic pain syndrome need to know that the condition is not contagious and does not cause cancer (Norris, 2018). Referral sources for information include Healthy Male (https://healthymale.org.au) and Healthdirect (https://www.healthdirect.gov.au).

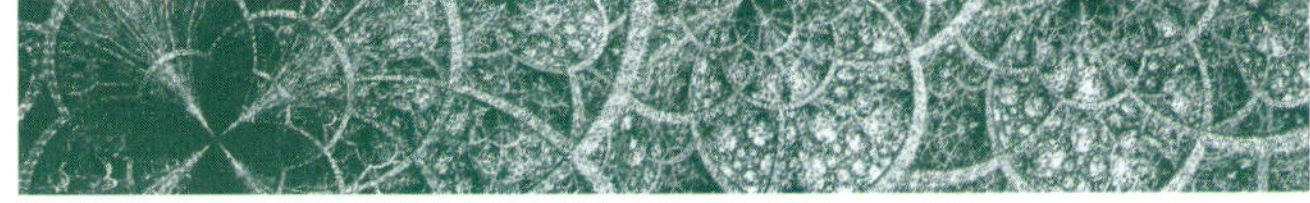

THE MAN WITH BENIGN PROSTATIC HYPERPLASIA

Benign prostatic hyperplasia (BPH), a non-malignant enlargement of the prostate gland, is a common disorder of the ageing male, thought to be associated with endocrine changes although its exact cause is unknown. The prostate, very small at birth, grows at puberty and reaches adult size around age 20. Almost 1 in 4 Australian men aged 40–49 years receive treatment for prostate problems, and this increases to 3 in every 4 men aged 70 years and older (Healthy Male, 2021c). Some men remain asymptomatic even though their prostate may have begun to grow larger. The problem that brings men to a healthcare provider is usually the associated urinary dysfunction.

Risk factors

Although the exact cause of BPH is unknown, risk factors include:

- age
- family history
- risk factors similar to heart disease (i.e. obesity, high blood pressure, type 2 diabetes mellitus)
- diet high in meat and fats (Healthy Male, 2021c).

Pathophysiology

The two necessary preconditions for BPH are age of 50 or greater and the presence of testes. Men who are castrated before puberty do not develop BPH. The androgen that mediates prostatic growth at all ages is dihydrotestosterone (DHT), which is formed in the prostate from testosterone. Although androgen levels decrease in ageing men, the ageing prostate appears to become more sensitive to available DHT. Oestrogen, produced in small amounts in men, appears to sensitise the prostate gland to the effects of DHT. Increasing oestrogen levels associated with ageing or a relative increase in oestrogen related to testosterone levels may contribute to prostatic hyperplasia.

> **FAST FACTS**
>
> Urinary problems with BPH:
>
> - A hesitant, interrupted weak stream.
> - Urgency with leaking or dribbling of urine.
> - More frequent urination in small amounts, especially at night (nocturia).

BPH begins as small nodules in the periurethral glands, which are the inner layers of the prostate. The prostate enlarges through formation and growth of nodules (hyperplasia) and enlargement of glandular cells (hypertrophy). These changes occur over a long period of time. The pathophysiological effects result from a combination of factors, including urethral resistance to the effects of BPH, intravesical pressure during voiding, detrusor muscle strength, neurological functioning and general physical health.

Manifestations

The expanding prostatic tissue compresses the urethra (see Figure 47.3) and causes partial or complete obstruction of the outflow of urine from the urinary bladder. The detrusor muscles hypertrophy to compensate for increased resistance

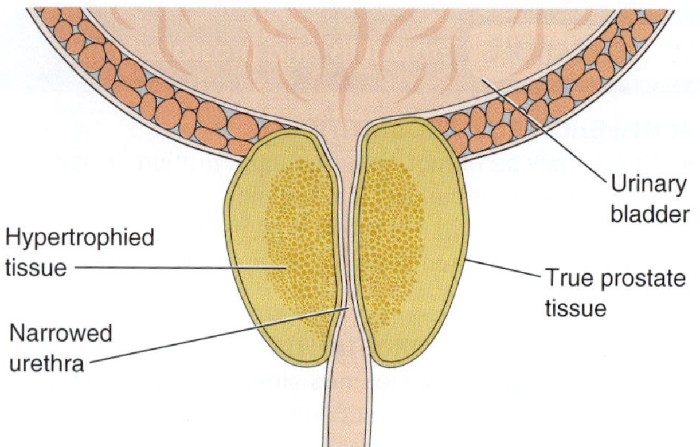

FIGURE 47.3 *Benign prostatic hyperplasia*

to urinary flow; however, eventually decreased bladder compliance and bladder instability result. As a result, the man with BPH has manifestations from obstruction (decreased force of stream, increased time to initiate and complete void, hesitancy, incomplete bladder emptying and post-void dribbling) and irritation (frequency, urgency, incontinence, nocturia, dysuria and bladder pain). Urinary retention may become chronic, resulting in overflow incontinence with any increase in intra-abdominal pressure. There is little correlation between the size of the prostate gland and the urinary manifestations. Manifestations of BPH are summarised in the 'Manifestations' box.

Complications

Unless the enlarging mass is reduced, multiple complications may occur. Acute urinary retention is quite common in men with BPH (Healthy Male, 2021c). As urine is retained in the bladder, increasing bladder distension occurs. Diverticula (outpouchings) on the bladder wall result from the distension. The distension may also obstruct the ureters. Infection, more common in retained urine and in diverticula, may ascend from the bladder to the kidneys. Hydroureter, hydronephrosis and renal insufficiency are possible complications. Renal calculi risk is increased in men with BPH, due to the alkalisation of the retained or residual urine.

> **MANIFESTATIONS Benign prostatic hyperplasia**
>
> - Diminished force of urinary stream
> - Hesitancy in initiating voiding
> - Post-void dribbling
> - Sensation of incomplete emptying
> - Urinary retention
> - Nocturia
> - Frequency
> - Urgency
> - Urge incontinence
> - Dysuria

INTERPROFESSIONAL CARE

Care of men with BPH focuses on diagnosing the disorder, correcting or minimising the urinary obstruction and preventing or treating complications. There is no way to reverse BPH. Treatment is often determined by the severity of the manifestations and the presence of complications. Mild cases are often monitored over time and may remain stable or improve.

Diagnosis

A diagnosis of BPH involves both physical examination and laboratory tests not only to diagnose the disease but also to differentiate it from prostate cancer. A digital rectal examination (DRE) is done to examine the external surface of the prostate; in BPH it is asymmetrical and enlarged. Examination of the creatinine levels of the blood is conducted to assess for kidney damage.

The urine is examined for WBCs, RBCs and bacteria. Urinary function is assessed by measuring residual urine (amount of urine remaining in the bladder after voiding) with ultrasonography or post-voiding catheterisation (more than 100 mL is considered high), and through uroflowmetry, which measures urine flow rate. Normal is greater than 14 mL/sec. A finding of less than 10 mL/sec indicates obstruction.

PSA levels are obtained to rule out prostate cancer. PSA may be slightly elevated but cannot be used to determine BPH. PSA is a glycoprotein produced only in the cytoplasm of benign and malignant prostate cells; the serum level corresponds with the volume of both benign and malignant prostate tissue. Further information is provided in the next section under diagnosis of prostate cancer.

In addition, the man's own subjective experiences with BPH are included in the diagnosis and treatment. For example, the International Prostate Symptom Score uses a scale of 0 (not at all) to 5 (almost always) to collect data about areas such as feeling as though the bladder did not empty with urinating, the need to urinate within 2 hours after urinating, starting and stopping the stream several times while urinating and straining to urinate. This questionnaire also asks how many times during the night the man gets up to urinate and how he feels about having the disorder.

Medications

Treatment with medications is based on two considerations: the hyperplastic tissue is androgen dependent and smooth muscle contraction within the prostate can exacerbate urinary obstruction. The first consideration is usually addressed by treatment for mild prostate enlargement with an anti-androgen agent such as finasteride (Proscar) that inhibits the conversion of testosterone to DHT and causes the enlarged prostate to shrink in size. These agents may cause impotence, decreased libido and decreased volume of ejaculate. Individual and family education includes the information that crushed tablets should not be handled by pregnant women because the drug may be absorbed through the skin and be harmful to a male fetus.

Excessive smooth muscle contraction in BPH may be blocked with the alpha-adrenergic antagonists such as terazosin (Hytrin) and tamsulosin (Flomaxtra). These medications relieve obstruction and increase the flow of urine. They may cause orthostatic hypotension. Individual and family education includes advice about making position changes slowly to avoid dizziness and accidental falls, how to take and record blood pressure, and to check with the healthcare provider before taking any medication for coughs, colds or allergies (because these over-the-counter medications may contain an adrenergic agent).

Surgery

Men who have urinary retention, recurrent urinary tract infection, haematuria, renal calculi or renal insufficiency secondary to BPH are candidates for surgical intervention. Surgical treatment may be performed by minimally invasive surgery or through transurethral surgery, open surgery or by laser surgery.

MINIMALLY INVASIVE SURGERY Because medications are not effective for all men, a number of procedures have been developed to relieve the manifestations of BPH that are less invasive than traditional surgery.

Transurethral microwave thermotherapy uses a transurethral probe to deliver microwaves directly to the prostate. It uses heat to destroy excess prostate tissue. During the procedure, a cooling system protects the urinary tract. The procedure takes about an hour and can be performed on an outpatient basis. Although microwave procedures do not cure BPH, they do reduce urinary manifestations. The procedures do not cause impotence or incontinence.

The *transurethral needle ablation* (TUNA) system uses low-level radio frequency through twin needles to burn away a region of the enlarged prostate. Shields protect the urethra. TUNA improves the flow of urine through the urethra. It does not cause impotence or incontinence.

TRANSURETHRAL SURGERY A *transurethral resection of the prostate (TURP)* is the most common surgical procedure used. Obstructing prostate tissue is removed using the wire loop of a resectoscope and electrocautery, inserted through the urethra (see Figure 47.4). No external incision is necessary. During the procedure, a resectoscope is used to remove obstructing tissue one piece at a time. The tissue is flushed into the bladder with fluid and then flushed out at the end of the operation. This surgery has potential risks, however, including postoperative haemorrhage or clot retention, inability to void and urinary tract infection. Other possible complications are incontinence, impotence and retrograde ejaculation.

In the *transurethral incision of the prostate* (TUIP) procedure, small incisions are made in the smooth muscle where the prostate is attached to the bladder. The gland is split to reduce pressure on the urethra. No tissue is removed, so this procedure is most appropriate for men with smaller prostate glands. TUIP can be done on an outpatient basis and has the additional advantage of less risk of postoperative retrograde ejaculation than is associated with TURP or other prostatectomy procedures.

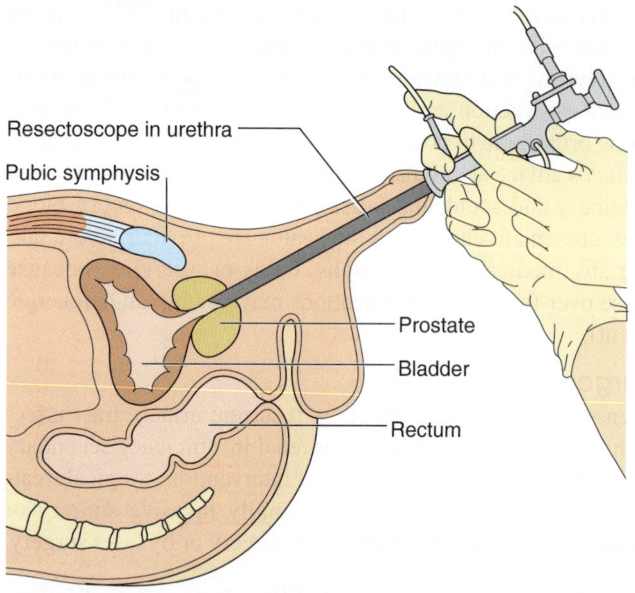

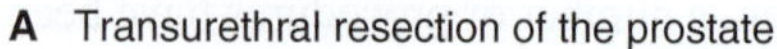

A Transurethral resection of the prostate

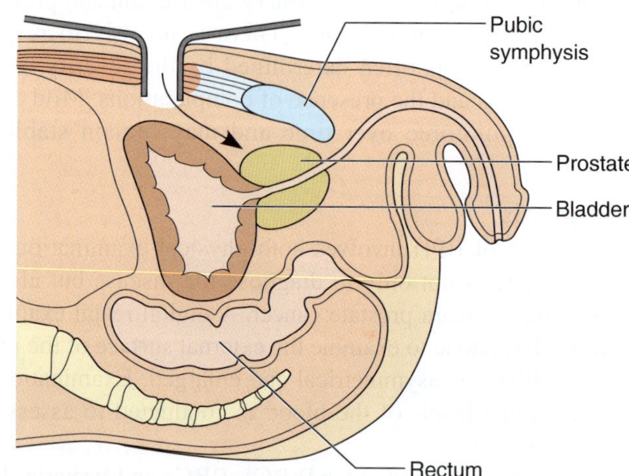

B Retropubic prostatectomy

FIGURE 47.4 ***A, In a transurethral resection of the prostate, a resectoscope inserted through the urethra is used to remove excess prostate tissue. B, In a retropubic prostatectomy, prostate tissue is removed through an abdominal incision***

LASER SURGERY Another minimally invasive procedure used to treat BPH is laser therapy. In laser surgery, a laser beam is delivered via a cystoscope transurethrally to cut, coagulate and vaporise excessive prostatic tissue with several short bursts of energy. An advantage of laser surgery is decreased blood loss and a more rapid recovery time. However, this method may not be as effective for larger prostates.

OPEN SURGERY When the prostate gland is very large, an open prostatectomy may be used. These procedures are discussed in the section on prostate cancer that follows. Nursing care for the man having prostate surgery (prostatectomy) is outlined in the accompanying box.

New treatments

Newer treatments for BPH include minimally invasive procedures such as balloon urethroplasty and placement of intraurethral stents to maintain patency of the urethra. Balloon urethroplasty is a simple procedure in which a balloon-tipped catheter is inserted into the narrowed portion of the urethra and inflated. Inflation of the balloon widens the urethra, relieving obstruction. These procedures can be done as outpatient surgery.

Alternative and complementary therapies

Phytotherapy is the use of plants or plant extracts for medical treatment. Several plant extracts have been used for years in Europe to treat BPH, including *Serenoa* (saw palmetto berry), the bark of *Pygeum africanum*, the roots of *Echinacea purpurea* and *Hypoxis rooperi* and the leaves of the trembling poplar. The mechanism of action of these extracts is unknown.

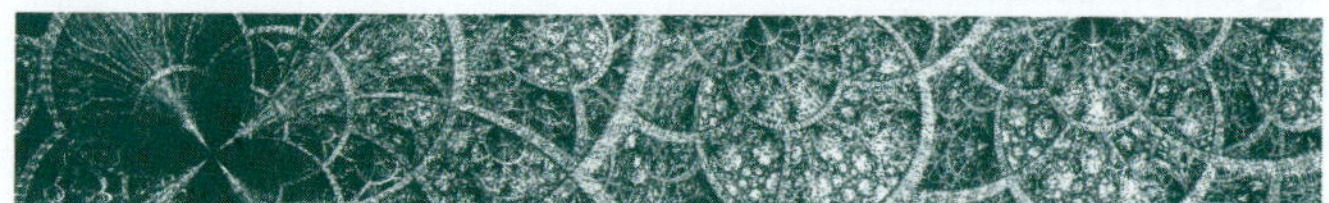

Nursing care

Most men are unsure of the function of the prostate gland and even of the prostate's exact location, though its relationship to sexual and urinary function is at least generally known. This lack of knowledge, coupled with the growing number of treatment options, is confusing to many men. There are many similarities between the nursing care of men with BPH and that of men with prostate cancer (see the prostate cancer section that follows).

Nursing interventions

This section provides interventions related to deficient knowledge, urinary retention, risk of infection and risk of imbalanced fluid volume.

Deficient knowledge

- Explain the anatomy and physiology of the prostate gland, as well as normal changes that occur with ageing. *Men must know about their bodies in order to make accurate decisions about treatment.*
- Discuss treatment options, including information about effects on erectile function, ejaculation and fertility. *Counsel the man to discuss specific concerns with his urologist. Many different treatment options are available; the choice should be a mutual decision between the man, his partner and the urologist.*

NURSING CARE OF THE MAN having a prostatectomy

PREOPERATIVE CARE

- Assess the man's and family's knowledge about the surgery. *Some men are confused about the surgical approach because there are several, quite different methods.*
- Inform the man that he will have a urinary catheter when he returns from surgery and he may have a drain(s) in his incision. He also will be wearing sequential pneumatic compression stockings. *This knowledge can reduce anxiety postoperatively and increase cooperation with postoperative care.*
- Ensure that a signed consent form is in the chart and that all other preoperative tasks outlined in the chapter 'Nursing care of people having surgery' are completed.
- Communicate willingness to address any concerns or anxiety. *Men may be anxious about the outcome of their surgery and potential long-term effects of the surgery on their sexuality. When a prostatectomy is performed for prostate cancer, additional fears include the extent of the cancer and surgery, chances for cure and possible end-of-life issues.*

POSTOPERATIVE CARE

- Maintain the usual postoperative assessments (see the chapter 'Nursing care of people having surgery') and follow aseptic techniques in urinary drainage and irrigation care. Monitor vital signs closely for the first 24 hours and regularly thereafter. *The man who has had prostate surgery is at risk of haemorrhage and infection. Vital sign changes may be early manifestations and can assist in recognising deterioration.*
- Maintain an accurate fluid balance chart, including amounts of irrigating solution used. Frequently assess patency of any catheters and drains. Monitor colour and character of urine. *Catheters may become occluded by blood clots or kinks, interfering with urinary drainage and increasing the risk of haemorrhage.*
- Assess and manage the man's pain. *The man may have at least three types of pain: incisional pain, bladder spasms and abdominal cramps due to intestinal gas. Analgesics and non-steroidal anti-inflammatory drugs (NSAIDs) are administered on a routine and prn basis to control incisional pain. Bladder spasms may be accompanied by strong urges to void and urine leakage around the catheter. Oral oxybutynin hydrochloride may be used to relieve bladder spasms.*
- Maintain anti-embolic stockings and pneumatic compression devices as ordered. Assist with leg exercises and ambulation as ordered. *The man who has had prostate surgery is at risk of developing thromboemboli; these are important preventive measures.*
- Encourage the man to maintain a liberal fluid intake of 2 to 3 L a day. *Increased fluids reduce burning on urination after catheter removal and the risk of urinary tract infection.*

THE MAN WITH A TRANSURETHRAL RESECTION OF THE PROSTATE (TURP)

- For the first 24 to 47 hours, monitor for haemorrhage, evidenced by frank blood in urinary output, presence of large blood clots, decreased urinary output, increasing bladder spasms, decreased haemoglobin and haematocrit, tachycardia and hypotension. Notify the doctor if any of these manifestations occur. *Postoperative haemorrhage may be either arterial or venous and may be precipitated by movement, bladder spasms or an obstructed urinary drainage system.*
- Instruct the man with a three-way indwelling catheter with traction to keep his leg straight while the traction is applied. An 18 Fr. to 22 Fr. three-way catheter with a 30 to 45 mL balloon usually is inserted following a TURP. *The inflated balloon is pulled down into the prostatic fossa and the catheter tubing is pulled down and taped to the man's leg to apply pressure against the operative site, preventing bleeding.*
- Explain that the presence of a urinary catheter will cause the sensation of needing to void, but it is important not to strain to try to void around the catheter or when having a bowel movement. Explain that bladder spasms—experienced as lower abdominal pressure or pain—and a desire to urinate may occur. Ensure that the man understands that this is an expected sensation and that medications can help alleviate this discomfort. *Pressure on the urethra by the large catheter and on the internal sphincter by the catheter's balloon stimulate the micturition reflex. Straining to void or to have a bowel movement may stimulate bladder spasms and increase pain; it also may increase the risk of bleeding. Administer pain medications at regular intervals.*
- If the man has continuous bladder irrigation (CBI), assess the catheter and the drainage tubing at regular intervals. Maintain the rate of flow of irrigating fluid to keep the output light pink or colourless. Assess the urinary output every 1 to 2 hours for colour, consistency, amount and presence of blood clots; assess for bladder spasms. *CBI is used to prevent the formation of blood clots, which could obstruct urinary output. Bladder distension resulting from output obstruction increases the risk of bleeding. Irrigating fluids are continuously infused and drained at a rate to keep urine light pink or colourless. Indicators of obstruction and bleeding are: urine has frank blood; urine contains multiple blood clots, decreased urinary output, or the man has bladder spasms.*
- Assess for fluid volume excess and hyponatraemia, called TURP syndrome, manifested by hyponatraemia, decreased haematocrit, hypertension, bradycardia, nausea and confusion. If these manifestations occur, notify the doctor. *TURP syndrome results from the absorption of irrigating fluids during and after surgery. Untreated, it may result in arrhythmias, seizures or both.*
- If the man does not have CBI, follow organisational policy and protocols for irrigating the indwelling catheter (usually when the urine contains frank blood or has numerous larger blood clots, or when bladder spasms increase). In most instances, using sterile technique, the catheter is gently irrigated with 50 mL of irrigating solution at a time, until the obstruction is relieved or the urine is clear. Ensure equal input and output of irrigating fluid. *Intermittent irrigation may be used to prevent obstruction of urinary drainage.*

(continued)

NURSING CARE OF THE MAN having a prostatectomy (continued)

- Following catheter removal, assess the amount, colour and consistency of urine. Explain to the man that he may experience burning on urination, that dribbling after urination is a common experience and that the urine may contain small blood clots after catheter removal. *The CBI and catheter usually are removed in the 24 to 48 hours following surgery. Urinary control may be improved by teaching the man to start and stop the urine stream several times during each voiding and by practising pelvic floor exercises. Regaining full control may take up to 1 year.*

THE MAN WITH A RETROPUBIC PROSTATECTOMY

- Assess the abdominal incision for the presence of urine. *Because the bladder is not entered during a retropubic prostatectomy, no urine should be found on the dressing.*
- Assess the abdominal incision for increased or purulent drainage and the man for an increased temperature and pain. *These manifestations indicate the presence of infection.*

THE MAN WITH A SUPRAPUBIC PROSTATECTOMY

- Assess urinary output from both the suprapubic and the urethral catheters. *The man with a suprapubic prostatectomy often has two separate closed drainage systems: one from the suprapubic incision and one from a urethral catheter.*
- Assess the abdominal dressing for urinary drainage and change saturated dressings frequently. Consult with a wound care specialist if necessary. *Urine is highly irritating to the skin.*
- Following removal of the urethral catheter (usually 2 to 4 days after surgery) and based on protocols, clamp the suprapubic catheter and encourage the man to void. Assess residual urine by unclamping the suprapubic catheter and measuring urinary output after voiding. *If residual urine is 75 mL or less with several voidings, the suprapubic catheter is removed.*

THE MAN WITH A PERINEAL PROSTATECTOMY

- Assess perineal incision for drainage and manifestations of infection. *Location of the incision in the perineum increases the risk of infection.*
- Do not take rectal temperatures or administer enemas. *Insertion of a thermometer or enema tubing into the rectum may precipitate bleeding.*
- Use a T-binder or padded scrotal support to hold the dressing in place. Following removal of the dressing and perineal sutures, heat lamps or sitz baths may be used. *The location of the dressing makes application difficult: heat lamps or sitz baths provide heat and promote healing.*
- Teach the man to perform perineal irrigations with sterile normal saline as ordered and after each bowel movement. *Because of the proximity of the incision to the anus, special wound care is necessary to prevent infection.*

- Discuss effects of prostate surgery, including urinary retention and urinary incontinence. *These common transient postoperative effects are related to the surgical procedure and the postoperative indwelling catheter.*
- Explain to the man having a TURP that a catheter will be placed into the bladder, with the tubing taped to his inner thigh, and that irrigation fluid will be infusing into and out of the catheter for the first 36 to 72 hours following surgery. *The catheter and irrigation are necessary to remove blood clots from the bladder and allow drainage of urine. Gentle traction is applied to the catheter to apply pressure to the operative site (prostatic fossa) and prevent excessive bleeding.*
- Explain that, following removal of the catheter, he will most likely have urinary frequency and urgency. He may also experience dribbling of urine after voiding. Stress the importance of increasing oral fluid intake and regular pelvic floor exercises. *Urinary manifestations are related to the surgical procedure and the indwelling catheter. Increased fluid intake helps decrease dysuria. Pelvic floor exercises strengthen periurethral muscles and decrease post-voiding urine leakage.*

Urinary retention

- Educate the man about the manifestations of acute urinary retention: dysuria, overflow incontinence, bladder pain and distension, no urine output. *Acute urinary retention is a potential complication of BPH, requiring immediate medical attention.*
- Provide health education about how the risk of developing urinary retention increases when the man with BPH takes over-the-counter (OTC) decongestant medications or prescription medications such as antidepressants, anticholinergics, calcium channel blockers, antipsychotics and medications to treat Parkinson's disease. *OTC decongestants may contain alpha-adrenergic agonists that increase smooth muscle tone of the prostate, bladder neck and proximal urethra. The prescribed medications may relax detrusor muscle contractions. Both actions may increase the risk of urinary retention.*
- Suggest avoiding intake of large volumes of liquid at any one time. *A single intake of a large volume of liquid results in rapid bladder filling and increases the risk of urinary retention.*
- Teach how to use the double-voiding technique: urinate, then sit on the toilet for 3 to 5 minutes, then urinate again. *This technique may relieve mild to moderate urinary retention.*

CONSIDERATION FOR PRACTICE

In addition to avoiding a large amount of fluids at one time, it is also important to teach the man to limit liquids that stimulate voiding, such as coffee, caffeine-containing beverages and alcoholic beverages.

Risk of infection

- Monitor WBC and vital signs. *Infection is indicated by an increase in WBCs, body temperature and pulse rate.*
- Maintain sterile procedures when changing irrigation fluids and emptying Foley catheter draining bag. *Sterile procedures are necessary to prevent infection.*

Risk of imbalanced fluid volume

A prostatectomy brings increased risk of imbalanced fluid volume as a result of excessive bleeding from the operative site (prostatic fossa) as well as absorption of irrigating fluid. Report manifestations indicating hypovolaemic shock, excess bleeding and/or TURP syndrome immediately.

- Monitor pulse and blood pressure. *Manifestations of hypovolaemic shock include an increasing pulse and a decreasing blood pressure.*
- Monitor colour of drainage in urinary drainage bag (see Table 47.2). *The appearance of dark or red-coloured urine and irrigation fluid in the urinary drainage bag is an excellent indicator of bleeding after a prostatectomy.*
- Monitor for manifestations of transurethral resection (TURP) syndrome: nausea and vomiting, confusion, hypertension, bradycardia and visual disturbances. *The absorption of isotonic bladder irrigating fluids during and after surgery may cause this hypervolaemic, hyponatraemic state. Treatment includes diuresis and, in severe cases, hypertonic saline administration (Papadakis, McPhee & Rabow, 2022).*
- Change from the daytime leg drainage bag to a larger night drainage bag. *A larger bag suspended from the bed frame at night permits gravity drainage of urine and prevents reflux of urine back into the bladder.*

TABLE 47.2 Significance of character of urine after prostatectomy and related nursing care

URINE COLOUR	NURSING IMPLICATIONS
Light red to red	Normal on day of surgery and first postoperative day.
Very dark red	May indicate increased venous bleeding or inadequate dilution. Catheter at risk of occlusion. Increase flow rate of irrigant. If urine does not clear, notify doctor.
Bright red	May indicate arterial bleeding. Increase flow rate of irrigant, monitor vital signs and notify doctor.
Contains blood clots	Occasional blood clot normal. If clots are frequent, catheter may become obstructed. Increase flow rate of irrigant.
Clear to light pink	Normal throughout hospitalisation.

Community-based care

Depending on the man's choice of treatment, the procedure may be performed on an outpatient basis. The man having a TURP, although hospitalised for the surgery, may be discharged quite quickly after surgery if there are no complications. Discharge instructions after prostate surgery are provided in the 'Meeting individualised needs' box. Home care often involves care of an indwelling urinary catheter. The nurse should educate the man how to care for the catheter and drainage bag, including the following information:

- Avoid strapping the leg bag on too tightly, which can decrease venous return and increase risk of thrombophlebitis and embolic complications such as pulmonary emboli.
- Place a soft cloth between the leg bag and thigh to decrease friction and absorb dampness under the bag, reducing the risk of skin irritation.

MEETING INDIVIDUALISED NEEDS Discharge instructions for men after prostate surgery

ACTIVITY

The healing period lasts from 4 to 8 weeks. Avoid strenuous activity and heavy lifting. Do not drive for 2 weeks. Take long walks; take stairs slowly and carefully. Continue exercises that you did in the hospital to prevent blood clots in the legs. You can take showers; avoid baths while the catheter is in place.

BLEEDING

Bleeding can occur any time after surgery. It is fairly common after a bowel movement, coughing or increased exercise. If you notice blood in the urine, increase fluids and rest until the urine is clear. If heavy bleeding blocks the catheter, call the doctor immediately. Avoid aspirin and NSAIDs (e.g. Nurofen) for at least 2 weeks.

BOWEL MOVEMENTS

Keep bowel movements regular and soft to avoid pressure on the prostate area. Drink fruit juices and take mild laxatives or stool softeners as ordered.

DIET

Resume your normal diet. Increase fluids to 10 glasses daily. Avoid alcohol unless otherwise advised by your doctor.

SEXUAL INTERCOURSE

Do not have sex for 6 weeks after surgery to avoid bleeding. You may still have erections even with the catheter in place. When you resume sex, ejaculate flows back into the bladder, so you will express little or no semen.

URINATION

After your catheter is removed, you may experience some burning, stinging or leakage for several weeks and you may pass small blood clots occasionally. These symptoms will disappear as the area heals. Use pads to control leakage.

WORK

If work is not strenuous, you may return in 4 weeks; otherwise, wait 6 to 8 weeks.

PLEASE CALL IMMEDIATELY IF:

- You are unable to urinate.
- Bleeding is not controlled by fluids and rest, or is excessive.
- You have chills and fever or severe abdominal pain.
- Your scrotum becomes swollen and tender.
- You have pain in one calf, chest pain or difficulty breathing.

- Empty the leg bag every 3 to 4 hours during waking hours to prevent overfilling.
- Promptly report any unexpected changes in urine colour, consistency or odour, haematuria, evidence of frank bleeding or large blood clots, as well as a lack of or significant decrease in urine output.

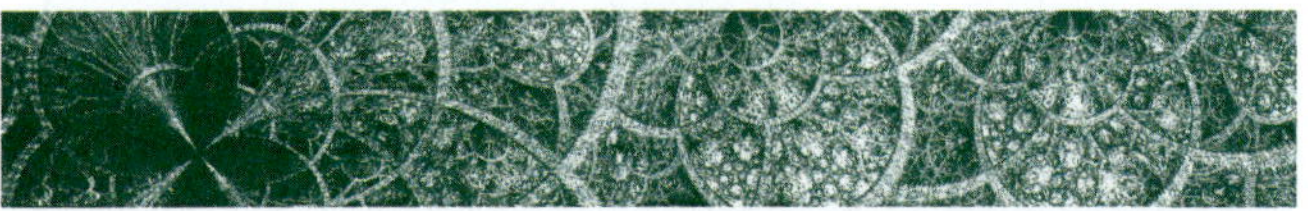

THE MAN WITH PROSTATE CANCER

Cancer of the prostate is the most common form of cancer present in Australian men over 50 (excluding some forms of skin cancer), with 24,217 men diagnosed in 2022, accounting for one-third of all new diagnoses of cancer in men (AIHW, 2021). It is the second most common cause of deaths from cancer in men, with 1 in 8 men developing prostate cancer in their lifetime (Cancer Australia, 2021). Men living in inner-regional areas of Australia have a higher age-standardised incidence rate for prostate cancer than men living in rural areas (AIHW, 2021). This is attributed to lack of awareness and education about prostate cancer, along with distances from testing and treatment, poor general practitioner awareness and limited access to specialists. The number of deaths annually from prostate cancer in men is equivalent to the number of women who die from breast cancer, approximately 3,102 (Cancer Australia, 2021).

When diagnosed early, prostate cancer is curable. If the man presents with metastatic prostate disease, it is incurable, so control of disease progression is key. The incidence of prostate cancer increases with age. Most diagnoses (85%) are made in men over 65 years of age (Cancer Council, 2022), with 1 in 8 men at risk up to age 85 (AIHW, 2021). In New Zealand, the incidence of prostate cancer is lower, with 1 in 13 men being diagnosed up to age 75 (Prostate Cancer Foundation of New Zealand, 2022). It is more prevalent in men in Western countries and less common in men from South-East Asia. This may be due to the extent to which PSA and digital rectal examination screening are used; hence, caution should be taken when interpreting variations in prevalence. Many men are found to have prostate cancer on autopsy; usually the cancer has produced no manifestations or complications.

Risk factors

In addition to age, other risk factors being investigated are as follows:

- genetic and hereditary factors, with risk increased in men who have a family history of the disease
- ethnicity—more common in Western countries and less common in Asian countries, particularly South-East Asia
- having a vasectomy, believed to increase the levels of circulating free testosterone
- dietary factors, including a diet high in animal fat and excessive supplemental vitamin A.

FOCUS ON CULTURAL DIVERSITY

Risk and incidence of prostate cancer

- The incidence of prostatic cancer is lower for Indigenous Australian men than it is for non-Indigenous men (AIHW, 2021).
- Prostatic cancer is the second most common cancer for Indigenous males, following lung cancer (AIHW, 2021).

Pathophysiology

The prostate gland consists primarily of glandular epithelial cells. The exact aetiology of prostate cancer is unknown, although androgens are believed to have a role in its development. Almost all primary prostate cancers are adenocarcinomas and develop in the peripheral zones of the prostate gland. This location increases the risk of local spread to the prostatic capsule. Despite its proximity to the rectum, metastasis to the bowel is uncommon because a tough sheet of tissue, Denonvilliers' fascia, acts as an effective physical barrier.

As the tumour enlarges, it may compress the urethra, obstructing urinary flow. The tumour may metastasise and involve the seminal vesicles or bladder by direct extension. Metastasis by lymph and venous channels is common.

Manifestations

Men with early-stage prostate cancer are often asymptomatic. Pain from metastasis to bones is often the initial manifestation noted. Urinary manifestations depend on the size and location of the tumour and the stage of the malignancy. They are often much like manifestations of BPH: urgency, frequency, hesitancy, dysuria and nocturia. The man may also notice haematuria or blood in the ejaculate (Norris, 2018). Manifestations of prostate cancer are summarised in the 'Manifestations' box.

Complications

Death usually occurs secondary to debility caused by multiple sites of skeletal metastasis, especially to the vertebrae. Compression fractures of the spine are common, resulting in the possible loss of mobility and bowel and bladder function. Tumours may eventually involve bone marrow, resulting in severe anaemias and impaired immune function.

INTERPROFESSIONAL CARE

Care of the man with prostate cancer focuses on diagnosis, elimination or containment of the cancer, and prevention or treatment of complications. There are currently no clinical strategies to prevent the development of prostate cancer. Therefore, early detection remains the main emphasis for intervention related to this disease.

MANIFESTATIONS Prostate cancer

GENITOURINARY
- Urinary symptoms—frequency, urgency, poor flow, difficulty commencing voiding, incomplete emptying
- Dysuria
- Haematuria
- Abnormal prostate on digital rectal examination
- Nocturia
- Haematospermia
- Erectile dysfunction

MUSCULOSKELETAL
- Bone or joint pain
- Migratory bone pain
- Back, hip and pelvic pain

NEUROLOGICAL
- Nerve pain
- Bilateral lower extremity weakness
- Bowel or bladder dysfunction
- Muscle spasms

SYSTEMIC
- Weight loss
- Fatigue

Diagnosis

Although an increasing number of men are now diagnosed with asymptomatic prostate cancer, many men with prostate cancer have either locally advanced cancer or distant metastasis at the time of diagnosis. The definitive diagnosis can be made only by biopsy (prostate biopsy is discussed in the chapter 'A person-centred approach to assessing the male and female reproductive systems'); however, other tests may suggest the presence of prostate cancer.

A digital rectal examination (DRE) is useful in assessing the prostate gland. Any hardness in the gland may indicate cancer; however, hardness may be a result of calcification due to prolonged inflammation or prostatic stones. DRE only allows the posterior surface of the gland to be palpated. Anterior lesions are not able to be detected using DRE. PSA levels are used to diagnose and stage prostate cancer and to monitor response to treatment. PSA is not a true tumour marker, but measurement of PSA has made dramatic differences to earlier diagnosis of prostate cancer in men. PSA levels rise in the presence of benign prostatic enlargement, prostatitis and other non-malignant conditions due to the fact that PSA is organ specific rather than cancer specific. Levels depend on age, and there is no specific normal or abnormal level. An increase over time is more significant than one reading. The PSA test is used with a DRE to help detect prostate cancer in men age 50 or older, and is also used to monitor effects of treatment.

While the normal range for PSA is 0–4.0 ng/mL, normal ranges for serum PSA for men of different ages in Western countries are as follows:

- 40–49 years: average 0.7 ng/mL, upper limit of normal 2.5 ng/mL
- 50–59 years: average 1.0 ng/mL, upper limit of normal 3.5 ng/mL
- 60–69 years: average 1.4 ng/mL, upper limit of normal 4.5 ng/mL
- 70–79 years: average 2.0 ng/mL, upper limit of normal 6.5 ng/mL (Healthy Male, 2021d).

Transrectal ultrasonography (TRUS) may be used when the DRE is abnormal or if the PSA is elevated. In this test, a small probe is inserted into the rectum. The probe gives off sound waves that create a picture of the prostate on a video screen. Guided by this picture, the doctor inserts a narrow needle through the rectal wall into the prostate gland and the needle removes a sample of tissue for examination. Other tests that may be ordered include a urinalysis or cystoscopy. Bone scan, magnetic resonance imaging (MRI) or CT scans may be performed to determine the presence of tumour metastasis.

Grade and stage help to determine prognosis and guide treatment decisions. Grade (cancer cell differentiation) is determined by the pathologist. Prostate cancer is staged with a variety of tests. Table 47.3 outlines treatment options according to the stage of the cancer.

TABLE 47.3 Prostate cancer staging and treatment

STAGE	DESCRIPTION	TREATMENT
Localised	Cancer is confined to prostate, non-palpable, focal involvement; well differentiated	Close observation and follow up Interstitial or external-beam radiation therapy Prostatectomy Brachytherapy (radioactive seeds implanted in prostate)
Locally advanced	Cancer has broken through the capsule of the prostate, palpable, involves one or both lobes; poorly differentiated	Careful observation in selected people Hormone therapy Prostatectomy Interstitial or external-beam radiation therapy Ultrasound-guided percutaneous cryosurgery
Advanced	Extension of the tumour outside the prostate capsule, possible seminal vesicle involvement, cancer has metastasised, often to bone or lymph nodes	Adjunctive hormone therapy Chemotherapy/interstitial radiation Steroids External-beam radiation therapy Radical prostatectomy Palliative surgery (TURP)

Diagnosis is reached following a combination of history taking, DRE, PSA testing and prostate biopsy or alternative.

Research for prevention

Toremifene (Fareston) to treat men with abnormal prostate growth might help prevent the growths from becoming malignant. The drug, which blocks some of the effects of oestrogen, had previously been used to treat advanced breast cancer in women. Men who have prostate intraepithelial neoplasia (PIN) have about a 30% chance of developing prostate cancer in 1 year and about a 65% chance within 2 years. A larger study is now in progress. In addition, other studies reported that men who took statins (to treat high cholesterol) were less likely to have prostate cancer. The drug abiraterone (Zytiga), developed by Cancer Research UK, has been found to extend the lives of some people with advanced prostatic cancer following chemotherapy.

Treatments

The treatment of prostate cancer is complex and depends on the grade and stage of the cancer, as well as the age, general health and preference of the man. In some cases—for example, when the man with a slow-growing tumour is elderly or has a limited life expectancy—watchful waiting is the treatment of choice. Treatments for prostate cancer include surgery, radiation therapy and hormone manipulation.

SURGERY Surgery for prostate cancer includes several types of prostatectomies. For very early disease in older men, cure may be achieved with a simple prostatectomy (such as TURP), discussed in the section on benign prostate hyperplasia.

- *Radical prostatectomy* involves removal of the prostate, prostate capsule, seminal vesicles and a portion of the bladder neck. The entire prostate gland with that component of the urethra within the gland and seminal vesicles is removed, so the urethra below the prostate is then connected to the bladder. The surgery can be performed by open surgery or by using laparoscopic surgery, where small incisions are made in the abdomen and a laparoscope is inserted and used to remove the prostate. Varying degrees of urinary incontinence are experienced by men following this surgery, with approximately 10% having ongoing incontinence 12 months on. Erectile dysfunction is commonly experienced by men following this surgery, with up to 85% of men having problems with getting and maintaining an erection. There are strategies to reduce this incidence and treatment if ED persists (Healthy Male, 2021a) (see Table 47.4). Some surgeons do the surgery from an area other than the operating room by using a robotic interface. Nursing research reporting men's satisfaction with a discharge program following a radical prostatectomy is discussed in the 'Translation to practice' box.
- *Retropubic prostatectomy* may be performed because it allows adequate control of bleeding, visualisation of the prostate bed and bladder neck, and access to pelvic lymph nodes.
- *Perineal prostatectomy* is often preferred for older men or those who are poor surgical risks. This approach requires less time and involves less bleeding.
- *Suprapubic prostatectomy* is rarely used, usually when problems with the bladder are expected. Control of bleeding is more difficult because the surgical approach is through the bladder.

For men with locally advanced (beyond the prostatic capsule) cancer, surgery is controversial because of the likelihood of hidden lymph node metastasis and relapse. TURP is not performed as curative therapy but may be used to relieve urinary obstruction for men with advanced disease.

Surgical intervention is now available for men with urinary sphincter insufficiency, which is the main cause of incontinence after prostatectomy. An artificial urinary sphincter is surgically

TABLE 47.4 Potential complications related to radical prostatectomy and radiation therapy

RADICAL PROSTATECTOMY	RADIATION THERAPY
Erectile dysfunction	Erectile dysfunction*
Urethral stricture	Urethral stricture
Fistula/rectal injury	Rectal/anal stricture*
Urinary incontinence	Cystitis
Surgical/anaesthetic risk	Diarrhoea
	Proctitis
	Rectal ulcer
	Bowel obstruction*
	Urinary incontinence

*Delayed complications; may appear months or years after completion of therapy.

Links to National Patient Safety Standards

NSQHS: Partnering with Consumers Standard

The intent of this standard is to create an organisation in which there are mutually valuable outcomes by having men with reproductive system and breast disorders and their families as partners in planning, design, delivery, measurement and evaluation of systems and services. It is desired that men and their families be partners in their own care, to the extent that they choose.

Source: ACSQHC (2021). *National Safety and Quality Health Service Standards* (2nd ed.). Sydney: ACSQHC.

TRANSLATION TO PRACTICE Evidence-based practice: improve discharge teaching

The period immediately after discharge for a radical prostatectomy is often a difficult time for men and their families as they cope with the emotional and physical demands of cancer surgery. Knowledge deficits about how long it will take to recover and how to provide care at home can significantly affect recovery. Nurses must recognise the need to provide thorough discharge teaching and communication prior to hospital discharge and make it part of actual practice for every man they treat. This will ensure timely, purpose-driven and effective communication and documentation that support continuous, coordinated and safe care to ensure that men with reproductive system and breast disorders get the most effective care possible both at home and in the community.

IMPLICATIONS FOR NURSING

Discharge education for men is essential and needs to include how to manage potential side effects following surgery, including urinary incontinence, ED and other side effects associated with radiotherapy and hormone therapy, such as bladder irritation and cystitis. Early discussion of side effects and clear management strategies are vital for men as they prepare to go home. Use of printed information sheets about preoperative and postoperative radical prostate surgery, along with a health education checklist and a discharge bag containing a urinary leg bag, urinary collection bag, wound supplies, incontinence product samples and a community resources brochure, are good strategies to ensure information is clear. It is important for nurses to partner with consumers in order to obtain the best person-centred outcomes.

Catheter care is one of the most valuable types of information required by men. Nurses are now, and will continue to be, challenged to provide the type and amount of information needed for self-care at home. Essential information that needs discussion and advice with the man following surgery is outlined below:

- pelvic floor exercises to promote continence and discussion about regular undertaking of the exercises
- education on preventing constipation and ensuring adequate fluid intake
- awareness and avoidance of bladder irritants such as tea, coffee, alcohol and diet soft drinks
- advice on how to source and use incontinence pads for men
- discussion with the doctor about medication to assist erections is important from a psychological, as well as a physical, perspective
- referral to support organisations.

CRITICAL THINKING IN PERSON-CENTRED CARE

1. You are caring for a 75-year-old man who has had a radical prostatectomy for prostate cancer. His husband tells you they have always had an active sex life and he hopes this surgery will not change that. What would you say to him?
2. Why is the risk of infection high for a man providing self-care at home following a radical prostatectomy? Which interventions would you suggest during health education to reduce this risk?
3. If you were developing a list of community resources for men following prostate surgery, what would you include? How would your list vary for the following situations?
   - a 64-year-old man with a wife and four married children who all live close
   - a 77-year-old man who lives alone and has no family
   - a 90-year-old man who will go to a residential care facility after discharge
   - a 56-year old homosexual man who lives with his partner.

implanted (see Figure 47.5). To be eligible, the man must be able to manipulate the pump placed in the scrotum and have adequate cognitive function to know when a problem with the appliance occurs.

RADIATION THERAPY Radiation therapy may be used as a primary treatment for prostate cancer. Long-term problems of impotence and urinary incontinence may be avoided and survival rates often are comparable. Radiation may be delivered either by external beam or interstitial implants of radioactive seeds of iodine, gold, palladium or iridium (*brachytherapy*). Brachytherapy is used when there are no major or acute lower urinary tract symptoms. Interstitial radiation has a lower risk of impotence and rectal damage than external-beam radiation. See the chapter 'Nursing care of people with cancer' for nursing care of the person receiving radiation therapy.

Radiation therapy has a palliative role for men with metastatic prostate cancer, reducing the size of bone metastasis, controlling pain and restoring some function, such as continence or the ability to ambulate for men with spinal cord compression.

HORMONAL MANIPULATION Androgen deprivation therapy is used to treat advanced prostate cancer by aiming to achieve castration and hence increase survival rate by suppressing testosterone, since prostate cancer is androgen dependent. Many cells in the growing tumour are androgen dependent and either cease to grow or die if deprived of androgens. Unfortunately, other cancer cells thrive without androgen and are unaffected by therapy to reduce circulating androgens. Therefore, the effects of hormone manipulations vary from complete but temporary regression of the tumour to no response at all. Strategies to induce androgen deprivation vary from orchidectomy to oral administration of hormonal agents. Table 47.5 compares surgical and hormone therapies. In addition, new drugs are being developed that block the effects of male hormones and research is being conducted to demonstrate what mix of hormones is best and at what time in the perioperative period they are most effective.

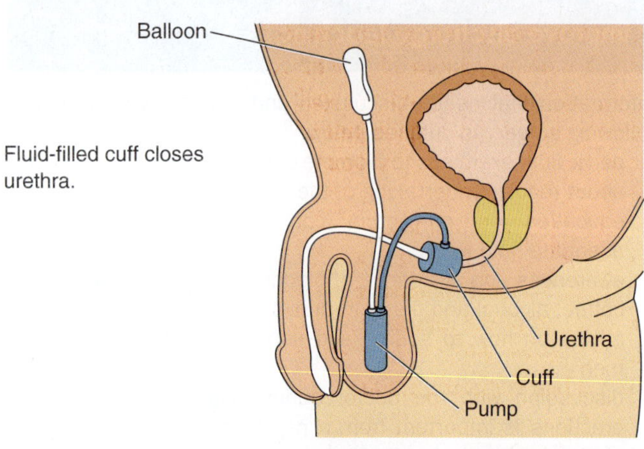

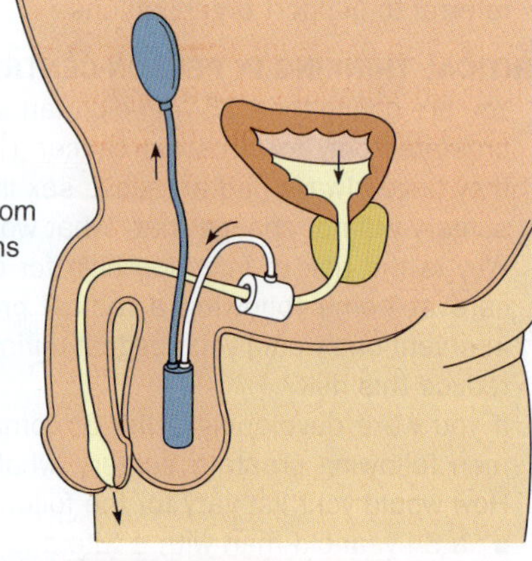

After voiding, fluid drains back to cuff, closing urethra.

FIGURE 47.5 ***Method of operation of an artificial urinary sphincter***

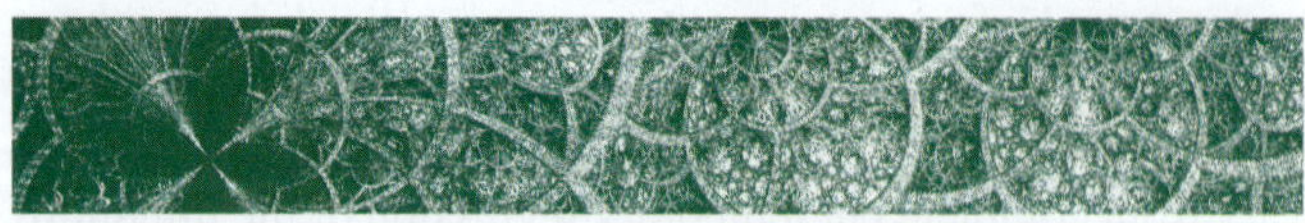

Nursing care

Nurses plan and provide interventions to help prevent prostate cancer and to facilitate a return to functional health status. Interventions may range from health education to using knowledge and skill in physical care following a radical prostatectomy. See the accompanying nursing care plan for a man with prostate cancer.

Health promotion

Nurses are in a unique position to increase public awareness about early detection of prostate cancer. Every encounter with men and their families—in clinics, hospital units or in the home—is an opportunity to provide information about early detection and identify needs. Several studies have shown a positive correlation between increased awareness of and participation in prostate cancer screening procedures. Organisations such as Cancer Council and Healthy Male have information about early detection of prostate cancer, which is useful in educating the public.

One risk factor that can be easily changed is diet. Men should know that they can lower their risk of prostate cancer by eating less red meat and fat, and increasing their intake of fruit and vegetables, particularly tomatoes, pink grapefruit and watermelon, as these are high in lycopenes, which help prevent damage to DNA and may help lower prostate cancer risk. Other substances that may help lower the risk are vitamin E and selenium.

All men should be given information about the limitations and benefits of testing for early detection and of treatment so they can make an informed decision. Currently, routine screening of PSA as a diagnostic tool for prostatic cancer is not recommended by Australian cancer authorities. An elevated PSA may indicate that there is a problem with the prostate; however, it may not be cancer. Factors such as the man's level of concern about having cancer, age and family history should be discussed prior to having a PSA level taken. Diagnosis of cancer is made following physical assessment and a transrectal ultrasound and biopsy of the prostate.

Assessment

Collect the following data through the health history and physical examination (see the chapter 'A person-centred approach to assessing the male and female reproductive systems'). Note that a digital rectal examination (DRE) is an advanced nursing assessment.

- *Health history*: risk factors, urinary elimination patterns and manifestations, haematuria, pain.
- *Physical assessment*: DRE to assess prostate size, symmetry, firmness and nodules.

Nursing interventions

The nursing care of men with prostate cancer must be holistic, sensitive and individualised. Nursing interventions discussed for the man with BPH may also be appropriate. This section focuses on problems with urinary incontinence, sexual function and pain.

Urinary incontinence (reflex, stress, total)

Urinary incontinence is a disturbing complication following treatment for prostate cancer. Both radical prostatectomy and external-beam radiation therapy can cause urinary incontinence, ranging from a few drops when the man lifts a heavy object (*stress incontinence*) to no control at all. Older men may experience *urge incontinence*, the involuntary passage of urine soon after a strong sense of urgency to void. Total and unpredictable loss of urine is classified as total incontinence.

TABLE 47.5 Surgical and hormone* therapy in the management of advanced prostate cancer

TREATMENT	ADVANTAGES	DISADVANTAGES
Orchidectomy	Inexpensive Immediate effect (i.e. men report diminished pain from metastasis in the OR recovery room)	Body image issues due to loss of testicles
Oestrogen compounds (diethylstilbestrol)	Inexpensive Effects reversible	Increased risk of cardiovascular problems (e.g. DVT) More likely to cause gynaecomastia, hypertrophy of breast tissue
Luteinising hormone-releasing hormone agonist (LHRH) (leuprolide)	Effects reversible No cardiovascular risk Monthly administration	Very expensive Subcutaneous injection route Slow onset: up to 3 weeks Can lead to exacerbation of clinical symptoms
Steroidal anti-androgens (megestrol acetate (Megace))	Effects reversible No cardiovascular risk Inexpensive Less risk of ED Less risk of osteoporosis	May not drop testosterone levels sufficiently Weight gain Increased risk of hepatotoxicity
Non-steroidal anti-androgens (flutamide; often used in conjunction with LHRH)	Do not alter circulating androgens Block some side effects of LHRH May be effective if other methods fail	Very expensive

*All hormonal manipulations have the potential disadvantage of loss of libido, erectile dysfunction, hot flushes and gynaecomastia.

NURSING CARE PLAN A man with prostate cancer

Bill Burns, a 76-year-old, lives with his wife in a small retirement community. His wife had a stroke 2 years ago and Mr Burns does all the cooking and housework. He has been in good health for most of his life, having only mild osteoarthritis in his knees and hands. He has noticed a gradual onset of urinary urgency and frequency over the past 2 years but has never had incontinence. During a routine check-up, the doctor at the local general practice performs a digital rectal examination and palpates a hard nodule on the surface of Mr Burns' prostate. Following discussion with Mr Burns and his wife, a PSA is performed. After his PSA is found to be elevated, Mr Burns is referred to a urologist, who diagnoses prostate cancer. Mr Burns chooses to have surgery, and a radical retropubic prostatectomy and lymph node dissection are performed. The lymph nodes are negative for metastasis. Following surgery, Mr Burns' recovery is uncomplicated. However, the nurse caring for him is concerned about his ability to care for his indwelling catheter because of his arthritis and his wife's physical disabilities from the stroke. The nurse makes a referral to community health to ensure he can manage his care at home. An initial home health assessment is scheduled for the day after Mr Burns is discharged from the hospital.

ASSESSMENT

The community health nurse notes that the house is clean and neat. Mr Burns is dressed, but still wearing his night urinary drainage bag, even though it is 1300 hrs. Mr Burns tells the nurse that his main problem is going to get groceries because he is embarrassed to be seen with the drainage bag. He says he has not been able to remove the drainage bag and attach the leg bag because of his arthritis. Physical assessment findings include the pelvic incision healing without signs of infection. There is no tenderness in his calves, chest pain or shortness of breath. The urine is yellow, without odour. Mr Burns states that he sees no need for the pelvic exercises since he is no longer in the hospital. He also expresses the belief that he is cured of cancer and questions the need for follow-up care.

NURSING CONCERNS

- *Risk of stress urinary incontinence* related to surgical procedure.
- *Ineffective health maintenance* related to inability to care for the urinary drainage system, not understanding the need for postoperative exercises and questions about follow-up care.

PLANNING

Establish realistic outcomes for Mr Burns through education and support.

Expected outcomes

- Regain urinary continence after catheter removal.
- Change the urinary drainage bag with the appropriate assistance.
- Verbalise the rationale for performing postoperative exercise.
- Verbalise the need for continued follow-up care.

IMPLEMENTATION

- Discuss the possibility of stress incontinence after the catheter is removed.
- Reinforce the need for ongoing pelvic floor exercises while the catheter is still in place.
- Explore Mr Burns' support system to identify people who could assist him with catheter care and arrange a teaching session with them.
- Teach Mr Burns the importance of follow-up care, relating the care to the history of the disease.

(continued)

NURSING CARE PLAN A man with prostate cancer (continued)

EVALUATION

Good friends from Mr Burns' bowling club have assisted him with care of his drainage bag and have reminded him to do his pelvic floor exercises several times a day while the catheter is in place. When the catheter is removed, Mr Burns has only a small amount of leaking of urine after voiding. He understands that it may take several weeks for this to resolve. Efforts to help him understand the need for continued medical care are less successful. He continues to state that he is cured, his wife needs him and he sees no need to see his doctor.

CRITICAL THINKING IN THE NURSING PROCESS

1 Outline a health education plan for Mr Burns related to the *Risk of altered skin integrity* related to urinary incontinence.
2 As a result of Mr Burns' refusal to have ongoing medical care, he might be labelled as non-compliant. Would you make this assumption? Why or why not?
3 If you were the community health nurse making a home visit and found that Mr Burns had no urinary drainage for 16 hours, which assessments would you make? How would you handle this problem?

REFLECTION ON THE NURSING PROCESS

1 Consider some strategies you might use to engage Mr Burns in understanding the need for ongoing medical care.
2 How would you know that your education strategies with Mr Burns were successful for the long term?

The man's reaction to incontinence may be severe even if the incontinence is not great. Many men have significant anxiety at the prospect of an incontinent episode in public because they feel shame and often guilt about the loss of control.

- Assess the degree of incontinence and its effects on lifestyle. *The nurse needs to determine previous urinary patterns and the type of incontinence currently being experienced to plan appropriate interventions.*
- Teach pelvic floor exercises to help restore continence and discuss regularity of performing the exercises. *Pelvic floor or Kegel exercises can almost always improve stress incontinence, with the possibility of eliminating it.*
- Teach methods to control dampness and odour from stress incontinence:
  - Do not attempt to prevent accidental voiding by restricting fluids. *Not only will the man continue to have incontinent episodes, but also his urine will become concentrated, exacerbating the problem with odour and increasing risk of UTI.*
  - Manage occasional episodes (one to three small-volume accidents per day) with an absorbent pad worn inside the underwear and changed as needed. Most pads are made with a polymer gel that controls odour. *Appropriate measures help promote good hygiene, decrease anxiety and increase comfort.*
- Refer to a physiotherapist or a continence specialist for additional measures to promote continence. *Special exercises, restricting some types of fluids and other measures such as bladder training can help the man deal with incontinence.*
- Explore options such as an external collection device (external catheter or suprapubic catheter) for the man with total incontinence. *This device may improve the man's self-esteem and allow resumption of social activities.*
- Encourage verbalising feelings about the impact of incontinence on quality of life. The degree of incontinence does not necessarily correlate with the perceived level of suffering. *Listening to these concerns with sensitivity can help the man work through these feelings and may allow him to move towards a healthy adaptation to his change in function.*

Sexual dysfunction

Surgical treatment for prostate cancer may cause erectile dysfunction and changes in ejaculatory function. Hormone therapy for advanced prostate cancer lowers libido and may also cause ED. The diagnosis of cancer and body image changes caused by hormone therapy may lower self-esteem, which in turn can diminish sexual desire and willingness to interact sexually with a partner. Most older men are active sexually and fully capable of sustaining an erection. They are likely to fear the effect of treatment on their sexual health. They may allow their anxiety to guide their decision about treatment or they may refuse all interventions because of this fear. Reactions vary greatly and the nurse must maintain a non-judgmental approach to education and support.

- Assess the man's pre-treatment sexual function. *Knowledge of previous sexual function is necessary to plan appropriate interventions.*
- Teach the man about the actual or potential effects of therapy on sexual function. *The incidence of ED varies with different therapies for prostate cancer.*
- Provide an opportunity for the man and his partner to discuss the implications of and their concerns about the diagnosis and treatment of sexual function. *The treatments for prostate cancer often affect the physiology of erection. The man and his partner need support and counselling during the period of adjustment. Sexual activity should not be resumed until 6–8 weeks following surgery. Stress and anxiety can exacerbate ED, so management of these need to be discussed and strategies put in place to manage them.*
- Discuss medical and surgical treatments for ED (see the first section of this chapter). *Many men are as devastated by the loss of erectile function as they are by the diagnosis of cancer. Information about achieving erection and maintaining sexual intimacy is essential to quality of life.*
- Refer for sexual counselling as appropriate. Refer to support groups. *The man and his partner may require therapy beyond that provided by nurses.*

CONSIDERATION FOR PRACTICE

A therapeutic approach to assessing how the man feels is to use an opening statement such as, 'Some men are very concerned about the effects of the treatment on their ability to have an erection. Tell me how you feel about it.'

Acute/chronic pain

There are many causes of pain in men with advanced prostate cancer. It is not unusual for a man to have three or four distinct pains simultaneously, all from different sources. The most common cause of pain is metastasis to the spinal column, usually the thoracic spine. Other sources of pain include fractures, lymphoedema of the lower extremities and muscle spasms. Because most men with prostate cancer are over the age of 65, many also have pain associated with pre-existing conditions, such as osteoarthritis, unrelated to the cancer.

- Assess the intensity, location and quality of the pain. A cardinal rule of successful pain management is the importance of reducing or eliminating the cause of pain. *Appropriate interventions are based on a careful assessment of the man's pain.*
- Provide optimal pain relief with prescribed analgesics. *It is important that the man and his family understand that pain medications should be used on a regular basis to maintain comfort and should not be delayed until pain is severe.*
- Teach the man and his family non-invasive methods of pain control. *Various modalities can be successful in alleviating pain or reducing its perception, thus enhancing the comfort of the person (see the chapter 'Nursing care of people in pain').*

Community-based care

Depending on the type of treatment, the following topics should be addressed in preparing the man and his family for home care:

- for the man having a surgical procedure: manifestations of infection and excessive bleeding, catheter care, wound care, pain management
- for the man receiving radiation therapy:
  - danger of radiation damage to others (sleep in a room alone for a week; and avoid close contact with pregnant women, infants and children)
  - condom use during sexual contact (ejaculate may be discoloured, distressing the sexual partner)
- the importance of keeping appointments with healthcare providers and having yearly PSA and rectal examinations
- if appropriate, community services, such as support groups, community-based nurses and hospice
- helpful resources:
  - Cancer Council: https://www.cancer.org.au
  - Prostate Cancer Foundation of Australia: https://www.prostate.org.au.

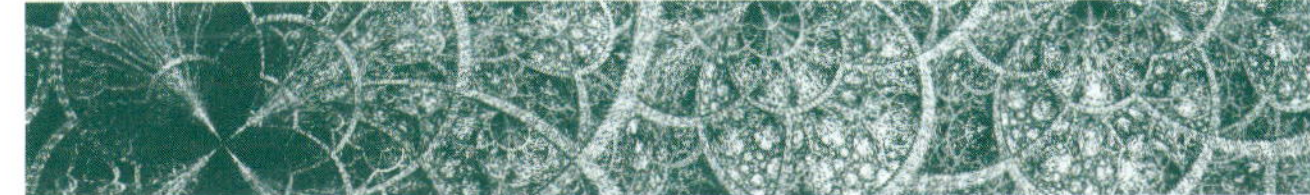

Male breast disorders

THE MAN WITH GYNAECOMASTIA

Gynaecomastia, the abnormal enlargement of the glandular tissue in the male breast, is thought to result from a change in the ratio of testosterone to oestrogen, where the level of oestrogen is elevated. It is common during puberty, affecting one breast in as many as 50% of adolescent males, but usually resolves within 1 to 2 years. Any condition that increases oestrogen activity or decreases testosterone production can contribute to gynaecomastia. Conditions that increase oestrogen activity include obesity, testicular tumours, kidney and liver disease, and adrenal carcinoma. Conditions that decrease testosterone production include chronic illness such as tuberculosis or Hodgkin's disease, injury, orchitis and some genetic conditions (such as Klinefelter's syndrome). Drugs can contribute to gynaecomastia, particularly certain antidepressants, antihypertensives, anabolic steroids, marijuana, opiates, extreme amounts of alcohol and chemotherapeutic agents. Gynaecomastia after adolescence is usually bilateral. If it is unilateral, biopsy may be necessary to rule out breast cancer.

No treatment is necessary for the transient gynaecomastia of puberty. If the condition becomes chronic, creating psychological discomfort, surgery may be necessary to remove the subcutaneous breast tissue. When related to an underlying disorder, treatment of that disorder is required. If the cause is due to drugs, ceasing that drug usually decreases the breast tissue within a month. Where there is no hormonal problem and in severe cases, tamoxifen can be given to decrease oestrogen activity. Tamoxifen is used in treating breast cancer and is not approved for management and treatment of gynaecomastia, although improvements have been reported by men taking the drug.

Nursing care for the man with gynaecomastia includes health education about the cause and treatment of the condition, and emotional support for the psychosocial implications of this condition.

THE MAN WITH BREAST CANCER

Although male breast cancer is rare, accounting for about 0.2% of all male cancer cases in Australia, it is as serious to the men who have it as it is to women. Breast cancer accounts for about 0.1% of all male cancer deaths in Australia (AIHW, 2021).

The aetiology of male breast cancer is unclear; hormonal, genetic and perhaps environmental factors appear to be important.

Male breast cancer is clinically and histologically similar to female breast cancer, although lobular cancer is rare in males. Most tumours are oestrogen-receptor positive. Because many men believe that breast cancer is only a woman's disease, they often delay seeking medical attention for symptoms, and thus may present with advanced disease.

Treatment of male breast cancer is much like the treatment of female breast cancer, beginning with modified radical mastectomy, node dissection and staging to determine the therapeutic options. Radiation, chemotherapy and hormonal therapy (usually tamoxifen) are the conventional adjuncts to surgery. Castration (surgical removal of the testes) is the most successful palliative measure in men with advanced breast cancer, resulting in tumour regression and prolonging life.

Nursing care for the man with breast cancer is essentially the same as for the woman with breast cancer (see the chapter 'Nursing care of women with reproductive system and breast disorders'). The nurse has an opportunity to help the man and his family cope with the psychosocial effects of having breast cancer. He may feel embarrassment or shame about his condition, as well as fear about the life-threatening nature of the disease. His family may share those feelings. By listening with understanding and empathy, the nurse can help the man and his family resolve their feelings and move towards healing.

CHAPTER HIGHLIGHTS

- Disorders of male sexual function include erectile dysfunction (ED) and ejaculatory dysfunction. Many different illnesses, medications and surgical procedures may affect male sexual function. Treatments include medications, mechanical devices and surgical procedures. It is important for nurses to initiate a discussion of sexual concerns during assessments and to recognise that many male reproductive treatments and surgeries may result in sexual dysfunction.
- Phimosis and priapism are disorders of the penis that can cause problems with urination and sexual activity and may, in some cases, be considered medical emergencies. The risk of cancer of the penis, although rare, is increased by phimosis, poor genital hygiene and viral HPV and HIV infections.
- Benign scrotal masses include hydrocoele, spermatocoele and varicocoele. Epididymitis may be associated with a urinary tract infection, prostatitis, urethral strictures or a sexually transmitted infection.
- The testes may be infected (orchitis), twisted (testicular torsion) or develop cancer. Testicular cancer is the most common cancer in men between the ages of 15 and 40. Monthly testicular self-examination is critical to early detection and treatment of cancer.
- The prostate gland may be inflamed or infected (prostatitis), enlarged (benign prostatic hyperplasia (BPH)) or develop cancer. BPH is a common disorder of the ageing male that causes problems with urination as the enlarging prostate gland constricts the urethra. Treatments include medications and various types of surgery, depending on the size of the prostate and the age and health status of the man.
- Cancer of the prostate is the most common type of cancer in Australian men. When diagnosed early, prostate cancer is curable. Diagnosis is often based on an increasing level of PSA and an abnormal DRE. The cancer is treated with surgery, radiation or hormonal manipulation.
- The male breast may become enlarged (gynaecomastia) or develop cancer.

CONCEPT CHECK

1 When conducting a health assessment, which of the following statements would most likely elicit information about sexual concerns?
1 'Following your prostate surgery, when did you first notice you had problems with sexual intercourse?'
2 'Why do you think you should be sexually active at your age?'
3 'Do you miss having sex?'
4 'Tell me about your experience with sexual function since you developed prostate enlargement.'

2 You are conducting a health education session for young men. Which topic would be appropriate to teach them about reducing the risk of cancer of the penis?
1 wearing a condom during sexual intercourse
2 retracting the foreskin of the penis when showering
3 avoiding tight pants and very hot showers
4 maintaining a regular testicular self-examination schedule

3 Which disease of the male reproductive system is a risk if a man also has a sexually transmitted infection (gonorrhoea)?
1 epididymitis
2 hydrocoele
3 erectile dysfunction
4 gynaecomastia

4 Which of the following statements is true of testicular cancer?
1 The incidence increases with age.
2 It occurs most between ages 15 and 40.
3 It rarely occurs in brothers.
4 Severe pain is the initial manifestation.

5 You are educating a man with chronic prostatitis how to care for himself at home. Which simple measures can be used to decrease discomfort?
1 take cold showers and restrict oral fluids
2 wear a scrotal support and take anti-inflammatory drugs
3 increase oral fluid intake to 3 L/day and void often
4 increase fibre intake and avoid sexual activity

6 Which diagnostic tests are used to differentiate BPH from prostate cancer? (Select all that apply.)
1 pelvic ultrasound
2 digital rectal examination
3 blood chemistry
4 PSA level
5 sperm count

7 The enlarging prostate in BPH typically is manifested by assessment of problems with:
1 bowel elimination
2 urinary elimination
3 peripheral vascular function
4 skin integrity

8 You are caring for a man who has returned to the unit from the recovery room following a TURP. His urinary drainage bag is filled with dark-red fluid with obvious clots. He is having painful bladder spasms. What would you do first?
1 assess his intake and output since surgery
2 administer pain medication in the form of oral oxybutynin hydrochloride
3 report your assessments to his urologist
4 nothing, because these manifestations are expected following a TURP

9 Which cancer is the most common malignancy in Australian men?
1 prostate cancer
2 testicular cancer
3 lung cancer
4 colon cancer

10 Which nutritional information should be included in a community program to reduce the risk of prostate cancer?
1 increase fibre intake
2 decrease lycopene intake
3 avoid foods high in sodium
4 decrease red meat and fat intake

BIBLIOGRAPHY

Akers, C. (2018). Aetiology, clinical presentation and treatment of testicular cancer. *Nursing Standard*, *32*(28), 50–61.

Australian Commission on Safety and Quality in Health Care (ACSQHC) (2021). *National Safety and Quality Health Service Standards* (2nd ed.). Sydney: ACSQHC.

Australian Institute of Health and Welfare (AIHW) (2021). *Cancer in Australia*. Retrieved from https://www.aihw.gov.au/

Cancer Australia (2021). *Prostate cancer*. Retrieved from https://canceraustralia.gov.au/

Cancer Council (2022). *Understanding prostate cancer*. https://www.cancer.org.au/

Cancer Council South Australia (2020). *Understanding testicular cancer.* Retrieved from https://www.cancersa.org.au/

Dreyer, D., Macfarlane, K. & Hendry, D. (2018). The testicular cancer nurse specialist: A pivotal role in patient care. *British Journal of Nursing*, *27*(18), S26–27. Retrieved from https://pubmed.ncbi.nlm.nih.gov/30281354/

Healthy Male (2021a). *Erectile dysfunction*. Retrieved from https://www.healthymale.org.au/

Healthy Male (2021b). *Penis cancer*. Retrieved from https://www.healthymale.org.au/

Healthy Male (2021c). *Prostate enlargement*. Retrieved from https://www.healthymale.org.au/

Healthy Male (2021d). *For health professionals: The evolution of PSA testing*. Retrieved from https://www.healthymale.org.au/

Lotti, F. & Maggi, M. (2018). Sexual dysfunction and male infertility. *Nature Reviews Urology*, *15*(5), 287–307.

Norris, T. L. (2018). *Porth's pathophysiology: Concepts of altered health states* (10th ed.). Philadelphia: Lippincott Williams & Wilkins.

Papadakis, M., McPhee, S. & Rabow, M. (2022). *Current medical diagnosis and treatment* (61st ed.). New York: McGraw-Hill Education.

Prostate Cancer Foundation of New Zealand (2022). *Prostate cancer*. Retrieved from http://prostate.org.nz/

Rupp, L. & Leslie, S. (2021). Epididymitis. *StatPearls*. Retrieved from https://www.ncbi.nlm.nih.gov/

WebMD (2021). *What can cause erectile dysfunction?* Retrieved from https://www.webmd.com/

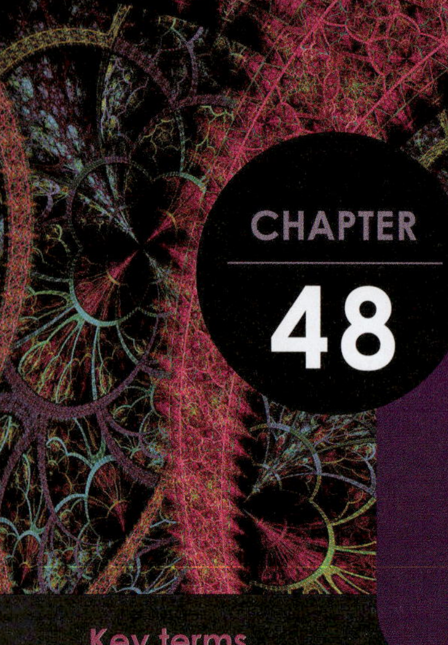

CHAPTER 48

Nursing care of women with reproductive system and breast disorders

Shahla Meedya

Key terms

amenorrhoea 1781
dysfunctional uterine bleeding (DUB) 1781
dysmenorrhoea 1779
endometriosis 1790
fibrocystic changes (FCCs) 1804
leiomyoma 1789
menopause 1801
menorrhagia 1781
metrorrhagia 1781
premenstrual syndrome (PMS) 1777

Learning outcomes

- Explain the pathophysiology, symptoms, complications, interprofessional care and nursing care of women with reproductive system and breast disorders.
- Discuss alternative and complementary therapies used by women to relieve symptoms associated with menstrual disorders.
- Compare and contrast the risk, incidence, pathophysiology, symptoms, diagnosis, treatment and nursing care for cancer of the cervix, endometrium, ovary and vulva.
- Describe the physiological process of menopause.
- Discuss treatment, including alternative and complementary therapies, used by women to relieve symptoms associated with menopause disorders.
- Discuss health education for women with disorders of the reproductive system and breast.
- Discuss cancer screening: the purposes, nursing implications, medications and treatments.

Clinical competencies

- Assess the functional status of women with reproductive system and breast disorders, and report, monitor and document abnormal symptoms.
- Use evidence-based research to design interventions to promote early diagnosis and treatment of women with cervical and breast cancer, with particular focus on the health disparities for women from areas of social disadvantage; for example, women living in remote and rural areas of Australia and Aboriginal and Torres Strait Islander women.
- Determine nursing priorities based on assessed data to select and implement individualised nursing interventions for women with reproductive system and breast disorders.
- Administer medications used to treat female reproductive system and breast disorders knowledgeably and safely.
- Provide skilled care for the woman having a cervical dilation and curettage (D&C), laparoscopy, hysterectomy, mastectomy and breast reconstruction.
- Integrate an interdisciplinary approach into the care of women with reproductive system and breast disorders.
- Provide health education appropriate for community-based self-care of female reproductive and breast disorders.
- Revise the plan of care as needed to provide effective interventions to promote, maintain or restore functional health status to women with reproductive system and breast disorders.

Disorders of the female reproductive system range from minor discomfort of menstrual cramps to life-threatening diseases such as cancer. Many of these disorders can occur at any point in a woman's adult life. They may affect her sexuality, ability to bear children and sense of wellbeing.

A holistic approach to meet the needs of women who experience reproductive system changes and disorders is required to ensure that their physical, emotional and educational needs are met. The ability to reproduce affects self-esteem, feelings of femininity and general health. Sensitivity and understanding from caregivers are essential. Often women are required to disclose personal information when providing a medical and family history and undergoing diagnostic tests. Women may find providing intimate information embarrassing and uncomfortable. When planning and implementing care, nurses must consider the woman within the context of her culture, socioeconomic and educational level, and lifestyle. It is also important that the nurse not make assumptions or judgments about sexual orientation.

In this chapter, disorders of the female reproductive system, physiological changes during menopause and breast disorders are discussed. Many of the disorders result in actual or potential health problems requiring nursing care that is evidence based. To avoid repeating strategies and interventions for each disorder, they have been divided between the nursing care discussions as appropriate. Treatment of cancer with chemotherapy and radiation is discussed in the chapter 'Nursing care of people with cancer'. Nursing care of women with reproductive system and breast disorders is complex and requires a holistic and well-coordinated approach that is in full collaboration with the woman and her significant others.

DISORDERS OF FEMALE SEXUAL FUNCTION

Two physiological sexual responses occur during sex: vasocongestion and myotonia. Sexual stimulation results in vasocongestion of the blood vessels surrounding the vagina, causing engorgement, increased lubrication, genital swelling and enlargement. Arousal, or myotonia, increases muscular tension, resulting in voluntary and involuntary muscle contraction. The sexual response cycle has four phases: excitement, plateau, orgasm and resolution. These phases always occur in the same sequence; however, the duration of each phase may vary. Sexual arousal typically ends in orgasm (climax), but not always. A refractory period, or period in which the sexual organs are incapable of responding to stimulus, does not occur in the female. Multiple orgasms are physically possible in all women. Women maintain the capacity for sexual activity and orgasm long after menopause (see the 'Meeting individualised needs' box).

MEETING INDIVIDUALISED NEEDS Sexual function in the ageing woman

The belief that older women are no longer interested in expressing their sexuality may occur within society. This view results from myths, taboos and stereotypical views held by some people. Two commonly held myths are that menopause causes the demise of a woman's sexuality and that hysterectomy results in the inability of a woman to function sexually. Loss of sexual function is not an inevitable result of ageing, although physical changes related to ageing do affect the female sexual response. These physical changes, along with chronic conditions common in ageing women, may alter a woman's sexual function. In addition, the sexual response can be altered by some medications used to treat the chronic conditions associated with ageing. Factors affecting women's sexuality are often not discussed or raised by health professionals. The role of the nurse is to provide information about the normal changes in women's sexual function and ways to achieve optimal sexual health, as well as educating women about the myths and misinformation around changes in sexual functioning.

PHYSIOLOGICAL CHANGES IN THE AGEING WOMEN

Changes in women's sexual function begin in the perimenopausal period as oestrogen levels decrease. Oestrogen-sensitive cells are found throughout the central nervous system and the cardiovascular system. These cells are involved in the female sexual response. With menopause comes a decrease in the levels of oestradiol, which affects nerve transmission and the response in the peripheral vascular system. As a result, the timing and degree of vasocongestion during the sexual response are affected.

Specific changes in the female sexual response occur in all phases. During the plateau phase, the capacity for vasocongestion decreases, as does muscle tension. In the orgasmic phase, the contractions are fewer and less intense. During the resolution phase, vasocongestion subsides more quickly.

NURSING CARE

The nursing role centres on educating women about the physiological and psychological changes associated with menopause and assisting women to reach optimal sexual functioning. Nurses should be able to obtain a sexual history without embarrassment, discuss sexual concerns with women and make appropriate referrals. Providing education on how the effects of chronic illness and the medications used to treat these illnesses can affect sexual functioning is important. Educating about the importance of maintaining a healthy lifestyle, which includes a balanced diet, weight-bearing and aerobic exercises, stress management and routine health examinations is essential.

For problems related to vaginal dryness and dyspareunia, water-soluble vaginal lubricants or vaginal gels can be used before intercourse. Intercourse on a regular basis and oestrogen replacement therapy can also be recommended. Women who experience joint pain or other musculoskeletal pain due to conditions such as arthritis can benefit from education on how to adapt positions for intercourse.

Links to National Patient Safety Standards

NSQHS: Partnering with Consumers Standard

The intention of this standard is to create an organisation in which there are mutually valuable outcomes by having the women as partners in planning, design, delivery, measurement and evaluation of systems and services and as partners in their own care, to the extent that they choose.

Source: Australian Commission on Safety and Quality in Health Care (ACSQHC) (2021). *National Safety and Quality Health Service Standards* (2nd ed.). Sydney: ACSQHC. © Australian Commission on Safety and Quality in Health Care.

Pathophysiology

Disorders of sexual function include dyspareunia, inhibited sexual desire and orgasmic dysfunction.

Dyspareunia

The woman with dyspareunia feels pain during intercourse and may find it difficult to express her feelings to her partner. This condition may manifest itself as decreased desire or inhibited orgasm.

The causes of dyspareunia range from organic to psychogenic. Physical conditions, such as imperforate hymen, vaginal scarring or vaginismus, may cause dyspareunia. *Vaginismus* is a rare condition where the vaginal muscles at the introitus contract so tightly that an erect penis cannot be inserted. An early traumatic event, such as sexual abuse, fear of men or rape, may contribute to this disorder. However, it is estimated that most dyspareunia is psychogenic in origin. The woman develops an anxiety–fear–guilt cycle in which negative thoughts become associated with the act of vaginal penetration, initiating a conditioned involuntary reflex. However, other sexual activity may be pleasurable. The woman's partner needs to be included in any discussion or education sessions to assist them to understand their partner's issues.

Inhibited sexual desire

Inhibited sexual desire is complex and may be a result of pathophysiological processes or may be psychogenic in origin. Inhibited sexual desire often is rooted deeply in personal experiences that may be too painful to recall. Cultural and religious values can also affect the processing of sexual stimuli. Fear of pregnancy or sexually transmitted infections (STIs) and depression can also contribute to decreased libido.

Orgasmic dysfunction

Female orgasm inhibition (anorgasmia) is the most prevalent sexual problem in women. However, fewer than 20% of cases are physiological in origin. It is estimated that between 8% and 15% of women have never experienced an orgasm in the waking state. Psychogenically induced anorgasmia may result from unresolved conflicts about sexual activity. Organic causes of anorgasmia include the presence of disease that results in general debilitation that affects the sexual response cycle, or the use of medications that depress the central nervous system (CNS).

Primary anorgasmia exists when a woman has never experienced an orgasm during the waking state, either through self-stimulation, partner stimulation or intercourse. Secondary anorgasmia exists when a woman who previously experienced orgasms is no longer able to do so.

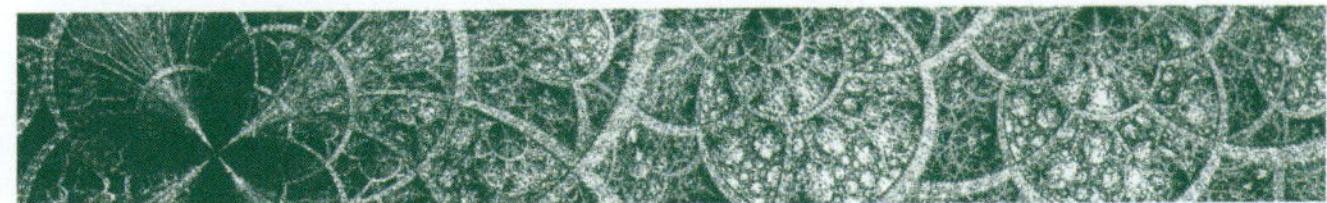

Nursing care

Nursing care focuses on identifying the type of sexual dysfunction with a thorough history, including onset, duration, frequency and context or situation in which the problem occurs. The woman's partner should be included in discussions.

The woman and her partner may require education about varied normal sexual responses. The goal is to increase self-awareness and understanding of communication and how this impacts on sexual desire. Differences in behaviours that men and women consider sexually stimulating may need to be discussed. Sex therapists may provide training in stimulation techniques (masturbation) after inhibitions about this practice are discussed. Group therapy may be encouraged to help the woman discuss her problem and to decrease the sense of isolation.

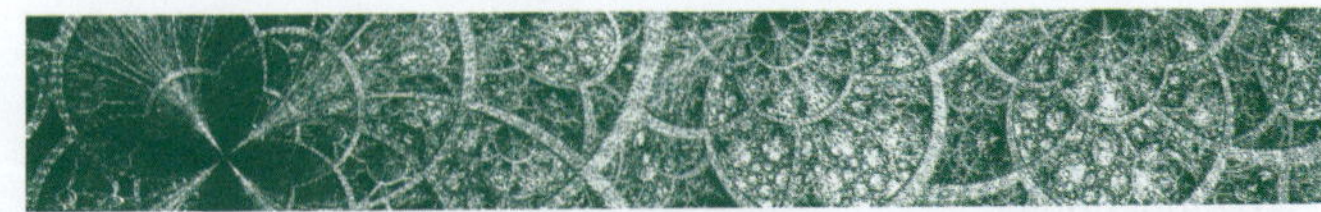

Menstrual disorders

Monthly menstruation normally involves some minor discomfort, including breast tenderness, feelings of heaviness and congestion in the pelvic area, uterine cramping and lower backache. Many women, however, experience more serious effects, both physiological and psychological. This section discusses premenstrual syndrome, dysmenorrhoea and abnormal uterine bleeding. (The menstrual cycle is discussed in the chapter 'A person-centred approach to assessing the male and female reproductive systems'.)

THE WOMAN WITH PREMENSTRUAL SYNDROME

Premenstrual syndrome (PMS) is a complex group of symptoms. Women can present with a range of these (e.g. mood swings, breast tenderness, fatigue, irritability, food cravings and depression) that are limited to 2 to 14 days before menstruation and relieved by the onset of menses. However, the usual time frame for symptoms to be present for most women who experience PMS is approximately 7 days a month. PMS is diagnosed if the woman reports the symptoms during 5 days before menses for at least three menstrual cycles (Women's Health & Research Institute of Australia, 2022). For a small number of women, PMS is so disabling that it is given the psychiatric label of premenstrual dysphoric disorder (PMDD).

The syndrome is seen less frequently during the teens and twenties and is more common in women aged between 30 and 45 years. The cause is unknown; however, it is linked to stress.

Pathophysiology

Although the pathophysiology of PMS is not clearly understood, hormonal changes such as altered oestrogen–progesterone ratios, increased prolactin levels and rising aldosterone levels during the luteal phase of the menstrual cycle may contribute to the problem. Increased aldosterone results in sodium retention and oedema. Decreased levels of monoamine oxidase in the brain are associated with depression, and reduced levels of serotonin can lead to mood swings.

Manifestations

Symptoms of PMS occur during the luteal phase of the menstrual cycle (7 to 10 days prior to the onset of the menstrual flow), abating when the menstrual flow begins. See 'Multisystem effects of PMS'. Although PMS may produce a variety of physiological and psychological symptoms, the exact nature of these symptoms and their intensity are individualised for each woman with this disorder. The symptoms may even differ from month to month in the same woman.

INTERPROFESSIONAL CARE

If no organic cause can be identified, the goals of care are to relieve symptoms and develop self-care patterns that will help the woman anticipate and cope more effectively with future episodes of PMS. There are no definitive diagnostic tests for PMS. The regular recurrence of symptoms preceding the onset of menses for at least 2 to 3 months leads to a diagnosis of PMS. The treatment of PMS integrates a self-monitored record of symptoms. Women can then be educated on ways of relieving symptoms, such as undertaking regular exercise, ensuring healthy eating patterns and reducing the level of stress in their lives. However, there are a variety of treatments available (Women's Health & Research Institute of Australia, 2022).

Medications

If the symptoms of PMS are severe or incapacitating, ovulation may be suppressed by the use of gonadotropin-releasing hormone (GnRH) agonists, oral contraceptives or danazol. Progesterone and antiprostaglandin agents such as non-steroidal anti-inflammatory drugs (NSAIDs) may help relieve cramping. Diuretics may be prescribed to relieve bloating. Selective serotonin reuptake inhibitors (SSRIs) such as fluoxetine (Prozac), sertraline (Zoloft) and paroxetine (Aropax) may be used to manage mood and some physical symptoms of PMS.

Alternative and complementary therapies

Alternative and complementary therapies the woman with PMS may find helpful focus on diet, exercise, relaxation and stress management.

- A diet high in complex carbohydrates with limited simple sugars and alcohol is recommended to minimise reactive hypoglycaemia, which can contribute to the symptoms of PMS.
- Reduced sodium intake helps minimise fluid retention.
- Increased intake of vitamin E, omega-3 fatty acids, vitamin B_1, vitamin B_6, calcium and magnesium supplements have been shown to reduce the symptoms of PMS (Mayo Foundation for Medical Education and Research, 2022).
- Caffeine should be restricted to reduce irritability.
- Herbal remedies include chasteberry (Premular), evening primrose oil and a bee pollen extract called Femal. Women are encouraged to talk to their doctors before taking any herbal remedies (Women's Health & Research Institute of Australia, 2022).
- Exercise is beneficial, but adequate rest also is necessary.
- Techniques for relaxation and stress management include deep abdominal breathing, meditation, muscle relaxation and guided imagery.

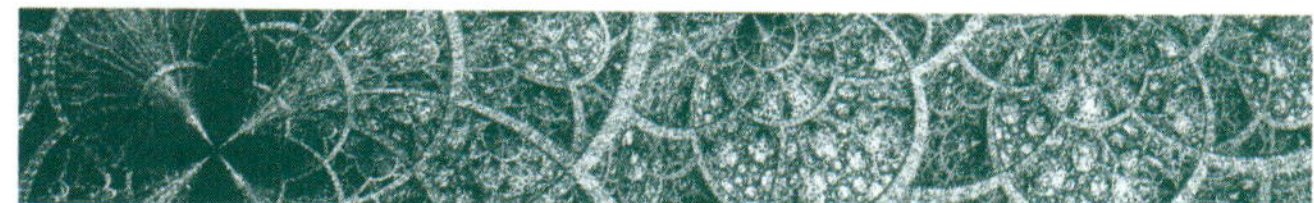

Nursing care

Nursing diagnoses and interventions

Nursing care for the woman with PMS focuses on relieving symptoms. Most women experiencing PMS require interventions to manage pain and enhance coping.

Acute pain

The woman with PMS may have pain from headache (including migraine), menstrual cramps, excessive fluid retention, breast swelling, joint and muscle pain, and backache.

- Teach effective pharmacological and non-pharmacological self-care measures to relieve pain: application of heat, relaxation techniques (such as breathing exercises, imagery techniques or meditation) and exercise. *Heat relieves muscle spasms and dilates blood vessels, increasing blood supply to the pelvis and uterine muscles. Relaxation and exercise aid the release of naturally produced pain relievers called endorphins.*

Multisystem effects of PMS

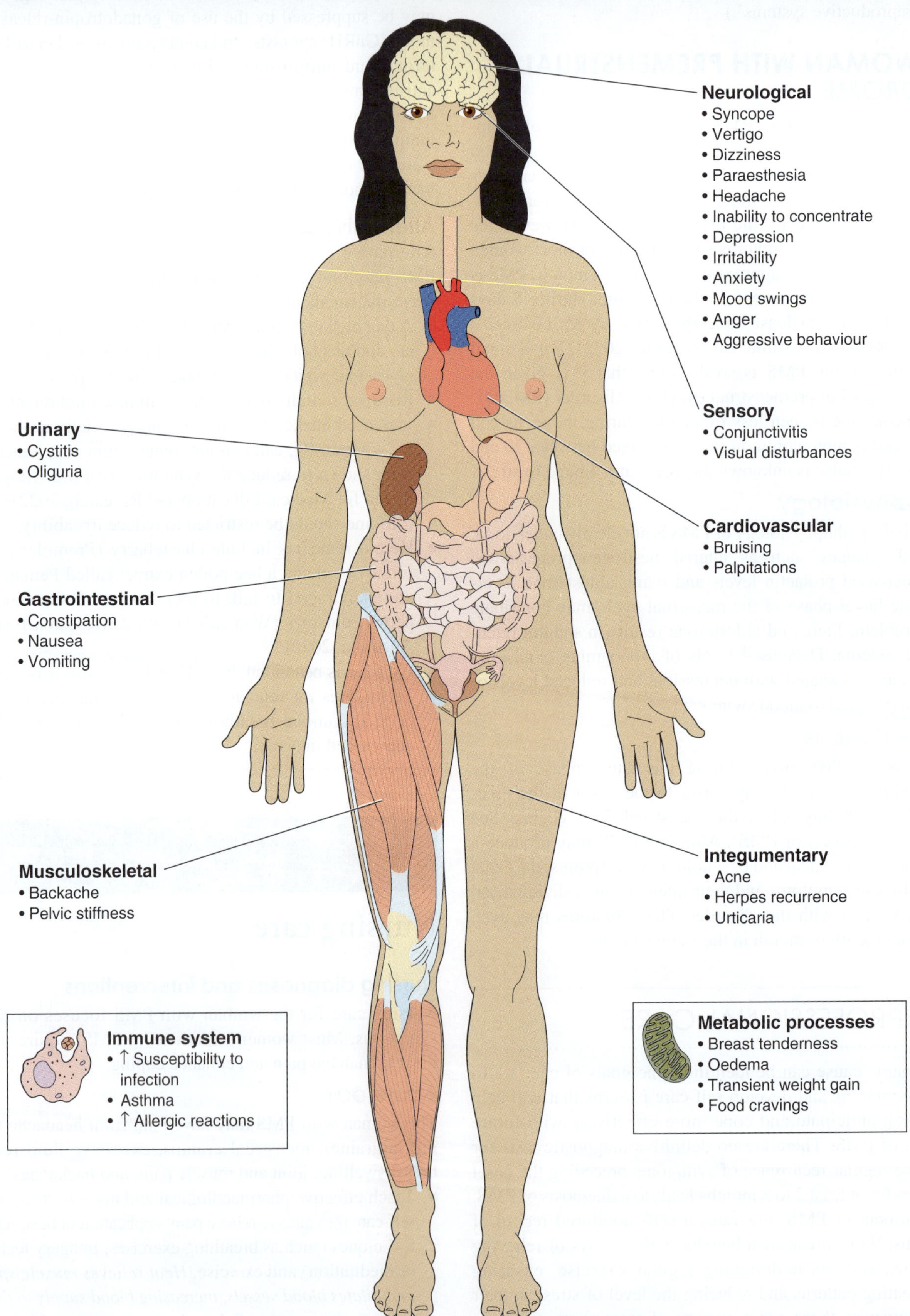

- Review daily activities and suggest ways to balance rest periods and activity. *During rest periods, energy and oxygen requirements decrease, increasing the amount of energy and oxygen available to muscles.*
- Review symptoms and, if possible, correlate these with dietary patterns and activity levels. Encourage the woman to keep a diary of PMS symptoms. *Maintaining a diary of PMS symptoms, activity and foods eaten can provide data to identify modifiable causes of discomfort.*
- If appropriate, suggest sexual activity as a way to lessen menstrual cramps. *Orgasm may help relieve dysmenorrhoea.*

Ineffective coping

Many women experience wide mood swings during episodes of PMS, sometimes exhibiting self-destructive or aggressive behaviours towards others. These mood swings can interfere with a woman's ability to manage her daily responsibilities.

- Encourage the woman to keep a journal of her menstrual cycle and to document her mood changes in the 7 to 10 days prior to menstruation. *Recognising the signs and timing of PMS is the first step in developing methods to cope with the problem.*
- Explore possible ways to rearrange or reschedule activities when experiencing PMS. *Planning ahead enables the woman to assume more control and promotes coping methods.*
- Explore what, if any, self-care measures have helped with mood alterations in the past. *Encourage healthful coping mechanisms, such as relaxation techniques and exercise. Some women may rely on alcohol or other medications during PMS, which only exacerbate the symptoms.*

Community-based care

Provide health education that enables the woman and her family to understand that PMS is not caused by a pathological process but is a physiological response to hormonal changes of the menstrual cycle. With an understanding of the condition, the woman is better able to manage anxiety and to become actively involved in techniques to reduce the symptoms. Education should also include dietary measures, relaxation techniques and exercise, stress-reduction techniques, mental health promotion and support systems.

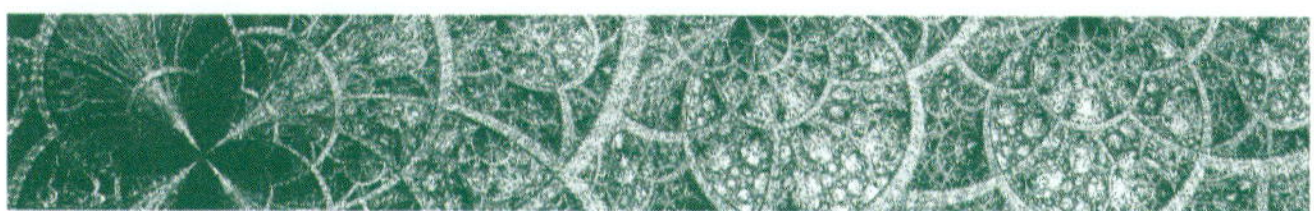

THE WOMAN WITH DYSMENORRHOEA

Dysmenorrhoea (pain or discomfort associated with menstruation) is experienced by a significant number of menstruating women. *Primary dysmenorrhoea* occurs without specific pelvic pathology and is most often seen in females who have just begun menstruating, becoming less severe after the mid twenties or giving birth. *Secondary dysmenorrhoea* is related to identified pelvic disease.

Pathophysiology

In primary dysmenorrhoea, excessive production of prostaglandins stimulates uterine muscle fibres to contract, meaning uterine circulation is compromised, resulting in uterine ischaemia and pain. These contractions range from mild cramping to severe muscle spasms. Psychological factors, such as anxiety and tension, may contribute to dysmenorrhoea. Secondary dysmenorrhoea is related to underlying organic conditions that involve scarring or injury to the reproductive tract. Endometriosis, fibroid tumours, pelvic inflammatory disease or ovarian cancer may result in painful menses.

MANIFESTATIONS Primary dysmenorrhoea

- Abdominal pain beginning with onset of menses and lasting 12 to 48 hours
- Pain radiating to lower back and thighs
- Headache
- Nausea
- Vomiting
- Diarrhoea
- Fatigue
- Breast tenderness

Manifestations

Symptoms of primary dysmenorrhoea (see the 'Manifestations' box) may be severe enough to disrupt activities of daily living, sexual function and even fertility.

INTERPROFESSIONAL CARE

Care of the woman with menstrual pain focuses on identifying the underlying cause, re-establishing functional capacity and managing pain.

A careful history is taken and a physical assessment is performed to rule out any underlying organic cause of dysmenorrhoea. If no organic cause can be found, the diagnosis is primary dysmenorrhoea. In addition, attitudes and expectations about menstruation and lifestyle disruption are identified and explored.

Diagnosis

Various diagnostic tests are performed to identify structural abnormalities, hormonal imbalances and pathological conditions that could cause menstrual pain. Diagnostic tests are described in the chapter 'A person-centred approach to assessing the male and female reproductive systems'.

Diagnosis is informed by a comprehensive history of signs and symptoms. As the onset of primary dysmenorrhoea usually occurs following the onset of menarche, the age group for this presentation is normally between 11 and 13 years. Therefore, it is not appropriate for a vaginal examination and pelvic ultrasound to be undertaken unless there are physical signs on abdominal palpation of ovarian masses. For this group of young teenagers, treatment with non-steroidal anti-inflammatory drugs (NSAIDs) is recommended.

The second group of women who experience primary dysmenorrhea is older teenage women who may be sexually active. Performing a vaginal examination for women in this age group needs to be carefully assessed on an individual basis. For this age group, treatment may be offered in the form of the combined oral contraceptive pill. If the young woman is sexually active, it is important to discuss the importance of cervical screening, contraception and STIs. If symptoms persist after commencing treatment, a pelvic examination and diagnostic procedures (including a cervical screening test (formerly Pap smear) and cervical and vaginal cultures; ultrasound of the pelvis and vagina; and computed tomography (CT) scan or magnetic resonance imaging (MRI) to detect structural abnormalities, malignancy or infections) are undertaken. Tests used to assess possible causes of dysmenorrhoea are as follows:

- *follicle-stimulating hormone (FSH)* and *luteinising hormone (LH) levels* to assess the function of the pituitary gland. The results are correlated with the time of the menstrual cycle
- progesterone and oestradiol levels to assess ovarian function
- thyroid function tests (T_3 and T_4) to assess thyroid function.

Laparoscopy is used to diagnose structural defects and blockages caused by scarring, endometriosis, tumours and cysts (see Figure 48.1). See the accompanying box for nursing care of the woman having a laparoscopy. A dilation and curettage (D&C) of the uterus may be performed to obtain tissue for evaluation or to relieve dysmenorrhoea and heavy menstrual bleeding. (This procedure is discussed later in this chapter.)

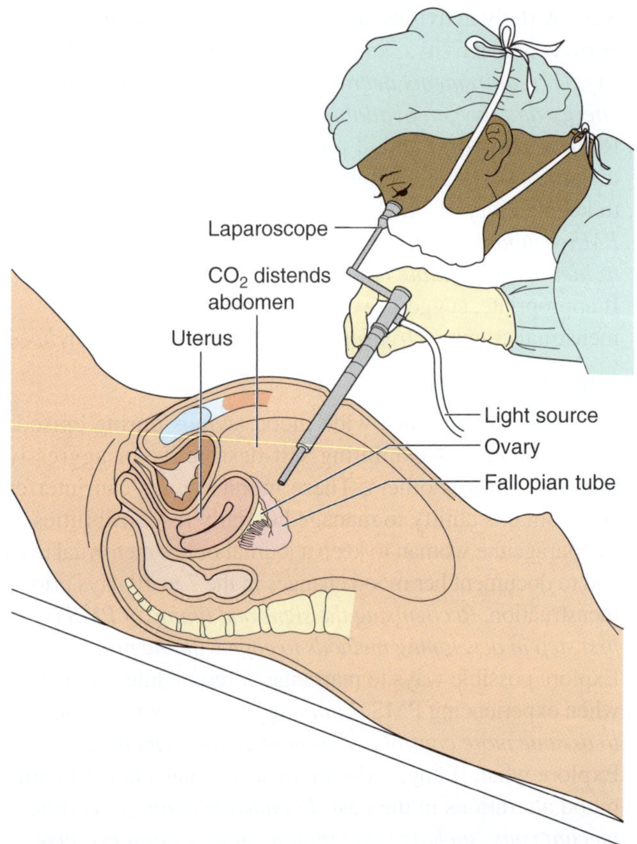

FIGURE 48.1 ***Laparoscopy. In this surgical procedure, a flexible, lighted instrument (laparoscope) is inserted through a periumbilical incision. Laparoscopy allows visualisation of the pelvic cavity***

Medications

Dysmenorrhoea may be treated with analgesics, prostaglandin inhibitors such as NSAIDs or oral contraceptives (see the 'Medication administration' box). A Cochrane review of 80 randomised control trials with 5820 women reported that NSAIDs are the best pain relief for primary dysmenorrhoea (Marjoribanks et al., 2015).

Alternative and complementary therapies

The complementary therapies listed for the woman with PMS may also be useful for the woman with dysmenorrhoea. Another helpful activity is regular and gentle physical exercise. Using a transcutaneous electrical nerve stimulation (TENS) machine, a heated pad on the abdomen or taking a warm bath also helps reduce pain.

NURSING CARE OF THE WOMAN having a laparoscopy

PREOPERATIVE CARE

- Orient the woman to the environment.
- Instruct the woman to empty the bladder prior to the procedure.
- Explain to the woman that referred shoulder pain or expulsion of gas through the vagina may occur postoperatively. *During the procedure, the woman's abdomen is insufflated with carbon dioxide gas to distend the abdomen and facilitate visualisation of the pelvic organs. The examination table is then tilted so that the intestines will fall away from the pelvic organs. Some carbon dioxide gas may remain in the abdomen after the procedure.*
- Explain that pain should be minimal. However, pain relief is available if required. Ask the woman to report excessive pain immediately. *Excessive pain signals infection or other postoperative complication.*

POSTOPERATIVE CARE

- Routine postoperative observations include pulse, blood pressure, respiratory rate, oxygen saturation level and consciousness.
- It is important to monitor vaginal bleeding. *Minor bleeding is normal; excessive bleeding may indicate haemorrhage.*
- Change the perineal pad, recording blood loss. Teach the woman proper perineal hygiene, emphasising the need to change pads at least every 4 hours. Keep a pad count to monitor blood loss. Proper perineal hygiene reduces the risk of postoperative infection. *Pad count is an indication of blood loss.*

MEDICATION ADMINISTRATION **The woman with dysmenorrhoea**

EXAMPLES OF ORAL CONTRACEPTIVES

Norethisterone and ethinylestradiol (Brevinor)
Ethinylestradiol (Microgynon 30)

Oral contraceptives inhibit ovulation and help reduce cramping and bleeding. Side effects include breast tenderness, weight gain, nausea, midcycle bleeding, mood swings, depression, chloasma (skin discolouration) on the face and chest, hypertension, vascular complications, vaginal candidiasis, migraines and glucose intolerance. Oral contraceptives are contraindicated in women with personal or family history of breast cancer in first-degree relatives, hypertension, history of stroke or transient ischaemic attack (TIA), smoking, history of oestrogen-dependent cancer, pregnancy, liver disease or thrombophlebitis.

Nursing responsibilities

- Assess the woman for potential contraindications to medication therapy.

Health education for the woman and family

- Take the medication as prescribed until otherwise indicated by a health professional or until side effects prevent continuation.
- If taking oral contraceptives, be sure to take them at the same time every day.
- Report any suspected pregnancy and any side effects such as nausea, rash, drowsiness, stomach pain, ringing in the ears, tenderness in the calf or shortness of breath.
- Do not smoke while taking oral contraceptives.
- Wear TED stockings when travelling long distances when you may not be very active, such as long plane flights or car travel.

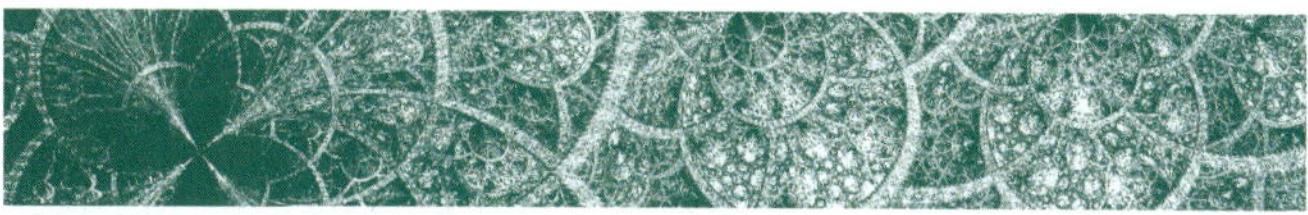

Nursing care

Nursing care for the woman with primary dysmenorrhoea focuses on controlling symptoms and providing health education about the normal physiology of the menstrual cycle and self-care measures. Care of the woman with secondary dysmenorrhoea varies according to the underlying cause and is discussed in this chapter within sections on specific disorders. Nursing interventions previously described for the woman with PMS are also appropriate for the woman with dysmenorrhoea.

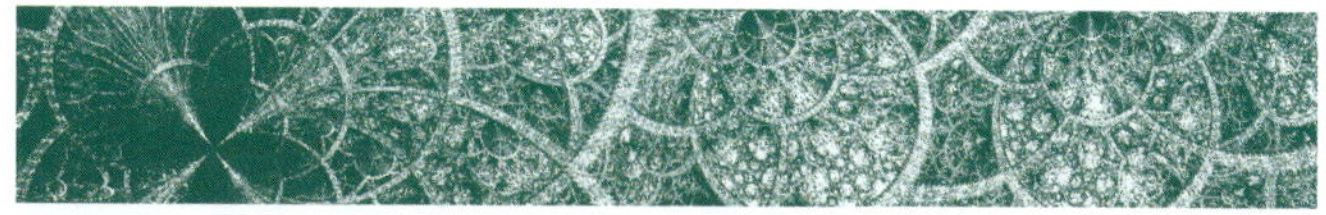

THE WOMAN WITH DYSFUNCTIONAL UTERINE BLEEDING

Dysfunctional uterine bleeding (DUB) refers to vaginal bleeding that is usually painless but is abnormal in amount, duration or time of occurrence. The types of DUB include primary and secondary amenorrhoea, oligomenorrhoea, menorrhagia, metrorrhagia and postmenopausal bleeding.

A number of factors may predispose a woman to DUB. These factors include stress, extreme weight changes, use of oral contraceptive agents or intra-uterine devices (IUDs), and postmenopausal status. DUB is usually related to hormonal imbalances or pelvic neoplasms, either benign or malignant.

Pathophysiology

The types of DUB outlined above will now be discussed.

- **Amenorrhoea** is the absence of menstruation. *Primary amenorrhoea*, absence of menarche by age 16 (or by age 14 if secondary sex characteristics fail to develop), may be caused by structural abnormalities, hormonal imbalances, polycystic ovary disease or an imperforate hymen. Because a certain percentage of body fat is required for menstruation to occur, anorexia nervosa, bulimia or excessive athletic training can also cause primary amenorrhoea. *Secondary amenorrhoea*, absence of menses for at least 6 months in a previously menstruating female, may also be caused by anorexia nervosa, excessive athletic activity or training, or a large weight loss. Other causes include hormonal imbalances and ovarian tumours. Normal (physiological) secondary amenorrhoea occurs during pregnancy, breastfeeding and menopause.
- *Oligomenorrhoea* (scant menses) usually is related to hormonal imbalances.
- **Menorrhagia** (excessive or prolonged menstruation) may result from thyroid disorders, endometriosis, pelvic inflammatory disease, functional ovarian cysts or uterine fibroids or polyps. Clotting disorders and anticoagulant medications also can cause menorrhagia.
- **Metrorrhagia** (bleeding between menstrual periods) may be caused by hormonal imbalances, pelvic inflammatory disease, cervical or uterine polyps, uterine fibroids or cervical or uterine cancer. Because cancer is a possible cause of metrorrhagia, early evaluation and treatment are extremely important. *Mittelschmerz* (midcycle spotting associated with ovulation) occurs in many women and is not considered metrorrhagia.
- *Postmenopausal bleeding* may be caused by endometrial polyps, endometrial hyperplasia or uterine cancer. The possibility of cancer makes early evaluation and treatment essential.

Hormonal imbalances, especially progesterone deficiency with relative oestrogen excess, result in endometrial hyperplasia. Oestrogen stimulates endometrial proliferation, but without the support provided by progesterone, sloughing occurs, resulting in vaginal bleeding that may be irregular, prolonged or profuse. Defects in the follicular phase shorten the proliferative phase of the menstrual cycle, resulting in spotting and breakthrough bleeding. Defects during the luteal phase result in excessive amount or duration of flow due to persistence of the corpus luteum. This leads to a deficiency of progesterone, resulting in vaginal bleeding. *Anovulation*, absence of ovulation, is associated with both oestrogen and progesterone deficiencies. Emotional upsets or stress can cause hormonal imbalances and thus affect menstruation. Pelvic neoplasms, discussed later, also cause abnormal bleeding.

INTERPROFESSIONAL CARE

The care of the woman with DUB focuses on identifying and treating the underlying disease. A careful history is taken and a physical examination is performed. Abdominal and pelvic examinations are performed to rule out abdominal masses. The woman may need to keep a menstrual history and basal body temperature chart for several months to determine whether ovulation is occurring.

Diagnosis

A variety of diagnostic tests are used to diagnose the cause of DUB. Diagnostic tests are discussed in the chapter 'A person-centred approach to assessing the male and female reproductive systems' and include a cervical screening test to rule out or identify cervical carcinoma, a pelvic ultrasound to identify luteal cysts, a hysteroscopy to detect abnormalities of the uterine cavity or an endometrial biopsy to obtain endometrial tissue for histological examination.

Laboratory studies may include:

- a *full blood count (FBC)* to rule out systemic disease as a contributing factor to DUB and to evaluate its effects.
- *thyroid function studies*, including measurement of tri-iodothyronine (T_3), thyroxine (T_4) and thyroid-stimulating hormone (TSH) levels, to rule out hyper- or hypothyroidism as a cause of DUB.
- *endocrine studies* to evaluate pituitary and adrenal function. Pituitary dysfunction may first be manifested by menstrual irregularities.
- *serum progesterone levels* to determine the level of progesterone deficiency.

Medications

For many women, hormonal agents can correct menstrual irregularities. For anovulatory DUB, oral contraceptives may be prescribed for 3 to 6 months. Progesterone or medroxyprogesterone also may be prescribed to regulate uterine bleeding. Ovulatory DUB may be treated with progestins during the luteal phase. Oral iron supplements may be prescribed to replace iron lost through menstrual bleeding.

Surgery

Surgical intervention emphasises the least invasive method that provides effective relief, beginning with a therapeutic dilation and curettage (D&C) procedure, then endometrial ablation and, finally, hysterectomy.

THERAPEUTIC D&C In a therapeutic D&C, the cervical canal is dilated and the uterine wall is scraped. D&C, the most frequently performed minor gynaecological surgical procedure, is used to diagnose and treat DUB and other disorders of the female reproductive system. It may be performed to correct excessive or prolonged bleeding. D&C is contraindicated in any woman who has been taking anticoagulant medications or whose condition precludes the use of regional or general anaesthesia. Nursing care of the woman having a D&C is described in the accompanying box.

ENDOMETRIAL ABLATION In an endometrial ablation, the endometrial layer of the uterus is permanently destroyed using laser surgery or electrosurgical resection. It is performed in women who do not respond to pharmacological management

NURSING CARE OF THE WOMAN having a dilation and curettage (D&C)

PREOPERATIVE CARE

- Orient the woman to the environment.
- Provide education and reassurance.
- If indicated and possible, ask the woman to come in 24 hours before surgery for insertion of a laminaria tent. *This device absorbs cervical secretions and slowly dilates the cervix.*
- Instruct the woman to remain nil by mouth after midnight on the day of surgery.

POSTOPERATIVE CARE

- Monitor circulation and sensation in the legs and avoid compression of the popliteal area. *The lithotomy position requires the woman's legs to be elevated, which can impair circulation.*
- Asses and monitor blood loss.
- Instruct the woman to use perineal pads and avoid using tampons for 2 weeks. *This reduces the risk of infection and allows tissues to heal.*
- Explain that the onset of the next menstrual period may be delayed.
- Explain that intercourse and anything inserted into the vagina should be avoided until after the postoperative checkup and after vaginal discharge has ceased. *This precaution reduces the risk of infection.*
- Instruct the woman to rest for several days after surgery, avoid heavy lifting and report any bleeding that is bright red or exceeds that of a normal menstrual period. *Vigorous activity, lifting or straining interferes with healing and may cause haemorrhage.*

or D&C. The woman needs to understand that this procedure ends menstruation and reproduction.

HYSTERECTOMY Hysterectomy, or removal of the uterus, may be performed when medical management of bleeding disorders is unsuccessful or malignancy is present, particularly if the woman no longer wishes to bear children. In premenopausal women, the ovaries are usually left in place; in postmenopausal women, a total hysterectomy, or panhysterectomy, may be performed; this procedure involves removal of the uterus, fallopian tubes and ovaries. However, removal of the ovaries may significantly impact on the woman's future cardiovascular, psychosexual, cognitive and mental health and, therefore, this needs to be considered before removing the ovaries.

FAST FACTS

- Hysterectomy is a commonly performed elective surgery.
- This surgery is most often performed in women who are between the ages of 40 and 44.
- Three conditions most associated with hysterectomy are uterine leiomyomas (fibroids), endometriosis and uterine prolapse.

Hysterectomy may involve an abdominal, vaginal or laparoscopic approach and depends on the underlying disorder, the need to explore the abdominal cavity and the preference of the surgeon and woman. Nursing care of the woman undergoing a hysterectomy is described in the accompanying box.

Abdominal hysterectomy is performed when a pre-existing abdominal scar is present, when adhesions are thought to be present or when a large operating field is necessary. The surgical incision may be either longitudinal, made in the midline from umbilicus to pubis, or a *Pfannenstiel incision*, also known as the bikini cut.

Vaginal hysterectomy, removal of the uterus through the vagina, is desirable when the uterus has descended into the vagina or if the urinary bladder or rectum have prolapsed into the vagina. Vaginal hysterectomy leaves no visible abdominal scar. Laparoscopy-assisted vaginal hysterectomy (LAVH) is most often performed.

Laparoscopic hysterectomy is when a hysterectomy is performed by making three to four incisions in the abdomen. The organs can then be viewed by inserting the laparoscope through one of the incisions; surgical instruments are inserted through the remaining incisions. The benefits of this procedure are a shorter hospital stay and quicker recovery.

NURSING CARE OF THE WOMAN **having a hysterectomy**

PREOPERATIVE CARE

- Assess the woman's understanding of the procedure. Provide explanation, clarification and emotional support as needed. Reassure that the anaesthesia will eliminate any pain during surgery and that medication will be administered postoperatively to minimise discomfort. *The woman who understands the procedure to be performed and what to expect after surgery will be less anxious.*
- Check that consent has been obtained.
- Perform preoperative procedures as per policy.
- Administer preoperative medications as indicated and provide psychological support.

POSTOPERATIVE CARE

- Assess for signs of haemorrhage. *Haemorrhage is more common after vaginal hysterectomy than after abdominal hysterectomy.*
- Monitor vital signs every 4 hours and measure intake and output. *These data are important indicators of haemodynamic status and complications.*
- Once the catheter has been removed, measure the amount of urine voided.
- Assess for complications, including infection, ileus, shock or haemorrhage, thrombophlebitis and pulmonary embolus.
- Assess vaginal discharge; provide health education about perineal care.
- Assess incision and bowel sounds regularly.
- Encourage turning, coughing, deep breathing and early ambulation.
- Encourage fluid intake.
- Teach to splint the abdomen and cough deeply. Heavy lifting, stair climbing, douching, tampons and sexual intercourse should be avoided. The woman should shower, avoiding tub baths, until bleeding has ceased. *Infection and haemorrhage are the greatest postoperative risks; restricting activities and preventing the introduction of any foreign material into the vagina helps reduce these risks.*
- Explain to the woman that she may feel tired for several days after surgery and needs to rest periodically.
- Explain that appetite may be depressed and bowel elimination may be sluggish. *These are after-effects of general anaesthesia, handling of the bowel during surgery and loss of muscle tone in the bowel while empty.*
- Teach the woman to recognise signs of complications that should be reported:
  a. temperature greater than 37.7°C
  b. vaginal bleeding that is greater than a typical menstrual period or is bright red
  c. urinary incontinence, urgency, burning or frequency
  d. severe pain.
- Encourage the woman to express feelings that may signal a negative self-concept. Correct any misconceptions and provide emotional support. *Some women believe that hysterectomy means weight gain, the end of sexual activity and the growth of facial hair.*
- Provide information on risks and benefits of hormone replacement therapy (HRT), if indicated. *If the ovaries have also been removed, the woman is immediately thrust into menopause and may want or need HRT.*
- Reinforce the need to obtain gynaecological examinations regularly, even after hysterectomy.

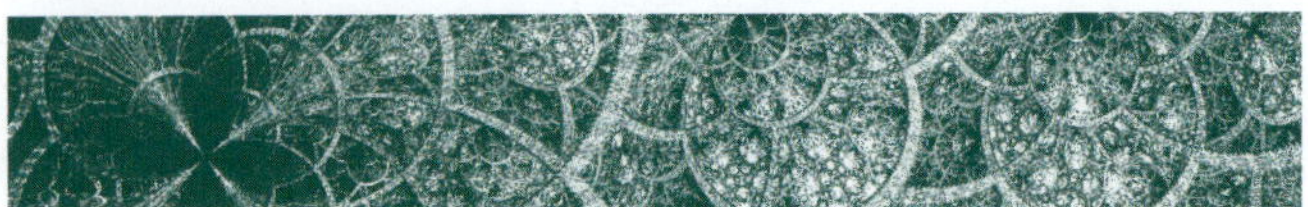

Nursing care

DUB usually causes anxiety. Self-image, sexuality or reproductive capacity may be threatened, and the woman may fear the possibility of cancer. She may be embarrassed to discuss her menstrual history and hygiene practices.

Nursing diagnoses and interventions

Interventions for the woman with DUB commonly address problems with anxiety and sexual function.

Anxiety

Anxiety associated with abnormal uterine bleeding can be intense. Until the cause of the bleeding is identified and has been addressed, the woman may fear cancer or other life-threatening conditions.

- Discuss the results of tests and examinations with the woman. *This allows for open exchange of information and correction of misconceptions.*
- Provide information about the causes, treatments, risks, long-term effects of treatments and prognosis. *This empowers the woman to assume responsibility for her own health and become involved in her own treatment plan.*
- Evaluate coping strategies and psychosocial support systems. Teach coping strategies if indicated. The possibility of surgery or cancer represents a crisis for the woman and her support system. *Support groups can provide assistance for the woman.*

Sexual dysfunction

The woman with DUB may be unwilling to express herself sexually, particularly if bleeding is frequent or heavy. Provide information about engaging in sexual activity during menstruation. Explain that conception is possible during this time (therefore birth control measures are required) and that orgasm may help relieve symptoms. *Orgasm causes a release of tension and vascular congestion, and frequently provides at least temporary relief of symptoms.*

- Provide an opportunity for the expression of concerns related to alterations in lifestyle and sexual functioning. Some women have had a prolonged period of sexual abstinence related to DUB. *Empowering women to verbalise concerns can assist them in working collaboratively with the healthcare provider to minimise the impact of illness and optimise function.*

CONSIDERATION FOR PRACTICE

Nurses should be open to discussing sexuality and sexual activities with women. If the nurse is not comfortable they cannot expect the woman to be.

Community-based care

Provide support, appropriate reassurance and information to help the woman and her family better understand her disorder and the therapeutic interventions indicated. Education should include:

- administration and side effects of prescribed medications, including iron
- the need to maintain a balanced diet, increasing iron-rich foods such as eggs, beans, liver, beef and shellfish. (Inform the woman that while orange juice may improve the absorption of iron, foods high in calcium and oxalic acid, such as spinach, may reduce its absorption)
- importance of maintaining a fluid intake of 2 to 3 L a day
- the need to immediately report recurring episodes of DUB, particularly in postmenopausal women, to the healthcare provider
- the importance of the woman looking after her mental health.

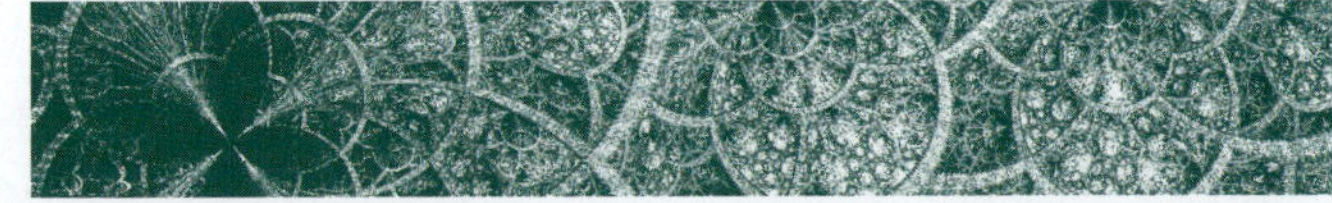

Structural disorders

Structural disorders of the female reproductive system include displacement disorders and fistulas.

THE WOMAN WITH A UTERINE DISPLACEMENT

The uterus may be displaced within the pelvic cavity or may descend into the vaginal canal. Displacement of the uterus within the pelvic cavity is classified according to the direction of the displacement (see Figure 48.2):

- *Retroversion* of the uterus is a backwards tilting of the uterus towards the rectum.
- *Retroflexion* involves a flexing or bending of the uterine corpus in a backwards manner towards the rectum.
- *Anteversion* is an exaggerated forwards tilting of the uterus.
- *Anteflexion* is a flexing or folding of the uterine corpus upon itself.

Prolapse of the uterus into the vaginal canal can vary from mild to complete prolapse outside of the body. First-degree, or mild, prolapse involves a descent of less than half the uterine corpus into the vagina. Second-degree, or marked, prolapse involves the descent of the entire uterus into the vaginal canal, so that the cervix is at the introitus to the vagina. Third-degree

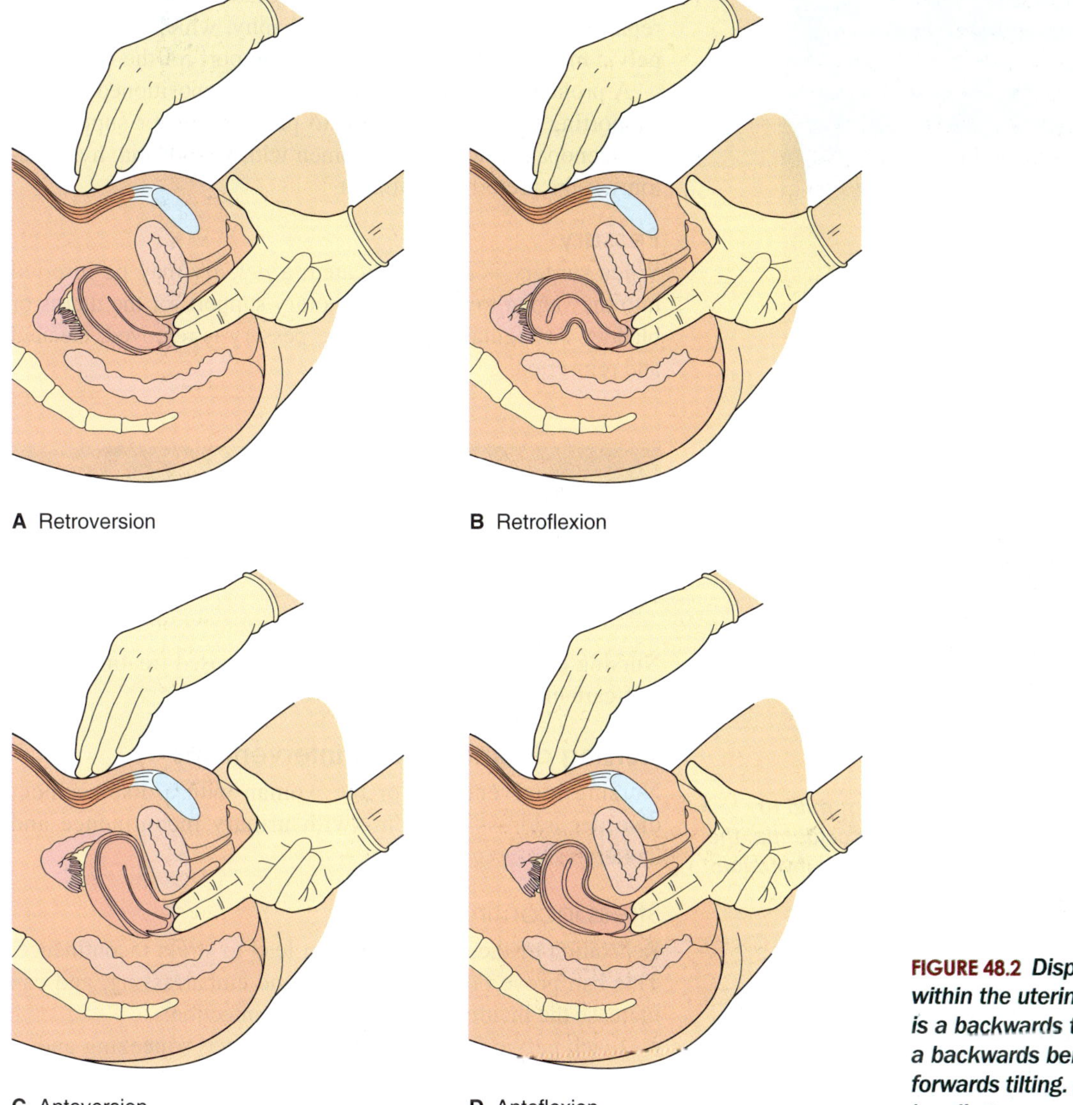

FIGURE 48.2 *Displacements of the uterus within the uterine cavity. A, Retroversion is a backwards tilting. B, Retroflexion is a backwards bending. C, Anteversion is a forwards tilting. D, Anteflexion is a forwards bending*

prolapse, or *procidentia*, is complete prolapse of the uterus outside the body, with inversion of the vaginal canal (see Figure 48.3). Prolapse of the uterus is often accompanied by *cystocoele* (herniation of the bladder into the vagina) or *rectocoele* (herniation of the rectum into the vagina).

Pathophysiology

Displacement or prolapse of the uterus, bladder or rectum can be a congenital or an acquired condition. Congenital tilting or flexion of the uterus is rare. More commonly, tilting or flexion disorders in which the uterus remains within the pelvic cavity are related to the scarring and inflammation of pelvic inflammatory disease, endometriosis, pregnancy and tumours.

Downwards displacement of the pelvic organs into the vagina results from weakened pelvic musculature, usually attributable to stretching of the supporting ligaments and muscles during pregnancy and childbirth. Unrepaired lacerations from childbirth, rapid deliveries, multiple pregnancies, congenital weakness or loss of elasticity and muscle tone may contribute to these disorders.

Manifestations

The symptoms of displacement disorders are listed in the 'Manifestations' box.

MANIFESTATIONS Displacement disorders

UTERINE DISPLACEMENT WITHIN THE PELVIC CAVITY

- Dysmenorrhoea
- Backache
- Dyspareunia
- Infertility

UTERINE PROLAPSE

- Backache
- Urinary incontinence
- Bearing-down sensation
- Haemorrhoids
- Constipation
- Dyspareunia

CYSTOCOELE/RECTOCOELE

- Bearing-down sensation
- Haemorrhoids
- Constipation
- Urinary incontinence
- Faecal incontinence

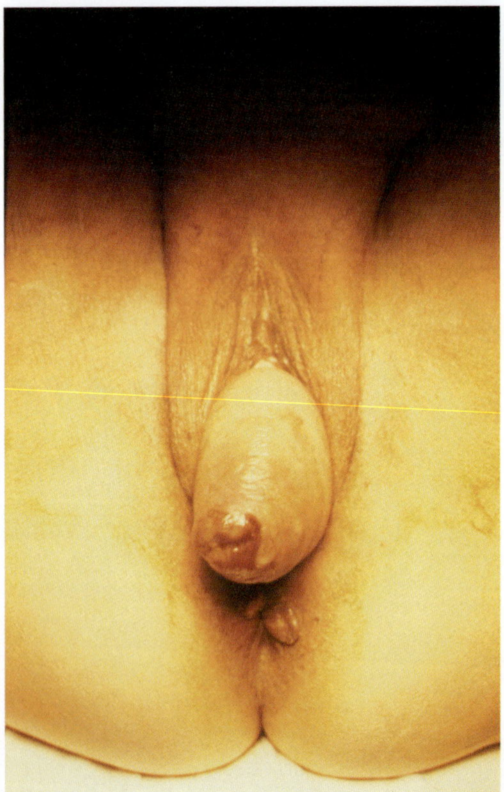

FIGURE 48.3 ***Prolapse of the uterus can vary from mild to complete. In third-degree uterine prolapse, or procidentia, the uterus prolapses completely outside the body, with inversion of the vagina***

Source: DELALANDE/BSIP SA/Alamy Stock Photo.

INTERPROFESSIONAL CARE

Interprofessional care focuses on identifying the cause of the structural disorder, correcting or minimising the condition, relieving pain, preventing or treating infection, and supporting and educating the woman.

A careful history is taken and a physical examination is performed. Diagnosis of uterine displacement is made after physical examination. If herniation of the rectum or bladder is suspected, the woman is asked to bear down or cough during the examination so the prolapse can be palpated and any leakage of urine or faeces visualised. A history of infections, multiple pregnancies in rapid succession and rapid labours support this diagnosis.

Treatment may include pelvic floor (Kegel) exercises to strengthen weakened pelvic muscles. Pelvic floor exercises can be useful in the early stages of downwards displacement. These exercises are discussed in the chapter 'Nursing care of people with urinary tract disorders'.

Surgery

Several surgical procedures are used to repair structural disorders. For women presenting with a cystocoele, *anterior colporrhaphy* (repair of the cystocoele) is the most common procedure. The anterior repair shortens the pelvic muscles, providing tighter support for the bladder. A rectocoele is repaired with a posterior colporrhaphy, which shortens the pelvic muscles, providing a tighter support for the rectum.

A prolapsed uterus may be surgically repositioned and the supporting muscles shortened to provide greater support. In postmenopausal women or women with procidentia, hysterectomy is the preferred treatment.

Pessary

When surgery is contraindicated, a *pessary* may be inserted into the vagina to provide temporary support for the uterus or bladder. At regular intervals, the pessary is removed, cleaned and reinserted.

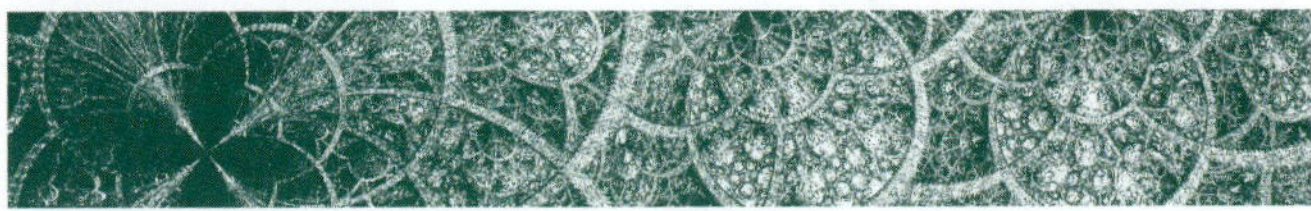

Nursing care

Nursing care focuses on education, proposed treatments and self-care measures for relief of symptoms.

Nursing diagnoses and interventions

Nursing interventions for the woman with a displacement disorder address problems with urinary incontinence and anxiety.

Stress incontinence

Relaxation of the pelvic floor can lead to stress incontinence. This can prove both troublesome and embarrassing, and can increase the incidence of urinary tract infection.

- Teach pelvic floor training that involves squeezing and lifting the muscles around back passage and vagina (Continence Foundation of Australia, 2022). These exercises strengthen perineal muscle tone, minimise urinary leakage and minimise descent of the bladder and rectum into the vagina. *In postmenopausal women, oestrogen supplements also can improve muscle tone in the perineal area.*
- Suggest the use of perineal pads (ranging from thin panty liners to full-thickness incontinence pads) or special underwear to absorb urine leakage. *Using pads or undergarments often allows the woman to once again take part in her usual social activities.*
- Explain perineal care and proper use of perineal pads. Cleansing the perineum from front to back and applying and removing perineal pads the same way minimises cross-infection from the anus to the vaginal and urethral openings. *Incontinence pads need to be changed frequently to minimise surface bacterial counts.*
- Suggest reducing or eliminating caffeine intake. *Reducing caffeine intake can reduce urinary frequency and urgency.*
- Stress the importance of cleaning the perineal area. *Urine is very irritating to the skin.*

Anxiety

Anxiety is common in women with a displacement disorder. Many women have a limited understanding of their reproductive anatomy, leading to anxiety. The nurse can use models or pictures to explain structural disorders and treatment options available.

- Encourage questions from the woman and her partner. *This helps assess the level of understanding so that health education can be more effective.*
- Explain that the relief from discomfort and fatigue may positively influence sexual expression and reassure the woman that the capacity for orgasm will not be affected. *Many women and their partners have major concerns about the effects of the disorder and its treatment on their sex life and capacity for sexual pleasure.*
- Explore coping mechanisms that have been previously successful. *This can help relieve anxiety and boost self esteem.*

Community-based care

If surgery is the treatment of choice, health education focuses on the preoperative and postoperative periods. If medical treatment is used initially, education focuses on measures to relieve the symptoms, such as pelvic floor exercises, use of incontinence pads or the use, care and insertion of a pessary.

As obesity is a risk factor associated with relaxation of the pelvic and abdominal muscles, dietary counselling may be indicated. Preoperatively, a diet high in fibre may alleviate constipation, a particular concern during the postoperative period.

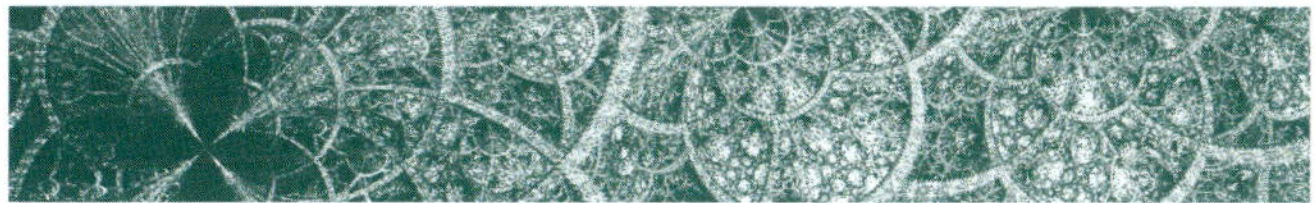

THE WOMAN WITH A VAGINAL FISTULA

A fistula is an abnormal opening or passage between two organs or spaces that are normally separated, or an abnormal passage to the outside of the body. Vaginal fistulas may be vesicovaginal or rectovaginal. A *vesicovaginal fistula* is an abnormal opening between the urinary bladder and the vagina, leading to incontinent leakage of urine through the vagina. A *rectovaginal fistula* (less common) is an abnormal opening between the rectum and vagina, causing incontinent leakage of stool or flatus through the vagina.

Vesicovaginal or rectovaginal fistulas may develop as a complication of childbirth, gynaecological or urological surgery, or radiation therapy for gynaecological cancer. Cancer of the bladder is sometimes involved. The woman with a vaginal fistula often presents with involuntary leakage of urine or flatus and symptoms of infection.

INTERPROFESSIONAL CARE

Fistulas are diagnosed by pelvic examination. Diagnosis of a vesicovaginal fistula can be made by instilling dye into the urinary bladder through a catheter and observing the vagina for leakage. If no leakage is detected, a tampon or vaginal pack is inserted into the vagina and the woman is asked to ambulate. If an abnormal opening is present, the tampon will absorb the dye. Dye may also be injected intravenously because it is excreted by the kidneys. Urine and vaginal cultures may be performed to rule out infections. Antibiotics are administered if infection is present.

A small vaginal fistula may resolve spontaneously. Otherwise, surgery is performed after inflammation has subsided—often a period of several months. Rarely, in the presence of a large, highly inflamed rectovaginal fistula, a temporary colostomy is performed, allowing inflammation and irritation to subside (see the chapter 'Nursing care of people with bowel disorders').

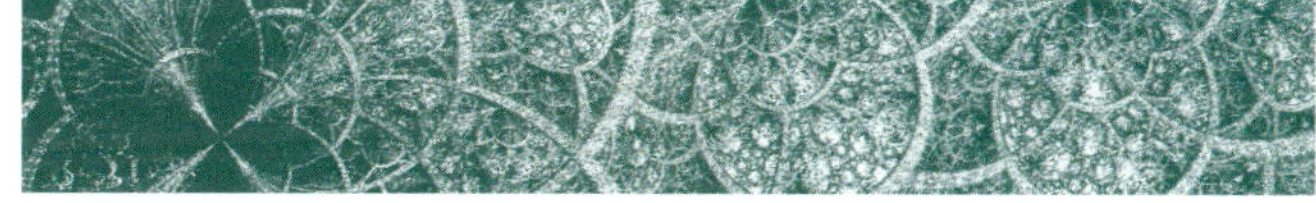

Nursing care

Nursing care for the woman with repair of a vaginal fistula is similar to that for the woman with a displacement disorder. Health education is an important component of nursing care. Stress the importance of careful perineal cleansing to reduce irritation and prevent further tissue breakdown. Perineal pads or special underwear may be used to absorb urine or faecal drainage. For the woman with a rectovaginal fistula, provide information about avoiding gas-forming foods to minimise embarrassment from odour.

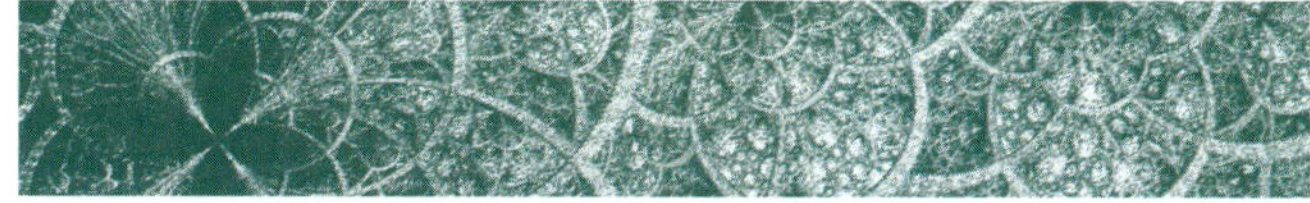

Disorders of female reproductive tissue

Both benign and malignant tissue disorders affect the female reproductive system. Benign tumours and cysts include Bartholin's gland cysts, cervical polyps, endometrial cysts and polyps, ovarian cysts and uterine leiomyomas (fibroids). Endometriosis is a condition in which endometrial tissue implants outside the uterus in various locations in the pelvic cavity. Malignant tumours of reproductive tissue include cervical, endometrial, ovarian and vulvar cancer.

THE WOMAN WITH CYSTS OR POLYPS

A *cyst* is a fluid-filled sac. A *polyp* is a highly vascular solid tumour attached by a pedicle or stem. Cysts or polyps of the female reproductive system can occur in the vulva, cervix, endometrium or ovaries.

Pathophysiology

Following are different types of female reproductive tissue cysts and polyps:

- *Bartholin's gland cysts* are the most common cystic disorder of the vulva. These cysts are caused by the infection or obstruction of Bartholin's gland.
- *Cervical polyps* are the most common benign cervical lesion in women of reproductive age. The polyps tend to occur in women over age 40 who have borne several children and have a history of using oral contraceptives. It is possible cervical polyps develop from endocervical hyperplasia. The polyp develops at the vaginal end of the cervix, has a stem and is highly vascular.
- *Endometrial cysts and polyps* are caused by endometrial overgrowth and are often filled with old blood. (The dark colour leads to the label 'chocolate cysts'.) Endometrial cysts are the result of endometrial implants on the ovary and are associated with endometriosis. Endometrial polyps, in contrast, are intrauterine overgrowths, similar to cervical polyps, and usually have a stalk.
- *Ovarian cysts* are classified as follicular cysts and corpus luteum cysts. Follicular cysts develop as a result of failure of the mature follicle to rupture or failure of an immature follicle to reabsorb fluid after ovulation. Corpus luteum cysts develop as a result of increased hormone secretion by the corpus luteum after ovulation. Most functional cysts regress spontaneously within two or three menstrual cycles.
- *Polycystic ovarian syndrome* (POS, also known as *Stein–Leventhal syndrome*) is an endocrine disorder characterised by an excess of androgens and a long-term lack of ovulation. The exact cause is unknown. As a part of the disease, as many as 8 to 10 cysts form in the ovaries from a failure to release ova. Symptoms include amenorrhoea or irregular menses, hirsutism, obesity, acne, hypertension, sleep apnoea and infertility. Women with POS often have insulin resistance and are at increased risk of early-onset type 2 diabetes, as well as heart disease, breast and endometrial cancer.

Manifestations and complications

The causes and symptoms of benign cysts and polyps of the female reproductive system are presented in Table 48.1. Complications associated with these disorders include infection, rupture, infertility, haemorrhage and recurrence.

INTERPROFESSIONAL CARE

Care focuses on identifying and correcting the disorder and preventing recurrence. A careful history is taken and physical examination performed, including inspection and visualisation. Examination of the reproductive tract reveals the presence of most cysts and polyps. The menstrual history may reveal menstrual irregularities.

Diagnosis

Diagnostic tests include laparoscopy to visualise ovarian cysts, ultrasound or x-ray to differentiate cysts from solid tumours and a pregnancy test when luteal cysts are suspected. Laboratory analysis will demonstrate elevated LH and testosterone levels, as well as a reverse in FSH/LH in the woman with POS.

Medications

Antibiotics are used to treat infection or abscess, and oral contraceptives are used to promote regression of functional ovarian cysts. Clomiphene (Clomid, Serophene) may be prescribed to stimulate ovulation in the woman with POS who wishes to become pregnant. Other hormones may be added to increase the likelihood of ovulation.

Surgery

Cervical polyps are visible through a vaginal speculum and usually are removed with a clamp, using a twisting motion. To remove endometrial cysts or polyps, a transcervical approach is used. The specimen is sent to the laboratory for evaluation and chemical or electrical cauterisation is applied after cyst removal. For Bartholin's gland cysts and any abscesses, the lesion is incised and drained and a drainage device is left in place. Follicular cysts may be punctured through laser surgery or a wedge resection of the ovary may be performed to restore ovulation. Rarely, *oophorectomy* (removal of the ovary) is performed if the cysts are very large.

TABLE 48.1 Benign cysts and polyps of the female reproductive system

SITE	TYPE	AETIOLOGICAL ORIGIN	SYMPTOMS
Ovary	Functional cysts	Ovulation–include follicular cysts and corpus luteum cysts	May resolve spontaneously; can cause pain, menstrual irregularity or amenorrhoea
	Polycystic ovarian syndrome	Unknown; possible hypothalamic-pituitary dysfunction	Hirsutism, obesity; amenorrhoea or irregular menses; hyperinsulinaemia; infertility
Vulva	Bartholin cysts	Obstruction or infection of Bartholin's gland	Pain, redness, perineal mass, dyspareunia
Endometrium	Chocolate cysts	Endometrial overgrowth; filled with old blood	Bleeding between periods
	Endometrial polyps	Unknown	
Cervix	Cervical polyps	Unknown	Bleeding after intercourse or between periods

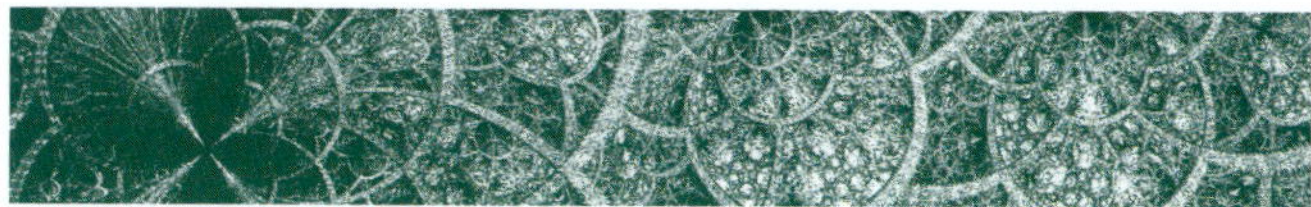

Nursing care

Nursing care focuses on relieving pain and preventing recurrence and complications. Address the following topics for self-care at home:

- the condition, its treatment and measures to relieve pain
- the importance of keeping follow-up appointments
- symptoms of infection (for post-surgical care) and the need to notify the health professional should they occur
- if cervical polypectomy is performed, advise use of external pads for 1 week. The woman must be able to state the signs of excessive bleeding and recognise that saturating more than one pad in an hour indicates the need for immediate follow up
- the importance of long-term follow-up care for the woman with POS.

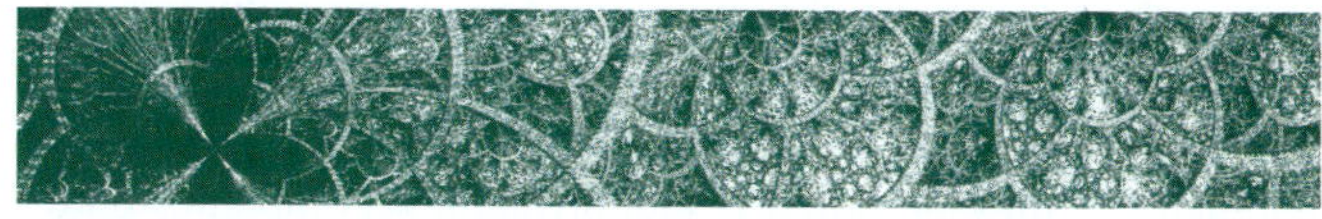

THE WOMAN WITH LEIOMYOMA

Leiomyomas (*fibroid tumours*) are benign tumours that originate from smooth muscle of the uterus. The prevalence of fibroid tumours with clinical symptoms ranges between 25% and 50% of the female population. Fibroids are very common among older women prior to the perimenopausal transition stage (Brito et al., 2019).

Pathophysiology

The cause of fibroid tumours is not clearly understood, but there is a strong association with oestrogen stimulation. Fibroid tumours usually develop in the uterine corpus and may be intramural, subserous or submucous (see Figure 48.4):

- *Intramural fibroid tumours* (the most common type) are embedded in the myometrium. They usually present as an enlargement of the uterus.
- *Subserous fibroid tumours* lie beneath the serous lining of the uterus and project into the peritoneal cavity. They may become pedunculated (on a stem) and displace or compress other tissues, such as the ureter or bladder.
- *Submucous fibroid tumours* lie beneath the endometrial lining of the uterus. They displace endometrial tissue and are more likely to cause bleeding, infection and necrosis than the other types.

Manifestations

Small tumours may be asymptomatic. The rate of growth varies but may increase in size during pregnancy or with use of oral contraceptives or HRT. Large fibroid tumours can crowd other organs, leading to pelvic pressure, pain, dysmenorrhoea, menorrhagia and fatigue. Depending on the location of the tumour, constipation and urinary urgency and frequency may occur. Most fibroid tumours shrink with menopause.

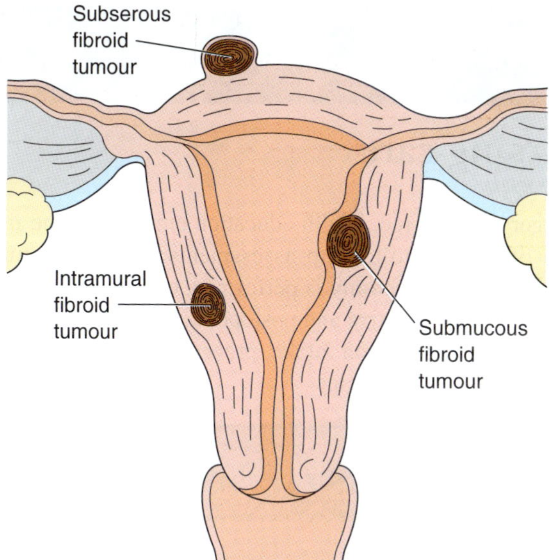

FIGURE 48.4 ***Types of uterine fibroid tumours (leiomyomas). Intramural fibroid tumours lie within the uterine wall. Subserous fibroid tumours lie beneath the serous lining of the uterus and project into the peritoneum. Submucous fibroid tumours lie beneath the endometrial lining of the uterus***

INTERPROFESSIONAL CARE

Treatment of the woman with uterine fibroids depends on the size and location of tumours, the severity of symptoms and her age and childbearing status. Tests to diagnose uterine fibroids may include ultrasound to differentiate leiomyoma from endometriosis, and laparoscopy to visualise subserosal leiomyomas.

In asymptomatic women who wish to bear children, the fibroid tumours are monitored. Follow up is recommended two to three times per year to monitor growth.

Medications

Hormonal contraceptives are used to decrease the size of the tumour if surgery is contraindicated or not desired. Gonadotropin-releasing hormone (GnRH) agonists are also administered.

Surgery

Myomectomy, removal of the tumour without removing the entire uterus, is the surgical procedure of choice for young women who wish to retain reproductive capability. Laparoscopic laser technique is used for many women. A hysterectomy is performed if tumours are large and if bleeding or other problems continue in perimenopausal women. A hysterectomy usually requires a hospital stay and a 6-week recovery time. A non-surgical method of treatment is a *uterine fibroid embolisation*. In this procedure, a catheter is guided through the femoral artery to the uterus, where tiny particles are injected into the artery supplying the fibroid to cut off the fibroid's blood supply.

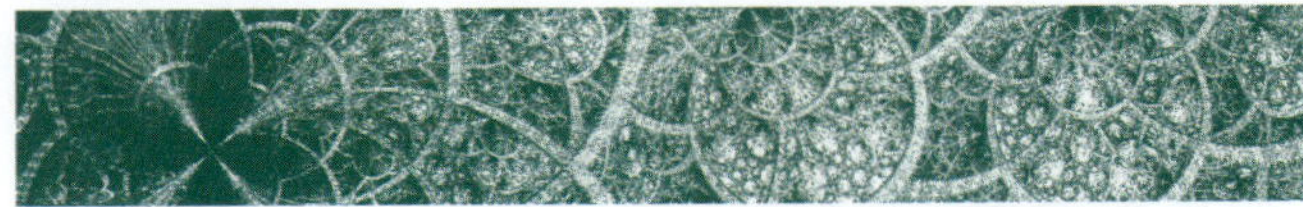

Nursing care

If surgery is deferred, health education emphasises the importance of regular follow-up assessments to monitor tumour growth. If a hysterectomy is performed, education emphasises appropriate preoperative and postoperative care. Dietary modifications to increase iron intake, prevent constipation and promote healing are important.

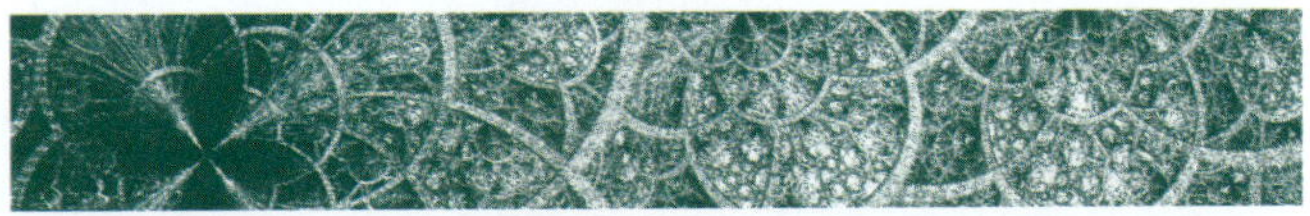

THE WOMAN WITH ENDOMETRIOSIS

Endometriosis is a condition in which multiple, small, usually benign implantations of endometrial tissue develop most commonly in the pelvic cavity, but also occasionally in other areas of the body, such as the lungs. Endometriosis affects 10–15% of women of childbearing age and is more common in women who postpone childbearing. Risk factors include early menarche, regular periods with a cycle of less than 27 days, menses lasting more than 7 days, heavier flow, increased menstrual pain and a history of the condition in first-degree female relatives.

Pathophysiology

The cause of endometriosis is unclear, but several theories have been proposed. The metaplasia theory asserts that endometrial tissue develops from embryonic epithelial cells as a result of hormonal or inflammatory changes. The theory of retrograde menstruation suggests that menstrual tissue backs up through the fallopian tubes during menses, implants on various pelvic structures and survives. The transplantation theory asserts that endometrial implants spread via lymphatic or vascular routes.

The abnormally located endometrial tissue responds to cyclical ovarian hormone stimulation, and bleeding at the time of menstruation occurs at the sites of implantation. Scarring, inflammation and adhesions may develop. Endometriosis is a slowly progressive disease, responsive to ovarian hormone stimulation. Thus, the implants regress during pregnancy and atrophy at menopause unless the woman is receiving HRT. Because progressive scarring may interfere with the ability to conceive, women with significant endometriosis are encouraged to have children early if they wish to do so.

Manifestations

Symptoms of endometriosis, which usually occur during the luteal phase of the menstrual cycle, are summarised in the 'Manifestations' box.

MANIFESTATIONS Endometriosis

- Heavy, throbbing pain of the lower abdomen and pelvis, radiating down the thighs and around the back. (The degree of pain is not indicative of disease severity.)
- Feeling of rectal pressure and discomfort when having a bowel movement.
- Dyspareunia.
- Dysfunctional uterine bleeding.
- Infertility.

INTERPROFESSIONAL CARE

Endometriosis may be difficult to diagnose, but a history of dysmenorrhoea, dyspareunia and infertility strongly suggests this diagnosis. Interventions depend on the severity of symptoms, the extent of the disease and the woman's age and desire for childbearing. Treatment goals focus on pain management and restoring fertility.

Diagnosis

Diagnostic tests are ordered to rule out other medical conditions and identify the endometrial implants. The tests include pelvic ultrasound and laparoscopy (see the chapter 'A person-centred approach to assessing the male and female reproductive systems'), as well as an FBC with differential to rule out pelvic abscesses and infectious processes. A low haemoglobin and haematocrit may be noted if menorrhagia accompanies endometriosis or tissue implants bleed significantly during menses. A definitive diagnosis can be made when a laparoscopy is performed and a biopsy of tissue is undertaken (Endometriosis Australia, 2022).

Medications

Medications include analgesics to control pain and prostaglandin synthesis inhibitors such as NSAIDs. Hormone therapy may include oral contraceptives or progesterone to induce pseudopregnancy. Intra-uterine devices (IUD) and implants can be used for long-term solutions. Danazol (Azol) is also used to induce amenorrhoea and involution of endometrial tissue. However, prolonged use of danazol may result in masculinising effects. GnRH is used to elevate levels of oestrogen and progesterone and minimise bleeding.

Surgery

Surgical interventions include laparoscopy with laser ablation (excision or removal) of endometrial implants. Refractory endometriosis may be treated with total hysterectomy.

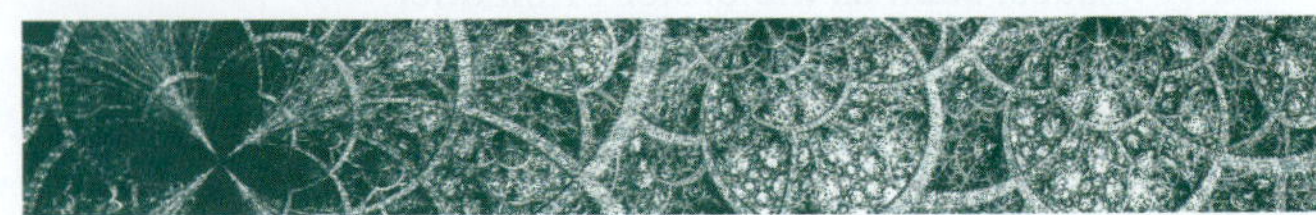

Nursing care

Nursing care includes providing pain relief, engaging the woman in health education about her condition and treatment options, and helping her identify strategies to cope with treatment outcomes. The severity of the disease and its symptoms are not necessarily related. Advanced disease may exhibit few symptoms, whereas early disease may be quite painful. See the accompanying nursing care plan for a woman with endometriosis.

NURSING CARE PLAN A woman with endometriosis

Joy Smith is a 29-year-old school teacher. She has been in a permanent relationship with her partner for the past 4 years. Joy describes a history of severe dysmenorrhoea and menorrhagia, a feeling of pelvic heaviness and pain that radiates down her thighs. Joy is seeking assistance for these symptoms, as she is not coping with the ongoing effect they have on her health and lifestyle. She also discusses her own and her partner's desire to have children. However, at the current time she is reluctant to have sex as she experiences severe discomfort and pain. Her partner has been supportive. However, it is affecting their relationship. Following review, endometriosis is suspected and a diagnostic laparoscopy has been scheduled.

ASSESSMENT

Registered Nurse and Nurse Practitioner Christian Bright interviews Joy and makes the following assessments: BP 110/70, P 68, R 18, T 36.7°C. Joy's weight is 59 kg and within normal limits for her height. Review of laboratory findings indicates a haemoglobin level of 98 g/L (normal range: 115 to 165 g/L) and a haematocrit of 33.1% (normal range: 38% to 47%). Physical examination reveals pelvic tenderness on manipulation of the cervix and small masses that are palpable on abdominal/pelvic examination.

DIAGNOSES

- *Chronic pelvic pain* related to the endometriosis and endometrial pelvic implants.
- *Anxiety* related to effect of endometriosis on fertility.
- *Deficient knowledge* related to diagnosis and treatment options.
- *Ineffective sexuality pattern* related to the symptoms of endometriosis.

PLANNING

- Identify the location, type, duration and history of the pain.
- Recommend analgesics and heat therapy.
- Provide information on biofeedback, relaxation and imagery to lessen pain.
- Discuss with Joy and her partner, David, the causes of endometriosis and its symptoms.
- Encourage Joy and David to discuss their feelings about the effect of the disease on their sex life, lifestyle and fertility.
- Refer the couple to appropriate counselling if required.
- Refer the couple to support organisations such as Endometriosis Australia https://www.endometriosisaustralia.org.

Expected outcomes

- Develop effective self-care measures to deal with the pain and discomfort.
- Verbalise decreased anxiety.
- Demonstrate understanding of the disease and treatment options.
- Verbalise an improvement in sexual functioning and a decrease in interpersonal stress between Joy and her partner.

IMPLEMENTATION

- Initiate each of the steps outlined in the planning section detailed above.
- Monitor the effectiveness of the plan by monitoring Joy's response to:
  - analgesics, heat therapy and biofeedback
  - relaxation and imagery to lessen pain.
- Ongoing discussion with Joy and David about their sexual relationship and infertility issues.

EVALUATION

Two years after the initiation of treatment, Joy and David have become parents of a baby girl. Joy states that the discomfort and other symptoms of endometriosis have eased. Relaxation and imagery have effectively minimised her pain and brought about improvement in her function as a mother and sexual partner. Counselling has improved the interpersonal and sexual relations between Joy and David. Dietary management has improved her anaemia, although the menorrhagia persists. Joy and David are trying to have a second baby. They will be followed up and referred to an infertility clinic if conception does not occur within 1 year.

CRITICAL THINKING IN THE NURSING PROCESS

1 Explain the pathophysiological basis for Joy's anaemia.
2 How would you handle the situation if Joy and David were extremely uncomfortable and embarrassed about discussing their sexual problems?
3 Develop a plan of care for Joy for *Situational low self-esteem* related to the symptoms of endometriosis.

REFLECTION ON THE NURSING PROCESS

1 Outline what you have learned from Joy's case study. How would you incorporate this into your future nursing practice?
2 Which strategies would you use in your future nursing practice to assist women who are experiencing endometriosis and subsequent infertility?

Nursing diagnoses and interventions

Interventions for pain, discussed previously, are also appropriate for the woman with endometriosis. A priority for care for women with this disorder is anxiety related to the risk of loss of reproductive function.

Anxiety

Anxiety about the unsure prognosis related to infertility is a particular problem for young women who plan to have a family in the future.

- Encourage expression of fears and anxiety about infertility and answer questions honestly and based on evidence. *Knowledge helps relieve anxiety and fear.*
- Provide information on fertility awareness methods, including measurement of basal body temperature and other techniques for recognising ovulation. *Understanding these techniques helps the woman optimise the conditions for conception.*

Community-based care

Explain the cause of the disorder and various treatment options, including side effects. Discuss fertility awareness methods and the risks and benefits of long-term use of oral contraceptives. Stress the importance of regular exercise, smoking cessation and weight control. If surgical treatment is chosen, provide preoperative and postoperative education.

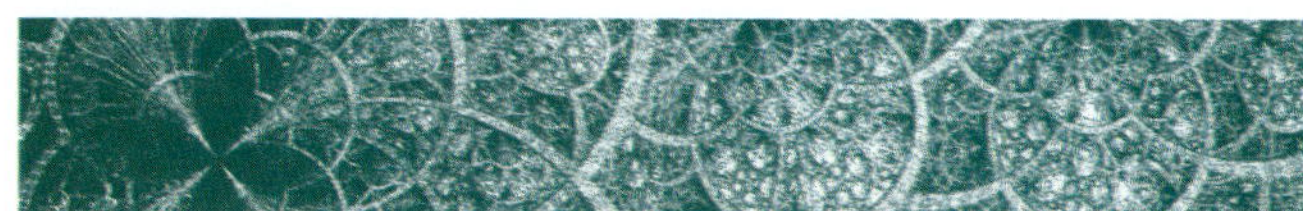

THE WOMAN WITH CERVICAL CANCER

Cancer of the cervix is the fourth most common cancer in women worldwide (World Health Organization, 2022) but is less common in women in Australia (Cancer Australia, 2022a). Only 1.3% of all new female cancer cases were diagnosed as cervical cancer in 2021. The lower incidence in Australia is primarily the result of screening with cervical screening tests and the introduction of the HPV vaccine Gardasil. Gardasil 9 has been shown to be 97% effective against nine types of HPV, which are responsible for 93% of cervical cancer cases in women (Australian Institute of Health and Welfare (AIHW), 2019a; National HPV Vaccination Program Register, 2018).

The incidence of diagnosis with cervical cancer prior to 85 years of age is 1 in 185 women (Cancer Australia, 2022a). However, it is important to remember that cervical cancer begins to appear in women in their twenties. According to the AIHW (2019a), effective screening with the cervical screening test and treatment have reduced the death rate in women as a result of cervical cancer. However, the mortality rate remains high for Aboriginal and Torres Strait Islander women (see 'Fast facts' box) and health professionals need to provide health education and work towards lowering this unacceptable mortality rate (AIHW, 2019b).

FAST FACTS

- The AIHW (2019a) reports that cervical cancer rates in Australia are at a historic low. Incidence rates have decreased since the introduction in 1991 of the National Cervical Screening Program (NCSP). However, for people from Aboriginal and Torres Strait Islander heritage, the incidence rates are double that of the non-Indigenous population. The mortality rate for cervical cancer is four times higher in Aboriginal and Torres Strait Islander women in comparison with the non-Indigenous population.
- Nearly 100% of women with cervical cancer have evidence of cervical infection with human papillomavirus (HPV) (see the chapter 'Nursing care of people who have sexually transmitted infections').
- The NCSP for Australian women recommends all women aged 25 to 69 years, whether vaccinated or unvaccinated, should have cervical screening by a cervical screening test every 5 years if the test is a primary HPV test with partial HPV genotyping and reflex liquid-based cytology (LBC) triage, with exit testing age of 70 to 74 (AIHW, 2019a).

Risk factors

Risk factors for cervical cancer include first intercourse before 16 years of age, multiple sex partners or male partners with multiple sex partners, a history of STIs and infection with HIV. The most important risk factor is infection with HPV. Other risk factors include smoking and poor nutritional status, family history of cervical cancer and exposure to diethylstilbestrol (DES) in utero.

Pathophysiology

Most cervical cancers (70%) are squamous cell carcinomas that begin as neoplasia in the cervical epithelium. *Precancerous dysplasia* (*cervical intraepithelial neoplasia (CIN), cervical carcinoma in situ*) is estimated to occur in 1 in 8 women before the age of 20 and is often associated with HPV infection. Studies have also found a strong association with reproductive infections with *Chlamydia trachomatis*. (These infections are discussed in the chapter 'Nursing care of people who have sexually transmitted infections'.) The precursor lesions may spontaneously regress, persist) or progress and undergo malignant change. Only about 1% become invasive. Systems of grading of dysplastic changes in the cervix use the term *cervical intraepithelial neoplasia (CIN)* or the Bethesda system (see Table 48.2). Carcinoma in situ is localised; invasive cancer spreads to deeper layers. The Bethesda system was modified to differentiate any suspected low-grade abnormalities from confidently predicted low-grade abnormalities, which is more suitable for the international terminology (Cancer Council, 2022a).

Cancer in situ most often develops in the transformation zone where the columnar epithelium of the cervical lining meets the squamous epithelium of the outer cervix and vagina. Squamous cell cancers spread by direct invasion of accessory

TABLE 48.2 Classification systems for cervical screening tests

DYSPLASIA/NEOPLASIA	CIN (CERVICAL INTRAEPITHELIAL NEOPLASIA)	BETHESDA SYSTEM	NUMERICAL
Benign	Benign	Normal	1
Benign with inflammation	Benign with inflammation	Normal Atypical squamous cells of undetermined significance (ASC-US)	2
Moderate dysplasia	CIN I	Low-grade squamous intraepithelial lesion (SIL)	3
Severe dysplasia	CIN II	High-grade SIL	3
Carcinoma in situ	CIN III	High-grade SIL	4
Invasive cancer	Invasive cancer	Invasive cancer	5

structures, including the vaginal wall, pelvic wall, bladder and rectum. Although metastasis is most frequently confined to the pelvic area, distant metastasis may occur through the lymphatic system.

Manifestations

Pre-invasive cancer is limited to the cervix and rarely causes symptoms. Invasive cancer causes vaginal bleeding after intercourse or between menstrual periods, and a vaginal discharge that increases as the cancer progresses. These changes are subtle and may be more readily noticed by postmenopausal woman. Symptoms of advanced disease include referred pain in the back or thighs, haematuria, bloody stools, anaemia and weight loss.

INTERPROFESSIONAL CARE

The goals of treatment are to eradicate the cancer and minimise complications and metastasis. Treatment depends on the degree of malignant change, the size and location of the lesion and the extent of metastasis.

Diagnosis

Diagnostic tests used to diagnose cervical cancer include a cervical screening test, colposcopy and cervical biopsy. A loop diathermy technique (loop electrosurgical excision procedure (LEEP) allows simultaneous diagnosis and treatment of dysplastic lesions found on colposcopy. This procedure is performed in the healthcare provider's office, using a wire for both cutting and coagulation during excision of the dysplastic region of the cervix. An MRI or CT of the pelvis, abdomen or bones may be performed to evaluate the spread of the tumour.

Medications

Chemotherapy is used for tumours not responsive to other therapy, tumours that cannot be removed or as adjunct therapy if metastasis has occurred (see the chapter 'Nursing care of people with cancer').

Surgery

When combined with colposcopy, laser surgery is a viable treatment method provided that the cancer is limited to the cervical epithelium. Cryosurgery, which involves the use of a probe to freeze tissue, causing necrosis and sloughing, is also used for non-invasive lesions. Conisation (see Figure 48.5) is performed to treat microinvasive carcinoma when colposcopy cannot define the limits of the invasion. For invasive lesions, hysterectomy or radical hysterectomy (removal of the uterus, fallopian tubes, lymph nodes and ovaries) is performed.

A *pelvic exenteration*, the removal of all pelvic contents including the bowel, vagina and bladder, is performed if the cancer recurs without involvement of the lymphatic system. An anterior exenteration is the removal of the uterus, ovaries, fallopian tubes, vagina, bladder, urethra, and lymphatic vessels and nodes. An ileal conduit is created for excretion of urine.

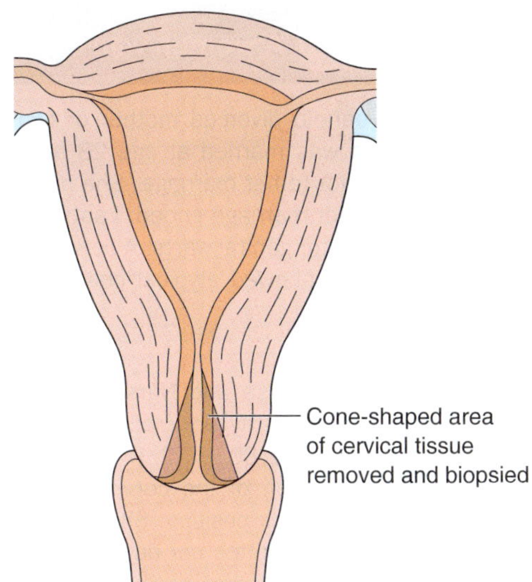

FIGURE 48.5 ***Conisation, the surgical removal of a cone-shaped section of the cervix, is used to treat microinvasive carcinoma of the cervix***

A posterior exenteration is the removal of the uterus, ovaries, fallopian tubes, bowel and rectum. A colostomy is created for excretion of faeces (see the chapter 'Nursing care of people with bowel disorders').

Radiation therapy

Radiation therapy is used to treat invasive cervical cancer. External radiation beam therapy and intracavity cesium irradiation can be used. Radiation is discussed in the chapter 'Nursing care of people with cancer'.

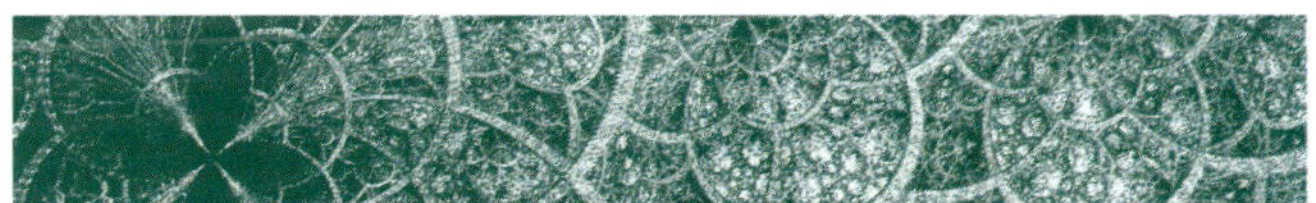

Nursing care

Nursing care involves helping the woman deal with the physical and psychological effects of a potentially life-threatening illness, providing information needed to make informed decisions and minimising the adverse effects of therapy. Pain relief measures are important, as is counselling for the woman and her family. The woman should be educated and encouraged to perform self-care activities and to resume normal everyday activities and sexual functioning to the extent possible. See the accompanying nursing care plan for a woman with cervical cancer.

Providing effective nursing care for the woman who has cancer involves a holistic and comprehensive approach.

Health promotion

The NCSP in Australia recommends that women should begin their screening for cervical cancer with the cervical screening test every 5 years from age 25. Women who are 70 to 74 years of age should have an exit test (AIHW, 2019a). Screening for

NURSING CARE PLAN A woman with cervical cancer

Kay Young is a 45-year-old divorced mother of two children aged 15 and 13. She was married at age 28 and had several sexual partners prior to her marriage. She has had three sexual partners since her marriage ended. Last year she was treated with cryosurgery for genital warts. A cervical screening test taken 2 weeks ago showed atypical cells and she has come in for a repeat test.

ASSESSMENT

Laura Jones, Registered Nurse and Nurse Practitioner, the admitting nurse, interviews Kay and records the following assessment findings: BP 130/80, P 72, R 18, T 37.3°C. Kay weighs 64.5 kg. Examination of the cervix reveals a large necrotic lesion at the 7 o'clock position. She has reduced her smoking to less than 10 cigarettes per day and she does not drink alcohol.

Kay is extremely fearful and anxious and has told no one about her abnormal cervical screening test. She reveals that she has had back pain radiating down her thighs for several months and a foul vaginal discharge that increases after intercourse. Until 2 weeks ago, she had not had a cervical screening test for 7 years. Laura Jones performs a cervical screening test, which is positive for squamous cell carcinoma of the cervix. A CT scan and lymphangiography are scheduled. Laparoscopy shows the disease to be widespread in the pelvic cavity.

DIAGNOSES

- *Personal distress* related to Kay having to make a decision about the various treatment options that she could undertake.
- *Chronic and acute pain* related to disease progress and the management of the metastasis, including recovering from surgery.
- *Risk of impaired skin integrity* related to side effects of the treatment options such as radiation.
- *Fear for her wellbeing and future* related to diagnosis and management of cervical cancer.
- *Anticipatory grieving* related to potential loss of life and the effect of this on her children.
- *Anxiety* related to her diagnosis and prognosis, and the future wellbeing of her two children.

PLANNING

- Discuss treatment alternatives, including the prognosis with each option.
- Administer pain medications as prescribed.
- Examine skin surfaces daily before and after radiation therapy.
- Provide information on biofeedback training and relaxation techniques for control of moderate pain.
- Refer to a local cancer support group so that she can interact with cancer survivors. (If in a rural or remote area provide resources and/or online and/or telephone contacts.)
- Refer Kay to a social worker in preparation for her altered level of functioning and for assistance with finding care for her two children while she is undergoing treatment. (Kay lives in an urban area in Australia. Social worker services might not be immediately available if Kay lived in a rural or remote rural area.)

Expected outcomes

- Gain knowledge to make informed decisions about treatment options.
- Develop strategies for pain control.
- Maintain skin and tissue integrity during radiation treatment.
- Express her feelings about the fear of cancer and death, and her concerns related to her children.
- Develop effective coping strategies for dealing with life-threatening illness and pain.

IMPLEMENTATION

- Initiate each of the steps outlined in the planning section detailed above.
- Monitor the effectiveness of the plan by monitoring Kay's response to:
  - analgesics
  - radiation therapy.
- Ongoing discussion with Kay about the implementation of the plan and her psychosocial wellbeing.

EVALUATION

Kay has begun radiation therapy following pelvic exenteration. She controls her pain with relaxation and imagery techniques, requiring only occasional analgesics. She uses a water-based lotion to soothe the skin surface and is careful not to remove the skin markings. She seems optimistic and has quit smoking. She and her family have continued to attend the cancer support group meetings. Kay is planning for the future and has talked with her children and extended family about what it means to live with cancer.

CRITICAL THINKING IN THE NURSING PROCESS

1 Compare and contrast your education plan for health promotion interventions to decrease the risks of cervical cancer for a young woman aged 17 and an older woman aged 70. Would they differ and, if so, how and why?

2 Develop an education plan to help Kay cope with the effects of treatment.

3 During a home visit, Kay informs the nurse that she has been so tired since beginning radiation treatments that all she can do is sit in her chair. Design a plan of care for assisting Kay to cope with *Fatigue*.

REFLECTION ON THE NURSING PROCESS

1 Outline what you have learned from Kay's case study. How would you incorporate this into your future nursing practice?

2 Which strategies would you use in your future nursing practice to assist women who are undergoing treatment for cervical cancer?

Links to National Patient Safety Standards

NSQHS: Comprehensive Care Standard

The intention of this standard is to ensure that women with reproductive system and breast disorders receive comprehensive care that is well coordinated and aligned with the woman's expressed goals of care and healthcare needs. The standard also intends nurses to consider the effect of the woman's health issues on her life and wellbeing, and to provide care that is clinically appropriate.

Source: ACSQHC (2021). *National Safety and Quality Health Service Standards* (2nd ed.). Sydney: ACSQHC. © Australian Commission on Safety and Quality in Health Care.

women who have had a total hysterectomy (including the cervix) is not recommended unless the surgery was done as a treatment for cancer. Women who have had a hysterectomy without removal of the cervix should continue to follow National Cervical Screening Program guidelines.

It is vital that nurses educate women of all ages about controlling risk factors for cervical cancer and about the importance of screening for this cancer throughout the lifespan. Educate young women about the relationship between early sexual activity, multiple partners and risk of STIs and cervical cancer. Discuss safer-sex alternatives and using condoms for protection. Emphasise the importance of continued screening examinations for women who may not see a health professional on a regular basis. Encourage women under the age of 26 to receive Gardasil 9, the vaccine described earlier. Gardasil 9 is given as three injections over a 6-month period and does not protect against HPV in a woman already infected. For this reason, the Therapeutic Goods Administration in Australia recommends that the vaccine be routinely given to girls and boys aged 12 and 13, which requires only two doses (National HPV Vaccination Program Register, 2018)

Assessment

Collect the following data through a health history and physical examination (see the chapter 'A person-centred approach to assessing the male and female reproductive systems'):

- *Health history*: history of STIs, sexual history, partner's sexual history, family history of cervical cancer, vaginal bleeding or discharge, smoking history, maternal treatment with DES.
- *Physical assessment*: pelvic examination, abdomen, lymph glands.
- *Psychological assessment*: anxiety, coping strategies and stress levels.

Nursing diagnoses and interventions

This section discusses nursing interventions for the woman who has been diagnosed with cervical cancer and requires surgical and/or radiation treatment. Other interventions that may be appropriate for the woman with cervical cancer are discussed in the sections on other female reproductive system cancers.

Fear

Many people believe that cancer equals death; however, this is no longer true in many cases, especially with early diagnosis. For cervical cancer diagnosed at an early stage (in women aged 25–29), the 5-year survival rate is 91.9% (AIHW, 2019b).

- Explain that 91.9% of women with cervical cancer survive for 5 years or more and that the earlier the cancer is detected, the better the prognosis. *This gives the woman hope, an essential ingredient in recovery.*
- Allow adequate time for the woman and her family to express their concerns and ask questions. *Unexpressed feelings and fears and lack of understanding may cause the woman to view the situation as worse than it is.*
- Refer to cancer counsellor or support groups for additional information. *Cancer survivors who visit people in the hospital provide proof that people can survive the diagnosis and treatment of cancer and lead normal, productive lives.*

Impaired tissue integrity

Surgery interrupts the integrity of the skin surface, providing a potential portal of invasion for bacteria. Radiation therapy causes an inflammatory response in the skin and mucous membranes within the field of radiation, creating further risk of tissue reaction and breakdown.

- Provide health education on wound and skin care, particularly if pelvic exenteration is performed. Irrigations with saline or other prescribed solutions can be performed at intervals. *Open and damaged tissue increases the risk of infection. Meticulous skin and wound care is necessary to prevent infection and further tissue destruction.*
- If appropriate, provide education on stoma care and care for the skin surrounding the stoma. (These procedures are discussed in the chapter 'Nursing care of people with bowel disorders'.) *Urine and stool are irritating to the skin. Without proper care, the skin surrounding the stoma can become excoriated.*
- Apply non-oil-based lotions to skin to help minimise itching and maintain integrity. *Oil-based lotions are not recommended for tissue undergoing radiation.*
- Educate the woman about the importance of the markings used to localise the radiation beam and not to remove them. *Markings are used in future radiation treatments.*
- Monitor for evidence of fistula formation and teach the woman to do the same. *Fistula formation is a potential complication of radiation to the pelvic or abdominal cavities.*

Community-based care

Health education varies according to the stage of the cancer and the treatment selected. Provide information concerning radiation, chemotherapy or surgery, as indicated. Preoperative health education focuses on postoperative expectations, including management of urinary or faecal diversion, if indicated (see the chapters 'Nursing care of people with bowel disorders' and 'Nursing care of people with urinary tract disorders') and psychological impacts of the diagnosis and surgery. Help the woman and family recognise signs of infection and understand the importance of follow-up care. In addition, suggest the following resources:

- ABC Health & Wellbeing: www.abc.net.au/health/conditions/cancer/default.htm
- Cancer Council support: www.cancer.org.au/about-cancer/patient-support/.

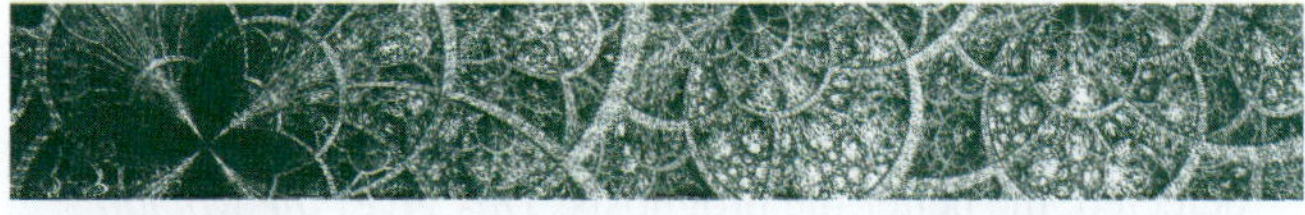

THE WOMAN WITH ENDOMETRIAL CANCER

Endometrial cancer is the most common invasive gynaecological cancer in Australia. The incidence rate of endometrial cancer is increasing due to the increased rate of obesity and the ageing population. In 2021, it was estimated that 4.6% of women were diagnosed with uterine cancer. When diagnosed and treated early in the disease, the 5-year survival rate is about 84% (Cancer Australia, 2022b).

Risk factors

A significant risk factor for endometrial cancer is prolonged oestrogen stimulation. Other factors that increase risk are obesity, anovulatory menstrual cycles, decreasing ovarian function (as from menopause), oestrogen-secreting tumours and unopposed oestrogen (e.g. oestrogen therapy without progesterone). Medical conditions that may alter oestrogen metabolism and increase the risk of endometrial cancer are diabetes mellitus, hypertension and polycystic ovarian syndrome. Tamoxifen, a medication that blocks oestrogen receptor sites and is used to treat breast cancer, has a weak oestrogenic effect on the endometrium and is also a risk factor.

Endometrial cancer is the most commonly inherited gynaecological cancer. A family history of hereditary non-polyposis colon cancer (HNPCC) may mean that a woman has an inherited mutation that is a mismatch of repair genes and has a 60% risk of endometrial cancer.

Pathophysiology

Most endometrial malignancies are adenocarcinomas that are slow to grow and metastasise. These cancers develop in the glandular cells or endometrial lining of the uterus (the same tissue that is shed each month during a normal menstrual period). Endometrial hyperplasia (excessive growth) is a precursor of endometrial cancer. These tumours tend to grow slowly in the early stages.

Tumour growth usually begins in the fundus, invades the vascular myometrium and spreads throughout the female reproductive tract. Metastasis occurs by means of the lymphatic system, through the fallopian tubes to the peritoneal cavity and to the rest of the body via the bloodstream. Target areas for metastasis include the lungs, liver and bone. The International Federation of Gynecology and Obstetrics (FIGO) (2009, p. 104) classification of endometrial cancer is presented in Table 48.3.

TABLE 48.3 FIGO staging classification for endometrial cancer

STAGE	DESCRIPTION
I	Tumour limited to endometrium or myometrium
II	Endocervical glandular involvement or invasion of cervical stroma
III	Metastasis or invasion of serosa, adnexae, vagina and pelvic or para-aortic lymph nodes
IV	Tumour invasion of bladder or bowel mucosa; distant metastases

Manifestations

The main manifestation of endometrial hyperplasia or overt endometrial cancer is abnormal, painless vaginal bleeding. In menstruating women, this bleeding is manifested as menorrhagia or metrorrhagia. In postmenopausal women, any bleeding is abnormal. Later symptoms include pelvic cramping, bleeding after intercourse and lower abdominal pressure. In advanced disease, lymph node enlargement, pleural effusion, abdominal masses and ascites may be present.

INTERPROFESSIONAL CARE

The goals of care for the woman with endometrial cancer are to eradicate the cancer and minimise complications and metastasis.

Diagnosis

Tests used to diagnose cancer of the endometrium include a vaginal or transvaginal ultrasound to determine endometrial thickening, which may indicate hypertrophy or malignant changes, or an endometrial biopsy or a dilation and curettage (D&C) to provide a definitive diagnosis. Other tests to determine the extent of the disease include chest x-ray, intravenous urography, cystoscopy, barium enema, sigmoidoscopy, MRI and bone scans.

Medications

Although the treatment of choice for primary endometrial carcinoma is surgery, progesterone therapy may be used for recurrent disease. About one-third of women respond favourably, primarily those with well-differentiated tumours. Chemotherapy is less effective than other forms of therapy, although cisplatin or combination chemotherapy may be used for women with disseminated disease.

Surgery

After the diagnosis is confirmed, a total abdominal hysterectomy and bilateral salpingo-oophorectomy is performed for stage I cancer. A radical hysterectomy with node dissection is performed if the disease is stage II or beyond.

Radiation therapy

Treatment with external and internal radiation may be performed as a preoperative measure or as adjuvant treatment in advanced cases.

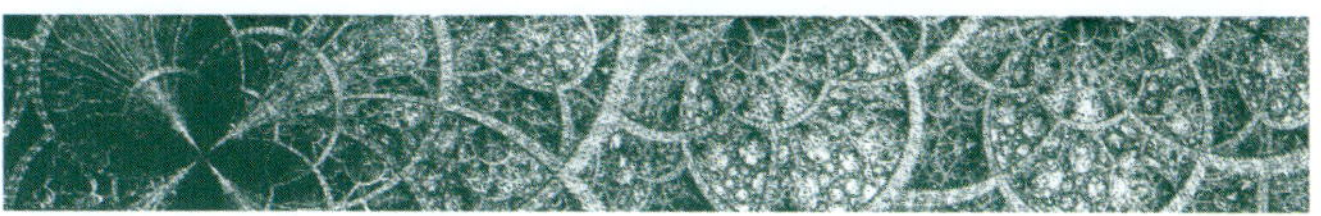

Nursing care

Health promotion

All women, including perimenopausal and postmenopausal women, need regular pelvic examinations. At the time of menopause all women should be informed of the risks and symptoms of endometrial cancer and strongly encouraged to report any unexpected bleeding or spotting to their healthcare provider. In addition, control of diseases such as diabetes mellitus and hypertension decreases the risk of endometrial hyperplasia.

Assessment

Undertake a health history and physical examination (see the chapter 'A person-centred approach to assessing the male and female reproductive systems'):

- *Health history*: abnormal vaginal bleeding, menstrual history, use of oestrogen (without progesterone) to treat menopausal symptoms, breast cancer treated with tamoxifen, childbearing status, presence of chronic illnesses, family history of hereditary non-polyposis colon cancer.
- *Physical assessment*: height and weight, pelvic examination, abdomen, lymph glands.
- *Mental health assessment*: anxiety, coping strategies, emotional wellbeing.

Nursing diagnoses and interventions

Nursing care involves supporting the woman to deal with the physical and psychological effects of a potentially life-threatening illness, make informed decisions and minimise the adverse effects of therapy. Pain relief is a key component of care, as is counselling for the woman and family. Encourage the woman to perform self-care and resume normal activities of daily living.

Acute pain

Total abdominal hysterectomy can involve severe and prolonged pain, not only from the surgical incision but also from the manipulation of internal organs during surgery. Abdominal viscera are highly vascular and are easily bruised by handling.

- Encourage the woman to report her pain. *This enables a nursing assessment to be undertaken and effective pain relief to be administered.*
- Administer analgesics. *Analgesics provide pain relief and promote early ambulation.*
- Encourage ambulation. *Ambulation facilitates the expulsion of flatus, which can cause distension as well as discomfort.*

Disturbed body image

For many women, side effects of cancer treatment can be almost as difficult and painful as the disease itself. Although side effects of the different therapies vary between individuals, the woman's body image and quality of life are always affected. Such side effects as alopecia (hair loss), nausea, vomiting, fatigue, diarrhoea, stomatitis and surgical scarring disturb body image.

- Encourage the woman to verbalise her feelings. *This allows the nurse to work with the woman on her emotional wellbeing and mental health.*
- Review the side effects of the proposed treatment regimen and assist the woman to develop a plan to deal with these effects. *This promotes a sense of control.*
- Suggest to the woman and family that side effects are usually manageable and may be temporary. *Over-the-counter agents can be used to alleviate stomatitis. Frequent rest periods can relieve fatigue. Medications can be prescribed for nausea, vomiting and diarrhoea.*

Ineffective sexuality pattern

Altered sexuality may result from a feeling of unattractiveness, fatigue or pain, and discomfort. The woman's partner may fear that sexual activity will be harmful.

- Encourage expression of feelings about the effect of cancer on their lives and sexual relationship. *Verbalising feelings helps relieve stress and maximises relaxation.*
- Suggest that the couple explore alternative sexual positions and coordinate sexual activity with rest periods and times that are relatively free from pain. *This creates a more favourable environment for satisfying sexual activity.*

Community-based care

Provide information about the specific treatment and prognosis for the cancer. Explain the expected side effects of radiation implant therapy (see the chapter 'Nursing care of people with cancer'). Pain control measures are also an essential part of the health education plan (see the chapter 'Nursing care of people in pain'). The resources listed for the woman with cervical cancer are also appropriate for the woman with endometrial cancer.

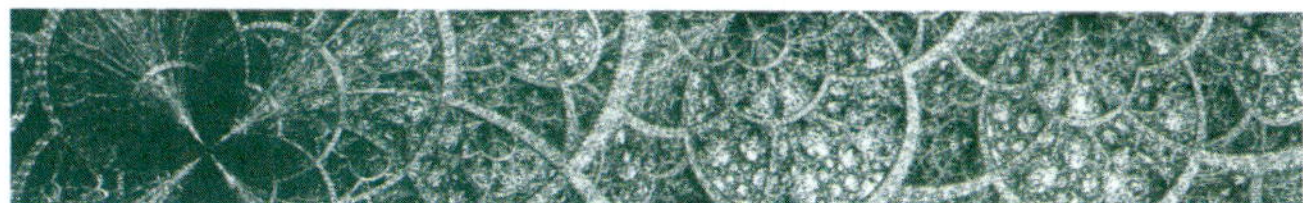

THE WOMAN WITH OVARIAN CANCER

Ovarian cancer is the 8th most common cancer diagnosed in women in Australia. There is a 1 in 85 chance of being diagnosed with ovarian cancer before the age of 85.

Risk factors

Most ovarian cancers have unknown causes, but women over 50 who have no menstruation have higher risk of ovarian cancer. Having a family history of first- or second-degree relatives with ovarian, breast, bowel and uterine cancers is one of the other risk factors. Other types of inherited risk are breast–ovarian cancer caused by a fault in the BRAC1 and BRAC2 genes and family cancer syndrome (Lynch syndrome II) (Cancer Council, 2022b).

Risk factors also include being overweight, smoking, early puberty, late menopause and using oestrogen-only HRT for 5 or more years. There is inconsistent and insufficient evidence to demonstrate an increased risk of ovarian cancer with exposure to talc powder (Berge et al., 2018) or asbestos (Slomovitz et al., 2021). Protective factors include breastfeeding, having children, using combined oral contraceptive, removing fallopian tubes or tubal ligation (Cancer Council, 2022b).

Pathophysiology

There are several types of ovarian cancers: epithelial, germ-cell and gonadal stromal tumours. Most ovarian cancers are epithelial tumours, originating from the surface epithelium of the ovary. Ovarian cancer usually spreads by local shedding of cancer cells into the peritoneal cavity and direct invasion of the bowel and bladder. Cancer cells in peritoneal fluid can implant in the intestines, bladder and mesentery. Tumour cells also spread through the lymph and blood to such organs as the liver and across the diaphragm to involve the lungs. Both pelvic and para-aortic lymph nodes may be involved and tumour cells can block lymphatic drainage from the abdomen, resulting in ascites. Staging for ovarian cancer is based on surgical and histological evaluation (see Table 48.4).

Manifestations

In early stages, ovarian cancer generally causes no warning signs or symptoms. When symptoms do develop, they are often vague and mild, such as indigestion, urinary frequency, abdominal bloating and constipation. Abnormal vaginal bleeding may occur if the endometrium is stimulated by a hormone-secreting tumour or if the tumour erodes the vaginal wall. Pelvic pain sometimes occurs. An enlarged abdomen with ascites signals later-stage disease.

TABLE 48.4 FIGO staging classification for ovarian cancer

STAGE	DESCRIPTION
I	Growth limited to the ovaries
II	Growth involving one or both ovaries with pelvic extension
III	Tumour involving one or both ovaries, with peritoneal implants outside the pelvis or positive retroperitoneal or inguinal nodes
IV	Growth involving one or both ovaries with distant metastasis

Complications

The complications of advanced ovarian cancer, with related nursing assessments and treatment, are outlined in Table 48.5.

INTERPROFESSIONAL CARE

As with other malignancies, care of the woman with ovarian cancer is focused on surgery to determine the stage of the tumour and to remove as much of the tumour as possible. Unfortunately, because there are no early symptoms, the disease is often well advanced prior to diagnosis. In younger women, an ovarian mass may be monitored for several menstrual cycles, but any ovarian mass must immediately be investigated in a postmenopausal woman.

Diagnosis

Tests used in the diagnosis of ovarian cancer may include transvaginal or abdominal ultrasound, a CT scan of the abdomen and pelvis and a blood test. A positron emission tomography (PET) scan can also highlight abnormal tissues in the body. Biopsy is the only way to confirm the diagnosis of an ovarian cancer. (See the chapter 'A person-centred approach to assessing the male and female reproductive systems' for further information about diagnostic tests.)

TABLE 48.5 Complications of advanced ovarian cancer

COMPLICATION	ASSESSMENTS	TREATMENT
Ascites (accumulation of fluid in the abdominal cavity; a form of third spacing)	• Abdominal distension • Shiny abdominal skin • Dullness on percussion of dependent areas • Dyspnoea, constipation • Abdominal pain	Paracentesis (removing fluid from the abdomen)
Intestinal obstruction	• Abdominal distension • Abdominal pain • Projectile vomiting • Constipation • Hyperactive bowel sounds	Nasogastric tube insertion, NBM
Deep venous thrombosis	• Leg oedema • Leg pain • Redness, warmth	Anticoagulants
Lymphoedema (leg)	• Oedema of leg • Decreased range of motion • Tight, shiny skin on leg	Skin care, range-of-motion (ROM) exercises, massage or physical therapy, compression bandaging

The blood test most useful is a CA-125 antigen level. CA-125 is a tumour marker that is highly specific to epithelial ovarian cancer. Transvaginal or transabdominal ultrasonography is used to measure ovarian size and detect small masses. These tests, however, are not appropriate screening measures because they cannot differentiate between cystic or benign ovarian masses and malignancy. Genetic testing may be considered to look for faulty genes that are known to cause ovarian cancer.

Medications

While surgery is the treatment of choice for ovarian cancer, chemotherapy may be used to achieve remission of the disease. Many women with ovarian cancer respond well to platinum-based chemotherapy such as cisplatin. However, in 1 year, the ovarian cancer cells become resistant to the platinum. Combining platinum-based medication with DNA repair inhibitors such as wortmannin enhances the result of chemotherapy (Zhang et al., 2018). Close monitoring of bone marrow and renal function is vital while the woman is on chemotherapy because these medications have significant toxic effects. Targeted therapy is also used in combination with chemotherapy. Targeted therapy drugs enter the cancer cells and block particular enzymes to stop the growth of the cancer cells.

Surgery

In young women with stage I disease who wish to have children, treatment may be limited to removal of one ovary. Usually, however, total hysterectomy with bilateral salpingo-oophorectomy (removal of the ovaries and fallopian tubes) and removal of the omentum are performed.

Radiation therapy

Radiation therapy using external-beam or intracavitary implants is performed for palliative purposes only and is directed at shrinking the tumour at selected sites.

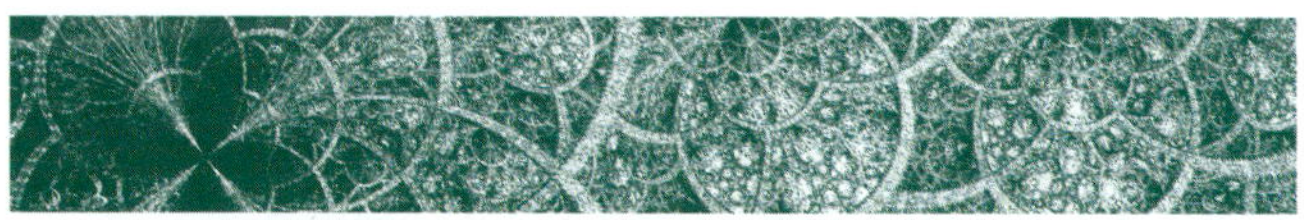

Nursing care

Nursing care for the woman with ovarian cancer is similar to nursing care for women with other gynaecological cancers. The side effects of treatment of cancer and generally poor prognosis diminish the woman's quality of life and involve major psychosocial implications (see the chapter 'Nursing care of people with cancer').

Community-based care

Address the following topics in preparing the woman and her family for self-care:

- If a positive family history of the disease or previous breast cancer exists, stress the importance of obtaining regular pelvic examinations. Inform women in this risk group that annual screening with transvaginal ultrasound and CA-125 measurements may be recommended.
- Educate about positive lifestyle such as healthy diet and physical activity.
- Long-term use of oral contraceptives may reduce the risk of developing ovarian cancer.
- It is crucial not to ignore symptoms such as indigestion, nausea or urinary frequency, because these seemingly unrelated symptoms may be early signs of ovarian tumours. Emphasise, however, that ovarian cancer usually is asymptomatic in early stages.
- Discuss treatment options and their side effects and provide information on ways to minimise or manage side effects.
- Refer to palliative services when appropriate. The resources suggested for the woman with cervical cancer are also appropriate for the woman with ovarian cancer.

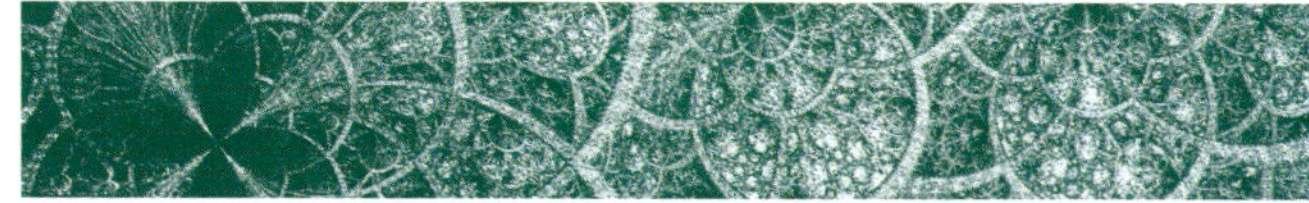

THE WOMAN WITH CANCER OF THE VULVA

Cancer of the vulva is rare, occurring in two in 100,000 women in Australia. It usually occurs in postmenopausal women. The prognosis of vulvar carcinoma depends on the degree of invasion, general health status of the woman, presence of chronic diseases and ability to withstand treatment.

Pathophysiology

The cause of vulvar cancer is unknown, but there is evidence to associate it with STIs, particularly HPV. Nearly 85% of malignant and premalignant cervical and vulvar lesions have been found to contain HPV DNA, HPV structural antigens or both. Herpes simplex type 2 (HSV2) infection has also been associated with vulvar cancer. Other risk factors include advanced age, diabetes and a history of leucoplakia (a precancerous lesion on the vulvar mucous membranes characterised by raised white patches).

Most vulvar cancers are epidermoid or squamous cell carcinomas. The primary site is usually the labia majora, but vulvar cancer is also found on the labia minora, clitoris, vestibule and occasionally in multiple locations. Metastasis occurs by direct extension into the vagina, perineal skin, anus and urethra. The cancer also spreads through the lymphatic system via the superficial and deep inguinal and femoral nodes and to the pelvic lymph nodes.

Manifestations

The woman with vulvar cancer is often asymptomatic and lesions are discovered on routine examination or self-examination. Discolouration can vary from white macular patches to red painless sores. Lesions may be *exophytic* (proliferating outwardly), *endophytic* (proliferating inwardly), *ulcerative* or *verrucous* (resembling a wart).

Pruritus (itching) is the most common manifestation and the woman often has had a history of prolonged vulvar irritation. Perineal pain and bleeding indicate large tumours and advanced disease. In very advanced disease, dysuria related to urethral involvement may be the presenting symptom.

INTERPROFESSIONAL CARE

The report of itching, burning or a sore on the vulva merits careful investigation and biopsy of any lesions found. Inguinal lymph nodes may be enlarged. The goal of care is to eradicate the lesion and reduce the risk of recurrence. Surgical resection is the preferred treatment. If lymph nodes are involved, radiation therapy is used postoperatively. Chemotherapy is reserved for distant metastases.

Diagnosis is based on the results of an excisional biopsy of the lesion. Metastasis, if suspected, can be evaluated by chest x-ray examination, barium enema, intravenous pyelogram, cystoscopy, CT and MRI scans, and proctoscopy. Lymphangiography can also be used.

Surgery is the most common treatment for vulvar cancer. The specific procedure depends on the stage of the cancer. Early, non-invasive lesions may be treated with laser surgery, cryosurgery or electrocautery. For more advanced disease, vulvectomy may be performed (see Figure 48.6). A simple vulvectomy involves the removal of the vulva, labia majora and minora, clitoris and prepuce. A radical vulvectomy is performed if invasion is suspected. This procedure involves removal of all the tissue in a simple vulvectomy, as well as the subcutaneous tissue and regional lymph nodes.

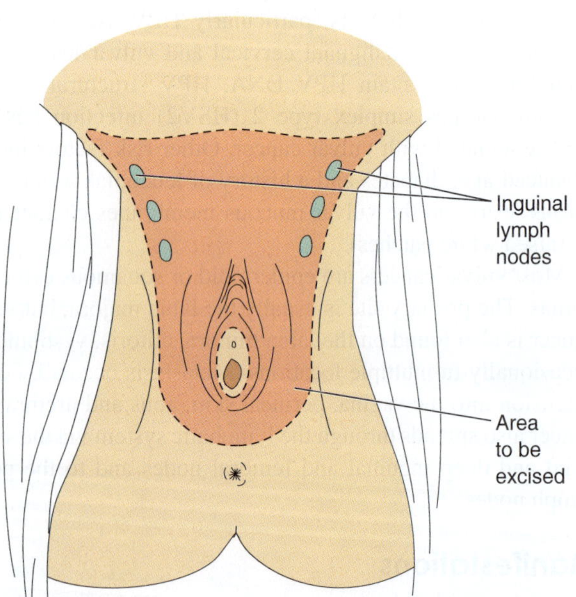

FIGURE 48.6 ***Vulvectomy for vulvar carcinoma. A radical vulvectomy involves removal of the vulva, labia majora, labia minora, clitoris, prepuce, subcutaneous tissue and regional lymph nodes***

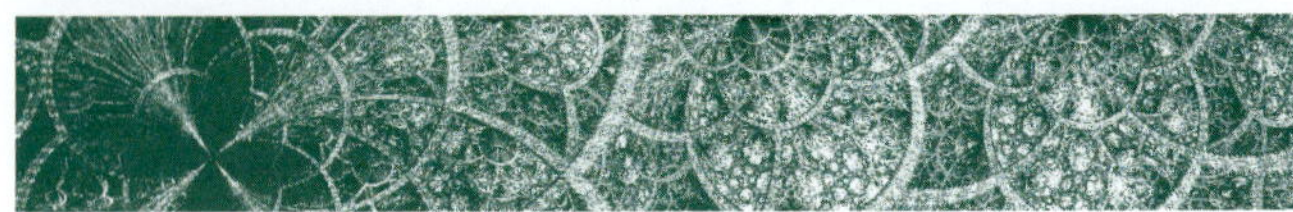

Nursing care

Nursing care is similar to that for the woman with endometrial cancer. The woman fears death as the ultimate outcome, as well as the possible pain and suffering that surgery and other treatments may cause. Radical surgery represents a great emotional loss to women of all ages.

Nursing diagnoses and interventions

Women who have been diagnosed with cancer of the vulva and are undergoing treatment will need to be supported. A mental health assessment for anxiety, coping strategies and emotional wellbeing is required. The disruption of perineal tissues is a priority issue for these women. Pain, discomfort and altered body image would also impact on the woman's wellbeing.

Impaired tissue integrity

The woman who has undergone a vulvectomy is at high risk of infection and impaired healing because of the proximity of the surgical site to urinary and anal orifices. In addition, the women are often older and may have age-related changes in healing and immune function.

- Educate the woman and/or her partner or other family member on the procedure for irrigation of the vulvectomy. If neither is able to perform this procedure, arrange for community health nursing. Irrigation helps prevent skin breakdown and infection.
- After irrigation, dry the area; a hairdryer on low heat may be used. Dry heat helps promote healing and comfort.
- Provide information on maintaining a diet high in protein, iron and vitamin C. These nutrients promote collagen formation and wound healing.

Community-based care

Health education for the woman undergoing a vulvectomy should emphasise the potential for skin breakdown, particularly with radiation therapy. Explain that removal of lymph nodes leads to lymphoedema and that recurrent cellulitis and sexual dysfunction are common complications of vulvar cancer.

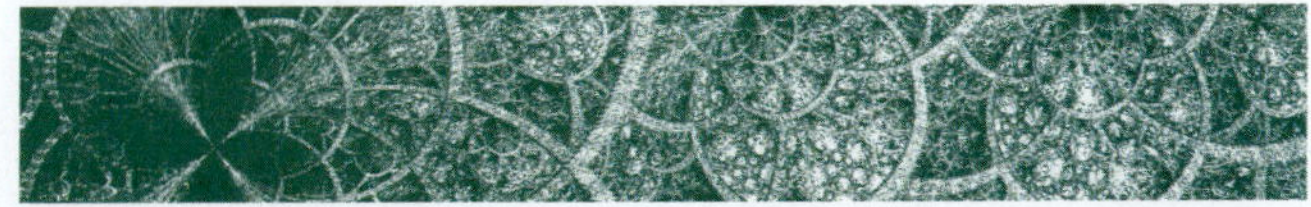

The perimenopausal woman

MENOPAUSE

Menopause is the permanent cessation of menses. The *climacteric*, or *perimenopausal*, period denotes the time during which reproductive function gradually ceases. For most women, the perimenopausal period lasts several years. It begins with a decline in the production of the hormone oestrogen, includes the permanent cessation of menstruation due to loss of ovarian function, and extends for 1 year after the final menstrual period, at which time a woman is said to be *postmenopausal*. On average, women live one-third of their lives after menopause.

Menopause is a normal physiological process. It is not a disease or a disorder. It is included here because it does increase the risk of physical disorders, as well as affecting various aspects of women's health. Many women welcome the freedom from monthly menstrual periods and have relatively minor physical effects from the reduction in oestrogen. However, the hormonal changes that occur can be accompanied by side effects. There is wide variation in how individual women experience these side effects. In Australia, most women cease menstruating between 48 and 55 years of age, with the average being about 50 or 51 years. Early menopause is when a woman stops menstruating before 45 years of age. In 50% of cases of early menopause, there are no known causes. However, early menopause is associated with surgical removal of the ovaries, chemotherapy and radiotherapy (Jean Hailes for Women's Health, 2017). After menopause certain health risks increase, including heart disease, osteoporosis, macular degeneration, cognitive changes and breast cancer.

The physiology of menopause

The menopausal period marks the natural biological end of reproductive ability. *Surgical menopause* occurs when the ovaries are removed in premenopausal women, dramatically reducing the production of oestrogen and progestins. *Chemical menopause* often occurs during cancer chemotherapy, when cytotoxic medications arrest ovarian function.

As ovarian function decreases, the production of oestradiol (E2) decreases, and is ultimately replaced by oestrone as the main ovarian oestrogen. Oestrone is produced in small amounts and has only about one-tenth the biological activity of oestradiol. With decreased ovarian function, the second ovarian hormone, progesterone, is also markedly reduced.

Manifestations

As oestrogen decreases, various tissues are affected, and breast tissue, body hair, skin elasticity and subcutaneous fat decrease. The ovaries and uterus become smaller and the cervix and vagina also decrease in size and become pale in colour. These changes may result in problems with vaginal dryness, dyspareunia, urinary stress incontinence, urinary tract infections (UTIs) and vaginitis. Hot flushes, palpitations, dizziness and headaches are often caused by vasomotor instability. Other problems resulting from vasomotor instability include insomnia, frequent awakening and perspiration (night sweats). The woman may experience irritability, anxiety and depression as a result.

Long-term oestrogen deprivation results in an imbalance in bone remodelling and osteoporosis, leading to fractures and kyphosis. The risk of cardiovascular diseases increases in response to an increase in atherosclerosis (from an increase in the LDL-to-HDL cholesterol ratio). Symptoms of the perimenopausal period are listed in the 'Manifestations' box. These symptoms vary widely. Some women experience few or no symptoms, others experience moderate symptoms and some women experience severe symptoms.

MANIFESTATIONS The perimenopausal period

- Menstrual cycles become unpredictable. Menstrual flow varies widely in amount and duration and eventually ceases.
- Vaginal, vulval and urethral tissues begin to atrophy.
- Vaginal pH rises, predisposing the woman to bacterial infections.
- Vaginal lubrication decreases and vaginal rugae decrease in number. This may result in dyspareunia, injury and fungal infections.
- Vasomotor instability due to a decrease in oestrogen may result in hot flushes and night sweats. A hot flush starts in the chest, moves upwards towards the face and may last from seconds to several minutes.
- Psychological symptoms may include moodiness, nervousness, insomnia, headaches, irritability, anxiety, inability to concentrate and depression.

INTERPROFESSIONAL CARE

Care of the woman experiencing menopausal symptoms focuses on relieving symptoms and minimising postmenopausal health risks.

Diagnosis

As oestrogen secretion diminishes, levels of FSH and LH rise and remain elevated. A woman who has not menstruated for 1 full year or who has an increased FSH blood level is considered menopausal.

Medications

Hormone replacement therapy may be prescribed to alleviate severe symptoms of menopause, but only for a limited amount of time and only after a woman has been provided with information about known risks. HRT may include oestrogen alone for women who have had a hysterectomy, or a combination of oestrogen and progestin for women who still have their uterus. The addition of progestin stimulates monthly shedding of the interuterine lining, decreasing the risk of uterine cancer. HRT relieves hot flushes and night sweats and decreases problems of vaginal dryness and urogenital tissue atrophy, which can lead to painful intercourse and urinary incontinence. A long-term HRT may increase the risk of breast cancer, ovarian cancer, stroke and venous thrombosis (Women's Health & Research Institute of Australia, 2022). However, women who have had a hysterectomy and take oestrogen alone do not have an increased risk of breast cancer (Lancet Oncology, 2012).

Selective oestrogen receptor modulators (SERMs), such as raloxifene (Evista) and tamoxifen, bind to oestrogen receptors and exert site-specific effects in different target tissues. Tamoxifen and toremifene (a derivative of tamoxifen) have a beneficial effect on bone mineral density, and serum lipids and decrease the risk of invasive breast cancer in women at high risk. They also provide an alternative to HRT for preventing osteoporosis.

Alternative and complementary therapies

Non-traditional or alternative therapies have become popular as a result of the controversy surrounding the use of HRT. The following complementary therapies are examples used by menopausal women to reduce associated discomfort:

- acupuncture
- auriculotherapy
- biofeedback
- massage
- meditation and yoga
- supplements such as vitamin E
- herbs such as *Cimcifuga racemosa* (black cohosh), flaxseed, evening primrose oil, soy protein and Chinese herbal medicine.

Evidence from systematic reviews demonstrated no significant effect on symptoms of menopause when women used black cohosh (Leach & Moore, 2012), alternative therapy (Nedrow et al., 2006) or Chinese medicine (Zhu et al., 2016). However, exercise such as yoga or walking may assist women to maintain a healthy lifestyle and may combat some of the side effects of menopause (Women's Health & Equality Queensland, 2017).

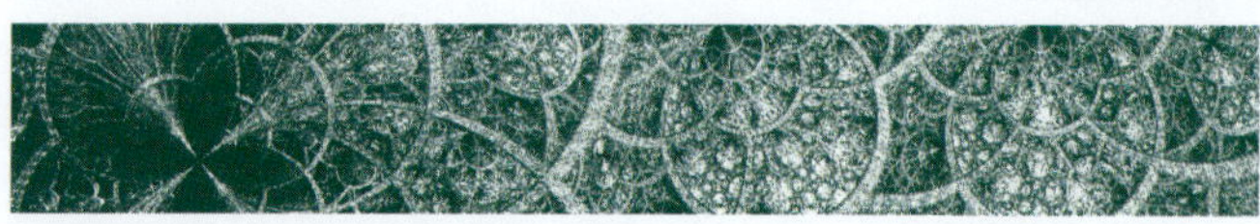

Nursing care

Nursing care focuses on implementing lifestyle changes that are important to the woman's health and wellbeing. These will assist to minimise the symptoms associated with hormonal changes, reducing the risk of cardiovascular disease, cancer and osteoporosis.

Health promotion

National screening programs are available in Australia for various cancers, such as breast, bowel and cervical. It is a good idea to have regular health assessments. A health assessment includes examination for cancers of the thyroid, ovaries, lymph nodes, oral cavity and skin. Other important health assessments include screening for cervical, breast and colorectal cancer. Health counselling should also include information about alcohol and tobacco use, sun exposure, diet and nutrition, exercise, risk factors, sexual practices, mental and emotional wellbeing, and environmental and occupational exposures. It is important to discuss the benefits of rest and exercise, as well as a diet that includes fruit, vegetables and fibre. In addition, suggest the following resources for further information:

- Women's Health Australia: www.alswh.org.au
- Australasian Menopause Society: www.menopause.org.au
- Jean Hailes for Women's Health: https://jeanhailes.org.au
- Women's Health & Equality Queensland: https://womhealth.org.au/.

Assessment

Undertake a thorough health history and physical examination. When assessing the older woman, be aware of normal changes with ageing, as outlined in the chapter 'A person-centred approach to assessing the male and female reproductive systems'.

- *Health history*: problems with urinary frequency, urgency or incontinence; menstrual history; sexual history; dyspareunia; use of alcohol, nicotine and illicit drugs; medications, sleep patterns, hot flushes, night sweats, changes in emotional responses.
- *Physical assessment*: height and weight; posture; vital signs; abdominal assessment; with verbal consent, breast examination and pelvic examination.

Nursing diagnoses and interventions

Although each nursing care plan must be individualised, interventions often focus on physical problems. There is often a lack of information on sexuality, self-esteem, mental health and body image.

Deficient knowledge

Menopausal symptoms vary widely. Well-informed women are better prepared to deal with the symptoms they experience.

Discuss physiological symptoms, such as hot flushes and night sweats. The underlying cause of hot flushes is not known. As previously discussed, many physiological effects of menopause are responsive to non-pharmacological methods of relief, such as lifestyle changes.

> **CONSIDERATION FOR PRACTICE**
>
> **When hot flushes occur at night and are accompanied by perspiration, they are called night sweats. Night sweats often interfere with normal sleep patterns, leading to increased tiredness and irritability.**

- Provide information to the woman about dietary recommendations. The recommended daily intake of calcium for women over 50 is 1,200 mg. *Some women need to use calcium supplements or calcium-containing antacid tablets to meet this requirement.*

- Emphasise the importance of weight-bearing exercise. *Weight-bearing exercise reduces the rate of bone loss, helps maintain optimum weight and reduces cardiovascular risk.*
- Provide information about the benefits and risks of HRT. Not every woman will need or want it. *Every woman needs to understand both the risks and the benefits before deciding whether to use HRT.* To assist health professionals and individuals to whom they provide care to make informed choices regarding HRT, there are various web-based resources available.
- Encourage the woman to perform monthly breast self-examination (BSE) on the same day each month, and to have a mammogram. Mammograms are recommended every 2 years for women aged between 50 and 74 (Cancer Council, 2022c).

Ineffective sexuality pattern

Vaginal dryness and atrophy, together with the emotional effects of menopause, can interfere with sexual expression and satisfaction. Suggesting measures to help the woman and her partner cope with these changes can enable them to continue or resume a mutually satisfying sexual relationship.

- Encourage expression of feelings and concerns about how menopause is changing the woman's sex life. *Many women are not comfortable discussing their intimate sexual behaviour.*
- Suggest ways to increase vaginal lubrication, such as spending more time in foreplay and/or using water-soluble gels (e.g. K-Y Jelly) for vaginal lubrication. A more leisurely approach to sexual activity can be mutually gratifying for both the woman and her partner. *Use of water-soluble gels can prevent vaginal pain and irritation and improve the quality of the sexual experience.*
- Explain that as women age, it may take longer for vaginal lubrication and orgasm to occur. *This information is important to prevent the woman from believing something is wrong with her, or her partner believing she is no longer interested or sexually exciting.*
- Inform about changes in the sexual responsiveness of male partners. Difficulty in achieving an erection or maintaining an erection occurs in 1 in 5 Australian men over the age of 40.

Situational low self-esteem

Each woman responds to the ageing process in her own way. Most women have coping skills that adequately equip them to deal with the gradual changes associated with ageing. Factors that may provoke a lowered self-esteem are the loss of youth, a sense of emptiness as children leave home and the need to redefine one's self-concept and roles as parenting becomes less important. Women who place a high value on their physical attractiveness may experience a negative psychological response to the physical changes of menopause.

- Encourage expression of fears and concerns related to changes in interpersonal and family functions. *Many women associate ageing with 'uselessness' and unattractiveness.*
- Suggest volunteer activities or employment for the woman who has extra time. *This enables the woman to increase her sense of self-worth.*
- Discuss the importance of a healthy lifestyle in maintaining physical attractiveness. Identify risk factors and high-risk behaviours. *Lifestyle habits and behaviours affect many body systems and physical appearance. For example, cigarette smoking and overexposure to the sun make the skin age faster, contributing to wrinkles.*

Disturbed body image

As women progress through the perimenopausal period, changes in appearance and the loss of childbearing ability may combine to make them feel vulnerable to community stereotyping of the 'older woman' as less attractive and unproductive. Although this is far from the truth, with women living at least one-third of their lives after menopause in productive careers and activities, it nevertheless is the perception of women as well as society. The physical changes a woman often experiences include growth of facial hair, excessive perspiration, flushing of the face and weight gain.

- Encourage the woman to describe her perceptions of her own body. *This information is necessary to obtain data to establish an individualised care plan.*
- Encourage verbalisation of feelings of concern, anger, anxiety, loss and fear over body changes. *Expressing these emotions can facilitate the grieving process and acceptance of change.*
- Stress that certain physical characteristics of a person cannot be changed; emphasise the importance of learning to recognise and appreciate one's own special strengths. *These help the woman gain acceptance and have a realistic appraisal of self.*
- Refer, as appropriate, for dietary management, exercise, sleep studies, stress management and cosmetic assistance (e.g. for aggravating facial hair). *These actions increase wellness and a positive sense of self.*

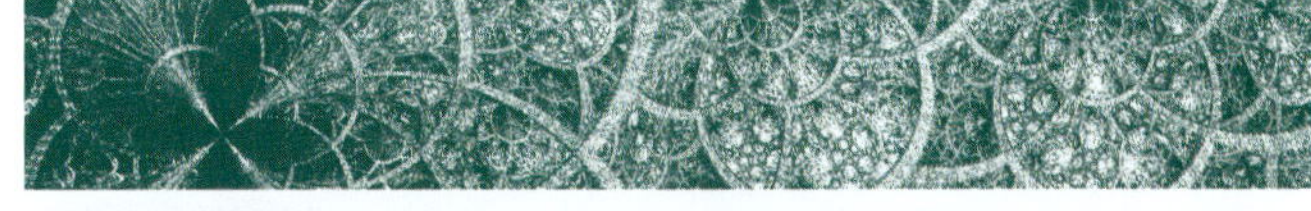

Disorders of the breast

Breast disorders are common conditions that primarily affect women. (Disorders of the male breast are discussed in the chapter 'Nursing care of men with reproductive system and breast disorders'.) When a woman discovers a breast lump, her first response is often fear: of breast cancer, of losing her breast and perhaps of losing her life. As many societies view the breast as a significant component of feminine sexuality, any problem that threatens it often strikes at the core of a woman's self-image.

Nurses play a critical role in the care of women experiencing breast disorders by providing education, support and advocacy. Part of the nurse's role is educating women about normal breast tissue, common benign breast disorders, available screening techniques and risk factors for breast cancer, and breast self-examination (BSE).

THE WOMAN WITH A BENIGN BREAST DISORDER

Benign breast disorders occur frequently in women and may be a source of anxiety. Changes in a woman's breast tissue often correspond to hormonal changes of the menstrual cycle. Most women notice increased tenderness and lumpiness prior to menses. (For this reason, it is best to perform BSE 7 to 10 days after the beginning of the menstrual period.) Breast tissue also changes in response to nutritional, physical and environmental stimuli. Benign breast disorders include fibrocystic breast changes, fibroadenomas, intraductal papillomas, duct ectasia, fat necrosis and mastitis (see Table 48.6).

Pathophysiology and manifestations

Fibrocystic changes

Fibrocystic changes (FCCs) (*fibrocystic breast disease*) are the physiological nodularity and breast tenderness that increase and decrease with the menstrual cycle. An estimated 60% of all women experience some of these changes, which include fibrosis, epithelial proliferation and cyst formation. FCC is most common in women 30 to 50 years of age (Centre of Health, 2022) and is rare in postmenopausal women who are not taking HRT.

FCC includes many different lesions and breast changes. The more common non-proliferative form does not increase the risk of breast cancer. The proliferative form, accompanied by giant cysts and proliferative epithelial lesions, does increase the risk of breast cancer.

Non-proliferative changes may be cystic or fibrous. Cystic change refers to the dilation of ducts in the subareolar, lobular or lobe areas. Cysts often go unnoticed unless pain and tenderness occur with menses. Fibrous changes are infrequent but can occur during the menstrual years. A firm, palpable mass, 2–3 cm in size, is typically located in the upper outer breast quadrant following an inflammatory response to ductal irritation.

Women with fibrocystic changes experience bilateral or unilateral pain or tenderness in the upper, outer quadrants of their breasts and report that their breasts feel particularly thick and lumpy the week prior to menses. Nipple discharge may be present. Pain is due to oedema of the connective tissue, dilation of the ducts and some inflammatory response; some women report an increase in breast size. Multiple, mobile cysts may form, usually in both breasts (see Figure 48.7). Fluid aspirated from these cysts ranges in colour from milky white to yellow, brown or green. If the fluid is tinged with blood, there is reason to suspect malignancy.

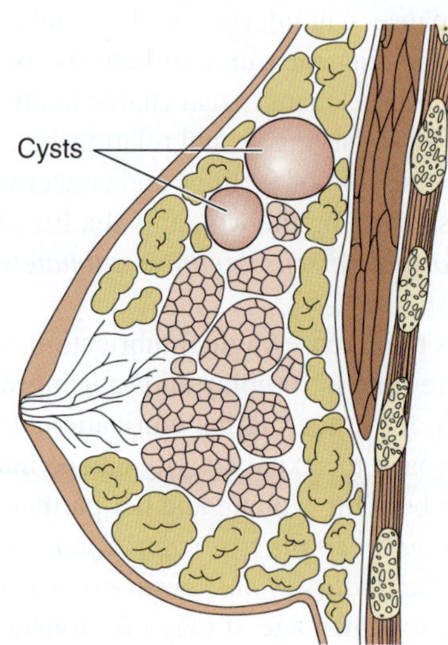

FIGURE 48.7 ***Fibrocystic breast changes***

TABLE 48.6 Summary of common breast disorders

CONDITION	AGE	PAIN	NIPPLE DISCHARGE	LOCATION	CONSISTENCY AND MOBILITY	DIAGNOSIS AND TREATMENT
Duct ectasia	35 to 55 years; median age 40	Burning around nipple	Sticky; multi-coloured; usually bilateral	No specific location	Retroareolar mass with advanced disease	Open biopsy; local excision of diseased portion of breast
Fibroadenoma	15 to 39 years; median age 20	No	No	No specific location	Mobile, firm, smooth, well-delineated mass	Mammography; surgical or needle biopsy; excision of the tumour
Fibrocystic changes (FCC)	20 to 49 years; median age 30 (may subside with menopause)	Yes	May occur	Upper outer quadrant	Bilateral multiple lumps influenced by the menstrual cycle	Needle aspiration; observation; biopsy if there is an unresolved mass or mammographic changes
Intraductal papilloma	35 to 55 years; median age 40	Yes	Serous or sanguineous; usually unilateral from one duct	No specific location	Usually soft, poorly delineated mass	Screen of nipple discharge; biopsy; wedge resection
Mastitis, acute	Childbearing years	Tenderness; pain	No	No specific location	Generalised redness of overlying skin	Antibiotic therapy; incision and drainage if mastitis progresses to an abscess
Mastitis, chronic	Any age	Tenderness, pain; headache; high fever	No	No specific location	Generalised redness and swelling	Antibiotics, usually penicillin
Fat necrosis	Any age	Tenderness	No	No specific location	Firm; irregular; palpable	Surgical biopsy to rule out cancer

Intraductal disorders

An *intraductal papilloma* is a tiny, wart-like growth on the inside of the peripheral mammary duct that causes discharge from the nipple. The discharge may be clear and sticky or bloody. When more than one of these growths is present, the condition is called *intraductal papillomatosis*. This condition is most common in women in their forties (Breast Cancer Care, 2022). The lesion must be investigated to rule out malignancy.

Mammary duct ectasia (*plasma cell mastitis*) is a palpable lumpiness found beneath the areola. Duct ectasia involves periductal inflammation, dilation of the ductal system and accumulation of fluid and dead cells that block the involved ducts. The condition usually occurs in perimenopausal women and is difficult to differentiate from cancer.

Symptoms of mammary duct ectasia include sticky, thick nipple discharge with burning and itching around the nipple and inflammation. The discharge may be green, greenish brown or bloody. Nipple retraction often is associated with duct ectasia in postmenopausal women.

INTERPROFESSIONAL CARE

Diagnosis of FCC is based on complete history, physical examination and imaging studies. A biopsy may be required for diagnosis.

Analysis of nipple discharge, mammography and possibly ductography may be used to diagnose ductal disorders. The affected duct is excised in an open biopsy procedure. Nursing care for the woman is similar to that for any person with an open biopsy. It also is important to reassure the woman that these disorders are not breast cancer.

Treatment is usually symptomatic. Cyst aspiration may relieve pain and allows examination of fluid to confirm the cystic nature of the disease. A well-fitting bra, one without underwire, that provides good support worn day and night helps relieve discomfort. Some women report that eliminating xanthines (found in coffee, tea, cola and chocolate) from the diet decreases symptoms. Aspirin, mild analgesics, local heat or cold, and vitamin E may help relieve breast pain. Hormone therapy is controversial because of the benign nature of the disease and potential adverse effects of therapy. Danazol, a synthetic androgen, may be prescribed for women with severe pain.

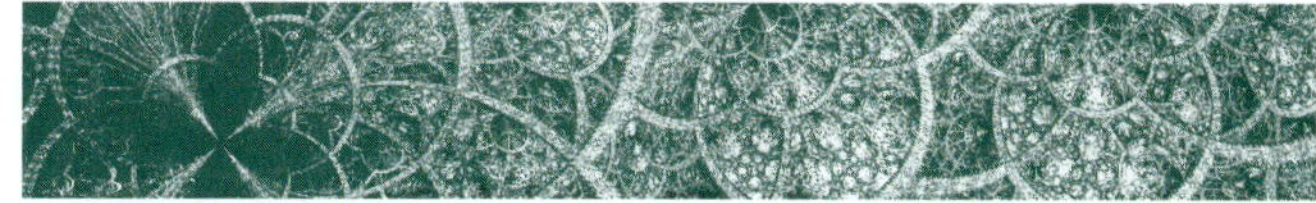

Nursing care

When a woman presents with a breast mass, nursing responsibilities include taking a careful physical and mental health history and facilitating follow-up care. If a palpable mass is present, it is important to ask how long the lesion has been present and whether the woman has noticed any pain associated with the mass, any change in its size and any changes in association with the menstrual cycle.

In many cases, definitive diagnosis of the breast disorder requires biopsy to rule out cancer. During the diagnostic process, the nurse should provide emotional support and health education about diagnostic and therapeutic procedures, self-care and comfort measures, and resources to help the woman discuss her feelings and cope with the experience.

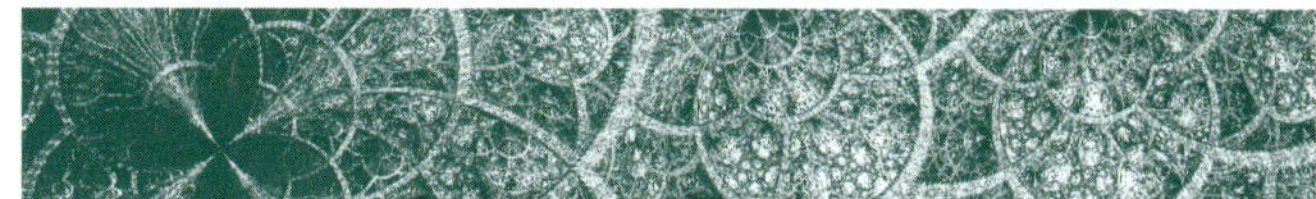

THE WOMAN WITH BREAST CANCER

Breast cancer is the unregulated growth of abnormal cells in breast tissue. Breast cancer is the second most common invasive cancer in Australia. One in 8 women (13%) and 1 in 829 men (0.12%) under the age of 85 are at risk of being diagnosed with breast cancer (Cancer Australia, 2022c). There are racial differences in the incidence and mortality of breast cancer (see the 'Focus on cultural diversity' box).

Risk factors

Of the various kinds of risk factors for breast cancer, some can be changed and some cannot. Those that cannot be changed are:

- *Age and gender.* Women are 100 times more likely to have breast cancer than men, with the risk increasing with age. See the 'Nursing care of the older woman' box.
- *Genetic risk factors.* (Discussed below in 'Pathophysiology'.)
- *Family history of breast cancer.* Relatives from either the maternal or the paternal side of the family. The risk is greater if two or more relatives have been diagnosed with

FOCUS ON CULTURAL DIVERSITY Incidence and mortality for breast cancer in women

- Breast cancer is more prevalent in non-Indigenous Australian women.
- Breast cancer is more prevalent in Caucasian women over the age of 40 years.
- Indigenous Australian women are more likely to die from breast cancer because they are often diagnosed at an advanced stage as they are less likely to participate in breast screening (Cancer Australia, 2022d).

breast cancer. Although women who have a first-degree relative who has experienced breast cancer are at an increased risk, most do not develop breast cancer. If these women do develop breast cancer, they are likely to be aged over 50. Having a male family member with breast cancer also poses an increased risk.

- *Personal history of breast cancer.* A woman with cancer in one breast has a three- to five-fold increase in risk of developing a new cancer in the other breast or in a different part of the same breast.
- *Previous breast biopsy.* If earlier breast biopsies were diagnosed as proliferative, then breast disease without atypical hyperplasia increases risk by 1.5 to two times. A previous biopsy of atypical hyperplasia increases risk by four to five times.
- *Previous chest irradiation.* Radiation of the chest as a child or young woman for other cancer (such as Hodgkin's disease) significantly increases the risk.
- *Menstrual history.* Women who begin menstruating before the age of 12 or who have menopause after the age of 50 are at a slightly higher risk.

Lifestyle-related factors and breast cancer risk include using oral contraceptives, not having children or having them after the age of 30, using HRT for more than 5 years, not breastfeeding, drinking alcohol (especially two to five drinks daily), obesity, high-fat diets, physical inactivity and (possibly) environmental pollution. Lower risk factors for breast cancer include breastfeeding, moderate or vigorous physical activity, and maintaining a healthy body weight.

Pathophysiology

Possible causes of breast cancer include environmental, hormonal, reproductive and hereditary factors. Two breast cancer susceptibility genes have been identified: BRCA1 on chromosome 17 and BRCA2 on chromosome 13. These genes may be responsible for the approximately 10% of women with hereditary breast cancer, with genetic mutations causing up to 80% of breast cancer in women younger than 50 years of age. A woman with identified mutations in BRCA1 (known to be involved in tumour suppression) has a lifetime risk of 56–85% for breast cancer and also has an increased risk of ovarian cancer. Mutations of a tumour suppressor gene are also linked to increased risk of breast cancer.

Cancer of the breast begins as a single transformed cell and is hormone dependent. Cancers of the breast are classified as non-invasive (in situ) or invasive, depending on the penetration of the tumour into surrounding tissue. Breast cancer may remain a non-invasive disease or an invasive disease without metastasis for long periods of time.

Breast cancer may be categorised as carcinoma of the mammary ducts, carcinoma of mammary lobules or sarcoma of the breast. Most breast cancers are adenocarcinomas and appear to arise in the terminal section of the breast ductal tissue. There are many histological types of breast cancer and only examples are described here. The most common type is *infiltrating ductal carcinoma.* Two atypical types of breast cancer are inflammatory carcinoma and Paget's disease. Inflammatory carcinoma of the breast, a systemic disease, is the most malignant form of breast cancer. Oedema with dimpling of the skin that results in the skin looking like the peel of an orange (*peau d'orange*) is usually present. *Paget's disease* is a rare type of breast cancer involving infiltration of the nipple epithelium.

Breast cancer can metastasise through the bloodstream or lymphatic system. The common sites of metastasis are bone, brain, lung, liver, skin and lymph nodes. Staging is a system of classifying cancer according to the size of the tumour, involvement of lymph nodes and metastasis to distant sites, and the presence/absence of distant metastasis (see Table 48.7). The staging of the breast cancer provides important information for making decisions about treatment options and is also used as a basis for prognosis.

NURSING CARE OF THE OLDER WOMAN with breast cancer

- Although the incidence of breast cancer is increasing in premenopausal women, it is still primarily a disease of older women. However, the needs of older women with breast cancer have been inadequately addressed in the professional literature and in the popular media.
- Women between the ages of 50 and 65 are the group most likely to benefit from screening mammography, yet many women in this age group have never had a mammogram. Failure of health professionals to refer older women for mammography is the reason most frequently cited for this statistic; nurse practitioners and female medical officers are more likely to refer women for mammography.
- For too long, mastectomy was perceived as the only treatment option open to most older women with breast cancer, even those with early-stage disease. Slowly that perception is changing as breast-conservation treatment gains greater acceptance. The choice of surgical treatment, particularly for older women, is highly individual. Many older women wish to preserve their breasts.
- Although older women with breast cancer may experience coexisting chronic illnesses and impaired physical function, research suggests that they show lower levels of emotional distress than younger women. Obviously the need for services such as personal care, shopping, housekeeping and transportation increases as the ages of the woman and the caregiver increase.

TABLE 48.7 Staging of breast cancer

STAGE	TUMOUR	NODE INVOLVEMENT	METASTASIS
0	Tis–Carcinoma in situ or Paget's disease of the nipple	N0–No regional lymph node metastasis	M0–No evidence of distant metastasis
I	T1–Tumour no larger than 2 cm	N0	M0
IIA	T0–No evidence of primary tumour T1	N1–Metastasis to movable ipsilateral axillary nodes	M0
	T2–Tumour no larger than 5 cm	N0	M0
IIB	T2	N1	M0
	T3–Tumour larger than 5 cm	N0	M0
IIIA	T0 T1 T2	N2–Metastasis to ipsilateral fixed axillary nodes	M0
	T3	N1	M0
		N2	M0
IIIB	T4–Tumour of any size with direct extension to chest wall or skin	Any N	M0
	Any T	N3–Metastasis to ipsilateral internal mammary lymph nodes	M0
IV	Any T	N0 and N1	M1–Distant metastasis

Manifestations

The symptoms of breast cancer may include a non-tender lump in the breast (most often in the upper outer quadrant, the area with the most glandular tissue), abnormal nipple discharge, a rash around the nipple area, nipple retraction, dimpling of the skin or a change in the position of the nipple (see the 'Manifestations' box). There may also be nipple pain, scaliness, ulceration, skin irritation or discharge. Breast cancer is usually painless, but some women report a burning or stinging sensation. Many women with breast cancer have no symptoms and their tumours are detected by mammography. However, most breast cancers are found by the women themselves (during BSE or a shower) or by their partners during sexual activity.

INTERPROFESSIONAL CARE

Diagnosis of breast cancer begins with detection of either asymptomatic lesions discovered through screening or symptomatic lesions discovered by the woman. Any palpable mass requires evaluation. Once the diagnosis is made, a number of treatment options are available. The choice of treatment depends on several factors, such as the stage of the cancer, the age of the woman, geographical location of the woman and related health services and the woman's preferences.

MANIFESTATIONS Breast cancer

- Breast mass or thickening
- Unusual lump in the underarm or above the collarbone
- Persistent skin rash near the nipple area
- Flaking or eruption near the nipple
- Dimpling, pulling or retraction in an area of the breast
- Nipple discharge
- Change in nipple position
- Burning, stinging or pricking sensation

Diagnosis

Early detection of breast cancer is possible with clinical breast examination (CBE) and mammogram (see the chapter 'A person-centred approach to assessing the male and female reproductive systems' for further information). Mammography can detect breast tumours 2 years before they reach palpable size; most of these tumours have been present for 8 to 10 years. The Cancer Council recommends mammograms every 2 years for women aged between 50 and 74, although women from 40 years of age onwards can have free mammograms (Cancer Council, 2022d). Magnetic resonance imaging (MRI) is used for women who are at high risk of breast cancer or have very dense breast tissue (Cancer Council, 2022d).

Other diagnostic tests include a percutaneous needle biopsy to define a cystic mass or fibrocystic changes and provide specimens for cytological examination and a breast biopsy. In aspiration biopsy or fine-needle aspiration biopsy, a needle is used to remove cells or fluid from the breast lesion (see Figure 48.8). The types of breast biopsy and related nursing care are described in the chapter 'A person-centred approach to assessing the male and female reproductive systems'. In many facilities, fine-needle aspiration biopsies are performed using a stereotactic biopsy device; mammography and a computer are used to guide the needle.

Medications

Tamoxifen citrate (Nolvadex) is an oral medication that interferes with oestrogen activity. It is used to treat advanced breast cancer, as an adjuvant for early-stage breast cancer and as a preventive treatment for women at high risk. Nursing implications for tamoxifen are presented in the 'Medication administration' box.

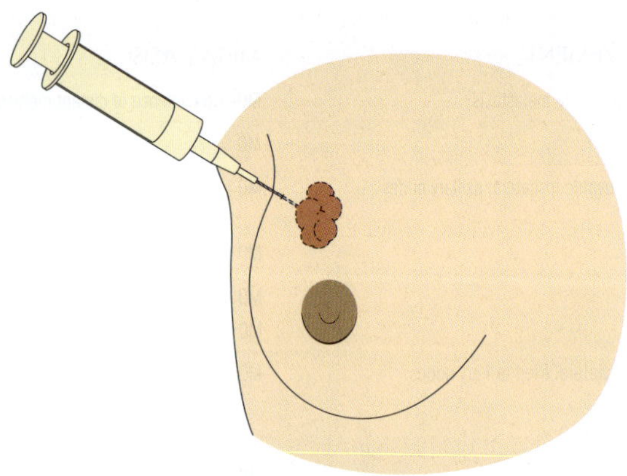

A Aspiration biopsy

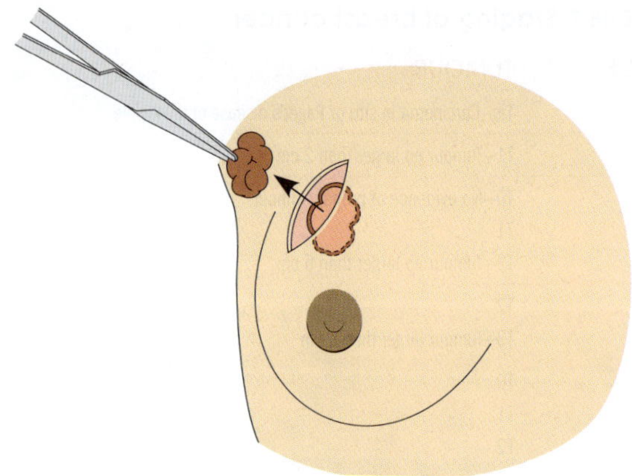

B Excisional biopsy

FIGURE 48.8 ***Types of breast biopsy. A, In an aspiration biopsy, a needle is used to aspirate fluid or tissue from the breast. B, In an excisional biopsy, tissue from the breast lesion is removed surgically***

Immunotherapy, using trastuzumab (Herceptin), is used to stop the growth of breast tumours that express the HER2/neu receptor (which binds an epidermal growth factor that contributes to cancer cell growth) on their cell surface. This medication is a recombinant DNA-derived monoclonal antibody that binds to the receptor, inhibiting tumour cell proliferation.

Chemotherapy has become the standard of care for the majority of breast cancer cases with axillary node involvement. In late metastatic disease, chemotherapy becomes the primary treatment to prolong the woman's life. Chemotherapy is discussed in the chapter 'Nursing care of people with cancer'. Adjuvant (additional) systemic therapy following primary treatment for early-stage breast cancer refers to the administration of chemotherapy and other pharmacological agents. This type of therapy reduces the rates of recurrence and death from breast cancer. For example, bevacizumab (Avastin), when combined with chemotherapy to treat metastatic breast cancer, has extended cancer-free survival; and letrozole (Femara) (an aromatase inhibitor) has reduced the risk of recurrence after surgery (in some cases, more effectively than tamoxifen).

Surgery

Until recently, the treatment of choice for breast cancer was a radical mastectomy. The trend now is towards more conservative surgery combined with chemotherapy, hormone therapy or radiation, depending on the stage of the tumour and the age of the woman.

MASTECTOMY There are various types of mastectomy for breast cancer. *Radical mastectomy* is the removal of the entire affected breast, the underlying chest muscles and the lymph nodes under the arms. *Simple mastectomy* is the removal of the complete breast only. *Segmental mastectomy* or *lumpectomy* (see Figure 48.9A) is the removal of the tumour and the surrounding margin of breast tissues. Modified radical mastectomy is the removal of the breast tissue and lymph nodes under the arm (axillary node dissection), leaving the chest wall muscles intact (see Figure 48.9B). See the accompanying box for the nursing care of a woman having a mastectomy.

Axillary node dissection is generally performed during surgery for all invasive breast carcinoma to stage the tumour. This

MEDICATION ADMINISTRATION Tamoxifen

TAMOXIFEN (NOLVADEX)

Tamoxifen is the most widely prescribed breast cancer medication, commonly given to prevent recurrence of oestrogen-positive breast cancer in postmenopausal women. It inhibits tumour growth by blocking the oestrogen receptor sites of cancer cells. Tamoxifen increases a woman's risk of developing endometrial cancer, deep venous thrombosis (DVT) and pulmonary embolism.

Nursing responsibilities

- Assess for potential contraindications to therapy.
- Assess liver function tests; tamoxifen may interfere with liver function.

Health education for the woman and family

- If in childbearing years, use a non-hormonal, barrier form of contraception; tamoxifen has adverse effects on the developing fetus.
- Take the medication as prescribed until the health practitioner indicates otherwise.
- Side effects such as hot flushes, vaginal dryness, irregular periods and weight gain are commonly experienced by women taking tamoxifen.
- If you are a smoker, stop. Smoking further increases the risk of DVT and is linked to the development of cancer.
- Promptly report any abnormal vaginal bleeding (non-menstrual bleeding, bleeding after menopause) to your primary care provider.

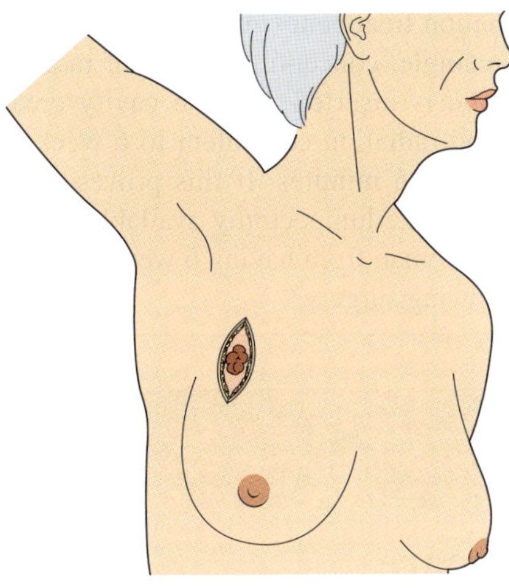
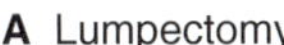
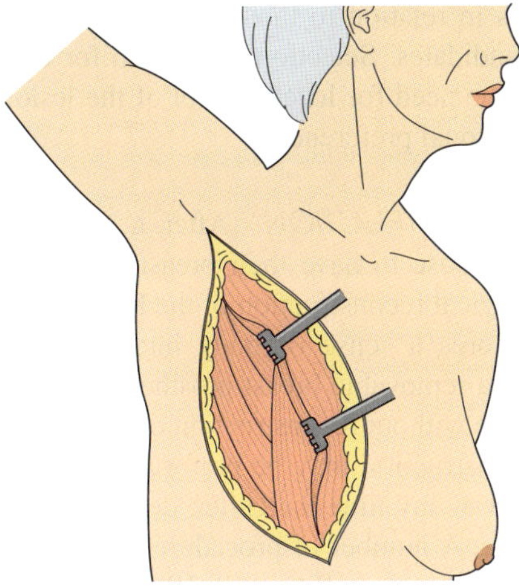

A Lumpectomy

B Modified radical mastectomy

FIGURE 48.9 *Types of mastectomy. A, In a lumpectomy, only the tumour and a small margin of surrounding tissue are removed. B, In a modified radical mastectomy, all breast tissue and the underarm lymph nodes are removed, but the underlying muscles remain*

NURSING CARE OF THE WOMAN having a mastectomy

PREOPERATIVE CARE

- Ensure that the woman or family member signs an informed consent form.
- See the chapter 'Nursing care of people having surgery' for preoperative preparation.

POSTOPERATIVE CARE

- Deep-breathing exercises are important because after general anaesthesia it is difficult for air to reach the lungs, particularly with restrictive surgical dressings that decreases chest expansion.
- A suction apparatus will be placed in the wound to allow drainage of excess body fluids that accumulate when the lymph nodes are removed. This device is usually removed 3 to 5 days after surgery.
- An IV line may be in place for fluid replacement and antibiotics to reduce the risk of postoperative infection.
- Control pain by using the patient-controlled analgesia device or requesting analgesics before pain becomes severe. Take analgesics as needed before performing recommended exercises to facilitate full movement.
- Note any signs of bleeding on the dressing or on the bedding.
- Numbness or feelings of 'pins and needles' in the axillary area are common.
- Lying on one's back or on the side not operated on helps fluid drain from the site.
- Moving the arm on the operated side helps regain mobility; specific exercises will be prescribed for increasing mobility after the incisions have healed.
- If fluid builds up after the drains have been removed, it can be aspirated by the surgeon.
- Use caution if lifting heavy objects with the arm on the operated side.
- Be careful about injury and infection on the affected side; wear rubber gloves when washing dishes, garden gloves when working outside. Request that caregivers not perform blood pressures or venipunctures on the operative side to reduce the risk of injury and infection.
- Feelings of anxiety, sadness and fear of looking at the incision are normal; mastectomy means abrupt change in body image. It is normal to mourn the loss of a breast and to fear the loss of one's life after a cancer diagnosis.
- Sexual intimacy can be affected by mastectomy; it often helps to be able to discuss potential sexual problems with one's partner, a counsellor or a breast cancer support group.

surgery can cause lymphoedema (accumulation of fluid in the soft tissues of the arm caused by removal of lymph channels), nerve damage and adhesions, and because of the role of the lymph nodes in immune system function, non-surgical methods of detecting lymph node involvement are used. Sentinel node biopsy prior to a node dissection is conducted by injecting a radioactive substance or dye into the region of the tumour. The dye is carried to the first (sentinel) lymph node to receive lymph from the tumour and would therefore be the node most likely to contain cancer cells if the cancer had metastasised. If the sentinel node is positive, more nodes are removed. If it is negative, further node evaluation is usually not indicated.

LUMPECTOMY Breast conservation surgery (*lumpectomy*) may be defined as excision of the primary tumour and adjacent breast tissue followed by radiation therapy. Many women are candidates for this procedure; however, women who have multicentric breast neoplasms and those who have large tumours in relation to their breast size are examples of unsuitable candidates. Selection of women for this procedure is guided by the need for local control of the lesion, cosmetic results and personal preference.

BREAST RECONSTRUCTION After a mastectomy, some women may choose to have their breast reconstructed. They report that surgical reconstruction of the breast simplifies their lives and restores a sense of body integrity. Other women choose to use a removable breast prosthesis and some women are comfortable without reconstruction or a prosthesis.

Breast reconstruction may be performed at the time of the mastectomy or at any time thereafter, depending on the woman's preference. A number of procedures may be used for the breast reconstruction (see Figure 48.10). These include placement of a submuscular implant, the use of a tissue expander followed by an implant, the transposition of muscle and blood supply from the abdomen or back, or using (most often) the transverse rectus abdominis myocutaneous (TRAM) free-tissue flap. Nursing implications for the care of women undergoing breast reconstruction surgery are summarised in the accompanying box.

Radiation therapy

Radiation therapy is typically used following breast cancer surgery to destroy any remaining cancer cells that could cause recurrence or metastasis. If a tumour is unusually large, radiation may be used to shrink the tumour prior to surgery. Radiation therapy is most commonly used in combination with lumpectomy for early stage (I or II) breast cancer. Palliative radiation therapy is also used to treat chest wall recurrences and some bone metastases to help control pain and prevent fractures. Radiation therapy is administered by means of an external beam or tissue implants.

A new radiation treatment (*intraoperative radiotherapy*) is provided by a single, concentrated dose of radiation. During surgery, a probe is inserted into the cavity created by the lumpectomy and radiation equivalent to 6 weeks of doses is emitted for about 25 minutes. If this proves successful, the treatment could make lumpectomy available to more women and prevent the woman from having 6 weeks of daily radiation treatments following surgery.

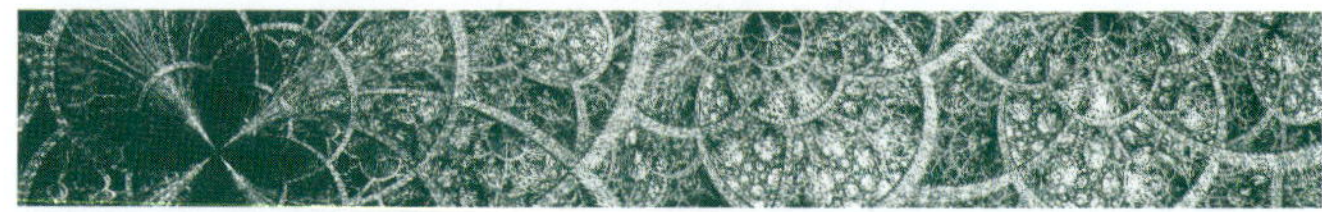

Nursing care

Breast cancer is not one disease entity, but many, depending on the affected breast tissue, the tissue's oestrogen dependency and the age of the person at onset. The psychological and social impact of breast cancer extends beyond the fear and threat of death. The diagnosis may transform the woman's sense of self and lead to reintegration or negotiation of family relationships. See the accompanying nursing care plan for a woman with breast cancer.

Health promotion

All women should be taught to perform BSE monthly (see Box 48.1). Premenopausal women should perform BSE between 7 and 10 days from the first day of their menstrual period, because hormonal changes increase breast tenderness and lumpiness prior to menses. Postmenopausal women should choose one date of the month (e.g. the first day of the month) for BSE.

Educational messages about breast cancer screening need to be culturally and age sensitive. Media campaigns promoting

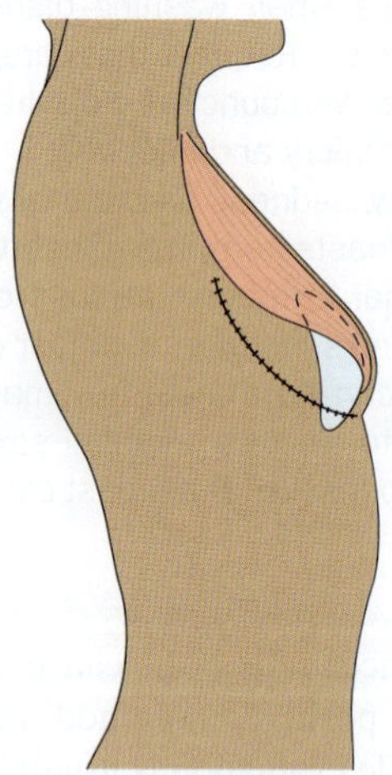

A Implant

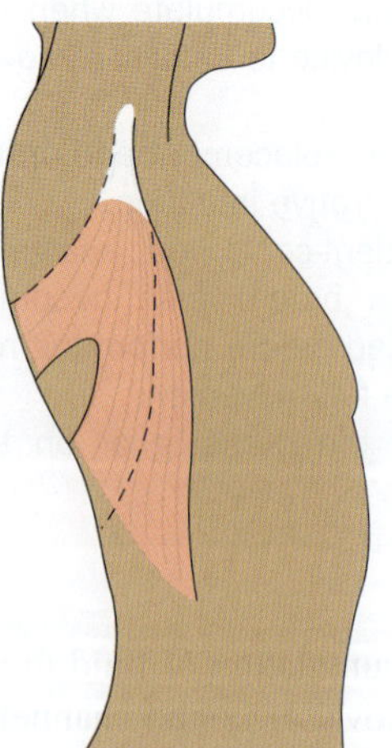

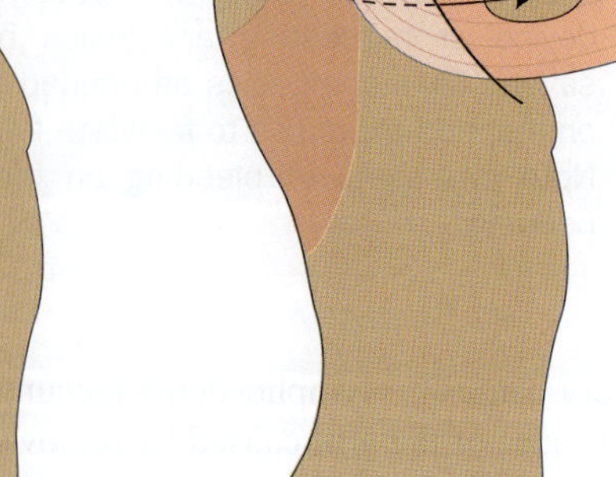

B Latissimus dorsi musculocutaneous flap

FIGURE 48.10 ***Types of breast reconstruction surgeries. A, A breast implant is inserted under the pectoris muscle. B, Autogenous procedures transfer a flap of skin, muscle and fat from the donor site on the woman's body to the mastectomy site. The most frequently used donor muscle sites are the latissimus dorsi and the rectus abdominis (the TRAM flap)***

NURSING CARE OF THE WOMAN having breast reconstruction

HEALTH EDUCATION FOR THE WOMAN AND FAMILY

- Reconstruction can be done immediately after a mastectomy or at any time later on. Some surgeons believe that delayed reconstruction offers better cosmetic results.
- Reconstructive surgery can create a natural-looking breast that makes clothes fit better. Since it has no nerve endings, however, the reconstructed breast has no feeling or sensations.
- If a simple mastectomy is done, an implant approximately the same size as the other breast is placed under the pectoral muscle on the operative side. This creates a breast mound that closely resembles the natural breast in shape and softness. If the implant is placed over the pectoral muscle, a high degree of firmness may occur.
- With a simple mastectomy or modified radical mastectomy, a tissue expander may be used to replace the breast. The tissue expander is placed under the pectoral muscle and gradually expanded with saline injections every 2 to 3 weeks to stretch the overlying skin and create a pocket. After a period of time, usually 1 to 2 months, the tissue expander is exchanged for a saline implant.
- With more extensive surgery such as radical mastectomy, a flap of skin, fat or muscle is transferred from a donor site to the operative area. A new nipple may be created by using tissue from the opposite nipple or from the inner thigh.
- Reconstructive surgery may require multiple surgeries, including all the risks associated with anaesthesia. As the complexity of the procedures increases, so does the risk of complications such as infection.
- To decrease the risk of a fibrous capsule forming around the implant, it is important to perform breast massage as instructed.

NURSING CARE PLAN A woman with breast cancer

Vanessa Cole is a 46-year-old mother of three—Sarah, aged 20, Rory, aged 18, and Jennifer, aged 16. Due to a family history of breast cancer, she has been closely monitored (annual mammograms and clinical breast examination, monthly BSE, a needle aspiration biopsy with negative findings) for 4 years prior to her diagnosis. Vanessa discovers a lump in her left breast during her monthly BSE. An incisional biopsy reveals invasive lobular carcinoma in the left breast. Vanessa is debating whether to have reconstructive breast surgery. One of her greatest concerns is how her illness will affect her ability to support and care for her family. The breast cancer diagnosis seems part of the family legacy. She wonders, 'When will it happen to Jennifer? To Sarah?'

ASSESSMENT

During the history, Marc Acut, RN, the admitting nurse, learns from Vanessa that her mother, two of her aunts and one sister had been diagnosed with breast cancer. Her mother and one of the aunts died before age 45. Physical assessment findings include T 37.0°C, BP 110/62, P 65, R 14. Her weight is 54 kg; she is 168 cm tall. Modified radical mastectomy is performed; histological examination shows a 3 cm tumour; axillary node dissection shows that 4 of 16 lymph nodes are positive.

DIAGNOSES

- *Infection risk* related to surgical incision.
- *Acute pain* related to surgery and postoperative recovery.
- *Body image altered* in response to loss of her breast.
- *Personal conflict* about treatment options, related to concerns about risks and benefits.
- *Personal fear* related to current and future wellbeing related to the disease process/prognosis.
- *Anxiety.*

PLANNING

- Educate Vanessa about handwashing and wound care.
- Assess her pain tolerance and administer analgesics as prescribed.
- Educate her to use caution when moving the arm on the operated side, to avoid lifting heavy objects and to wear gloves when gardening.
- Encourage her to discuss her thoughts and feelings about her body changes.
- The Breast Cancer Network Australia (https://www.bcna.org.au) or her state/territory Cancer Council can also be a good source of support; also social work or community health referral to assist with care of her children while undergoing treatment. If Vanessa lives in a rural or remote rural area of Australia, her family may need to be temporarily relocated to be with her.
- Assess her interest in support agencies and refer if appropriate.
- Discuss the use of a temporary prosthesis and later the fitting of a permanent prosthesis (6 to 8 weeks after surgery), the need to be fitted by an experienced person and health insurance reimbursement for the prosthesis.
- Discuss the possibility of attending a breast cancer support group where she can draw on the experiences of other women who have undergone mastectomy, chemotherapy or radiation.
- Encourage her to verbalise her fears about her own prognosis and about her daughters' future risk of breast cancer; assess the need/interest for referral to psychological counselling in the future. However, these services may not be readily available in some geographical regions of Australia. Registered Nurses as health professionals can provide information, education and reassurance.

Expected outcomes

- Remain free of infection.
- Experience minimal pain or discomfort during her recovery.
- Maintain a positive body image, regardless of her decision about reconstruction.
- Evaluate the treatment options in relation to personal values and decide on a course of action.

(continued)

NURSING CARE PLAN A woman with breast cancer (continued)

- Identify the sources of her fear and demonstrate behaviours that may reduce fears.

IMPLEMENTATION

- Initiate each of the steps outlined in the planning section detailed above.
- Monitor the effectiveness of the plan by monitoring Vanessa's response to:
  - surgery
  - pain management.
- Engage in ongoing discussion with Vanessa about the implementation of the plan and her psychosocial wellbeing.

EVALUATION

At discharge, Vanessa has no signs of physical complications and is looking forward to being at home with her daughters as temporary caregivers. Vanessa contacted a Breast Cancer Network volunteer, who sent her a temporary prosthesis and booklets about postmastectomy exercises, chemotherapy and breast reconstruction. The volunteer also referred her to a local cancer support group. Vanessa has talked about her concerns related to breast reconstruction. 'I want to avoid anything that would increase the risk of complications. The possibility of recurrence and my fear for my daughters' future health are more than enough to worry about.'

CRITICAL THINKING IN THE NURSING PROCESS

1 What role could genetic counselling play in helping Vanessa and her daughters better understand the daughters' risk of breast cancer?
2 Describe the types of mastectomies and their implications for nursing care.
3 Which medications might help minimise the side effects of chemotherapy?
4 Develop a plan of care for Vanessa for her *Disturbed sleep pattern*.

REFLECTION ON THE NURSING PROCESS

1 Outline what you have learned from Vanessa's case study. How would you incorporate this into your future nursing practice?
2 Which strategies would you use in your future nursing practice to assist women who are undergoing treatment for breast cancer?

BOX 48.1 Breast self-examination (BSE)

- Observe your breasts for any visual changes.
- Lie down on your back and place your right arm behind your head. (BSE should be done while lying down because this position spreads breast tissue evenly over the chest wall, making it easier to feel all the breast tissue.)
- Use the finger pads of the middle fingers on your left hand to feel for lumps in the right breast. Use overlapping 20-cent-sized circular motions of the finger pads to feel the breast tissue.
- Use three different levels of pressure to feel all the breast tissue. Light pressure is needed to feel the tissue closest to the skin; medium pressure to feel a little deeper; and firm pressure to feel the tissue closest to the chest and ribs. A firm ridge in the lower curve of each breast is normal. Use each pressure level to feel the breast tissue before moving on to the next spot.
- Move around the breast in an up and down pattern starting at an imaginary line drawn straight down your side from the underarm and moving across the breast to the middle of the chest bone (sternum, breastbone). Be sure to check the entire breast area before going down until you feel only ribs and up to the neck or collar bone.
- Repeat the exam on your left breast, using the finger pads of your right hand.
- Stand in front of the mirror with your hands pressing firmly down on your hips. Look at your breasts for any changes in size, shape, contour or dimpling.
- Examine your underarm while sitting or standing and with your arm only slightly raised.
- If you find any changes, see your healthcare provider as soon as possible.

mammography often show young white women, an approach that has proved ineffective for Aboriginal and Torres Strait Islander women (see the 'Translation to practice' box). By working with women from culturally and linguistically diverse (CALD) backgrounds, nurses can help make breast cancer education more meaningful to women in these groups.

Assessment

Undertake a thorough health history and physical examination (see the chapter 'A person-centred approach to assessing the male and female reproductive systems'). Further focused assessments are described with nursing interventions.

- *Health history*: family history of breast cancer, breast changes, nipple discharge, use of HRT, personal history of breast cancer, previous diagnostic tests and treatment for cancer, menstrual history, pregnancies, alcohol intake, physical activity, dietary history.
- *Physical assessment*: height and weight, breasts, lymph glands.
- *Mental health assessment*: anxiety, coping strategies, emotional wellbeing.

Nursing diagnoses and interventions

Although each woman has individual needs, nursing priorities prior to surgery are concerned with *Anxiety*, *Decisional conflict*, *Grief*, *Risk of infection*, *Risk of injury* and *Disturbed body image* over the loss of a breast. As the typical hospital stay is short, preoperative education is often done on an outpatient basis.

Anxiety

The woman with breast cancer is often anxious about the diagnosis, the surgery, the outcome of surgery if nodal involvement is found and the possible changes in sexual and family relationships. Studies show that young women with breast cancer, a growing population, are particularly vulnerable to anxiety and other psychosocial effects, as are their spouses and their children.

TRANSLATION TO PRACTICE Evidence-based practice: breast and cervical cancer in Aboriginal and Torres Strait Islander women

Despite efforts to improve both the diagnosis and treatment of women with breast and cervical cancer, Aboriginal and Torres Strait Islander women experience a higher incidence of cervical cancer (Diaz et al., 2018) and have poorer outcomes for breast and cervical cancer than non-Indigenous women (AIHW, 2019b). Data show that Aboriginal and Torres Strait Islander women experience less incidence of breast cancer than non-Indigenous women, yet the survival outcome is poorer (AIHW, 2019b; Supramaniam et al., 2014). It is believed that this statistic is the result of Aboriginal and Torres Strait Islander women's advanced stage of disease at diagnosis, primarily due to a delay in seeking treatment. Seeking treatment is difficult in rural and remote areas of Australia where health services are few or non-existent (AIHW, 2019b; Sabesan et al., 2012).

Reath and Carey (2008) found that partnership between the Aboriginal and Torres Strait Islander community and health workers, in addition to the availability of a female general practitioner, were the key elements to improving Aboriginal and Torres Strait Islander women's participation in cervical and breast screening processes.

IMPLICATIONS FOR NURSING

Nurses must consider multiple factors when considering what may or may not influence Aboriginal and Torres Strait Islander women to delay diagnosis and treatment for cervical and breast cancer, including intra- and intercultural differences and similarities, as well as perceptions and health beliefs. Nurses need to conduct accurate assessments and design interventions based on considerations of both individual and group cultural differences. Culturally safe and appropriate healthcare is paramount.

CRITICAL THINKING IN PERSON-CENTRED CARE

1 Which barriers to cervical and breast cancer screening in women of all cultures and ethnicities can you identify? Do you think these barriers differ based on culture, race or socioeconomic level? Why or why not?
2 Are there barriers to cervical or breast cancer screening that might be unique to Aboriginal and Torres Strait Islander women?
3 What type of questions would you include in a health assessment to identify if an Aboriginal or Torres Strait Islander woman may be worried about cervical or breast cancer, but has not sought diagnosis?

- Provide opportunities to express thoughts and feelings. In this process, the woman can name her fears. *Once the fears are named, the nurse may simply listen, educate or dispel fears that stem from lack of understanding.*
- Discuss with the woman her knowledge of breast cancer. *Assessing the woman's knowledge of breast cancer helps the nurse plan more effective health education.*
- Encourage discussion relating to immediate concerns about resuming her life at home and the changes she must make. *Anticipatory guidance can help plan for and cope with changes in her life and relationships.*
- Explain the surgical procedure, including information about preoperative medications, anaesthesia and recovery. *Knowing what to expect helps to decrease anxiety.*
- Explain that it is normal to have decreased sensation in the surgical area. *Severed or damaged nerves reduce sensation.*

Decisional conflict

The woman with breast cancer must make life-changing decisions about treatment within a relatively brief and highly stressful time. Her age, menopausal status, relationships and stage of cancer are only some of the factors that affect her decisions. Culture, values, lifestyle, socioeconomic status and self-esteem also are considered.

- Provide an opportunity for the woman to ask questions; answer them as simply and directly as possible. Make eye contact as appropriate and pay attention to body language. *During this time, the woman can process information and make informed decisions.*
- Focus on immediate concerns and provide up-to-date written material for the woman to review. *Written material provides easy reference to information not processed immediately because of anxiety and stress.*
- Listen to the woman in a non-judgmental and respectful manner during her decision-making process. *Non-judgmental, empathic listening helps the woman process information and make informed decisions. Only she knows the context of her life.*
- If the woman wishes, provide opportunities for her to meet with other women who have had breast cancer surgery. *Not all women are ready to meet others in their situation, but opening the door to this resource is appropriate. The woman may choose to talk with these women after the surgery.*
- Facilitate a team approach with the surgeon, anaesthetist, oncologist, plastic surgeon and other health professionals. *Being the woman's advocate during this time of anxiety and decision making reduces the stress of coordinating multiple healthcare provider schedules.*

Anticipatory grieving

Breast surgery, even lumpectomy, alters the appearance of the breast. This loss is expressed through grief and anger.

- Listen attentively to expressions of grief and watch for non-verbal cues (failure to make eye contact, crying, silence, anger, bargaining). *Not all women will express grief clearly or openly; sometimes unspoken grief is the most painful. Grief is best relieved only when expressed in a non-threatening environment.*
- Allow time to interact and do not rush interactions. *Taking time to be with the woman communicates caring.*

- Explain that it is normal to have periods of depression, anger and denial after breast surgery. *All these feelings are appropriate expressions of grief.*
- If the woman wishes to do so, involve the partner in helping her cope with her grief. Remember that the partner may also be grieving. *Not all women want to share their grief and not all partners are interested and supportive.*

Risk of infection

Like any person undergoing surgery, the woman who has breast surgery is at risk of infection. Removal of lymph nodes and the presence of a draining wound increase the risk.

- Assess the surgical dressings for bleeding, drainage, colour and odour every 4 hours for 24 hours and document your findings. Circle any visible bleeding and drainage on the dressing as a baseline for subsequent assessment. *Excessive bleeding or drainage signals postoperative complications that may require emergency attention.*
- Observe the incision and IV sites for pain, redness, swelling and drainage. Assess the drainage system for patency and adequate suction; note the colour and amount of drainage. *Careful observation for any signs of infection is essential because the woman's immune system is compromised. IV catheters should be placed on the uninvolved side only.*
- Change dressings and IV tubing using aseptic technique. Moist dressings and intravenous tubing provide sites for bacterial growth. *Routine dressing and IV tubing changes using aseptic technique reduce the risk of infection.*
- Encourage a protein-rich diet. Discuss the woman's nutritional status with the dietitian and request a consultation for the woman. *Adequate nutrition promotes healing and boosts the immune system.*
- Teach the woman how to care for the drainage system, if present. (Clean the site, empty the device and record the amount, colour and type of drainage.) *The woman is often discharged prior to removal of the drainage system and dressings, and needs health education to provide self-care.*
- At discharge, educate the woman how to recognise and report to her healthcare provider the symptoms of infection: fever, redness or hardness at the surgical site or purulent drainage. Any of these symptoms should be reported to the physician/surgeon. *Knowing the signs and symptoms of infection prepares the woman to seek prompt treatment if infection occurs.*
- Explain that she may experience scaling, flaking, dryness, itching, rash or dry desquamation of the skin, particularly after radiation therapy. *Impaired skin integrity increases the risk of infection.*
- Tell the woman to avoid deodorants and talcum powder on the affected side until the incision is completely healed. *These substances may irritate the skin and impede healing.*

Risk of injury

Removal of the lymph nodes puts the woman at risk of injury and long-term complications such as lymphoedema and infection.

- When obtaining blood pressure and starting IVs, use the non-surgical side. *Compression of the arm on the surgical side may cause lymphoedema.*
- Elevate the affected arm higher than the shoulder on a pillow, but do not abduct it; the hand should be higher than the elbow. *Elevating the arm permits drainage, prevents swelling and promotes circulation.*
- Encourage ROM exercises in the affected arm. *Exercise helps develop collateral drainage.*
- Explain that lymphoedema massage and an elastic compression bandage may help control the swelling after she has recovered from surgery. *It is important that women know about the resources available after recovery.*

Disturbed body image

Breast surgery can change the woman's body image. The surgical changes may be compounded by weight gain and other side effects of chemotherapy or hormone therapy. Self-esteem also affects adjustment to a changed body image.

- Assess how the woman views her body. Discuss what image of herself she had prior to surgery. *Self-image is related to self-esteem. Discuss whether her self-image has changed.*
- Explain that redness and swelling in the scar will fade with time. *The knowledge that the scar will fade may give the woman a more realistic view of the changes.*
- Include the partner and family if possible when discussing the plan of care and activities of daily living (ADLs). Request consultation with a mental health professional if the woman is interested. *Discussion with the partner and family can facilitate the woman's emotional healing process.*

> **CONSIDERATION FOR PRACTICE**
>
> **Offer referral to support groups with women experiencing similar problems. Some women may prefer one-on-one counselling. However, these services may not readily available in some geographical regions of Australia. Registered Nurses as health professionals can provide information, education and reassurance.**

- Offer pamphlets and suggest books and DVDs and appropriate websites that might increase knowledge about what lies ahead. *Knowing what to expect can help the woman cope.*
- Encourage the woman to look at her incision when she feels ready; often the reality is not as frightening as she had imagined. Explain that it is normal to be afraid to look. *Reassurance that her behaviour is normal decreases anxiety.*
- If the woman is interested in breast reconstruction, provide written material and encourage her to talk (in person, telephone or online) with a plastic surgeon and with women who have had reconstruction. *It is important for the woman to be fully informed about available options to make an informed decision.*

Community-based care

The woman with breast cancer and her family have much to learn to provide self-care at home. Address the following topics in preparation for home care:

- Symptoms of infection and the need to report any that occur to her healthcare provider.
- The importance of ADLs, such as eating properly, combing her hair and washing her face.

- Postmastectomy exercises and lymphoedema care (see Figure 48.11), as discussed with physicians and physical therapists.
- The need for adequate rest and emotional support.
- Participation in a breast cancer support group and online information services and bulletin boards for sources of education and support.

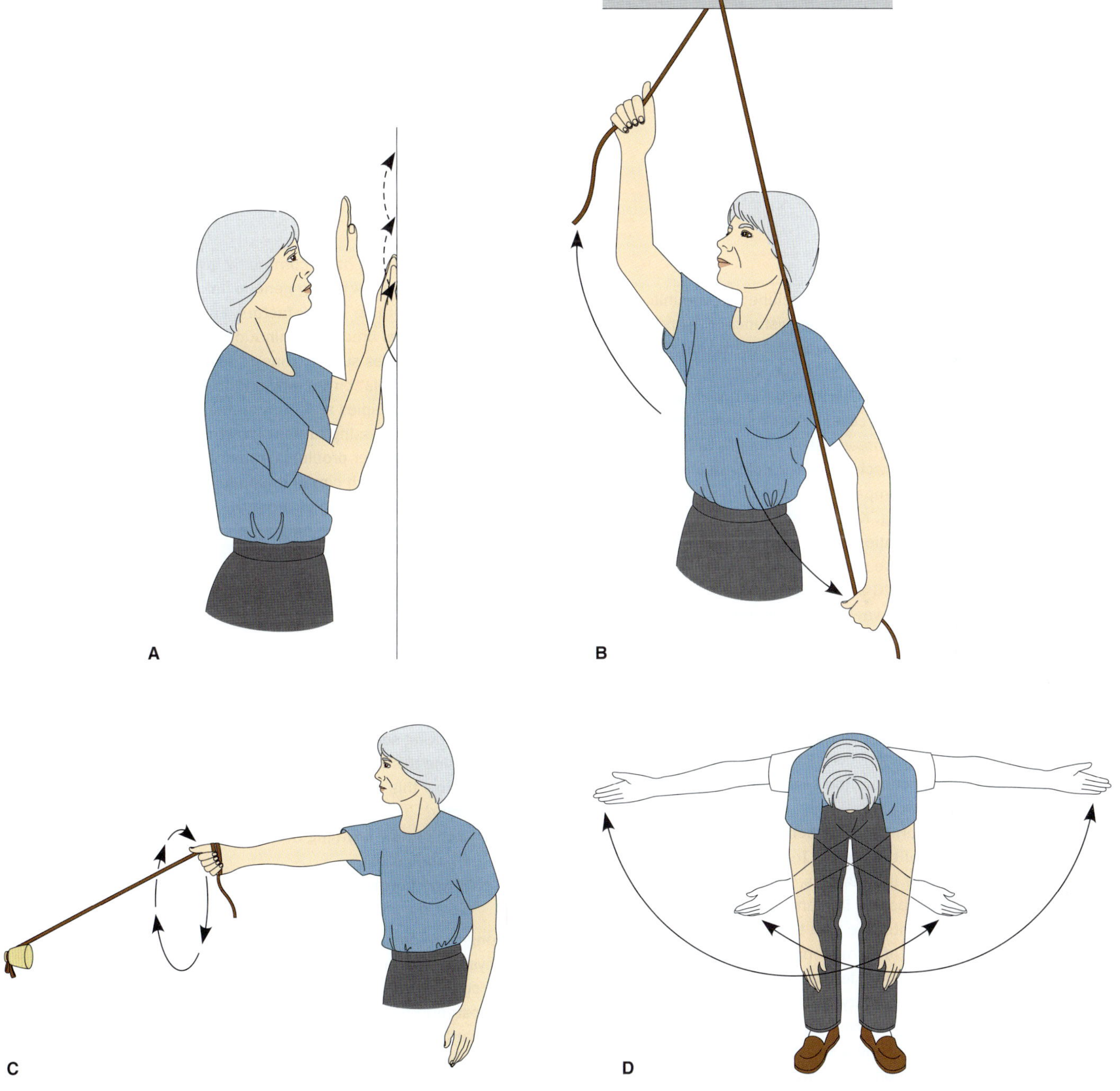

FIGURE 48.11 *Postmastectomy exercises. A, Wall climbing: stand facing wall with toes 15 to 30 cm from wall. Bend elbows and place palms against wall at shoulder level. Gradually move both hands up the wall parallel to each other until incisional pulling or pain occurs. (Mark that spot on wall to measure progress.) Work hands down to shoulder level. Move closer to wall as height of reach improves. B, Overhead pulley: using operated arm, toss 1.8-metre rope over shower curtain rod (or over top of a door that has a nail in the top to hold the rope in place for the exercise). Grasp one end of rope in each hand. Slowly raise operated arm as far as comfortable by pulling down on the rope on opposite side. Keep raised arm close to your head. Reverse to raise unoperated arm by lowering the operated arm. Repeat. C, Rope turning: tie rope to door handle. Hold rope in hand of operated side. Back away from door until arm is extended away from body, parallel to floor. Swing rope in as wide a circle as possible. Increase size of circle as mobility returns. D, Arm swings: stand with feet 20 cm apart. Bend forwards from waist, allowing arms to hang towards floor. Swing both arms up to sides to reach shoulder level. Swing back to centre, then cross arms at centre. Do not bend elbows. If possible, do this and other exercises in front of a mirror to ensure even posture and correct motion*

- Prosthesis management, if this option is chosen. (A temporary lightweight prosthesis may be worn immediately after the drains and sutures have been removed from the surgical site. Due to prostheses being expensive, a permanent one should not be purchased until the wound has completely healed. Prostheses are available at medical stores and many larger department stores. Most health insurance policies pay for the first prosthesis.)
- Helpful resources:
  - Breast Cancer Network Australia: https://www.bcna.org.au
  - Cancer Council—*After a diagnosis*: https://www.cancer.org.au/about-cancer/after-a-diagnosis/
  - Breast cancer survival for Indigenous women: https://www.cancercouncil.com.au/aboriginalcancer/research-information-findings/publications/breast-cancer-survival-comparison/.

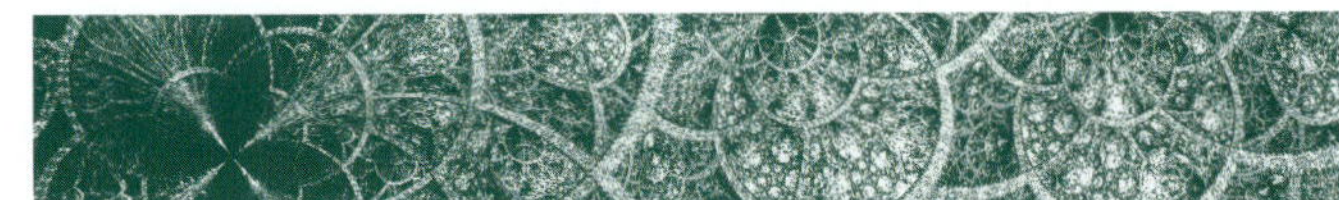

CHAPTER HIGHLIGHTS

- Disorders of female sexual function include dyspareunia, inhibited sexual desire and orgasmic dysfunction. Nurses should obtain a sexual history, discuss sexual concerns and make appropriate referrals without embarrassment.
- Menopause, a normal physiological event in the lifespan of a woman, is the permanent cessation of menses. Loss of oestrogen results in widespread tissue changes and increases the risk of osteoporosis, fractures and cardiovascular disease.
- Menstrual disorders encompass PMS, dysmenorrhoea and abnormal uterine bleeding. Nursing interventions are focused on providing health education about good health practices and interventions to relieve symptoms. Interprofessional care includes a therapeutic D&C and hysterectomy.
- Uterine displacement and vaginal fistulas are structural disorders. Uterine displacements may be treated surgically or with a pessary and may include education about pelvic floor exercises to minimise urinary leakage. Fistulas may spontaneously resolve if small or may be surgically repaired.
- There are both benign and malignant disorders of female reproductive tissue, including cysts or polyps, leiomyomas, endometriosis and cancers of the cervix, endometrium, ovaries and vulva.
- Leiomyomas (fibroid tumours) are benign tumours that originate from smooth muscle of the uterus. Treatment depends on the size and location of the tumours. Both leiomyomas and endometrial implants (benign implants of endometrial tissue in the pelvic cavity) may interfere with the ability to have a child and are reduced in size after menopause.
- Cervical cancer is a common female reproductive system cancer, but the incidence and mortality has been greatly reduced by the cervical screening test for early diagnosis.
- Endometrial cancer is the most common invasive gynaecological cancer in Australia, with one in 69 women being affected by the age of 75 years. The main manifestation is abnormal, painless vaginal bleeding (menorrhagia or metrorrhagia in menstruating women). Postmenopausal women should have annual pelvic examinations and report any unexpected vaginal bleeding to their healthcare provider.
- Ovarian cancer increases in incidence with ageing; one in 78 women will be diagnosed prior to the age of 85. In early stages, there are generally no warning signs.
- Benign breast disorders in women include fibrocystic changes and intraductal disorders. Both treatment and nursing care are primarily symptomatic.
- Breast cancer is the most commonly invasive cancer in Australian women. A strong genetic link has been identified, as have a large number of risk factors. Early diagnosis is possible with BSE, clinical breast examination and mammograms. Treatment includes surgery (one of several types of mastectomy, lumpectomy), radiation therapy and chemotherapy. Both combination therapies and immunotherapy are proving to be effective in suppressing tumour growth and facilitating longer life. Along with other problems, mastectomy and radiation therapy interfere with lymph drainage on the affected side, leading to lymphoedema of the arm.
- Appropriate preoperative nursing diagnoses for the woman with breast cancer include anxiety and fear, decisional conflict and anticipatory grieving. Following surgery, interventions focus on risk of infection, risk of injury, pain and disturbed body image.

CONCEPT CHECK

1 During a health assessment, a woman in her fifties tells you that she is having some pain with intercourse. You are uncomfortable discussing this topic with her. What would you say?
1 'I know this can be a problem; please discuss it with your doctor.'
2 'I don't know anything about that; you'll have to ask someone else.'
3 'Do you normally enjoy sexual activity?'
4 'What do you think is causing your problem?'

2 Long-term oestrogen deprivation results in an increased risk of physical disorders. What are these? (Select all that apply.)
1 colon cancer
2 osteoporosis
3 cardiovascular disease
4 fractures
5 cervical cancer

3 You are conducting a health education seminar for postmenopausal women. When discussing calcium intake, you recommend ________ mg per day.

4 An intervention for the woman with a uterine displacement disorder is to teach pelvic floor exercises. These exercises may help reduce:
1 stress incontinence
2 menorrhagia
3 vaginal discharge
4 retroversion

5 Which of the following topics would you include in a health-promotion seminar to reduce the risk of cervical cancer?
1 weight loss
2 safer-sex methods
3 yearly mammograms
4 a diet high in iron

6 When discussing dietary guidelines with a woman with PMS, you recommend she reduce her sodium intake. What is your rationale?
1 Sodium increases reactive hypoglycaemia, increasing physical symptoms.
2 Sodium increases thirst, thereby facilitating increased oral fluid intake.
3 In and of itself, sodium is not harmful, but it may increase cancer risk.
4 Sodium restriction helps minimise fluid retention.

7 What happens to endometrial implantations after menopause?
1 They tend to become malignant.
2 They tend to atrophy and disappear.
3 The number of implants increases.
4 Each implant enlarges.

8 You are designing an education plan for home care for a woman who had an abdominal hysterectomy. Which interventions should be included? (Select all that apply.)
1 Restrict heavy lifting for 4 to 6 weeks.
2 Take tub baths until bleeding has stopped.
3 Report an increase in temperature or severe pain.
4 Take regular rest periods.
5 Avoid coughing and deep breathing at home.

9 Of the following women, which one would be most at risk of breast cancer?
1 age 23, two children
2 age 33, never pregnant
3 age 45, very thin
4 age 64, positive family history

10 You are caring for a woman who is scheduled to have a mastectomy for breast cancer. She is crying. Why might this be so?
1 *Disturbed body image*
2 *Fatigue*
3 *Anticipatory grieving*
4 *Risk of injury*

BIBLIOGRAPHY

Australian Commission on Safety and Quality in Health Care (ACSQHC) (2021). *National Safety and Quality Health Service Standards* (2nd ed.). Sydney: ACSQHC.

Australian Institute of Health and Welfare (AIHW) (2019a). *Cervical screening in Australia 2019*. Canberra: AIHW.

Australian Institute of Health and Welfare (AIHW) (2019b). *Cancer in Australia*. Canberra: AIHW.

Berge, W., Mundt, K., Luu, H. & Boffetta, P. (2018). Genital use of talc and risk of ovarian cancer: A meta-analysis. *European Journal of Cancer Prevention*, 27(3), 248–257. Retrieved from https://www.cancerwa.asn.au/

Breast Cancer Care (2022). *Intraductal papilloma*. Retrieved from https://www.breastcancercare.org.uk/

Brito, L. G., Stewart, E. A., Olivi Chaim, S. O., Martins, W. P. & Farquhar, C. (2019). Interventions for uterine fibroids: An overview of Cochrane Reviews. *Cochrane Database of Systematic Reviews, 2019*(9). https://doi.org/10.1002/14651858.CD013426

Cancer Australia (2022a). *Cervical cancer in Australia*. Retrieved from https://cervical-cancer.canceraustralia.gov.au/

Cancer Australia (2022b). *Uterine cancer (C54-C55)*. Retrieved from https://gynaecological-cancer.canceraustralia.gov.au/

Cancer Australia (2022c). *Breast cancer in Australia*. Retrieved from https://breast-cancer.canceraustralia.gov.au/

Cancer Australia (2022d). *Aboriginal and Torres Strait Islander health professionals*. Retrieved from https://canceraustralia.gov.au/

Cancer Council (2022a). *Understanding cervical cancer. A guide for people with cancer, their families and friends*. Retrieved from https://www.cancercouncil.com.au/

Cancer Council (2022b). *Understanding ovarian cancer*. Retrieved from https://www.cancer.org.au/

Cancer Council (2022c). *Diagnostic tests for breast cancer*. Retrieved from https://www.cancercouncil.com.au/

Cancer Council (2022d). *Breast cancer*. Retrieved from https://www.cancercouncil.com.au/

Centre of Health (2022). *Fibrocystic breast disease*. Retrieved from http://thecentreofhealth.com.au/

Continence Foundation of Australia (2022). *Pelvic floor muscles in women*. Retrieved from https://www.continence.org.au/

Diaz, A., Baade, P. D., Valery, P. C., Whop, L. J. & Moore, S. P. (2018). Comorbidity and cervical cancer survival Indigenous and non-Indigenous Australian women: A semi-national registry-based cohort study (2003–2012). *PLOS ONE, 13*(5), e0196764. https://doi.org/10.1371/journal.pone.0196764

Endometriosis Australia (2022). *About endometriosis*. Retrieved from https://www.endometriosisaustralia.org/

International Federation of Gynecology and Obstetrics (FIGO) (2009). Retrieved from https://www.figo.org/

Jean Hailes for Women's Health (2017). *Menopause: Fact sheet*. Retrieved from https://jeanhailes.org.au/

Lancet Oncology (2012). *Study finds oestrogen-only HRT continues to protect women against breast cancer long after they have stopped taking the treatment*. Press release. Retrieved from https://www.menopause.org.au/

Leach, M. J. & Moore, V. (2012). Black cohosh (*Cimicifuga* spp.) for menopausal symptoms. *Cochrane Database of Systematic Reviews, 2012*(10), CD007244. https://doi.org/10.1002/14651858.CD007244.pub2

Marjoribanks, J., Ayeleke, R. O., Farquhar, C. & Proctor, M. (2015). Nonsteroidal anti-inflammatory drugs for dysmenorrhoea. *Cochrane Database of Systematic Reviews, 2015*(7). doi: 10.1002/14651858.CD001751.pub3

Mayo Foundation for Medical Education and Research (Mayo Clinic) (2022). *Premenstrual syndrome (PMS)*. Retrieved from https://www.mayoclinic.org/

National HPV Vaccination Program Register (2018). *HPV and the new vaccine*. Retrieved from http://www.hpvregister.org.au/

Nedrow, A., Miller, J., Walker, M., Nygren, P., Huffman, L. H. & Nelson, H. D. (2006). Complementary and alternative therapies for the management of menopause-related symptoms: A systematic evidence review. *Archives of Internal Medicine, 166*(14), 1453–1465. https://doi.org/10.1001/archinte.166.14.1453

Reath, J. & Carey, M. (2008). Breast and cervical cancer in Indigenous women: Overcoming barriers to early detection. *Australian Family Physician, 37*(3), 178–182.

Sabesan, S., Larkins, S., Evans, R., Varma, S., Andrews, A., Beuttner, P., Brennan, S. & Young, M. (2012). Original research telemedicine for rural cancer care in North Queensland: Bringing cancer care home. *Australian Journal of Rural Health, 20*, 259–264.

Slomovitz, B., de Haydu, C., Taub, M., Coleman, R. L. & Monk, B. J. (2021). Asbestos and ovarian cancer: Examining the historical evidence. *International Journal of Gynecological Cancer, 31*(1), 122–128. doi: 10.1136/ijgc-2020-001672

Supramaniam, R., Gibberd, A., Dillon, A., Goldsbury, D. E. & O'Connell, D. L. (2014). Increasing rates of surgical treatment and preventing comorbidities may increase breast cancer survival for Aboriginal women. *BMC Cancer, 14*, 163. https://doi.org/10.1186/1471-2407-14-163

Women's Health & Equality Queensland (2017). *Alternatives to HRT*. Retrieved from https://womhealth.org.au/

Women's Health & Research Institute of Australia (2022). *Managing PMS and PMDD*. Retrieved from https://www.whria.com.au/

World Health Organization (2022). *WHO updates recommendations on HPV vaccination schedule*. Retrieved from https://www.who.int/

Zhang, M., Hagan, C. T., Min, Y. et al. (2018). Nanoparticle co-delivery of wortmannin and cisplatin synergistically enhances chemoradiotherapy and reverses platinum resistance in ovarian cancer models. *Biomaterials, 169*, 1–10.

Zhu, X., Liew, Y., Liu, Z. L. & Zhu, X. (2016). Chinese herbal medicine for menopausal symptoms. *Cochrane Database of Systematic Reviews, 2016*(5), CD009023–CD009023. https://doi.org/10.1002/14651858.CD009023.pub2

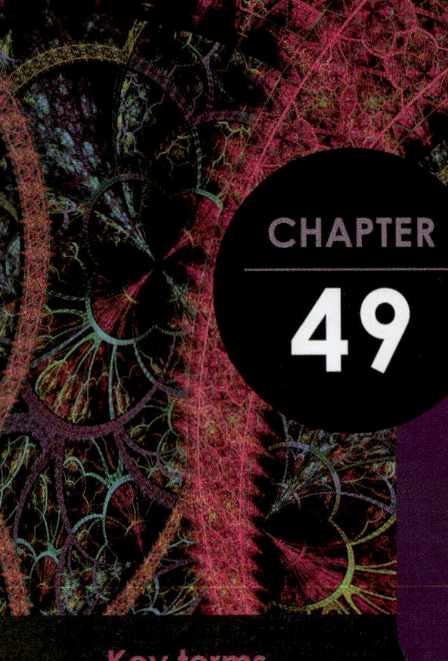

CHAPTER 49

Nursing care of people who have sexually transmitted infections

Heidi Green

Key terms

Learning outcomes

- Explain the incidence, prevalence, characteristics and prevention/control of sexually transmitted infections (STIs).
- Compare and contrast the pathophysiology, manifestations, interprofessional care and nursing care of genital herpes, genital warts, vaginitis, chlamydia, gonorrhoea, syphilis and pelvic inflammatory disease.
- Explain the risk factors for and complications of STIs.
- Discuss the effects and nursing implications of medications and treatments used to treat STIs.

Clinical competencies

- Assess the functional health status of people living with an STI and monitor, document and report clinical indicators.
- Determine nursing priorities and select and implement individualised nursing interventions for people living with an STI.
- Administer treatment, including medications, knowledgeably and safely.
- Provide nursing care for people living with an STI.
- Provide education appropriate for prevention, management and self-care of STIs.
- Revise plans of care as needed to provide effective interventions to promote, maintain or restore functional health status for people living with an STI.
- Provide emotional support for the person living with an STI.

Infections transmitted by vaginal, oral and anal intimate contact and intercourse are referred to as **sexually transmitted infections (STIs)**. Infections transmitted by sexual intercourse are also sometimes known as *sexually transmitted diseases (STDs)* or *venereal diseases*. The most contemporary and acceptable term is STI. A person can have an STI before having symptoms of the disease. STIs also include systemic diseases (such as tuberculosis, hepatitis and HIV/AIDS) that can be transmitted from one infected person to another. This chapter discusses STIs that involve the urogenital system, as well as vaginal infections.

Overview of sexually transmitted infections

Sexually transmitted infections include those caused by bacteria, viruses, fungi, protozoa and parasites. Portals of entry for these agents of transmission include the mouth, genitalia, urinary meatus, anus, rectum, skin and from mother to baby. STIs have many consequences and nurses have a responsibility to provide health education on the prevention of STIs to people, regardless of their gender, age or sexual orientation. Nurses have a critical role in the prevention of STIs by providing accurate information about these diseases, their prevention, treatment and potential complications. Nurses should be aware of policies, protocols and health promotion strategies that apply to STIs. These include Australia's *Fourth National Sexually Transmissible Infections Strategy 2018–2022* (Department of Health, 2018), *Australian STI Management Guidelines for Use in Primary Care* (ASHM, 2022) and the World Health Organization (WHO) *Global Health Sector Strategies on, Respectively, HIV, Viral Hepatitis and Sexually Transmitted Infections 2022–2030* (WHO, 2022).

Incidence and prevalence

Sexually transmitted infections are a major public health issue. STIs have reached epidemic proportions in many countries and are on the increase worldwide. The WHO estimates that a total of 374 million new cases of chlamydia, gonorrhoea, syphilis and trichomoniasis occur globally each year (WHO, 2021). In addition to this, the WHO estimates that more than 500 million people aged 15 to 49 years are infected with the sexually transmitted virus herpes simplex type 2, and approximately 300 million women have the human papillomavirus.

Accurate information about infection rates is difficult to obtain, especially for many developing countries, and the available information is often at least 3 to 4 years old. There is no one organisation that regularly collates all global STI statistics, although the WHO does try. To complicate matters further, different countries have different types and levels of reporting. It is thought that many reports substantially underestimate the number of new STI cases because of social stigma and other factors, such as poverty, that prevent people seeking healthcare.

Women are disproportionately affected by STIs. Many STIs are more easily transmitted from a man to a woman than they are from a woman to a man due to anatomical differences. Women are less likely to experience symptoms of common STIs, delaying diagnosis and treatment. Furthermore, women are at greater risk of complications of STIs such as pelvic inflammatory disease (PID), infertility and genital cancers.

Several factors may help explain the escalating incidence of STIs. The 'sexual revolution' of the 1960s and 1970s, fuelled by 'the pill' and the freedom this gave women from unplanned pregnancy, led to more permissive attitudes about sexual freedom and increases in sexual activity and the number of sexual partners. When hormonal contraceptives became available in Australia in the 1960s, they replaced the condom as the predominant means of birth control. However, unlike condoms, oral contraceptives do not protect against STIs, a fact of increasing public health importance.

STIs affect men and women of all ages, backgrounds and socioeconomic levels. Individual factors related to the contraction of STIs are risk-taking behaviours such as drug abuse, sex with multiple or new partners, sex with high-risk partners, unprotected sex, sex while intoxicated and sex in exchange for money. Another factor contributing to the increasing incidence of STIs is that people are becoming sexually active younger and committing to one partner later. As a result, sexually active people today are more likely to have multiple sex partners in their lifetime and are potentially at higher risk of STIs. Also, gonorrhoea has progressively developed a resistance to prescribed antibiotics (Centers for Disease Control and Prevention (CDC), 2022a).

The emergence of HIV/AIDS created an 'epidemiological synergy' between all STIs. Other STIs, such as syphilis, herpes simplex virus (HSV) and chancroid, facilitate the transmission of HIV/AIDS, and the immunosuppression caused by HIV potentiates the infectious process of other STIs. People who are infected with STIs are at greater risk of acquiring HIV if they are exposed to the virus. This is the result of genital ulcers creating a portal of entry for HIV, non-ulcerative STIs increasing the concentration of cells in genital secretions that can be targets for HIV and infection with both an STI and HIV resulting in an increased likelihood of having HIV in genital secretions and semen.

Pathophysiology, manifestations and nursing care

Although STIs are caused by a variety of organisms, they have several common characteristics:

- Most can be prevented by the use of latex condoms.
- They can be transmitted during sexual activities, including non-penetrating intimate exposure.
- For treatment to be effective, sexual partners of the infected person must also be treated.
- Two or more STIs frequently coexist in the same person.

FAST FACTS

- The majority of STIs are present without symptoms.
- More than 1 million people acquire an STI every day.
- Each year, an estimated 374 million people become ill with one of four STIs: chlamydia, gonorrhoea, syphilis and trichomoniasis.
- More than 500 million people (aged 15–49 years) have a genital infection with herpes simplex virus (HSV2).
- More than 300 million women have a human papillomavirus (HPV) infection. HPV causes 570,000 cases of cervical cancer and 311,000 cervical cancer deaths each year.
- STIs can have serious consequences beyond the immediate impact of the infection itself, through mother-to-child transmission of infections and chronic diseases.
- Drug resistance, especially for gonorrhoea, is a major threat to reducing the impact of STIs worldwide.
- In developing countries, STIs and their complications rank in the top five disease categories for which adults seek healthcare.
- The WHO reports fewer people are dying of HIV-related causes, with 680,000 deaths in 2020.
- According to estimates from the WHO (2021), around 37.7 million people were living with HIV in 2020. The number of people newly infected with HIV in 2020 was 1.5 million.
- The number of new HIV diagnoses in Australia has declined by 36% since 2016, with 1,012 in 2016 and 6,333 in 2020.
- In 2020, an estimated 29,090 people were living with an HIV diagnosis in Australia.
- Since 2016, infectious syphilis notifications have increased. Large outbreaks are ongoing in northern, central, western and southern Australia among young Aboriginal and Torres Strait Islander people aged 15 to 34 years, which has contributed to the signification increase.
- Between 2016 and 2020, HIV notifications among Aboriginal and Torres Strait Islander people decreased by 18% and decreased by 9% in the Australian-born non-Indigenous population.
- Chlamydia was the most common STI notification in Australia, with a total of 103,000 notifications in 2019.
- In 2020, there were 29,516 gonorrhoea notifications in Australia which was a 14% decrease from 2019. Indigenous Australians are over-represented in STI notification data.
- One in 2 sexually active people will contract an STI by age 25.

Sources: WHO (2021); Kirby Institute (2021); Department of Health and Aged Care (2022).

The complications of STIs in women include pelvic inflammatory disease, ectopic pregnancy, infertility, chronic pelvic pain, neonatal illness and death, and genital cancer. Some bacterial STIs can be treated through appropriate early intervention with antibiotics. Others, like genital herpes, are chronic conditions that can be managed but not cured because they are caused by viruses. The most serious STI is HIV/AIDS, which currently does not have a cure. HIV/AIDS is discussed in the chapter 'Nursing care of people with altered immunity'. Treatment guidelines for STIs are updated regularly and are available from the WHO website and at https://sti.guidelines.org.au.

Prevention and control

Prevention and control of STIs are based on the principles of education, early detection, diagnosis and treatment of infected people and evaluation, treatment and counselling of sexual partners of people who are infected. This implies comprehensive care that is well coordinated.

The skill of the healthcare provider in managing care and obtaining an accurate sexual history is essential to prevention and control efforts. One approach to collecting accurate information about key areas was summarised in the CDC (2022b) guide to taking a sexual history. It includes the '5 Ps': partners, practices, protection from STIs, past history of STDs and prevention of pregnancy. Suggested questions to use are found on the CDC website at https://www.cdc.gov/std/treatment/sexualhistory.htm

It is recommended that all partners be tested for STIs, including HIV, before beginning to have sexual intercourse. If a person chooses to have intercourse with an infected partner or one whose infection status is unknown, a new condom should be used for each act of intercourse (CDC, 2022b). See Table 49.1 for STI barrier guidelines.

Links to National Patient Safety Standards

NSQHS: Comprehensive Care Standard

The intent of this standard is to ensure that the person with an STI receives comprehensive and coordinated care that is aligned with the person's expressed goals of care and healthcare needs and which considers the effect of the person's health issues on their life and wellbeing and is clinically appropriate.

Source: Australian Commission on Safety and Quality in Health Care (ACSQHC) (2021). *National Safety and Quality Health Service Standards* (2nd ed.). Sydney: ACSQHC.

TABLE 49.1 STI barrier guidelines

BARRIER PROTECTION	HEALTH EDUCATION
Male condoms	• Use a new condom for each act of sexual intercourse. • Handle carefully to avoid damaging the condom. Condoms are affected adversely by heat—keep them in a cool place. • Be sure no air is trapped in the end of the condom. • Put the condom on when the penis is erect and before genital contact with partner. • Ensure adequate lubrication exists during intercourse, using only water-based lubricants (e.g. K-Y jelly) and latex condoms. Oil-based lubricants, such as petroleum jelly, massage oil, mineral oil or body lotions can weaken latex and should not be used. • Ensure adequate lubrication during vaginal and anal sex. • Withdraw while the penis is erect and hold the condom firmly against the base of the penis during withdrawal.
Female condoms	• The female condom is a lubricated polyurethane sheath with a ring on each end that is inserted into the vagina. It is an effective mechanical barrier to viruses.
Dental dam	• The dental dam is a latex or polyurethane sheet used between the mouth and vagina or rectum during oral sex. It reduces the risk of STIs.
Vaginal spermicides, sponges, diaphragms	• Spermicides used alone without condoms do not reduce the risk of cervical gonorrhoea, chlamydia or HIV infection. • Diaphragms protect against cervical gonorrhoea, chlamydia and trichomoniasis, but not HIV.

Health education for the person who is an injection drug user includes:

- Enrol or continue in a drug treatment program.
- Do not use injection equipment that has been used by another person. If equipment is shared, first clean the syringe and needle with bleach and water (to reduce the rate of transmission).
- Use clean needles.
- Dispose of used needles safely and appropriately.

Syringe disposal containers are located in many public places including shopping centres, public toilets, airports, cinemas and universities.

Eliminating further transmission and reinfection of STIs is critical for control. For treatable STIs, this means that referral of sexual partners for diagnosis, treatment and counselling is essential. Most STIs, including HIV/AIDS, are a reportable disease in every state and territory in Australia. See https://www.health.gov.au/initiatives-and-programs/nndss#diseases-on-the-national-notifiable-disease-list. When an infected person is referred, every effort is made to identify and contact sexual partners. Reports of STI and HIV infections are maintained in the strictest confidence and are protected by law from subpoena. Suggested resources for people with STIs are listed in Box 49.1.

BOX 49.1 Resources for people who have STIs

- **Sexual Health and Family Planning Australia: http://www.shfpact.org.au**
- **Australian Society for HIV, Viral Hepatitis and Sexual Health Medicine (ASHM): https://www.ashm.org.au/resources/**
- **Department of Health and Aged Care: https://www.health.gov.au/health-topics/sexual-health/resources**
- **Healthdirect: https://www.healthdirect.gov.au/safe-sex-overview**
- **Australian Federation of AIDS Organisations (AFAO): https://www.afao.org.au**
- **Young Deadly Free: https://youngdeadlyfree.org.au/**

THE PERSON WITH GENITAL HERPES

Genital herpes is caused by the HSV1 and HSV2. Like most STIs, genital herpes is most commonly found in young, sexually active people and is associated with early onset of sexual activity and multiple sexual partners. In Australia, 1 in 8 adults have genital herpes. Genital herpes is twice as common in adult women as in adult men and is most prevalent in women aged 35–44 (Sexual Health Australia, 2018). Currently there is no cure and the treatments are primarily symptomatic.

Pathophysiology

HSV1 and HSV2 are transmissible via direct contact. HSV1 is associated with cold sores but may be transmitted to the genital area by oral intercourse or by self-inoculation through poor handwashing practices. HSV2 is the virus that causes genital herpes and is transmitted by sexual activity or during childbirth. HSV infections begin with exposure to the virus by contact with infectious lesions or secretions. The virus then moves into the stratified squamous epithelium, stimulating the replication of the epithelium and infecting the neurons that innervate the area. HSVs are neurotropic viruses, meaning that they grow in neurons and can maintain their disease potential even when there are no manifestations. The virus ascends through the peripheral nerves to the dorsal root ganglia, where it can remain dormant. For unknown reasons, the virus may reactivate and return to the nerve root of the skin, causing lesions. During dormancy, the virus is impervious to treatment. The incubation period ranges from 6 weeks to 8 months.

Manifestations

Within 2 to 10 days after exposure to the herpesvirus, painful red vesicles appear in the genital area. In men, the lesions generally occur on the glans or shaft of the penis and men may present with recurrent anogenital ulcers, erythema, urethritis or proctitis (CDC, 2021a). In women, the lesions commonly occur on the labia, vagina and cervix. Women may also experience cervicitis and proctitis. Anal intercourse or oral–anal sex may also result in lesions in and around the rectum (CDC, 2021a).

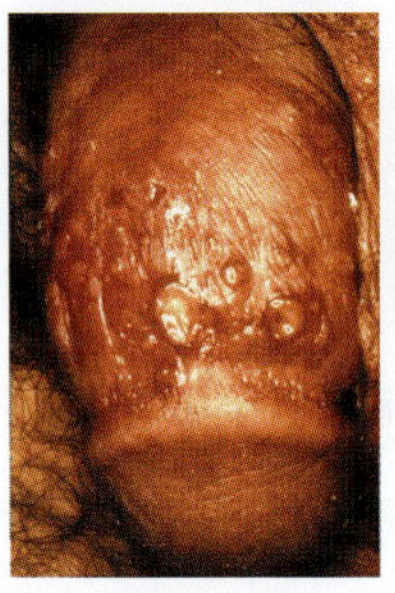
A

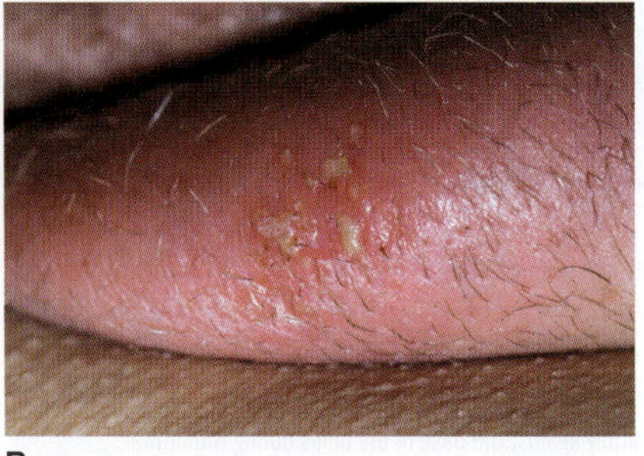
B

FIGURE 49.1 ***Genital herpes on A, the penis and B, the labia***

Sources: A, Dr N.J. Flumara, Dr Gavin Hart/CDC; *B*, SneSivan/Shutterstock.

Soon after the vesicles appear, they form small painful blisters filled with clear fluid containing virus particles (see Figure 49.1). The blisters break, shedding the highly infectious virus and creating patches of painful ulcers that last approximately 2–4 weeks (or longer if they become infected). Touching these blisters and then rubbing or scratching in another place can spread the infection to other areas of the body (*autoinoculation*).

The first outbreak of herpes lesions is called *first-episode infection*, with an average duration of 12 days. Subsequent occurrences, usually less severe, are termed *recurrent infections* (average duration of 4–5 days). The period between episodes is called *latency*, during which time the person remains infectious even though no symptoms are present. During latency, the virus withdraws into the nerve fibres that lead from the infected site to the lower spine, remaining dormant until recurrence, at which time it retraces its path to the genital area.

The manifestations of genital herpes are presented below. Prodromal symptoms of recurrent outbreaks of genital herpes can include burning, itching, tingling or throbbing at the sites where lesions commonly appear. These sensations may be accompanied by pain in the legs, groin or buttocks. Some research suggests that prodromal symptoms signal increased levels of infectiousness, during which sexual contact should be avoided.

MANIFESTATIONS Genital herpes

- Herpetic lesions
- Regional lymphadenopathy
- Headache
- Fever
- General malaise
- Dysuria
- Urinary retention
- Vaginal discharge
- Urethral discharge (men)

INTERPROFESSIONAL CARE

Presumptive diagnosis of genital herpes is based on history and physical examination of the person, including lesions and patterns of recurrence. Because there is no cure for genital herpes, treatment focuses on relieving symptoms and preventing the spread of the infection. Health education is essential to prevent further transmission of the disease and to help the person integrate chronic disease management into their life.

Diagnosis

Definitive diagnosis requires isolation of the virus in tissue culture. Ideally, tissue specimens should be obtained within 48 hours of the appearance of the blisters. Diagnostic tests are described in the chapter 'A person-centred approach to assessing the male and female reproductive systems'.

Medications

Valaciclovir and aciclovir are common antiviral drugs used in the treatment of HSV 1 and 2 (ASHM, 2022). Valaciclovir is recommended as an initial treatment, with aciclovir as an alternative treatment to slow the growth and spread of the herpes virus so the body can fight off the infection. Neither valaciclovir nor aciclovir will cure herpes, but they can help reduce the length and severity of the first episode and lessen the symptoms of the infection. The oral form of valaciclovir is considered most effective for first-episode infections, as well as for recurrent infections, and is given for 5 to 10 days or until lesions heal (ASHM, 2022). Drug resistance to aciclovir is commonly seen in people with HIV. In most cases, foscarnet will be used as an alternative.

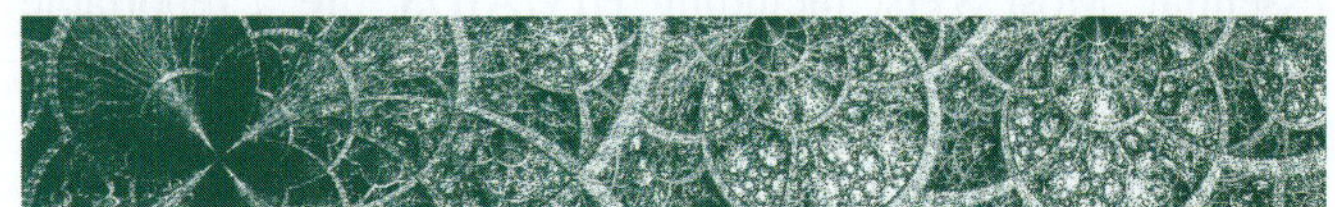

Nursing care

Planning and implementing nursing care for the person who has genital herpes requires consideration of short- and long-term implications. Although the immediate priority is symptom relief and prevention of further transmission, the person will need help to formulate strategies to deal with the life-changing diagnosis of living with a chronic disease. Stigma is also an important consideration; therefore, nurses need to be aware of the person's psychological, as well as physical, needs.

Nursing diagnoses and interventions

Nursing interventions in this section focus on pain and sexual dysfunction.

Acute pain

Herpetic lesions are very painful and can become infected. Because the virus resides in the nerve ganglia, pain may also occur in the legs, thighs, groin or buttocks. While valaciclovir and aciclovir diminish the pain of herpes and accelerate the healing process, additional measures can relieve the discomfort further.

- Educate the person on how to keep herpes blisters clean and dry. A solution of warm water and soap can be used to cleanse the lesions two to three times daily. Lesions can be dried using a hair dryer turned to a cool setting. It is important to wear loose cotton clothing that will not trap moisture and avoid wearing items such as lycra, pantyhose and tight jeans. *Keeping the lesions clean and dry reduces the possibility of secondary infection and speeds the healing process.*
- For dysuria, suggest the person pours water over their genitals while urinating. Drinking additional fluids (particularly water) also helps dilute the acidity of the urine. Fluids that increase acidity, such as cranberry juice, should be avoided. *These measures dilute the acid content of urine and thereby reduce the burning sensation.*
- Suggest the person has sitz baths, where only the buttocks and hips are immersed in tepid water for 15–30 minutes several times a day. *The warm water is soothing and decreases pain from ulcers and an irritated urethral meatus. It also facilitates wound healing.*

Sexual dysfunction

Some people who learn that they are infected with an incurable STI may believe they can no longer have a normal sex life. Fortunately, many people have learned to live with and manage genital herpes without infecting their partners and/or children.

- Provide a supportive, non-judgmental environment so feelings can be discussed and questions asked freely about what this diagnosis means for future sexual relations. *Feelings of guilt, shame and anger are natural responses and can lead to a total avoidance of sexual intimacy.*
- Provide information about support groups and other resources for people with herpes. *Information about how others cope with this disease can offset feelings of shame and hopelessness.*

Community-based care

Health education for people who are living with genital herpes involves supporting them to manage this chronic disease with the least possible disruption to their lifestyle and relationships. Understanding the disease process and factors that affect it helps the person regain a sense of control and see the potential for future sexual intimacy without transmission of infection. The following topics should be discussed:

- how to recognise prodromal symptoms of recurrence and factors that seem to trigger recurrences (e.g. emotional stress, acidic food, sun exposure)
- the need for abstinence from sexual contact from the time prodromal symptoms appear until 10 days after all lesions have healed
- use of latex condoms or dental dams, due to viral shedding at any time, and careful hygiene practices (such as not sharing towels or other personal items) even during latency periods.

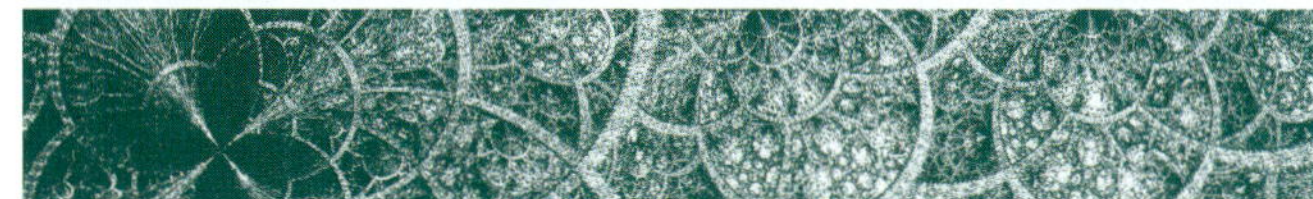

THE PERSON WITH GENITAL WARTS

Genital warts (*condylomata acuminata*), caused by the human papillomavirus (HPV), are one of the most common sexually transmissible genital infections and are considered epidemic. Genital warts are chronic and, in many people, largely asymptomatic. Currently, treatment is cosmetic rather than curable.

Genital warts are often described as fleshy growths or bumps seen mostly in areas around the genitals and anus. HPV is spread through genital-to-skin contact during sexual activity with a person infected with HPV through tiny breaks in the skin. This can occur even when there are no visible warts, explaining why genital HPV infection spreads easily. HPV may also be passed from mother to baby during childbirth. The virus can live on the skin for many years and during that time can be passed on through sexual contact.

Warts that occur elsewhere on the body are caused by different types of HPV. Contact with these warts is not known to cause genital warts.

Prevention

Some types of HPV infection can be prevented by new vaccines which have been registered for use in Australia. The use of condoms and dental dams for all sexual contact can reduce the transmission of HPV.

Women are at greater risk of HPV genital infections because they have a larger mucosal surface area exposed in the genital area. Most HPV infections are asymptomatic or unrecognised.

HPV infection rates vary greatly between geographical regions and population groups. Almost all cervical cancer is caused by HPV. HPV 16 and 18 are the two most common forms and are known to cause over 70% of cervical cancers. While vaccines are available that prevent infection from both HPV 16 and 18, they do not treat an existing infection.

HPV and cervical cancer

For maximum benefit, the HPV vaccine should be administered prior to the commencement of sexual activity to adolescents aged 12–13 years (National Centre for Immunisation Research and Surveillance (NCIRS), 2022). This includes male-to-female and female-to-female and male-to-male contact. Regular cervical screening is still recommended every 5 years, or more frequently if abnormalities are detected. The Gardasil 9 vaccine is indicated for females aged 9 to 26 years for the prevention of cervical, vulvar, vaginal and anal cancer, precancerous or dysplastic lesions, genital warts and infection caused by HPV (NCIRS, 2022). Gardasil 9 is also indicated for males aged 9 to 26 for the prevention of anal cancer, precancerous or dysplastic lesions, external genital lesions and infection caused by HPV. HPV types 16 and 18 are linked to 80% of cervical cancers in Australia; types 6 and 11 are linked to approximately 90% of genital warts cases (Cancer Australia, 2021). The National HPV Vaccination Program is ongoing for 12- to 13-year-old girls and boys and provides free vaccination through a school-based program. For information about the program, see the position statement on HPV at http://www.ncirs.org.au/public/ncirs-position-statement-hpv-vaccination.

FAST FACTS

- Prevalence of HPV is declining due to the success of the HPV vaccination program (NCIRS, 2022).
- Most people with a genital HPV infection do not know they are infected; most women are diagnosed by cervical cancer screening (CDC, 2022c).

The vaccine will not prevent all types of HPV that cause cervical cancer, nor can it 'cure' an HPV infection if it has been acquired previously. There are many different types of the HPV virus that can affect various parts of the body.

Although the majority of infected people are asymptomatic, some experience frequent recurrences. Other than recurrences, men are not likely to experience serious physical complications from genital warts. Women, however, have an increased risk of cervical cancer, with HPV DNA having been identified in almost all cervical cancers worldwide, and in approximately 50–80% of vaginal, vulvar and anogenital cancers.

Pathophysiology

Genital warts, sometimes called venereal warts, are caused by HPV and are transmitted by genital, oral or anal intercourse. The incubation period is between 1 and 20 months (South Australia Health, 2022).

Manifestations

Although some people with HPV may not have manifestations, others exhibit characteristic lesions: single or multiple painless, soft, moist, pink or flesh-coloured swellings in the vulvovaginal area, perineum, penis, urethra, anus, groin or thigh (see Figure 49.2). In women, the growths may be in the vagina or on the cervix and be apparent only during a pelvic examination.

The four types of genital warts are:

1. *Condyloma acuminata*: cauliflower-shaped lesions that appear on moist skin surfaces such as the vagina or anus.
2. *Keratotic warts*: thick, hard lesions that develop on keratinised skin such as the labia major, penis or scrotum.
3. *Papular warts*: smooth lesions that also develop on keratinised skin.
4. *Flat warts*: slightly raised lesions, often invisible to the naked eye, that also develop on keratinised skin.

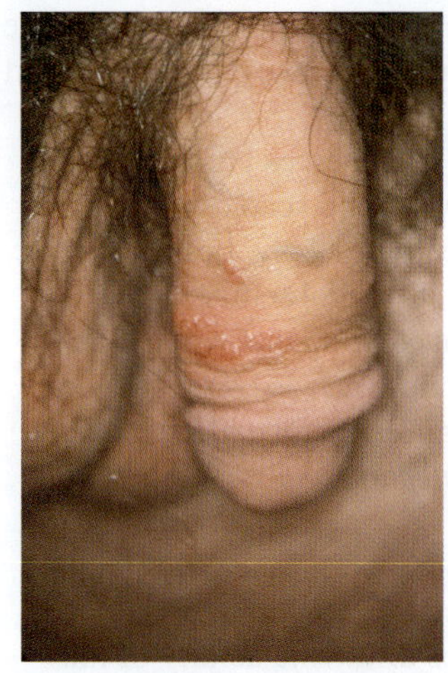

A

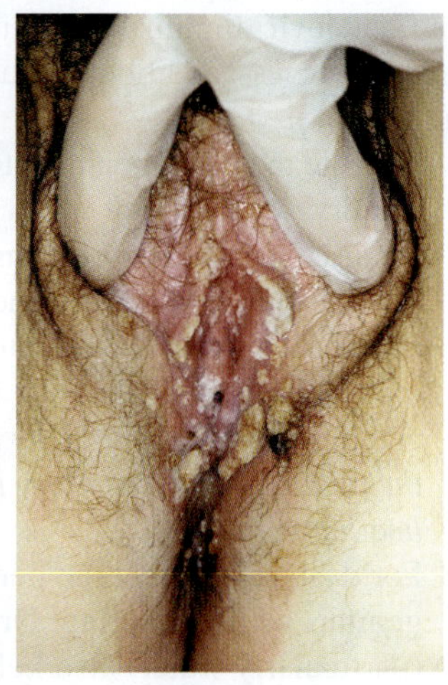

B

FIGURE 49.2 ***Genital warts (condyloma acuminata) on A, the penis and B, the vulva***

Sources: A, Dr M.F. Rein/CDC; B, Joe Millar/CDC.

INTERPROFESSIONAL CARE

Treatment is directed at removal of warts, relief of symptoms and health education to reduce the risk of recurrence and future transmission. Infection with HPV is considered chronic. Research has shown that for about 90% of women, cervical HPV becomes undetectable within 2 years (CDC, 2022c).

Genital and anal warts are diagnosed primarily by clinical appearance. An HPV DNA test is specific for diagnosis in women. There are currently no HPV tests for men.

Medications

Topical agents can be used to treat genital warts and include podofilox and imiquimod (both can be applied by the person), or podophyllin and trichloroacetic acid (which is administered by health professionals). Podophyllin is contraindicated during pregnancy and can have side effects ranging from nausea, diarrhoea and lethargy to paralysis and coma (see the 'Medication administration' box). Gardasil 9 is administered by two intramuscular injections given over a 6- to 12-month period.

Other treatments

Genital warts may also be removed by cryotherapy, electrocautery, laser vaporisation or surgical excision. Carbon dioxide laser surgery is becoming increasingly common for removal of extensive warts.

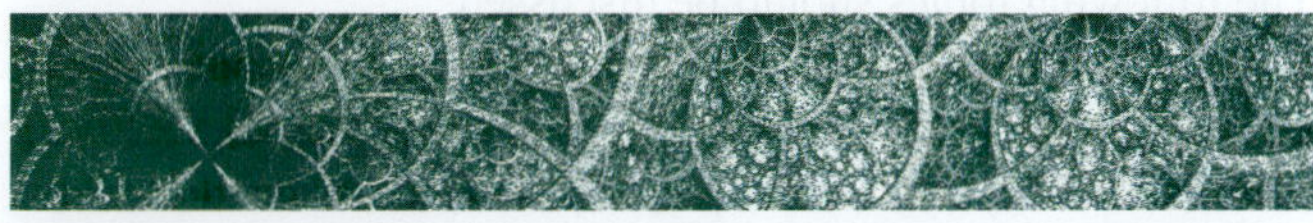

Nursing care

Health promotion activities should include information about the causes, treatments and prevention of HPV infections.

MEDICATION ADMINISTRATION The person who has genital warts

TOPICAL APPLICATIONS
Podophyllin
Trichloroacetic acid
Although cryotherapy using liquid nitrogen or a cryoprobe is commonly used to treat genital warts, podophyllin preparations are recommended. Podophyllin is applied topically to the warts twice a day for 3 days, then 4 days off. This can be repeated weekly for 4–6 cycles until resolved.

Podophyllin is contraindicated during pregnancy; the alternative is cryotherapy, although this can have a poor response. Podophyllin is also contraindicated in cervical, urethral and anorectal warts. It is important to avoid contact of podophyllin resin with the eyes. Adverse effects of podophyllin include local irritation, severe ulceration of surrounding tissue, nausea, diarrhoea, lethargy, paralysis and coma.

Nursing responsibilities
- As per the National Safety and Quality Health Service Preventing and Controlling Infections Standard and Medication Safety Standard (ACSQHC, 2021), wear appropriate personal protective equipment (PPE) when applying topical treatment and ensure the individual's information needs are met.
- Undertake a health assessment to establish baseline data, including mental status, vital signs and weight. All health assessments should be in partnership with the individual, as per the Partnering with Consumers Standard (ACSQHC, 2021).
- Document and report any existing lesions (genital, anal or oral). All documentation must be accurately recorded so critical information and risks are communicated to ensure the person's safety—Communicating for Safety Standard (ACSQHC, 2021).
- Cover the tissue surrounding the warts with a protective barrier cream or a paste of baking soda and water to protect the tissue from the caustic treatment solution.

Health education for the infected person and their significant others
- Wash off the treated area thoroughly within 1–4 hours after the first application; gradually increase this period to 6–8 hours after the second and subsequent applications.
- Return for regular treatment until warts are gone.
- Refer partners for examination and any necessary treatment.
- Report any adverse effects (nausea, diarrhoea, local irritation, lethargy, numbness).
- Avoid sexual activity until the person and their partners have been free of disease for 1 month.
- Use condoms to prevent future infections.
- Return for cervical cancer screening.

Nursing diagnosis and interventions

Nursing interventions primarily involve health education, and discussions on stigma, fear and anxiety. People are often acutely embarrassed.

Knowledge deficits

HPV is spread by contact with infectious lesions or secretions. Up to 70% of genital warts are spread by people who do not know they have the infection. Although there is currently no known cure, it is essential to prevent secondary infections.

- Discuss the need for prompt treatment, and the necessity for sexual abstinence until lesions have healed or using a condom while lesions are present. *This reduces the risk of reinfection and further transmission of the disease. Using condoms promotes the regression of HPV lesions in both men and women.*
- Discuss the increased risk of cervical cancer and the importance of cervical cancer screening. *Understanding the risk, the person will be more motivated to seek screening.*
- Stress the importance of thorough handwashing. Demonstrate an appropriate handwashing technique. *Appropriate handwashing is essential to prevent the spread of HPV.*

Fear

Surgery creates some degree of fear in most people: fear of the procedure itself and/or of pain and possible complications. Surgery or cryotherapy in the genital area involves these fears plus fear of possible impaired sexual function, as well as stigma.

- Provide opportunities for the person to express their fears and feelings about the procedure. Explain the procedure, approximate recovery time, possible complications and ways to avoid them, and ways to cope with complications that do occur. *Knowing what to expect reduces the person's fear and helps them feel a greater sense of control.*
- Explain that the procedure is performed with a local anaesthesia. *Being awake during surgery gives the person a greater sense of partnership in the treatment process.*

Anxiety

A pregnant woman with an HPV infection faces an increased risk of infection of her neonate during delivery. The neonatal infection can range from asymptomatic to widely disseminated fatal disease. Transmission occurs during passage through the birth canal. The risk is highest during the first episode of infection.

- Discuss with women of childbearing age that caesarean delivery can prevent transmission of infection to the neonate. In women without manifestations of recurrence, vaginal delivery is possible. *Understanding that infection of the neonate can be prevented helps relieve anxiety.*

Community-based care

Health education emphasises the need for the infected person and their infected sexual partners to return for regular treatment until lesions have resolved and to use condoms to prevent reinfection. Annual cervical cancer screening is essential for infected females due to the increased risk of cervical cancer.

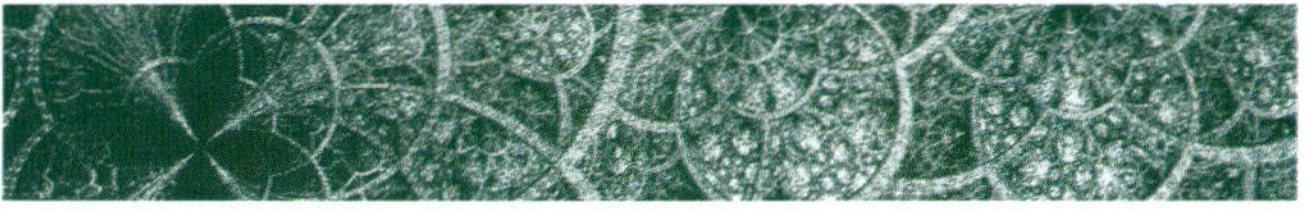

THE PERSON WITH A VAGINAL INFECTION

The vagina may be infected by yeasts, protozoa or bacteria. These infections can be sexually transmitted, but the male partner does not usually have manifestations of the infection. Risk factors include the use of hormonal contraceptives or broad-spectrum antibiotics, obesity, diabetes, pregnancy, unprotected sexual activity and multiple sexual partners, particularly if unprotected sex has been practised. Manifestations of vaginal infections are outlined in Table 49.2.

Preventive measures include education about the need for high standards of personal hygiene and safe sex practices. Women should avoid frequent douching and wearing nylon underwear, lycra and/or tight jeans or trousers. Unprotected sexual activity, particularly with multiple partners, increases the risk of vaginal infections.

Pathophysiology and manifestations

Alterations in pH, changes in the normal flora and low oestrogen levels are conducive to the development of vaginal infections. When conditions are favourable, microorganisms invade the vulva and vagina.

Bacterial vaginosis

Bacterial vaginosis (non-specific vaginitis) is the most common cause of vaginal infection in women of reproductive age. *Gardnerella vaginalis* is one of the causative organisms, but others are also implicated. The relationship of sexual activity to this infection is not clear. The primary manifestation is a vaginal discharge that is thin and greyish and has a foul, fishy odour. Complications include pelvic inflammatory disease, preterm labour, premature rupture of the membranes and postnatal endometritis. The infection is treated with oral or intravaginal antibacterial agents.

Candidiasis

Candidiasis (moniliasis or yeast infection) is caused by the organism *Candida albicans*, which has several strains of different virulence. Candida organisms are part of the normal vaginal environment in up to 50% of women, causing problems only when they multiply rapidly. When increased oestrogen levels, antibiotics, diabetes mellitus, faecal contamination or other factors alter the normal vaginal flora, the organism proliferates, resulting in a yeast infection. The manifestations include an odourless, thick, white vaginal discharge (see Figure 49.3). This is often accompanied by itching and irritation of the vulva and vagina, dysuria and dyspareunia. Uncircumcised men may develop a yeast infection over the glans penis, manifested by itching and dysuria. The infection is treated with oral medications or, for women, intravaginal antifungal agents.

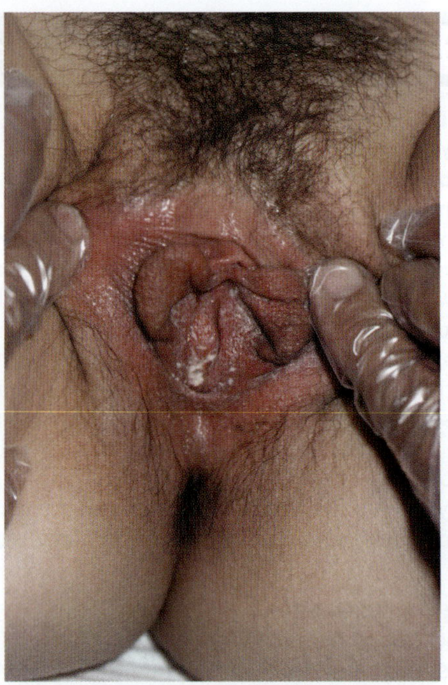

FIGURE 49.3 *Yeast infection on female genitalia*

Source: Biophoto Associates/Science Source.

Trichomoniasis

Trichomoniasis is caused by *Trichomonas vaginalis*, a protozoan parasite. It is the most common STI worldwide but is curable. It affects mostly women and is common in Australia. Women who have unprotected sex with multiple partners are at higher risk. Rates of trichomoniasis are endemic in some Aboriginal and Torres Strait Islander communities (ASHM, 2022). Symptoms usually appear within 5 to 28 days of exposure. It most commonly infects the vagina in women and

TABLE 49.2 Vaginal infections

INFECTION	TYPE OF DISCHARGE	TYPICAL MANIFESTATIONS	NURSING CARE
Candidiasis (*Monilia*, yeast)	Thick white patches adhering to cervix and vaginal wall, resembling cottage cheese; little odour	Itching of vulva and vaginal area, redness, painful intercourse	Teach perineal hygiene and proper use of vaginal applicators. Instruct the person to complete the entire treatment.
Simple vaginalis (bacterial vaginosis, *Gardnerella vaginalis*)	Thin, white, 'milk-like', or grey with fishy odour, especially when mixed with potassium hydroxide	None to mild itching or burning in vulvar area; clue cells on microscopic examination	Educate the person about proper perineal hygiene. Instruct the person to complete treatment. Inform the person about the relationship of infection to pelvic inflammatory disease.
Trichomoniasis	Frothy, yellow or white, foul odour	Burning and itching of vulva	Provide health education about perineal hygiene.
Atrophic vaginitis (senile vaginitis)	Thin, opaque discharge, occasionally blood tinged, odourless; pale, smooth, thin, dry vaginal walls	Painful intercourse, itching, vaginal dryness	Inform the person about symptoms of menopause and sexual techniques to minimise trauma.

the urethra in men. Most men are asymptomatic, but when symptomatic may complain of dysuria and urethral discomfort. Women have a frothy, green-yellow vaginal discharge with a strong fishy odour, often accompanied by itching and irritation of the genitalia. A woman with HIV who becomes infected has an increased risk of transmitting HIV to her sexual partner.

Trichomoniasis is treated with 7 days of BD metronidazole orally with food. These antibiotics are effective against anaerobic bacteria and certain parasites. Anaerobic bacteria are single-celled, living organisms that thrive in environments in which there is little oxygen (anaerobic environments). They selectively block some of the functions within the bacterial cells and the parasites, resulting in their death.

INTERPROFESSIONAL CARE

Interprofessional care focuses on identifying and eliminating the infection and preventing recurrence.

Diagnosis

Diagnostic tests vary with the suspected organism. Cervical cultures are used to diagnose the causative organism. *Trichomonas* is identified by microscopically examining a specimen of vaginal discharge in saline. Ten per cent potassium hydroxide is used to identify spores and filaments of candida. Diagnostic tests are described in the chapter 'A person-centred approach to assessing the male and female reproductive systems'.

Medications

Pharmacological treatments vary with the organism. Sexual partner/s of a woman who has a *Trichomonas* infection must also be treated to prevent reinfection. Some antifungal agents are available without prescription, which can sometimes lead to self-medication with the incorrect agent or allow repeated infections to go unreported.

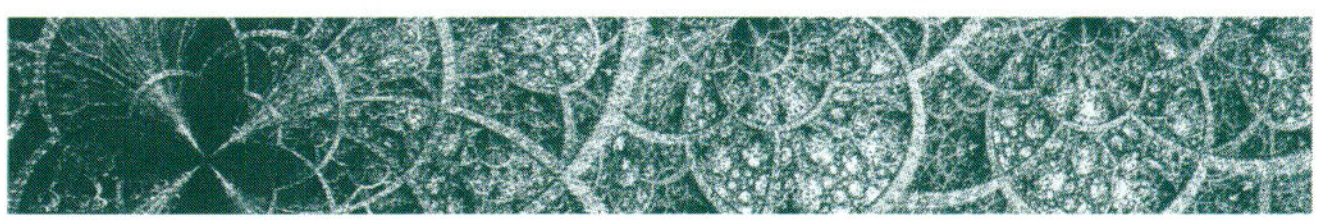

Nursing care

Engaging the infected woman in health education and, if necessary, her sexual partner/s to comply with the treatment regimen and using safer sex practices, can prevent future transmission of the infection. Careful history taking may reveal high-risk sexual practices that require intervention, particularly if the woman has had repeated infections. The initial presenting symptom for many HIV-positive women is vaginal candidiasis which may not respond to over-the-counter treatments. Treatment with some antibiotics destroys normal vaginal flora, also resulting in superinfection with yeast.

Nursing interventions

- Reflecting the Patient Safety Competency Framework for Nursing Students (Levett-Jones et al., 2017), undertake a health assessment to establish baseline data, including partner history, mental status, vital signs and weight. All health assessments should be in partnership with the woman, as also outlined in the Partnering with Consumers Standard (ACSQHC, 2021).
- Consistent with the Communicating for Safety Standard, maintain accurate documentation so critical information and risks are communicated to ensure the person's safety (ACSQHC, 2021).
- Integrate screening and assessment in collaboration with the individual to develop a goal-directed comprehensive care plan as outlined in the Comprehensive Care Standard (ACSQHC, 2021).
- Although each care plan must be individualised, priorities for care that often apply to women with vaginal infections are *Health education* and *Acute pain.*

Health education

Health education focuses on eliminating the infection, preventing further disease transmission and relieving discomfort associated with the condition. Educating the woman and her partner/s about safe sex and improved genital hygiene practices can reduce the incidence of recurrence.

Many women are unaware of the causes of vaginal infections and the self-care measures to prevent and treat these infections. If possible, both the woman and her sexual partner/s should be provided with information.

- As outlined in the Patient Safety Competency Framework for Nursing Students (Levett-Jones et al., 2017), provide appropriate education. Explain the transmission of the infection and check that you are understood. Many infections are transmitted most easily during menstruation; some can also be transmitted by towels or other inanimate objects, or by certain types of sexual activity. *An open discussion of disease transmission and prevention with the woman and her partner/s can reduce the risk of reinfection.*
- Explain the need to complete the entire course of treatment. *Many infections are asymptomatic in one partner. Incomplete treatment allows for recurrence of the infection and reinfection of the partner.*

Acute pain

The symptoms of vaginitis can include dysuria, painful excoriation or ulceration of tissue, and painful intercourse (dyspareunia). Often these symptoms can be relieved by relatively simple self-care measures. See Box 49.2 for additional comfort measures.

- Suggest the use of cool compresses. *Cool compresses relieve itching.*
- Recommend warm, not hot, sitz baths to alleviate discomfort. *Sitz baths cleanse the perineal area and the warmth is soothing to inflamed, irritated skin and membranes.*

BOX 49.2 Self-care comfort measures

- Do not wear pantyhose, nylon or lycra; wear loose-fitting trousers, shorts, skirts or dresses.
- Double-rinse underwear; do not use fabric softener.
- Do not use bubble bath, perfumed soaps or perfumed feminine hygiene products.
- Use 100% cotton menstrual pads and/or tampons.
- Use unscented toilet paper.
- Use a water-soluble lubricant for intercourse.
- Apply ice or a frozen gel pack wrapped in a towel to the vulva after intercourse to relieve burning. Ensure the towel is cleansed properly or disposed of.
- Rinse vulva with cool water after voiding and intercourse.

- Wear cotton underwear. *Cotton absorbs moisture and allows better air circulation than other types of material.*
- If infected with *Trichomonas*, avoid sexual contact until treatment is completed. *Treatment of the infected woman and her partner/s, as well as sexual abstinence, are necessary to facilitate healing and to prevent reinfection.*

Community-based care

Health education

Health education focuses on eliminating the infection, preventing further disease transmission and relieving discomfort associated with the condition. Educating the woman and her partner/s about safe sex and improved genital hygiene practices can reduce the incidence of recurrence.

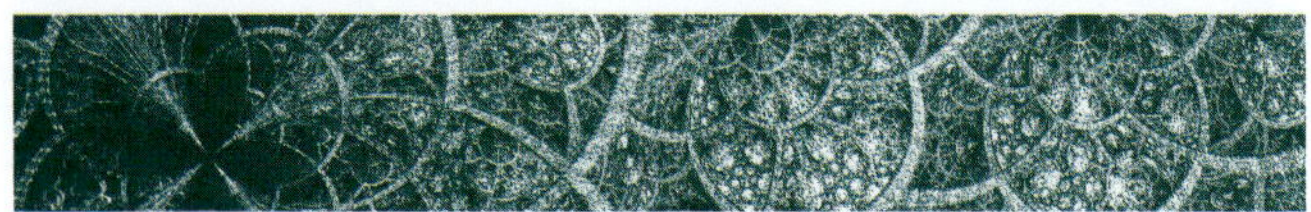

THE PERSON WITH CHLAMYDIA

Chlamydia is a group of STIs caused by *Chlamydia trachomatis*, a bacterium that behaves like a virus, reproducing only within the host cell. The bacterium is spread by any sexual contact and to the neonate from an infected mother during childbirth. The infections caused by chlamydia include acute urethral syndrome, non-gonococcal urethritis, mucopurulent cervicitis and pelvic inflammatory disease.

Chlamydia is the most commonly reported bacterial STI in Australia, with 416.8 cases per 100,000 people each year (Kirby Institute, 2018). Of that number, 73% of reported cases occur in people aged between 15 and 29 years. Risk factors for chlamydia are listed in Box 49.3.

Because chlamydia is asymptomatic in most women until the uterus and fallopian tubes have been invaded, treatment may be delayed, resulting in devastating long-term complications. Nearly one-third of men with urethral chlamydia are also asymptomatic. Chlamydia is a leading cause of preventable blindness in the newborn.

BOX 49.3 Higher risk factors for chlamydial infection

- Young sexually active people
- Previous history of STI
- Homosexually active men and men who have sex with men (MSM)
- Indigenous Australian people
- Oral contraceptive use
- Unprotected sexual activity
- Multiple sexual partners

Pathophysiology

C. trachomatis is an intracellular bacterial pathogen that resembles both a virus and a bacterium. The organism enters the body as an elementary body, a form in which it can enter uninfected cells. The infection begins when the organism enters a cell and changes into a reticulate body. The reticulate body divides within the cell, bursting the cell and infecting adjoining cells.

Manifestations

The incubation period is poorly defined but is probably from 1 to 3 weeks. Chlamydia may be present for months or years without producing noticeable symptoms in women. It typically invades the same target organs as gonorrhoea (cervix and male urethra) and results in similar manifestations (dysuria, urinary frequency and discharge). People with the infection may be asymptomatic. However, they are still potentially infectious.

Complications

If a chlamydial infection in women is not treated, it ascends into the upper reproductive tract, causing complications such as pelvic inflammatory disease, which includes endometritis and salpingitis. Chronic pelvic pain may result. These infections are a major cause of infertility and ectopic pregnancy, which are potentially life threatening. Complications of chlamydial infections in men include pelvic inflammatory disease, epididymitis, prostatitis, sterility and Reiter's syndrome. Reiter's syndrome is a form of reactive arthritis; it is relatively uncommon but can be a debilitating syndrome that follows a gastrointestinal or genitourinary infection. Routine screening for sexually active adolescents and young adults is encouraged to minimise these serious complications in asymptomatic people.

INTERPROFESSIONAL CARE

C. trachomatis is treated with medications to eradicate the infection. Its prevalence, particularly in younger populations, makes widespread screening necessary if the disease is to be controlled. Because chlamydia is often asymptomatic, treatment is often begun on a presumptive basis. Chlamydial infections are notifiable in Australia and must be reported in the National Notifiable Disease Surveillance System (NNDSS) (Department of Health and Aged Care, 2022).

Diagnosis

The diagnostic tests that may be ordered include Gram stain of discharge from the female endocervix and urethra or from the male urethra to look for polymorphonuclear leucocytes (considered evidence of infection).

Tests for antibodies to chlamydia, such as the direct fluorescent antibody (DFA) test and an enzyme-linked immunosorbent assay (ELISA), as well as polymerase chain reaction (PCR) or ligase chain reaction (LCR) tests, are highly sensitive and specific tests performed on cervical and urethral swab specimens. Nucleic acid amplification tests (NAATs), also performed on cervical and urethral swab specimens, are currently the diagnostic method of choice.

Medications

Treatment for chlamydial infections in men and non-pregnant women is doxycycline BD, orally for 7 days, or azithromycin, orally in a single dose. All sexual partners must be treated simultaneously or prior to resuming sexual intercourse.

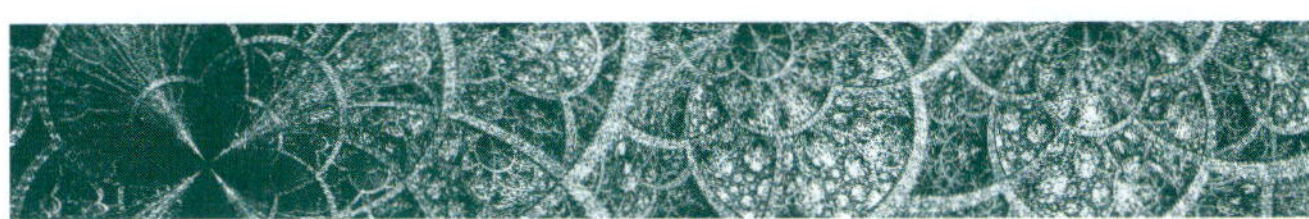

Nursing care

Nursing care of the person who has chlamydia focuses on eliminating the infection, prevention of future infections and management of any chronic complications. Nursing priorities and care for the person who has chlamydia are the same as for anyone with any STI. Interventions are similar to those described for gonorrhoea and genital herpes.

- Reflecting the Patient Safety Competency Framework for Nursing Students (Levett-Jones et al., 2017), use therapeutic communication to build trust and maintain a non-judgmental stance.
- Undertake a health assessment to establish baseline data, including partner history, mental status, vital signs and weight. All health assessments should be in partnership with the individual and reflect the Partnering with Consumers Standard (ACSQHC, 2021), and educate the individual about health promotion and prevention.
- All documentation must be accurately recorded so critical information and risks are communicated to ensure the individual's safety—Communicating for Safety Standard (ACSQHC, 2021).
- Integrate screening and assessment in collaboration with the individual to develop a goal-directed comprehensive care plan as outlined in the Comprehensive Care Standard (ACSQHC, 2021).

Community-based care

Health education for the person who has chlamydia focuses on adherence with the treatment regimen, referring partners for testing and necessary treatment, and the use of condoms to avoid reinfection. If the infection has progressed to pelvic inflammatory disease (discussed later), the person will require additional information on self-care and health promotion. Annual screening for chlamydia for people who are young, sexually active and do not use condoms correctly with every act of sexual intercourse is recommended.

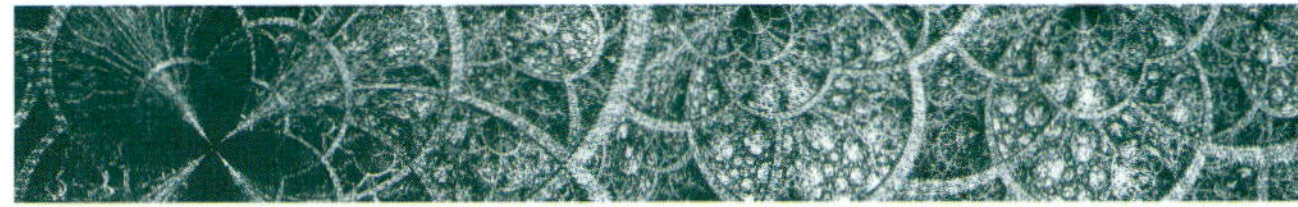

THE PERSON WITH GONORRHOEA

Gonorrhoea, also known as 'GC' or 'the clap', is caused by *Neisseria gonorrhoeae*, a Gram-negative intracellular diplococci bacterium. Gonorrhoea is the second most reported STI in Australia. The estimated annual global incidence of gonorrhoea is 78 million people (WHO, 2021).

In Australia in 2020, there were 29,516 new cases of gonorrhoea (Department of Health, 2021a). More than three-quarters of gonorrhoea notifications were in males. Infection rates are higher in the Aboriginal and Torres Strait Islander population (135.9 per 100,000) than in the non-Indigenous population (95.6 per 100,000) (Department of Health, 2021a). Risk factors include residing in large urban areas, being transient, early onset of sexual activity, multiple serial or consecutive sexual partners, illicit drug use, alcohol misuse, prostitution and previous gonorrhoeal or concurrent STIs.

Pathophysiology

The causative organism of gonorrhoea is a pyogenic (pus-forming) bacterium that causes inflammation characterised by purulent exudate. Humans are the only host for the organism. Gonorrhoea is transmitted by direct sexual intercourse and perinatally from mother to baby during childbirth. The portal of entry can be the genitourinary tract, eyes, oropharynx, anorectum or skin. The incubation period is 2 to 7 days after exposure. The organism initially targets the female cervix and the male urethra. Without treatment, the disease ultimately spreads widely to other organs. In men, gonorrhoea can cause acute, painful inflammation of the prostate, epididymis and periurethral glands, and can lead to sterility. In women, it can cause pelvic inflammatory disease, endometritis, salpingitis and pelvic peritonitis.

Manifestations

Manifestations of gonorrhoea in men include dysuria and serous, milky or purulent discharge from the penis. Some men also experience regional lymphadenopathy. About 20% of men and 80% of women remain asymptomatic until the disease is advanced. Women with symptoms experience dysuria, urinary frequency, abnormal menses (increased flow or dysmenorrhoea), increased vaginal discharge and dyspareunia (difficult or painful sexual intercourse).

Anorectal gonorrhoea is seen most often in people who practise anal sex. The manifestations include pruritus, mucopurulent rectal discharge, rectal bleeding and pain, and constipation. Gonococcal pharyngitis occurs primarily in people after oral sex (fellatio) with an infected partner. The manifestations include fever, sore throat and enlarged lymph glands.

Complications

The complications of untreated gonorrhoea in both men and women may be permanent and serious. They include:

- pelvic inflammatory disease in women, leading to internal abscesses, chronic pelvic pain, ectopic pregnancy and infertility
- blindness, infection of joints and potentially lethal infections of the blood in the newborn, contracted during delivery
- epididymitis and prostatitis in men, resulting in infertility and dysuria
- spread of the infection to the blood causing disseminated gonococcal infection (DGI)
- increased susceptibility to and transmission of HIV.

INTERPROFESSIONAL CARE

The goals of treatment for the person who has gonorrhoea include elimination of the organism and any coexisting disease and prevention of reinfection and transmission. It is important to emphasise the importance of medication adherence and abstaining from sexual contact until the infection is cured in both the person and their partner/s. Condom use to prevent future infections is essential, particularly for pregnant women whose partner/s may be infected. Gonococcal infections are notifiable in Australia and must be reported in the National Notifiable Disease Surveillance System (NNDSS) (Department of Health and Aged Care, 2022).

Diagnosis

Diagnosis of gonorrhoea is based on cultures from the infected mucous membranes (cervix, urethra, rectum or throat), examination of urine from an infected person and a Gram stain to visualise the bacteria under the microscope. Testing for other STIs (especially chlamydia and syphilis) at the same time is recommended. Pregnant women are routinely screened during their first prenatal visit. Diagnostic tests are described in the chapter 'A person-centred approach to assessing the male and female reproductive systems'.

Medications

The first-line treatment of *N. gonorrhoeae* is a single dose of IMI ceftriaxone 500 mg plus a single dose of oral azithromycin 1 g. The alternative treatment is with a single dose of oral ciprofloxacin 500 mg. Fluoroquinolone therapy (such as with ciprofloxacin or levofloxacin) is often prescribed because it is inexpensive, oral and single dose. Because of increased prevalence of fluoroquinolone-resistant *N. gonorrhoeae* in Asia, the Pacific Islands and California in the US, this therapy is no longer recommended for use in treating gonorrhoea in those areas. A single dose of IMI ceftriaxone 500 mg plus a 7-day course of oral doxycycline (Vibramycin, Vivox) is usually added to treat any coexisting chlamydial infection. All sexual partners also need to be treated within 60 days of diagnosis of the infection.

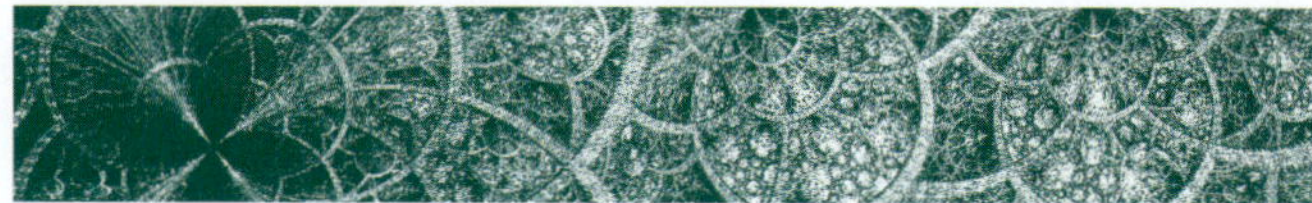

Nursing care

In planning and implementing care for the person who has gonorrhoea, the student nurse uses clinical reasoning to consider the possible coexistence of other STIs and the implications of these (Levett-Jones et al., 2017). These may include syphilis and HIV, the impact of the disease and its treatment on the person's lifestyle and emotional wellbeing, and the likelihood of noncompliance.

- As with other STIs, the nurse will undertake a health assessment in partnership with the individual to establish baseline data, including partner history, mental status, vital signs and weight (ACSQHC, 2021).
- All documentation must be accurately recorded so critical information and risks are communicated to ensure the individual's safety—Communicating for Safety Standard (ACSQHC, 2021).

See the nursing care plan for the person who has gonorrhoea.

Nursing interventions

Nursing priorities discussed in this section focus on non-adherence with treatment and social isolation.

Noncompliance

Although one-time treatment with the recommended antibiotic is highly effective in curing gonorrhoea, non-adherence with the doxycycline regimen may leave any coexisting chlamydial infection unresolved. Noncompliance with recommendations for abstinence, follow up or condom use fosters a high rate of reinfection. Failure to refer partners for examination and treatment also leads to reinfection.

- Reinforce the need to take all medications as directed and to keep follow-up appointments to be sure no reinfection has occurred. Discuss the prevalence of gonorrhoea and the potential complications if it is not cured. *The person who understands the complications of incomplete or failed treatment is more likely to adhere to the medication regimen.*
- Discuss the importance of sexual abstinence until the infection is cured, referral of partners and condom use to prevent reinfection. *Understanding that cure is possible and reinfection is avoidable helps the person cope with the disease and its treatment, and is likely to increase compliance.*
- Explain to women that condoms must be used during treatment, even if other methods of birth control are used. *Oral contraceptives increase the alkalinity of the vaginal pH, facilitating the growth of the gonococcal bacteria, and intrauterine devices alter the endometrial barrier, favouring persistent gonococcal infections.*

Social isolation

Diagnosis of any STI can make people feel 'dirty', ashamed and guilty about their sexual behaviours, and unworthy of being with others.

NURSING CARE PLAN The person with gonorrhoea

Joaddie Deall is a single 26-year-old Assistant in Nursing who lives in a high-density metropolitan apartment. Ms Deall is currently dating Angus Penting, who lives nearby. Ms Deall visits her gynaecologist because her periods have become irregular and she is experiencing pelvic pain. She also complains of an abnormal amount of vaginal discharge. Recently she has developed a sore throat. The pelvic pain has begun to disrupt her sleeping pattern and she is concerned that she might have cancer because her mother recently died of ovarian cancer.

ASSESSMENT

When Ms Deall arrives for her appointment at the gynaecologist's office, Bradley Terr, the Nurse Practitioner (NP), respectfully and non-judgmentally interviews her. Mr Terr undertakes a thorough medical and sexual history, including gathering information about Ms Deall's menstrual periods, pain associated with urination or sexual intercourse, urinary frequency, most recent Pap smear, birth control method, history of STI and drug use, and types of sexual activity. Ms Deall tells the NP her symptoms and her concerns about possible ovarian cancer. She also indicates that she is taking oral contraceptives and therefore sees no need for Angus to use a condom. She believes their relationship to be monogamous.

Physical examination reveals both pharyngeal and cervical inflammation and lower abdominal tenderness. Her temperature is 37.2°C. There are no signs or symptoms of pregnancy.

A Pap smear is ordered and cultures of the cervix, urethra and pharynx to evaluate for gonorrhoea and chlamydial infection. Mr Terr, the NP, takes blood for a white cell count. Test results are positive for gonorrhoea and negative for chlamydia. The white cell count is slightly elevated, indicating possible salpingitis. Because Angus has been Ms Deall's only sexual partner, it is clear that he is the source of infection and also requires treatment.

DIAGNOSES

- *Acute pain* related to the infectious process.
- *Anxiety* related to fear about possible cancer.
- *Low self-esteem* related to shame and guilt because of having an STI.
- *Altered sexuality patterns* related to the impaired relationship and fear of reinfection.

PLANNING

Reflecting the Patient Safety Competency Framework for Nursing Students (Levett-Jones et al., 2017):

- Establish a therapeutic relationship that is respectful and non-judgmental.
- Maintain Ms Deall's dignity and privacy.
- Confirm her understanding of the situation.
- Encourage participation in decision making.
- Discuss with Ms Deall which tests and investigations will be ordered and why.
- In collaboration with Ms Deall, set goals and priorities for care and treatment.
- Health assessments and interventions should be in partnership as outlined in the Partnering with Consumers Standard (ACSQHC, 2021).

Expected outcomes

- A therapeutic relationship is established and Ms Deall feels as though she was treated with respect and dignity.
- Ms Deall receives education regarding tests and investigations and understands why they have been ordered.
- A care plan is jointly established and agreed upon.
- Ms Deall experiences relief of pain, indicating that the infection has been eliminated.
- Ms Deall understands that she has nothing to be ashamed of and that she was wise to seek treatment as soon as her symptoms occurred.
- Ms Deall understands her diagnosis and the implications of the illness.
- Ms Deall understands the need for her and her partner to use condoms during future sexual activity.

IMPLEMENTATION

- Administer ceftriaxone IMI.
- Emphasise the need for regular cervical screening and pelvic examinations because of the family history of ovarian cancer.
- Discuss feelings and concerns about the diagnosis of gonorrhoea. Stress that such a diagnosis is not a reflection on her worth as a person.
- Educate how to talk with sexual partner/s about condom use.

EVALUATION

A week later, during her follow-up visit, Ms Deall states that she is feeling much better and sleeping well at night since the pain has ended. She has terminated her relationship with Mr Penting and is considering joining a health club in the hope of increasing her level of fitness and perhaps meeting someone new.

CRITICAL THINKING IN THE NURSING PROCESS

1 In what ways are Ms Deall's manifestations related to the infectious process of gonorrhoea?
2 Should the nurse have suggested that Ms Deall also be tested for HIV? Why or why not?
3 Develop a care plan for Ms Deall related to social isolation.
4 Consider the stages of grieving regarding the break-up of a relationship.

REFLECTION ON THE NURSING PROCESS

1 Why is it so important that a therapeutic relationship be established and that the nurse is non-judgmental and respectful?
2 Which aspects of health education should the nurse focus on?

- Provide privacy, confidentiality and a safe, non-judgmental environment for expression of concerns. Support the person to gain an understanding that gonorrhoea is a consequence of sexual behaviour, not a punishment, and that it can be avoided in the future. *Being treated with respect and privacy helps the person realise that the disease does not change an individual's worth as a person. This knowledge enhances the person's ability to relate to others.*

Community-based care

Health education focuses on supporting people to understand the importance of: (1) taking all prescribed medication, (2) referring sexual partners for evaluation and treatment, (3) abstaining from all sexual contact until the person and their partners are cured, and (4) using a condom to avoid transmitting or contracting infections in the future. Individuals also need to understand the need for a follow-up visit 4 to 7 days after treatment is completed.

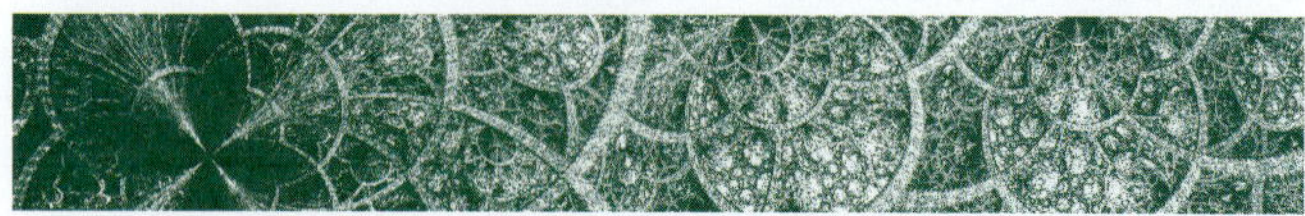

THE PERSON WITH SYPHILIS

Syphilis is a complex systemic STI caused by the spirochaete *Treponema pallidum*. It can infect almost any body tissue or organ and is transmitted from open skin lesions and mucous membranes during any sexual contact (anal, oral or vaginal intercourse). Vertical transmission can also occur during any stage of pregnancy (congenital syphilis). Less commonly, syphilis can be transmitted by infected blood or other body fluid, such as saliva, due to being able to survive in fluids for days. The incubation period ranges from 10 to 90 days, averaging 21 days. If not treated appropriately, syphilis can lead to blindness, paralysis, stillbirth, cardiovascular damage and death. Syphilis often occurs with one or more other STIs, such as HIV/AIDS or chlamydial infection.

Famous people suspected of having syphilis include Charles VIII of France, Adolph Hitler, Mussolini and Leo Tolstoy. Those suspected of dying from the disease include Christopher Columbus, George Washington, Napoleon Bonaparte and Franz Schubert. It is posited that 'the pox', as syphilis is sometimes called, was spread worldwide by Christopher Columbus and his men.

Syphilis remains a significant public health problem, with high rates in certain geographical regions and specific populations. There is an ongoing outbreak among Aboriginal and Torres Strait Islander people aged 15 to 34 years in northern, central, western and southern Australia. Infection rates in major cities are also increasing, especially among men who have sex with men (MSM). The incidence of primary and secondary syphilis is highest in people 20 to 39 years of age (Department of Health, 2019).

In 2020–2021, Aboriginal and Torres Strait Islander people continued to be disproportionately represented in the syphilis notifications, with reported rates among males of 155.2 per 100,000, compared to 31.1 per 100,000 in non-Indigenous males. In 2020–2021, notification rates of syphilis among Aboriginal and Torres Strait Islander females increased by 16%, compared to non-Indigenous females with a 4% decrease in notifications (Department of Health, 2021b).

Pathophysiology

Any break in the skin or mucous membrane is vulnerable to invasion by the spirochaete. Upon entering the system, the spirochaete spreads through the blood and lymphatic system. Congenital syphilis is transferred to the fetus through the placental circulation.

Manifestations

Syphilis is generally characterised by three clinical stages: primary, secondary and tertiary. Each stage has characteristic manifestations (see Table 49.3). The person who has syphilis also may experience a latency period when no signs of the disease are evident.

Primary syphilis

The primary stage of syphilis is characterised by the appearance of a **chancre** (see Figure 49.4) and by regional enlargement of lymph nodes; little or no pain accompanies these warning signs. The chancre appears at the site of inoculation (such as the genitals, anus, mouth, breast, fingers) 3 to 6 weeks after the infectious contact. In women, a genital chancre may go unnoticed, disappearing within 4 to 6 weeks. In both primary and secondary stages, syphilis remains highly infectious, even if no symptoms are evident.

Secondary syphilis

Manifestations of secondary syphilis may appear any time from 4 weeks to 12 weeks after the initial chancre disappears. Symptoms can include a headache, low-grade fever, skin rash, especially on the palms of the hands or soles of the feet; mucous patches in the oral cavity; sore throat; lymphadenopathy; condylomata lata (large, raised, flat-topped lesions found in moist areas) and alopecia. These manifestations generally disappear within 2 to 6 weeks and an asymptomatic latency period begins.

Latent and tertiary syphilis

The latent stage of syphilis begins 2 or more years after the initial infection and can last up to 50 years. During this stage, no symptoms of syphilis are apparent and the disease is not transmissible by sexual contact. It can be transmitted by infected blood. Therefore, all prospective blood donors are screened for syphilis. In two-thirds of all cases, the latent stage persists without further complications. Unless treated, the remaining one-third of infected people progress to late-stage or tertiary syphilis. In the presence of HIV infection, disease progression seems to be more rapid.

Two types of late-stage syphilis occur. Benign late syphilis, of rapid onset, is characterised by localised development of infiltrating tumours (*gummas*) in skin, bones and liver, generally responding promptly to treatment. A more insidious onset involves a diffuse inflammatory response that involves the central nervous and cardiovascular system. Though the disease can still be treated at this stage, much of the cardiovascular and central nervous system damage is irreversible.

TABLE 49.3 Manifestations of syphilis

SYSTEM	PRIMARY	SECONDARY	TERTIARY
Reproductive	Genital chancre (may be internal in female)	Condylomata lata	
Integumentary		Rash on palms of hands and soles of feet	Granulomatous lesions involving mucous membranes and skin
Gastrointestinal	Loss of appetite Oral mucous patches		
Neurological		Asymptomatic Meningitis Headache Cranial neuropathies	Asymptomatic Tabes dorsalis Neurosyphilis Seizures, hemiparesis, hemiplegia Personality changes, hyperactive reflexes, Argyll Robertson pupil, decreased memory, slurred speech, optic atrophy
Musculoskeletal		Arthralgia Myalgia Bone and joint arthritis Periostitis	Gummas
Cardiovascular			Aortic insufficiency Aortic aneurysm Stenosis of openings to coronary arteries
Renal		Glomerulonephritis Nephrotic syndrome	
Other	Regional lymphadenopathy	Generalised lymphadenopathy Fever Hepatitis Malaise Alopecia	

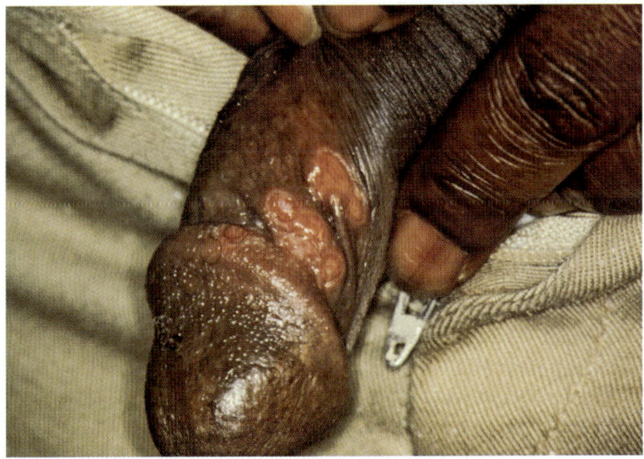

FIGURE 49.4 ***Chancre of primary syphilis on the penis***

Source: CDC/M. Rein.

INTERPROFESSIONAL CARE

The goals of treatment are to inactivate the spirochaete and provide health education about how to prevent reinfection or further transmission. Treatment includes antibiotic therapy and identification and referral of partners for testing and treatment if necessary, follow-up testing and education about condom use to prevent reinfection of self and transmission of disease to partners. In addition, people with syphilis should also be screened for chlamydial infection and advised to have an HIV test.

Diagnosis

Diagnosis of syphilis is complex because it mimics many other diseases. A careful history and physical examination are required, as well as laboratory evaluations of lesions and blood. Diagnostic tests are described in the chapter 'A person-centred approach to assessing the male and female reproductive systems'.

People with syphilis become positive about 4 to 6 weeks after infection. However, these tests are not specific for syphilis and other diseases may also cause positive results. Additional tests are required for a definitive diagnosis.

The treponemal test is specific for *T. pallidum* and uses agglutination assay to detect *T. pallidum* particle agglutination (TPPA). A non-treponemal test called rapid plasma regain (RPR) can also be used; however, this test does not detect an antibody to *T. pallidum* but to regain, which is a useful indicator of disease activity. Point-of-care testing is also available in Australia using Determine Syphilis TP™.

Medications

The treatment of choice for all stages of syphilis is benzathine penicillin 1.8 g, given IM in a single dose. People who are allergic to penicillin are given oral doxycycline for 14 days.

Treatment of syphilis may result in a severe reaction called the *Jarisch–Herxheimer reaction*, involving fever, musculoskeletal pain, tachycardia and sometimes hypotension. This is not a reaction to the penicillin itself, but to the sudden and massive destruction of spirochaetes by the penicillin and the resulting release of toxins into the bloodstream. The Jarisch–Herxheimer reaction generally begins within 24 hours of treatment and subsides in another 24 hours. Treatment should not be discontinued unless symptoms become life threatening.

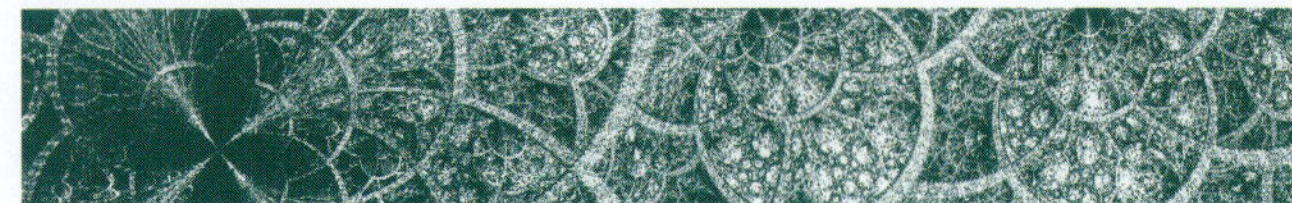

Nursing care

In planning and implementing nursing care for the person who has syphilis, the nurse needs to consider the person's age, their lifestyle, access to healthcare and their educational level. The Patient Safety Competency Framework for Nursing Students (Levett-Jones et al., 2017) requires pre-registration nursing students to:

- Demonstrate the ability to conduct a culturally appropriate assessment.
- Avoid generalisations and stereotypes.
- Adapt practice to accommodate the individual's cultural needs and values.
- Educate the individual about prevention strategies.

See the nursing care plan for a person who has syphilis.

Nursing diagnoses and interventions

Nursing priorities discussed in this section focus on the *Risk of injury*, *Anxiety* and *Low self-esteem.*

Risk of injury

If syphilis is not diagnosed and treated promptly and effectively, it can have devastating effects on all body systems, particularly the neurological and cardiovascular systems, eventually leading to a painful death.

NURSING CARE PLAN A person who has syphilis

Nate Elgmisson, aged 24, works as a butcher. For the past year he has shared a house with Callie Lincoln, who is 5 months pregnant with his child. Although he intends to marry Callie before the baby is born, he has continued to have a sexual relationship with a previous partner named Joshua Sorronsoin. His sexual activities with Joshua have increased in frequency as Ms Lincoln's pregnancy has advanced. Recently, Mr Elgmisson has noticed a swelling in his groin and a sore on his penis.

ASSESSMENT

When Mr Elgmisson comes to the community health centre, he is interviewed by the Nurse Practitioner (NP), Mary Pertolloti. Mary establishes a therapeutic relationship and gathers a thorough medical and sexual history, including information about drug use, allergies, difficulty with urination, urinary frequency, itching or discharge from the penis, recent sexual activities, precautions taken against infection, history of STIs and sexual function. Mary determines that Mr Elgmisson has been having unprotected sex with both Ms Lincoln and Mr Sorronsoin. Nate thinks that Joshua is not having sex with anyone except him but he is not sure.

Physical assessment reveals a classic syphilitic chancre on the shaft of the penis and regional lymphadenopathy. A specimen of exudates from the chancre is sent for dark-field examination. Ms Pertolotti discusses with Mr Elgmisson the likelihood that he has syphilis and the need to tell both Ms Lincoln and Mr Sorronsoin so that they can be tested and, if necessary, treated. Ms Pertolotti also suggests that Mr Elgmisson be tested for HIV since he has been having unprotected sex with two people, at least one of whom may be sexually active with other partners. He agrees and blood is drawn for an ELISA test. Dark-field analysis of the chancre exudate confirms the diagnosis of syphilis; the ELISA results are negative for HIV.

DIAGNOSES

- *Risk of injury* to the person, his partners and the infant, related to the disease process.
- *Lack of knowledge* about the disease process, its transmission and the need for treatment.
- *Anxiety* related to the effects of the infection on the unborn child and discussing the diagnosis with partners.
- *Possible relationship breakdown* related to diagnosis of syphilis and non-monogamous sexual activity.

PLANNING

- Establish a therapeutic relationship based on respect and a non-judgmental attitude as outlined in the Partnering with Consumers Standard (ACSQHC, 2021) and the Patient Safety Competency Framework for Nursing Students (Levett-Jones et al., 2017).
- Accurately document critical information as outlined in the Communicating for Safety Standard (ACSQHC, 2021).
- Explain the diagnosis and what having this illness means for the person.
- Establish a collaborative care and treatment plan.
- Explain tests and interventions (e.g. the ELISA test).
- Collaboratively identify coping strategies.

Expected outcomes

- Therapeutic relationship and rapport established.
- Prompt treatment will cure the syphilis.
- The person understands the need to abstain from sexual contact during treatment, complete all medications, return for follow-up visits and use condoms to prevent reinfection.
- The person can identify strategies to cope with the effect of diagnosis and treatment on their relationship/s.
- Decreased anxiety following health and psychosocial education and treatment.
- Penicillin administered.
- Follow-up appointments made.
- Health education material provided and any questions and concerns answered and clarified.
- Sexual partners notified that they need to attend the clinic for testing.
- Confirmed and probable cases of infectious (i.e. primary, secondary, early latent) syphilis and congenital syphilis are entered into jurisdictional notifiable conditions databases within 1 day of confirmation (Department of Health, 2019).

NURSING CARE PLAN A person who has syphilis (continued)

IMPLEMENTATION

- Administer IM injection of benzathine penicillin.
- Discuss the importance of Mr Elgmisson and his partners abstaining from sexual activity for 5 days post treatment or until symptoms are resolved (whichever is longer), and of using condoms to prevent reinfection.
- Explain the need to return for follow-up testing in 3 months and again at 6 months. Provide a copy of the STI prevention checklist, and document that reminders need to be sent at 3- and 6-month intervals.
- Notify sexual partners that they need to be tested.
- Provide counselling about the effect of the disease on relationships.
- Provide health education regarding the importance of treatment to the health of the infant.

EVALUATION

At the 3-month follow-up visit, the chancre on Mr Elgmisson's penis has healed and he reports that he is using a condom whenever he has sex. Ms Lincoln also tested positive for syphilis and negative for HIV, so she, too, is given penicillin and verbal and written follow-up instructions, including follow up until the infant is born. The couple is meeting every second week with a relationship counsellor and say that, although strained, the relationship is improving. Mr Sorronsoin has received similar test results and is given a prescription for doxycycline because he is allergic to penicillin.

CRITICAL THINKING IN THE NURSING PROCESS

1. Which manifestations might a person with early syphilis experience?
2. List some appropriate questions for taking a sexual history when you suspect the presence of one or more STIs.
3. How might you support Mr Elgmisson to help him break the news of his diagnosis to his sexual partners, especially Ms Lincoln?

REFLECTION ON THE NURSING PROCESS

1. Which relationship issues will the couple have to deal with?
2. Would your thoughts about Mr Elgmisson's behaviour affect the way you interact with him?

- Educate the person about the importance of taking any prescribed medication. *Taking the prescribed antibiotic is important to ensure eradication of the infecting organism.*
- Encourage referral of any sexual partners for evaluation and any necessary treatment. *Without treatment of all partners, reinfection can occur or the disease may be transmitted to other people through sexual activity.*
- Educate about why the person needs to abstain from sexual contact until they and their partner/s are cured, and why they should use condoms to prevent future infections. *Abstinence until the organism is eliminated prevents reinfection. Condoms provide barrier protection, reducing the risk of infection during sexual activity.*
- Emphasise the importance of returning for follow-up testing at 3- and 6-month intervals for early syphilis and at 6- and 12-month intervals for late latent syphilis. *Follow-up testing is performed to ensure eradication of the disease.*
- Provide information about manifestations of reinfection. *Successful treatment of the disease does not prevent possible subsequent infections.*

Anxiety

The diagnosis of syphilis understandably causes the person significant levels of anxiety, not only about personal wellbeing but also about the wellbeing of partners and, in the expectant woman, her fetus.

- Emphasise that syphilis can be effectively treated, preventing the serious complications of late-stage disease. *This information provides a sense of control and can help decrease anxiety.*

Links to National Patient Safety Standards

NSQHS: Partnering with Consumers Standard

The intent of this standard is to ensure that the person with an STI is a partner in planning, design, delivery, measurement and evaluation of systems and services that provide care and that they are partners in their own care, to the extent that they choose.

Source: ACSQHC (2021). *National Safety and Quality Health Service Standards* (2nd ed.). Sydney: ACSQHC.

- Educate the pregnant woman about taking medications as directed and that returning each month for follow-up testing will help ensure the wellbeing of her baby. *Knowing that treatment can reduce the risk to her baby relieves anxiety and possibly increases compliance.*

Low self-esteem

Living with any chronic disease can be damaging to someone's self-esteem. The person who has syphilis needs additional support to cope with the stigma of this kind of disease. Unfortunately, people who are most affected by STIs often lack family and other social support networks.

- Create an environment where the person feels respected and safe to discuss questions and concerns about the disease and its effect on their life. *Being treated with respect helps enhance self-esteem.*
- Provide privacy and confidentiality. *People are often embarrassed to discuss the intimate details of their sex lives.*
- Let the person know that the nurse and other healthcare providers care about them and the successful treatment of their disease. *Feeling valued enhances self-esteem.*

Community-based care

Health and psychosocial education is an essential part of nursing care for someone who has an STI. The nurse emphasises that syphilis is a chronic disease that can be spread to others even though no symptoms are evident. The following topics need to be discussed:

- taking all prescribed medication
- referring sexual partners for evaluation and treatment
- abstaining from all sexual contact
- using a condom to avoid transmitting or contracting infections in the future
- the need for follow-up testing (at 3 and 6 months for people with primary or secondary syphilis, and at 6 and 12 months for those with late-stage disease). If the person is also HIV positive, follow-up visits are recommended 1, 2, 3, 6, 9 and 12 months after treatment.

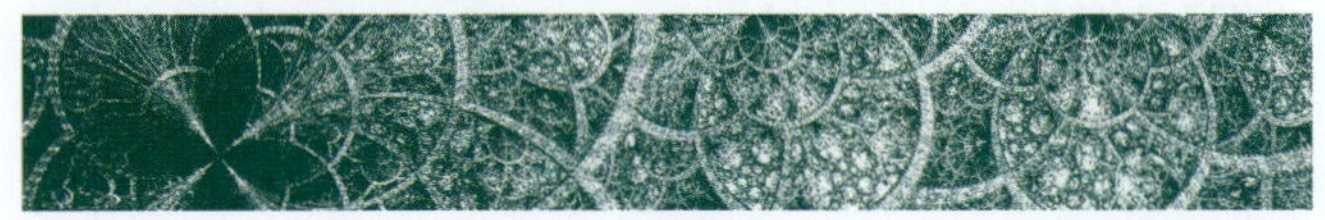

THE PERSON WITH PELVIC INFLAMMATORY DISEASE

Pelvic inflammatory disease (PID) is a term used to describe infection of the pelvic organs, including the fallopian tubes (*salpingitis*), ovaries (*oophoritis*), cervix (*cervicitis*), endometrium (*endometritis*), pelvic peritoneum and the pelvic vascular system. PID can be caused by one or more infectious agents, including *Neisseria gonorrhoeae*, *Chlamydia trachomatis*, *Mycoplasma genitalium* and *Trichomonas vaginalis*. *C. trachomatis* is responsible for 50% of PID while *N. gonorrhoeae* is responsible for 25%.

Pelvic inflammatory disease is not a reportable disease in Australia. PID is most common among sexually active women aged 20 to 24 years and approximately 1 in 8 Australian women will experience PID in their lifetime (Healthdirect, 2021). Up to 40% of women may experience infertility after three recurring episodes of PID, and ectopic pregnancies occur at up to six times the frequency of women who report no episodes of PID (CDC, 2021b). The disease may also cause pelvic abscesses and chronic abdominal pain.

Sexually active women aged 16 to 24 years are most at risk, with risk factors including a history of STI (especially gonorrhoea and chlamydia), bacterial vaginosis, multiple sex partners, douching and previous PID. Barrier contraceptive devices such as condoms reduce the risk of PID.

Prognosis depends on the number of episodes, promptness of treatment and modification of risk-taking behaviours. Prevention includes health education, especially for young women, regarding the causes and transmission of infection and methods of self-protection, such as avoiding unprotected sexual activity.

Pathophysiology

Pelvic inflammatory disease is usually polymicrobial (caused by more than one microbe) in origin, with *N. gonorrhoeae* and *C. trachomatis* being common causative organisms. Pathogenic microorganisms enter the vagina and travel to the uterus during intercourse or other sexual activity. They can also gain direct access to the uterus during childbirth, insertion of intrauterine devices (IUD), termination of pregnancy and surgery of the reproductive tract. The organisms ascend from the endocervical canal to the fallopian tubes and ovaries.

Manifestations

Manifestations of pelvic inflammatory disease include fever, purulent vaginal discharge, severe lower abdominal pain and pain during sex. However, manifestations may be so mild that the infection is not recognised.

Complications

Complications include pelvic abscess, infertility, ectopic pregnancy, miscarriage, chronic pelvic pain, pelvic adhesions, dyspareunia and chronic pelvic pain. Abscess formation is common.

INTERPROFESSIONAL CARE

The goals of treatment are to eliminate the infection and prevent complications and recurrence. The physical examination may reveal abdominal, adnexal and cervical pain.

Diagnosis

Tests used in the diagnosis of PID may include a full blood count with differential, which will show a markedly elevated white blood cell count and increased sedimentation rate. A laparoscopy or laparotomy may reveal inflammation, oedema or hyperaemia of the fallopian tubes or tubal discharge and, possibly, generalised pelvic involvement, abscesses and scarring.

Medications

Combination antibiotic therapy with a single dose of ceftriaxone 500 mg IM, plus metronidazole 400 mg orally for 14 days, plus doxycycline 100 mg orally for 14 days is the typical treatment for PID. In severe cases, the person may be hospitalised. Analgesics are given, and antibiotics and fluids are administered intravenously. Nursing implications for antibiotics are discussed in the chapter 'Nursing care of people with infections'.

Surgery

A drain may be inserted into an abscess, if present, and any adhesions may be removed. If the person does not respond to conservative therapy, surgical removal of the uterus, fallopian tubes and ovaries may be necessary.

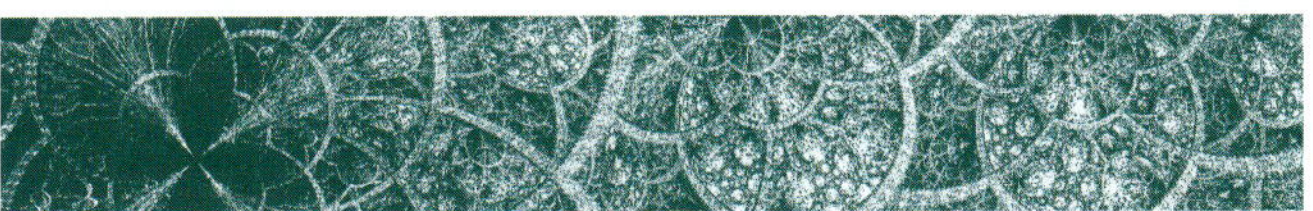

Nursing care

The goals of nursing care are to treat the infection and to prevent complications, such as scarring and infertility. The person who is hospitalised maintains bed rest in the semi-Fowler's position to promote drainage and to localise the infectious process in the pelvic cavity.

Nursing interventions

Nursing priorities that apply to the person with PID include: *Risk of injury* and *Health education*.

Risk of injury

Pelvic inflammatory disease can have severe, even life-threatening, complications. Scarring of fallopian tubes can lead to ectopic pregnancy or pelvic abscess. Infertility is a common complication, as are recurrent or chronic PID, chronic abdominal pain, pelvic adhesions, premature hysterectomy and depression. Severe infection and manifestations may require hospitalisation.

- Administer antibiotic therapy and monitor closely for adverse effects. *Antibiotics used in acute PID are potent agents; some can have serious side effects.*
- Demonstrate effective handwashing and strict adherence to universal precautions when handling perineal pads and linen (Levett-Jones et al., 2017). Appropriate disinfection of bedpans, toilet seats, linen and utensils is also important. *These practices help avoid transmitting the infection to others.*

Health education

Pelvic inflammatory disease is most common in young women, who often do not understand their own anatomy and physiology or STIs. Diagnosis and treatment of PID provides an opportunity to increase that understanding, thereby preventing complications and recurrent infection. The pre-registration nurse can apply the Patient Safety Competency Framework for Nursing Students (Levett-Jones et al., 2017) by demonstrating communication skills that avoid jargon and complex terms. The pre-registration nurse should also educate the individual about safe medication compliance and the transmission of infection.

- Explain how infection is spread and which measures to take to prevent future infection. *Understanding can improve adherence with treatment regimens and perhaps change high-risk behaviour.*
- Explain the need to complete the treatment regimen and the importance of follow-up visits. If the person or their partner/s fail to take all of the medication as prescribed, the infection may not be completely cured. *Noncompliance and recurrence are common, particularly if follow-up appointments are not kept.*
- Provide education about proper perineal care, especially wiping from front to back. *This reduces transmission of faecal organisms to reproductive tissues and reduces the incidence of urinary tract infections.*
- Caution the person about using tampons. Educate the person about why it is important to change tampons or pads at least every 4 hours. *Menstrual flow and other discharges provide a favourable environment for microorganisms to multiply.*
- Provide information about safe sex practices and family planning. Support the person to understand that they need to remove diaphragms within 6 hours after use. IUDs are contraindicated. Latex condoms offer the most effective protection against infection. *These measures help prevent recurrence of infection.*
- Educate the person to recognise and report any unusual vaginal discharge or odour to the healthcare provider. *Treatment is most effective early in the disease process.*
- Provide emotional support.

Community-based care

Provide general information related to STIs. Discuss ways to eliminate the infection and prevent recurrence, and support the person to identify strategies to deal with the physical and psychosocial implications of treatment, including possible infertility. Inform the person that the patency of the fallopian tubes can be evaluated after several menstrual cycles; this delay allows for complete resolution of the inflammatory process.

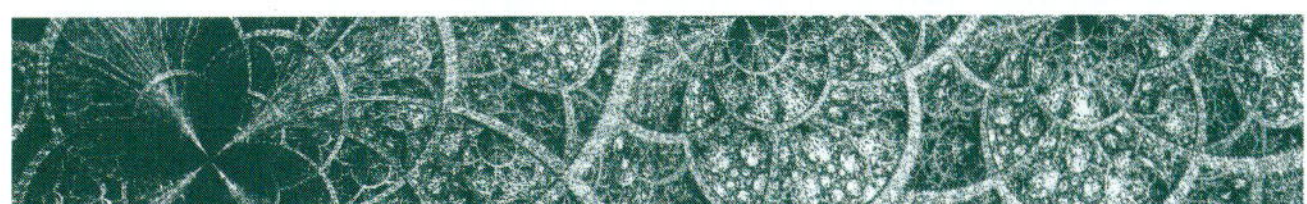

CHAPTER HIGHLIGHTS

- Sexually transmitted infections (STIs) are infections transmitted by sexual contact, including vaginal, oral and anal intercourse. STIs affect women and infants more than men, and are more common in people who have multiple sex partners, abuse drugs or are of a lower socioeconomic status.
- STIs can coexist in the same person and are transmitted by sexual contact. Effective treatment mandates that all sex partners be treated. Most STIs can be prevented by using latex condoms.
- Genital herpes, caused by an infection with an HSV virus, is a commonly occurring STI in teens and young adults. There is currently no cure and treatment is primarily symptomatic. Nursing care is directed towards relieving the pain of the lesions, mitigating sexual dysfunction and relieving anxiety.
- Genital warts, caused by the human papillomavirus (HPV), are a chronic, incurable STI. They are manifested by warts of various forms or may be present without manifestations. Infection with HPV poses a major risk of cervical cancer. A vaccine against the virus has been developed and is recommended.
- Urogenital infections include vaginal infections (bacterial vaginosis, candidiasis and trichomoniasis), chlamydia, gonorrhoea, syphilis and pelvic inflammatory disease (PID).
- Chlamydia, occurring most in young adults under age 25, is a bacterial infection that can spread to the uterus and fallopian tubes in women, causing PID, infertility and ectopic pregnancy. Untreated chlamydia in men may result in epididymitis, prostatitis, sterility and Reiter's syndrome.
- Gonorrhoea (caused by a bacteria) and syphilis (caused by a spirochaete) affect both men and women and may infect the newborn as it moves through the birth canal in an untreated woman. Syphilis, if untreated, exists in the body in three stages, with the third stage lasting up to 50 years. Both of these STIs are treated with antibiotics. Nursing care focuses on education, preventing injury from complications, relieving anxiety and supporting self-esteem.
- Pelvic inflammatory disease is an infection of the female pelvic organs and may be caused by one or more infectious agents. Sexually active young women between the ages of 16 and 24 are most at risk. The prognosis depends on the number of episodes, promptness of treatment and modification of risk-taking behaviours. The goals of nursing care are to treat the infection and prevent complications.

CONCEPT CHECK

1 Which population is most often affected by STIs?
1 men
2 women and infants
3 adolescent males
4 older adults

2 Which of the following statements indicates that a person understands how they should treat an STI?
1 'My sex partner and I must both take medications.'
2 'I know I can never have sex again.'
3 'I will douche after every sexual encounter with my partner.'
4 'My sex partner does not have an infection, so won't need medications.'

3 When providing a man with information about using condoms to prevent STI, which topics should be included? (Select all that apply.)
1 Use a new condom with each sex act.
2 Ensure a small amount of air is in the tip.
3 Use oil-based lubricants, such as petroleum jelly.
4 Handle carefully to ensure no damage.
5 Withdraw when the penis is erect.

4 You are assessing a young male. He has both blisters and ulcerations on the shaft of his penis. What is he most likely to have contracted?
1 chlamydia
2 gonorrhoea
3 genital warts
4 genital herpes

5 Of the following statements about genital warts, which one is not true?
1 The infection is caused by a yeast organism.
2 The infection can be spread by any type of intercourse.
3 The infection may be transmitted to the fetus.
4 The infection cannot be cured.

6 You are counselling a young woman with an HPV genital infection. Which screening test would you recommend she have every year?
1 breast exam and mammogram
2 stool for occult blood
3 full blood count (FBC) to detect anaemia and infection
4 pelvic exam and Pap smear

7 Which of the following symptoms would most commonly be elicited as part of a health assessment for a woman who has a vaginal infection?
1 pain
2 itching
3 nausea
4 diarrhoea

8 When providing health education to a woman with an STI who has severe genital discomfort, what is one simple recommendation that may relieve her discomfort?
1 Wear nylon pantyhose.
2 Cut fingernails short.
3 Wear cotton underwear.
4 Don't have sex anymore.

9 The infective organism responsible for gonorrhoea initially targets which body parts?
1 male urethra and female cervix
2 female vulva and vagina
3 male prostate
4 male and female external genitalia

10 When providing health education to a person with syphilis, what would you say?
1 Syphilis is caused by a virus.
2 Syphilis is a local genital infection.
3 Syphilis is a systemic infection.
4 Syphilis has no effect on the developing fetus.

BIBLIOGRAPHY

ASHM (Australasian Society for HIV, Viral Hepatitis and Sexual Health Medicine) (2022). *Australian STI management guidelines for use in primary care*. Retrieved from https://www.sti.guidelines.org.au/

Australian Commission on Safety and Quality in Health Care (ACSQHC) (2021). *National Safety and Quality Health Service Standards* (2nd ed.). Sydney: ACSQHC.

Cancer Australia (2021). *Cervical cancer*. Retrieved from https://www.canceraustralia.gov.au/

Centers for Disease and Control and Prevention (CDC) (2021a). *Genital herpes*. Retrieved from https://www.cdc.gov/

Centers for Disease and Control and Prevention (CDC) (2021b). *Pelvic inflammatory disease*. Retrieved from https://www.cdc.gov/

Centers for Disease Control and Prevention (CDC) (2022a). *Antibiotic-resistant gonorrhoea*. Retrieved from https://www.cdc.gov/

Centers for Disease Control and Prevention (CDC) (2022b). *Sexually transmitted diseases (STDs)*. Atlanta: CDC. Retrieved from https://www.cdc.gov/

Centers for Disease Control and Prevention (CDC) (2022c). *Human papillomavirus*. Retrieved from https://www.cdc.gov/

Department of Health (2018). *Fourth national sexually transmissible infections strategy 2018–2022*. Retrieved from https://www.health.gov.au/

Department of Health (2019). *National response to syphilis*. Retrieved from https://www.health.gov.au/

Department of Health (2021a). *Australian gonococcal surveillance programme annual report, 2020*. Retrieved from https://www.health.gov.au/

Department of Health (2021b). *National syphilis surveillance report 2021*. Retrieved from https://www.health.gov.au/

Department of Health and Aged Care (2022). *Australian national notifiable diseases and case definitions*. Canberra: Department of Health. Retrieved from https://www.health.gov.au/

Healthdirect (2021). *Pelvic inflammatory disease*. Retrieved from https://www.healthdirect.gov.au/

Kirby Institute (2018). *HIV, viral hepatitis and sexually transmissible infections in Australia: Annual surveillance report 2018*. Sydney: UNSW. Retrieved from https://kirby.unsw.edu.au/

Kirby Institute (2021). *HIV, viral hepatitis and sexually transmissible infections in Australia: Annual surveillance report 2021*. Sydney: UNSW. Retrieved from https://kirby.unsw.edu.au/

Levett-Jones, T., Dwyer, T., Reid-Searl, K., Heaton, L., Flenady, T., Applegarth, J., Guinea, S. & Andersen, P. (2017). *Patient Safety Competency Framework (PSCF) for Nursing Students*. Sydney. Retrieved from http://psframework.wpengine.com/

National Centre for Immunisation Research and Surveillance (NCIRS) (2022). *Human papillomavirus (HPV) vaccine for Australians*. Retrieved from http://www.ncirs.org.au/

Sexual Health Australia (2018). *General*. Retrieved from https://www.sexualhealthaustralia.com.au/

South Australia Health (2022). *Human papillomavirus (HPV)*. Retrieved from https://sahealth.sa.gov.au/

World Health Organization (WHO) (2021). *Global progress report on HIV, viral hepatitis and sexually transmitted infection, 2021*. Geneva, Switzerland: WHO. Retrieved from http://www.who.int/

World Health Organization (WHO) (2022). *Global health sector strategies on respectively, HIV, viral hepatitis, and sexually transmitted infections 2022–2030*. Geneva, Switzerland: WHO. Retrieved from https://who.int/

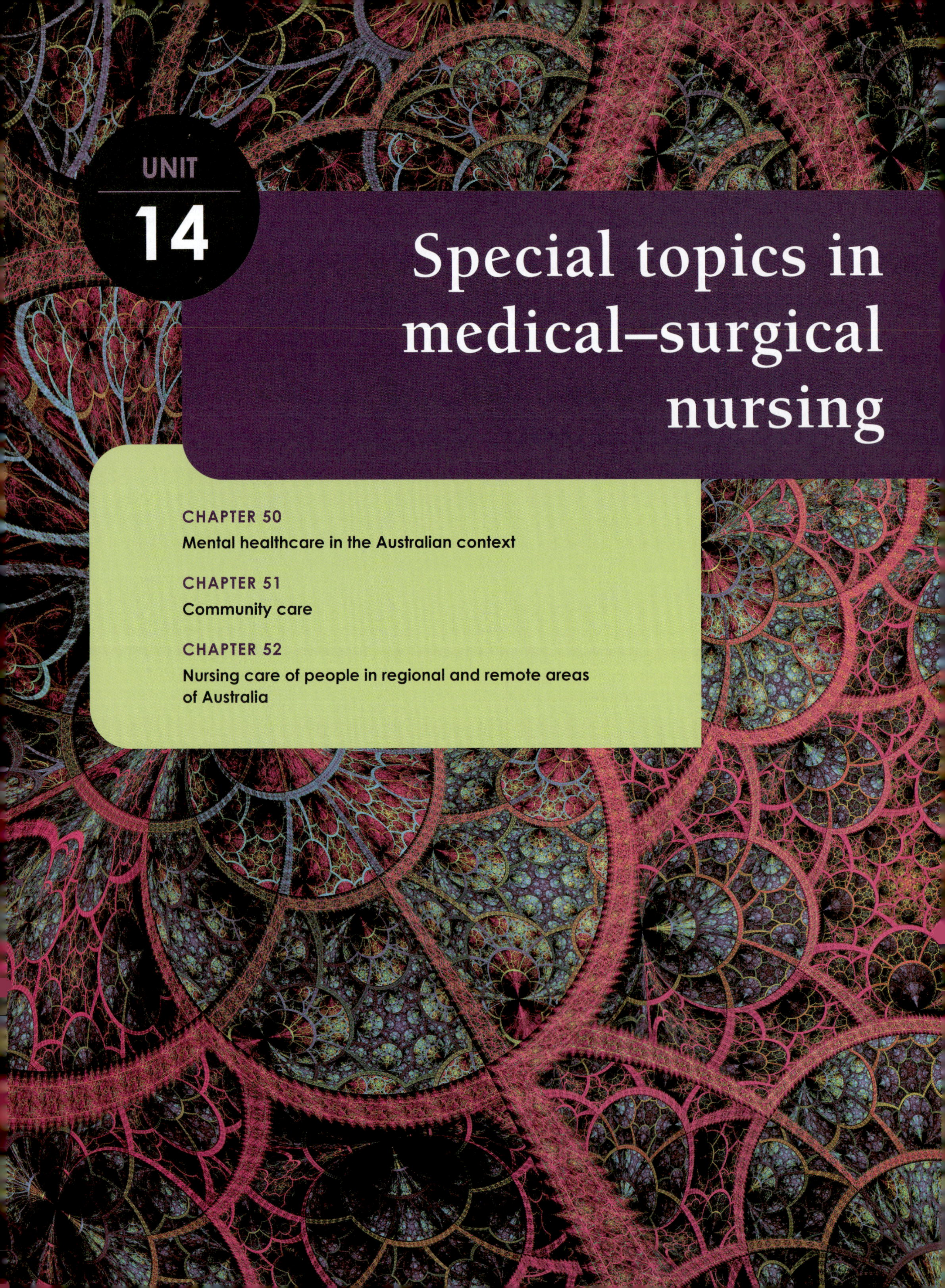

UNIT

14

Special topics in medical–surgical nursing

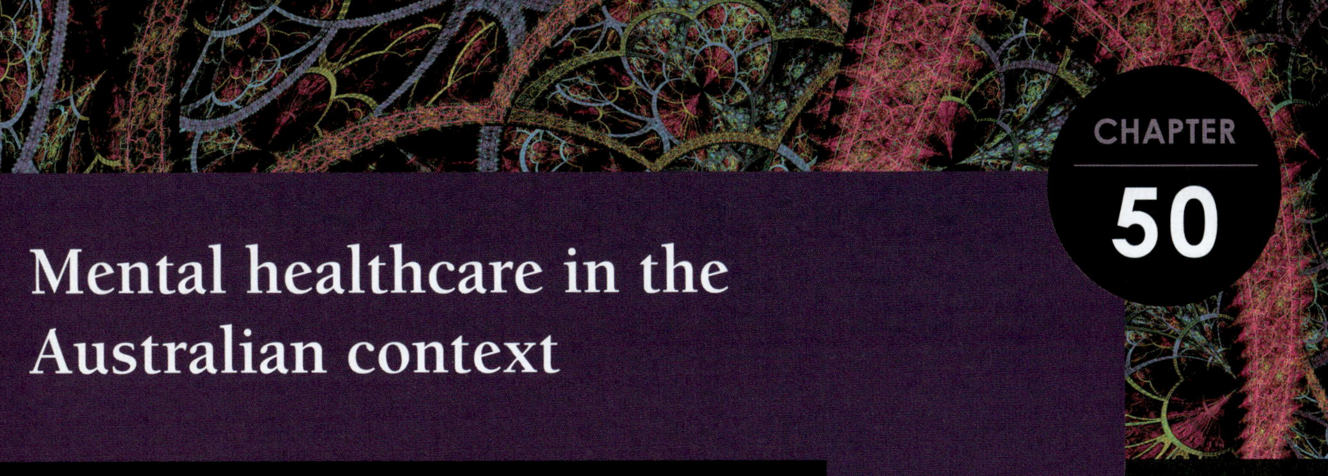

CHAPTER 50

Mental healthcare in the Australian context

Lorna Moxham, Paul Robson, Christopher Patterson

Learning outcomes

- Understand the complexity of definitions related to mental health and mental illness.
- Understand the specialised role of the mental health nurse.
- Appreciate the importance of the personal recovery approach within mental healthcare.
- Identify legislation pertaining to the provision of care for people who have a mental illness.
- Understand the symptoms and signs of psychotic and non-psychotic disorders.

Clinical competencies

- Conduct a mental state examination (MSE) on a person who is thought to have a mental health issue.
- Use an evidence-based approach to design interventions that promote personal recovery.
- Determine priority nursing care, based on assessed data and evidence, to select and implement individualised nursing interventions for the person living with a mental health issue.
- Provide skilled mental health nursing care for people who live with a mental illness.
- Integrate mental health nursing care into an interprofessional focus for people who live with a mental illness.
- Provide education and advocacy to decrease the stigma associated with mental illness.

Key terms

There is no health without mental health! Having good mental health means an increased ability to function, connect, cope and thrive, but mental health exists on a complex continuum, with experiences ranging from optimal states of wellbeing to debilitating states of distress and immense emotional pain (World Health Organization (WHO), 2022a).

In all countries, mental health conditions are highly prevalent. They vary with sex and age. Depressive and anxiety disorders are the most common in both males and females (WHO, 2022a). The incidence of mental ill health is growing—during the first year of the COVID-19 pandemic, rates of already common conditions such as depression and anxiety went up by more than 25% (WHO, 2022a). In Australia, as many as 1 in 4 people are now thought to have a mental health issue. As the burden of mental disorders continues to grow globally, impacts on health and major social, human rights and economic consequences increase.

Mental health knowledge and skills, as well as understanding and acknowledging what we believe and assume (sometimes referred to as mental health literacy), are therefore necessary for nurses working in all areas of nursing practice. Increasing mental health literacy will aid in recognition, management and prevention. Nurses meet and provide care and treatment in a variety of environments, including emergency department (ED), drug and alcohol services, surgical and medical units, critical care units (CCUs), maternity, outpatients, day surgery, baby health clinics, schools, GP surgeries, paediatrics, intensive care units (ICUs), community health, sexual health clinics, pathology and x-ray departments. Mental healthcare is needed everywhere, in all settings and all geographical locations.

Holistic and comprehensive care

Mental health, as an integral part of a person's general health and wellbeing, is a basic human right. Even though a nurse may not undertake practice within a specialised mental health setting, it is highly likely they will provide care for a person with a mental health issue, and the care should be comprehensive and clinically appropriate. It may not be the actual person who is the recipient of direct care; it may be their partner, friend or family member. As nurses, we are beholden to provide the best care we can to all people we interact with. In mental healthcare, the involvement of carers and family is very important and significant others should be included wherever possible. Nurses provide holistic care, across the entire lifespan, which means people are cared for in an inclusive and respectful way, and without judgment. Care and treatment should not 'split' people into physical, social, spiritual or mental health 'parts'—nursing does not compartmentalise. Comprehensive care can be challenging and nurses cannot be expected to be experts in every nursing specialty.

Nurses do, however, need to have an understanding of many discipline areas. In this regard, it is important to be aware that there are a number of different types of knowledge bases that contribute to understanding and knowledge. Figure 50.1 demonstrates where our **knowledge resource base** comes from. In the mental health context, the knowledge resource base is founded on recognition of diversity, mental health literacy, an enriched range of services and supports, and social acceptance and inclusion.

As Figure 50.1 shows, knowledge and beliefs about mental health issues are acquired in different ways. Despite recognising multiple ways of knowing and doing, mental health service provision in Australia is still largely based on the medical model. However, with more consumers and carers gaining a legitimately stronger voice, a social position is being strengthened, with nurses also advocating for a more holistic approach. Nurses need to appreciate that a balanced understanding of a person's mental health does not come only from medical or clinical knowledge. This is important as mental healthcare needs to be seen through many different lenses and, significantly, the lived experience perspective is imperative.

Because of the widespread nature of mental health issues, it is necessary to identify some trends around mental health and illness across Australia (see the 'Fast facts' box).

MENTAL HEALTH AND MENTAL ILLNESS

Mental health and *mental illness* can be difficult terms to understand because there are no universally agreed definitions. While such ambiguity can be frustrating, there are many reasons. One key reason arises from the impossibility of separating mind from body; another results from the many unique and individual ways that humans express themselves. Mental illness, as an expression,

Links to National Patient Safety Standards

NSQHS: Comprehensive Care Standard

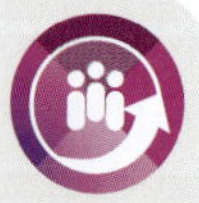

The intention of this standard is to ensure that comprehensive care is provided to the person that is well coordinated and aligned with the person's expressed goals of care and healthcare needs. This standard considers the effect of the person's health issues on their life and wellbeing and is clinically appropriate.

Source: Australian Commission on Safety and Quality in Health Care (ACSQHC) (2021). *National Safety and Quality Health Service Standards* (2nd ed.). Sydney: ACSQHC.

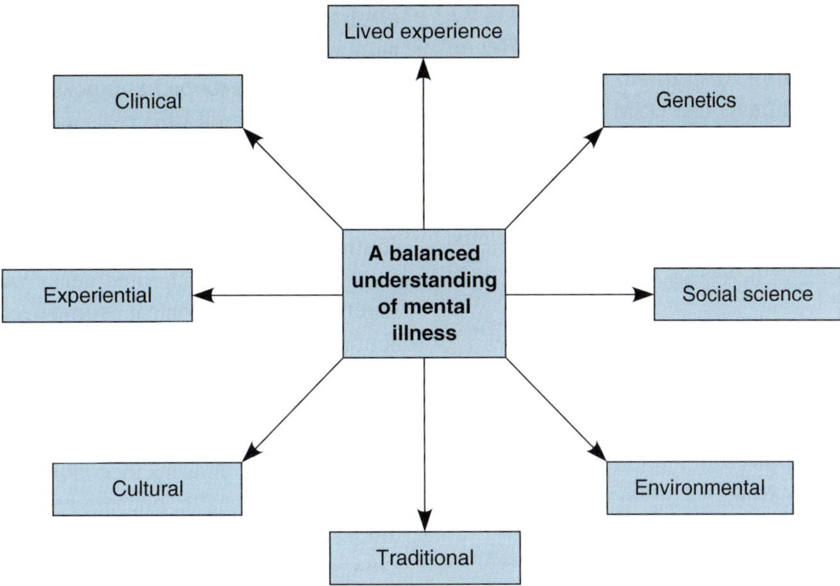

FIGURE 50.1 *Knowledge resource base*

Links to National Patient Safety Standards

NSQHS: Partnering with Consumers Standard

Partnership with consumers applies to every aspect of care and this standard is applicable to all interactions and should be considered when considering nursing treatments and interventions throughout this chapter. In mental health, the saying 'Nothing about me without me' directly links to this standard.

Source: ACSQHC (2021). *National Safety and Quality Health Service Standards* (2nd ed.). Sydney: ACSQHC. © Australian Commission on Safety and Quality in Health Care.

FAST FACTS

The 2021 National Study of Mental Health and Wellbeing (ABS, 2022) estimated that:

- Over 2 in 5 (43.7%) Australians aged 16–85 had experienced a mental disorder during their lifetime.
- Anxiety disorders were the most prevalent type of disorder (16.8%), followed by affective disorders (7.5%) and substance use disorders (3.3%).
- A higher proportion of females than males (44.6% compared with 42.7%) had experienced a mental disorder in their lifetime.
- 16–24-year-olds (39.6%) were most likely to have experienced symptoms of a mental disorder in the previous 12 months, while those aged 75–85 years were the least likely (3.7%).

is also culturally linked and determined, so what might be deemed mental illness in one culture might not be in another.

While it is difficult to arrive at succinct, yet meaningful, definitions of mental illness and mental health, many attempts have been made to conceptualise them. These include:

- lived experience perspectives (expert by experience)
- the medical model (which emphasises processes of diagnosis and treatment and is based on traditional reductionist models of science)
- the psychoanalytical or psychodynamic approach
- neurobiological theories
- cognitive behavioural perspectives
- lay views
- the legal framework
- sociological stances (including social causation, social reaction (labelling theory), holism and the social model of disability).

Just as the definitions of mental health and mental illness are not clear, so too are the causes and then associated nursing care and medical treatments. This makes mental health nursing both complex and challenging. Modern multidisciplinary mental health practice synthesises the application of understandings that are derived from the various conceptual approaches listed above. Despite this, treatment and management often remains heavily dominated by medical models and medical discourse. This is because psychiatrists, as specialist medical practitioners, are trained to identify sick individuals (diagnose), predict the future course of their illness (provide a prognosis), speculate about the cause (identify aetiology), then prescribe a response to the condition, either to cure it or ameliorate its symptoms (medicate).

Diagnosis

The diagnosis of mental illness occurs as a result of an assessment process. The American Psychiatric Association

(APA, 2022) established a set of diagnostic criteria, known as the **DSM** *(Diagnostic and Statistical Manual of Mental Disorders)*. The DSM is used in Australia to diagnose a person thought to have mental illness. The DSM 5 is the current edition.

Another set of diagnostic criteria that is used is called the **International Classification of Diseases (ICD)**, which is the global standard to report and categorise diseases, health-related conditions and external causes of disease and injury. The most recent version is the ICD-11.

Both classification systems are constantly revised and are used by nurses, medical officers, researchers, health information managers, medical coders, policy makers, insurers and health service user organisations.

Psychiatrists are often in powerful and dominant positions within mental health settings (they are often the directors of mental health services at local, state, territory and national levels). As such, medical opinion remains at the fore of any debate about mental health/mental illness. As a result of their medical training, many psychiatrists principally view people through an illness lens when they encounter variations in conduct or when they have to assess someone who is 'different'. The concept of illness—and its associated language, symptoms, therapies and the people who are living with the illness, who are invariably known as 'patients'—legitimises and perpetuates the prevailing public perceptions and attitudes, often at the expense of other possible frameworks.

Significant debate therefore still exists about what constitutes mental health or mental illness. One of the places where discussion occurs is the **Australian College of Mental Health Nurses (ACMHN)**. This college is the peak professional body for mental health nurses in Australia and is overseen by a Board of Directors elected by college members. The ACMHN is recognised as representing the specific interests of mental health nurses in Australia. The ACMHN hosts an annual international conference during which issues such as mental health, mental illness, treatment, policy and particularly mental health nursing practice and research are discussed and debated.

Defining mental health and mental illness

Despite there being no specific universal definition, mental health can be described as a positive state in which the person is responsible, self-directive, displays self-awareness and is generally accepted within a group. Numerous factors impact on mental health, such as genetics, childhood nurturing and life circumstances, including trauma. The nature/nurture debate continues in the field of mental health.

Nature refers to inherited genes and characteristics that are totally out of one's control. Nurture refers to parent–child interactions, sibling interactions and early communication patterns. Positive childhood nurturing refers to the child feeling loved, secure and accepted.

Life circumstances from birth also influence one's mental health. These include socioeconomic status, quality of relationships, physical health, housing and educational success or failure. If influencing factors are positive, a person is more likely to experience positive mental health and a sense of wellbeing.

Mental health is generally defined by essential characteristics rather than a set of statements about a state of health. In order to understand mental health, comparisons are often made between mental health and mental illness. This is done in an attempt to distinguish the 'normal' from the 'abnormal'. In the absence of a universal definition, Figure 50.2 describes the factors that influence a person's mental health, while Table 50.1 offers a set of indicators for mental health.

Stigma

Stigma is still the single most difficult issue that people with a mental illness face (Perlman et al., 2020). When society or communities consistently stigmatise people with mental illness, as has been the case for hundreds of years, such attitudes become internalised. Internalised stigma is a process whereby people with mental illness endorse stereotypes, anticipate social rejection, consider stereotypes to be self-relevant and believe they are devalued members of society. Sensationalist media headlines lead to a perpetuation of such stigma (see Box 50.1).

As the scenario in Box 50.1 demonstrates, *reactions* as a result of this event were considered 'over the top'. Thanks to

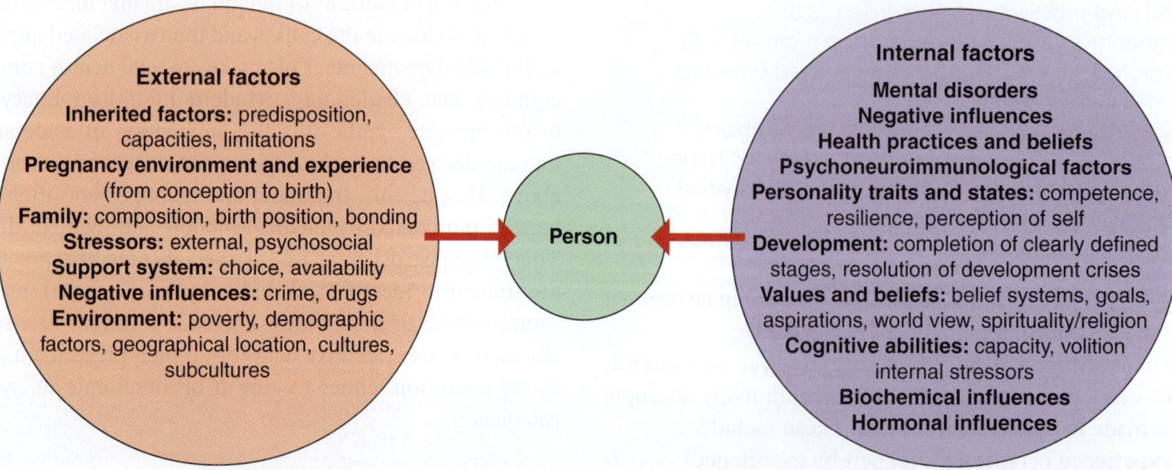

FIGURE 50.2 *Influencing factors for mental health or illness*

TABLE 50.1 Components of mental health

SELF-AWARENESS AND DEVELOPMENT	ENGAGEMENT WITH AND RESPECT FOR OTHERS	ADAPTABILITY AND RESILIENCE	CLARITY AND INSIGHT
Attain and maintain positive self-esteem: • Self-concept • Self-image • Self-esteem Involve self in purposeful, meaningful life work Maintain reasonable expectations concerning self and others Seek self-actualisation Learn from experiences Use talents to fullest Maintain wholesome values and belief system Develop and demonstrate appropriate sense of humour Attain self-defined spirituality	Respect societal rules and sanctions Accept self and others as uniquely different but humanly similar Engage in play Relate to others: • Form relationships • Maintain close, meaningful, loving, adaptive relationships • Work and play well with others • Be intimate, appropriately and selectively • Respond to others in need • Feel and exhibit compassion and empathy towards others • Demonstrate culturally and socially acceptable interpersonal interactions • Manage interpersonal conflict constructively • Give and receive gracefully • Learn from and teach others • Function interdependently	Adapt to social environment Function interdependently Return to usual or higher function after crises Be optimistic Be resilient Find beauty, joy and goodness in self, others and the environment Appreciate life Negotiate each development stage Cope with internal and external stressors in constructive and adaptive ways	Ability to: • Demonstrate mental and physical competence and skills • Perceive self, others and events correctly • Recognise own strengths, weaknesses, capabilities and limitations • Separate fantasy from reality Think clearly: • Problem solve • Use good judgment • Reason logically • Reach insightful conclusions
SELF-CONTROL	**INDEPENDENCE**	**SELF-EXPRESSION**	**PHYSICAL HEALTH**
Control impulses and behaviour Delay gratification	Accept responsibility for actions Function independently	Be creative Express emotions Exhibit congruent thoughts, feelings and behaviours	Presence of anatomical and physiological components necessary to function in the world Absence of signs and symptoms of mental disorder Freedom from excessive mental and emotional disability and pain

BOX 50.1 The story of a person with a mental illness

Consider the case of a person in Queensland, Australia. The person was described on the front page of the *Courier-Mail* (a Queensland newspaper) as 'a paranoid schizophrenic who hacked off his clergyman father's head' (*Courier-Mail*, 23 January 2002). He had left his ward, which was within the grounds of a large psychiatric rehabilitation facility, without permission. Eighty-four hours later, a tired, hungry and thirsty man quietly returned to his ward after having spent the entire time under a cricket shed in the grounds of the psychiatric institution.

In the meantime, following what was reported as 'extensive searching', a maelstrom erupted; the resultant media coverage could be described as nothing less than a feeding frenzy. The man appeared to represent everything that society feared about mental illness—namely, that all people with mental illness are dangerous and unpredictable. In a sense, this man became stigma personified and for weeks people in Queensland were bombarded with news of other 'mentally ill people' on the run. 'Dangerous', 'violent', 'criminal', 'escapees' and 'killer' were all used to describe people who had a mental illness but were currently, and for numerous valid reasons, not in psychiatric hospitals at all. The relentless media barrage, particularly the insinuation that members of the general public were in danger from these 'killers at large', resulted in a reaction few would have expected. First, an inquiry was held to quantify how many 'patients' who were deemed to be criminally insane were absent without leave (AWOL) from mental health facilities. Recommendations from this inquiry included the 'capture' of these so-called AWOL patients. Surprisingly and controversially, given the ethical nature of the issue, the then state premier ordered the release of photographs of 15 'patients' who were described as AWOL; these pictures were published in the *Courier-Mail*. Second, any person then under a forensic order (FO) who was living in the community, despite the fact that their leave had been granted by the treating psychiatrist and the then Patient Review Tribunal (now the Mental Health Review Tribunal), was taken back to hospital under an Involuntary Treatment Order (ITO). Many people who were well and residing in the community were returned to hospital as a result of this unprecedented over-reaction. Others feared that they, too, would be 'taken back to hospital'. Would anyone contemplate doing this to people who have a physical illness, such as a person with diabetes who was not adhering to their insulin regimen?

The tragedy of this so-called 'escape' and its aftermath reached far beyond the city where it occurred. It was acutely felt by people living with mental health issues across the country. The stigma extended to families and their friends, many of whom have also struggled with the discrimination that having a family member with mental health issues brings.

Perhaps media reporting has changed over the years? To critique the evidence, see Chen and Lawrie's (2017) article, Newspaper depictions of mental and physical health. *BJPsych Bulletin, 41*(6), 308–313.

sensationalist media reporting, which still persists, common public perception remains that innocent individuals may become the victim of random acts of violence perpetuated by people with mental health issues.

Generally, people perceive those with mental illness to be dangerous. This perception underpins some destructive stereotypes. Evidence demonstrates that people with mental illness are no more violent than other members of society. In fact, they are often frightened and are among the most vulnerable members of society. That is not to say, though, that they do not get frustrated and angry with things that happen as part of everyday life (as we all do). The media have promulgated negative stereotypes. Public perception is largely influenced by media sources (Burns et al., 2021), and negative portrayals have negative impacts on people who live with mental illness and their family.

Most people living with mental illness do not need inpatient treatment. If they do, admissions are often brief. Effective treatments have removed the need for isolation and confinement in asylums—a common occurrence in the past (see Figure 50.3). The attitude of family, friends and the community towards people with mental illness plays a critical part in determining their quality of life. Attitudes that people, including nurses hold, have a major effect on how the people feel about themselves and on their recovery. Many people with mental illness face isolation and discrimination simply for having an illness, but this is not often the case for people with a physical illness. People with cancer, diabetes, asthma, multiple sclerosis, Alzheimer's disease, Parkinson's disease and heart diseases such as cardiomyopathy are often met with sympathy, but people with mental illnesses are often the butt of jokes, innuendos and scaremongering.

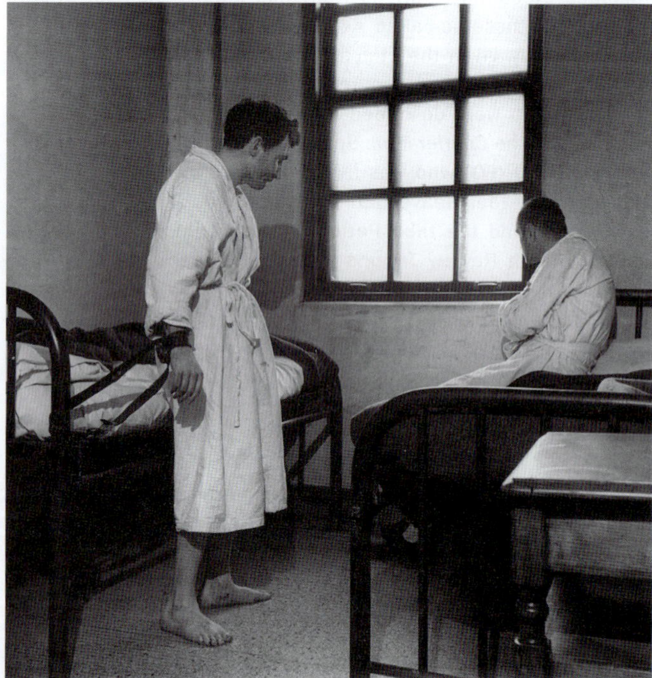

FIGURE 50.3 ***Isolation and confinement in asylums was common treatment for mental illness prior to the 1950s***

Source: Jerry Cooke/Science Source.

Who would get your donation? An organisation that works with people who have cancer, or one that works with people who have a mental illness? Why is it that people donate more for physical conditions when mental health problems affect at least 25% of the population?

The role of the mental health nurse

The role of the mental health nurse is multifaceted, specialised and dynamic. The ACMHN says that:

> *mental health nursing is a specialised field of nursing which focuses on working with consumers to meet their recovery goals. Mental health nurses consider the person's physical, psychological, social and spiritual needs, within the context of the individual's lived experience and in partnership with their family, significant others and the broader community.* (ACMHN, 2022)

Mental health nurses support consumers and their families during life crises and transition periods. They liaise discreetly and efficiently with a range of healthcare providers, provide information and education on mental health maintenance and restoration, coordinate care and provide talking therapy.

Mental health nurses work across the full range of clinical and service settings and across metropolitan, regional and remote areas. They play a significant role in the healthcare system and have the qualifications, skills and experience to provide high-quality mental health nursing care in all contexts (see Figure 50.4). The mental health nursing workforce needs to be flexible and responsive, and able to work with people across the lifespan in a variety of workplace settings.

Mental health nurses' skills, and the roles that they perform, vary according to the context of practice and the level of education, training and experience of the individual nurse.

If you would like to hear about mental health nursing, you can read some testimonials located on the ACMHN website at https://acmhn.org/what-mental-health-nurses-do/.

Mental health nursing has long been recognised as one of the three specialist nursing areas. Psychiatric nursing had separate registration or endorsement in Australia. Previously, students could enter directly into a 3-year hospital-based psychiatric nursing course, graduating with a certificate in psychiatric nursing and registering as a Registered Psychiatric Nurse (RPN). This changed when nursing education moved to the higher education sector. Today, baccalaureate programs (BN) prepare the comprehensive nurse for 'beginning level' practice in all health settings, but many BN students have only limited clinical placements in mental health settings and some get no placements at all in mental health. Some education providers have a 'major' in mental health nursing, where the student nurse can start to specialise, usually in the second year of their BN. For the most part, specialist mental health nursing is now a postgraduate area where RNs undertake a graduate certificate (GradCert), graduate diploma (GradDip), master's, professional doctorate or PhD.

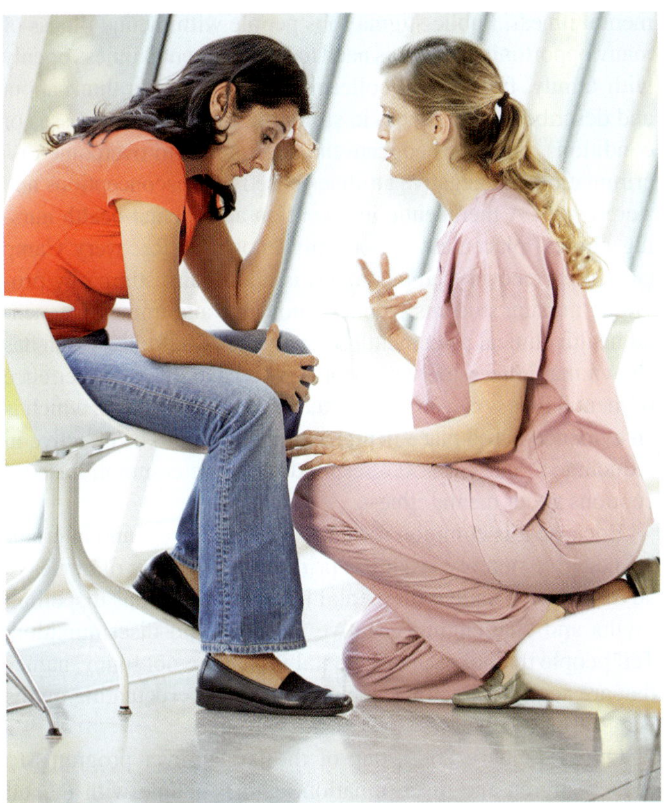

FIGURE 50.4 ***Mental health nurses provide care for people whose lives are affected by mental illness***

Source: Monkey Business Images/Shutterstock.

Mental health nursing in practice

Mental health nurses can aptly be described as the eyes and ears of the multidisciplinary team. Nurses interact with people on a continual basis, observing ADLs and social functioning, monitoring effects (positive and negative) of medication and treatment, and working closely with people and their significant others in a therapeutic manner toward Recovery. Such a person-centred therapeutic relationship places nurses in excellent positions to work collaboratively with the person and their family to provide care. This may include:

- planning, implementing and evaluating interactions to help the person achieve the highest possible quality of life using a Recovery focus (see below)
- the establishment and maintenance of the therapeutic relationship
- monitoring the person's response to nursing and other interventions, including medication efficacy.

Mental health nursing is founded upon a **therapeutic relationship**, a rapport based on empathy and trust with the person, family and significant others. There is increasing evidence suggesting that a positive therapeutic relationship contributes significantly to *recovery*. Mental health nurses are central in forming and maintaining the therapeutic relationship and play a pivotal role in the *recovery* of a person who is living with mental illness. The essence of mental health nursing is therefore not the tasks that are performed, but the positive relationship(s) the nurse develops and maintains. Nursing focus should not be on the illness (the diagnosis that has been given) but on how the person manages on a daily basis. People living with a mental illness are more focused on day-to-day living than the label they have been given.

AREAS OF PRACTICE **Acute inpatient units** could be described as the mental health service's equivalent of high-dependency nursing, but it is important to note that within an inpatient unit in many Australian settings, there are also high-dependency units (for people who are even more acutely unwell). These can be equated to critical or intensive care units in general hospitals. Mental health nurses in these settings need highly developed expertise and skills in observation, assessment, negotiation, de-escalation and milieu management.

Intake team or *acute care team nurses* are often considered the 'gatekeepers' to mental health services. This type of mental health nursing is also acute care. In these settings, the mental health nurse provides short-term interventions and requires highly specialised skills in assessment, psychopharmocology and observing. Mental health nurses on these teams can be required to do their 'work' via the telephone when people call mental health services in crisis. It takes special expertise to be able to conduct an accurate assessment without face-to-face interaction. The role of mental health nurses in this setting is also to be aware of and to liaise with other services and agencies.

Community care coordinators are mental health nurses who undertake their nursing practice by providing continuing care and follow up of people in the community. They used to be called 'case managers', but consumers say, and rightly so, they are not 'cases' to be 'managed'. Care coordinators often have many people to work with and undertake duties such as psychosocial support, psychotherapy and assisting with medication management. Assisting people find accommodation

Links to National Patient Safety Standards

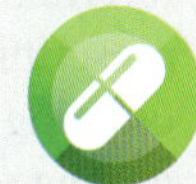

NSQHS: Medication Safety Standard

The intention of this standard is to ensure clinicians 'are competent to safely prescribe, dispense and administer appropriate medicines and to monitor medicine use' and to 'ensure consumers are informed about medicines and understand their individual medicine needs and risks' (ACSQHC, 2021, p. 33).

Source: ACSQHC (2021). *National Safety and Quality Health Service Standards* (2nd ed.). Sydney: ACSQHC. © Australian Commission on Safety and Quality in Health Care.

and employment, as well as linking people in with therapeutic leisure and recreation activities, are also part of the role. **Community mental health nurses** also provide family support and work with the broader community in mental health promotion, advocacy and education. Increasingly, they assist people with National Disability Insurance Scheme (NDIS) applications and packages. Information about the NDIS can be accessed from https://www.ndis.gov.au.

Forensic mental health nurses practise in a range of settings that include courts, police custody centres, prisons, secure hospitals and the community. In 2012, the *Forensic Mental Health Standards of Practice* were published. These can be found at https://www.forensicare.vic.gov.au/wp-content/uploads/2021/08/Forensic-Mental-Health-Nursing-Standards-2012.pdf.

Consultation liaison (CL) nurses have different approaches depending on the setting in which they are practising. This area of mental healthcare is rapidly expanding as a result of the number of people within generalist care settings who also have a mental illness. One approach is having CL nurses in the emergency department (ED) to provide specialist care for someone with a mental health problem. Another CL approach is where the CL nurse provides care to people who are admitted to a general hospital for a non-psychiatric condition. The CL nurse in this instance usually gets a referral from their general nursing or medical colleagues and provides direct consultation with the person or indirect consultation through support, education and advice for colleagues. CL nurses have high-level assessment and interpersonal skills and broad nursing knowledge that enable them to rule out physical causes and work with complex health issues.

A **Mental Health Nurse Practitioner (MHNP)** is a specialist mental health nurse with qualifications at master's degree level. MHNPs are educated and endorsed to function autonomously and collaboratively in advanced and extended clinical roles, and can work in public, private, community and primary healthcare settings. MHNPs are clinical leaders who work from an evidence base and possess advanced skills in clinical leadership, evidence-based practice, health assessment, diagnostic skills, therapeutic management, psychopharmacology, evaluation and collaboration in care. According to the ACMHN, people who see a MHNP can receive additional clinical services associated with the extensions to practice that the Nurse Practitioner role allows. These can include:

- advanced mental health assessment
- clarification and confirmation of diagnosis
- a wide range of treatment options within the Nurse Practitioner's scope of practice
- referrals to specialists
- prescribing medications
- ordering diagnostic investigations
- issuing sick certificates.

STIGMA AND THE ROLE OF THE NURSE As Box 50.1 shows, the general public continues to receive a very distorted picture of people with mental health problems. Sensationalist reporting exacerbates discriminatory attitudes and stigmatising viewpoints that society in general holds towards people with mental illness. Public stigma robs people with mental illness of many opportunities. Nurses need to discuss mental illness openly with family, friends and colleagues. When nurses think about and describe mental illness in similar terms to other illnesses or conditions, this helps educate the community to overcome discrimination and negative attitudes based on misconceptions and stereotypes. A therapeutic intervention and mental health nursing clinical placement opportunity known as Recovery Camp (see http://recoverycamp.com.au) is addressing stigma by providing nursing students with an innovative and immersive mental health clinical placement (Goman et al., 2020). Research has shown that immersion with people who have a lived experience of mental illness can change attitudes. Recovery Camp, which is an evidence-based placement, has been shown to be effective in reducing stigma. Box 50.2 responds to some common misconceptions about mental illness.

Because it is common for individuals to accept and internalise negative stereotypes, it is a prime responsibility of nurses to advocate for people with mental illness. This means dispelling myths and challenging negative attitudes and discrimination. Tell people that jokes about mental illness are not funny, names that are negative are not acceptable and that perpetuating myths is harmful.

On 21 January 2009, one of the largest ever programs to reduce stigma and discrimination against people with mental illness was launched. It was called Time to Change and was UK based. The initiative was funded with £18 million and run by three charities: Mental Health Media, MIND and Rethink. Despite the formal campaign concluding in 2011, two of the charities involved, MIND and Rethink Mental Illness, have continued to evolve the campaign. Importantly, the campaign continues to advocate for changes in community and individual behaviour and not just attitudes toward people with mental illness. You can access the Time to Change website at http://www.time-to-change.org.uk and research about the impact of the campaign at https://www.ncbi.nlm.nih.gov/pmc/articles/PMC7292343/ (Henderson, Potts & Robinson, 2020).

MENTAL HEALTH PROMOTION AND THE ROLE OF THE NURSE Nurses have an important role in promoting mental health. This can be achieved by nurturing healthy attitudes and coping mechanisms through early childhood and adult life. Nurses can empower people by helping them develop appropriate and effective ways to deal with trauma in relationships, situations and events. All nurses, no matter what their discipline area, should provide high-quality support and treatment services that enable people with mental illness to participate fully in all aspects of their life (Recovery-focused care). Even when not on duty, nurses can encourage and assist friends and relatives who may have a mental illness to seek care and obtain treatment. The nurse can then follow up by encouraging engagement and fulfilment of the treatment regimen, just as they would with a person who has a physical illness, disease or injury that requires professional healthcare.

Nurses should encourage, support and undertake research related to mental health. Research contributes to evidence-based practice and helps the community understand causes of mental

BOX 50.2 The facts about mental illness and violence

Are people with mental illness violent?
Having a mental illness does not mean someone will be violent. People receiving treatment for mental illness are no more violent or dangerous than anyone else. To make this clear, it has been calculated that the lifetime risk of someone with an illness such as schizophrenia seriously harming or killing another person is just 0.005%.

Is there a link between mental illness and violence?
Research suggests that people with mental illness are more likely to be victims of violence. Violent behaviour is slightly more likely among people with a psychotic illness, especially in the first episode of illness. It may also be associated with other factors, including the type of person they were before the illness and if they have been violent in the past. It is also associated with drug use such as ice.

Does having an illness such as schizophrenia mean someone will be violent?
Violence is not a symptom of psychotic illnesses, such as bipolar disorder and schizophrenia.

There is a slightly increased possibility someone with a psychotic illness may be violent if they are not receiving treatment, have a previous history of violence or are abusing alcohol or drugs.

Symptoms of psychotic illnesses may include frightening hallucinations and delusions, as well as paranoia. This means there is a small chance someone who is experiencing them may become violent when they are scared and misinterpret what is happening around them. If a person is being effectively treated for psychotic illness and is not abusing alcohol or drugs, there is no more risk they will be violent than anyone else.

Who is most likely to be violent in our society?
Research by the Australian Institute of Criminology indicates the vast majority of violence is committed by males aged 18 to 30. This is more likely when someone has exhibited highly aggressive behaviours previously and has a history of alcohol and/or drug abuse. People in this group are far more likely to be violent than someone with a mental illness.

Where do people learn about mental illness?
The media plays a big part in the way we think about mental illness. Sadly, media often make the link between mental illness and violence appear stronger than it is. There is actually a weak link between mental illness and violence, but many people wrongly believe all people with mental illness are violent.

What can be done to help?
Mental health workers, people with mental illness and their families all agree the most important step is making sure people receive effective treatment. Mental health workers need to know who is most at risk of being violent or of being a victim of violence. Ensuring people receive the right treatment as quickly as possible requires early intervention, especially in the first episode of illness, and ongoing treatment for as long as required. It is also important for everyone to understand that mental illness is not a choice and could happen to anybody.

Source: SANE Australia: https://www.sane.org. Reproduced with permission of SANE Australia, the national mental health charity.

illness; how these illnesses affect people, their families and the community as a whole; how people manage their illness; and how mental illness can be prevented. Importantly, lived experience should be an integral part of mental health nursing research.

Mental health legislation

In 1901, Australia became a federation: a country with different local, state, territory and federal governments. State and territory differences occur in school curricula and holidays, number plates, pension entitlements and laws. Often terminology is also different between jurisdictions. Definitions about mental health and mental illness also differ between jurisdictions. These definitions are outlined in the various **Mental Health Acts** (see Box 50.3) and further demonstrate the complex nature of mental illness and mental healthcare and treatment. Why is it that the states and territories do not differ in their approach to broken legs, appendicitis or aneurysms? Why is mental healthcare different?

Why is mental illness treated so differently?

The various definitions indicate that what *is not* a mental illness is just as important as what *is* a mental illness. This again shows the complexity of defining a mental illness; in fact, some of the mental health legislation does not actually define mental illness.

BOX 50.3 State and territory mental health legislation

Australian Capital Territory—*Mental Health Act 2015.* Available at https://www.legislation.act.gov.au/a/2015-38
New South Wales—*Mental Health Act 2007.* Available at https://legislation.nsw.gov.au/view/html/inforce/current/act-2007-008
Northern Territory—*Mental Health and Related Services Act 2004.* Available at https://legislation.nt.gov.au/en/LegislationPortal/~/link.aspx?_id=73F8E04941FF41BEB5A839A60CCBBEB9&_z=z
Queensland—*Mental Health Act 2016.* Available at https://www.legislation.qld.gov.au/view/pdf/asmade/act-2016-005
South Australia—*Mental Health Act 2009.* Available at https://www.sahealth.sa.gov.au/wps/wcm/connect/public+content/sa+health+internet/about+us/legislation/mental+health+act+2009
Tasmania—*Mental Health Act 2013.* Available at https://www.legislation.tas.gov.au/view/html/inforce/current/act-2013-002
Victoria—*Mental Health Act 2014.* Available at https://www.legislation.vic.gov.au/in-force/acts/mental-health-act-2014/022
Western Australia—*Mental Health Act 2014.* Available at https://www.legislation.wa.gov.au/legislation/statutes.nsf/law_a147019.html

Although mental health legislation across various Australian jurisdictions has similar intent, the differences create major challenges for mobile populations, including nurses. Mental health nurses need to understand and implement different Mental Health Acts as they move across borders when changing jobs. Subtle differences also make it more complicated for people who are managing their own journey of recovery, particularly if they also wish to travel interstate and are subject to an order set down within a Mental Health Act.

The concept of **Recovery** is a recognised and accepted paradigm that has significant implications for people who have mental illness, their carers, mental health professionals and mental health services. Traditional models of mental health service delivery were not focused on Recovery; rather, they focused on containment and control of the individual. The notion of Recovery is embedded in the very personal journey of the person, which is, of course, unique. Research has shown that people with a mental illness can and do recover but Recovery does not necessarily mean a cure; nor does it necessarily mean a return to a pre-illness state. Hope energises the Recovery process and lays the groundwork for the healing process to begin.

Recovery

Contemporary mental healthcare now incorporates Recovery models of care in practice. The Australian Government is committed to the notion of Recovery as a process not an end point. The following information about the Recovery model was sourced from the excellent booklet *Sharing responsibility for recovery: Creating and sustaining recovery oriented systems of care for mental health*: https://www.wmhi.com.au/wp-content/uploads/2013/10/Sharing-Responsibility-For-Recovery.pdf.

Recovery, as it is used in mental health, is the journey towards a valued sense of identity, role and purpose outside the parameters of mental illness. Recovery is about living well despite the limitations resulting from illness, its treatment and personal and environmental conditions. Mental health services that are Recovery focused are underpinned by a fundamental shift in power, attitude and beliefs regarding the prognosis for a person who has been diagnosed with a mental illness. A Recovery approach emphasises mutual respect and collaboration between providers and service users as opposed to individual dependency on the system and a profound loss of personal autonomy.

Recovery-focused service providers create environments that nurture recovery and facilitate the process of recovery, rather than determining its direction. Recovery is considered a journey not an outcome.

The Recovery journey is a unique and personal experience (see Figure 50.5). It has often been said to be about gaining and retaining hope, understanding of one's abilities and limitations, engagement in an active life, personal autonomy, social

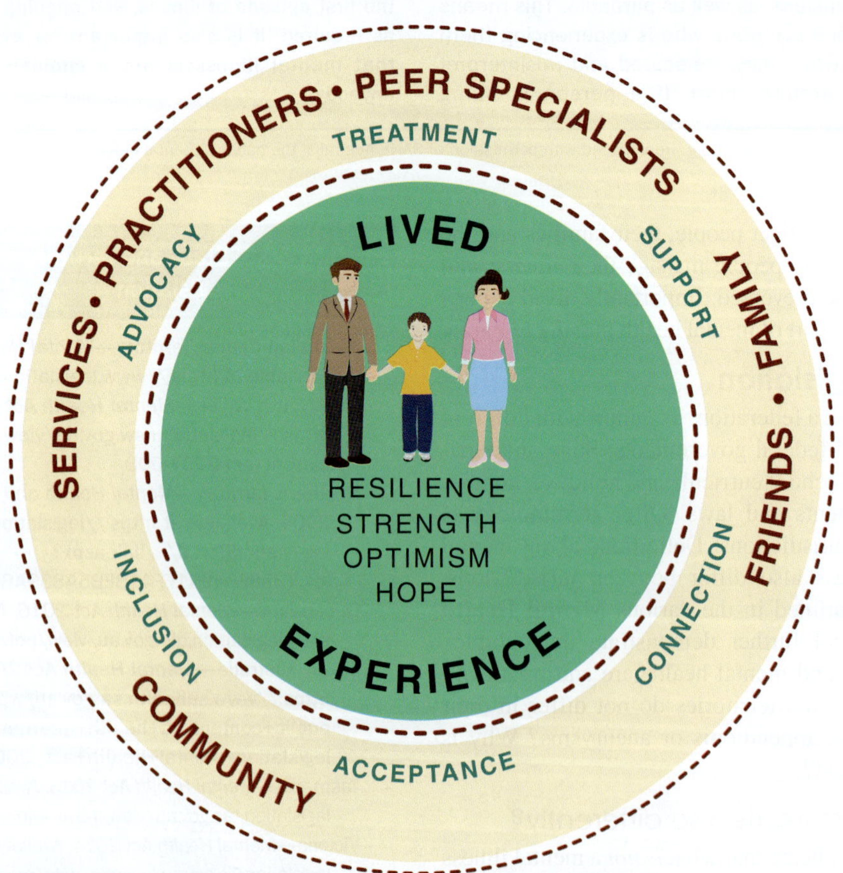

FIGURE 50.5 ***The concept of Recovery***

Source: Glover (2012). Recovery, life long learning, social inclusion and empowerment: Is a new paradigm? In P. Ryan, S. Ramon & T. Greacen, *Empowerment, lifelong learning and recovery in mental health: Towards a new paradigm*. Palgrave Publishers. Figure 2, p. 12. © 2013 Commonwealth of Australia.

identity, meaning and purpose in life, and a positive sense of self. Essentially, the personal view of Recovery is about a life journey of living a meaningful and satisfying life (New South Wales Consumer Advisory Group, 2022).

The New South Wales Consumer Advisory Group explains moving Recovery-oriented service provision from policy to practice on its website, available from https://nswcag.org.au.

HOPE **Hope** is the foundation or guiding principle of Recovery. Hope is the belief that things do not have to remain the same and that change for the better can and does happen. Hope instils the belief that it is possible for someone to have a meaningful life while living with a mental illness. An approach based on hope concentrates on a person's strengths, with a focus on the future. Nurturing hope celebrates all successes rather than expecting and insisting on large and rapid change. Setting smaller goals means they are realistic and much more likely to be achieved. Positive reinforcement occurs because change has happened. This in turn provides future hope. Hope is about being positive and is important for the person to hold on to, but is equally important for others to have for the person. The positive impact that the hope of others can have on an individual with mental illness, when all seems bleak, cannot be underestimated. What do we have if we have no hope?

CONSIDERATION FOR PRACTICE

Mental health nurses can be the holders of hope. When a person expresses little or no hope, offer to hold their hope in your hands. Explain how you will care for it and nurture it and when they are ready, you will hand it back.

ACTIVE SENSE OF SELF For some people with mental illness, their sense of self can become lost and their identity can revolve around their illness. It is very important that mental health nurses do not perpetuate this by referring to the person as 'the schizophrenic' or 'the depressive'. This kind of language is easy to fall into, but what it does is put the illness first, in front of the person. It is very disempowering and serves to help destroy an already fragile sense of self. It is also stigmatising.

Nurses need to remember that having an illness is only one part of a person. Having a positive self-image comes from being treated as a whole person instead of just a part—this is called an **active sense of self**. Imagine if you were to be compartmentalised by only being referred to as a 'redhead' or a 'waiter'. There is far more to a person than the colour of their hair or their job. It devalues the complex person we all are if only a single component of us is referred to. Recovery, then, goes beyond just merely functioning. It is the development of meaningful existence and a sense of purpose. Everyone needs a reason to get up in the morning and our sense of purpose is developed through things such as relationships and work.

DISCOVERY In mental health, **discovery** means that peo-ple with mental illness deserve equality and respect. People who live with mental illness struggle every day with stereotypes that are perpetuated in the media (see Mindframe: https://mindframe.org.au). They are the most stigmatised and discriminated group in society. Unconditional positive regard is what nurses should afford people.

CONNECTEDNESS Recovery is a social process and correlates to the strength of people's social networks. It involves being with other people and connecting with the world. There are times when we all enjoy solitude, but mostly humans are social creatures and need company. Humans actually need interpersonal relationships in order to be mentally healthy. To make social connections, social roles must be established. This is often hard for the person who has a mental illness as society is not very accepting of '**differentness**' and, as we have already discussed, subscribes to myths and stereotypes that are simply untrue.

In fostering social connectedness, issues relating to community integration and full community participation need to be considered. Community integration is a concept drawn from the larger disability and civil rights movements and is founded upon the belief that all people have a right to full community participation and full community membership. This includes jobs, relationships with people who don't have a mental illness and appropriate and affordable housing.

PERSONAL RESPONSIBILITY It is the people who are affected by the mental health problem who hold the key to their own recovery, not service providers. Service providers such as mental health nurses need to ensure that people with mental health problems are recognised as whole people who are self-determining, able to make their own choices and able to take **personal responsibility** and live with the consequences of their decisions. Service providers, who are often risk averse, can find handing responsibility to the person a challenge. Recovery occurs when people are empowered to take ownership and when they can take an active role in their own recovery process. **Empowerment** is vital for correcting the learned helplessness that many people experience as a result of long-term interactions with a mental health system. The importance of people participating in their own healthcare has long been recognised as an essential element of effective service provision. This right is included in the WHO *Declaration of Alma-Ata* (1978). It is also consistent with the principles stated in the *National Standards for Mental Health Services 2010*, the *Fifth National Mental Health and Suicide Prevention Plan* and Vision 2030, which shapes the national direction for mental health and wellbeing in Australia. These each serve to highlight the need for care to be focused on the needs of the individual, rather than the service.

In 2012, The Council of Australian Governments (COAG) released the *Roadmap for National Mental Health Reform 2012–2022*. This document, often simply referred to as 'The Roadmap', reaffirmed a commitment by state and territory governments to support the federal initiatives with a shared vision for mental health reform. The *National Mental Health and Suicide Prevention Plan* (COAG, 2022) has five pillars based on the principles of Prevention, Compassion and Care (see https://www.health.gov.au/sites/default/files/documents/2021/05/the-australian-government-s-national-mental-health-and-suicide-prevention-plan-national-mental-health-and-suicide-prevention-plan.pdf).

While much attention has been placed on national initiatives in recent years, individual state and territory governments have also implemented their own suite of state/territory-specific mental health action plans and initiatives. Mental health is, and will remain for many years to come, a national health priority area.

The Commonwealth Government, having acknowledged the full significance of growing national mental health issues, committed to a raft of new and expanded mental health reforms. This includes increased expenditure, which is needed given that billions of dollars are spent annually in Australia on mental-health-related services. While a considerable sum by any standards, it is, however, a lot less than the amount spent on physical illnesses, despite the fact that mental illness in the community is growing, especially as a result of COVID-19. Perhaps we need to ask why governments continue to concentrate their funding on physical illnesses while acknowledging that mental health is a national priority.

Recovery versus rehabilitation

The following sums up the difference between rehabilitation and Recovery:

> *Rehabilitation refers to the services and technologies that are made available to disabled persons so that they may learn to adapt to their world. Recovery refers to the lived or real-life experience of persons as they accept and overcome the challenge of the disability.* (Deegan, 1988)

The aim of rehabilitation is the restoration of function and the minimisation of disability. Rehabilitation does this through the development of strengths, restoration of hope, environmental modifications, enhancement of vocational potential and maximisation of social and recreational networks.

Recovery therefore forms the basis upon which rehabilitation services can be developed, but rehabilitation services should not be considered the only vehicle for Recovery. Rather, rehabilitation services are just one component in a framework that ensures hope, respect and pathways to community participation within a comprehensive service system that collectively works towards the individualised goal of Recovery.

Assisting Recovery

People with mental illness describe helpful strategies. These include:

- *ventilation*: being able to converse with others; sharing concerns
- *reality testing*: having people assist in maintaining clear distinctions between reality and distortions of thought
- *material support*: help with financial, housing and transport issues
- *social approval and integration*: receiving reassurance that people are accepting them and providing a sense of belonging
- *constancy*: associating with people they knew before they became unwell, connecting current identity with 'illness' identity
- *motivation*: receiving encouragement to achieve higher levels of occupational and social functioning
- *role modelling*: observing the behaviour of others and incorporating appropriate behaviour into own lifestyle
- *symptom monitoring*: having others alert them to manifestations of symptoms
- *problem solving*: discussing problems and getting concrete, solution-focused feedback
- *empathic understanding*: being understood by people important to them
- *reciprocal relating*: becoming an equal partner, able to share and be of assistance to others
- ***insight***: acquiring more complete and accurate understanding of themselves.

Part of the nursing processes that all nurses need to appreciate is the importance of gathering sound data and undertaking an assessment that provides enough information to collaboratively establish a beginning path of action. Probably the most common of these, and one that all nurses should have a good understanding of and be competent in, is the mental state assessment.

Assessing people for signs of mental illness

MENTAL STATE EXAMINATION (MSE)

A **mental state examination (MSE)** is a systematic assessment that provides a picture of what a nurse observes and hears during an interaction or interview with a person (see Box 50.4). The MSE is for that particular interaction only. It is important to remember that a person's mental state can often change. An MSE can help recognise deterioration that the mental health nurse can then respond to.

An MSE is not only undertaken by specialist mental health clinicians. Nurses use their skills to conduct MSEs in many healthcare settings. In fact, you are probably applying some of the elements of an MSE already. When you first meet someone, you 'assess' them: who you decide to sit next to on the bus or train or in the movie theatre; when you see an old friend after a time apart, you check out what they are wearing, how they are behaving, what sort of things they are talking about, how their mood seems. All of these are elements of an MSE.

The MSE is part of a bigger picture. A more complete, holistic (biopsychosocial) assessment needs to be undertaken while being mindful of the context of the person's presentation and their history. Think of someone's life as a jigsaw—it is made up of many pieces. A full mental health assessment includes

BOX 50.4 Components of a mental state assessment

Identifying information
Name
Preferred pronouns
Age
Gender/identity
Sexual orientation
Occupation/income
Cultural affiliation
Religion/spirituality
Next of kin/emergency contact

Presenting problem
What brought the person to seek help?
What do they see as the problem?
Appearance
Hygiene
Grooming and dress
Posture
Eye contact
Scars/marks/tattoos/piercing/ needle sites
Appearance versus stated age
Overall appearance

Behaviour
Tics/tremors
Calm
Agitated
Hyperactive
Rigidity
Facial movements
Unusual movements or gestures
Catatonia

Speech (assessment of the person's ability to communicate vocally)
Tone
Rapid/slow
Pressured
Loud/soft
Fluency (hesitant, mute)
Repetition

Attitude to interview
Cooperative
Hostile
Friendly
Combative
Aloof
Suspicious
Guarded
Apathetic
Distant

Thought processes
Blocking
Flight of ideas
Clang associations
Tangentiality
Loose associations
Circumstantiality
Echolalia
Word salad
Concrete thinking

Thought content
Delusions
Paranoia
Phobias
Magical thinking
Poverty of speech
Obsessions
Risk:
- Self-harm
- To others
- To reputation
- Of dependence/institutionalisation

Mood (objective—ask the person to describe their mood). Use the person's words to describe what they feel is:
- Sad
- Elated
- Fearful
- Worried
- Angry
- Guilty
- Happy
- Hopeless
- Irritable
- Mixed (anxious and depressed)

Affect (subjective—the clinician's view) = What do you observe?
Is the person:
- Flat
- Blunted
- Diminished
- Appropriate
- Inappropriate

Perceptual disturbances
Hallucinations
Visual
Auditory:
- Command
- Loud/soft
- Commenting
- Discussing
- Tactile
- Olfactory
- Gustatory
- Illusions
- Depersonalisation

Memory/cognition
Orientation (time, place and person)

Memory (ability to store, retain and recall information, both recent and remote)
General: alertness and cooperation
Attention: WORLD backwards and serial sevens (consider education level)
Language: naming and repetition
Calculation: division and subtraction
Abstraction: proverbs and similarities

Insight and judgment
Awareness of illness
- Do you consider that you are ill in any way?
- What has brought you here today?
- Do you have a physical or a mental illness?
- Are you suffering from a mental health problem? What is it?
- Correct labelling of abnormality:
- You described several things that are happening. These are ...
- What is your explanation of these experiences?

Willingness to take treatment:
- How do you feel about being in hospital ... coming to the clinic ...?
- How do you feel about taking medication?
- Has the medication been helpful?
- Have any other treatments been helpful?
- What helps you remain well?
- What supports do you have?

Impulse control
- Can the person control urges of anger, laughter, self-harm?

information about why a person has sought help, any significant mental health or medical history, current medications, drug or alcohol use, family history and current family circumstances, developmental history, their social situation and current level of functioning, including sleep, self-care, spirituality, diet and sexual health.

People often present for help as a result of the impact that their symptoms are having on their level of functioning. This frequently includes situations where things feel overwhelming such as when a person's mood is so low they wish they could die, or their **anxiety**—excessive worry about everyday life events with no obvious reasons for this worry—has become so great they cannot leave home without having a panic attack. Health practitioners, however, are often focused on the need for a diagnosis. While diagnosis can be important, the 'label' is not what

Links to National Patient Safety Standards

NSQHS: Recognising and Responding to Acute Deterioration Standard

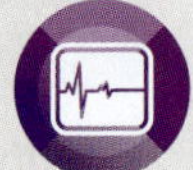

The intent of this standard is to 'ensure that a person's acute deterioration is recognised promptly and appropriate action is taken. Acute deterioration includes physiological changes, as well as acute changes in cognition and mental state' (ACSQHC, 2021). The latter can be assessed by a nurse conducting a thorough MSE.

Source: ACSQHC (2021). *National Safety and Quality Health Service Standards* (2nd ed.). Sydney: ACSQHC. © Australian Commission on Safety and Quality in Health Care.

the person is concerned with. People with mental illness, like all of us, generally just want their life to improve. The needs of the person seeking help should be at the forefront of all nursing care.

The process of assessment is in itself an intervention. This is because the nurse is spending time engaging with the person. An MSE has formal terms and processes that we will now examine. A framework for conducting the assessment is also outlined. There are many assessment tools in use. The following outlines the main components. It is beholden upon the nurse conducting an MSE to make the person feel comfortable about expressing their thoughts and feelings without fear of negative judgment. A conversational approach, rather than a set of formal closed questions, is likely to make the person feel calmer and less anxious. This will result in greater rapport with the nurse and therefore better information. Use open-ended questions and be conscious of your own non-verbal responses and body language. People can tell if you have a genuine interest in them or are just 'going through the motions'. People with mental illness are no less sensitive to this. Validating feelings is always helpful. Where possible, sit with the person and/or their family.

The assessment process cannot be rushed. Often people who have mental illness feel anxious, afraid and vulnerable, and may fear that nurses will judge them negatively. The more patience and respect shown, the faster the nurse will gather information and the more accurate it will be. Accurate information is needed to form the basis of a comprehensive and holistic assessment.

TYPES OF MENTAL ILLNESS

The brevity of this chapter does not allow for an in-depth examination of the various types of mental illness. Broadly speaking, mental illness falls into two groupings—psychotic disorders and non-psychotic disorders.

Psychotic disorders

Psychosis describes a state in which a person's reasoning and thinking (**cognition**) are distorted, leading to a loss of contact with reality. Psychosis, like most mental illnesses, is episodic in nature. People who experience psychotic disorders are not out of touch with reality all the time. Instead, when someone is experiencing psychosis, they are having what is known as a psychotic episode. Such an occurrence describes the state of mind that the person is currently in.

A psychotic episode can occur in different contexts; for example, in schizophrenia, as part of a drug-induced state, in affective illnesses such as depression or mania, and where there is an established physically defined brain disease or impairment, including brain tumours or even epilepsy.

A psychotic episode can be a frightening and confusing event for the person experiencing it, and for their carers and friends. Approximately 3 in every 100 people will experience a psychotic episode at some time, and a psychotic episode usually first occurs between the ages of 15 and 35 years. Of this group, fewer than 4.5 people per 1,000 will seek contact with specialised public mental health services. Sometimes a psychotic episode has a rapid onset (a few days), but often the onset of a psychotic episode is more gradual, over a period of weeks or months. When the onset is more gradual, individuals and their families will often describe how things 'haven't been quite right' for some time. A psychotic episode requires treatment, with studies showing that the earlier the intervention, the better the outcome for the person.

The main distinguishing feature of a psychotic disorder is the person's loss of contact with reality. The person may not be aware of this, however. Two of the key symptoms that a nurse might observe in a person who is experiencing a psychotic disorder are delusions and hallucinations.

Delusions

Delusions are fixed false beliefs that are not a normal part of the person's cultural or religious/spiritual environment and that cannot be altered by logic. A person who has a delusion is absolutely convinced that what they think is true. It cannot be argued with. A nurse who tries to dispel the delusion and argues with the person runs the risk of becoming incorporated into the delusion and being perceived as combative. Delusions are often complex and can be difficult to comprehend, especially when they incorporate very unusual beliefs. Delusions can manifest as a person who believes they have chips inserted into their brain to track their thoughts and feelings, or that they were attached to a genetic line of descendants from gangsters located in spy organisations, or that they are working for prime ministers, ASIO or presidents. Delusions that involve the belief that the person is being followed, controlled or watched are common. Such beliefs can be very distressing and cause the person to act in ways they would not normally act. There are many different types of delusions. Some include:

- *delusions of grandeur*: beliefs of great importance or extraordinary powers or abilities (e.g. the person believes they are royalty, the president or a superhero)

- *somatic delusions*: beliefs that something odd is happening to their body, that they have a disease or that part of their body is missing or has been changed in some way, despite medical evidence to the contrary (e.g. the person believes they have no stomach)
- *delusions of reference*: beliefs that the behaviour of others, events, objects or information such as television, songs or newspapers contain messages that are specifically meant for them (e.g. the person believes that car number plates send special messages)
- *delusions of persecution/paranoia*: beliefs of being pursued, watched, tracked or followed (e.g. the person believes that a government agency is following them).

Hallucinations

A **hallucination** is an alteration in sensory perception. It occurs when a person experiences a sensation of something that is not objectively present. A person can experience hallucinations in any of the senses—auditory (hearing), visual (sight), olfactory (smell), tactile (touch) and gustatory (taste).

- *Auditory*: the most common type of hallucination relates to hearing something that others cannot. The sounds (voices, music, tapping etc.) can be 'inside' or 'outside' the head. They are real and should never be dismissed as a joke. What the person hears can be of any nature. Auditory hallucinations can be pleasant but can also be frightening, threatening or critical. Voices may comment on what the person is doing or tell them they are wrong or that they should be doing something else or that they are worthless. On the other hand, the voices may be kind, comforting or neutral. Sometimes voices command a person to do something. The name given to this is *command hallucinations* and, depending on what the voices are commanding the person to do, they can pose a threat to the safety of the person or to others. It is very important that the nurse establishes what it is that the person is being commanded to do. Refer back to the MSE and note that when assessing perceptual disturbances, it is important to ascertain the content of the voices. Yet other voices may repeat the person's thoughts. Sometimes the person may hear two or more voices having a conversation about them, or several voices at once shouting or yelling at them. Sometimes it may not be a voice/s. People have described hearing an orchestra, birds, animals, drums and all manner of sounds. As with voices, these sounds are not imagined and brain-imaging studies suggest that voices arise from parts of the brain in the left temporal lobe that are ordinarily involved in perceiving spoken speech.
- *Visual*: things or people are seen that cannot be seen by others. Hallucinations are not illusions. An accurate assessment (MSE) will ascertain the difference. An **illusion** is a distortion of sensory perception and, therefore, reality. It is a misinterpretation of a true sensation and is shared by most people.
- *Olfactory*: if a person experiences olfactory hallucinations, they smell things that others cannot. These smells may be good or bad and can have an effect on what the person eats.
- *Gustatory*: if a person experiences gustatory hallucinations, food may taste as if it is bad, contaminated or poisoned. If this is the case, the nurse has to be very skilful in order to get the person to have enough sustenance.
- *Tactile*: with this type of hallucination, sensations are experienced that have not actually occurred or are sensed differently from the way they usually are—for example, the person may feel as though spiders, bugs or ants are crawling over their skin, or that they are being touched by someone. Tactile hallucinations are said to be common in people who use the methamphetamine ice.

Types of psychotic disorders

DRUG-INDUCED PSYCHOSIS Using certain drugs, coming down from them or withdrawing can precipitate psychotic symptoms. It is common to see people who have a drug-induced psychosis present with delusions and hallucinations. Sometimes these symptoms wane within a few days as the effects of the substances wear off, and the person may not experience another episode unless they continue to use drugs. However, for some people the effects can last for a long time, even after abstinence. If someone has an underlying vulnerability to a psychotic disorder such as schizophrenia, the psychotic episode can last much longer, and may be triggered by the initial substance use. Drugs such as methamphetamines are often linked to psychotic episodes. See also Lowe et al. (2019) for a review of cannabis and mental illness.

ORGANIC PSYCHOSIS The importance of ascertaining possible physical causes of what may appear to be a mental illness cannot be underestimated. Sometimes a physical injury or disease that affects the brain can be the cause of an organic psychosis. Such conditions include brain tumours and infections, dementia, delirium, cardiovascular accident and some vitamin deficiencies. Treating the underlying physical problem is the main intervention.

BRIEF REACTIVE PSYCHOSIS A traumatic or very stressful event in someone's life, such as the death of a loved one, a physical or sexual assault, or a natural disaster, can cause a psychotic episode. During a brief reactive psychosis the symptoms can be severe and appear quickly. Symptoms can also rapidly abate.

DELUSIONAL DISORDER In a delusional disorder, the main sign is that the person has a strong belief in something that is not true (see previous examples of delusions). People who have a delusional disorder may not experience any other symptoms of mental illness. If the delusions do not affect their lives as such, they can usually continue to manage their responsibilities, and their behaviour may not be very different from usual. Some delusions may not interfere with life as much as others. For example, a delusion where a person believes that all women who have purple hair, wear green Versace jeans and are very tall are dangerous is not likely to cause alarm because meeting a person who fits this description is not very likely. However, if a person believes that men under 25 who drive white cars are dangerous, then this is likely to have an impact on the person's life because it is highly probable they will encounter this scenario. The effect is dependent on the nature and content of the delusion.

SCHIZOPHRENIA **Schizophrenia** is a mental illness that affects approximately 1 person in every 100. People who live with this psychotic disorder often experience hallucinations, delusions and thought disorder (see Figure 50.6). The onset of schizophrenia can be rapid, with acute symptoms developing quickly, or it may be slower, developing over months or even years. Some people experience only one episode, but for others it is a lifelong condition. First onset is often in adolescence and early adulthood, but it can occur for the first time in older people. Schizophrenia refers to a change in a person's mental function. A person who has schizophrenia does not have a 'split personality' although this is how this condition is often described, especially in the media. People with schizophrenia may experience changes to their own personality as a result of disturbed perceptions and thoughts.

There are different types of schizophrenia, but it normally has three phases:

1. *Prodromal phase*: early warning signs are present; something is 'not quite right'.
2. *Acute phase*: symptoms of a psychosis are observed, such as hallucinations and/or delusions and/or thought disorder.
3. *Recovery phase*: people return to their day-to-day lives, with the help of treatment.

BIPOLAR AFFECTIVE DISORDER is the name given to what was previously known as manic depressive psychosis. Bipolar disorder describes recurrent episodes of 'up and down' mood swings. These can range from elation and excitement to sadness and depression. When people experience extremes in mood it can be difficult for them to manage day-to-day responsibilities such as work, finances and family commitments. Episodes of mania (see Box 50.5) and episodes of depression (see Box 50.6) can last for a short time (days) or for a longer time (months). There are four basic types of bipolar disorder, all of which involve clear changes in mood, energy and activity levels:

1. Bipolar I disorder involves periods of severe mood episodes from mania to depression.
2. Bipolar II disorder is a milder form of mood elevation, involving milder episodes of hypomania alternating with periods of severe depression.
3. Cyclothymic disorder describes brief periods of hypomanic symptoms alternating with brief periods of depressive symptoms that are not as extensive or as long lasting as seen in full hypomanic episodes or full depressive episodes.
4. Mixed features refers to the occurrence of simultaneous symptoms of opposite mood polarities during manic, hypomanic or depressive episodes. It is marked by high energy, sleeplessness and racing thoughts. At the same time, the person may feel hopeless, despairing, irritable and suicidal.

Rapid cycling describes having four or more mood episodes within a 12-month period. Episodes must last for a minimum number of days in order to be considered distinct episodes. Some people also experience changes in polarity from high to low or vice versa within a single week, or even within a single day.

People who have bipolar disorder can experience psychotic episodes. The symptoms usually match the person's current mood. If a person is depressed, they might hear voices that tell

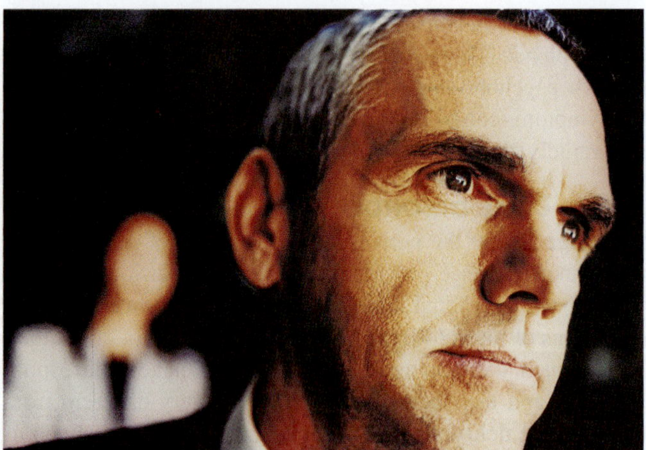

FIGURE 50.6 ***Some people with schizophrenia experience hallucinations and delusions***

Source: © Triangle Images/Getty Images.

BOX 50.5 Symptoms of mania

- An elated, happy mood or an angry, irritated mood
- Increased energy or activity levels
- Decreased sleep/less need for sleep/difficulty getting to sleep
- Increased talking, and talking louder and faster than usual
- More thoughts, and faster thinking than usual
- Overly ambitious plans and reckless behaviour (e.g. overspending or engaging in careless or potentially dangerous behaviour)
- Grandiose delusions

BOX 50.6 Signs and symptoms of depression

- Feelings of sadness, dejection, indifference or despondency
- Reduced motivation, apathy and low energy
- Changes in sleep patterns
- Changes in appetite or weight
- Poor concentration and memory
- Reduced capacity to enjoy life—nothing is pleasurable
- Feelings of guilt and worthlessness
- Reduced libido
- Suicidal thoughts

them they are horrible or no good, or direct the person to hurt themself. A person who is manic, however, might believe that they are very special and can do remarkable things (delusions of grandeur).

Some famous people who are thought to have had bipolar disorder include Andrew Johns, Catherine Zeta-Jones, Mariah Carey, Jimi Hendrix, Russell Brand, Edgar Allen Poe, Jean-Claude Van Damme, Sinéad O'Connor, Selena Gomez and Kanye West.

PSYCHOTIC DEPRESSION People who experience psychotic depression may have many of the same symptoms that people with bipolar disorder experience when they are depressed (see Figure 50.7). People who have psychotic depression, though, do not experience periods of elation or mania. When people have psychotic depression they tend to experience symptoms that match their mood; for example, they might hear voices that tell them to kill themselves, or voices that make fun of them, or they may experience delusions.

Non-psychotic disorders

Throughout life, at some point we all experience strong feelings of sadness, tension or fear. For some people though, these feelings are so overpowering they have difficulty coping with everyday activities, including those that they have been successfully managing for years. The processes of going to work, enjoying leisure time and maintaining relationships become so intense the person is unable to perform them.

Such all-consuming feelings are not often evident to others. For the person experiencing them, they can cause considerable personal distress and anguish. Such mental illnesses are labelled as non-psychotic illnesses. They are common for many people and the list below demonstrates how widespread and prevalent they are. It is highly likely that someone with one of these illnesses will require care within the general nursing setting. Nurses themselves can also have these illnesses. Given that mental illness affects 1 in 4 people, it is highly likely that someone you know, are related to, study with or work with has a mental health issue. Maybe it is even you!

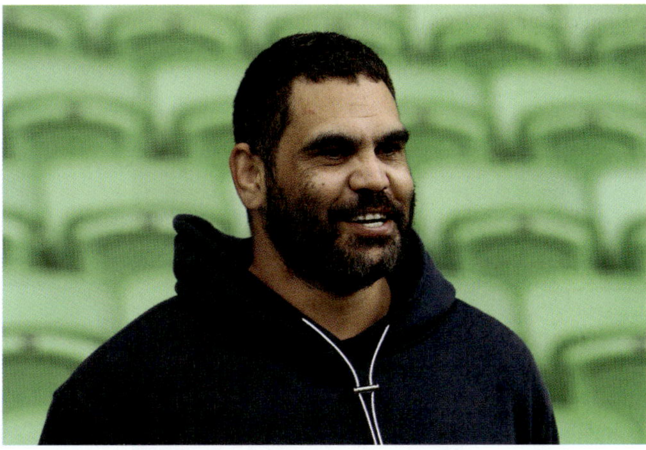

FIGURE 50.7 ***Highly successful individuals, like the former NRL player Greg Inglis, are not immune from mental illness. Nurses conducting an MSE need to make the person feel comfortable expressing their thoughts and feelings without fear of negative judgment***

Source: Kelly Defina/Getty Images.

- Adjustment disorder
- Anxiety disorders
- Post-traumatic stress disorder
- Phobias
- Obsessive compulsive disorder
- Dissociative disorders
- Eating disorders:
  - Bulimia nervosa
  - Anorexia nervosa
- **Impulse control** disorders:
  - Pyromania
  - Kleptomania
  - Pathological gambling
- Mood disorders
- Sexual disorders:
  - Paedophilia
  - Necrophilia
  - Fetishism
- Sleep disorders:
  - Night terror disorder
  - Insomnia
  - Narcolepsy
- Sexual dysfunctions:
  - Gender identity disorder
  - Sexual aversion disorder
  - Premature ejaculation
- Somatoform disorders:
  - Hypochondriasis disorder
  - Pain disorder
- Substance use disorders:
  - Substance abuse
  - Substance dependency
- Personality disorders:
  - Antisocial personality disorder
  - Narcissistic personality disorder
  - Borderline personality disorder.

Most non-psychotic illnesses can be effectively treated, usually with a combination of medication and psychotherapies. Treatment helps the person understand their illness and gain insight into what exacerbates their symptom. This assists with management strategies and recovery.

The most common type of non-psychotic disorder is depression. Depression is so commonplace that, globally, more than 300 million people are thought to have the illness (WHO, 2022b).

Depression

We have all felt sad or 'blue' sometimes. Having a low mood can result from something we have experienced: a loss, relationship difficulties, trauma or an event to which we can attribute feeling down. Sometimes people experience low moods for no apparent reason. Feeling 'down' can, though, become an illness. Indications that a person may have a depressive illness include when a low mood becomes very severe and lasts for 2 weeks or more, and when the low mood interferes with the person's ability to function.

Depression affects both physical and psychological functions. A person with depression may have difficulty getting out of bed, be unable to care for their ADLs, have difficulty coping at work and have constipation (related to not eating; lack of mobility). Many famous people are said to have had depression: Schumann, Virginia Woolf, Rachmaninov, Tchaikovsky, Dwyane Johnson, Billy Joel, Buzz Aldrin, Katy Perry, Kurt Cobain, Vincent van Gogh, Lady Gaga, Winston Churchill, Sheryl Crow, Gwyneth Paltrow and Rosie O'Donnell, to name but a few.

The signs and symptoms listed in Box 50.6 is not exhaustive and having one or two symptoms is not necessarily indicative of a depressive illness. The nurse needs to ascertain thoughts of self-harm, which then need to be further explored so that risk can be properly assessed.

Treatments in mental health

Treatments for mental illness are as varied and diverse as the illnesses themselves but largely fall into two categories: physical treatments and psychological therapies.

Physical treatments

There are a number of types of physical treatments. The most common is medication.

MEDICATIONS One of the roles of a mental health nurse is to administer, monitor and evaluate drug therapy. Medications are used widely for many different mental health issues. Medications fall broadly into a number of categories, including antidepressants, anxiolytics, antipsychotics and mood stabilisers (see Figure 50.8). The mental health nurse needs to engage with the person regarding their pharmacological treatment and provide psychoeducation with the aim of medication management.

BRAIN STIMULATION THERAPIES Brain stimulation therapies involve activating or touching the brain directly with electricity, magnets or implants. These therapies are usually focused on mood and anxiety-type disorders. Brain stimulation therapies include vagus nerve stimulation, repetitive transcranial magnetic stimulation, magnetic seizure therapy and deep brain stimulation. Some of these are relatively new and are currently considered experimental methods.

ELECTROCONVULSIVE THERAPY (ECT) is considered particularly useful for someone who is suffering with severe depression or life-threatening mania. Before ECT is administered, the person is sedated with a general anaesthetic and given a muscle relaxant. This prevents jerking and movement during the procedure. As with all general anaesthetics the person's breathing, heart rate and blood pressure are closely monitored throughout the procedure.

Electrodes are placed on the person's temples, bilaterally or unilaterally, and an electric current is applied through the brain. The person under anaesthesia does not feel this impulse, and a mild convulsion is induced. In contemporary practice, this convulsion is barely visible and usually lasts only a few seconds. This is in stark contrast to the early days of ECT treatment where the person often thrashed about violently on the procedure table. The most common side effects associated with ECT are headache, upset stomach and muscle aches. Some people may also experience memory problems, especially around the time of the treatment. People may also have trouble remembering information learned shortly after the procedure, but this difficulty usually disappears over the days and weeks following the end of an ECT course. ECT is usually done in a course of treatments that are individualised for the person.

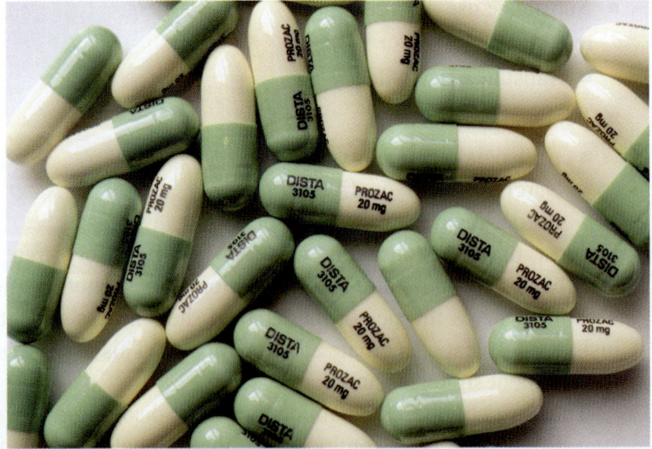

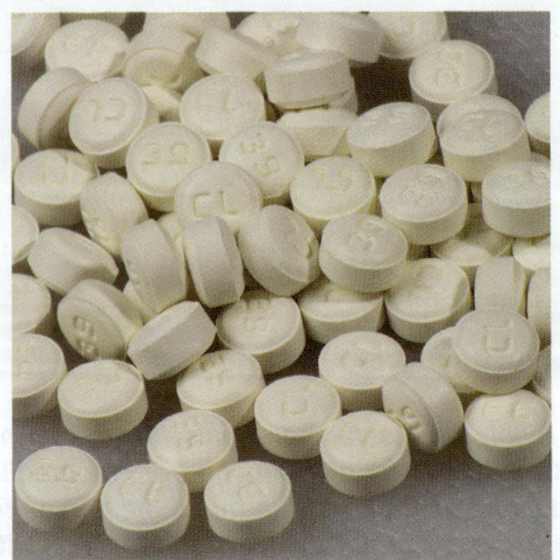

FIGURE 50.8 *Types of medications: A, an antidepressant, B, an antipsychotic*

Sources: *A*, Scott Camazine/Alamy Stock Photo; *B*, Ray Geiger/Shutterstock.

Psychological therapies

Psychological therapies are a major benefit in the Recovery journey of a person who has a mental illness. The most important of these is the development and maintenance of a therapeutic relationship. The importance of this relationship is the subject of many research papers written by mental health service users, their carers and clinicians.

COGNITIVE BEHAVIOURAL THERAPY (CBT) Along with a therapeutic relationship, CBT can also be useful. CBT aims to work closely with the person in order for them to see the links between their moods and their thinking. The aim is to get the person to think in ways that are more positive.

INTERPERSONAL THERAPY (IPT) aims to help the person identify current life factors that are leading them to experience a mental illness. IPT is founded upon the assumption that a person's vulnerabilities lead them to an illness. The aim is to strengthen the vulnerable parts of the person's personality.

NARRATIVE THERAPY (NT) places its main emphasis on a person's strengths. Narrative therapists listen closely to the person's life story and help them recognise times when they have solved problems with a positive outcome. Past situations and circumstances are thus learned from and built upon, ready to be used in future situations.

All therapies and treatments work best when the person is part of collaborative care. See Box 50.7 for the SANE checklist to determine whether someone should see a mental health practitioner. Psychological therapies will not work if the person does not trust the therapist. Once again, the importance of developing and maintaining a therapeutic relationship is at the fore.

BOX 50.7 A SANE checklist

- Are you worried about someone whose behaviour has changed? If someone you know has become confused, avoids people or has developed strange ideas that are not shared by others, it is important they talk to a mental health nurse or doctor to get help. The reason for this change may be that they have an illness.

Checklist

Encourage someone to seek help if anything on this checklist describes how they feel or act:

- They stop talking to family and friends.
- They become afraid or suspicious for no reason.
- They sleep poorly or often are awake all night.
- They develop strange ideas.
- They hear voices no one else can hear.
- They feel they have special powers.
- They have difficulty concentrating.
- They say or write things that don't make sense.
- They abuse drugs or alcohol.

How to get help

- Encourage the person to see a doctor.
- Offer to go with them, as a support.
- Ask for a longer appointment so there is sufficient time to explain concerns.
- Suggest you write some notes together to help explain things to the doctor.
- If the person is reluctant to seek help, visit the doctor yourself to ask for advice.

CHAPTER HIGHLIGHTS

- The global burden of mental illness accounts for 32.4% of years lived with disability (YLDs) and 13.0% of disability-adjusted life years (DALYs). In Australia, mental disorders are the third leading cause of overall disease burden.
- Mental health has been a national priority health area in Australia since 1996.
- All nurses need the skills and knowledge to provide safe and effective care for the large number of people affected by mental illness.
- The care that people who have a mental illness receive should be no less evidence based than the care that is provided to people who have a physical illness or injury.
- Nurses' attitudes towards people who have a mental illness should be respectful and non-judgmental; the nurse should show positive regard and be professional at all times.
- There is a difference between clinical recovery and personal recovery. Care should always be collaborative.

CONCEPT CHECK

1 There are two main diagnostic criteria used internationally:
1 DSN and ICD
2 DSM and ICC
3 DSM and ICD
4 DMM and ICD

2 The American Psychiatric Association *Diagnostic and Statistical Manual of Mental Disorders*:
1 assists with diagnosis
2 sets nursing priorities
3 establishes appropriate treatment regimes
4 ensures accurate epidemiological data is collected

3 Antonio has altered thought processes. An appropriate nursing response would be to:
1 explore his delusions with him
2 redirect his attention back to the here and now
3 point out gently the way in which his thinking is altered by giving examples
4 ensure you speak loudly enough so that he can hear you above his hallucinations

4 Bipolar disorder is:
1 a non-reactive set of depressive symptoms
2 a common disorder in young males
3 a psychotic disorder
4 a hereditary mental illness

5 People with bipolar disorder have:
1 delusions and spatial disruption
2 positive and negative symptoms
3 mood swings
4 hallucinations and thought blocking

6 Manic symptoms associated with bipolar disorder include:
1 little eye contact
2 speaking one's mind
3 no time for conversations
4 feeling really good

7 The following is not an example of a perceptual disturbance:
1 delusion
2 seeing things
3 hearing voices
4 feeling things on your skin

BIBLIOGRAPHY

American Psychiatric Association (APA) (2022). *Diagnostic and statistical manual of mental disorders DSM-5-TR* (5th ed.). Washington, DC: American Psychiatric Association.

Australian Bureau of Statistics (2022). *National study of mental health and wellbeing*. Retrieved from https://www.abs.gov.au/statistics/

Australian College of Mental Health Nurses (ACMHN) (2022). Retrieved from www.acmhn.org

Australian Commission on Safety and Quality in Health Care (ACSQHC) (2021). *National Safety and Quality Health Service Standards* (2nd ed.). Sydney: ACSQHC.

Burns, S., Tapsell, A., Perlman, D., Patterson, C. & Moxham, L. (2021). Stigma in the media: Investigating journalism students' attitudes towards mental illness. *International Journal of Mental Health Nursing, 31*(1), 104–110.

Chen, M. & Lawrie, S. (2017). Newspaper depictions of mental and physical health. *BJPsych Bulletin, 41*(6), 308–313.

Council of Australian Governments (COAG) (2012). *Roadmap for national mental health reform 2012–2022*. Retrieved from https://www.coag.gov.au/

Council of Australian Governments (COAG) (2022). *Fifth national mental health and suicide prevention plan*. Retrieved from http://www.coaghealthcouncil.gov.au/

Deegan, P. E. (1988). Recovery: The lived experience of rehabilitation. *Psychosocial Rehabilitation Journal, 11*(4), 11–19.

Glover, H. (2012). Recovery, life long learning, social inclusion and empowerment: Is a new paradigm? In P. Ryan, S. Ramon & T. Greacen, *Empowerment, lifelong learning and recovery in mental health: Towards a new paradigm*. UK: Palgrave Publishers.

Goman, C., Patterson, C., Moxham, L., Harada, T. & Tapsell, A. (2020). Alternative mental health clinical placements: Knowledge transfer and benefits for nursing practice outside mental health care settings. *Journal of Clinical Nursing, 29*(17–18), 3236–3245.

Henderson, C., Potts, L. & Robinson, E. J. (2020). Mental illness stigma after a decade of Time to Change England: Inequalities as targets for further improvement. *European Journal of Public Health, 30*(3), 497–503.

Lowe, D. J. E., Sasiadek, J. D., Coles, A. S & George, T. P. (2019). Cannabis and mental illness: A review. *European Archives of Psychiatry and Clinical Neuroscience*, 269, 107–120.

New South Wales Consumer Advisory Group (2022). *Mental health awareness*. Retrieved from http://www.nswcag.org.au/

Perlman, D., Moxham, L., Patterson, C., Cregan, A., Alford, S. & Tapsell, A. (2020). Mental health stigma and undergraduate nursing students: A self-determination theory perspective. *Collegian, 27*(2), 226–231. SANE Australia. Retrieved from https://www.sane.org

SANE Australia. Retrieved from https://www.sane.org.

World Health Organization (WHO) (1978). *Declaration of Alma-Ata*. Retrieved from http://www.who.int/

World Health Organization (WHO) (2022a). *World mental health report: Transforming mental health for all*. Geneva. Retrieved from http://www.who.int/

World Health Organization (WHO) (2022b). *Depression, key facts*. Retrieved from https://www.who.int/

CHAPTER 51

Community care

Gemma McErlean, Catherine Stephen, Liz Halcomb

Learning outcomes

- Describe the background and contemporary context of community care in Australia.
- Differentiate the health models underpinning and influencing community care services in Australia.
- Compare individualist and structuralist–collectivist approaches to health promotion.
- Discuss the evidence for social determinants of health as factors that affect the health of communities.
- Differentiate between primary healthcare and primary care and identify their relationships to community care approaches.
- Explain the role and contribution of nurses in community care, including intersectoral partnerships.

Clinical competencies

- Understand the health of communities in conjunction with the health of individuals.
- Apply the social determinants of health in relation to the health of individuals and communities.
- Collaborate with health and non-health professionals intersectorally to promote health, prevent illness/injury and restore health for individuals and communities.
- Utilise culturally safe approaches to care within primary healthcare and primary care services.
- Utilise partnership approaches to facilitate consumer-directed care.

Key terms

INTRODUCTION

The health of the community requires a whole-of-society approach to ensure that every individual can access the healthcare they need and maintain a healthy lifestyle via access to secure food, shelter and clean water. Primary healthcare (PHC) encompasses the continuum of healthcare from health promotion and prevention to treatment, rehabilitation and palliative care (World Health Organization (WHO) & United Nations Children's Fund (UNICEF), 2018). Countries with strong PHC systems have better health outcomes and often reduced health costs, as costly hospital admissions are avoided by care delivered within the community (WHO & UNICEF, 2018).

In Australia, a range of government and non-government organisations provide PHC services in the community. These organisations aim to support and improve health by providing a universal point of access to the health system, promoting health and preventing illness, providing high-quality healthcare across the lifespan and ensuring continuity of care (Australian Productivity Commission, 2022). Nurses play an important role in the delivery of care in these organisations, ranging from early childhood assessment to occupational health services, chronic disease management and prevention of disease or injury. Another important role of nurses is to identify and address social, environmental and political factors that impact on the health of individuals and communities (WHO & UNICEF, 2018). As the population ages and rates of chronic and complex disease continue to rise, nurses will increasingly be in demand to deliver healthcare in the community (Guzys et al., 2020).

This chapter introduces the concepts that facilitate an understanding of PHC services in Australia and provides examples of nursing practice in this sector. It is important to appreciate the interrelated nature of each concept to understand the contribution of PHC organisations to the health of people and populations and how PHC services work with but differ from provided acute care services. Community care organisations are characterised by their diversity, ranging from state/territory- and Australian-Government-funded health services to not-for-profit, private businesses and volunteer organisations. Many of these organisations are not recognised as formal healthcare organisations but nevertheless play a vital role in supporting the health of the Australian community (Australian Productivity Commission, 2022). In addition, key nursing concepts, such as culturally safe care and critical thinking, are covered in this chapter as they apply to nursing in community. To begin to understand how community care organisations work and the concepts that guide nurses working in this sector, the term community is clarified.

WHAT IS A COMMUNITY?

When considering communities and their health, it is helpful to reflect on what is meant by the term **community**. In the healthcare context, it may be defined as *community as place* and *community as relationships* (Guzys et al., 2020; Yerkes, Hoogenboom & Javornik, 2020). *Community as place* refers to the geographical location that people share with others (e.g. town, city or suburb), reflecting the impact of people's environment and its resources on health. *Community as relationships* refers to the human interactions and social connections that unite people (Guzys et al., 2020). Different communities of people therefore have different attributes, making it important not to assume communities are the same; that is, by thinking they have close-knit relationships or shared values and interests (Taylor et al., 2020). Each community is likely to have subcommunities, such as school communities and inner- and outer-town communities, based on relationships, cultural and religious backgrounds, interests or localities, creating a complex and dynamic whole. Based on these meanings, the health of a community is a synthesis of people interacting or relating within their locality (Taylor et al., 2020).

COMMUNITY CARE IN AUSTRALIA

To achieve the goals of community health and to meet the needs of groups within the population, community care services are provided in a variety of settings, by a range of people and organisations, and are funded through a range of different sources (Australian Institute of Health and Welfare (AIHW), 2022a). Complex networks of organisations exist, which together support the health of the community and its people. These networks involve interaction between community care organisations and those of the acute or hospital system, as well as interaction between formal health services and other organisations which address the social determinants of health or public health and safety. Figure 51.1 describes service network connections between general and specialist community services and acute care services. Some examples are listed in Table 51.1.

The complex funding structure and areas of responsibility of Australia's health system are illustrated in Figure 51.2. This figure shows the network of health system services, including community and public health services. Note that health services comprise a mix of public and private sector involvement, with funding from the Australian Government, the state and territory governments and private funders. The two largest areas of health that were funded in 2019–2020 were hospitals ($83.5 billion) and PHC ($66.9 billion). This equates to an

TABLE 51.1 Community groups: needs and services

COMMUNITY GROUP	SERVICE ACTIVITY
Community members not at risk of ill health/injury	Health promotion
Community members at risk of developing a health problem	Prevention and early detection
Community members who present with a health problem	Assessment and investigation that does not require access to special technology
Community members with a confirmed problem	Community treatment
Community members with chronic consequences arising from a health problem	Continuing care

Source: Eagar et al. (2008). *Community health at the crossroads: Which way now? Final report of the NSW Community Health Review*. Wollongong: Centre for Health Service Development, University of Wollongong.

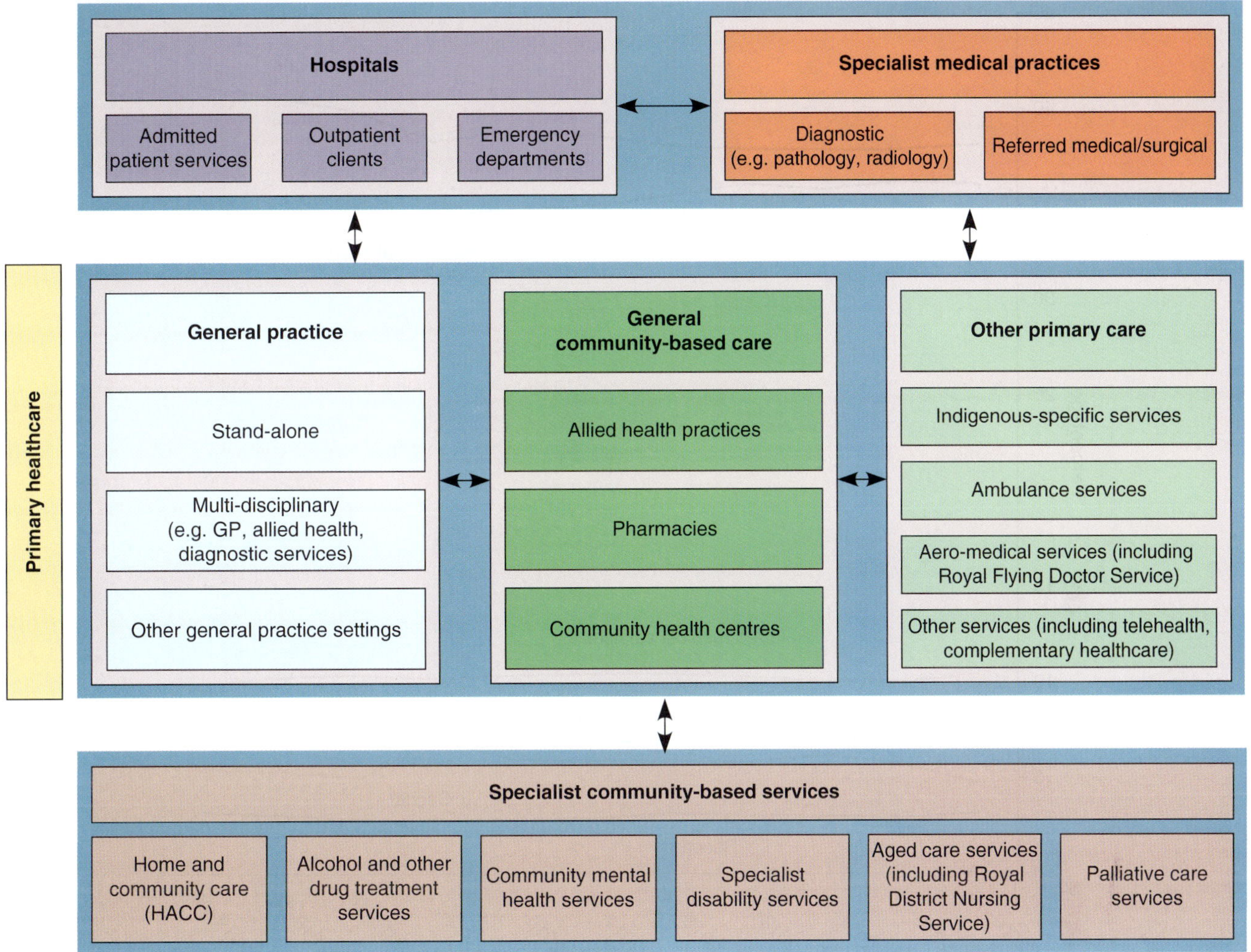

FIGURE 51.1 ***Community health service network connections***

Source: AIHW (2014). *Australia's health 2014*. Chapter 8: Treating and preventing ill health. Retrieved from http://www.aihw.gov.au/australias-health/2014/ preventing-ill-health/#t3.

expenditure of some $7,926 (an increase of 0.2% per year) on acute health services alone (AIHW, 2021). This cost does not account for any community care funding.

Community health services work in partnership with health and other services within the community to ensure the health of the population. They work with many government and non-government organisations and services which are funded outside the health system and which make significant contributions to the health of the population, particularly disadvantaged groups (e.g. people who are homeless). This is known as **intersectoral** collaboration. Examples of these organisations include religious organisations; specific interest groups such as Diabetes Australia, Australian Breastfeeding Association and SIDS and Kids; and income-support organisations. Some other partners that are needed to develop and sustain healthy communities are listed in Box 51.1.

Many of the major issues for the future attainment of community health involve strategies that promote effective links within and beyond the services of the health system, so that a reorientation of health services and expenditure to primary health can be achieved (WHO & UNICEF, 2018). People within communities move between community organisations and acute care services at some time in their life, further highlighting the need for partnerships between services in each setting and recognition of the contribution each makes to the health of individuals and communities across the lifespan. While community organisations and the services they deliver are important, they cannot function without each other to achieve health for people and communities.

The complex nature of the community health system is also characterised by a tension between providing a comprehensive, participatory and health promoting approach and a need to provide community-based direct care and interventions that are efficient, sustainable and future focused (Department of Health, 2021). Compounding this complexity is a view that community care services should provide the full range of services from prevention to palliation where people live. At the same time, these services are expected to cater for the needs of hospitals under stress from the impact of factors such as pandemics, climate disasters and the increasing incidence of chronic diseases

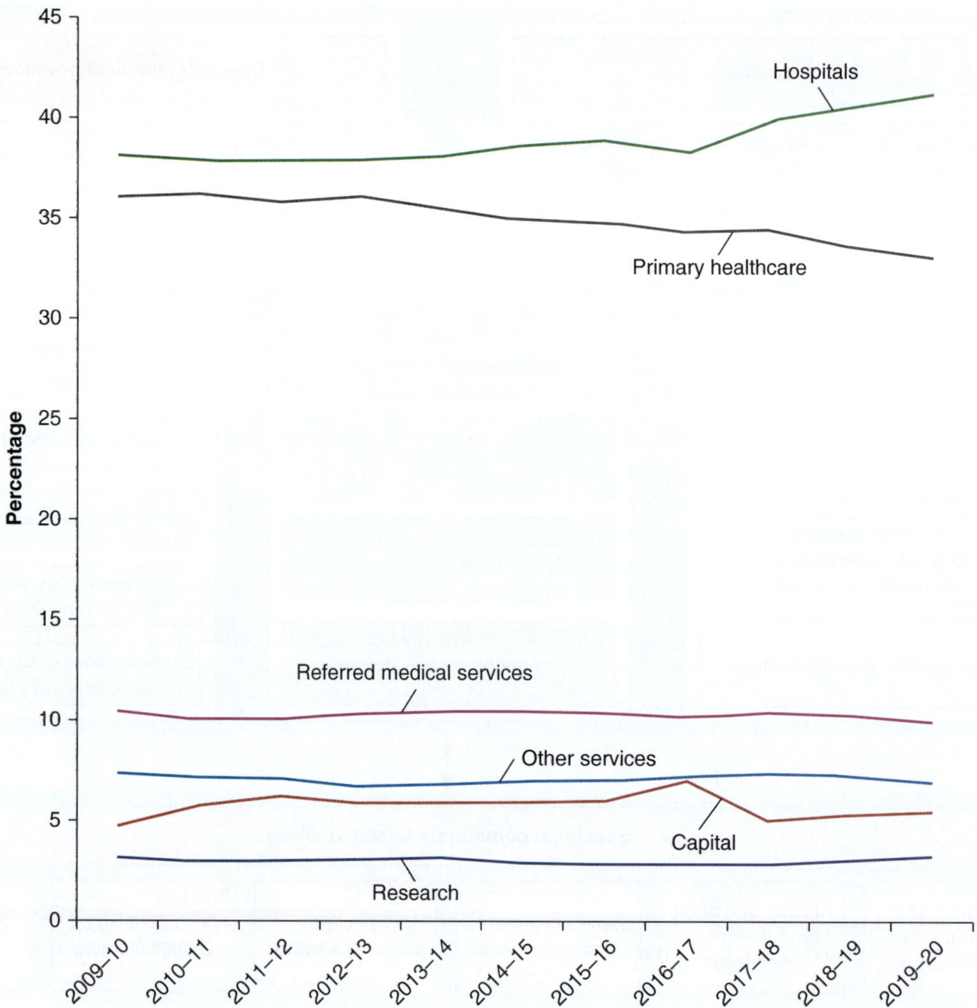

FIGURE 51.2 ***Proportion of total health spending, by area of expenditure, current prices, 2009–2010 to 2019–2020***

Source: AIHW (2021). *Health expenditure Australia 2019–20*. Retrieved from https://www.aihw.gov.au/reports/health-welfare-expenditure/health-expenditure-australia-2019-20/contents/trends-by-area-of-spending. AIHW Health Expenditure Database (Table 28). Licensed under the Creative Commons Attribution 4.0 International License, https//creativecommons.org/licenses/by/4.0/.

BOX 51.1 Possible partners in the healthcare continuum

Community health partners include, but are not limited to, the following:

Health promotion
Public health units, local government, schools, other state government departments, non-government organisations (NGOs), community groups and consumers.

Prevention and early detection
Schools, GPs, General Practice Nurses (GPNs), Nurse Practitioners, other state government departments, NGOs, community groups and consumers.

Assessment and investigation
GPs, GPNs, Nurse Practitioners, allied health professionals, community nurses (general, child and family, and mental health), schools, other state government departments, Commonwealth-funded services such as aged care assessment teams (ACATs), NGOs and consumers.

Community treatment
GPs, practice nurses, Nurse Practitioners, allied health professionals, community nurses (general, child and family, and mental health), pharmacies, NGOs and consumers.

Continuing care
GPs, practice nurses, Nurse Practitioners, hospitals, other state government departments (particularly ageing, disability and home care, community services, housing and police), home care services and Commonwealth-funded services such as community aged care packages (CACPs), NGOs/charities and consumers.

Source: Adapted from Eagar et al. (2008). *Community health at the crossroads: Which way now? Final report of the NSW Community Health Review*. Wollongong: Centre for Health Service Development, University of Wollongong. p. 7. Reproduced by permission, NSW Ministry of Health © 2016.

and their complications (e.g. diabetes and respiratory diseases) (Eagar et al., 2008; Kadandale et al., 2020; Kearon & Risdon, 2020). See Figure 51.3.

There is also increasing emphasis on working in partnership with the people, or consumers, who use community services. This shift responds to consumers' calls for models of care which are consumer driven and oriented, and is reflected in the introduction of services underpinned by **consumer-directed care** (CDC) philosophies. These CDC services aim to increase consumer control over care, increase consumer satisfaction and improve health outcomes (Aged Care Guide, 2022; COTA, 2023; WHO & UNICEF, 2018). A collaborative approach also aligns with the National Safety and Quality Health Service Partnering with Consumers Standard and Comprehensive Care Standard (Australian Commission on Safety and Quality in Health Care (ACSQHC), 2021).

Community programs based on the CDC model have been available in the Australian disability sector for some time, and more recently in the community aged care sector. In Australia, community aged care CDC refers to enhancing service users' autonomy by enabling and optimising consumer goal setting and control over the care they receive and the providers who deliver their services (AIHW, 2018).

Community care initiatives based on CDC have similarities with the NSQHS Partnering with Consumers Standard. However, community-based aged care and disability service CDC extend consumer choice, control and responsibility further, placing care outcomes in the hands of consumers by enabling consumer decision making regarding care goals, which services are provided, who provides them and how each consumer's individual service budget is spent (ACSQHC, 2021; COTA, 2023).

Another issue associated with the achievement of the goals of community care in Australia is continuity of care (AIHW, 2018). Increasingly, community care is using digital

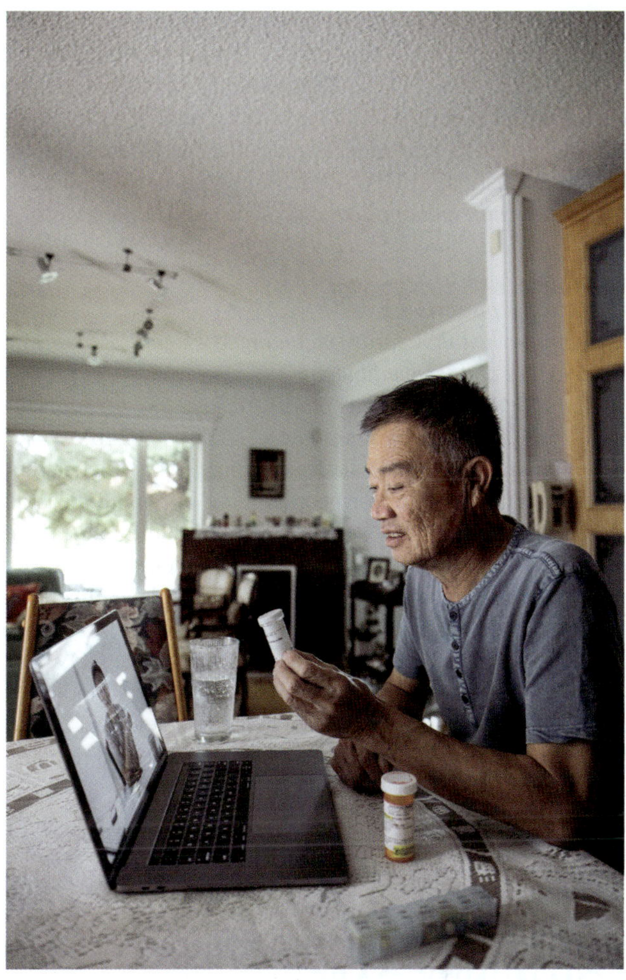

FIGURE 51.3 ***Community care has become increasingly important for those in rural and remote areas during the COVID-19 pandemic***

Source: Hero Images Inc./Alamy Stock Photo.

Links to National Patient Safety Standards

NSQHS: Partnering with Consumers Standard

The intention of this standard is to create a health service that partners with consumers when planning, designing and delivering care, and also in the measurement and evaluation of care. Partnerships between clinicians and patients must include respectful, equal information sharing and decision making in care planning.

Source: ACSQHC (2021). *National Safety and Quality Health Service Standards* (2nd ed.). Sydney: ACSQHC. © Australian Commission on Safety and Quality in Health Care.

Links to National Patient Safety Standards

NSQHS: Comprehensive Care Standard

The intention of this standard is to ensure that comprehensive care is provided to the person that is well coordinated and aligned with the person's expressed goals of care and healthcare needs. This standard considers the effect of the person's health issues on their life and wellbeing and is clinically appropriate.

Source: ACSQHC (2021). *National Safety and Quality Health Service Standards* (2nd ed.). Sydney: ACSQHC. © Australian Commission on Safety and Quality in Health Care.

technologies to improve continuity by increasing access to information and contact between the service and the consumer (James, Ashley et al., 2021). **Telehealth** is one of these technologies. **Digital health** refers to a broad 'range of technologies that can be used to treat patients and collect and share a person's health information' (AIHW, 2022b). It includes:

- *mobile health and applications (such as SMS reminders via mobile messaging, wellness apps, Medicare Online and COVID check-in apps)*
- *electronic prescribing*
- *electronic health records (including My Health Record)*
- *telehealth and telemedicine*
- *wearable devices (such as fitness trackers and monitors)*
- *robotics and artificial intelligence*. (AIHW, 2022b)

Community care will increasingly rely on telehealth to deliver community care for people living in remote areas and others, especially older people, who have difficulties with transportation. Telehealth also enables the delivery of a more cost effective and efficient service for people with chronic conditions to manage their health (AIHW, 2022b). Given the need to rapidly expand telehealth as a result of the COVID-19 pandemic, significant advances have been made in models of telehealth across the community (James, Ashley et al., 2021). As we emerge from the pandemic, many of these will remain as an adjunct to face-to-face care.

The model of health embraced by community organisations is reflected in the types of services they provide.

MODELS OF HEALTH AND COMMUNITY CARE

Each community organisation is based on a model of health which influences how healthcare is defined and provided. It also affects when and how the factors that affect health are addressed. In the following sections three models of health are discussed and presented sequentially, representing a continuum which illustrates a move from medical to social orientations to health, and individual to population health concerns. While there are many other models of health, those presented here are a useful introduction to community organisations and the services they provide. The use of different models across health organisations does, however, mean that there can be tensions around the focus of healthcare for individuals, the interventions used and how care is ultimately delivered. In community care, the biomedical and social models of health are often integrated (Taylor et al., 2020).

The biomedical model of health

The **biomedical model of health**, also known as the medical model, defines health as the absence of disease. Health is primarily understood as an individual responsibility determined by biology and lifestyle choices (Germov, 2019). In services where this is the predominant model, the psychological and social dimensions of health are not priority concerns for organisations or practitioners and may be overlooked in favour of biomedical investigations and individual behaviour change interventions. In contrast, in community and primary care settings, the broader psychological and social dimensions of health are prime considerations. It is argued that community care services need to move beyond this model and embrace psychological and social dimensions of health as important considerations (WHO & UNICEF, 2018).

As a reaction to the dominance of biomedicine and its orientation to health, a biopsychosocial movement developed. This is a modification of the biomedical model which incorporates the concept of holistic wellbeing. It can be seen as an intermediate or middle-of-the-road model which lies between the biomedical and social models of health.

The biopsychosocial model of health

The **biopsychosocial model** defines health as holistic wellbeing within an individual (Taylor, 2015). It argues that a focus on disease is too narrow, and that health services need to assess psychological and social functioning and social and personal resources, as well as physical capacities (Taylor, 2015). In this model, health is a dynamic concept influenced by multiple interacting factors that change over time. It reasserts a connection between mind and body, seeing the individual's mental state as influencing biological processes and thus susceptibility to disease (Germov, 2019). However, it shares many key assumptions and characteristics of the biomedical model, including the focus on individual diagnosis and treatment, so that it is individualistic even if it includes emotional and social factors.

The social model of health

The **social model of health**, also referred to as new public health or the social ecological model (Germov, Freij & Richmond, 2019), sees health as multifaceted, with a focus on social rather than biological determinants of health. This model emphasises health equity and prevention of illness or injury, as well as collaboration and empowerment (Taylor et al., 2020).

> *The social model locates people in social contexts, conceptualises the physical environment as socially organised, and understands ill health as a process of interaction between people and their environments.* (Broom cited in Germov, 2019, p. 16)

The social model focuses on the interrelationship between human interaction, social organisation and natural environment and sees health as a resource within individuals, communities and the population as a whole. It underpins many health policies on a national and global scale. For instance, the WHO's Commission on Social Determinants of Health's 2008 report *Closing the gap in a generation: Health equity through action on the social determinants of health* argues that the 'high burden of illness... arises in large part because of the conditions in which people are born, grow, live, work and age—conditions that together provide the freedom people need to live lives they value' (WHO, 2008). In the Commission's view the biomedical approach, while important, downplays the significance of influences on health that lie beyond the health sector—otherwise known as social determinants of health (AIHW, 2022c; Keleher & MacDougall, 2021). Also ignored in the biomedical approach are values, vested interests, politics and context (Baum, 2016).

The social model of health makes a link between individual problems, such as obesity, diabetes or unemployment, and social issues, such as transport options, food availability, government policy and globalisation (Germov, 2019). This alerts us to the fact that individuals often share problems, including health problems. Problems then may have a common cause, which may be solved through collective action. Health and illness, in this view, are not simply an individual concern but the result of wider social conditions, known as social determinants.

SOCIAL DETERMINANTS AND COMMUNITY HEALTH

The AIHW (2018) calls the factors that affect the health of people '**health determinants**'. There is a growing body of evidence which shows that understanding the full range of health determinants is the key to understanding the health of a community, promoting health and providing healthcare (Baum, 2016). In particular, the **social determinants of health** are central to understanding the health of a community and the role of community organisations which embrace the social model of health.

Social determinants of health 'are the conditions in which people are born, grow, live, work and age, including access to the health system. These circumstances are shaped by the distribution of money, power and resources at global, national and local levels' (WHO & UNICEF, 2018). The social determinants are increasingly recognised as the key to the health of people and communities because of the evidence that social conditions, specifically where people are born, live and work, determine people's chances of good health and a long life (WHO & UNICEF, 2018). Despite increasing levels of affluence in modern communities, people who are disadvantaged still have poorer health (AIHW, 2022c). Figure 51.4 shows that people with the lowest socioeconomic status die at a higher rate than people with fewer disadvantages. These differences are explained by the social determinants approach.

There are several ways of thinking about social determinants of health. For instance, Wilkinson and Marmot (2003) refer to a list of social determinants which continue to influence health outcomes in Australia (AIHW, 2022c) (see Box 51.2). Others have developed models to describe the social processes and elements that influence health. All such models attempt to map a number of common and interconnected dimensions that

BOX 51.2 WHO social determinants of health

- Social gradient
- Stress
- Early life
- Social exclusion
- Work
- Unemployment
- Social support
- Addiction
- Food
- Transport

Sources: Adapted from Wilkinson & Marmot (2003). *Social determinants of health: The solid facts* (2nd ed.). Denmark: WHO; AIHW (2022c). *Social determinants of health*. Retrieved from https://www.aihw.gov.au/.

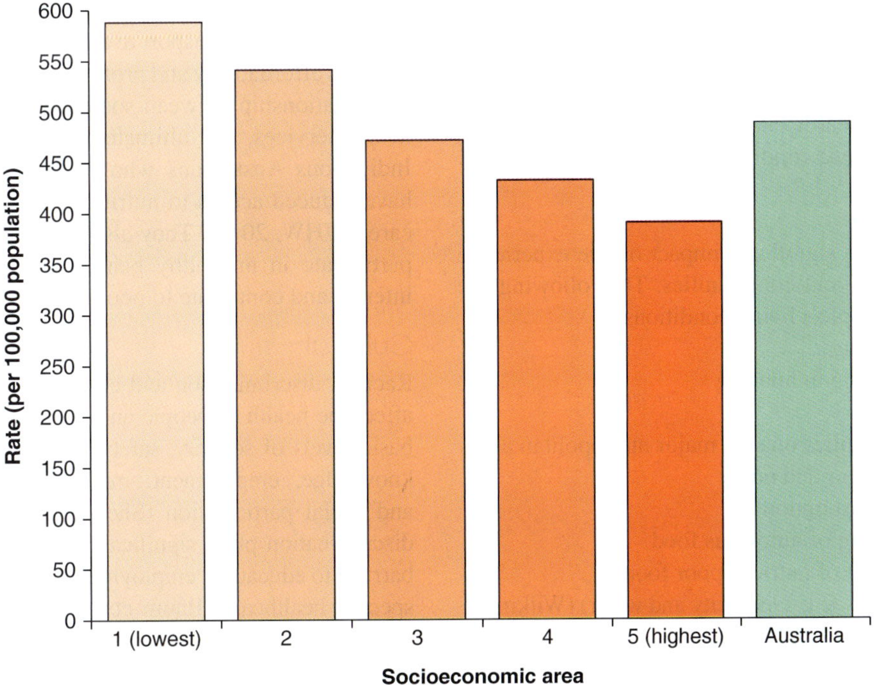

FIGURE 51.4 ***All-cause mortality rate by socioeconomic area, 2020***

Source: AIHW (2022d). *Health across socioeconomic groups*. Retrieved from https://www.aihw.gov.au/reports/australias-health/health-across-socioeconomic-groups#_Toc30611177. Licensed under the Creative Commons Attribution 4.0 International License, https//creativecommons.org/licenses/by/4.0.

operate as an intricate web of influence on people and their lives, acting on individuals and the population as a whole (Baum et al., 2017).

Early life factors

Early life factors influence a person's experience of health. For example, an adult's health is adversely influenced by physiological or emotional deprivation in early childhood and/or before birth (AIHW, 2022c; Wilkinson & Marmot, 2003). When a child is emotionally deprived, brain development can be adversely affected, which in turn can lead to low levels of educational attainment, problem behaviour and social exclusion in later life. Physical deprivation such as lack of nourishment in a child is associated with decreased development and function of major organs, which increases the risk of ill health in later life (AIHW, 2022c).

Some models include genetics as a social determinant of health because social factors interact with each other and with the individual's genetic composition. Others exclude genetics on the grounds that even though a person's genetic susceptibility to disease produces ill health, this health change is not a product of the social environment.

Income and socioeconomic conditions

Income and socioeconomic conditions are one of the key social determinants of health (Baum et al., 2017). People with higher incomes are often healthier and live longer lives than people who have middle and lower incomes (AIHW, 2018; Marmot, 2002). Health and wellbeing improve as people's income and social position move upwards—a concept known as the social gradient (Baum et al., 2017). The more people live in difficult financial and social circumstances, the greater the risks to their short and long-term health (WHO & UNICEF, 2018). Income and social conditions act in relation to one another and, at times, it is not only a lack of material resources that affects health but also the social (dis)advantages associated with these conditions.

Living conditions

Living conditions have a significant impact on the experience of health by individuals and communities. The following are important aspects of people's living conditions:

- affordability of housing
- degree of overcrowding in housing
- design of cities
- liveability of communities outside major metropolitan areas
- degree of pollution—air and noise
- availability of transport options
- availability and pricing of nutritious food
- exposure to marketing of nutrient-poor foods
- affordability of utilities (e.g. electricity and water) (Wilkinson & Marmot, 2003; WHO & UNICEF, 2018).

The cost of living is increasing in Australia, particularly for housing, food and utilities. As a result, people reliant on government benefits and on low incomes are experiencing erosion of their living conditions and are subsequently at an increased risk of ill health.

Other factors

Education

Levels of education, health literacy, behaviours and lifestyle factors are intrinsically linked to health. Education provides the basis for employment and generating an income. It also enables people to engage with health information and to take the appropriate actions to maintain their health. This engagement is referred to as *health literacy* (Nutbeam & Lloyd, 2020). When a person does not have sufficient education they are more likely to be health illiterate. Education and health literacy also influence a person's behaviours and lifestyle. With good health literacy, there is an increased likelihood that people will be able to address behaviours or lifestyle factors that adversely impact on health. Regular tobacco use, poor food choices and low exercise levels are significantly greater in the lowest socioeconomic groups in Australia (AIHW, 2018).

Access to services

The equitable distribution of resources, such as health services, is another key social determinant of health (WHO & UNICEF, 2018). Access to and use of health services influences the health of a person and a community. Comprehensive accessible healthcare should be available to all Australians based on their need, not the ability to pay. However, access to health services is affected by many factors including socioeconomic status, geographical location, cultural background and intellectual or other disabilities. While most Australians benefit from our universal healthcare system, equity of access to healthcare remains an issue for immigrants, asylum seekers, refugees and Indigenous Australians (Au et al., 2019). For example, access to health services is lower for Indigenous people than non-Indigenous people because of proximity, availability, cultural appropriateness, transport availability, health insurance, health services affordability and proficiency in English (AIHW, 2018). The relationship between socioeconomic status and access to health services, and ultimately to health, is well established. Indigenous Australians who have low socioeconomic status have reduced access to nutritious food, education and healthcare (AIHW, 2018). They also live in risky environments and participate in unhealthy behaviours. All these social factors interact and contribute to poor health.

Cultural

Racism, discrimination and culture are also known factors that affect the health of people and communities, as these influence basic levels of security, safety, hygiene, housing, nourishment, knowledge, employment, medical care, community support and social participation (Shepherd et al., 2018). Racism and discrimination place significant pressure on people by creating barriers to education, employment and culturally appropriate and specific healthcare (Baum et al., 2017). Many people are culturally, socially and economically disadvantaged simply because of cultural difference. Cultural difference may place people at increased risk of disease for a range of reasons including identity, misunderstanding and perceived threats to personal safety.

The concept of cultural safety (see the chapter 'Medical–surgical nursing') is an attempt to respond to these factors.

Cultural safety is concerned with developing ways of addressing the historical, social and political injustice responsible for health inequity in Indigenous cultural communities (Taylor & Guerin, 2019). Practising cultural safety means ensuring quality in healthcare through culturally appropriate communication and ensuring equity and access to health services. It implores us to reflect on our attitudes and values, respect difference, recognise power differentials in relationships and act upon these. The idea of cultural safety recognises the unique power imbalances that exist in healthcare relationships between a professional and a consumer. Cultural safety is about respect, shared meaning, knowledge and experience (Williams, Dune & McLeod, 2021).

Social connection

Social interaction and support at an individual and community level increase a sense of belonging and social connectedness that has been linked to positive physical and psychological health (Halcomb et al., 2022). Social exclusion leads to loss or lack of connection to the community in which a person lives. This exclusion is linked to psychological stress, depression, smoking, use of illicit drugs, and alcohol misuse and dependence (AIHW, 2018). Therefore, when engagement and interaction between individuals and communities is lacking, people experience ill health. To facilitate interaction and engagement, health services need to embrace body, mind, spirit, land, environment, culture, customs and socioeconomic status, and be accessible to all individuals and communities as close as possible to where they live.

Levels of determinants and interventions

Some social determinants of health have a more direct effect on health than others and hence they can be viewed on a continuum from proximal to distal (Keleher & MacDougall, 2021). **Distal determinants** of health tend to be stable and concern historical, national, institutional, political, legal and cultural factors; for example, anti-discrimination law, changes in taxation or changes to the provision of government income support. The influence of distal determinants is often mediated through more proximal determinants (Keleher & MacDougall, 2021). **Intermediate determinants** concern community infrastructure, personal wealth or access to resources, and natural, physical and built environments. This level also includes access to healthcare and health systems (Keleher & MacDougall, 2021). **Proximal determinants** have a more direct impact on health, and include lifestyle and behavioural factors as well as underlying health conditions (Keleher & MacDougall, 2021).

Different community organisations address the determinants of health in different ways. Health promotion based on the social model of health focuses on distal or upstream factors and seeks to address health equity, social inequality, working conditions or the effects of rapid social change by changing environments and introducing legislation (Froehlich-Grobe et al., 2021). Examples of this include campaigns for legislation on food labelling, changes in environmental legislation such as those that have banned smoking from public places or, on a smaller scale, the introduction of harm-reduction strategies, such as needle-exchange programs and early intervention programs for families. Organisations that are grounded in social determinants aim to undertake advocacy, intersectoral collaboration and community development. Health promotion based on the biomedical model concentrates on proximal or downstream factors such as screening for high cholesterol levels and treating people with lifestyle changes or drugs (Johnson et al., 2022). Organisations using the biopsychosocial model, the middle-of-the-road model of health that includes psychological and social factors, often focus prevention on intermediate factors or midstream factors.

PRIMARY HEALTHCARE

Primary healthcare

The philosophy of **primary healthcare (PHC)** originates from the WHO. As an agency of the United Nations, the WHO was established to address international health issues and aims to achieve worldwide health (Taylor et al., 2020). In 1978, 134 nations attended the WHO's International Conference on Primary Health Care as a response to growing concern about the world's health in terms of its people and healthcare systems (WHO, 2008). This conference was marked by the *Declaration of Alma-Ata*, a declaration that articulates PHC as the guiding philosophy for health development across the world and as a vision for the future (WHO, 2008). Since this Declaration, the concept of PHC has been refined and debated. In 2018, the WHO and UNICEF jointly hosted the Astana conference in Kazakhstan. At this conference, the Astana Declaration was made to redefine PHC and emphasise the need for governments across the world to prioritise PHC. The Declaration stated:

> *PHC is a whole-of-society approach to health that aims at ensuring the highest possible level of health and well-being and their equitable distribution by focusing on people's needs and as early as possible along the continuum from health promotion and disease prevention to treatment, rehabilitation and palliative care, and as close as feasible to people's everyday environment.* (WHO & UNICEF, 2018, p. xii)

The goal of PHC, underpinned by the principles of social justice, empowerment/community participation and equity, is 'Health for All' (WHO, 1978). It advocates community services that promote community participation and ensures access to health-related services for all people and the provision of services at a cost that is affordable and as close as possible to where people live (WHO, 1978). The philosophy of PHC is also underpinned by the tenets of cultural safety. Guided by a PHC philosophy, community organisations work in partnership with people and communities to enable and empower change that is local, affordable and sustainable (Taylor et al., 2020). The focus is on addressing the social determinants of health experienced by people and communities, reducing the effects of disadvantage and health inequality (Taylor et al., 2020).

To practise in a way consistent with PHC, community organisations need to focus on addressing social determinants of health and to encompass strategies that address the underpinning principles noted previously, including cultural safety. The minimum activities for PHC described by the WHO (1978) are listed in Box 51.3. Intersectoral collaboration, a strategy to address social determinants of health and structural barriers to health, refers to **transdisciplinary** partnerships, with the needs of the community dictating which are the most appropriate services and service relationships. Transdisciplinary care goes beyond past models of multidisciplinary or interprofessional care and facilitates intersectoral relationships which value expertise in areas beyond those addressed by traditional health disciplines. This might include partnerships with services that provide education, transport or income support, reflecting an understanding of the social determinants of health. These approaches are central to PHC and have been identified as key processes for closing the gap between the health of Indigenous and non-Indigenous people in Australia (Milroy & Bandler, 2021). An exemplar of an Australian community service based on the philosophy of PHC is detailed later in this chapter.

The WHO outlined three components of PHC as key to its vision: (1) integrated health services, (2) multi-sectoral policies and action, and (3) empowered people and communities (WHO & UNICEF, 2018). In terms of integrated services, PHC involves 'the delivery of quality health services that respond to the needs and preferences of people, at both the population and individual level' p. 13). PHC delivers care both across the community, in terms of population-based health services, and within the community, through primary care. Multi-sectorial policies and actions refer to the actions of non-health sectors that impact on the health of people and their communities, such as urban planning, education and transport. The final component espoused by the WHO is empowering people and communities. This involves health professionals and people working together as equal partners to plan and integrate actions that enhance the health of the community. People can do this by acting as advocates for policy and action, co-developers of health services and carers of themselves and others.

Primary care

Primary care, often called *family practice* or *general practice*, is a person's initial point of contact with the health system. While historically this had often been a medical model of care, increasingly, multidisciplinary primary care teams work with people to identify and prioritise their health goals. Primary care clinicians, such as doctors, nurses and allied health professionals, assess individual health needs and provide evidence-based treatment or referral to specialist services as required (WHO & UNICEF, 2018). As people often visit the same primary care setting over time, they develop a level of continuity of care with health professionals that enables the building of trust and rapport. A key role of primary care, particularly when multiple providers are involved, is to identify the range of needs and coordinate the care of individuals. Such coordination is important at transition points, such as hospital discharge, where there is a risk if fragmentation of care occurs.

BOX 51.3 Minimum activities for primary healthcare

- Education concerning prevailing health problems and the methods of preventing and controlling them.
- Promotion of food supply and proper nutrition.
- Provision of an adequate supply of safe water and basic sanitation.
- Provision of maternal and child healthcare, including family planning.
- Immunisation against major infectious diseases.
- Prevention and control of locally endemic diseases.
- Appropriate treatment of common diseases and injuries.
- Provision of essential medication.

Source: WHO (1978). *The Declaration of Alma-Ata, International Conference on Primary Health Care*. Retrieved from http://www.who.int/publications/almaata_declaration_en.pdf.

Population-based services

Population-based services are informed by a public health approach to address health and wellbeing issues across the community. This includes activities such as disease prevention, health promotion, surveillance and emergency response (WHO & UNICEF, 2018). These activities seek to provide services and opportunities for individuals and communities to enhance their health and reduce lifestyle behaviours that increase risk of poor health. Strategies can focus on specific population groups (selective) or take a whole-of-community approach (comprehensive).

HEALTH EDUCATION AND HEALTH PROMOTION

Health promotion, illness/injury prevention and health education are the cornerstones of PHC and community care. **Health promotion**, incorporating illness/injury prevention, is described in the *Ottawa Charter for Health Promotion* as the process of enabling people to increase control over and improve their health (WHO, 1986). **Health education** is often used interchangeably with health promotion; however, health education refers to an individualist model which focuses on the individual and individual strategies to improve health by increasing knowledge or influencing attitudes to alter behaviours and lifestyle, such as health counselling and health education (WHO & UNICEF, 2018). PHC, which focuses on the determinants of health, is aligned with population-focused strategies for health promotion, known as structuralist–collectivist health promotion (SCHP), a model that involves community engagement and capacity building.

Individualist health promotion

The individualist model of health promotion focuses on changing individual behaviour and lifestyle, and rests on the assumption that individuals harm their health by engaging in unhealthy living (i.e. smoking, eating fatty foods, not exercising and drinking alcohol). It aims at improving health by focusing on risk factors, particularly those identified as precursors to disease (Germov et al., 2019). In this model, disease and illness are seen as a consequence of failure to comply with healthy lifestyle choices; in an individualist society, this is difficult to challenge because it appears to make sense. However, it is a single-cause approach which emphasises individual choices associated with risk factors rather than the underlying social conditions that influence choice and behaviours. Most factors affecting illness and health lie outside the control of individuals, and lifestyles are powerfully influenced, if not fully determined, by the social organisation in which they are embedded (Germov et al., 2019).

Individualist health promotion (IHP) is promoted as being successful and cost effective, but adequate evaluation is lacking (Baum & Fisher, 2014). Few programs succeed for any length of time and many are either unsuccessful or cater only for the well motivated (e.g. weight loss programs). Exaggerated in this case is the ease with which individuals make connections between knowledge and behaviour, when there is a complex interaction between knowledge, attitude and practice/behaviour change (Taylor et al., 2020). Education alone does not necessarily lead to behaviour change and approaches that rely only on education underestimate the impact of social factors on health and illness or injury.

While IHP is a dominant model and can be useful, it is often too narrow in its focus and ignores the broader context in which health and wellbeing are situated. It also risks leading to victim blaming; if an individual is sick, it is because they have not complied with health advice. In short, if people took better care of themselves, they would not have the health problems they have. The person who develops lung cancer and is also a smoker is an obvious example. IHP programs do nothing to alter the structural causes or determinants of ill health or injury and can be paternalistic and patronising (Taylor et al., 2020). For example, people on low incomes may not be able to afford the most nutritious foods, irrespective of their health education. In this example, it is not so much ignorance that is the problem but inadequate employment opportunities and/or welfare allowances. Healthy choices are not easy choices for the disadvantaged; people with little choice about their lives often regard immediate comfort to be more important than end-stage health (James, Halcomb et al., 2021). All these situations highlight issues and concerns for healthcare which is experienced as culturally safe.

Effective health promotion must also consider social situations and available resources. In particular, attention to the social determinants of health can bridge the disparity between 'knowing' and 'doing' by empowering people to make healthier choices. This can involve small-scale local interventions as well as broader national or global social change. Table 51.2 lists the characteristics of individualist health promotion, including its relationship to models of health and PHC.

Structuralist–collectivist health promotion

In accordance with the Ottawa Charter, and in alignment with the WHO's PHC approach, health priorities should be community-based, reflect the concern of particular communities and be 'bottom up' (WHO, 1978, 1986). Often, though, structuralist–collectivist health promotion (SCHP) is less about structural change and more about health education in disguise by imposing policies or legislation on communities without adequate consultation. A barrier to SCHP approaches is that some interventions are highly politicised (such as food advertising to children) (Germov et al., 2019).

The Ottawa Charter (WHO, 1986) aims to integrate individualist and SCHP approaches by focusing on 'positive' health, improving the settings for decision making on health and rewarding health professionals for their involvement in health promotion. Figure 51.5 illustrates a continuum of health promotion approaches and Table 51.2 contrasts characteristics of individualist health promotion and SCHP. The 'Translation to practice' box describes the development of a community care model, based on CDC, which led to educational resources aimed at supporting implementation of the model in community practice. For health education to be effective, culturally safe approaches are necessary.

NURSES AND COMMUNITY CARE

To cater for the diverse communities and complex health needs of Australian people, a broad range of community care

TABLE 51.2 Individualist and structuralist–collectivist health promotion

	INDIVIDUALIST HEALTH PROMOTION (IHP)	STRUCTURALIST–COLLECTIVIST HEALTH PROMOTION (SCHP)
Model of health	Biomedical or biopsychosocial model	Social model
Target level	Individuals Operates at point of entry, screening, advice Downstream determinants	Community Active care recipients and communities, social change Upstream determinants
Focus of education	Individual focus, expert-led, passive person Lifestyle, risk taking	Participatory, legislation, bureaucratic intervention Community engagement, advocacy, enabling, mediating, organisational development, builds healthy policies
Aim	Persuade individual change Improve physiological risk factors and personal behaviours	Invoke population change Address determinants of health, redress inequities
Examples	Healthy eating campaigns Safe-driving campaigns Brief intervention strategies Quit campaign	Needle exchange Legislation (e.g. banning smoking in public places, compulsory wearing of seat belts) Health services offered by Indigenous health workers working with Indigenous communities
Relationship to PHC	Selective PHC or primary care	Comprehensive PHC or primary care

Sources: Based on Richmond & Germov (2014). A sociology of health promotion. In J. Germov (ed.) *Second opinion: An introduction to health sociology* (5th ed.). Melbourne: Oxford University Press; Keleher & MacDougall (eds) (2016). *Understanding health* (4th ed.). Melbourne: Oxford University Press.

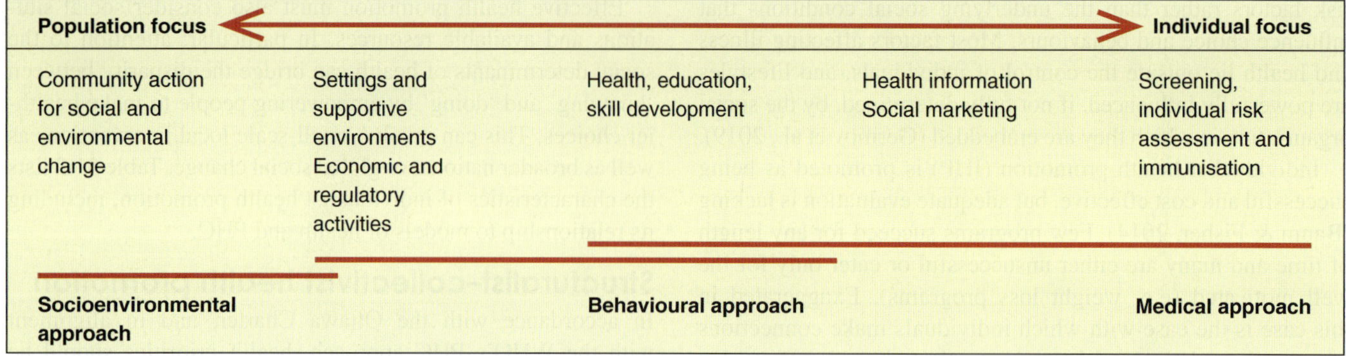

FIGURE 51.5 *Continuum of health promotion approaches*

Sources: Taylor et al. (2020). *Promoting health: The primary health care approach* (7th ed.). Sydney: Elsevier Churchill Livingstone; adapted from Labonte (1992). Heart health inequalities in Canada: Models, theory and planning. *Health Promotion International*, 7(2), 119–121.

services are needed, many of which are characterised by innovative approaches. Nurses in the community work in a range of clinical and non-clinical roles and settings (Australian Primary Health Care Nurses Association (APNA), 2017). Table 51.3 provides an insight into some of the different community settings in which nurses work.

Irrespective of the specific setting or the work performed, the goal of all primary care nurses is to improve the health and wellbeing of people, families or communities. These services care for people and communities where they live, work and gather, and this may include homes, caravans, outback campsites, schools and workplaces. Examples of some Australian community nursing services follow. Each is in the community and demonstrates aspects of primary care or PHC. They aim to meet the specific health needs of their population and each contributes to ensuring the health of its community in a different way. Reading each example should promote reflection on the key concepts discussed earlier in this chapter and how these are enacted in practice by community nurses.

Initiating courageous end-of-life conversations in the community

Conversations around death and dying can be confronting for many members of the community. These conversations may be delayed or avoided to prevent emotional distress. However, discussion or even planning for end of life ensures a person's needs and preferences are respected. Nurses within the community, especially those working in general practice settings, are ideally placed to guide individuals through these discussions and plans (Nagarajan et al., 2022a).

TRANSLATION TO PRACTICE Applying evidence about CDC to community aged care practice

Between 2010 and 2012, a major trial of aged care CDC in Australia, the People at Centre Stage (PACS) project, addressed obstacles for successful CDC reported previously by international researchers, and gathered evidence about CDC implementation in Australia (Ottmann & Mohebbi, 2014). In the PACS trial, a 'case management led capacity building and restorative health approach' (p. 600) was applied in conversations with older people to set health priorities and goals, and to support three levels of self-direction: level 1, where the older person participated in care planning; level 2, where the older person assumed both care planning and care coordination responsibility; and level 3, where the older person performed the activities of level 2 but also administered and budgeted care using a voucher option with a small cash component. Overall, the PACs model resulted in most older people reporting increased satisfaction with care and decision processes, improved health, sense of engagement and community connectedness (Ottmann, Laragy & Allen, 2012, p. 24).

Evidence obtained from the PACS trial led to the development of practical resources and tools for community aged care providers delivering CDC-based services to older Australians. These materials, referred to as the 'choices' model of CDC, provide services with materials to address the distinctive needs of older Australians while implementing CDC, including restorative health and capacity building; goal-directed care planning; individualised budgets; self-direction and mentoring; enabling risk; community connectors; and planning ahead. Resources can be obtained at the COTA website: https://www.cota.org.au/information/home-care-today/.

IMPLICATIONS FOR NURSING

- To provide CDC, nurses need to work in partnership with individuals to enable consumer choice and control about all aspects of their care.
- Community care nurses need to work with older individuals to identify their care goals as well as choose care options that match the individual's preferences for community care.

CRITICAL THINKING IN PERSON-CENTRED CARE

1 How might person-centred care be different from consumer-directed care?
2 Why might consumer direction and control be important for community-based individuals?
3 How can nurses enable consumer choice and control of community care?

TABLE 51.3 Common community nursing settings

SETTINGS	
Community settings	Include community-controlled health services, correctional facilities (including juvenile and adult), refugee health, the community health sector and roles within social service settings
Medical rooms	GPs' rooms, specialist clinics
Domiciliary settings	In the home, including residential aged care, custodial/detention settings, boarding houses and outreach to homeless people
Educational settings	Preschool, primary and secondary school, vocational and tertiary education settings
Occupational settings	Occupational health and safety and workplace nursing
Informal and unstructured settings	Include ad hoc roles in daily life, such as sports settings and community groups

Source: Guzys et al. (2020). *An introduction to community and primary health care* (3rd ed.). Melbourne: Cambridge University Press.

Advance care planning (ACP)

Advance care planning involves reflective, pragmatic discussion that enables a person to plan the type of healthcare they would or would not like to receive at the end of life. This plan is then used to inform care provision in the event of a person being unable to make or communicate health decisions for themselves (Royal Australian College of General Practitioners (RACGP), 2020). See Box 51.4.

General practice nursing

One of the largest groups of nurses working in the community are general practice nurses (see Figure 51.6). These nurses deliver nursing services in a general practice setting, mainly employed by the many private businesses and corporate chains that operate general practices across Australia (Lane et al., 2017). This role has developed due to a combination of factors, including inadequate numbers of general practitioners in the primary care sector, a renewed focus on health promotion and increased need for chronic disease management in the community (Halcomb & Ashley, 2019). A significant driver for nurse employment in general practice, particularly for the development of the nursing role in chronic disease management, has been the Nursing in Primary Health Care (NiPHC) Program funded by the Department of Health and Aged Care. While this program has evolved as more nurses are employed in general practice, the funding of nurses remains a key barrier to nurses working to the extent of their scope of practice (James, Halcomb et al., 2021).

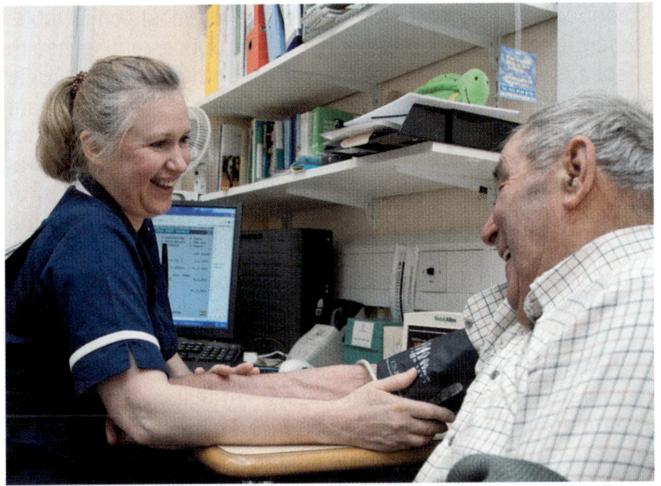

FIGURE 51.6 ***Nurses work in community-based general practices in Australia***

Source: © Life in View/Science Photo Library/Alamy Stock Photo.

The introduction in 2017 of a pilot program across Australia, the Health Care Homes model, is another initiative that supported the role of nurses in general practice. A **Health Care Home (HCH)** is defined as 'a general practice that coordinates care for people with chronic and complex conditions' (Department of Health, 2018). In an HCH, a team of health professionals, which includes a general practitioner, practice nurses and allied health, work together with the person to develop a care plan that is shared. HCH resulted in the expansion of the practice nurse role to include care coordination, chronic disease management and nurse-led services (Pearse et al., 2022).

The *National Practice Standards for Nurses in General Practice* are important in that they articulate aspects of the nursing role unique to the context of general practice, as distinct from those expected of the nurse in other clinical settings (Australian Nursing and Midwifery Federation, 2014). The 22 standards are presented in four domains: professional practice, nursing care, the general practice environment and collaborative practice. They also distinguish between the roles of the Enrolled Nurse, Registered Nurse and Advanced Practice Nurse.

BOX 51.4 Values of person-centred advance care planning

Person-centred advance care planning:

- is based on fundamental principles of self-determination, dignity and the avoidance of suffering
- promotes the expression of a person's values, beliefs and life goals
- ensures that a patient's expressed wishes remain the focus of decisions made about their care
- enhances ongoing and end-of-life care, along with personal and family satisfaction
- aids decision making for healthcare professionals and organisations
- reduces unnecessary transfers to acute care and unwanted treatment
- can be incorporated into routine general practice in the community setting.

Source: Based on RACGP (2020). *Advance care planning*. Retrieved from https://www.racgp.org.au/running-a-practice/practice-resources/practice-tools/advance-care-planning.

TRANSLATION TO PRACTICE The Advance Project

THE ADVANCE PROJECT

The Advance Project (www.theadvanceproject.com.au) seeks to enhance general practice nurses' ability to implement and initiate ACP and palliative care (PC) into everyday practice. Nagarajan et al. (2022b) undertook a qualitative study of the Advance Project using semi-structured interviews and thematic analysis. The Project provided practical, evidence-based resources and training funded by the Australian Government. Nurses received a toolkit of resources and multi-component training involving online modules and face-to-face workshops. This training enhanced nurses' ability to provide person-centred ACP in a location where people felt most comfortable: their community. Nurses initiated ACP during routine health assessments with older people and those with chronic conditions, and assessed patients palliative/supportive care needs. Over time, the Project expanded to include the wider general practice team, with education provided to general practitioners and practice managers. Additionally, four champion primary health networks (PHNs) implemented the Project throughout their region, assisting practices with ongoing trainer development, workshop delivery and support.

IMPLICATIONS FOR NURSING

On evaluation, the Advance Project enhanced nurses' competency and confidence when implementing ACP in practice (Nagarajan et al., 2022b). As with all new innovations, implementation into regular routine will take time and ongoing practical support for nurses is essential for sustainability in the short term and long term. Despite the emotional and professional challenges presented by ACP in practice, the Advance Project highlights the valuable contribution nurses make in supporting the community in end-of-life decisions.

CRITICAL THINKING IN PERSON-CENTRED CARE

1 What are your patient's values and preferences for end-of-life care? How can you incorporate them into their care plan?
2 What are your patient's goals for their remaining time? How can you support them in achieving those goals?
3 What are your patient's cultural, spiritual or religious beliefs that may impact their preferences for end-of-life care? How can you respect and incorporate those beliefs into their care plan?

Recently, the contribution of general practice nurses to mental health care has been identified. To that end, the *Mental Health Practice Standards for Nurses in Australian General Practice*, authored by Halcomb et al. (2018), was produced by the Australian College of Mental Health Nurses. These standards highlight the important role of the general practice nurse in assessment, triage and either intervention or referral. As we see increasing numbers of people experiencing mental health sequelae following the COVID-19 pandemic, the importance of this role is magnified (Halcomb et al., 2021).

Managing acute illness at home

Community nurses work in a range of contexts, including people's homes and community health centres. They can either be generalist nurses or provide specialty services (e.g. palliative care, heart failure). Community nurses are generally employed by the Local Health District or non-government organisations (e.g. McGrath Breast Care). For the community nurse, contact with people is initiated for many reasons. In the following exemplar, nursing assistance was sought because of an acute illness. It demonstrates a nursing focus beyond the individual to the family, and to health beyond the immediate health issue. Assessing the needs of the person in their own environment and within their normal family relationships highlights the importance of being holistic in the way health is considered. The following narrative provides an example of primary care which extends beyond the biomedical model.

Jed, a community nurse working in a new local multipurpose centre, has been asked to see Mr Louis Spelt, aged 72 years. The reason given for the referral from a hospital ward is care of a wound with a vacuum-assisted closure (VAC) system and continuous IV antibiotic therapy administered via a Baxter pump into a peripheral intravenous catheter (PIC) line. Mr Spelt has returned home from the local private hospital following revision surgery of his tibia. He originally had a benign tumour removed near his knee but an infection developed and required further removal of bone, and debridement of the original wound.

Jed arrives at Mr Spelt's home and notices it has four steps at the entry. Mr Spelt's husband answers the door and invites Jed into their home. Jed finds Mr Spelt in his dressing gown and waiting in the living room. The room is very comfortable but is cluttered. Jed proceeds to complete their assessments and, in consultation with Mr Spelt and his husband, identifies that Mr Spelt will need nursing care every morning to renew the Baxter infusion and to monitor the VAC dressing, also allowing time for carer support for Mr Spelt's husband, Jim, and health education as their situation changes.

During the holistic assessment Jim assists, describing himself as 'Louis' full-time carer at the moment. He really can't do much for himself.' Before Jed completes the consultation, they are able to discuss with Mr Spelt some of his other needs and what support Jim needs in his caring role. Jed discusses pain management and completion of activities of daily living. Mr Spelt is mobilising with a single crutch and has an exercise program that he doesn't think is important. Jed, Louis and Jim review the program and work out an achievable plan to follow. Jed also discusses ways of reducing the risk of falls, including the removal of some occasional tables in the living room. They further express a concern about the entry steps, but Jim assures Jed that Louis would only use them when he is there to assist.

One week passes and Jed arrives to change the VAC dressing for the third time. Jed no longer changes the Baxter unit daily as they have been able to educate Louis and Jim to attend to this independently; every morning after his shower they do this together. Jim is proud that he can help and they are pleased, because once the Baxter is changed, they are free to continue their day and no longer need to wait for the nurse to arrive. Although there is still the dressing, life is returning to normal for them.

Today while Jed is changing the VAC dressing, they reflect on the changes that have occurred over the past week. Louis met them at the door and was dressed in casual clothes ready for a trip to his friend's house. He was relaxed and chatting about a cruise they were going to book once his leg had healed. The living room was free of clutter and Jim was hanging out the washing.

Jed's narrative shows how individual and family wellbeing are facilitated despite significant illness. Mr Spelt's clinical recovery has been supported by the community nurse's actions, for him as an individual and as a couple. The community nurse's role has been described as one where '... you are very much involved in a person's life, not just their condition... In this kind of nursing one must consider all of the influences in a client's situation' (Adrian, 2009, p. 43).

THE WAY FORWARD

Revision and reorientation of the Australian healthcare system towards a more comprehensive PHC approach is required in response to increasing social and demographic factors, such as health system burdens from chronic conditions, an ageing population and a need to manage increasing healthcare costs (Department of Health, 2022). The complexity and volume of care delivered also continues to increase due to factors such as reduced hospital stay duration, increased focus on ageing in place and care at home, and de-institutionalisation processes (Department of Health, 2021). Governments across Australia are now focused on developing capacity in the prevention and management of chronic conditions. In particular, the recently developed National Preventive Health Strategy (Department of Health, 2021) and Primary Health Care 10 Year Plan (Department of Health, 2022) set out the roadmap for developing PHC in Australia. The goals of this health reform have been a reorientation of services toward increased PHC and include increased service access, strengthened prevention and early intervention, improved management of chronic conditions, integrated delivery and cross-disciplinary team-based care (AIHW, 2018). Central to these developments is a desire to shift the emphasis of the system from narrow hospital-based care, treatment and cure of already established disease to the promotion of health across the lifespan; prevention of injury/disease; effective management of chronic disease; and the reduction of health inequalities. This inherently emphasises the importance of integrated systems including strong primary care and population-based services, making them linchpins of the health system. To achieve this outcome, more nurses will be needed, with nurses working in diverse community roles and in ways that harness the benefits of a PHC approach (APNA, 2017).

This expectation that PHC will become increasingly important in Australia is reflected in the revision of the *Code of Conduct for Nurses*, where Principle 7 focuses on health and wellbeing (Nursing and Midwifery Board of Australia (NMBA), 2018). Not only the nurses working in community settings, but all nurses have a responsibility to improve the health of the community. See Box 51.5 for Principle 7 of the *Code of Conduct for Nurses*.

Choosing to work as a nurse in the community is an exciting decision and a step towards a challenging and rewarding career. In community care, the community as a whole and the person are both privileged, no matter whether they are a child, a family, a work team or a school. It is important to acknowledge that community members have the potential to make their own decisions about their health and healthcare. The challenge is to work in a sustained way with individuals, groups and organisations to assist community members, their families and community groups to prevent illness and injury, and to lead healthy and rewarding lives. Optimising health for the community is about ensuring a quality of life that is consistent with the individual's and community's needs and values and is within the WHO's framework for 'Health for All' (WHO, 1978).

BOX 51.5 *Code of Conduct for Nurses* Principle 7: Health and Wellbeing

Principle 7: Health and Wellbeing

Nurses have a responsibility to improve population health and hold views complementary to the philosophies of primary healthcare. They are ideally placed to contribute to this reform and the health of communities. Nurses promote health and wellbeing for people and their families, colleagues, the broader community and themselves and in a way that addresses health inequality.

Source: NMBA (2018). *Code of Conduct for Nurses*. Retrieved from https://www.nursingmidwiferyboard.gov.au/.

CHAPTER HIGHLIGHTS

- The factors that determine the health of a community include societal, environmental and socioeconomic factors, as well as the knowledge, values, beliefs and health behaviours of individuals and the community as a whole.
- Different models of health underpin the way community organisations contribute to the health of individuals and communities.
- In Australia, community services are underpinned by the biomedical, psychosocial and social models of health. Those services underpinned by a social model of health will approach health differently from acute care services based on the biomedical or psychosocial model.
- Community care is delivered in a diverse range of settings, to diverse populations and by a range of different people/services.
- Cultural safety is integral to community care in all settings.
- Community care is provided in partnership with the person and their family, and a range of government and non-government organisations.
- Health promotion and health education are based on different models of health and contribute in different ways to achieving community health. Structural–collectivist approaches to health promotion support primary healthcare.
- Many community organisations in Australia approach community care service provision using a primary care approach rather than a primary healthcare approach.

CONCEPT CHECK

1 Social determinants of health are:
1 all biological and environmental conditions that affect the health of people and communities
2 the conditions in which people are born, grow, live, work and age
3 the biological factors that cause ill health in people
4 none of the above

2 Which factors are considered important social determinants of the health for an individual or group in a community? (Select all that apply.)
1 presence of disease
2 unemployment
3 attitudes
4 genetics
5 life skills

3 Primary healthcare is described by the World Health Organization as essential healthcare based on practical, scientifically sound and socially acceptable methods, which is affordable and is delivered to individuals and families in the community.
1 true
2 false

4 Match the following terms to as many models as needed for each term.

Terms
a Primary healthcare
b Primary care

Models
1 Social model of health
2 Biomedical model of health
3 Biopsychosocial model of health

5 What are the principles that underpin a primary healthcare orientation to community health? (Select all that apply.)
1 social justice
2 medical expertise
3 equity
4 responsiveness to need
5 community participation

6 Which of the following are characteristics of primary care? (Select all that apply.)
1 reduction of specific disease and a technical focus
2 based on the biomedical model of health
3 involvement of sectors other than health
4 focus on curative care, with some attention to prevention and promotion
5 limited community engagement

7 Which of the following are characteristics of primary healthcare? (Select all that apply.)
1 improvement in overall health of the community and individuals, and 'Health for All' as overall social and political goal
2 based on the socioecological model of health
3 strong focus on health sector with very limited involvement from other sectors
4 comprehensive strategy with curative, rehabilitative, preventive and health promotion that seeks to remove root causes of health
5 engaged participation that starts with community strengths and the community's assessment of health issues, is ongoing and aims for community control

8 Which of the following are drivers to reorienting community service organisations towards primary healthcare? (Select all that apply.)
1 One-quarter of the total population suffers from chronic disease which will never be cured.
2 Medical and social aspects of health are so interrelated that they require teams of health and welfare professionals to assist.
3 Behaviour and attitudes of people influence their health. Prevention can be encouraged in the community.
4 Demand for greater provision and variety of primary health services.

9 In health, two common ways of understanding what is meant by 'community' are:
1 community as relationships
2 community as politics
3 community as locality
4 community as health

10 On the continuum of interventions using social determinants, which of the following levels of health determinant have a more direct effect on the health of an individual?
1 distal and proximal determinants
2 proximal and intermediate determinants
3 distal and intermediate determinants
4 none of the above

11 Intersectoral collaboration refers to:
1 health professionals' interaction within community organisations
2 health professionals' interaction within their own organisation
3 health professionals' interaction with non-health organisations
4 none of the above

BIBLIOGRAPHY

Adrian, A. (2009). *Primary health care in Australia: A nursing and midwifery consensus view*. Royal College of Nursing Australia. Retrieved from https://www.anf.org.au/

Aged Care Guide (2022). Retrieved from https://www.agedcareguide.com.au/

Au, M., Anandakumar, A. D., Preston, R. et al. (2019). A model explaining refugee experiences of the Australian healthcare system: A systematic review of refugee perceptions. *BMC International Health and Human Rights, 19*, 22. https://doi.org/10.1186/s12914-019-0206-6

Australian Commission on Safety and Quality in Health Care (ACSQHC) (2021). *National Safety and Quality Health Service Standards* (2nd ed.). Sydney: ACSQHC

Australian Institute of Health and Welfare (AIHW) (2014). *Australia's health 2014*. Australia's health series no. 14. (Cat. no. AUS 178.) Canberra: AIHW.

Australian Institute of Health and Welfare (AIHW) (2018). *Australia's health 2018*. Australia's health series no 16. (Cat no. AUS 221.) Canberra: AIHW.

Australian Institute of Health and Welfare (AIHW) (2021). *Health expenditure Australia 2019–20*. Retrieved from https://www.aihw.gov.au/

Australian Institute of Health and Welfare (AIHW) (2022a). *Australia's health 2022*. Retrieved from https://www.aihw.gov.au/

Australian Institute of Health and Welfare (AIHW) (2022b). *Digital health*. Retrieved from https://www.aihw.gov.au/

Australian Institute of Health and Welfare (AIHW) (2022c). *Social determinants of health*. Retrieved from https://www.aihw.gov.au/

Australian Institute of Health and Welfare (AIHW) (2022d). *Health across socioeconomic groups*. Retrieved from https://www.aihw.gov.au/

Australian Nursing and Midwifery Federation (2014). *National Practice Standards for Nurses in General Practice*. Melbourne: Australian Nursing and Midwifery Federation.

Australian Primary Health Care Nurses Association (APNA) (2017). *Improving patient outcomes: Primary health care nurses working to the breadth of their scope of practice. Position statement.* Melbourne: APNA.

Australian Productivity Commission (2022). *Report on government services.* Ch. 10: Primary and community health. Retrieved from https://www.pc.gov.au/

Baum, F. (2016). *The new public health* (4th ed.). Melbourne: Oxford University Press.

Baum, F. & Fisher, M. (2014). Why behavioural health promotion endures despite its failure to reduce health inequities. *Sociology of Health and Illness, 36*(2), 213–225. doi: 10.1111/1467-9566.12112

Baum, F., Delany, T., MacDougall, C. et al. (2017). Ideas, actors and institutions: Lessons from South Australian health in all policies on what encourages other sectors' involvement. *BMC Public Health, 17*(811), 1–16.

COTA (2023). *What is CDC?* Retrieved from https://www.cota.org.au/

Department of Health (2018). *Health Care Homes.* Retrieved from http://www.health.gov.au/

Department of Health (2021). *National Preventive Health Strategy 2021–2030.* Retrieved from http://www.health.gov.au/

Department of Health (2022). *Australia's Primary Health Care 10 Year Plan 2022–2032.* Retrieved from http://www.health.gov.au/

Eagar, K., Owen, A., Cranny, C., Thompson, C. & Samsa, P. (2008). *Community health at the crossroads: Which way now? Final report of the NSW Community Health Review.* Wollongong: Centre for Health Service Development, University of Wollongong.

Froehlich-Grobe, K., Douglas, M., Ochoa, C. & Betts, A. (2021). Social determinants of health and disability. In D. J. Lollar, W. Horner-Johnson & K. Froehlich-Grobe (eds), *Public health perspectives on disability: Science, social justice, ethics, and beyond* (2nd ed., pp. 53–89). New York: Springer.

Germov, J. (2019). Imagining health problems as social issues. In J. Germov (ed.), *Second opinion: An introduction to health sociology* (6th ed.). Melbourne: Oxford University Press.

Germov, J., Freij, M. & Richmond, K. (2019). A sociology of health promotion. In J. Germov (ed.), *Second opinion: An introduction to health sociology* (6th ed.). Melbourne: Oxford University Press.

Guzys, D., Whitehead, D., Brown, R. & Halcomb, E. J. (2020). *An introduction to community and primary health care* (3rd ed.). Melbourne: Cambridge University Press.

Halcomb, E. & Ashley, C. (2019). Are Australian general practice nurses underutilised? An examination of current roles and task satisfaction. *Collegian, 26*(5), 522–527.

Halcomb, E., McInnes, S., Moxham, L. & Patterson, C. (2018). *Mental Health Practice Standards for Nurses in Australian General Practice.* Canberra: ACMHN.

Halcomb, E., McInnes, S., Patterson, C., Moxham, L. & Bird, S. (2021). Australian general practice nurse involvement in mental health: A descriptive survey. *Collegian, 29*(4), 448–455.

Halcomb, E., Thompson, C., Tillott, S., Robinson, K. & Lucas, E. (2022). Exploring social connectedness in older Australians with chronic conditions: Results of a descriptive survey. *Collegian, 29*(6), 860–866.

Home Care Today (2022). *Home Care Package basics.* Retrieved from https://www.cota.org.au/

James, S., Ashley, C., Williams, A. et al. (2021). Experiences of primary health care nurses in using telehealth during COVID-19: A qualitative study. *BMJ Open, 11*(8), 1–7.

James, S., Halcomb, E., Desborough, J. et al. (2021). Barriers and facilitators to lifestyle risk communication by Australian general practice nurses. *Australian Journal of Primary Health, 27*, 30–35.

Johnson, M. I., Bonacaro, A., Georgiadis, E. & Woodall, J. (2022). Reconfiguring the biomedical dominance of pain: Time for alternative perspectives from health promotion? *Health Promotion International, 37*(4), daac128.

Kadandale, S., Marten, R., Dalglish, S. L., Rajan, D. & Hipgrave, D. B. (2020). Primary health care and the climate crisis. *Bulletin of the World Health Organization, 98*(11), 818–820. doi: 10.2471/BLT.20.252882

Kearon, J. & Risdon, C. The role of primary care in a pandemic: Reflections during the COVID-19 pandemic in Canada. *Journal of Primary Care and Community Health, 11*, 2150132720962871. doi: 10.1177/2150132720962871.

Keleher, H. & MacDougall, C. (eds) (2016). *Understanding health* (4th ed.). Melbourne: Oxford University Press.

Keleher, H. & MacDougall, C. (2021). *Understanding health* (5th ed.). Melbourne: Oxford University Press.

Labonte, R. (1992). Heart health inequalities in Canada: Models, theory and planning. *Health Promotion International, 7*(2), 119–121.

Lane, R. et al. (2017). Advancing general practice nursing in Australia: Roles and responsibilities of primary health care organisations. *Australian Health Review, 41*(2), 127–132.

Marmot, M. (2002). The influence of income on health: Views of an epidemiologist. *Health Affairs, 21*(2), 31–46.

Mllroy, T. & Bandler, L. G. (2021). Closing the Gap: Where to now? *Medical Journal of Australia, 214*(5), 209–210.

Nagarajan, S. V., Lewis, V., Halcomb, E. et al. (2022a). Barriers and facilitators to nurse-led advance care planning and palliative care practice change in primary healthcare: A qualitative study. *Australian Journal of Primary Health, 28*(2), 151–157. doi: 10.1071/PY21081

Nagarajan, S. V., Lewis, V., Halcomb, E. et al. (2022b). Australian general practice experiences of implementing a structured approach to initiating advance care planning and palliative care: A qualitative study. *BMJ Open, 12*, e057184. doi: 10.1136/bmjopen-2021-057184

Nursing and Midwifery Board of Australia (NMBA) (2018). *Code of Conduct for Nurses.* Retrieved from https://www.nursingmidwiferyboard.gov.au/

Nutbeam, D. & Lloyd, J. E. (2020). Understanding and responding to health literacy as a social determinant of health. *Annual Review of Public Health, 42*, 159–173.

Ottmann, G., Laragy, C. & Allen, J. (2012). *People at centre stage: Evaluation summary report.* Melbourne: UCCO/Deakin University QPS.

Ottmann, G. & Mohebbi, M. (2014). Self-directed community services for older Australians: A stepped capacity-building approach. *Health and Social Care in the Community, 22*(6), 598–611. doi: 10.1111/hsc.12111

Pearse, J., Mazevska, D., McElduff, P. et al. (2022). *Health Care Homes trial final evaluation report.* Volume 1: Summary report. St Leonards, NSW: Health Policy Analysis.

Richmond, K. & Germov, J. (2014). A sociology of health promotion. In J. Germov (ed.), *Second opinion: An introduction to health sociology* (5th ed.). Melbourne: Oxford University Press.

Royal Australian College of General Practitioners (RACGP) (2020). *Advance care planning.* Retrieved from https://www.racgp.org.au/

Shepherd, S. M., Willis-Esqueda, C., Paradies, Y., Sivasubramaniam, D., Sherwood, J. & Brockie, T. (2018). Racial and cultural minority experiences and perceptions of health care provision in a mid-western region. *International Journal for Equity in Health, 17*(1), 33. doi: 10.1186/s12939-018-0744-x

Taylor, J. (2015). *Working with communities.* Melbourne: Oxford University Press.

Taylor, J., O'Hara, L., Talbot, L. & Verrinder, G. (2020). *Promoting health: The primary health care approach* (7th ed.). Sydney: Elsevier Churchill Livingstone.

Taylor, K. & Guerin, P. (2019). *Health care and Indigenous Australians: Cultural safety in practice* (3rd ed.). London: Macmillan.

Wilkinson, R. & Marmot, M. (2003). *Social determinants of health: The solid facts* (2nd ed.). Denmark: WHO. Retrieved from http://www.euro.who.int/

Williams, R., Dune, T. & McLeod, K. (2021). Principles of cultural safety. In T. Dune, K. McLeod & R. Williams (eds), *Culture, diversity and health in Australia: Towards culturally safe health care* (pp. 55–72). UK: Routledge.

World Health Organization (WHO) (1978). *The Declaration of Alma-Ata, International Conference on Primary Health Care.* Retrieved from http://www.who.int/

World Health Organization (WHO) (1986). *Ottawa Charter for Health Promotion.* Retrieved from http://www.who.int/

World Health Organization (WHO) (2008). *Closing the gap in a generation: Health equity through action on the social determinants of health (Commission on Social Determinants of Health Final Report).* World Health Organization. Retrieved from http://www.who.int/

World Health Organization (WHO) & United Nations Children's Fund (UNICEF) (2018). *A vision for primary health care in the 21st century: Towards universal health coverage and the Sustainable Development Goals.* Retrieved from http://www.who.int/

Yerkes, M. A., Hoogenboom, M. & Javornik, J. (2020). Where's the community in community, work and family? A community-based capabilities approach. *Community, Work & Family, 23*(5), 516–533. doi: 10.1080/13668803.2020.1818547

USEFUL WEBSITES

Australian Government Department of Social Services, a national service that supports both consumers and home care providers to work together to implement consumer-directed care through Home Care Packages: https://homecaretoday.org.au

Australian Health Promotion Association: https://www.healthpromotion.org.au

Australian Indigenous Health*InfoNet*: https://healthinfonet.ecu.edu.au

Australian Women's Health Network: www.awhn.org.au

Centre for Culture, Ethnicity & Health: https://www.ceh.org.au

Community Health Nurses, Western Australia: https://cahs.health.wa.gov.au/For-health-professionals/Resources/Community-Health-Clinical-Nursing-Manual

Department of Health and Aged Care: www.health.gov.au

National Health and Medical Research Council: https://nhmrc.gov.au

Palliative Care Australia: https://palliativecare.org.au

Primary Health Care Research & Information Service: www.phcris.org.au

World Health Organization: https://www.who.int/en

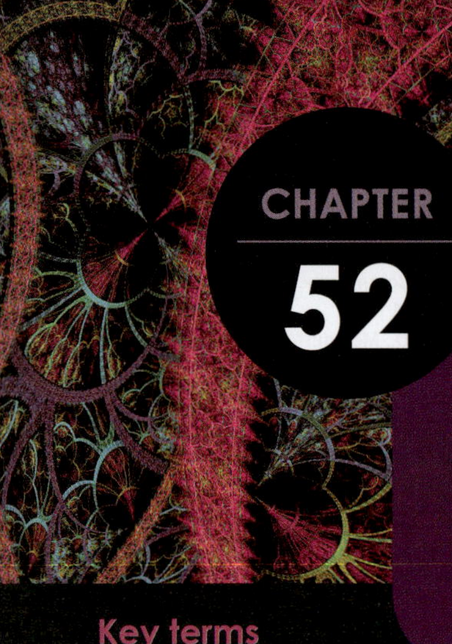

CHAPTER 52

Nursing care of people in regional and remote areas of Australia

Helen Pratt, Heidi Green

Key terms

continuum of care 1892
discharge planning 1892
Indigenous health 1883
primary healthcare 1882
referral 1891
regional and remote health workforce 1884
retrieval 1887
social determinants of health 1883
triage in regional and remote areas 1888

Learning outcomes

- Discuss the challenges faced in providing nursing care in regional and remote communities.
- Discuss the rewards of nursing in regional and remote areas.
- Identify the determinants of regional and remote classification in Australia.
- Identify the determinants of regional and remote health.
- Describe nursing in remote Indigenous communities with regard to cultural awareness, cultural safety and the rights of people living in these communities.
- Describe the role of the nurse in regional and remote healthcare.
- Discuss the barriers to healthcare for people living in regional and remote communities.

Clinical competencies

- Use evidence-based practice guidelines and clinical assessment skills to inform clinical decision making.
- Provide timely and accurate person-centred assessment.
- Incorporate an understanding of the local determinants of healthcare provision in regional and remote areas into quality nursing care.
- Use evidence-based nursing practice to provide quality nursing care in acute and non-acute situations, including health promotion and prevention strategies.
- Incorporate the principles of primary healthcare into the provision of nursing care in regional and remote settings.
- Provide culturally safe nursing care.
- Use professional communication skills to develop therapeutic relationships and establish professional boundaries when working in regional and remote communities.
- Use assessment findings to determine initial nursing care, referral and transfer as deemed necessary.
- Recognise and work within the interdisciplinary team locally and in distance mode.
- Incorporate all available resources, including technological resources, to maximise health outcomes.
- Recognise special considerations for people from regional and remote areas in the discharge planning process.

Note on clinical competencies

This chapter relates regional and remote nursing in Australia to the Nursing and Midwifery Board of Australia (NMBA) *Registered Nurse Standards for Practice* (2016a). The *Registered Nurse Standards for Practice* are used in conjunction with other NMBA standards, codes and guidelines to ensure that nursing practice is safe and coordinated. Additionally, the standards for practice facilitate quality nursing that includes comprehensive assessment, planning, implementation and evaluation of care that is provided.

The terms 'regional' and 'remote' imply geographical distance; however, the communities, people and available health services in these areas can vary greatly. So, too, do the responsibilities, roles and philosophies employed when providing nursing care for people in these areas. Therefore, any discussion about regional and remote nursing requires acknowledgement that there is no single definition of 'regional' or 'remote' and an awareness of the specific areas being discussed to ensure accurate and consistent representation.

Understanding regional and remote nursing is not exclusively the domain of the local workforce, health department officials or government policy advisers. All nurses, including those working in large metropolitan areas, need to possess a sound knowledge of the associated challenges and barriers. However, with the introduction of technology in healthcare, those challenges are much fewer than ever before.

Nurses provide a greater percentage of healthcare than any other health-related discipline (Department of Health, 2021a), and regional and remote nursing encompasses a vast range of nursing skills, including the ability to accurately identify and assess the health needs of people in these communities and to refer and/or transfer people to major health centres as appropriate. Nurses working in referral centres also face unique challenges when caring and planning discharge for people who reside in regional or remote areas.

This chapter discusses the nursing care of people in regional and remote areas from two perspectives: first, the challenges, opportunities and rewards associated with nursing in regional and remote Australia; and second, the provision of nursing care for people from those areas.

CHALLENGES AND REWARDS

Nurses choose to work in remote areas for many reasons. The reason that brings them to the community can be the same reason they leave, including partner employment, family commitments, end of employment contract and change in life expectations. Leaving remote communities can be a distressing time for the nurse, colleagues and community members. The situation can be compounded if there is difficulty in filling the vacant nursing position.

Working in regional and remote areas can be extraordinarily challenging while at the same time being immensely rewarding. Nursing practice in regional and remote areas is holistic. A nurse who works in a small community for many years may provide nursing care for several generations of a family, providing holistic care from the excitement of birth to challenges of chronic illness and impacts of death.

THE DIFFERENCES BETWEEN 'REGIONAL' AND 'REMOTE'

One of the most complex tasks when discussing regional and remote issues is to identify common definition. To assist in providing a consistent guide, the Australian Government uses classifications that combine many of the factors impacting on an individual's access to services based on location. These classifications are the Accessibility/Remoteness Index of Australia (ARIA+) (University of Adelaide, 2021) and the Australian Statistical Geography Standard (ASGS) (Australian Bureau of Statistics (ABS), 2021). The ASGS is divided into two sections: the ABS, which provides statistical information, and non-ABS structures (see Figure 52.1).

There is a complex and dynamic method of determining remoteness areas (RAs) in Australia. Remoteness is measured by the ARIA+, with the approach that over time population centres change size and, as road networks are established, the boundaries of remoteness are changed (ABS, 2018). Australia is divided into five geographical boundaries that include Major Cities, Inner Regional Australia, Outer Regional Australia, Remote Australia and Very Remote Australia. See Figure 52.2.

Nurses require knowledge of the RAs for a range of reasons. Of great importance is the statistical evidence that people who live in Remote and Very Remote Australia have overall poorer mortality (up to 1.5 times higher) and morbidity than those who live in major cities (Australian Institute of Health and Welfare (AIHW), 2021a). Aboriginal and Torres Strait Islander people make up a higher proportion (up to 32%) of the Remote and Very Remote area population than the Major Cities population. Indigenous people in regional and remote areas are also over-represented in poorer health outcomes data overall. This is consistent with the lower life expectancy rates for Indigenous people in Australia: 71.6 years for Indigenous males compared to 80.2 years for non-Indigenous males and 75.6 years for Indigenous females compared to 83.4 years for non-Indigenous females (AIHW, 2021a). Indigenous Australians are also twice as likely to die from suicide (AIHW, 2021a). The Council of Remote Area Nurses of Australia (CRANAplus) explains that working in remote areas can present its own set of challenges for nurses (CRANAplus, 2021). This can be due to factors such as geography causing difficult access, extreme distance and variations in weather conditions. The population is scattered, with people from different cultures and groups requiring care for challenging health conditions. Lack of resources and a highly itinerant group of health professionals also impact on delivery of quality health services to people in regional and remote areas of Australia (CRANAplus, 2021). A nurse working in a remote

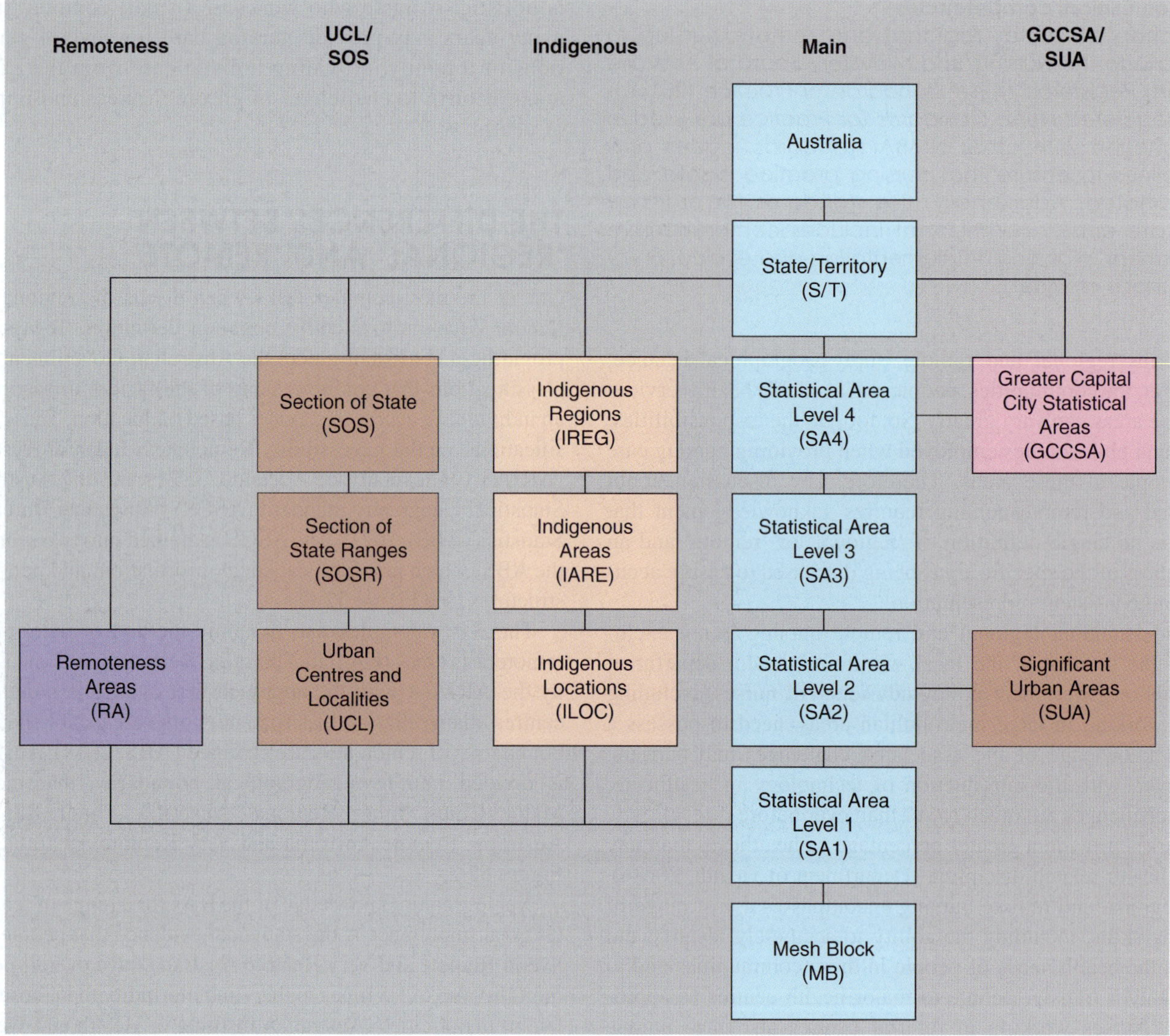

FIGURE 52.1 ***ASGS ABS structure***

Source: ABS (2018). *1270.0.55.005 Australian Statistical Geography Standard (ASGS): Volume 5—Remoteness structure, July 2016*, Diagram 1. Retrieved from https://www.abs.gov.au/ausstats/abs@.nsf/mf/1270.0.55.005.

location gains significant knowledge and experience as a generalist nurse; however, recognition of this role is severely lacking (Muirhead & Birks, 2019).

Regional and remote nursing

In Australia, nursing is one of the most stable and equally distributed healthcare disciplines, with many nurses working in a diverse range of settings within regional and remote areas. However, the nursing workforce in Very Remote Australia, just like the rest of Australia, is ageing (Collett, Fraser & Thompson, 2020). Nurses and midwives working in Very Remote Australia have an average age of 47.5 years, whereas the average age of nurses and midwives working in Major Cities is 42.6 years, and the overall average is 43.1 years (Department of Health, 2021a). A high 89.0% of the nurse workforce employed in Remote/Very Remote areas is women (Department of Health, 2018a), with only 1.3% of the workforce identifying as Indigenous (Department of Health, 2021a). Nurses and midwives working in Very Remote areas work the greatest number of hours: 40.1 hours per week compared with the national average of 33.5 hours per week (Department of Health, 2018a). Many Remote communities rely on health professionals who have not trained in Australia and on locums or fly-in/fly-out (FIFO) healthcare providers who do not have an ability to provide health services that are culturally responsive and culturally safe (AIHW, 2022a).

CRANAplus (see https://crana.org.au) describes Remote Area Nurses (RANs) as working in a multitude of settings such as Aboriginal and Torres Strait Islander communities, outback and isolated towns, farm communities, islands, tourist locations, mines and railways. They must have skills that facilitate a primary healthcare response ranging from covering an emergency to administering a variety of medications

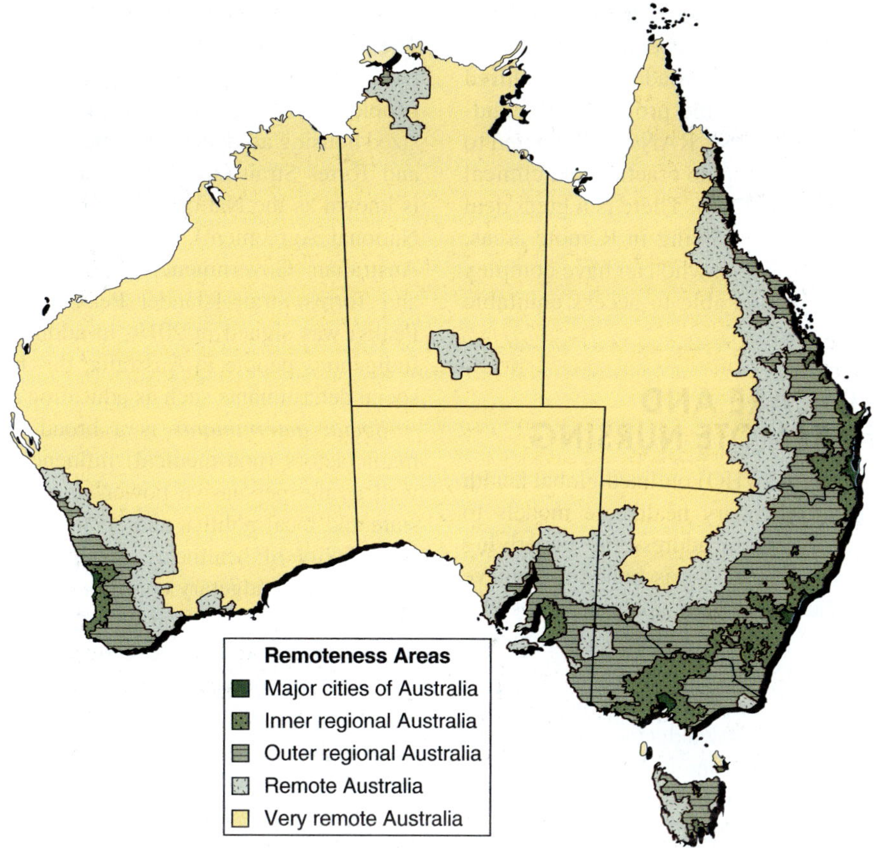

FIGURE 52.2 ***Map of the 2016 remoteness areas for Australia***

Source: ABS (2018). *1270.0.55.005 Australian Statistical Geography Standard (ASGS): Volume 5—Remoteness structure, July 2016*. Retrieved from https://www.abs.gov.au/ausstats/abs@.nsf/mf/1270.0.55.005. © Commonwealth of Australia, Australian Bureau of Statistics. Licensed under the Creative Commons Attribution 4.0 International License, https//creativecommons.org/licenses/by/4.0.

FAST FACTS

- Approximately 72.6% of the Australian population resides in Major Cities (ABS, 2017).
- Approximately 1.4 % of the population lives in Remote or Very Remote Australia (ABS, 2017).
- The Northern Territory has the largest percentage of people (59.5%) living in Outer Regional areas (including Darwin), and Remote (19.5%) and Very Remote (21%) areas (ABS, 2022a).
- The life expectancy for Aboriginal and Torres Strait Islander men is estimated to be 10.6 years lower than for non-Indigenous men (AIHW, 2021a).
- The life expectancy for Aboriginal and Torres Strait Islander women is 9.5 years lower than for non-Indigenous women (AIHW, 2021a).
- The mortality rate of Indigenous Australians is nearly twice that of non-Indigenous Australians and five times higher for Indigenous people aged 35 to 44 years (AIHW, 2021a).
- The rate of dying due to a land transport accident is approximately four times higher in Remote and Very Remote areas compared with all of Australia (AIHW, 2022b).
- The suicide rate for Remote and Very Remote areas is 2–2.9 times higher compared with all of Australia (AIHW, 2022b).
- Homelessness is an issue not only in major cities. There are high rates of homelessness in regional and remote areas due to family and domestic violence, housing affordability stress, financial difficulties, mental illness and drug and alcohol misuse (AIHW, 2021b). The total number of Aboriginal and Torres Strait Islander people who received support from specialist homelessness services (SHS) in 2020–2021 increased three times faster than for the non-Indigenous population (AIHW, 2021b).
- Of the proportion of people living in Very Remote and Remote areas, the Aboriginal and Torres Strait Islander population is high, with 12% living in Very Remote, compared to 0.5% of non-Indigenous Australians, and 6.7% in Remote areas, compared to 1.0% of non-Indigenous Australians (ABS, 2017).
- The nursing workforce in Australia increased by 14.1% from 2015 to 2020 (AIHW, 2022c).

to providing health education. The scope of practice required of an RAN can be quite diverse and, depending on a number of factors, can become quite broad when required (CRANAplus, 2021). In addition to the professional standards expected of any Registered Nurse, RANs are expected to adhere to their own standards of remote practice and clinical governance guide (CRANAplus, 2018). There is a great deal to know about the health of people living in Remote areas, particularly about Indigenous people, who can have complex health issues but who may be less able to access equitable health services.

PRIMARY HEALTHCARE AND REGIONAL AND REMOTE NURSING

The World Health Organization (WHO) outlined global health strategies ranging from early primary healthcare models to more specific strategies designed to address the underlying factors that affect health outcomes. This is hoped to achieve defined healthcare goals. These healthcare goals, as defined by the United Nations (UN), are supported by the 17 Sustainable Development Goals (SDGs) (UN, 2022).

The delivery of any health service based on **primary healthcare** principles includes acknowledgement of the individual and often specialised needs of the community. Primary healthcare is taken seriously in Australia, as demonstrated by the introduction of the Primary Health Network (PHN) in 2016, a Commonwealth Government initiative that works collaboratively with healthcare providers in the local community to increase the effectiveness of healthcare for the community (Department of Health and Aged Care, 2022a). The PHN considers an interdisciplinary approach, addressing all aspects of healthcare, from prevention and early detection to curative, rehabilitative and palliative services. Therefore, the role of the nurse in these areas has evolved. An example of this is the Nurse Navigator program that was first introduced to Queensland in 2016. The role is recognised as that of an advanced clinical practitioner who is able to provide a person with complex needs with other community links so that there is ongoing support with their general health and wellbeing (Queensland Government, 2019). Further examples are the level of care that can be provided by nurse and midwifery practitioners who are able to diagnose and treat illness independently as well as with medical practitioners and other allied healthcare team members (Department of Health, 2021b).

Through the Stronger Rural Health Strategy and the Rural Health Stakeholder Roundtable, a number of programs have been implemented to increase training and education in order to expand the regional and remote workforce in Australia, such as GP, medical student, nursing and allied health training incentives and scholarships (Department of Health, 2021c).

Primary healthcare and social determinants of health

In 2008, the WHO generated a report on the social determinants of health, highlighting the issue of inequity in healthcare globally. The report identified that health equity and social justice were imperative to assisting in closing the gap in a generation. The Australian Government made a commitment to work with in partnership with Aboriginal and Torres Strait Islander people to achieve health equality by increasing appropriately sized housing and increasing the life expectancy for Aboriginal and Torres Strait Islander people by 2031. This commitment is known as the National Agreement on Closing the Gap (the National Agreement). The National Agreement between all Australian Governments and the Coalition of Aboriginal and Torres Strait Islander Peak Organisations (Coalition of Peaks) was signed in 2019. In addition to health equality for Indigenous people in Australia, this health plan targets other social determinants such as education and employment.

Social determinants is a broad term that describes the main factors (non-medical) influencing health outcomes. As well as the persuasive power of global economics, national, state and local politics and economics influence the access to and quality of healthcare services. All governments, policy advisers and budgetary committees must be prepared to invest in the future health of all of their citizens in order to achieve the goals outlined by the United Nations Declaration on the Rights of Indigenous Peoples (UN, 2007) and the Close the Gap Statement of Intent (WHO, 2008).

Distance impacts on access to comprehensive healthcare services for people living in regional and remote areas because Australia is a vast country. Economic viability and sustainability are immense challenges to implementing higher-level health services in those areas. The health demands of people in regional and remote areas will never be as great as those in Major Cities, where a much greater percentage of the population resides. This not only substantially impacts on people who live in regional and remote areas, but also has significant implications for the clinical practice of health professionals. New levels of technology, such as telehealth, increase the ability of people who live and work in regional and remote areas to access healthcare services.

The role of the education provider should not be overlooked. Institutions providing courses for health professionals must address the health issues and concerns inherent in these communities. Graduates need to be encouraged to work in regional and remote areas; having a clinical placement opportunity in these areas can facilitate this.

There are a number of scholarship or intern schemes for all health disciplines that aim to recruit and retain staff in regional and remote areas. Some examples of these are the opportunities provided by the Australian College of Nursing (ACN) for nurses to participate in a regional or remote placement. Most state health departments also offer such opportunities. There are a number of incentives programs available to support medical, nursing and allied health students (Department of Health, 2021c).

Many education providers also offer courses that incorporate regional and remote health in Australia. Many universities offer clinical placements for regional and remote health. The importance being placed on regional and remote considerations is demonstrated by the forming of a number of centres for regional health at various universities throughout Australia.

The staff in these centres undertake research into issues such as mental health, Indigenous health, aged care, health workforce and health and wellbeing for people living and working in regional and remote communities.

INDIGENOUS HEALTH CONSIDERATIONS IN REGIONAL AND REMOTE AREAS

Aboriginal and Torres Strait Islander people are over-represented in mortality and morbidity statistics (AIHW, 2022a). These poorer health outcomes are an indicator of very complex issues relating to Australia's First Nation peoples, requiring greater consideration than a simple set of health problems. As mentioned previously, one of these strategies is the Closing the Gap campaign. See https://www.closingthegap.gov.au/.

The current estimate of the differences in life expectancy of Aboriginal and Torres Strait Islander people compared with non-Indigenous Australians is listed in the earlier 'Fast facts' box. Indicators that may cause a reduction in life expectancy are the principal reason for admission to hospital, numbers of current daily smokers, average daily alcohol consumption, levels of obesity, levels of physical activity and ability to access healthcare compared with need (AIHW, 2022a).

The *Closing the Gap in a Generation* (WHO, 2008) report calls for health equity through action on the **social determinants of health**. The social determinants of health are the circumstances relating to dealing with illness. The WHO (2012) states that regardless of where people are born, live or work, or who the government that rules on the day is, all people are entitled to equality in healthcare services. Low levels of health literacy are also seen as an issue that affects the health and wellness of lower socioeconomic groups, with many of these groups living in regional and remote areas (AIHW, 2022d).

Some of the relevant issues include improving access to health prevention and screening strategies, improving access to quality health services and improving the recruitment and retention of **Indigenous health** workers and professionals. The Australian Commission on Safety and Quality in Health Care (ACSQHC) has released a group of resources to improve healthcare for Aboriginal and Torres Strait Islander people, including health service standards, setting goals, cultural competence, improving identification rates, creating safe and welcoming environments, effective and safe communication and comprehensive care. Specific actions and best practice care have also been incorporated into the National Safety and Quality Health Service (NSQHS) Standards (ACSQHC, 2021).

Working in an Indigenous community

Nurses working with Aboriginal and Torres Strait Islander people in Indigenous communities must earn acceptance and respect by demonstrating cultural safety. This entails building trust and gaining relationships by having clear communication and adhering to cultural protocol (ACSQHC, 2021). Cultural safety follows the principles of reciprocity, respect, equality, responsibility and integrity. This approach goes at least some way to ensuring that the community members are not passive recipients of care and enables the health service provider to address the overarching health issues by actively addressing community-identified needs. It is essential that a consultative, respectful approach be taken to ensure that health strategies are embedded within the community structure in a sustainable manner.

The process of partnering with consumers and consultation aligns with the principles of respect and acknowledgement of traditional beliefs and practices. Aboriginal and Torres Strait Islander people hold a holistic view that considers the social, emotional and cultural wellbeing of the whole community. Aboriginal and Torres Strait Islander people's health needs are not sufficiently met through the biomedical model of healthcare. The long-term effects of implementing a community-driven healthcare service include improved mortality and morbidity statistics, a reduction in the representation of Indigenous people in relation to poor health outcomes and the ongoing world presence of a traditional culture for generations to come. Additionally, active consultation and consistent demonstration of cultural respect are safe cultural practice. All health professionals working for health service organisations have a responsibility to ensure that staff working in Indigenous communities complete professional development courses in cultural awareness and cultural competence prior to going to a community (ACSQHC, 2017).

Aboriginal or Torres Strait Islander Health Workers (ATSIHWs) employed in each Indigenous community are the foundation of the health service (see Figure 52.3). The ATSIHWs, as respected community members, often live within the community and have established links that are invaluable to engaging members of the community in healthcare issues. The professional relationship between the nurses and the health workers is a symbiotic one, in which each role relies upon the other to achieve stated outcomes. In summary, a mutually respectful, collaborative, collegial interdisciplinary team approach underpins the success of health initiatives in Indigenous communities (National Aboriginal and Torres Strait Islander Health Worker Association (NATSIHWA), 2021).

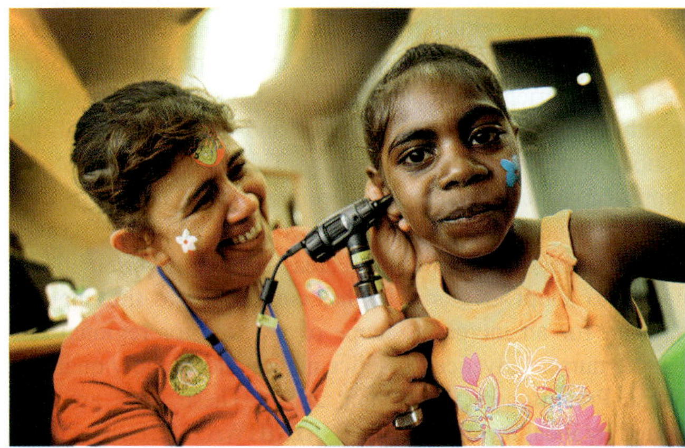

FIGURE 52.3 ***An Aboriginal and Torres Strait Islander Health Worker***

Source: © AAP Image/Clive Hyde, Northern Territory Government.

Links to National Patient Safety Standards

NSQHS: Comprehensive Care Standard

The intention of this standard is to ensure that comprehensive care is provided to the person that is well coordinated and is aligned with the person's expressed goals of care and healthcare needs. This standard considers the effect of the person's health issues on their life and wellbeing and is clinically appropriate.

Source: ACSQHC (2021). *National Safety and Quality Health Service Standards* (2nd ed.). Sydney: ACSQHC. © Australian Commission on Safety and Quality in Health Care.

THE REGIONAL AND REMOTE NURSING WORKFORCE

The roles of nurses in regional and remote communities differ from the roles of their city counterparts. However, regional and remote nurses can also find that their practice can vary greatly from location to location, depending on the economic, geographical, social, spiritual, cultural and political identity of the individual community. Regional and remote nurses can experience feelings of isolation and stress related to community demography, lack of multidisciplinary and interdisciplinary support, resource un/availability and the nurses' in/ability to meet the complex health requirements of the communities in which they work. The specific needs of the community, exacerbated by the degree of isolation that can be felt, require nurses to adopt more flexible and creative approaches to clinical problem solving.

Globally, the nursing workforce is ageing. The most recent statistics from the Department of Health (2021a) indicate that the average age of nurses working outside Major Cities is slightly higher than that of their Remote/Very Remote counterparts. Detailed statistics of the **regional and remote health workforce** show that the number of clinicians in Remote and Very Remote areas is decreasing, particularly for general practitioners (GPs), whose rate is lower than the national average of 114.5 per 100,000 population (Department of Health, 2021a). This means the number of practising GPs is not sufficient for demand in regional and remote areas, and this implies an increased workload for the nurses in those communities (AIHW, 2021a). The gap in health service provision is often met by experienced nurses adopting a greater role in local health services. Historically, nurses and GPs in regional and remote areas work collaboratively. The loss of professional support may lead to increased feelings of isolation, scope of practice issues and ethical dilemmas for the nurses. The lack of GPs in regional and remote areas and the requirement for nurses to adopt greater roles has contributed to the ongoing demand for an increased scope of practice for regional and remote nurses, advanced practice nurses and suitably qualified Nurse Practitioners (McKenna, 2019). These roles are supported by local health workers (NATSIHWA, 2021). The number of registered Aboriginal and Torres Strait Islander health practitioners in Australia rose from 474 in 2016 to 913 in 2021, with the majority of staff working in Outer Regional, Remote and Very Remote areas (AIHW, 2022c).

It is a common generalisation that people residing in regional and remote areas are resilient. This perceived resilience may relate to people 'living on the land' having to deal with extremes such as bushfire, drought and flood. It can also be expected that these generalisations extend to nurses in these areas, who deal with what has to be done with often limited resources. However, for some nurses, the stressors associated with practising in such difficult circumstances can lead to burnout. This can occur in health professionals due to an overwhelming anxiety resulting from the ongoing expectations and responsibility to people in their care (National Rural Health Alliance, 2019). While burnout is not specific to remote practice, it is unfortunately common in nurses who try to work harder and longer to fulfil the expectations of what can be sometimes unrelenting community demands. This can lead to increasing job dissatisfaction, increased stress levels, work/life imbalance, professional relationship breakdown, personal relationship breakdown and physical deterioration. Such professional side effects have the further potential to negatively impact on nurses in small communities, exacerbated by their high visibility and the overlap between personal and professional identity (National Rural Health Alliance, 2021) (see Figure 52.4).

Recruiting new nurses to regional and remote areas can be challenging for a number of reasons, such as a lack of connection with the community, a change in lifestyle, worries about physical security and a lack of personal support. New graduates may also not possess the advanced clinical competencies required to practise in a regional/remote setting that has limited resources (Calleja, Adonteng-Kissi & Romero, 2019; Terry et al., 2020). See the 'Translation to practice' box.

Competency to practise

Advanced and competent physical and mental health (given suicide rates) assessment skills are required for nurses working in regional and remote areas. Skills must include the ability to perform the assessment, note and interpret physical abnormalities and difference in mental state, initiate treatment, initiate communication with emergency transport and personnel as required, and refer to other health professionals locally if available. The nurse in this setting will also initiate access to professional guidance from a distant provider when necessary. A high level of responsibility is placed on nurses in these situations, with the experience

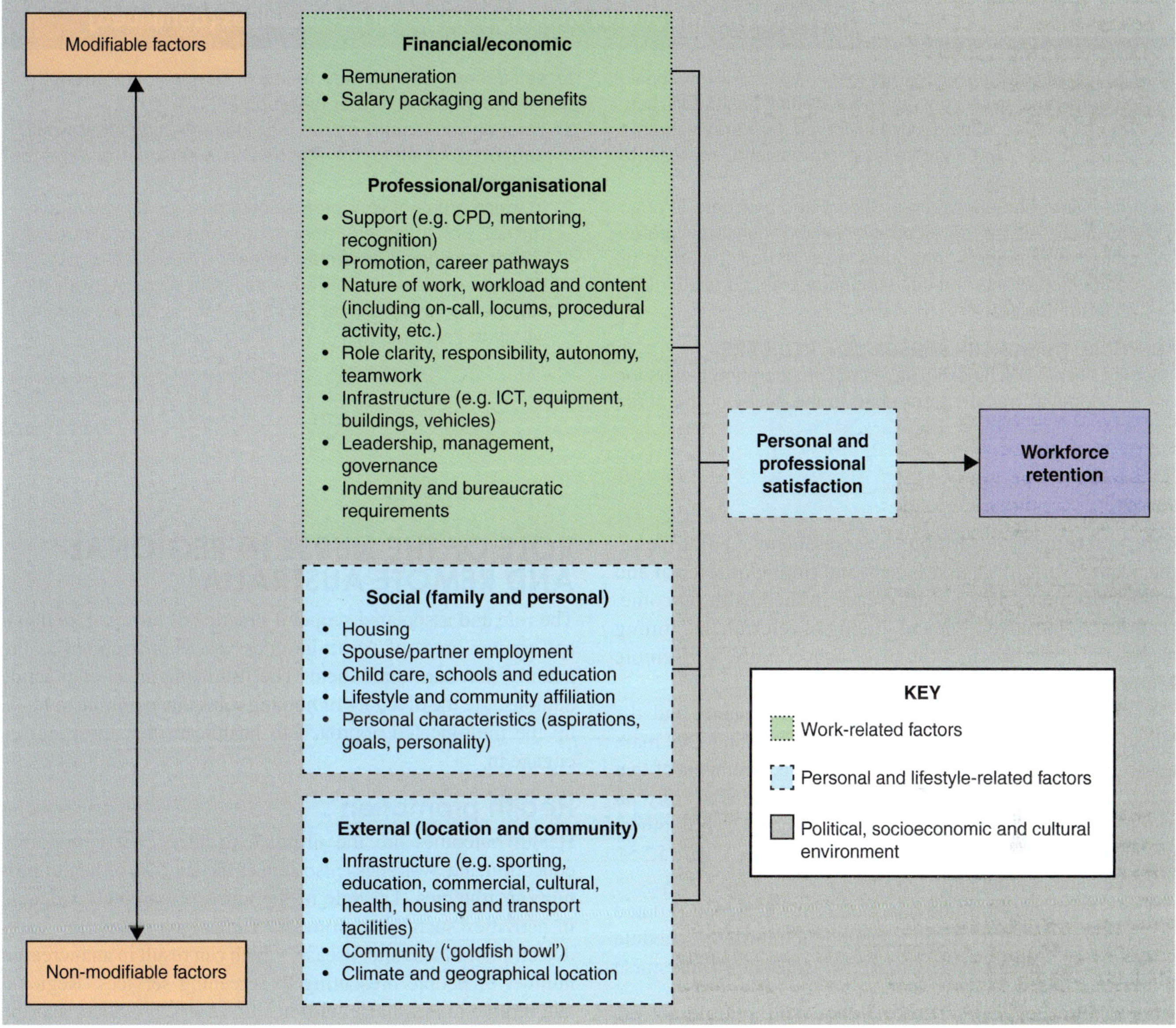

FIGURE 52.4 ***Factors affecting retention of health workers in regional and remote areas***

Source: Humphreys et al. (2009). *Retention strategies & incentives for health workers in rural & remote areas: What works?* Retrieved from aphcri.anu.edu.au/sites/aphcri.jagws03.anu.edu.au/files/research_project/292/international_retention_strategies_research_pdf_10642.pdf. Figure 1 Factors affecting renention, Australian Primary Health Care Research Institute, Nov. 2009, p. 9.

TRANSLATION TO PRACTICE New nursing graduates working in regional communities

Calleja et al. (2019) reported that factors such as personal and professional expectations, unusual workloads and varying levels of support available to staff can cause staff to leave regional and remote areas. McCullough et al. (2022) supported this by explaining that issues such as lack of cultural awareness, inadequate resources, role confusion and limited social support make working in regional and remote areas challenging. Although it is recognised that new graduate nurses may find the transition into the workplace challenging, with ongoing support from employers, obstacles can be overcome. The researchers found that issues such as understanding expectations, having social support and reviewing workloads should be an integral part of educating and preparing nurses for practice in regional and remote communities. With the current workforce shortages in regional and remote areas, it is imperative that these recommendations are acknowledged and incorporated in education programs and recruiting processes.

IMPLICATIONS FOR NURSING

- Resource planning by health services should individualise the health service to meet the specific needs of the

(*continued*)

TRANSLATION TO PRACTICE **New nursing graduates working in regional communities (continued)**

communities for which they are responsible. Skill-mix considerations need to be considered for staffing health facilities.

- These findings should be considered by nursing professional bodies when addressing professional representation and development needs of the nurses.
- Pre-registration education providers and providers of ongoing professional development should consider professional requirements, attributes expected of graduates on completion of their pre-registration degree, curriculum and program design.

CRITICAL THINKING IN PERSON-CENTRED CARE

Some critical-thinking skills linked to consideration of working in a regional or remote area relate to the ability of the nurse to self-assess and identify areas of professional strengths and areas requiring further development.

1 What do you identify as the individual strengths that would support your ability to practise in a regional or remote setting?
2 In which areas of your professional practice do you require further enhancement prior to embarking on a nursing career in regional or remote areas?
3 What do you see as the advantages of engaging with the community to identify the attributes of the nurses working within the community?

of the practitioner performing the assessment a major factor. The accuracy of initial assessment and timing of referral and transfer can make a major difference in the health outcome. Accuracy of initial assessment, timing of referral, and timing of transfer directly affect the prognosis (Centre for Remote Health, 2017).

Regional and remote areas are not all the same, and the individual characteristics of the region, including the main industries, will contribute to the healthcare requirements of that region. For example, some regional and remote areas rely on farming and agriculture for their local economy, while others may have a mixture of agriculture and mining (see Figure 52.5), or tourism and ecotourism.

The NMBA provides the opportunity for nurses in isolated areas to be endorsed to obtain, supply or administer a schedule 2, 3, 4 and 8 medicine as a regional and isolated practice nurse (NMBA, 2016b).

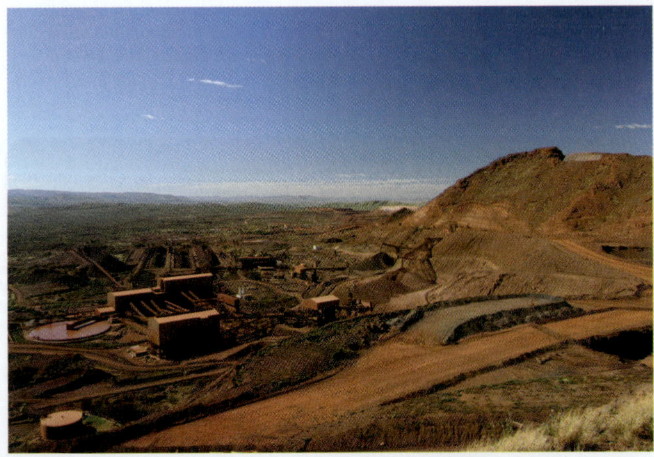

FIGURE 52.5 ***Mining is one of the main economic activities for regional and remote communities***

Source: STRINGER Image/Shutterstock.

ROLE OF THE NURSE IN REGIONAL AND REMOTE AUSTRALIA

The role and associated scope of practice of nurses in regional and remote areas of Australia is as vast and divergent as the country that surrounds them. The following areas of practice demonstrate the diversity of nursing roles that combine to make up the multifaceted approach to healthcare that these nurses engage in.

Health promotion

Health outcomes are the ultimate deciders, but community education and awareness also reflect the success of health promotion strategies. The role of the nurse is extremely valuable in activities such as multimedia campaigns promoting early detection of illness and disease, which can result in an increased number of people presenting to screening services. Regional and remote nurses liaise with health service providers and the community; advocate for individuals and for the community regarding access, which may include, for example, the arrival of a breast screen bus; coordinate the local application of service provision and accessibility for community members (ramps, signs); actively promote the event; recruit from the targeted population and facilitate follow-up care as necessary. When the initial health promotion strategy has been completed, the nurse, as part of the interdisciplinary team, is required to evaluate the program and ensure that people requiring further investigation or treatment gain referral to the appropriate service.

Regional and remote nurses actively participate in health promotion in individual, small group or community sessions, or by providing education sessions in the hospital or community setting. Furthermore, it is extremely difficult for nurses in small communities not to be identified as a nurse, so often their professional expertise and advice will be sought during their off-duty hours (e.g. at the local shop), extending their ongoing commitment to the provision of accurate health advice.

Governments and health providers organise national and state-wide rollouts of specific health promotion campaigns that include smaller regional/remote communities. Some of these campaigns will be specifically aimed at residents of country areas; for example, the *Close the Gap* campaign directed at Indigenous health inequality and the Care for Kids' Ears campaign aimed at highlighting the risk of hearing loss associated with ear disease in Aboriginal and Torres Strait Islander people. Nurses in these communities are actively involved in the planning, implementation and evaluation of the programs. This has further implications for practice, ongoing professional development and workload, and also requires that the nurses have up-to-date knowledge of the campaign content and the health promotion approach.

Screening and prevention strategies

Health screening programs globally are based on the principle of early detection leading to early intervention, which leads to improved health outcomes for individuals and communities. As previously stated, residents in regional and remote areas of Australia have statistically poorer outcomes for many diseases. This may be partially due to a lack of participation in screening programs, which in turn may be due to a lack of awareness or inability to access screening points. There are several reasons—not only confined to regional and remote communities—why people do not participate in screening programs. However, when geographical and cultural isolation are factored in, Australia suffers from a 'tyranny of distance', and there is an increased risk of non-participation. In many cases, strategic planning and service development address this through specialised, localised screening and detection programs, bringing the screening points to the community where possible. For example, in sparsely populated areas in Australia, mobile women's health nurses ensure that all women have access to regular, timely screening for breast and cervical cancers, among other health screening services. This model of health screening has also been used in other preventive health strategies, some of which are provided by community organisations as a not-for-profit community service.

Acute assessment

Nurses intending to work in regional and remote settings need to be cognisant of their individual scope of practice and seek to address limitations prior to embarking upon this field of nursing. This may necessitate gaining additional experience and education in areas such as aged care, paediatrics, people who live with mental health problems, or primary health screening.

Nurses working in small communities, either in health centres or in hospitals, must be competent to practise in emergency situations. In many instances, the nurse will be working alone or with only limited support from other health professionals. Some of the skills required in emergency situations are outlined below.

Unexpected illness, trauma or distress are main reasons why people living in sparsely populated areas seek healthcare. Road trauma, farm/workplace injuries and mental health issues require the nurse on duty to have a high level of competence in acute health assessment, including physical and mental health assessment, and an in-depth understanding of the types of injuries and presentations associated with these conditions. Injuries received in motor vehicle accidents can range from minor to life threatening, requiring immediate intervention. In a regional or remote area, the availability and timely response of emergency assistance is variable. Therefore, many regional and remote residences are equipped with emergency medical kits, provided through organisations such as the Royal Flying Doctor Service (RFDS). Medical advice can also be sought through radio or telephone contact: a suitably qualified professional will instruct the person at the site of the emergency what to do. Nurses in regional and particularly remote areas can be called upon to receive the person in the local health service clinic or hospital; or to assist in the **retrieval** process; or they can be called upon in their role as neighbour and community member.

Nurses working in regional and remote areas must be prepared to provide care for people with a broad spectrum of clinical presentations including mental illness. In Australia in 2020–2021, 43.7% of the adult population reported that they had experienced a mental disorder at some time in their life (ABS, 2022b), so the probability that the nurse will care for someone with a mental health issue is very high. While it is not feasible for any one person to know each and every possible clinical presentation, nurses must be able to identify deviations from normal and seek appropriate assistance in a timely manner to ensure optimal outcomes for the person presenting for help. In all areas of nursing practice, irrespective of the context, assessment forms the cornerstone of best practice. In regional and remote areas, enhanced assessment skills are the basis upon which management of the person and significant clinical decisions are made. Astute assessment provides the nurse with the requisite decision-making capacity. It is essential to be able to assess, plan, implement and evaluate treatment based on psychological, physiological and pathophysiological knowledge. Nurses are expected to identify and interpret data before responding appropriately. The presenting problem of the person will guide the order and priority of the type of assessment to be undertaken but will not limit the extent to which the nurse will perform a full physical and psychological assessment. For example, while some individuals will not present with any obvious physical injury or psychological dysfunction, they may exhibit signs of distress, altered mental health state and/or drug and alcohol issues. Acute presentation of injuries or illnesses acquired may be further complicated by comorbidities or by combinations of two or more problems (e.g. trauma and drug or alcohol problems). In addition to the varied physical and psychological presentations, nurses will be required to provide care to people who come from diverse cultural backgrounds and from across the lifespan.

Emergency nursing care

Triage

In remote communities and health sites across Australia, some degree of emergency care for communities is provided. The health outcomes are influenced in part by the large distances to travel, the time taken for retrieval and emergency stabilisation, and the emergency skills of the local practitioners. Those living in Very Remote areas are more than six times more likely to die due to a road accident than those living in Major Cities (AIHW, 2022e). People in regional and remote Australia are more likely to engage in behaviours associated with poorer health such as smoking, drinking alcohol, being overweight or obese, and having lower levels of exercise (AIHW, 2018). Australians living outside Major Cities are more likely to suffer from chronic illnesses, such as arthritis, asthma and diabetes, all of which can require episodes of hospitalisation and/or ongoing treatment (AIHW, 2018, 2022f). For **triage in regional and remote areas**, nurses may use the Australasian Triage Scale (ATS, see Table 52.1), but this may be quickly followed by the nurses themselves initiating emergency treatment. In situations such as this, the ATS is applied according to nurse waiting times.

TABLE 52.1 The Australasian Triage Scale

ATS CATEGORY	RESPONSE	DESCRIPTION OF CATEGORY	CLINICAL DESCRIPTORS (INDICATIVE ONLY)
Category 1	Immediate simultaneous assessment and treatment	**Immediately life threatening** Conditions that are threats to life (or imminent risk of deterioration) and require immediate aggressive intervention.	• Cardiac arrest • Respiratory arrest • Immediate risk to airway–impending arrest • Respiratory rate < 10/min • Extreme respiratory distress • BP < 80 (adult) or severely shocked child/infant • Unresponsive or responds to pain only (GCS < 9) • Ongoing/prolonged seizure • IV overdose and unresponsive or hypoventilation • Severe behavioural disorder with immediate threat of dangerous violence
Category 2	Assessment and treatment within 10 minutes (assessment and treatment often simultaneous)	**Imminently life threatening** The individual's condition is serious enough or deteriorating so rapidly that there is the potential of threat to life, or organ system failure, if not treated within 10 minutes of arrival or **Important time-critical treatment** The potential for time-critical treatment (e.g. thrombolysis, antidote) to make a significant effect on clinical outcome depends on treatment commencing within a few minutes of the individual's arrival in the ED or **Very severe pain** Humane practice mandates the relief of very severe pain or distress within 10 minutes	• Airway risk–severe stridor or drooling with distress • Severe respiratory distress • Circulatory compromise – Clammy or mottled skin, poor perfusion – HR < 50 or > 150 (adult) – Hypotension with haemodynamic effects – Severe blood loss • Chest pain of likely cardiac nature • Very severe pain–any cause • BSL < 3 mmol/L • Drowsy, decreased responsiveness–any cause (GCS < 13) • Acute stroke • Fever with signs of lethargy–any age • Acid or alkali splash to eye–requiring irrigation • Suspected endophthalmitis post eye procedure (pos cataract, post intravitreal injection), sudden onset pain, blurred vision and red eye • Major multi-trauma–requiring rapid organised team response • Severe localised trauma–major fracture, amputation • Suspected testicular torsion • High-risk history: – Significant sedative or other toxic ingestion – Significant/dangerous envenomation – Severe pain suggesting PE, AAA or ectopic pregnancy • Behavioural/psychiatric: – violent or aggressive – immediate threat to self or others – requires or has required restraint – severe agitation or aggression
Category 3	Assessment and treatment start within 30 minutes	**Potentially life threatening** The patient's condition may progress to life or limb threatening, or may lead to significant morbidity, if assessment and treatment are not commenced within 30 minutes of arrival or **Situational urgency** There is potential for adverse outcome if time-critical treatment is not commenced within 30 minutes or Humane practice mandates the relief of severe discomfort or distress within 30 minutes	• Severe hypertension • Moderately severe blood loss–any cause • Moderate shortness of breath • Seizure–now alert • Persistent vomiting • Dehydration • Head injury with short LOC–now alert • Suspected sepsis (physiologically stable) • Moderately severe pain–any cause–requiring analgesia • Chest pain likely non-cardiac and moderate severity • Abdominal pain without high-risk features–moderately severe or patient age > 65 years • Moderate limb injury–deformity, severe laceration, crush • Limb–altered sensation, acutely absent pulse • Trauma–high-risk history with no other high-risk features • Stable neonate • Child at risk of abuse/suspected non-accidental injury

TABLE 52.1 The Australasian Triage Scale (continued)

ATS CATEGORY	RESPONSE	DESCRIPTION OF CATEGORY	CLINICAL DESCRIPTORS (INDICATIVE ONLY)
			• Behavioural/psychiatric: – very distressed, risk of self-harm – acutely psychotic or thought disordered – situational crisis, deliberate self-harm – agitated/withdrawn – potentially aggressive
Category 4	Assessment and treatment start within 60 minutes	**Potentially serious** The individual's condition may deteriorate, or adverse outcome may result, if assessment and treatment is not commenced within 1 hour of arrival in ED. Symptoms moderate or prolonged. or **Situational urgency** There is potential for adverse outcome if time-critical treatment is not commenced within 1 hour or **Significant complexity or severity** Likely to require complex work-up and consultation and/or inpatient management or Humane practice mandates the relief of discomfort or distress within 1 hour	• Mild haemorrhage • Foreign body aspiration, no respiratory distress • Chest injury without rib pain or respiratory distress • Difficulty swallowing, no respiratory distress • Minor head injury, no loss of consciousness • Moderate pain, some risk features • Vomiting or diarrhoea without dehydration • Eye inflammation or foreign body–normal vision • Minor limb trauma–sprained ankle, possible fracture, uncomplicated laceration requiring investigation or interventionNormal vital signs, low/moderate pain • Tight cast, no neurovascular impairment • Swollen 'hot' joint • Non-specific abdominal pain • Behavioural/psychiatric: – Semi-urgent mental health problem – Under observation and/or no immediate risk to self or others
Category 5	Assessment and treatment start within 120 minutes	**Less urgent** The individual's condition is chronic or minor enough that symptoms or clinical outcome will not be significantly affected if assessment and treatment are delayed up to 2 hours from arrival or **Clinico-administrative problems** Results review, medical certificates, prescriptions only	• Minimal pain with no high-risk features • Low-risk history and now asymptomatic • Minor symptoms of existing stable illness • Minor symptoms of low-risk conditions • Minor wounds–small abrasions, minor lacerations (not requiring sutures) • Scheduled revisit (e.g. wound review, complex dressings) • Immunisation only • Behavioural/psychiatric: – Known patient with chronic symptoms – Social crisis, clinically well individual

GSC = Glascow Coma Scale; BSL = blood sugar level; PE = pulmonary embolism; AAA = abdominal aortic aneurysm; LOC = level of consciousness

Source: Australasian College for Emergency Medicine (ACEM) (2005). *G24 guidelines for the implementation of the Australasian Triage Scale in emergency departments.* Revised November 2016. Retrieved from https://www.acem.org.au. Reproduced with permission.

The ATS categories determine the urgency with which the person's presenting problem must be treated. In regional and remote areas, the deterioration of the person's condition must be considered with regard to the response time of appropriate personnel and the needs of the individual being triaged. Therefore, the category may be higher in anticipation of the challenges of assembling qualified personnel and required equipment. The triage categories are based on the presumption of morbidity if treatment is not initiated within the identified time to treatment. The categories also include behavioural or mental health disorders, which pose a threat of danger to self or others. Triage of people experiencing mental health illness can be supported further with the use of a mental health triage tool which includes further cues into observed or reported behaviours (Department of Health, 2013). This can help to ensure appropriate levels of care such as the need for 1:1 observation, urgent medical review and ensuring the safety of both the person presenting and the staff.

Triage depends on context and the attending nurse will use advanced decision-making processes to determine the person's need for emergency care and put in place the resources available to expedite time-critical interventions.

PRIMARY SURVEY A primary survey focuses on identifying life-threatening conditions and the need for emergency first aid. In the regional and remote context, nurses may be called to a scene to provide assistance or they may be the only staff member in the healthcare facility. In these situations, having the means by which to summon assistance is also a priority, requiring the nurse to be competent at emergency transmission via the telephone or by radio.

Understanding the principles of Danger, Response, Send for help, Airway, Breathing, Circulation, Disability (neurological) and Exposure is essential in the provision of safe and effective care. To provide appropriate and expedient care the nurse must possess effective assessment skills and be able to interpret findings accurately, in addition to having a working knowledge of all resources available. This includes awareness of where to locate, and how to use, emergency resuscitation equipment.

Some members of the community require special consideration during primary survey and physical assessment. Care of children in emergent situations requires more than merely size modification of adult assessment and management. Children are more susceptible to heat loss, and their fluid and medication requirements are different from adults. During the primary survey, nurses must incorporate knowledge of the physical, cognitive, emotional and behavioural stage of development into the interpretation of findings. Likewise, the older adult has altered states resulting from the normal ageing processes or disease processes that will influence the interpretation of assessment findings. This group is also at higher risk of complications from comorbidities or as a result of concurrent treatment regimens. The older adult and the child are only two examples that demonstrate the breadth of clinical practice needed by nurses working in regional and remote areas.

SECONDARY SURVEY A secondary survey is performed after the primary survey has been completed, findings have been interpreted and documented, and the prioritised interventions implemented. It is generally accepted that the secondary survey entails a comprehensive head-to-toe physical assessment. This physical assessment includes inspection, palpation, auscultation and percussion of the body systems.

Physical assessment is not the only form of assessment that nurses working in regional and remote areas must be proficient in performing. Mental health assessment is also frequently performed and requires the nurse to possess a sound understanding of assessment processes, manifestations of mental illness and treatment strategies. True holistic person-centred care includes acknowledgement of the whole person as well as the lifestyle factors influencing the person's health and wellbeing.

Depression has been recognised as a major health issue in Australia and is a health priority area nationally. Global statistics of suicide in young men living in regional areas show consistently higher rates in this demographic than in the general population (Elov, 2022; Fitzpatrick et al., 2022; Yip, Zheng & Wong, 2022). Both younger people (15–24 years) and those aged 75–84 years have significantly higher suicide rates in rural Australia than in metropolitan settings (Fitzpatrick et al., 2021). There are a range of factors that may influence the rates of suicide in men living in regional and remote areas, including mental illness, physical illness, unemployment, financial stress, isolated residence, increased availability of lethal means, male stereotyping and reluctance to seek help. High rates of suicide in Australian farming communities are significant, with farmers reporting changes in rural communities, community attitudes and stigma around mental health, and issues in relationships all impacting on suicide risk (Perceval et al., 2018). These issues are often exacerbated by variations in mental health services in these areas (AIHW, 2022b).

The *2019 Australian National Drug Strategy Household Survey* (AIHW, 2020) revealed that people living in Remote and Very Remote areas, unemployed people and Indigenous Australians are more likely than any other population to smoke daily and use illicit drugs. These data provide essential background knowledge for nurses working in these areas, to ensure that they possess the critical-thinking ability to assess each individual situation. The data may be relevant to opportunistic intervention and treatment, early detection and accurate monitoring and management of symptoms.

TYPES OF QUESTIONING In emergency situations, specific closed questioning is often appropriate. For example, when the person is short of breath and complaining of pain, the nurse should use closed questions to extract the relevant information in the shortest time (see Box 52.1 for examples).

Open questions require the person to respond in more than one word, allowing greater depth of information to be obtained (see Box 52.2). Open questions are the style predominantly used for mental health assessments where in-depth information is required in order to gain a comprehensive understanding of the presenting problem or issue. Try not to ask two questions as one, such as 'What car were you driving and was it yours?' These types of 'two in one' questions are confusing and should be asked separately.

In all aspects of nursing care in all settings—metropolitan, regional or remote—nurses must be proficient communicators to gain relevant information for care planning and to establish a supportive relationship with the person, their family and/or their carers. Often, if the person or their significant other is distressed, the empathetic presence of the nurse to listen and provide support is invaluable.

Establishing boundaries

Nurses working in small regional and remote communities are less anonymous than their urban counterparts, a consequence of which may be that a more considered commitment to the protection of each person's privacy and confidentiality is required. Personal communication can be either a barrier or a bridge in these communities. One of the most important factors in establishing a professional therapeutic relationship is that of trust. The person must feel comfortable discussing their personal information and health history with the nurse providing care. This can be difficult in small communities where the nurse may know the person through social and community interactions. While it is also possible for this to occur in larger towns or cities, it is far more likely to occur in communities

BOX 52.1 Closed questions

- Where is the pain?
- On a scale of 1–10, how much does it hurt?
- Does your arm hurt?
- Does it hurt when you breathe in?
- Does it hurt when you breathe out?
- Is the pain any better now?
- Have you had this pain before?

BOX 52.2 Open questions

- What brought you to hospital today?
- Can you describe what the pain is like?
- Tell me what were you doing when this pain started?
- What have you done since the pain started?
- Which types of pain relief have you tried?

where the population is smaller and the possibility of crossing paths in various roles is greater. For example, the person may be the manager of the local bank that holds the mortgage over the nurse's property. As in all professional interactions, the person requires reassurance that they will be treated with dignity, integrity and professionalism in the course of receiving healthcare—expectations which may be intensified and become challenging in smaller communities. It is thought that some people in small communities have sought healthcare away from their home areas to minimise the chance of knowing their care provider socially. Therefore, it is imperative that the nurse can reassure the person by verbal and non-verbal means during any interactions that they will always uphold confidentiality.

Subjective data on individuals are obtained through a range of clinical approaches which are each contingent upon the clinical context specific to the person. Both over-familiarity and failure to acknowledge the person may be perceived as equally offensive. The degree of familiarity will depend on each individual and the type of healthcare they require. Nurses will have to use their judgment and exercise it for each individual circumstance. One way to approach this is for the nurse to actually ask the person what degree of familiarity they would like. An example of this would be: 'If I see you in the shops, how would you like me to behave? Do you want me to say hello or would you prefer I just went about my business without acknowledging you?' Establishing mutually agreed upon boundaries can prevent uncomfortable situations.

The type and manner of the interview will depend largely on the information required. If the person is already known to the nurse, the beginning phase may be briefer. In many cases, it may be advisable to approach the interaction as if beginning a new relationship. Gaining the relevant information should not be influenced by previous interactions because each occasion where the person is seeking healthcare is a new and slightly different occasion. Closing the interview may involve reference to seeing the person in the community but should clearly reinforce the respect for confidentiality.

Teleconsultations/videoconsultations

The *Millennium Development Goals Report 2015* (UN, 2015) states that with regard to achieving the millennium goals related to the improvement of mortality and morbidity statistics, the global use of mobile communication services has been growing at a fast rate and is seen to be a major contributor to the success of the initiative. Access to information has the ability to increase the knowledge of individuals and communities, leading to improved, informed decision making and, ultimately, improved health outcomes—empowerment through knowledge. The objectives of these goals continues with 17 new sustainable goals to be developed by 2030 (UN, 2015).

An unexpected outcome of COVID-19 was the rapid expansion of telehealth, with the pandemic necessitating a governmental response to provide non-contact telehealth care for all Australians (Department of Health, 2021d). This enhanced the ability of a person in a regional or remote area to consult via phone or video with GPs, medical specialists and nursing, midwifery and allied health services, and is immensely valuable. The telehealth services introduced as a response to COVID-19 will now be ongoing (Department of Health and Aged Care, 2022b), and the establishment of universal telehealth may go some way to bridging the health access gap between urban and regional and remote communities. The financial savings of a video or phone link are immense compared to the cost of the person and carer travelling to the service for their appointment, and their accommodation.

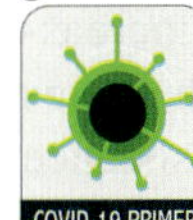

If travel is necessary, patient transport schemes do not cover all expenses. They usually only partially subsidise the person's costs, with most people who do have to travel to access healthcare being financially disadvantaged. The humanitarian savings of telehealth are immeasurable: the person is not removed from their home area; they remain with family, friends and support networks; and they do not have the burden of finding someone to care for family, property, animals or business for the period of their absence.

From a nurse's perspective, having access to clinical expertise while geographically isolated is reassuring. An example of this is the access to emergency mental healthcare in regional and remote emergency departments in Australia. Staff at remote locations have access to a telepsychiatry program to assist with emergency mental health issues (Noble, Haveland & Islam, 2022).

The introduction of telehealth to provide specialist advice to people living in regional or remote areas of Australia has been quite an achievement. A **referral** to a specialist can be from a nurse or medical practitioner, midwife, practice nurse or Aboriginal or Torres Strait Islander Health Worker on behalf of a medical practitioner. Among other potential benefits, telehealth enhances a sense of professional support for nurses and other health professionals in regional and remote settings.

The provision of professional support not only provides timely guidance but may well impact on recruitment and retention issues surrounding nursing in regional and remote areas. Nurses in these areas report a perception of professional isolation as a contributing factor to leaving these roles. The provision of professional support is extended to include online access to professional databases for current publications and best practice guidelines. The practitioner needs to be motivated to access, interpret and adopt current practice standards, which can be more difficult for nurses who may already be feeling mentally, emotionally and physically fatigued. Many professional groups and colleges offer online professional development opportunities for nurses in a vast range of specialties. The ability to access specialist health professionals in Major City locations via telehealth is helpful for people suffering health conditions as well as the health professionals situated in regional and remote areas. The expansion of the use of telehealth means more specialties are available online with, for example, emergency and ongoing mental health, specialist medical clinics, and oncology and palliative clinic consultations available by telemedicine (Adams et al., 2021; Burbury et al., 2021). The Royal Flying Doctor Service (RFDS) also provides telehealth medical consultation to people living or travelling in regional and remote Australia (RFDS, 2018a).

Liaison and advocacy

Nurses working in regional and remote areas of Australia must possess a high standard of interpersonal skills and be able to communicate effectively with their community, nursing colleagues, members of the interdisciplinary team, local health service providers, tertiary referral centres, retrieval teams and other organisations involved in the transfer of people in their care (e.g. the RFDS). In remote Indigenous communities, local health workers form the backbone of the health service, integrating community knowledge, cultural knowledge and health knowledge into individualised person-centred care. It is therefore imperative that nurses in these areas work closely with other health workers to ensure that the healthcare provided is culturally safe and acceptable to the community.

Referral and retrieval

Preparing a person for referral to a tertiary-level health service is a part of the daily routine for regional and remote nurses, especially when dealing with acute illness or trauma.

Public hospitals in central Australia are noticeably absent, but the RFDS is notable for its broad range of services throughout Australia, including in sparsely populated areas. The RFDS began in 1928 when Reverend John Flynn initiated a flying medical service to isolated inland communities (RFDS, 2018b). The service has continued to grow and is funded by the Australian Government to provide aeromedical transport and healthcare services to people living in regional and remote areas. The RFDS provides a 24-hour medical evacuation service, staffed by highly skilled flight nurses, midwives and medical practitioners; primary, oral and mental health clinics; and undertakes research that benefits regional and remote residents (RFDS, 2018b). It also provides remote consultations via phone or radio by medical practitioners or nurses and supplies medical chests for emergency use (RFDS, 2018b). The RFDS played an important role in ensuring COVID-19 vaccine availability and delivery to rural and remote communities (RFDS, 2021).

Access to services in regional and remote regions is improving due to the National Strategic Framework for Rural and Remote Health; however, the RFDS can provide invaluable support for practitioners where there are gaps in service provision. In many cases, the RFDS provides essential lifelines for the practitioners and communities where there are reduced or no services (Department of Health, 2018b).

Ensuring that transfer and retrieval guidelines and policy are followed is extremely important so that the process proceeds smoothly. Such professional actions may not be noticeable until after the transfer is complete. All centres have criteria for transfer, clearly articulated in policies and procedures, often with quick reference guides for use in emergent situations. The accurate handover of relevant information is essential to the provision of appropriate care during transfer and on arrival at the destination. In some cases, the nurse will escort the person to the referral centre. However, in other instances, the transfer will be by outside organisations such as ambulance or emergency services, or the RFDS. Nurses working in these areas must be cognisant of these transfer procedures prior to an emergency, as it is not the right time to be reading policies when dealing with a critically ill or injured person who requires immediate attention.

Discharge planning and continuum of care

When providing nursing care to a person in a health facility in any community, it is imperative that **discharge planning** is incorporated into all aspects of person-centred care. Commencement of discharge planning at the initial point of contact is a fundamental nursing consideration, whether the person presents with a chronic condition, acute illness or because of trauma. The role of the nurse is to assist the person to return to their home having regained their former level of independence, if possible, or having achieved an optimal level of independence or mental health recovery resulting from their altered physical, psychological or cognitive ability.

Discharge of a person within a regional or remote community or back to a regional or remote community from a tertiary facility must acknowledge the individuality of the person and their needs. It must also consider the resources and support available in their community when they return. If the discharge process is not performed appropriately, the chance of readmission is increased by limited availability of follow up, contact with health professionals and access to healthcare facilities.

Provision of care for the person from a regional or remote area

Nurses provide care for people who have had to travel, sometimes long distances, for treatment. These people have a unique set of challenges for inpatient treatment, upon discharge and for the **continuum of care** and need to be considered.

Considerations

The person is likely to feel isolated and lonely. Their support systems are often hundreds of kilometres away, which impacts on their mental health and their ability to heal. When a person is from a regional or remote area, discharge planning becomes even more significant in the overall care of the individual. When preparing to transfer a person back to their home, nurses must ensure that they take all aspects of transport into consideration (see Box 52.3).

Financial costs associated with transport must be incorporated into care and discharge planning. All states and territories have implemented a specific model of patient travel subsidy, identified by different titles according to whichever jurisdiction is the place of origin. In contemporary healthcare, with the continuous state of reduced bed availability, it is not uncommon for people to be transferred across jurisdictional borders to receive specialised medical care.

In some cases, the person may be required to fund their return home and claim expenses later. Claiming back the costs may be time consuming and exhausting for a person who may still be recuperating from significant illness or injury. Therefore, the cost of transport becomes increasingly important. Examples include the New South Wales Isolated Patients Travel and Accommodation Assistance Scheme (IPTAAS) (NSW Government, 2022) and the

BOX 52.3 Considerations when discharging or transferring a person

Transport availability

What type of transport is available?

- Private motor vehicle
- Aircraft (commercial)
- Aircraft (specialist provider)
- Bus
- Train
- Marine transport (some island communities are only accessible by water)

How frequently does this service run?

- Some services run only twice a week or weekly
- On demand

Will this cost money?

- How much?
- Who will pay?

Is the person able to travel via this mode of transport?

Can they spend long periods of time sitting?
Are they able to mobilise as necessary?
Can they board the transport?
Do they require a stretcher/lift to board?
If travelling by air, can the person tolerate the pressure changes?
Can this mode of transport accommodate the person's needs?

Carer support

Can the person travel unaccompanied?
Will the person require a nursing or medical escort?
Can the carer/escort travel with the person?

Patient Assistance Travel Scheme in the Northern Territory (NT Government, 2016). These schemes or others like them are available to all people living in regional and remote Australia in each state and territory. The cost of transport for a carer is often covered by the transport scheme, but this can vary. If there is more than one support person, individuals may be required to pay the full costs. For example, this may be a problem if the person has a great distance to travel, is required to change modes of transport at some stage during the journey and the carer is not physically able to assist. In these cases, there is an increased need for the assistance of another support person or carer. In the case of the transfer of a child, there may be two parents to accompany the child, one of whom will travel with the child regardless of transport and the remaining parent who will need to organise their own transport and perhaps that of other children. This may also occur when an older parent is travelling with their spouse and an adult child is required to be a further support person. There are support groups or volunteer organisations that can assist with emergency funding in times of financial difficulty for people and their families. Transport for treatment or returning home from treatment is deemed eligible for this purpose in many instances.

The person returning home will also need to have adequate supplies of medications and medical supplies, as access to a supplier may be limited (Pharmaceutical Society of Australia, 2021). Contact should also be made with the pharmacy in the person's local area to give sufficient time for ordering and receiving supplies.

In many regional and remote areas, residents and services are often restricted by seasonal weather patterns. For example, in the northern areas of Australia, the wet season between November and March can significantly impact on the mobility of the population and access to services. The coming of the rains usually brings great anticipation to the residents of the outback, especially those reliant on the water for crops, stock, replenishing water supplies and rejuvenating the bush flora. However, while the rains are essential to the lifeblood of the community, the associated flooding or limiting of access can range from being mildly frustrating to intensely problematic (see Figure 52.6). The lack of access can affect the ability of the person requiring healthcare to access the relevant services and limit the ability of the health service to discharge the person.

Community care

Hospitals are fast becoming places for people who are treated for acute illnesses and conditions. Many people are now treated at home for conditions that restrict their normal daily living or who are living with a disability. There are also services for frail older people with dementia, those who are financially disadvantaged or those in remote or isolated areas still living in their home. There are resources available through community care services such as in-home services; community-based clinical, counselling and respite services; and carer support. People who are having difficulty with their daily activities of living and are at risk of losing their independence are eligible for these services. The National Disability Insurance Scheme (NDIS) is an established national scheme providing referrals and support services for people with a disability so that they can achieve their goals and be in a better position to enjoy their lives (NDIS, 2021).

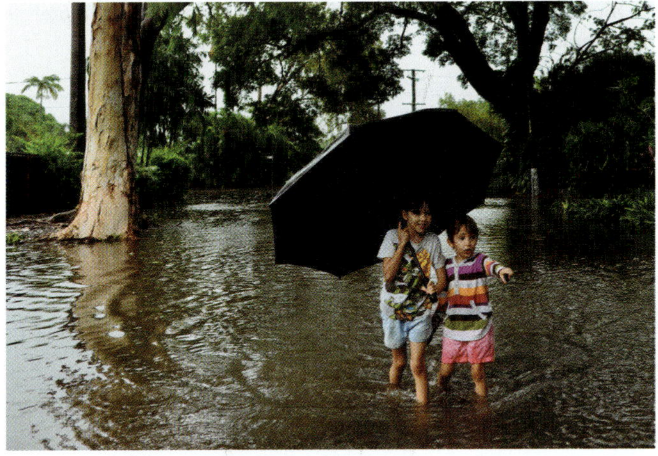

FIGURE 52.6 ***Rain is necessary for survival but it can isolate people and communities. Children often make the most of being restricted to the home area***

Source: P&F Photography/Alamy Stock Photo.

TRANSLATION TO PRACTICE The perceptions of people living in regional and remote areas

A review by Taylor, Thackrah and Thompson (2022) on palliative care in the Top End of the Northern Territory described the improvements in services. The review demonstrated that despite the establishment of the Allan Walker Cancer Care Centre, there was a lack of access to healthcare professionals to provide palliative care outside urban areas. Territory Palliative Care (TPC) is the sole provider of palliative care services in the Top End. This impacts on the level of care and support that can be provided prior to death. The review aligned with a recent WHO study indicating that it is taking too long for people to be diagnosed and receive palliative care before they die.

In rural New South Wales, the development of an older people's mental health program greatly enhanced access to older people's specialist mental health care (Jackson, Roberts & McKay, 2019). This service recognised the difficulties associated with travel for medical consultation or for long-term treatment (Van Spijker et al., 2019). It also highlighted the need for continuity of care across health services and the need for consideration of this to be incorporated into the care received in the referral centre, and that the support services needed are actually available.

IMPLICATIONS FOR NURSING PRACTICE

Research projects such as these provide significant evidence of the importance of more timely responses by healthcare teams that are sufficiently staffed to meet the needs of the community. People in regional and remote areas require appropriate levels of physical and psychosocial support to manage their illness and recover. The provision of support measures adapted for use in regional and remote areas is not insurmountable.

The difficulties associated with living in regional and remote areas are exacerbated in times of extreme vulnerability related to serious illness. The role of the nurse can impact positively and result in improved quality of life for people and their families.

CRITICAL THINKING IN PERSON-CENTRED CARE

1 Using your current knowledge about holistic person-centred care, how can a perceived lack of psychosocial support influence the person's response to treatment?
2 As a nurse working with people in this or similar situations, what are some strategies you could implement to meet the psychosocial needs of the person and their families?
3 People in these situations require significant support from their local community, but confidentiality is often a concern. Can you identify some community-based initiatives that would contribute to the overall wellbeing of these people?

CHAPTER HIGHLIGHTS

- **The formal acknowledgement of the specialised nature of regional and remote nursing is continuing to drive the adoption of greater clinical responsibility and advanced practitioner roles.**
- **Community-driven healthcare addressing the needs of the community, as identified by the community, is a key feature of healthcare provision in regional and remote areas.**
- **Equity in access to quality healthcare in a timely manner is the foundation for improving health status in regional and remote communities.**
- **Health promotion, including early detection and prevention strategies, is a vital component in regional and remote healthcare provision.**
- **Incorporating regionality into the provision of nursing care is not the sole domain of the regional and remote nursing workforce.**
- **Factors impacting on the continuum of care for people living in regional and remote areas must be addressed within the care and management provided by all nurses, regardless of location.**

CONCEPT CHECK

1 When triaging a person, the primary survey includes:
1 rescue, retrieval and response
2 assessment of danger, response, send for help, airway, breathing, circulation, disability, exposure
3 calling for immediate transfer
4 assessment of available resources

2 The 2016 National Drug Strategy Household Survey showed that people living in Remote and Very Remote areas, unemployed people or Indigenous Australians were more likely to consume alcohol at which level?
1 low
2 moderate
3 moderate–high
4 risky–high risk

3 The considerations for discharge planning for people from a regional or remote area:
1 are the same as those for all people regardless of location
2 include access to follow-up care and support services
3 include the assumption that the person will return home by the same means as they arrived
4 are the domain of the home health service

4 The challenges faced by regional and remote communities in accessing healthcare:
1 are driven only by economic forces
2 are contingent upon the local weather at the time
3 are the same as those faced by all communities in Australia
4 represent a multi-level, multifaceted integration of diverse influences

5 Community engagement with regional and remote health services is vital because:
1 the community should like whoever is working for them
2 it makes the people feel better even though the health service knows best
3 the community will vote for the government that gives the most money
4 the sustainability of a service depends on community involvement

6 Three of the five principles of working with Indigenous people are:
1 reciprocity, respect, equality
2 spirituality, respect, equality
3 economics, culture, demographics
4 spirituality, culture, demographics

7 Nurses working in regional and remote areas are predisposed to burnout as a result of:
1 community support
2 the opportunity to develop a broad range of clinical skills
3 the building of professional relationships with a smaller group of co-workers
4 longer work hours because the available resources are limited

8 Establishing and maintaining a therapeutic relationship with a person is:
1 easier in a small community because the nurse knows everyone already
2 more difficult in a small community where everyone knows everyone else
3 easier in a small community because the patients are the same ones all the time
4 more difficult in a small community because nurses cannot ethically provide care for people they already know

9 Clinical competency in regional and remote areas is:
1 directly linked to all domains of the NMBA *Registered Nurse Standards for Practice* (2016)
2 directly linked to all domains of the National Health and Medical Research Council guidelines
3 not very important because all of the high-level cases are transferred to larger centres
4 defined by a specific set of regional and remote competencies

BIBLIOGRAPHY

Adams, L., Lester, S., Hoon, E. et al. (2021). Patient satisfaction and acceptability with telehealth at specialist medical outpatient clinics during the COVID-19 pandemic in Australia. *Internal Medicine Journal*, *51*, 1028–1037. https://doi-org.ezproxy.uow.edu.au/10.1111/imj.15205

Australasian College for Emergency Medicine (ACEM) (2005). *G24 guidelines for the implementation of the Australasian Triage Scale in emergency departments*. Retrieved from https://www.acem.org.au/

Australian Bureau of Statistics (ABS) (2017). *Census of population and housing—Counts of Aboriginal and Torres Strait Islander Australians*. Retrieved from https://www.abs.gov.au/

Australian Bureau of Statistics (ABS) (2018a). *1270.0.55.005 Australian Statistical Geography Standard (ASGS): Volume 5—Remoteness structure, July 2016*. Retrieved from https://www.abs.gov.au/

Australian Bureau of Statistics (ABS) (2021). *Australian Statistical Geography Standard (ASGS) Edition 3, July 2021*. Retrieved from https://www.abs.gov.au/

Australian Bureau of Statistics (ABS) (2022a). *Regional population*. Retrieved from https://www.abs.gov.au/

Australian Bureau of Statistics (ABS) (2022b). *National study of mental health and wellbeing 2020–2021*. Retrieved from https://www.abs.gov.au/

Australian Commission on Safety and Quality in Health Care (ACSQHC) (2017). *Improving care for Aboriginal and Torres Strait Islander people*. Retrieved from https://www.safetyandquality.gov.au

Australian Commission on Safety and Quality in Health Care (ACSQHC) (2021). *National Safety and Quality Health Service Standards* (2nd ed.). Sydney: ACSQHC.

Australian Institute of Health and Welfare (AIHW) (2018). *Australia's health 2018: In brief*. Cat. no. AUS 222. Retrieved from aihw.gov.au

Australian Institute of Health and Welfare (AIHW) (2020). *National drug strategy household survey 2019*. Retrieved from aihw.gov.au

Australian Institute of Health and Welfare (AIHW) (2021a). *Life expectancy and deaths*. Retrieved from https://www.aihw.gov.au/

Australian Institute of Health and Welfare (AIHW) (2021b). *Specialist homelessness services annual report 2020–21*. Retrieved from aihw.gov.au/

Australian Institute of Health and Welfare (AIHW) (2022a). *Indigenous Australians and the health system*. Retrieved from https://www.aihw.gov.au/

Australian Institute of Health and Welfare (AIHW) (2022b). *Rural and remote health*. Retrieved from https://www.aihw.gov.au/

Australian Institute of Health and Welfare (AIHW) (2022c). *Health workforce*. Retrieved from https://www.aihw.gov.au/

Australian Institute of Health and Welfare (AIHW) (2022d). *Health literacy*. Retrieved from https://www.aihw.gov.au/

Australian Institute of Health and Welfare (AIHW) (2022e). *Transport accidents*. Retrieved from https://www.aihw.gov.au

Australian Institute of Health and Welfare (AIHW) (2022f). *Chronic conditions and multimorbidity*. Retrieved from https://www.aihw.gov.au

Burbury, K., Wong, Z.-W., Yip, D. et al. (2021). Telehealth in cancer care: During and beyond the COVID-19 pandemic. *Internal Medicine Journal*, *51*, 125–133. https://doi-org.ezproxy.uow.edu.au/10.1111/imj.15039

Calleja, P., Adonteng-Kissi, B. & Romero, B. (2019). Transition support for new graduate nurses to rural and remote practice: A scoping review. *Nurse Education Today*, *76*, 8–20.

Centre for Remote Health (2017). *CARPA standard treatment manual* (7th ed.). Retrieved from https://www.crh.org.au/

Collett, M. J., Fraser, C. & Thompson, S. C. (2020). Developing the future rural nursing workforce: Report on a nursing roundtable. *Collegian*, *27*(4), 370–374.

CRANAplus (2018). *CRANAplus framework for remote and isolated practice*. Retrieved from https://crana.org.au/

CRANAplus (2021). *What influences nurses' decisions to work in rural and remote settings? A systematic review and meta-synthesis of qualitative research*. Retrieved from https://crana.org.au/

Department of Health (2013). *Mental health triage tool*. Retrieved from https://www1.health.gov.au/

Department of Health (2018a). *Australia's future health workforce—Nurses*. Retrieved from http://www.health.gov.au/

Department of Health (2018b). *Royal Flying Doctor Service (RFDS) program*. Retrieved from https://www.health.gov.au/

Department of Health (2021a). *Health workforce data. Summary statistics: Remoteness area statistics 2020*. Retrieved from https://hwd.health.gov.au/

Department of Health (2021b). *Nurses and midwives in Australia*. Retrieved from https://www.health.gov.au/

Department of Health (2021c). *Rural health workforce*. Retrieved from https://www.health.gov.au/

Department of Health (2021d). *Ongoing telehealth: Strengthening primary care*. Retrieved from https://www.health.gov.au/

Department of Health and Aged Care (2022a). *Primary Health Networks (PHNs)*. Retrieved from https://www.health.gov.au/

Department of Health and Aged Care (2022b). *MBS specialist telehealth services from 1 July 2022*. Retrieved from http://www.mbsonline.gov.au/

Elov, Z. S. (2022). Suicide as a global problem facing humanity. *Science and Education*, *3*(2), 1247–1252.

Fitzpatrick, S. J., Brew, B. K., Handley, T. & Perkins, D. (2022). Men, suicide, and family and interpersonal violence: A mixed methods exploratory study. *Sociology of Health & Illness*, *44*, 991–1008.

Fitzpatrick, S. J., Handley, T., Powell, N. et al. (2021). Suicide in rural Australia: A retrospective study of mental health problems, health-seeking and service utilisation. *PLOS ONE*, *16*(7), e0245271. https://doi.org/10.1371/journal.pone.0245271

Humphreys, J., Wakerman, J., Pashen, D. & Buykx, P. (2009). *Retention strategies & incentives for health workers in rural & remote areas: What works?* Retrieved from aphcri.anu.edu.au/sites/

Jackson, K., Roberts, R. & McKay, R. (2019). Older people's mental health in rural areas: Converting policy into service development, service access and a sustainable workforce. *Australian Journal of Rural Health, 27*, 358–365. https://doi.org/10.1111/ajr.12529

McCullough, K., Bayes, S., Whitehead, L., Williams, A. & Cope, V. (2022). Nursing in a different world: Remote area nursing as a specialist-generalist practice area. *Australian Journal of Rural Health, 30*(5), 570–581. https://doi.org/10.1111/ajr.12899

McKenna, L. (2019). Improving health outcomes in rural and remote Australia: Optimising the contribution of nurses. *Collegian, 26*. https://doi.org/10.1016/j.colegn.2019.03.002

Muirhead, S. & Birks, M. (2019). Roles of rural and remote registered nurses in Australia: An integrative review. *Australian Journal of Advanced Nursing, 37*(1), 21–33.

National Aboriginal and Torres Strait Islander Health Worker Association (NATSIHWA) (2021). *National Framework for Determining Scope of Practice for Aboriginal and Torres Strait Islander Health Worker and Health Practitioner Workforce*. Retrieved from https://www.natsihwa.org.au/

National Disability Insurance Scheme (NDIS) (2021). Retrieved from https://www.ndis.gov.au/

National Rural Health Alliance (2019). *Nurses in rural, regional and remote Australia*. Retrieved from https://www.ruralhealth.org.au/

National Rural Health Alliance (2021). *Rural health in Australia snapshot 2021*. Retrieved from https://www.ruralhealth.org.au/

Noble, D., Haveland, S. & Islam, M. S. (2022). Integrating telepsychiatry based care in rural acute community mental health services? A systematic literature review. *Asia Pacific Journal of Health Management, 17*(2).

NSW Government (2022). *Isolated Patients Travel and Accommodation Assistance Scheme (IPTAAS)*. Retrieved from https://www.health.nsw.gov.au/

NT Government (2016). *Patient Assistance Travel Scheme*. Retrieved from https://nt.gov.au/

Nursing and Midwifery Board of Australia (NMBA) (2016a). *Registered Nurse Standards for Practice*. Retrieved from https://www.nursingmidwiferyboard.gov.au/

Nursing and Midwifery Board of Australia (NMBA) (2016b). *Registered Nurse—Supply scheduled medicines (rural and isolated practice)*. Retrieved from https://www.nursingmidwiferyboard.gov.au/

Perceval, M., Ross, V., Kõlves, K. et al. (2018). Social factors and Australian farmer suicide: A qualitative study. *BMC Public Health, 18*, 1367. https://doi.org/10.1186/s12889-018-6287-7

Pharmaceutical Society of Australia (2021). *Medicine safety: Rural and remote care*. Retrieved from https://www.psa.org.au

Queensland Government (2019). *Queensland Health. Nurse Navigators*. Retrieved from https://www.health.qld.gov.au/

Royal Flying Doctor Service (RFDS) (2018a). *Telehealth*. Retrieved from http://yourhealth.flyingdoctor.org.au/

Royal Flying Doctor Service (RFDS) (2018b). *Our history*. Retrieved from https://www.flyingdoctor.org.au/

Royal Flying Doctor Service (RFDS) (2021). *COVID-19: Responding to need*. Retrieved from https://www.flyingdoctor.org.au/

Taylor, E. V., Thackrah, R. D. & Thompson, S. C. (2022). Improving access to cancer treatment services in Australia's Northern Territory—History and progress. *International Journal of Environmental Research and Public Health, 19*(13), 7705.

Terry, D. R., Peck, B., Smith, A., Stevenson, T., Nguyen, H. & Baker, E. (2020). What Australian nursing students value as important in undertaking rural practice. *Online Journal of Rural Nursing and Health Care, 20*(1), 32–56.

United Nations (UN) (2007). *United Nations Declaration on the Rights of Indigenous Peoples*. Retrieved from https://www.un.org/

United Nations (UN) (2015). *The millennium development goals report 2015*. Retrieved from www.un.org/millenniumgoals/

United Nations (UN) (2022). *Sustainable Development Goals*. Retrieved from https://sdgs.un.org/

University of Adelaide (2021). *Accessibility/Remoteness Index of Australia (ARIA)*. Hugo Centre for Population and Migration Studies. Retrieved from https://www.adelaide.edu.au/

Van Spijker, B. A., Salinas-Perez, J. A., Mendoza, J. et al. (2019). Service availability and capacity in rural mental health in Australia: Analysing gaps using an Integrated Mental Health Atlas. *Australian & New Zealand Journal of Psychiatry, 53*(10), 1000–1012.

World Health Organization (WHO) (2008). *Closing the gap in a generation: Health equity through action on the social determinants of health. Final report of the Commission on Social Determinants of Health*. Retrieved from https://www.who.int/

World Health Organization (WHO) (2012). *Social determinants of health*. Retrieved from https://www.who.int/

Yip, P. S. F., Zheng, Y. & Wong, C. (2022). Demographic and epidemiological decomposition analysis of global changes in suicide rates and numbers over the period 1990–2019. *Injury Prevention, 28*(2), 117–124.

UNIT 14 BUILDING CLINICAL COMPETENCE

Special topics in medical–surgical nursing

Case study 1

A Registered Nurse with 2 years' postgraduate experience commenced working at a small regional hospital 2 weeks ago. This is her second afternoon shift in charge of the hospital's 10 beds, of which five are occupied by long-term residents. A very experienced Enrolled Nurse is working alongside her and has been a great source of advice and information on where to find things and who to contact.

The dreary day outside has suddenly turned violent with gale-force winds, intermittent hail and torrential rain. The lights flickered into a brief moment of total darkness before the hospital generators kicked in. The ageing phone system is not working, so it appears that the Registered Nurse and the Enrolled Nurse are isolated at this time.

At first the knock on the door sounds like trees or doors banging in the wind, but when the Registered Nurse goes to investigate, there are three young men at the door in various states of distress and with obvious physical injuries. One of the young men appears to have a head injury, is being held up by his mates and is losing consciousness as the nurse watches. The Registered Nurse calls out to the Enrolled Nurse who brings the trolley to transport the man into the assessment area. The man with the head injury is now not responding to verbal commands and requires assistance to maintain his airway. As the communication lines are down, and the man's mates are injured, the Enrolled Nurse runs to the nearby doctor's residence to request medical assistance.

Critical-thinking questions

1. If you were the Registered Nurse in this situation, how do you think you would react?
2. How would you ensure that you are still working within your scope of practice?
3. What are some of the ethical considerations of this case study? Does this constitute a professional dilemma? How did you come to this conclusion?
4. What do you think are some of the contributing factors to the above decisions being made?
5. If you think that this is not the right way to address this situation, what could the nurses have done differently?

Case study 2

Maryanne Freeman, aged 69 years, and her husband, James, 72 years, prepared to travel from their home in Remoteville to the nearest tertiary-level hospital in Cityton, where Maryanne is to undergo removal of a cataract and implantation of an intraocular lens to her right eye. Maryanne has a history of type 2 diabetes and osteoarthritis. James has a history of pacemaker insertion and congestive cardiac failure, and he and Maryanne manage independently. The couple are fortunate that the RFDS clinic run is able to transfer them to Cityton. While Maryanne is hospitalised, James is able to stay in hospital accommodation.

The operation goes smoothly and Maryanne remains as an inpatient for 3 days postoperatively. Maryanne is seen by the ophthalmic surgeon on the third morning and is cleared for discharge. The attending nurse provides education to both Maryanne and James, instructing them on how to instil eye drops, the need for Maryanne to cover her eyes at night and the need to continue wearing dark glasses. James becomes concerned and asks the nurse how they will get back home. The nurse contacts the hospital social worker who books two bus tickets for the journey and a taxi voucher for transfer from the hospital to the bus depot. James then asks if they could go back with the RFDS as the road journey is a 10-hour trip and he is concerned that Maryanne cannot sit that long on the bus. The social worker does not think that returning with the RFDS is possible. As the bus was to depart at 7 am, James became quite anxious that they would miss it and that they would need to leave the hospital at 6 am before Maryanne had had breakfast. The pharmacy organised discharge medications the night before.

The bus departed at 7 am and the couple endured the 10-hour journey home.

Critical-thinking questions

1. What are some of the practical concerns with this case study?
2. Were James's concerns valid and/or acknowledged?
3. Was the discharge planning individualised for Maryanne?
4. Can you identify any other considerations the nurse and the social worker should have included in their provision of care?

Appendix

Essentials for nurses: COVID-19

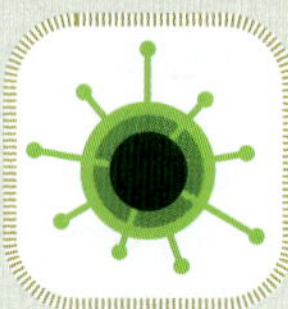

Stay current: knowledge about COVID-19 is changing daily. Check the following sources regularly for the latest information:

- **Australian Commission on Safety and Quality in Health Care:** https://www.safetyandquality.gov.au/covid-19-resources
- **Australian Government:** refer to relevant state or territory health departments for further details.
- **Australian Government:** refer to relevant state or territory health departments for further details on long COVID clinics.
- **Centers for Disease Control and Prevention (CDC):** https://www.cdc.gov/coronavirus/2019-ncov/index.html
- **Children and COVID-19:** refer to relevant state or territory children's hospitals for further details
- **Department of Health and Aged Care:** https://www.health.gov.au
- **Healthdirect:** https://www.healthdirect.gov.au/covid-19
- **Palliative Care Australia:** https://palliativecare.org.au/covid-19-updates/
- **Therapeutics Goods Administration (TGA):** https://www.tga.gov.au/
- **World Health Organization (WHO):** https://www.who.int/health-topics/coronavirus

PATHOPHYSIOLOGY AND TRANSMISSION

COVID-19 is a novel coronavirus, which means that it is a new virus not previously seen in humans. It is considered infectious and is caused by the SARS-CoV-2 virus (WHO, 2022a). The full name of this disease is coronavirus disease 2019. In the abbreviation COVID-19, *CO* represents *corona*, *VI* is *virus*, *D* is *disease* and *19* is *the year* it was identified (CDC, 2021a).

In the asymptomatic phase of COVID-19, the virus enters the nose and starts to replicate. In this stage, the person is infectious even though the viral burden is low. The virus is covered with spiked surface proteins that attach to receptors on cells, particularly in the lungs. It enters healthy cells through ACE2 receptors and destroys the cells. Over the next few days, the virus moves down the respiratory tract, which has a greater concentration of ACE2 receptors, and triggers an inflammatory response and respiratory symptoms. About 80% of individuals have mild symptoms. In the other 20% of individuals, shortness of breath develops in 5–8 days, followed by acute respiratory distress syndrome (ARDS) (Jackson et al., 2022; Mason, 2020).

Older adults and individuals with chronic illness are at greatest risk of developing symptoms and complications of COVID-19. At the time of writing, people aged 65 years and older and those who reside in aged care homes or long-term care facilities have had the greatest risk of mortality (National Institutes of Health (NIH), 2021). In Australia, the highest number of COVID-19 deaths was among those aged 80–89 years (85.2 years for males, 88.4 years for females).

Children may have asymptomatic infection or tend to experience similar, but milder, clinical manifestations that resemble a cold or flu (CDC, 2021a; Department of Health and Aged Care, 2022a). Some children develop a rare condition known as multisystem inflammatory syndrome that affects the heart, lungs, brain, skin, eyes and gastrointestinal tract (CDC, 2021b).

COVID-19 can be transmitted by both asymptomatic and symptomatic individuals. The incubation period for this virus (time from exposure to virus to onset of symptoms) is between 1 and 14 days, with a median onset of symptoms 5–6 days after exposure to a person with COVID-19 (CDC, 2021a; Healthdirect, 2022a).

COVID-19 spreads from the infected individual to another person primarily through respiratory droplets sprayed from the infected individual during coughing, sneezing, speaking, singing and breathing. The droplets range from large particles to smaller aerosols that may be inhaled into the lungs or land on another person's face, eyes, nose or mouth. The disease may also be transmitted by touching the face, mouth, nose or eyes with infected hands. The likelihood of transmission by droplets is greater when people are within 1.5–2 metres of each other (CDC, 2021c; Department of Health and Aged Care, 2022a; WHO, 2022a).

Viral shedding occurs when someone 'sheds' COVID-19 by breathing, sneezing, coughing or through their faeces and urine. It may occur up to several weeks after symptoms resolve. Some people continue to have non-infectious fragments which may still return a positive result when tested (CDC, 2021d; Department of Health and Aged Care, 2022a). The immune response and duration of immunity of individuals who have been infected with COVID-19 is not clearly understood and continues to be researched (CDC, 2021e).

At the time of writing, 13 variants of SARS-CoV-2 have been identified as causing COVID-19; however, only five (and their sub-variants such as XBB) continue to be classified as variants of concern—Alpha, Beta, Delta, Gamma and Omicron (Department of Health and Aged Care, 2022a; WHO, 2022a). Since 2019, the number of cases have risen significantly and continue to fluctuate due to these variants, which have caused severe illness in both vaccinated and unvaccinated people. It is thought that vaccinated people can carry and spread these variants to others. Although vaccinated people who contract one of these variants seem to have the same high amount of the virus, in most cases, they appear to have a milder case.

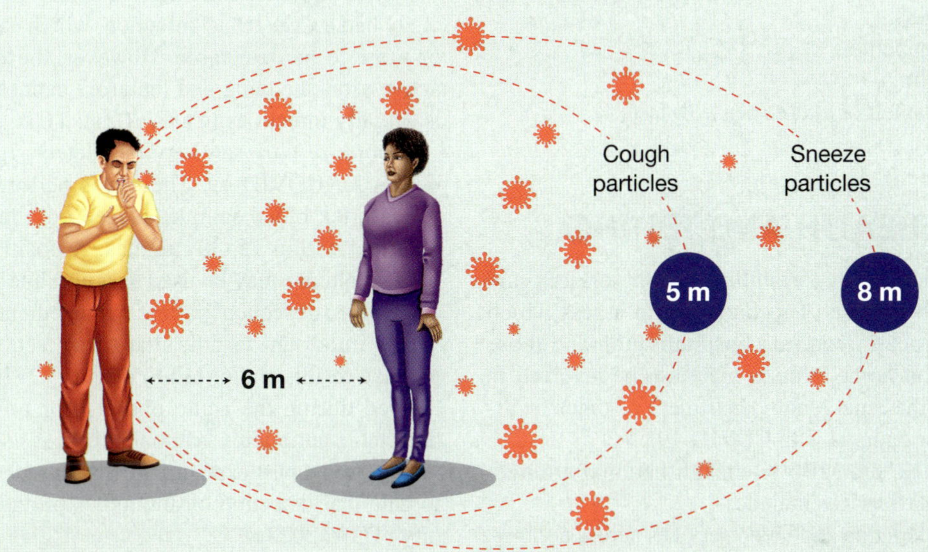

REDUCING AND PREVENTING SPREAD OF INFECTION

In the community: community spread of COVID-19 can be reduced or prevented by doing the following:

- placing at least 1.5 metres distance between people
- washing hands regularly with soap and water or hand sanitiser 70% + alcohol for a minimum of 20 seconds
- wearing a facemask in areas where it is a requirement, including healthcare settings, aged care facilities, doctors' surgeries and allied health clinics, public transport etc.
- sneezing or coughing into the elbow or a tissue if a mask is not being worn
- avoiding touching the face, eyes, nose and mouth
- receiving a vaccination against COVID-19
- disinfecting commonly touched surfaces and items.

In healthcare settings: spread of COVID-19 in healthcare settings can be reduced or prevented by:

- following policy for donning, doffing and disposing of PPE
- performing hand hygiene before entering a patient's room and/or donning PPE (gown, face shield or goggles and mask)
- correctly removing and disposing of PPE when leaving a patient's room followed by hand hygiene. (The Department of Health and Aged Care (2022b) and the Australian Commission on Safety and Quality in Health Care (ACSQHC) (2020) provide guidelines and resources about donning and doffing PPE in various healthcare settings.)
- avoiding touching the face and eyes
- washing hands frequently with soap and water for 20 seconds and/or using approved antimicrobial solutions
- taking breaks and eating food in designated areas away from the patient care unit.

In the home: nurses can reduce transmission of COVID-19 to family and others who share their living space by (American Nurses Association Enterprise, 2020):

- changing clothes and shoes before leaving work, if possible
- always washing hands before leaving work
- cleaning objects that are used at home and work, such as mobile phones, before leaving work
- removing shoes and clothing worn at work before entering the house and placing in a plastic bag or box
- washing hands before entering or immediately after entering the home
- washing scrubs/work clothes in hot soapy water and avoid mixing them with other clothing; discarding the plastic bag that held the contaminated items and washing hands
- leaving items such as stethoscope and pens at work.

SIGNS AND SYMPTOMS

Individuals with COVID-19 can present with various signs and symptoms; the most common are similar to cold and flu (CDC, 2021a; Department of Health and Aged Care, 2022a) including:

- fever
- coughing
- sore throat
- shortness of breath.

Other symptoms experienced include:

- runny nose or congestion
- headache or fatigue
- muscle or joint pains
- nausea or loss of appetite
- diarrhoea or vomiting
- temporary loss of smell or altered sense of taste.

TRIAGE, TELEHEALTH AND TESTING

Nurses are using telehealth (providing health services and information through the use of technology) to assess which patients need urgent care requiring hospitalisation and those who can be treated at home. Nurses may also be involved in triaging patients in the emergency department or other facilities set up to care for patients with COVID-19.

As of January 2022, the MBS telehealth national arrangements are permanent. Services include:

- a wide range of telephone and video services across a number of healthcare professionals (e.g. GPs, NPs, allied health, mental health, specialists)
- longer phone consultations for patients who have received a positive COVID-19 test (introduced in July 2022)
- electronic prescriptions.

All MBS telehealth services are informed by the relevant MBS Review Taskforce Principles in order to support safe and equitable services (Department of Health and Aged Care, 2022c). When using telehealth, it is important to:

- ***Prioritise!*** If the patient is experiencing a life-threatening emergency, advise the individual to call **000** and tell the operator if they have been in contact with or are experiencing symptoms of COVID-19 (Department of Health and Aged Care, 2022a).
- Ask patients if they have travelled to a place with a COVID-19 outbreak.
- Ask about vaccination status, signs and symptoms of the virus and any medical conditions that place individuals at high risk, such as chronic obstructive pulmonary disease (COPD), asthma, heart failure, diabetes, compromised/impaired immunity, liver disease, chronic kidney disease, obesity, neurological conditions and pregnancy.

The nurse will then direct patients to the appropriate level of care based on the severity of symptoms, other medical conditions and exposure. If patients are recommended to go to the hospital emergency department and/or a healthcare provider, they must review the relevant website and/or call to confirm any additional requirements prior to attending (e.g. face mask, RAT etc.).

A *polymerase chain reaction* (PCR) or *rapid antigen test* (RAT) may be performed to determine whether an individual currently has a COVID-19 infection. There are a variety of RATs available; their accuracy varies as they may not detect COVID-19 immediately. A PCR is recommended for confirmation (Department of Health and Aged Care, 2022c).

A number of laboratory-based serology immunoassay tests and point-of-care serology tests have also been approved by the TGA for use in Australia (TGA, 2022a).

An *antibody test* determines whether an individual has previously had a COVID-19 infection, which can take up to 2 weeks or more to be detectable. However, these tests do not detect active viral shedding and therefore cannot detect if the person is actually infectious (CDC, 2021f; TGA, 2022a).

A *point-of-care* serology test detects IgG and/or IgM antibodies for COVID-19. The test is performed from venous or finger prick blood samples placed on a test strip, with results obtained within 15–30 minutes. A positive test along with a clinical picture may be used as a possible positive diagnosis to determine subsequent patient management (TGA, 2022a).

It is important to note that these tests may produce false-positive results and/or fail to detect COVID-19 if they are performed during the acute phase prior to the development of detectable antibodies. Although these tests provide information on a person's past exposure to COVID-19, there is no evidence to date that detection of antibodies provides protective immunity (TGA, 2022a).

HOME CARE FOR PATIENTS WITH COVID-19

Individuals who are experiencing severe symptoms of COVID-19 should call **000**. Those who are experiencing mild symptoms should ideally speak to their healthcare professional and have either a telehealth or an in-person assessment (NIH, 2021). Suggested care for the patient with mild symptoms of COVID-19 includes the following:

- Stay home, even if no symptoms are present.
- Drink plenty of fluids to stay hydrated.
- Cough medicine may provide relief for dry and productive cough—take as per manufacturer recommendations.
- Take paracetamol for fever and/or pain as per manufacturer recommendations.
- Non-steroidal anti-inflammatory drugs (NSAIDs) such as ibuprofen (Nurofen) have also been reported to decrease signs and symptoms—take as per manufacturer recommendations.
- Continue to monitor for signs and symptoms that require calling **000**, including breathing difficulties, shortness of breath, pain or pressure in the chest that persists, confusion, inability to awaken and cyanosis (blue lips or face) (Department of Health and Aged Care, 2022a; CDC, 2021a).

- Monitor oxygen saturation (SpO_2) at home if a pulse oximeter is available. Advise the patient to use a warm finger and to notify their healthcare professional or **000** if the value is repeatedly (not one time) below 95% (NIH, 2021).
- Try resting in the prone (face-down) position if feeling short of breath (NIH, 2021).
- Stay away from other people as much as possible and wear a face mask when around others both in and outside the home.
- Wash hands often using soap and water or antimicrobial gel and disinfect common surfaces regularly.
- Do not share dishes and utensils.
- If possible, use a separate bathroom and bedroom. If this is not possible, improve ventilation such as by opening windows and disinfecting after use.

Nurses should educate patients staying at home about the signs and symptoms that require calling **000** and should provide or refer patients to the relevant federal, state or territory health department site for additional information.

HOSPITAL CARE FOR PATIENTS WITH COVID-19

The pandemic has and continues to have a profound impact on all private and public hospital activities including emergency departments, elective surgery and overall patient admissions (Australian Institute of Health and Welfare (AIHW), 2022).

The majority of people with COVID-19 will not require hospitalisation or any additional treatments, particularly if they have been vaccinated (AIHW, 2022). Individuals who are at high risk for serious COVID-19 and those with moderate to severe symptoms require close monitoring since there is a risk of them becoming critically ill and being admitted to ICU as soon as 1 week following the onset of symptoms (CDC, 2021d). However, where appropriate and available, individuals will be cared for on the ward in rooms with negative pressure or airflow that will lower the risk of transmission (Healthdirect, 2022b).

COVID-19 is a respiratory illness that weakens the immune system, causing inflammation, and leads to poor respiratory outcomes including pneumonia and secondary infections (Australian Bureau of Statistics (ABS), 2022).

The time taken to develop severe symptoms, such as dyspnoea and ARDS, and to be admitted to ICU varies among individuals depending on their current health, co-morbidities, vaccination status and other factors. At the time of writing, Australia had over 11 million total reported cases of COVID-19 and almost 18,000 deaths due to COVID-19, most of which had laboratory confirmation that they had died *with or from* the virus (ABS, 2022).

The Australian and New Zealand Intensive Care Society (ANZICS) has developed COVID-19 guidelines providing recommendations and suggestions to ensure the continued delivery of high-quality care in the ICU (adults and paediatric patients) and to its workforce (ANZICS, 2021).

LONG COVID OR POST-COVID CONDITIONS

The majority of people who contract COVID-19 will have symptoms for a short period of time and usually recover within a few weeks. However, some may continue to experience symptoms for weeks, months or sometimes years after diagnosis (WHO, 2022a).

A person is considered to have long COVID if symptoms have continued for more than 12 weeks after their initial infection (Healthdirect, 2022c). Although many long-term side effects remain unknown, common symptoms (Department of Health and Aged Care, 2022d, 2022e) include:

- extreme fatigue
- persistent cough, hoarse voice
- shortness of breath, heart palpitations, chest pains
- numbness, ‘pins and needles’ and joint or muscle pain
- issues with sleeping
- change in sense of taste or smell, reduced appetite and weight loss
- changes in mood such as anxiety, stress and depression
- cognitive dysfunction
- low-grade fever and rash
- headaches.

Research to date has identified that those who are at greater risk of long COVID varies and includes:

- those with underlying conditions (e.g. respiratory disease, diabetes, hypertension, chronic cardiovascular disease, chronic kidney disease, active cancer etc.)
- those who initially had mild illness which was managed at home
- those who suffered a severe illness during the initial phase of COVID-19
- those who were admitted to ICU
- those over 35 years of age
- females.

A Global Technical Network for Clinical Management of COVID-19 has been established by the WHO to undertake studies of patients in order to understand the proportion of patients experiencing long-term effects, how long they persist and why they occur in order to develop further guidance for patient care for both adults and children (WHO, 2022a).

At the time of writing, no specific treatment has been identified for long COVID. States and territories have opened long COVID clinics to specifically support those with ongoing symptoms, including personalised treatment plans requiring support from a range of healthcare professionals (Department of Health and Aged Care, 2022b, 2022c, 2022f; Healthdirect, 2022c).

DRUG THERAPY FOR COVID-19

According to the *Australian Guidelines for the Clinical Care of People with COVID-19*, treatment for patients is based on illness severity and monitoring of clinical progression markers (e.g. SpO_2, respiratory failure, sepsis etc.), particularly during days 5–10 of symptom onset (Department of Health and Aged Care, 2022g).

Patients with hypoxaemia despite increasing levels of oxygen supplementation may benefit from a trial of awake prone positioning. Careful positioning and protection are needed to avoid peripheral nerve and skin injury in the prone position (NIH, 2021). This position should not be used in patients who are haemodynamically unstable, in respiratory distress and who require imminent intubation (NIH, 2021).

In 2020 and 2021, the TGA provisionally approved the following drugs for the use in COVID-19 treatment:

- tixagevimab and cilgavimab (Evusheld)
- sotrovimab (Xevudy)
- remdesivir (Veklury).

In January 2022, the TGA also provided provisional approval for the first oral drug treatments—molnupiravir (Lagevrio®) and nirmatrelvir + ritonavir (Paxlovid®).

The Australian Guidelines provide a list of drug treatments recommended for use and those that are not recommended—detailed information is provided in the guidelines found at https://www.health.gov.au/health-alerts/covid-19/treatments/about.

The WHO continues to update and release new versions related to therapeutics and the role of medication management in COVID-19 patient treatment (Department of Health and Aged Care, 2022g; WHO, 2022b).

INDEPENDENT NURSING INTERVENTIONS

Nursing care for patients with COVID-19 focuses on supportive care, such as:

- monitoring vital signs, capillary refill and oxygen saturation levels (SpO_2)
- monitoring cardiac, respiratory, neurological, renal and other body systems for complications such as pneumonia, hypoxia, sepsis and septic shock, arrhythmias, cardiomyopathy, acute renal failure, thromboembolism and ARDS
- teaching patients to use a face mask when in contact with healthcare professionals
- turning and positioning patients, including the prone position
- providing psychosocial support to the patient and family
- providing care for patients requiring endotracheal intubation and mechanical ventilation.

Nurses are advocates for patients who are unable to express their own wishes and for family members who cannot be present with their loved ones. Nurses often create the technological connection between patients and families to say their goodbyes, explain care to families and provide both patients and families with end-of-life support. Nurses can also call on team members, such as chaplains and social workers, to provide patient and family support (Delgado, 2020; Palliative Care Australia, 2020).

Nurses who work with or need help having difficult conversations with patients and families may find the following resources useful:

- Palliative Care Australia, COVID-19 resources: https://palliativecare.org.au/covid-19-updates/
- VitalTalk, COVID-19 Ready Communication Playbook: https://www.vitaltalk.org/covid-resources/.

COLLABORATIVE CARE

Successfully dealing with any pandemic requires a multifaceted approach and strategies. This includes both clinical and non-clinical support as well as personal, cultural and socioeconomic mitigation measures (Lim et al., 2022; NIH, 2021) such as:

- administering supplemental oxygen, such as high-flow nasal cannula or non-invasive positive pressure ventilation
- administering medications, as prescribed, such as:
  - paracetamol for fever control
  - NSAIDs for pain relief
  - anticoagulants for thromboembolic prophylaxis
  - antibiotics for bacterial pulmonary infection
  - (See *Australian Guidelines for the Clinical Care of People with COVID-19* (Department of Health and Aged Care, 2022g) for recommended drug treatments: https://www.health.gov.au/health-alerts/covid-19/treatments/about.)
- consulting with healthcare providers and pharmacists before administering medications and treatments that are not yet TGA approved or are investigational/experimental to learn about factors such as indications, side effects and criteria to monitor
- assessing and managing fluid volume
- using prone position in patients with dyspnoea and mechanically ventilated patients with refractory hypoxaemia (NIH, 2021)
- using collaborative models and pathways of care that are supported by primary care and community organisations to alleviate pressure on hospitals so they can provide care for those with more severe illness or with risk factors for disease progression (Lim et al., 2022).

COVID-19 VACCINATIONS

There are currently four COVID-19 vaccines that are authorised by the TGA in Australia and recommended by the Australian Technical Advisory Group on Immunisation (ATAGI) for use (TGA, 2022b). See https://www.health.gov.au/our-work/covid-19-vaccines/advice-for-providers/clinical-guidance/doses-and-administration.

Viral vector, protein-based and mRNA vaccines work in different ways to protect against COVID-19. The *viral vector* vaccine uses recombinant viral vectors that do not replicate in the host but do induce an immune response. The *protein-based vaccine* contains part of the coronavirus spike protein. The immune system cells recognise the spike protein as a threat and begin building an immune response against it. The *mRNA* vaccine works by inserting fragments into the cells of the body to reprogram them to make antigens against the pathogen. The antigen then triggers an immune response (Department of Health and Aged Care, 2022h).

Common side effects that may occur following vaccination include pain, redness or swelling around the injection site. The person may also report fatigue, headache, muscle pain, chills, fever and nausea.

Side effects from the second dose may be more intense than following the first dose or there may be none at all (CDC, 2021g). The third booster dose and forth dose are recommended for those in high-risk categories—see ATAGI recommendations (TGA, 2022b).

Blood clots have been reported following viral vector vaccination (AstraZeneca). Severe allergic reaction (anaphylaxis) and myocarditis and pericarditis have been reported following protein-based vaccination (Novavax) (Department of Health and Aged Care, 2022i). Myocarditis and pericarditis have also been reported following mRNA vaccinations (Pfizer and Moderna), especially in adolescents and young adults (CDC, 2021h). These cases were predominantly in males aged 16 and older, within several days of being vaccinated, and often after the second dose. Be alert to shortness of breath, chest pain and palpitations in this age group following vaccination.

Children infected with the COVID-19 virus can become sick and can spread the virus to others. Please refer to ATAGI recommendations for further information regarding children and vaccine recommendations.

VACCINE HESITANCY

Many people have been hesitant to receive the COVID-19 vaccine and boosters. Reasons for this hesitancy include being against vaccines in general, believing the vaccines are not safe due to rushed production and lack of trust of authorities, government and science (Kaufman, Tuckerman & Danchin, 2022; Troiano & Nardi, 2021).

Other factors that may affect decisions about accepting the vaccine include cultural, social and political considerations (CDC, 2021c), along with potential allergic reactions (e.g. anaphylaxis) to any components or contraindications to the vaccines.

The first step in overcoming vaccine hesitancy is to listen to understand the person's concerns. Talk to the person who has vaccine concerns in an objective manner. Provide accurate and honest information to dispel the myths about the vaccines (CDC, 2021i; Department of Health and Aged Care, 2022j). There is a lot of misinformation in the media and online about the vaccines. Always choose a reliable source of information.

SELF-CARE FOR NURSES

This is an especially tough time for nurses and other healthcare professionals as they navigate the numerous stresses and detrimental impacts of the pandemic. Frontline healthcare workers have and continue to experience increased personal and professional challenges (Lewis et al., 2022; US Department of Veterans Affairs (DVA), 2020), including:

- risk in relation to the uncertainty and vulnerability of becoming infected and transmitting the virus to family and friends
- managing the strain of donning and doffing PPE over long periods of time
- managing the stress of restrictions and lockdowns
- mental and physical health issues such as anxiety, emotional distress and exhaustion, moral distress, palpitations, fatigue, burnout, feelings of anger and guilt, disruptions in usual self-care and coping strategies
- working with limited resources, both human and equipment, to ensure the delivery of safe, quality patient care.

Healthcare professionals have been faced with making difficult ethical decisions about who received care and who did not. Using an *egalitarian* approach, each patient has an equal chance to receive care. The *utilitarian* approach looks at who will benefit the most from receiving care. The *prioritarian* approach selects the sickest person first. These difficult and controversial decisions contribute to moral distress (Australian College of Nursing (ACN), 2020; Lewis, et al., 2022; US DVA, 2020).

There are significant challenges for healthcare organisations in recognising and supporting the wellbeing of frontline staff. Self-care actions that nurses who are engaged in patient care can take to manage stress and work demands (ACN, 2020; Lewis, et al., 2022) include:

- taking breaks, going outside and practising relaxation techniques (e.g. breathing exercises, meditation, short walks, listening to music)
- paying attention to bodily needs, such as using the bathroom, keeping hydrated and eating healthy food at regular intervals
- recognising strengths and maintaining strong boundaries to be more effective
- resting, engaging in regular exercise and enjoyable relaxation activities
- working as a team and supporting co-workers
- checking in regularly with colleagues (e.g. R U OK).

The following actions may be helpful to reduce the negative effects of moral distress (ACN, 2020; American Psychiatric Nurses Association, 2020; Greenberg et al., 2020):

- Engage in debriefing sessions to provide support and to help team members cope with the physical and emotional stress they are experiencing.
- Seek peer support and communicate with colleagues who can validate feelings.
- Engage in self-care activities such as journalling, meditating, breathing exercises and walking outside.
- Seek professional assistance to develop healthy coping mechanisms and process experiences.
- Check in regularly with colleagues on their mental wellbeing.

Discussion questions for nursing students

After you have read the news report and journal article, consider the following questions:

- Bernstein, L. & Gerberg, J. (2020). *A Brooklyn ICU amid a pandemic: Patients alone, comforted by nurses and doctors.* https://www.washingtonpost.com/national/health-science/in-the-icu-health-care-workers-with-little-to-offer-covid-19-

patients-soldier-on/2020/04/04/16face9e-74f3-11ea-a9bd-9f8b593300d0_story.html

- Raper, R. (2021). The implications of living with COVID-19 for intensive care in Australia. *Medical Journal of Australia, 215*(11), 511–512. doi: 10.5694/mja2.51332
- ***Discussion 1***: There are seven patients with COVID-19 in the emergency department who need a ventilator, but the hospital has only four available ventilators. Taking into consideration severity of COVID-19 symptoms, age, health, family role (e.g. mother of three young children), quality of life and other variables, how do you decide who receives ventilatory treatment?
- ***Discussion 2***: Think of the conversations you might have with patients and family members of those who will not receive ventilatory treatment due to lack of availability. Role-play these conversations with other group members.
- ***Discussion 3***: The intensive care unit at Best Hospital only has a 10-bed ICU capacity. Discuss ways to expand ICU capacity. What education and training will be necessary to make this change? Consider the changes that affect nurses as well as the interprofessional team.
- ***Discussion 4***: The nurses on a COVID unit are concerned about bringing the virus home to their families. Discuss measures that nurses can take to reduce virus spreading. Consider both your workplace and home resources and environment in your response.
- ***Discussion 5***: Experts are talking about a possible resurgence of COVID-19 infections in the next 1–2 years. Consider the resources in your workplace, community and at state/territory and federal levels and develop three changes that could be implemented as part of an overall plan to meet the predicted surge.
- ***Discussion 6***: You hear friends or family discussing their reluctance to be vaccinated against COVID-19 or hear them spreading misinformation about the disease. Think about how you will respond to these individuals. Practise role-playing your conversation with another student and have them give you feedback on your ability to listen and be objective.

Bibliography

American Nurses Association Enterprise (2020). *Keeping yourself and your family safe*. Retrieved from https://www.nursingworld.org/

American Psychiatric Nurses Association (2020). *Managing stress & self-care during COVID-19: Information for nurses*. Retrieved from https://www.apna.org/

Australian and New Zealand Intensive Care Society (ANZICS) (2021). *COVID-19 guidelines* (4th ed.). Retrieved from https://www.anzics.com.au

Australian Bureau of Statistics (ABS) (2022). *COVID-19 mortality in Australia, deaths registered to 31 January 2022*. Retrieved from https://www.abs.gov.au/

Australian College of Nursing (ACN) (2020). *Self-care resources*. Retrieved from https://www.acn.edu.au/

Australian Commission on Safety and Quality in Health Care (2020). Retrieved from https://www.safetyandquality.gov.au/

Australian Institute of Health and Welfare (AIHW) (2022). *Australia's hospitals at a glance*. Retrieved from https://aihw.gov.au/

Bernstein, L. & Gerberg, J. (2020). *A Brooklyn ICU amid a pandemic: Patients alone, comforted by nurses and doctors*. Retrieved from https://www.washingtonpost.com/

Centers for Disease Control and Prevention (CDC) (2021a). *Coronavirus disease 2019 (COVID-19). Frequently asked questions*. Retrieved from https://www.cdc.gov/

Centers for Disease Control and Prevention (CDC) (2021b). *For parents: Multisystem inflammatory syndrome in children (MIS-C) associated with COVID-19*. Retrieved from https://www.cdc.gov/

Centers for Disease Control and Prevention (CDC) (2021c). *Building confidence in COVID-19 vaccines*. Retrieved from https://www.cdc.gov/

Centers for Disease Control and Prevention (CDC) (2021d). *Interim clinical guidance for management of patients with confirmed coronavirus disease (COVID-19)*. Retrieved from https://www.cdc.gov/

Centers for Disease Control and Prevention (CDC) (2021e). *Clinical questions about COVID-19: Questions and answers*. Retrieved from https://www.cdc.gov/

Centers for Disease Control and Prevention (CDC) (2021f). *Testing for COVID-19*. Retrieved from https://www.cdc.gov/

Centers for Disease Control and Prevention (CDC) (2021g). *Possible side effects after getting a COVID-19 vaccine*. Retrieved from https://www.cdc.gov/

Centers for Disease Control and Prevention (CDC) (2021h). *Myocarditis and pericarditis following mRNA COVID-19 vaccination*. Retrieved from https://www.cdc.gov/

Centers for Disease Control and Prevention (CDC) (2021i). *How to talk to your patients about COVID-19 vaccination*. Retrieved from https://www.cdc.gov/

Delgado, S. (2020). End-of-life care during the COVID-19 pandemic. *AACN blog*. Retrieved from https://www.aacn.org/

Department of Health and Aged Care (2022a). *COVID-19 signs and symptoms*. Retrieved from https://www.health.gov.au/

Department of Health and Aged Care (2022b). *COVID-19—Donning and doffing personal protective equipment in primary care*. Retrieved from https://www.health.gov.au/

Department of Health and Aged Care (2022c). *Providing health care remotely during the COVID-19 pandemic*. Retrieved from https://www.health.gov.au/

Department of Health and Aged Care (2022d). *Getting help for long COVID*. Retrieved from https://www.health.gov.au/

Department of Health and Aged Care (2022e). *Long-term effects of COVID-19*. Retrieved from https://www.health.gov.au/

Department of Health and Aged Care (2022f). *Protect yourself and others from COVID-19*. Retrieved from https://www.health.gov.au/

Department of Health and Aged Care (2022g). *Treatments: Australian guidelines* (V65.2). Retrieved from https://www.health.gov.au/

Department of Health and Aged Care (2022h). *Approved COVID-19 vaccines*. Retrieved from https://www.health.gov.au/

Department of Health and Aged Care (2022i). *Nuvaxovid (Novavax)*. Retrieved from https://www.health.gov.au/

Department of Health and Aged Care (2022j). *Is it true? Get the facts on COVID-19 vaccines*. Retrieved from https://www.health.gov.au/

Greenberg, N., Docherty, M., Gnanaoragasam, S. & Wessely, S. (2020). Managing mental health challenges faced by healthcare workers during COVID-19 pandemic. *British Medical Journal*, *368*, m1211.

Healthdirect (2022a). *Symptoms of COVID-19 and when to seek medical advice*. Retrieved from https://www.healthdirect.gov.au/

Healthdirect (2022b). *Hospital and intensive care for COVID-19*. Retrieved from https://www.healthdirect.gov.au/

Healthdirect (2022c). *Understanding post COVID-19 symptoms and long COVID*. Retrieved from https://www.healthdirect.gov.au/

Jackson, C. B., Farzan, M., Chen, B. & Choe, H. (2022). Mechanisms of SARS-CoV-2 entry into cells. *Natural Review Molecular Cell Biology*, *23*, 3–20. https://doi.org/10.1038/s41580-021-00418-x

Kaufman, J., Tuckerman, J. & Danchin, M. (2022). Overcoming COVID-19 vaccine hesitancy: Can Australia reach the last 20 percent? *Expert Review of Vaccines*, *21*(2), 159–161. https://doi.Org/10.1080/14760584.2022.2013819

Lewis, S., Wills, K., Bismark, M. & Smallwood, N. (2022). A time for self-care? Frontline health workers' strategies for managing mental health during the COVID-19 pandemic. *SSM Mental Health*, *2*, 100053. doi: 10.1016/j.ssmmh.2021.100053

Lim, S. M., Allard, N. L., Devereux, J. et al. (2022). The COVID Positive Pathway: A collaboration between public health agencies, primary care and metropolitan hospitals in Melbourne. *The Medical Journal of Australia*, *216*(8), 413–419.

Mason, R. (2020). Pathogenesis of COVID-19 from a cell biology perspective. *European Respiratory Journal*, *55*. Retrieved from https://erj.ers-journals.com/

National Institutes of Health (NIH) (2021). *Coronavirus disease (COVID-19) treatment guidelines*. Retrieved from https://www.covid19treatmentguidelines.nih.gov/

Palliative Care Australia (2020). *Palliative care and COVID-19: Grief, bereavement and mental health*. Retrieved from https://palliativecare.org.au/

Raper, R. (2021). The implications of living with COVID-19 for intensive care in Australia. *Medical Journal of Australia*, *215*(11), 511–512. doi: 10.5694/mja2.51332

Therapeutic Goods Administration (TGA) (2022a). *COVID-19 testing in Australia—Information for health professionals*. Retrieved from https://www.tga.gov.au/

Therapeutic Goods Administration (TGA) (2022b). *Approved COVID-19 vaccines*. Retrieved from https://www.health.gov.au

Troiano, G. & Nardi, A. (2021). Vaccine hesitancy in the era of COVID-19. *Public Health*, *194*, 245–251.

US Department of Veterans Affairs (DVA) (2020). *Managing healthcare workers' stress associated with the COVID-19 virus outbreak*. Retrieved from https://www.ptsd.va.gov/

VitalTalk (2020). *COVID-19 Ready Communication Playbook*. Retrieved from https://www.vitaltalk.org/

World Health Organization (WHO) (2022a). *Coronavirus disease (COVID-19)*. Retrieved from https://www.who.int/

World Health Organization (WHO) (2022b). *Therapeutics and COVID-19: Living guideline*. Retrieved from https://www.who.int/

Glossary

abrasion Partial-thickness denudation of an area of integument, generally resulting from falls or scrapes.

accommodation The ability of the eye to adjust to variations in distance.

achalasia Absence of peristalsis of the oesophagus and high gastro-oesophageal sphincter pressure resulting in dilation and loss of tone in the oesophagus.

acidosis The condition in which the hydrogen ion concentration increases above normal (reflected in a pH below 7.35).

acid A substance that releases hydrogen ions in solution.

acne Disorder of the pilosebaceous (hair and sebaceous gland) structure, resulting in eruption of papules or pustules.

acoustic neuroma (schwannoma) Benign tumour of cranial nerve VIII.

acquired immune deficiency syndrome (AIDS) A specific group of diseases or conditions that are indicative of severe immunosuppression related to infection with the human immunodeficiency virus.

acromegaly Meaning literally 'enlarged extremities', this is a condition resulting from excessive growth hormone secretion during adulthood.

actinic keratosis Also called senile or solar keratosis, this is an epidermal skin lesion directly related to chronic sun exposure and photo damage.

active immunity Production of antibodies or development of immune lymphocytes against specific antigens.

active sense of self The development of meaning, purpose and direction in one's life.

active transport Movement of molecules across cell membranes and epithelial membranes against a concentration gradient; requires energy.

acute coronary syndrome (ACS) A general term used to describe the effects of coronary heart disease, including angina and myocardial infarction.

acute gastritis A benign, self-limiting disorder associated with ingestion of gastric irritants such as aspirin, alcohol, caffeine or foods contaminated with certain bacteria.

acute illness An illness that occurs rapidly, lasts for a relatively short time and is self-limiting.

acute inpatient unit A ward in a mental health facility that admits people who are generally very mentally unwell.

acute kidney injury (AKI) Kidney injury characterised by a rapid onset of symptoms that are potentially reversible with prompt intervention that addresses the initial cause of the injury.

acute myocardial infarction (AMI) Necrosis (death) of myocardial cells.

acute pain Usually temporary, localised and of sudden onset; it lasts for less than 6 months and has an identifiable cause, such as trauma, surgery or inflammation.

acute respiratory distress syndrome (ARDS) Non-cardiac pulmonary oedema and progressive refractory hypoxaemia.

acute tubular necrosis (ATN) A syndrome of abrupt and progressive decline in tubular and glomerular function.

adaptive immune response A specific and systemic immune response initiated by and directed against particular antigens.

addiction Dependency on a drug, which can be either physical or psychological.

Addisonian crisis A rare, life-threatening response to acute adrenal insufficiency; occurs in about 25% of patients.

Addison's disease A rare endocrine disorder wherein the adrenal glands produce insufficient steroid hormones.

adrenal crisis A constellation of symptoms that indicate severe adrenal insufficiency caused by insufficient levels of the hormone cortisol.

advance directive Also called a *living will*, this is a document in which a person formally states preferences for healthcare in the event that he or she later becomes mentally incapacitated, and names a person who has durable power of attorney to serve as a substitute decision maker to implement the patient's stated preferences.

afterload The resistance the ventricles must overcome to eject their blood volume; the pressure in the arterial system ahead of the ventricles.

agnosia The inability to recognise one or more subjects that were previously familiar; agnosia may be visual, tactile or auditory.

albuminuria Albumin (protein) in the urine.

alcohol An organic compound obtained by substituting a hydroxyl group for a hydrogen on a hydrocarbon.

alcoholic cirrhosis (Laënnec's cirrhosis) The end result of alcoholic liver disease.

alkalis Substances that accept hydrogen ions in solution.

alkalosis The condition where the hydrogen ion concentration decreases below normal (reflected in a pH above 7.45).

alleles Different forms of a gene or DNA occupying the same place on a pair of chromosomes; an allele for each gene is inherited from each parent.

allergy A hypersensitivity response to environmental or exogenous antigens.

allografts Grafts between members of the same species but who have different genotypes and HLA antigens. See also *homograft*.

alopecia Loss of hair; baldness.

Alzheimer's disease (AD) A form of dementia characterised by progressive, irreversible deterioration of the general intellectual functioning.

amenorrhoea Absence of menstruation.

amputation Partial or total removal of a body part.

anaemia An abnormally low number of circulating red blood cells, haemoglobin concentration or both.

anaesthesia State produced by medications given intravenously, intraspinally, subcutaneously or by inhalation to create temporary partial or total loss of sensation and consciousness in a person for invasive procedures such as surgery or painful diagnostic tests.

analgesic A medication that reduces or eliminates the perception of pain.

anaphylactic shock Shock resulting from a widespread hypersensitivity reaction (called *anaphylaxis*). The pathophysiology in this type of shock includes vasodilation, pooling of blood in the periphery and hypovolaemia with altered cellular metabolism.

anaphylaxis An acute systemic type I response that occurs in highly sensitive people following injection of a specific antigen.

anaplasia The regression of a cell to an immature or undifferentiated cell type.

anasarca Severe, generalised oedema.

androgens Hormones synthesised in the testes, ovaries and adrenal cortex that promote expression of male sex characteristics.

anergy Inability to react to specific antigens.

aneurysm Abnormal dilation of a blood vessel, commonly at a site of a weakness or tear in the vessel wall.

angina pectoris (angina) Chest pain resulting from reduced coronary blood flow that causes a temporary imbalance between myocardial blood supply and demand.

angioma (haemangioma) Benign vascular tumour.

anion gap The difference between the sum of two measured anions, chloride and bicarbonate, and the principal measured cation, sodium.

ankylosing spondylitis (AS) A chronic inflammatory arthritis that primarily affects the axial skeleton, leading to pain and progressive stiffening and fusion of the spine.

anorexia Loss of appetite.

anorexia nervosa An eating disorder characterised by a body weight less than 85% of expected for age and height, and an intense fear of gaining weight.

anorgasmia Absence of orgasm.

anosmia Inability to smell.

antibodies Immunoglobulin molecules that bind with an antigen to inactivate it.

antibody-mediated (humoral) immune response Activation of B cells to produce antibodies to respond to antigens such as bacteria, bacterial toxins and free viruses.

anticipatory grieving A combination of intellectual and emotional responses and behaviours by which people adjust their self-concept in the face of a potential loss.

antigen A substance capable of evoking a specific immune response; usually a protein, which the body recognises as foreign, causing an immune response to be stimulated.

anxiety An unpleasant feeling that is typically associated with uneasiness, apprehension, fear or worry.

aortic valve The semilunar valve between the left ventricle of the heart and the aorta in the heart. It prevents blood from flowing backwards into the ventricle.

aphasia Defective or absent language function.

apical impulse A normal, visible pulsation (thrust) in the area of the midclavicular line in the left fifth intercostal space. It can be seen on inspection in about half of the adult population.

aplastic anaemia A condition manifested by failure of the bone marrow to produce all three types of blood cells.

apnoea Cessation of breathing lasting from a few seconds to a few minutes.

appendicitis Inflammation of the vermiform appendix.

apraxia The inability to carry out a motor pattern (such as drawing a figure) even when strength and coordination are adequate.

arrhythmia Abnormal heart rate or rhythm.

arterial blood gas (ABG) A laboratory test used to evaluate acid–base balance and gas exchange.

arthritis Joint inflammation.

ascites Excess fluid in the peritoneal cavity.

asphyxiation Oxygen deprivation.

asthma Chronic inflammatory disorder of the airways that is characterised by recurrent episodes of wheezing, breathlessness, chest tightness and coughing.

astigmatism A condition that develops with abnormal curvature of the cornea or eyeball, causing the image to focus at multiple points on the retina.

ataxia Uncoordinated, irregular gait and muscle movement; weakness.

atelectasis Collapse of lung tissue following obstruction of the bronchus or bronchioles.

atherosclerosis A form of arteriosclerosis in which deposits of fat and fibrin obstruct and harden the arteries.

atrial natriuretic peptide (ANP) A hormone released by atrial muscle cells in response to distension from fluid overload.

atrioventricular block A block in the normal conduction pathways.

Australian College of Mental Health Nurses (ACMHN) Peak professional college for mental health nurses in Australia.

autograft Transplant of the person's own tissue; the most successful type of tissue transplant.

autoimmune disorder Failure of the immune system to recognise itself, resulting in normal host tissue being targeted by immune defences.

autonomic dysreflexia Exaggerated sympathetic response that occurs in people with spinal cord injuries at or above the T6 level.

autosome A single chromosome from any one of the 22 pairs of chromosomes not involved in sex determination (X or Y); humans have 22 pairs of autosomes.

B lymphocytes (B cells) Bursa-equivalent lymphocytes responsible for synthesising humoral antibody.

bacterial vaginosis Non-specific vaginitis.

bactericidal agent Capable of killing an organism without immune system intervention. These include the penicillins, cephalosporins and aminoglycoside antibiotics.

bacteriostatic agent Inhibits the growth of a microorganism, leaving its destruction to the host's immune system.

balloon tamponade The application of pressure to stop oesophageal bleeding using an inflatable balloon.

bariatric care The branch of healthcare that deals with the causes, prevention and treatment of obesity. The term *bariatrics* was created around 1965, from the Greek root *bar-* ('weight' as in barometer), suffix *-iatr* ('treatment' as in paediatrics) and suffix *-ic* ('pertaining to'). The field encompasses dieting, exercise and behavioural therapy approaches to weight loss, as well as psychotherapy, pharmacotherapy and surgery.

basal cell carcinoma (BCC) Epithelial tumour that is believed to originate either from the basal layer of the epidermis or from cells in the surrounding dermal structures. These tumours are characterised by an impaired ability of the basal cells of the epidermis to mature into keratinocytes, with mitotic division beyond the basal layer.

basal metabolic rate (BMR) The energy used when the body is at rest.

base excess (BE) A calculated value also known as buffer base capacity. Base excess reflects the degree of acid–base imbalance by indicating the status of the body's total buffering capacity.

bases (or alkalis) Substances that accept hydrogen ions in solution.

Bell's palsy (facial paralysis) Disorder of the facial nerve (seventh cranial nerve), characterised by unilateral paralysis of the facial muscles.

benign prostatic hyperplasia (BPH) Enlargement of the prostate gland.

benzodiazepines Minor tranquillisers belonging to the sedative–hypnotic group of drugs that have a CNS depressant effect through action at the gamma-aminobutyric acid (GABA) receptor sites.

bile A greenish, watery solution containing bile salts, cholesterol, bilirubin, electrolytes, water and phospholipids.

biliary colic A severe, steady pain in the epigastric region or upper right quadrant of the abdomen.

binge-eating disorder An eating disorder characterised by recurrent episodes of eating an excessive amount of food during a defined period of time, and a sense of lack of control over eating during binge episodes.

biofilms Polymicrobial microbial communities that proliferate and are encased in a protective glycocalax matrix.

biomedical model of health A model of health that mainly focuses on biological health determinants and broadly views health as the absence of disease. This model is also known as the medical model.

biopsychosocial model of health The biopsychosocial model of health broadly views health as individual holistic wellbeing.

biotherapy Treatment that modifies the biological processes that result in malignant cells, primarily through enhancing the person's own immune responses.

bitemporal homonymous hemianopia Loss of vision in each temporal visual field (outer half of vision) resulting from compression of the optic chiasm.

blood flow The volume of blood transported in a vessel, in an organ or throughout the entire circulation over a given period of time.

blood glucose levels (BGLs) The amount of glucose present in blood.

blood pressure The tension or pressure exerted by blood against arterial walls.

blunt trauma The type of trauma that occurs when there is no communication from the damaged tissues to the outside environment.

body mass index (BMI) Used to identify excess adipose tissue, BMI is calculated by dividing the weight (in kilograms) by the height (in metres squared, m^2).

bone marrow transplant (BMT) Infusion of bone marrow cells to restore bone marrow function after chemotherapy or radiation; allogeneic BMT uses donor bone marrow cells from a donor; autologous BMT uses the person's own bone marrow.

borborygmus Hyperactive high-pitched, tinkling, rushing or growling bowel sound.

botulism A severe, life-threatening form of food poisoning caused by *Clostridium botulinum*.

bradypnoea Abnormally low respiratory rate.

brain death The cessation of cerebral blood flow with global brain infarction and permanent loss of all brain function.

brain death criteria Clinical signs used to determine whether a comatose person is brain dead.

breakthrough pain A sudden flare or increase in pain despite comfort with or without baseline analgesia.

bronchiectasis Permanent abnormal dilation of one or more large bronchi and destruction of bronchial walls, usually accompanied by infection.

bronchitis Inflammation of the bronchi.

bruit An adventitious sound heard during auscultation; of venous or arterial origin.

buffer A substance that prevents major changes in pH by removing or releasing hydrogen ions.

bulimia nervosa An eating disorder characterised by recurring episodes of binge eating followed by purge behaviours such as self-induced vomiting, use of laxatives or diuretics, fasting or excessive exercise.

burn An injury resulting from exposure to heat, chemicals, radiation, cold injuries or electric current.

burn shock Hypovolaemic shock resulting from the shift of a massive amount of fluid from the intracellular and intravascular compartments into the interstitium following burn injury.

bursitis Inflammation of the bursa.

cachectic The state of very poor health and malnourishment in a person.

cachexia The wasted physical appearance characteristic of cancer and other chronic illnesses. It is characterised by rapid depletion of the body's protein, particularly in skeletal muscle, with less rapid loss of fat.

caffeine A bitter, white crystalline xanthine alkaloid that is a psychoactive stimulant drug.

calculi An abnormal concentration in the body, commonly called a stone; occur in the kidneys, ureters, bladder or urethra.

cancer A family of complex diseases with manifestations that vary according to body system and type of tumour cells involved; marked by uncontrolled growth and the spread of abnormal cells.

cancer pain A common condition of people suffering with advanced cancer, it is often persistent and arises from a number of factors.

candidiasis Infection of mucous membranes caused by *Candida albicans*, a yeast-like fungus.

cannabis The general name given to the psychoactive substances found in the marijuana plant, Cannabis sativa, the main active constituent being delta 9-tetra-hydrocannabinol (THC).

carbuncle A group of infected hair follicles.

carcinogen Cancer-causing agent.

carcinogenesis The production or origin of cancer.

cardiac arrest Sudden failure of the heart to pump.

cardiac index Cardiac output adjusted for body size.

cardiac output (CO) The amount of blood pumped by the ventricles into the pulmonary and systemic circulations in 1 minute.

cardiac rehabilitation A long-term program of medical evaluation, exercise, risk factor modification, education and counselling designed to limit the physical and psychological effects of cardiac illness and improve the person's quality of life.

cardiac reserve The ability of the heart to respond to the body's changing need for cardiac output.

cardiac tamponade Compression of the heart due to pericardial effusion, trauma, cardiac rupture or haemorrhage.

cardiogenic shock Shock that occurs when the heart's pumping ability is compromised to the point that it cannot maintain cardiac output and adequate tissue perfusion.

cardiomyopathy Primary abnormality of the heart muscle that affects its structural or functional characteristics.

cardiovascular disease (CVD) Generic term for disorders of the heart and blood vessels.

carpopedal spasm Involuntary flexion and contraction of the wrist and ankle joints.

carrier Any individual who carries a single copy of an altered gene or mutation for a recessive condition on one chromosome of a chromosome pair and an unaltered form of that gene on the other chromosome; a carrier generally is not affected by the gene alteration; on average, each person in the general population is a carrier of five or six gene mutations for recessive disorders.

catabolism Biochemical process involving the breakdown of complex structures into simpler forms.

cataract Opacification (clouding) of the lens of the eye.

cell cycle The four phases that occur during growth and development of a cell.

cell-mediated (cellular) immune response Direct or indirect inactivation of antigen by lymphocytes.

cellulitis A localised infection of the dermis and subcutaneous tissue.

central nervous system (CNS) depressants Drugs that can be used to slow down brain activity.

central obesity Obesity characterised by a waist-to-hip ratio of greater than 1 in men or 0.8 in women.

central pain Related to a lesion in the brain that may spontaneously produce high-frequency bursts of impulses that are perceived as pain.

cerebral oedema An increase in the volume of brain tissue due to abnormal accumulation of fluid.

cerumen Earwax.

chalazion Granulomatous cyst or nodule of the eyelid.

chancre Hard, syphilitic primary ulcer.

cheilosis Painful lesions at corners of mouth.

chemotherapy Cancer treatment involving the use of cytotoxic medications to decrease tumour size, adjunctive to surgery or radiation therapy, or to prevent or treat suspected metastases.

chlamydia A group of syndromes caused by *Chlamydia trachomatis*, a bacterium that behaves like a virus spreading within a host cell; spread by sexual contact and to the neonate by passage through the birth canal of an infected mother.

cholecystitis Inflammation of the gallbladder, usually associated with stones in the cystic or common bile duct.

cholelithiasis Formation of stones (calculi) within the gallbladder or biliary duct system.

chromosome Genetic material carried by each cell; found in the cell nucleus.

chronic bronchitis Excessive secretion of bronchial mucus characterised by a productive cough lasting 3 or more months in 2 consecutive years.

chronic condition A disease involving a long course in its development or its symptoms.

chronic gastritis Disorders characterised by progressive and irreversible changes in the gastric mucosa.

chronic hepatitis Chronic infection of the liver.

chronic kidney disease The presence of impaired or reduced kidney function that lasts longer than 3 months.

chronic obstructive pulmonary disease (COPD) Chronic airflow obstruction due to chronic bronchitis and/or emphysema.

chronic sorrow A cyclical, recurring and potentially progressive pattern of pervasive sadness experienced in response to continual loss, throughout the trajectory of an illness or disability.

chronic venous insufficiency A chronic disorder of inadequate venous return.

Chvostek's sign Contraction of the lateral facial muscles in response to tapping the face in front of the ear; caused by decreased blood calcium levels.

circulating nurse Assists scrub nurses and surgeons during surgery.

cirrhosis A progressive, irreversible disorder, eventually leading to liver failure; the end stage of chronic liver disease.

claudication Cramping, aching pain in the calves, thighs and buttocks that occurs with a predictable level of activity and is relieved by rest.

clinical governance A system of policies, processes and accountabilities that is directed at improving patient safety and the quality and effectiveness of patient care within a health service.

clinical pathway A healthcare plan designed to provide care with a multidisciplinary, managed-action focus; developed for specific diagnoses, usually those that are high volume, high risk and high cost.

clinical reasoning The process by which nurses (and other clinicians) collect cues, process the information, come to an understanding of a person's problem or situation, plan and implement interventions, evaluate outcomes, and reflect on and learn from the process.

cocaine An illegal drug extracted from a cocoa leaf that is white, odourless, and takes the form of a crystalline powder.

cognition The ability to process information and apply knowledge.

cold sore See *herpes simplex*.

colectomy Surgical removal of the colon.

collateral vessels Accessory pathways connected to the smaller arteries in the coronary system.

colostomy Ostomy made in the colon.

comedones Non-inflammatory acne lesions.

communication The exchange of information between two or more people, groups or entities. It involves verbal and written exchanges, as well as body language, attitude and tone.

community A collection of people who share some attribute of their lives.

community mental health nurse A nurse in mental health nursing who works with consumers who are living in the community. They are often involved in case management.

compartment syndrome Condition in which excess pressure constricts the structures within a compartment and reduces circulation to muscles and nerves.

concussion Injury resulting from a violent jar, shake or impact with an object.

conjunctivitis Inflammation of the conjunctiva.

consciousness A condition in which a person is aware of self and environment and is able to respond appropriately to stimuli; full consciousness requires both normal rousal and full cognition.

constipation The infrequent (two or fewer bowel movements weekly) or difficult passage of stools.

consultation liaison (CL) A specialist mental health nurse who is the interface between medicine and psychiatry.

consumer-directed care A model of service delivery designed to give more care choice and flexibility to consumers. This model provides consumers with more control over the types of care and services they access, and the delivery of those services, including who delivers the services and when they are delivered.

continuum of care The provision of ongoing quality healthcare in acute and community settings to optimise quality of life for people, underpinned by an interprofessional consultative team approach.

contractility The inherent capability of the cardiac muscle fibres to shorten.

contracture Permanent shortening of connective tissue.

contralateral deficit Manifestations of a stroke on the side of the body opposite the side of the brain that is damaged.

contusion Superficial tissue injury resulting from blunt trauma, such as a kick or blow from an object, that causes the breakage of small blood vessels and bleeding into the surrounding tissue.

convergence Moving inward of the eyes to see an object close to the face.

cor pulmonale Condition of right ventricular hypertrophy and failure that results from longstanding pulmonary hypertension.

corneal reflex Closure of eyelids (blinking) due to corneal irritation.

corneal ulcer Local necrosis of the cornea, may be caused by infection, exposure trauma or the misuse/overuse of contact lenses.

coronary heart disease (CHD) Heart disease caused by impaired blood flow to the myocardium.

coryza (rhinorrhoea) Profuse nasal discharge.

COVID-19 COVID-19 is a novel coronavirus, which means that it is a new virus not previously seen in humans. It is considered infectious and is caused by the SARS-CoV-2 virus.

crackles Discontinuous lung sound heard by auscultation; can be fine or coarse. Produced by air passing over airway secretions or the opening of collapsed airways.

creatinine The end product from the breakdown of creatine phosphate in muscles.

crepitation A grating sound heard on movement of a joint.

Creutzfeldt–Jakob disease (CJD, spongiform encephalopathy) Rare, progressive neurological disease that causes brain degeneration without inflammation.

critical thinking Self-directed thinking that is focused on what to believe or do in a specific situation.

Crohn's disease (regional enteritis) Chronic, relapsing inflammatory disorder affecting the gastrointestinal tract.

cultural competence Practising in a way that demonstrates the importance of social and cultural influences on patients' health beliefs and behaviours, and devising interventions that take these issues into account.

cultural safety The effective nursing practice of a person or family from another culture, as determined by that person or family.

culture A learned world viewpoint or paradigm shared by a population or group and transmitted socially. It influences values, beliefs, customs and behaviours, and is reflected in the language, dress, food, materials and social interactions of a group.

Curling's ulcers Acute ulcerations of the stomach or duodenum that form following a burn injury.

Cushing's disease One form of Cushing's syndrome caused by a functioning pituitary adenoma, leading to increased secretion of adrenocorticotropic hormone (ACTH), causing excessive cortisol levels.

Cushing's syndrome A chronic disorder in which hyperfunction of the adrenal cortex produces excessive amounts of circulating cortisol or adrenocorticotropic hormone (ACTH).

Cushing's ulcers Stress ulcers occurring as sequelae of head injury or central nervous system surgery.

cyanosis A bluish discolouration of the skin and mucous membranes due to oxygen deficiency.

cyst A sac containing fluid or semisolid fluid.

cystectomy Complete surgical removal of the urinary bladder and adjacent muscles and tissues.

cystic fibrosis (CF) Inherited disorder of the exocrine glands that results in the secretion of abnormal amounts of mucus.

cystitis Inflammation of the urinary bladder.

cytokines Hormone-like polypeptides produced primarily by monocytes, macrophages and T cells. Cytokines act as messengers of the immune system, facilitating communication between the cells to adjust or vary the inflammatory reaction or to initiate immune cell proliferation and differentiation.

dawn phenomenon A rise in blood glucose between 4 am and 8 am that is not a response to hypoglycaemia.

day surgery units/centres Facilities where surgery is performed and the person is discharged on the same day.

death Irreversible cessation of circulatory and respiratory functions or irreversible cessation of all functions of the entire brain, including the brainstem.

death anxiety Worry or fear related to death or dying.

debridement Process of removing dead tissue from a wound.

decerebrate posturing Abnormal posture with the neck extended; the jaw clenched; arms pronated, extended and close to the sides; legs extended and feet plantar flexed. Results from lesions of the midbrain, pons or diencephalons.

decorticate posturing Abnormal posture with the upper arms close to the sides; the elbows, wrists and fingers flexed; the legs extended and internally rotated; and the feet plantar flexed. Results from lesions of the corticospinal tracts.

deep venous thrombosis (DVT) Blood clot (thrombus) formation and inflammation within a deep vein, usually in the pelvis or lower extremities; a common complication of hospitalisation, surgery and immobilisation.

dehiscence An unintended separation of wound margins due to incomplete healing.

dehydration Loss of water.

delegation Assigning appropriate work activities to other members of the healthcare team. When the nurse delegates nursing care activities to another person, that person is authorised to act in the place of the nurse, while the nurse retains the accountability for the activities performed.

delusion A fixed false belief that is firmly sustained despite what constitutes incontrovertible and obvious proof or evidence to the contrary. The belief is not one ordinarily accepted by other members of the person's culture or subculture.

dementia A global impairment of cognitive function that usually is progressive and may be permanent; interferes with normal social and occupational activities.

dermatitis Acute or chronic inflammation of the skin characterised by erythema and pain or pruritus.

dermatophytoses Superficial fungal infection of the skin; also called *ringworm*.

determinants of health Factors that influence health in either a positive or a negative way. Some of these function on an individual level (e.g. health behaviours such as smoking or exercise, or our genetic make-up). Others function at a broader societal level, such as the availability of health services, vaccination programs or clean drinking water and healthy food.

diabetes insipidus (DI) The result of antidiuretic hormone insufficiency.

diabetes mellitus (DM) Group of chronic disorders of the endocrine pancreas, all categorised under a broad diagnostic label. The condition is characterised by inappropriate hyperglycaemia caused by a relative or absolute deficiency of insulin or by a cellular resistance to the action of insulin.

diabetic ketoacidosis (DKA) A form of metabolic acidosis induced by stress in a person with type 1 diabetes mellitus.

diabetic nephropathy A disease of the kidneys characterised by the presence of albumin in the urine, hypertension, oedema and progressive renal insufficiency.

diabetic neuropathies Disorders of the peripheral nerves and the autonomic nervous system manifesting one or more of the following: sensory and motor impairment, muscle weakness and pain, cranial nerve disorders, impaired vasomotor function, impaired gastrointestinal function and impaired genitourinary function.

diabetic retinopathy The collective name for the changes in the retina that occur in the person with diabetes. The retinal capillary structure undergoes alterations in blood flow, leading to retinal ischaemia and a breakdown in the blood retinal barrier.

***Diagnostic and Statistical Manual of Mental Disorders* (DSM)** A manual that is published by the American Psychiatric Association that provides common language and standard criteria for the classification of mental disorders.

dialysate Dialysis solution.

dialysis The diffusion of solute molecules across a semipermeable membrane from an area of higher concentration to one of lower concentration.

diaphoresis Copious production of sweat.

diarrhoea An increase in the frequency, volume and fluid content of the stool.

diastolic blood pressure The minimum pressure maintained by elastic arterial walls during diastole (cardiac relaxation) to maintain blood flow through capillary beds; averages 80 mmHg in a healthy adult.

differentiation A process occurring over many cell cycles that allows cells to specialise in certain tasks.

'differentness' Being different from another person or group of people.

diffuse oesophageal spasm Non-peristaltic contraction of oesophageal smooth muscle.

diffusion The process by which solute molecules move from an area of high solute concentration to an area of low solute concentration to become evenly distributed.

digital health A broad range of technologies that can be used to treat patients and collect and share a person's health information.

dilemma A choice between two unpleasant, ethically troubling alternatives.

diplopia Double vision.

disaster Event that requires extraordinary efforts beyond those needed to respond to everyday emergencies.

discharge planning A planned process beginning with the person's initial presentation, considering the needs of the unique individual, based upon the availability of, and access to, support and resources. This process ensures that these needs are met through ongoing assessment and consultation involving the relevant healthcare professionals, patient, family, carers and community services.

discovery Encompasses equality and respect. Equality is the belief that all people ought to be treated equally. Respect is esteem for, or a sense of the worth or excellence of, a person, a personal quality, ability or a manifestation of a personal quality or ability.

disease Literally meaning 'without ease', this term describes alterations in structure and function of the body or mind. Diseases may have mechanical, biological or normative causes.

dislocation Separation of contact between two bones of a joint.

dissection (aortic) A life-threatening emergency caused by a tear in the intima of the aorta with haemorrhage into the media.

disseminated intravascular coagulation (DIC) A disruption of haemostasis characterised by widespread intravascular clotting and bleeding; a syndrome that develops as a complication of many other disorders.

distal determinants Determinants of health that tend to be stable and concern historical, national, institutional, political, legal and cultural factors.

distributive shock Also called *vasogenic shock*, this includes several types of shock that result from widespread vasodilation and decreased peripheral resistance.

diverticulitis Inflammation in and around the diverticular sac; typically affects only one diverticulum, usually in the sigmoid colon.

diverticulosis Indicates the presence of diverticula.

DNA-based tests Tests that incorporate new, sophisticated technology that permits the examination of the DNA itself, obtained from blood, bone marrow, amniotic fluid, fibroblast cells of the skin or buccal cells from the mouth.

do-not-resuscitate (DNR) directive Usually written by the doctor for the person who has a terminal illness or is near death, this order is usually based on the wishes of the person and family that no cardiopulmonary resuscitation be performed for respiratory or cardiac arrest.

Down syndrome A human genetic disease caused by the presence of an extra chromosome 21; characterised by mental retardation and heart and respiratory defects.

dumping syndrome Complication of partial gastrectomy characterised by nausea, weakness, sweating, palpitation, syncope, sensation of warmth and occasionally diarrhoea.

duodenal ulcers Peptic ulcer disease affecting the duodenum.

dwarfism A medical disorder, the term being used to describe a person of short stature.

dysarthria Difficulty speaking.

dysfunctional uterine bleeding (DUB) Vaginal bleeding that is usually painless but abnormal in amount, duration or time of occurrence.

dysmenorrhoea Pain associated with menstruation.

dyspareunia Painful intercourse.

dysphagia Difficulty swallowing.

dysphonia Change in the tone of voice.

dysplasia The loss of DNA control over differentiation occurring in response to adverse conditions.

dyspnoea Difficult or laboured breathing.

dysuria Painful urination.

ecchymosis A flat, irregularly shaped lesion of varying size with no pulsation; caused by blood collecting under the skin.

ectopic beats Impulses originating outside normal conduction pathways of the heart.

ejection fraction (EF) The percentage of total blood remaining in the ventricle at the end of diastole (relaxation); normal is 50–70%.

electrolytes Substances that dissociate in solution to form charged particles called ions.

electronic medical records (EMRs) Electronic (digital) collections of medical information about a person that are stored on a computer. An electronic medical record includes information about a patient's health history, such as diagnoses, medicines, tests, allergies, immunisations and treatment plans. It can be seen by all healthcare providers who are taking care of a patient and can be used by them to help make recommendations about the patient's care. Also called EHR and electronic health record.

embolism Sudden obstruction of a blood vessel by debris.

emphysema Destruction of the walls of the alveoli, with resulting enlargement of abnormal air spaces.

empowerment Developing confidence in one's own capacities.

empyema Accumulation of purulent exudate in the pleural cavity.

encephalitis An acute inflammation of the parenchyma of the brain or spinal cord.

end-of-life care Care provided in the final weeks of life when death is imminent.

endocarditis Inflammation of the endocardium.

endogenous insulin The insulin the pancreas makes.

endometriosis A condition in which multiple, small implants of endometrial tissue develop throughout the pelvic cavity.

endotoxins Found in the cell wall of Gram-negative bacteria, endotoxins are released only when the cell is disrupted. They act as activators of many human regulatory systems, producing fever, inflammation and potentially clotting, bleeding or hypotension when released in large quantities.

end-stage kidney disease (ESKD) The final stage of chronic kidney failure in which the kidneys are unable to excrete metabolic wastes and regulate fluid and electrolyte balance adequately; characterised by a glomerular filtration rate of less than 5% of normal.

enduring power of attorney A document that can delegate the authority to make health, financial and/or legal decisions on a person's behalf. It must be provided in writing and state that the designated person is authorised to make healthcare decisions.

enophthalmos Sunken appearance of the eyes.

enteral nutrition Administration of liquid nutritional formulas to meet kilojoule and protein needs in people unable to consume adequate food; also called *tube feeding*.

enucleation Surgical removal of an eye.

epidemic A widespread occurrence of an infectious disease (biological), localised to a particular community, region or population.

epididymitis Infection or inflammation of the epididymis.

epidural haematoma (extradural haematoma) A collection of blood between the dura and the skull.

epilepsy Chronic seizure activity.

epistaxis Nosebleed.

erectile dysfunction Inability of the male to attain and maintain an erection sufficient to permit satisfactory sexual intercourse.

erosive gastritis Inflammation and superficial erosions of the gastric mucosa that may occur as a complication of other life-threatening conditions such as shock, severe trauma, major surgery, sepsis, burns or head injury.

erysipelas Infection of the skin most often caused by group A streptococci.

erythema A reddening of the skin.

erythropoiesis Red blood cell production.

eschar Hard, leathery crust that covers a burn wound and harbours necrotic tissue.

escharotomy Surgical removal of eschar from the torso or extremity to prevent circumferential constriction.

euthyroid The state of having normal thyroid gland function.

evisceration Protrusion of body contents through a surgical wound.

exogenous insulin The insulin people inject or infuse via an insulin pump.

exophthalmos Protrusion of the eyeballs.

exotoxins Soluble proteins secreted into surrounding tissue by the microorganism. Exotoxins are highly poisonous, causing cell death or dysfunction.

extracorporeal shock wave lithotripsy (ESWL, transcutaneous shock wave lithotripsy) Non-invasive technique for fragmenting kidney stones using shock waves generated outside the body.

faecal impaction A rock-hard or putty-like mass of faeces in the rectum.

family Two or more people who are emotionally involved with each other.

fascial excision (fasciectomy) Process of excising the wound to the level of fascia.

fasciculations Involuntary twitching.

fat embolism syndrome (FES) Characterised by neurological dysfunction, pulmonary insufficiency and a petechial rash on the chest, axilla and upper arms due to fat globules lodged in the pulmonary vascular bed or peripheral circulation.

fibrocystic changes (FCCs) Physiological nodularity and breast tenderness that increase and decrease with the menstrual cycle.

fibroid tumours (uterine leiomyomas) See *leiomyomas*.

fibromyalgia A common rheumatic syndrome characterised by musculoskeletal pain, stiffness and tenderness.

filtration The process by which water and dissolved substances (solutes) move from an area of higher hydrostatic pressure to an area of lower hydrostatic pressure.

flaccidity Decreased muscle tone in disease or trauma of the lower motor neurons.

flail chest Free-floating segment of the chest wall, resulting from two or more consecutive ribs fractured in multiple places.

flatus Gas in the digestive tract.

fluid resuscitation Replacement of the extensive fluid and electrolyte losses associated with major burn injuries.

fluid volume deficit (FVD) A decrease in intravascular, interstitial and/or intracellular fluid in the body.

fluid volume excess (FVE) Excess extracellular fluid resulting from retention of both water and sodium in the body.

focused assessment A physical assessment that concentrates on the part of the body that may be affected by disease or injury.

folliculitis Bacterial infection of the hair follicle, most commonly caused by *Staphylococcus aureus*.

forensic mental health A subspecialty of mental health in which scientific and clinical expertise is applied in legal contexts, combining civil, criminal, correctional and legislative matters.

fracture A break in a bone, usually due to trauma.

friction rub The sound heard when two dry surfaces are rubbed together.

full-thickness avulsion injuries Injuries that result in loss of all of the layers of the skin, causing fat and muscle to be exposed.

full-thickness burn A burn that involves all layers of the skin, including the epidermis, dermis and epidermal appendages.

fulminant hepatitis Hepatitis with a rapid and severe onset and course.

furuncle Often called a boil; an inflammation of the hair follicle.

gamma hydroxybutyrate (GHB) A dissociative anaesthetic agent; another of the newer drugs diverted to illicit use.

gastric mucosal barrier A protective barrier consisting of lipids, bicarbonate ions and mucous gel that protects the stomach lining from the damaging effects of gastric juices.

gastric outlet obstruction Obstruction of the pyloric region of the stomach and duodenum that impairs gastric outflow; a potential complication of peptic ulcer disease.

gastric ulcers Ulcers of the stomach lining, usually in the lesser curvature and antrum; more common in older adults.

gastritis Inflammation of the stomach lining.

gastroduodenostomy (Billroth I) Excision of the pylorus of the stomach with the anastomosis of the upper stomach to the duodenum; commonly used partial gastrectomy procedure.

gastroenteritis Inflammation of the gastrointestinal tract; not a specific disease, but a group of syndromes or a collection of related manifestations.

gastrojejunostomy (Billroth II) Subtotal excision of the stomach with closure of the duodenum and side-to-side anastomosis of the jejunum to the stomach; commonly used partial gastrectomy procedure.

gastro-oesophageal reflux Backward flow of gastric contents into the oesophagus.

gastro-oesophageal reflux disease (GORD) Causes heartburn, usually after meals, when bending over or reclining.

gene A sequence of DNA on a chromosome that represents a fundamental unit of heredity; occupies a specific spot on a chromosome (gene locus).

gene expression When the protein product of a gene is visible (e.g. through the presence of a body structure or identifiable through biochemical tests such as insulin or phenylalanine levels).

general anaesthesia Deep sedation, which includes analgesia and muscle paralysis. This type of anaesthesia requires respiratory maintenance without the aid of the person's respiratory musculature.

genetic locus The term used to describe a gene's location on a specific chromosome.

genetics The scientific study of heredity and hereditary variation.

genital herpes (herpes simplex genitalis) An infection of the external genitalia caused by herpes simplex genitalis; transmitted by vaginal, anal or oral–genital contact.

genital warts (*condyloma acuminatum*, venereal warts) A sexually transmitted condition caused by the human papillomavirus.

genomics The study of whole sets of genes and their interactions.

genotype The genes and the variations therein that a person inherits from his or her parents.

gigantism Occurs when growth hormone hypersecretion begins before puberty and the closure of the epiphyseal plates, leading the person to become abnormally tall.

gingivitis Inflammation of the gums, characterised by inflammation, redness and bleeding.

glaucoma Condition characterised by increased intraocular pressure of the eye and a gradual loss of vision.

glomerular filtration rate (GFR) The rate at which plasma is filtered through the glomeruli of the kidney.

glomerulonephritis Inflammation of the capillary loops of the glomeruli.

glossitis Inflammation of the tongue.

glucagon Hormone that stimulates the liver to breakdown glycogen into glucose and to synthesise glucose from lactic acid and non-carbohydrate molecules.

gluconeogenesis Formation of glucose from fats and proteins.

glucosuria Excessive glucose in urine.

glycogenolysis Breakdown of liver glycogen to glucose.

goitre An enlarged thyroid gland. Enlargement results from both inadequate and excessive synthesis of thyroid hormones.

gonorrhoea (GC, clap) An infection caused by *Neisseria gonorrhoeae* that is transmitted by direct sexual contact or by delivery of a neonate by an infected mother.

gout A syndrome that occurs from an inflammatory response to the production or excretion of uric acid resulting in high levels of uric acid in the blood (hyperuricaemia) and in other body fluids, including synovial fluid.

Graves' disease Caused by a defect in immunoregulation in genetically predisposed individuals, leading to production of thyroid-stimulating antibodies.

grief The emotional response to loss and its accompanying changes.

grieving The internal process the person uses to work through the response to loss.

Guillain–Barré syndrome (GBS) Acute demyelinating disorder of the peripheral nervous system characterised by progressive, usually rapid muscle weakness and paralysis.

gynaecomastia Breast enlargement in men.

haemangioma See *angioma*.

haematemesis Blood in the vomit.

haematochezia Blood in the stool.

haematopoiesis Blood cell formation.

haematuria Blood in the urine.

haemodialysis A procedure in which electrolytes, waste products and excess water are removed from the body by diffusion and ultrafiltration as blood passes by an artificial semipermeable membrane outside the body.

haemolysis The process of red blood cell destruction.

haemolytic anaemia Premature destruction (lysis) of red blood cells.

haemophilia A group of hereditary clotting factor disorders that lead to persistent and potentially severe bleeding.

haemoptysis Bloody sputum.

haemorrhage Rapid or excessive bleeding.

haemorrhagic stroke (intracranial haemorrhage) Cerebrovascular accident (CVA) occurring when a cerebral blood vessel ruptures.

haemorrhoids (piles) Clusters of dilated veins in swollen anal tissue.

haemostasis Control of bleeding.

haemothorax Blood in the pleural space.

halitosis (bad breath) A common condition caused by an increase in sulfur-producing bacteria in the oral cavity.

hallucination An alteration of sensory perception in the absence of a stimulus.

hallucinogens Drugs that produce hallucinations.

harm reduction A way of reducing the impact of drug- and/or alcohol-related harm to individuals and the community through a range of cost-effective public health policies, strategies and practices.

Hashimoto's thyroiditis An autoimmune disorder caused by the development of antibodies that destroy thyroid tissue.

health As defined by the World Health Organization, 'a state of complete physical, mental and social well-being, and not merely the absence of disease or infirmity'.

Health Care Home (HCH) A general practice that coordinates care for people with chronic and complex conditions.

health determinants Factors that affect the health of people.

health education Individualistic strategies to improve health, often by increasing knowledge or influencing attitudes to alter behaviours and lifestyle. Health education is often used interchangeably with health promotion although they are not the same.

health promotion Any activity undertaken for the purpose of achieving a higher level of health and wellbeing.

healthcare-associated infection (HAI) An infection contracted during residence in a hospital or extended care facility.

heart failure Inability of the heart to pump adequate blood to meet the metabolic demands of the body.

hemianopia The loss of half of the visual field of one or both eyes.

hemiparesis Weakness of the left or right half of the body.

hemiplegia Paralysis of the left or right half of the body.

hepatitis Inflammation of the liver, usually caused by a virus; may be acute or chronic.

hepatorenal syndrome Renal failure accompanied by azotaemia, sodium retention, oliguria and hypotension in people with cirrhosis and ascites.

hernia A defect in the abdominal wall that allows abdominal contents to protrude out of the abdominal cavity.

herpes simplex (fever blister, cold sore) Acute viral infections of the skin and mucous membranes caused by two types of herpes virus: HSV I and HSV II.

herpes zoster (shingles) Viral infection of a dermatome section of the skin caused by varicella zoster, the same herpes virus that causes chickenpox.

heterograft (xenograft) Skin obtained from an animal, usually a pig.

heterozygous Non-identical copies of a particular gene (different alleles) on the paired chromosomes.

hiatal hernia Protrusion of part of the stomach through the oesophageal hiatus of the diaphragm into the mediastinal cavity.

hirsutism Increased growth of coarse hair, usually on the face and trunk.

histocompatibility The ability of cells and tissues to survive transplantation without immunological interference by the recipient.

Hodgkin's disease Develops in a single lymph node or chain of nodes and spreads to adjoining nodes. Involved lymph nodes contain *Reed–Sternberg cells* (malignant cells) surrounded by host inflammatory cells. These malignant cells secrete inflammatory mediator substances, attracting inflammatory cells to the tumour site. They may invade almost any tissue in the body.

holistic healthcare Care in which all aspects of a person (physical, psychosocial, cultural, spiritual and intellectual) are considered as essential components of individualised care.

homeostasis The body's tendency to maintain a state of physiological balance in the presence of constantly changing conditions.

homograft (allograft) Human skin that has been harvested from cadavers.

homologous chromosomes Chromosomes that are members of the same pair and normally have the same number and arrangement of genes; usually one copy is from the mother and the other copy is from the father.

homozygous Identical copies of a particular gene (same alleles) on both paired chromosomes.

hope A belief in a positive outcome related to events and circumstances in one's life; the foundation of recovery from mental illness.

hordeolum (sty) Staphylococcal abscess that may occur on either the external or internal margin of the lid.

hospice care The delivery of care for terminally ill people either in healthcare facilities or in the person's home.

human genome The total amount of the DNA (genes) in an individual's cells.

human immunodeficiency virus (HIV) Virus responsible for AIDS.

Huntington's disease Progressive, degenerative, inherited neurological disease characterised by increasing dementia and chorea.

hydrocephalus An abnormal accumulation of cerebrospinal fluid within the cranial vault and dilation of the ventricles.

hydrocoele Fluid-filled mass within the scrotum.

hydronephrosis Distension of the urinary tract with urine behind an obstruction.

hyperglycaemia Elevated blood glucose levels (above 126 mg/dL), which causes osmotic diuresis and, if chronic, damages vessel epithelium and renal glomeruli.

hyperopia (farsightedness) The condition in which the eyeball is short, causing the image to focus behind the retina.

hyperosmolar hyperglycaemic state (HHS) A condition of very high blood glucose with adequate insulin to prevent ketosis, but which does cause diuresis.

hyperparathyroidism Results from an increase in the secretion of parathyroid hormone, which regulates normal serum levels of calcium and phosphate.

hyperplasia An increase in the number or density of normal cells.

hypersensitivity Exaggerated response of the immune system to an antigen.

hypertension Excess pressure in the arterial portion of systemic circulation.

hyperthyroidism A disorder caused by excessive delivery of thyroid hormone to the peripheral tissues. Also called thyrotoxicosis.

hypertrophic scar Overgrowth of dermal tissue that remains within the boundaries of the wound.

hyphaema Bleeding into the anterior chamber of the eye, possibly as the result of blunt eye trauma.

hypoglycaemia Low blood glucose levels; deficiency of blood sugar.

hypoparathyroidism A condition that results from abnormally low parathyroid hormone levels, causing hypocalcaemia and an elevated blood phosphate level.

hypothyroidism A disorder that results when the thyroid gland produces an insufficient amount of thyroid hormone.

hypovolaemic shock Shock caused by a decrease in intravascular volume of 15% or more. This form of shock is caused by the loss of whole blood, blood plasma or extracellular fluid.

hypoxaemia Decreased oxygen concentration in the blood, measured by PaO_2.

ileostomy An ostomy made in the ileum of the small intestine.

illness–wellness continuum A continuum representing health as a dynamic process, with high-level wellness at one extreme of the continuum and death at the opposite extreme.

illusion A distortion of the senses.

immunity The protection of the body from disease.

immunocompetent Possessing an immune system that can identify antigens and effectively destroy or remove them.

immunoglobulin (Ig) A protein that functions as an antibody.

immunosuppression Inability of the immune system to respond to an antigen. Occurs in response to disease or medications; may be intentional to prevent rejection of transplants or a side effect of some medications.

impetigo Infection of the skin caused by either *Staphylococcus aureus* or beta-haemolytic streptococci.

impotence Inability to achieve or maintain an erection.

impulse control The ability to control behavioural impetuosity.

increased intracranial pressure (IICP, intracranial hypertension) Sustained elevated pressure (10 mmHg or higher) within the cranial cavity.

Indigenous health A broad term which generally refers to the health status and health outcomes of the Aboriginal and Torres Strait Islander population of Australia.

infection Colonisation by and multiplication of an organism within a host. The host can be any organism capable of supporting the nutritional and physical growth requirements of the microorganism—for example, humans.

inflammation A complex, non-specific, adaptive response to injury that brings fluid, dissolved substances and blood cells into the interstitial tissues where the invasion or damage has occurred.

inflammatory bowel disease (IBD) Chronic inflammation of the bowel common to a group of conditions that includes Crohn's disease and ulcerative colitis.

influenza Highly contagious viral respiratory disease characterised by coryza, fever, cough and constitutional manifestations such as headache and malaise.

informed consent Disclosure of risks associated with the intended procedure or operation to the patient. The language of the document varies according to statutory and common law of each state.

innate immunity Specific and non-specific responses that prevent or limit the entry of invaders into the body, thereby limiting the extent of tissue damage and reducing the workload of the adaptive immune system.

insight The degree to which a person has an understanding of their illness or disorder.

instrument nurse The nurse primarily responsible for manual dexterity and in-depth knowledge of the anatomical and mechanical aspects of a particular surgery. The instrument nurse handles sutures, instruments and other equipment immediately adjacent to the sterile field.

insulin A hormone that facilitates entry of glucose into fat and muscle cells for energy.

insulin reaction Hypoglycaemia in people with type 1 diabetes mellitus.

intermediate determinants Determinants of health that concern community infrastructure, personal wealth or access to resources, natural, physical and built environments. This level also includes access to healthcare and health systems.

International Classification of Diseases (ICD) Classification of diseases, functioning and disability.

interprofessional care Care provided by an interprofessional team where two or more professions work together as a team with a common purpose, commitment and mutual respect (Freeth et al. 2005, cited in Dunston et al., 2009, p. 6).

intersectoral Working with more than one sector of society to take action on an area of shared interest, such as health.

intracerebral haematomas A collection of blood in the brain tissue, most often located in the frontal or temporal lobes.

intracranial aneurysm Saccular outpouching of a cerebral artery that occurs at the site of a weakness in the vessel wall.

intraoperative phase The time during surgery, from beginning to end.

iron deficiency anaemia The most common type of anaemia; results from inadequate iron for optimal red blood cell formation.

irritable bowel syndrome (IBS) A motility disorder of the gastrointestinal tract characterised by alternating periods of constipation and diarrhoea.

ischaemia Deficient blood flow to tissue.

ischaemic Deprived of oxygen.

isograft Tissue transplant where the donor and recipient are identical twins.

jaundice Yellow-to-orange colour visible in the skin and mucous membranes; most often the result of a hepatic disorder.

Kaposi's sarcoma (KS) A vascular malignancy (a tumour of the endothelial cells lining small blood vessels) that presents as vascular macules, papules or violet lesions affecting the skin and viscera. It is often the presenting symptom of AIDS.

keloid Elevated, irregularly shaped, progressively enlarging scar arising from excessive amounts of collagen in the stratum corneum during scar formation in connective tissue repair.

keratin A fibrous, water-repellent protein that gives the epidermis its tough, protective quality.

keratitis Inflammation of the cornea.

keratosis Any skin condition in which there is a benign overgrowth and thickening of the cornified epithelium.

ketamine A central nervous system depressant, best described as a dissociative anaesthetic agent.

ketonuria The presence of ketones in the urine.

ketosis An accumulation of ketone bodies produced during the oxidation of fatty acids.

kidney replacement therapy Therapy provided through haemodialysis, peritoneal dialysis or kidney transplantation.

kinaesthaesia The ability to perceive movement and sense of position.

Klinefelter's syndrome A syndrome in which males have an extra X chromosome in most of their cells (also known as the XXY condition).

knowledge resource base Ways in which knowledge is developed.

Korotkoff's sounds Sounds heard during auscultation of blood pressure.

kyphosis Exaggerated thoracic curvature of the spine common in older adults.

labyrinthitis Inflammation of the inner ear.

laceration Open wound that results from sharp cutting or tearing. Injuries to the integument are at risk of contamination from dirt, debris or foreign objects.

laminectomy Removal of the lamina of the vertebrae.

laparoscopic cholecystectomy Removal of the gallbladder using an endoscope.

laryngectomy Removal of the larynx.

laryngitis Inflammation of the larynx.

leiomyomas Solid, pedunculated benign tumours.

leucocytes Also called white blood cells, these are the primary cells involved in both non-specific and specific immune system responses. These cells isolate the infecting organism or injury, destroy pathogens and promote healing.

leucocytosis An increase in the number of leucocytes in the blood (above $10{,}000/mm^3$), usually caused by infection.

leucopenia Abnormal decrease of circulating leucocytes, usually below $5{,}000/mm^3$; occurs when bone marrow activity is suppressed, or when leucocyte destruction increases.

leucoplakia Formation of white patches or spots on the mucous membranes or tongue; these lesions may become malignant.

leukaemia ('white blood') A group of chronic malignant disorders of white blood cells (WBCs) and WBC precursors; characterised by replacement of bone marrow by malignant immature WBCs, abnormal immature circulating WBCs and infiltration of malignant cells into other tissues.

libido Instinctive drive associated with sexual desire.

life-limiting illness An illness where it is expected that death will be a direct consequence of the specified illness.

lipoatrophy Atrophy of subcutaneous tissue.

lipodystrophy Hypertrophy of subcutaneous tissue that may result if the same injection sites are used repeatedly, especially with porcine and bovine insulins.

lithiasis Stone formation.

lithotripsy Crushing of renal calculi.

liver transplantation Surgery to remove a diseased liver and transplant a healthy liver (whole or segment) from another person.

locked-in syndrome Person is alert and fully aware of the environment, but is unable to communicate through speech or movement as a result of blocked efferent pathways to the brain.

lordosis Increased lumbar curve.

loss An actual or potential situation in which a valued object, person, relationship, body part or emotion that was formerly present is lost or changed and can no longer be seen, felt, heard, known or experienced.

lung abscess Localised area of lung destruction or necrosis and pus formation.

lung compliance Distensibility of the lungs.

lymphadenopathy The enlargement of lymph nodes (over 1 cm) with or without tenderness. It may be caused by inflammation, infection or malignancy of the nodes or the regions drained by the nodes.

lymphocytes Account for 20–40% of circulating leucocytes. Lymphocytes are the principal effector and regulator cells of specific immune responses.

lymphoedema Extremity oedema due to accumulated lymph; may be primary or secondary, resulting from inflammation, obstruction or removal of lymphatic vessels.

lymphomas Malignancy of lymphoid tissue.

macrophages Monocytes mature into macrophages after settling into tissue. Macrophages are large phagocytes. They are important in the body's defence against chronic infections.

macular degeneration Destructive changes in the macula due to injury or gradual failure of the outer pigmented layer of the retina (the retinal layer adjacent to the choroid), which removes cellular waste products and keeps the retina attached to the choroid.

major trauma Serious single-system injury (such as the traumatic amputation of a leg) or multiple-system injuries. Also known as multiple trauma.

malabsorption A condition in which nutrients are ineffectively absorbed by the intestinal mucosa, resulting in their excretion in the stool.

malignant melanoma Skin cancer that arises from melanocytes.

malnutrition Inadequate nutrient intake to meet body needs; may include deficiency of major nutrients (kilojoules, carbohydrates, proteins and fats) or micronutrients such as vitamins and minerals.

man-made disasters Either accidental or intentional, they are complex emergencies, technological disasters, material shortages and other disasters not caused by natural hazards.

mass casualty incident (MCI) An event that generates more patients at one time than locally available resources can manage using routine procedures.

mastoiditis Bacterial infection of the mastoid process.

mean arterial pressure (MAP) The average pressure in the arterial circulation throughout the cardiac cycle; the product of cardiac output and systemic vascular resistance (SVR).

medical–surgical nursing The health promotion, healthcare and illness care of adults, based on knowledge derived from the arts and sciences and shaped by knowledge (the science) of nursing.

meiosis A modified type of cell division in sexually reproducing organisms consisting of two rounds of cell division but only one round of DNA replication. It results in cells with half the number of chromosome sets as the original cell.

melaena Black, tarry stool that contains blood.

melanin Skin pigment that forms a protective shield to protect keratinocytes and nerve endings in the dermis from the damaging effects of ultraviolet light.

memory The ability to store, retain and recall information.

Ménière's disease Chronic disorder of unknown cause characterised by recurrent attacks of vertigo with tinnitus and a progressive unilateral hearing loss.

meningitis Inflammation of the meninges of the brain and spinal cord.

menopause Permanent cessation of menses.

menorrhagia Excessive or prolonged menstruation.

menstrual cycle Cyclic build up of the uterine lining, ovulation and sloughing of the lining occurring approximately every 28 days in non-pregnant females.

menstruation Periodic shedding of the uterine lining in a woman of childbearing age who is not pregnant.

Mental Health Act Mental health legislation.

Mental Health Nurse Practitioner (MHNP) A specialist mental health nurse with qualifications at master's degree level.

mental state examination (MSE) A clinical assessment that describes the sum total of the examiner's observations at the time of the interview or interaction.

metabolic syndrome A cluster of manifestations often associated with type 2 diabetes. Includes insulin resistance, hypertension, low high-density lipoprotein cholesterol and high triglycerides.

metabolism The breakdown of complex structures into simpler forms to produce energy (catabolism) and the combination of simpler molecules to produce and maintain more complex structures necessary to living organisms (anabolism).

metaplasia A change in the normal pattern of differentiation such that dividing cells differentiate into cell types not normally found in that location in the body.

metastasis Secondary tumour; the process by which spreading of malignant neoplasms occurs; the transfer of disease from one organ or part to another not directly connected with it.

metrorrhagia Bleeding between menstrual periods; may be caused by hormonal imbalances, pelvic inflammatory disease, cervical or uterine polyps, uterine fibroids or cervical or uterine cancer.

microalbuminuria Protein in the urine.

micturition Releasing urine from the urinary bladder (voiding).

minor trauma Injury to a single part or system of the body, usually treated in the hospital or emergency department.

mitigation The action taken to prevent or reduce the harmful effects of a disaster on human health or property; it involves future-oriented activities to prevent subsequent disasters or to minimise their effects.

mitochondria Provide the energy a cell needs to move, divide, produce secretory products and contract.

mitosis A process of nuclear division in eukaryotic cells conventionally divided into five stages: prophase, prometaphase, metaphase, anaphase and telophase. Mitosis conserves chromosome numbers by allocating replicated chromosomes equally to each of the daughter nuclei.

mitral valve (bicuspid valve) Valve between the left atrium and ventricle in the heart; prevents blood from flowing backwards into the atrium.

monosomy (monosomic) When one member of the chromosome pair is missing—for example, in Turner syndrome (45, XO).

mood The way in which a person describes their feelings at a particular time.

morbid obesity Weight greater than 100% over ideal body weight.

motor neurone disease (MND) Progressive, degenerative neurological disease characterised by weakness and wasting of the involved muscles, without any accompanying sensory or cognitive changes; also called *Lou Gehrig's disease*.

mourning The actions or expressions of the bereaved, including the symbols, clothing and ceremonies that make up the outward manifestations of grief.

multifactorial Health conditions determined by multiple factors, including genetic and environmental factors, each having an additive effect.

multiple myeloma A malignancy in which plasma cells multiply uncontrollably and infiltrate the bone marrow, lymph nodes, spleen and other tissues.

multiple sclerosis (MS) A chronic demyelinating neurological disease of the CNS (brain, optic nerves and spinal cord), associated with an abnormal immune response to an environmental factor.

multiple trauma Most often the result of a motor vehicle crash, this type of trauma requires immediate intervention specifically focused on ensuring survival.

murmurs Sounds made by turbulent blood flow through the heart.

muscular dystrophy (MD) A group of inherited muscle diseases that cause progressive muscle degeneration and wasting.

myasthenia gravis Chronic, progressive neuromuscular disorder characterised by fatigue and severe weakness of skeletal muscles.

myocarditis Inflammatory disorder of the heart muscle.

myopia (nearsightedness) A condition in which the eyeball is elongated, causing the image to focus in front of the retina instead of on it.

myringotomy Incision of the tympanic membrane.

myxoedema An alternative term for severe or advanced hypothyroidism.

myxoedema coma A life-threatening complication of longstanding, untreated hypothyroidism usually triggered by an acute illness or trauma.

naevi (moles) Flat or raised macules or papules with rounded, well-defined borders.

natural disasters Disasters caused by acts of nature or emerging diseases. Some are unexpected, and some are predictable through advanced meteorological technologies.

natural killer cells (NK cells) Large, granular lymphocytes (found in the spleen, lymph nodes, bone marrow and blood) that provide immune surveillance and resistance to infection, and play an important role in the destruction of early malignant cells.

nausea An unpleasant sensation usually followed by vomiting.

neglect syndrome (unilateral neglect) A disorder of attention. In this syndrome, the person cannot integrate and use perceptions from the affected side of the body or from the environment on the affected side and, hence, ignores that part.

neoplasm A mass of new tissue (a collection of cells) that grows independently of its surrounding structures and has no physiological purpose.

nephrectomy Removal of the kidney.

nephrotic syndrome A condition marked by massive proteinuria, hypoalbuminaemia, hyperlipidaemia and oedema.

neurogenic bladder Dysfunctional urinary bladder due to lesion of central or peripheral nervous system.

neurogenic shock Shock resulting from an imbalance between parasympathetic and sympathetic stimulation of vascular smooth muscle. If parasympathetic overstimulation or sympathetic understimulation persists, sustained vasodilation occurs and blood pools in the venous and capillary beds.

neuropathic pain Pain caused by a lesion or dysfunction in the nervous system from the primary afferent conducting mechanism to the central nervous system.

nicotine An alkaloid found in the nightshade family of plants (*Solanaceae*) which constitutes approximately 0.6–3.0% of the dry weight of tobacco, with biosynthesis taking place in the roots and accumulating in the leaves.

nociception The physiological processes related to pain perception.

nociceptors Sensory nerve fibres that conduct pain impulses from the periphery to the central nervous system.

nocturia Voiding two or more times at night.

nondisjunction An error in meiosis or mitosis in which members of a pair of homologous chromosomes or a pair of sister chromatids fail to separate properly from each other.

non-Hodgkin's lymphoma (NHL) Lymphoid tissue malignancies that do not contain Reed–Sternberg cells.

non-union A state that exists when the ends of a fracture fail to heal together.

normal sinus rhythm (NSR) Normal heart rhythm, in which impulses originate in the sinus node and travel through normal conduction pathways without delay.

nursing process The series of critical-thinking activities nurses use as they provide care to patients; this logical approach to care ensures that patients receive comprehensive and effective care.

nutrients Substances found in food that are used by the body to promote growth, maintenance and repair.

nutrition The process by which the body ingests, absorbs, transports, uses and eliminates food.

nystagmus Rapid involuntary eye movements.

obesity An excess of body fat (adipose tissue).

obstructive shock Shock caused by an obstruction in the heart or great vessels that either impedes venous return or prevents effective cardiac pumping action.

occult bleeding Hidden bleeding.

oedema Accumulation of fluid in the body's tissues; an excess accumulation of fluid in the interstitial space.

oesophageal varices Enlarged, thin-walled veins that form in the submucosa of the oesophagus.

oesophagojejunostomy Removal of the entire stomach with anastomosis of the distal oesophagus to the jejunum.

oestrogen Hormone produced by the ovary.

oliguria Urine output of less than 400 mL in 24 hours.

oncogene Gene capable of triggering cancerous characteristics.

oncology The study of cancer.

opioid A chemical that works by binding to opioid receptors, which are found principally in the central nervous system and the gastrointestinal tract.

oral mucositis Inflammation and ulceration of the oral mucosa.

orchitis Infection or inflammation of the testicle.

orthopnoea Difficulty breathing when supine.

orthostatic hypotension A decrease in systolic blood pressure of more than 10 to 15 mmHg and a drop in diastolic blood pressure on standing.

osmosis The process by which water moves across a selectively permeable membrane from an area of lower solute concentration to an area of higher solute concentration.

ossification The process of bone formation.

osteoarthritis (OA) (degenerative joint disease) The most commonly occurring of all forms of arthritis. This disease is characterised by loss of articular cartilage in articulating joints and hypertrophy of the bones at the articular margins.

osteomalacia (adult rickets) Metabolic bone disorder characterised by inadequate mineralisation of bone matrix.

osteomyelitis Infection within the bone that can lead to tissue death and necrosis.

osteoporosis Literally defined as 'porous bones', a metabolic bone disorder characterised by loss of bone mass, increased bone fragility and an increased risk of fractures.

ostomy General term for an operation in which an artificial opening is created.

otitis externa Inflammation of the ear canal, commonly known as *swimmer's ear*.

otitis media Inflammation or infection of the middle ear.

otosclerosis Abnormal bone formation in the osseous labyrinth of the temporal bone causing the footplate of the stapes to become fixed or immobile in the oval window. The result is a conductive hearing loss.

ovarian cycle The female cycle that occurs from puberty until menopause in which the production of ova occur.

oxyhaemoglobin The combined form of haemoglobin and oxygen; found in arterial blood, it carries oxygen to body tissues.

pacemaker A pulse generator used to provide an electrical stimulus to the heart when the heart fails to generate or conduct on its own a rate that maintains the cardiac output.

$PaCO_2$ Partial pressure of carbon dioxide in arterial blood.

Paget's disease A skeletal disorder that results from excessive osteoclastic activity. Paget's disease is characterised by bone deformity, especially of the long bones of the lower limbs, the pelvis, the lumbar vertebrae and the skull.

pain tolerance The amount of pain a person can endure before responding to it.

palliative care An area of care that has evolved out of the hospice experience, but exists outside of hospice programs and is not restricted to the end of life. Palliative care is focused on the relief of physical, mental and spiritual distress for individuals who have an incurable illness and is used earlier in the disease experience than hospice care. The goal of palliative care is to prevent and relieve suffering by early assessment and treatment of pain and other physical, psychosocial and spiritual needs to improve the person's quality of life.

pallor Lack of colour; paleness of skin.

pancreatitis Inflammation of the pancreas.

pandemic The worldwide spread of a disease.

PaO_2 Partial pressure of oxygen in arterial blood.

paracentesis Aspiration of fluid from the peritoneal cavity.

paralytic ileus Impaired propulsion or forward movement of bowel contents.

paraplegia Paralysis of the lower portion of the body, sometimes involving the lower trunk.

parenchyma The key elements of an organ essential to its functioning, as distinct from the capsule that encompasses it and other supporting structures.

parenteral nutrition (PN) Intravenous administration of carbohydrates (high concentrations of dextrose), protein (amino acids), electrolytes, vitamins, minerals and fat emulsions.

Parkinson's disease (PD) Progressive, degenerative neurological disease characterised by non-intention tremor, bradykinesia and muscle rigidity.

paroxysmal nocturnal dyspnoea (PND) Attacks of acute shortness of breath that occur at night, waking up the person.

partial gastrectomy Removal of a portion of the stomach, usually the distal half to two-thirds.

partial-thickness burn Burn that involves the entire dermis and the papillae of the dermis (superficial partial-thickness burn) or extends into the hair follicles (deep partial-thickness burn).

passive immunity Temporary protection—provided by antibodies produced by other people or animals—against disease-producing antigens. Protection is gradually lost when these acquired antibodies are used up either by natural degradation or by combining with the antigen.

pathogens Virulent organisms rarely found in the absence of disease.

pediculosis An infestation with lice, parasites that live on the blood of an animal or human host.

pelvic inflammatory disease (PID) A term used to describe infection of the pelvic organs.

penetrance The percentage or likelihood that an individual who has inherited a gene mutation will actually express the disease signs and symptoms in his or her lifetime.

penetrating trauma Occurs when a foreign object enters the body, causing damage to body structures.

peptic ulcer An ulcer that occurs in any area of the gastrointestinal tract exposed to acid-pepsin secretions, including the oesophagus, stomach or duodenum.

peptic ulcer disease (PUD) A break in the mucous lining of the gastrointestinal tract where it comes in contact with gastric juice.

perforation Penetration of ulcer through mucosal wall.

pericarditis Inflammation of the pericardium.

perioperative nursing A highly skill, specialised area of nursing practice incorporating a number of sub-specialties.

peripheral obesity Obesity characterised by a waist-to-hip ratio of less than 0.8, more commonly seen in women.

peripheral vascular disease (PVD) Impaired blood supply to peripheral tissues, particularly the lower extremities.

peristalsis Alternating waves of contraction and relaxation of involuntary muscle.

peritoneal dialysis Procedure in which electrolytes, waste products and excess water are removed from the body by diffusion using the peritoneum surrounding the abdominal cavity as the dialysing membrane.

peritonitis Inflammation of the peritoneum.

pernicious anaemia Anaemia resulting from failure to absorb dietary vitamin B_{12} due to lack of intrinsic factor.

persistent (chronic) pain Ongoing and prolonged pain, not always associated with an identifiable cause but often arising from an acute cause.

persistent vegetative state (PVS) Condition of complete unawareness of self and the environment.

personal responsibility Admitting responsibility for choices made.

person-centred care A holistic approach to the planning, delivery and evaluation of healthcare that is grounded in mutually beneficial partnerships between healthcare professionals, patients and families. Person-centred care is underpinned by the principles of trust, empathy, dignity, autonomy, respect, choice, transparency and desire to help individuals lead the life they want.

pertussis (whooping cough) A highly contagious acute upper respiratory infection cause by the bacterium *Bordetella pertussis*.

phagocytosis A process by which a foreign agent or target cell is engulfed, destroyed and digested. Neutrophils and macrophages, known as phagocytes, are the primary cells involved in phagocytosis.

phantom limb syndrome (phantom pain) A confusing pain syndrome that occurs following surgical or traumatic amputation of a limb. The person experiences pain in the missing body part even though there is complete mental awareness that the limb is gone.

pharmacogenetics The study of how genetic factors influence drug action.

pharyngitis Acute inflammation of the pharynx.

phenotype The expression of a person's entire physical, biochemical and physiological make-up, as determined by the individual's genotype and environmental factors.

pheochromocytoma Tumours of chromaffi in tissues in the adrenal medulla. These tumours, which are usually benign, produce catecholamines (adrenaline or noradrenaline, also known as epinephrine and norepinephrine) that stimulate the sympathetic nervous system.

phimosis Constriction of the foreskin so that it cannot be retracted over the glans penis.

photophobia Sensitivity to light.

plasmapheresis (plasma exchange) Removal of the plasma component from whole blood.

pleural effusion Collection of excess fluid in the pleural space.

pleuritis Inflammation of the pleura.

pneumonia Inflammation of the lung parenchyma (the respiratory bronchioles and alveoli).

pneumothorax Results when air enters the pleural space due to blunt and penetrating injuries to the chest.

polycystic kidney disease (PKD) A hereditary disease characterised by cyst formation and massive kidney enlargement.

polycythaemia (erythrocytosis) Excess red blood cells characterised by a haematocrit higher than 55%.

polydipsia Excessive thirst.

polymorphisms DNA sequences that have many forms but give the genetic 'directions' for the same thing.

polymyositis A systemic connective tissue disorder characterised by inflammation of connective tissue and muscle fibres leading to muscle weakness and atrophy.

polyphagia Excessive eating.

polyuria A condition where increased blood volume increases renal blood flow and the hyperglycaemia acts as an osmotic diuretic, thereby increasing urine output.

portal hypertension Elevated pressure in the portal venous system that causes rerouting of blood to adjoining lower pressure vessels.

portal systemic encephalopathy Impaired consciousness and mental status due to the accumulation of toxic waste products in the blood (ammonia in particular) as blood bypasses the congested liver.

positioning Exposes the operative site in conjunction with access for anaesthesia administration. Proper positioning is imperative to prevent injury to the person.

postoperative phase Period when a procedure or surgery has been completed and the person is recovering from the stress associated with the surgery.

postpoliomyelitis syndrome A complication of a previous infection by the poliomyelitis virus.

preload The amount of cardiac muscle fibre tension or stretch that exists at diastole, just before ventricular contraction.

premenstrual syndrome (PMS) Complex of symptoms characterised by irritability, depression, oedema and breast tenderness preceding the monthly menses.

preparedness Having a comprehensive disaster plan in place that coordinates efforts among many people, agencies and levels of government.

preoperative phase Time when preparation of the person for surgery is conducted and completed.

presbycusis Age-related loss of the ability to hear high-frequency sounds; may occur because of cochlear hair cell degeneration or loss of auditory neurons in the organ of Corti.

presbyopia Impaired near vision resulting from a loss of elasticity of the lens related to ageing.

prescription medication misuse Non-medical use of pharmaceuticals or use for genuine medical purposes but without a valid prescription, or when prescribed in excessive quantities or frequencies, or when an iatrogenic dependence has developed.

pressure injury Ischaemic lesion of the skin and underlying tissue caused by external pressure that impairs the flow of blood and lymph.

pretibial myxoedema Also known as thyroid dermopathy, pretibial myxoedema refers to lesions of the skin resulting from the accumulation of hyaluronic acid, as a result of thyroid disease.

priapism Sustained, painful erection that lasts at least 4 hours and is not associated with sexual arousal.

primary care A clinical perspective that provides first contact services for individuals and families.

primary healthcare (PHC) Involves communities, public policy and social and environmental determinants of health.

primary hypertension (idiopathic, essential) A persistently elevated systemic blood pressure.

primary survey An initial assessment of a person to determine if there is serious compromise to airway, breathing or circulation.

procedural pain A type of breakthrough pain that is predictable because it is associated with movement such as turning or coughing.

progesterone Hormone produced by the ovary; works with oestrogen to control the menstrual cycle.

proptosis Forward bulging of one or both eyes.

prostatitis Inflammation of the prostate gland.

protein energy malnutrition (PEM) The state of decreased body pools of protein with or without fat depletion or a state of diminished functional capacity, caused at least partly by inadequate nutrient intake relative to nutrient demand, and/or which is improved by nutritional repletion.

proteinuria Abnormal proteins in the urine.

proximal determinants Determinants that have a more direct impact on health, and include lifestyle and behavioural factors as well as underlying health conditions.

pruritus Subjective itching sensation producing an urge to scratch.

psoriasis Chronic, non-infectious skin disorder that is characterised by raised, reddened, round circumscribed plaques covered by silvery white scales.

psychosis A mental health condition in which there is a loss of contact with reality.

psychostimulants A diverse group of natural and synthetic drugs with a wide range of psychological and physical effects, including euphoria, increased energy and irregular heartbeat.

ptosis Drooping of the eyelid.

pulmonary embolism Sudden occlusion of a pulmonary artery resulting in disruption of blood supply to the lung parenchyma.

pulmonary hypertension Condition in which the pulmonary arterial pressure is elevated to an abnormal level.

pulmonary oedema An abnormal accumulation of fluid in the interstitial tissue and alveoli of the lung.

pulmonic valve One of the semilunar valves, separating the ventricles from the great vessels.

pulse Rhythmic pressure waveform that can be felt over an artery.

pulse pressure The difference between the systolic and diastolic blood pressure.

puncture wound Wound that occurs when a sharp or blunt object penetrates the integument.

pupillary light reflex Reflex in which the pupil contracts in response to a bright light.

pyelonephritis Upper urinary tract inflammation affecting the kidney and renal pelvis.

pyuria (bacteriuria) Pus in the urine.

quadriplegia Injury to cervical segments of the cord thus impairing function of the arms, trunk, legs and pelvic organs.

rabies Viral (rhabdovirus) infection of the central nervous system transmitted by infected saliva that enters the human body through a bite or an open wound.

radiation therapy Therapy that uses radiation to kill a tumour, to reduce its size, to decrease pain or to relieve obstruction.

rapid cycling Having four or more mood episodes within a 12-month period.

Raynaud's disease Disorder characterised by episodes of intense vasospasm in the small arteries and arterioles of the fingers and possibly the toes; has no identifiable cause.

Raynaud's phenomenon Disorder characterised by episodes of intense vasospasm in the small arteries and arterioles of the fingers and possibly the toes; occurs secondarily to another disease.

reactive arthritis (Reiter's syndrome) An acute, non-purulent inflammatory arthritis that complicates a bacterial infection of the genitourinary or gastrointestinal tracts.

recovery The final phase of an emergency; the period when the emergency is under control and the community starts to rebuild.

Recovery A recognised and accepted paradigm, related to a personal journey, that has significant implications for people who have mental health problems, their carers, mental health professionals and mental health services.

referral Timely consultation and handing over of clinical care of people to the appropriate personnel and facility for ongoing management.

reflux, urinary Backflow of urine towards the kidneys.

refraction The bending of light rays as they pass from one medium to another medium of different optical density.

regional anaesthesia Anaesthesia that desensitises a particular area but does not involve the full central nervous system or cause sedation.

regional and remote health workforce A statistical representation of nurses working in identified regional and remote areas which includes the number of currently employed nurses, acknowledging their age, experience and qualifications.

regurgitation (valvular) Backflow of blood through an incompletely closed valve into the area it just left.

renal artery stenosis Narrowing of the renal artery.

renal colic Acute, severe, intermittent pain in the flank and upper outer abdominal quadrant generally associated with acute obstruction of a ureter and resulting ureteral spasm.

renal insufficiency Any condition in which the kidneys are unable to remove accumulated metabolites from the blood, leading to altered fluid, electrolyte and acid-base balance.

respiratory failure Inability of lungs to oxygenate the blood and remove carbon dioxide adequately to meet the body's needs, even at rest.

response Occurs in the emergency stage and after a disaster event has occurred.

retinal detachment Separation of the retina or sensory portion of the eye from the choroid.

retrieval Specialised transfer of people with needs exceeding the capacity of their current location to a clinical facility providing a higher level of specialised healthcare.

retrograde ejaculation Seminal fluid discharged into the bladder.

rheumatic disorders Refers to diseases of the muscles and bones as well as the joints.

rheumatic fever A systemic inflammatory disease caused by an abnormal immune response to pharyngeal infection by group A beta-haemolytic streptococci. The condition is characterised by acute inflammation, joint pain, fever and cardiac valve scarring.

rheumatic heart disease (RHD) Slowly progressive valvular deformity following acute or repeated attacks of rheumatic fever; characterised by rigid and deformed valve leaflets; fused valve commissures and fibrosis of chordae tendineae.

rheumatoid arthritis A chronic systemic autoimmune disease that causes inflammation of connective tissue, primarily in the joints.

rhinitis Inflammation of the nasal cavities.

rhinoplasty Surgical reconstruction of the nose.

risk factors Defined as individual or environmental variables that are related to the increased likelihood that a negative outcome will occur.

sarcoidosis Systemic disease characterised by granulomas in the lungs, lymph nodes, liver, eyes, skin and other organs.

scabies Parasitic infestation caused by the mite *Sarcoptes scabiei*.

schizophrenia A mental disorder characterised by abnormalities in the perception or expression of reality.

sciatica Pain over the sciatic nerve.

scleroderma Hardening of the skin; a chronic condition characterised by the formation of excess fibrous connective tissue and diffuse fibrosis of the skin and internal organs.

scoliosis A lateral curvature of the spine.

scope of practice The roles, functions, responsibilities, activities and decision-making capacity that nurses are educated, competent and authorised to perform.

sebum An oily substance secreted from sebaceous glands; softens and lubricates the skin and hair, and decreases water loss from the skin in low humidity. Sebum also protects the body from infection by killing bacteria.

secondary hypertension Elevated blood pressure resulting from an identifiable underlying process.

secondary survey A head-to-toe assessment of a person that includes all body systems.

seizure An episode of excessive and abnormal discharge of electrical activity within the central nervous system.

semen Contains sperm and fluids secreted by the male reproductive system glands.

septic arthritis Develops when a joint space is invaded by a pathogen.

septic shock One part of a progressive syndrome called systemic inflammatory response syndrome. Beginning with an infection, septic shock progresses to bacteraemia, then sepsis, then septic shock and finally multiple organ failure syndrome.

septicaemia Systemic disease associated with the presence of bacteria or their toxins in the blood.

seroconversion Antibody response to a disease or vaccine.

serum bicarbonate (HCO_3^-) Reflects the renal regulation of acid–base balance. It is often called the metabolic component of arterial blood gases.

severe acute respiratory syndrome (SARS) Lower respiratory illness of unknown aetiology; spread by close person-to-person contact.

sex chromosome A chromosome responsible for determining the sex of an individual.

sexually transmitted infection (STI, sexually transmitted disease, venereal disease) Any infection transmitted by sexual contact, including vaginal, oral and anal intercourse.

shingles See *herpes zoster*.

shock A clinical syndrome characterised by a systemic imbalance between oxygen supply and demand. This imbalance results in a state of inadequate blood flow to the peripheral tissues, causing life-threatening cellular dysfunction, hypotension and oliguria.

sickle cell anaemia A hereditary, chronic haemolytic anaemia characterised by episodes of sickling, during which red blood cells become abnormally crescent shaped.

sinusitis Inflammation of the mucous membranes of one or more of the sinuses.

Sjögren's syndrome An autoimmune disorder that causes inflammation and dysfunction of exocrine glands throughout the body.

skin tear A traumatic wound occurring principally on the extremities of older adults, as a result of friction alone or shearing and friction forces that separate the epidermis from the dermis (partial-thickness wound), or which separate both the epidermis and the dermis from underlying structures (full-thickness wound).

sleep apnoea Absence of airflow through the upper airways for 10 or more seconds.

social determinants of health The social factors that influence the health status and health outcomes of individuals and communities.

social model of health A model of health which views health as multifaceted, focusing on social rather than biological determinants of health. This model emphasises health equity and prevention of illness or injury, as well as collaboration and empowerment. The social model of health is also referred to as new public health or the social ecological model.

solvents Produce a depressant effect on the central nervous system and comprise a range of products producing vapours which, when inhaled through the nose or mouth, may cause an intoxicated feeling and lead to an altered state of consciousness.

somatic cell Any cell in the body that is not a sex cell (ova and sperm).

Somogyi phenomenon A morning rise in blood glucose to hyperglycaemic levels following an episode of nocturnal hypoglycaemia and a counter-regulatory hormone response.

spasticity Increased muscle tone in disease of the corticospinal motor tract.

spermatocoele A mobile, usually painless mass containing dead spermatozoa that forms in the epididymis.

spinal cord injury (SCI) Injury to spinal cord, usually due to trauma and classified according to systems.

spinal shock Temporary loss of reflex function below the level of injury.

sprain Tearing or stretching of a ligament that results from a twisting motion.

sprue A chronic primary disorder of the small intestine in which the absorption of nutrients, particularly fats, is impaired.

squamous cell carcinoma Malignant tumour of the squamous epithelium of the skin or mucous membranes.

starvation Inadequate dietary intake; the condition of being without food for long periods of time.

status asthmaticus Severe, prolonged asthma that does not respond to routine treatment. Without aggressive therapy, status asthmaticus can lead to respiratory failure with hypoxaemia, hypercapnia and acidosis.

steatorrhoea Greasy, frothy, yellow stools resulting from excess fat in the faeces.

stem cells (haemocytoblasts) Bone marrow precursor cells for all blood cells.

stem cell transplant (SCT) Infusion of donor stem cells to replace the recipient's blood cell lines (white blood cells, red blood cells and platelets).

stenosis Condition where valve leaflets fuse together and are unable to open or close fully.

steroids Often used illegally to build muscles and enhance exercise performance; also known as performance- and image-enhancing drugs (PIEDs).

stigma Severe social disapproval.

stoma Surface opening.

Strain Stretching injury to a muscle or a muscle–tendon unit caused by mechanical overloading.

stress-induced (erosive) gastritis See *erosive gastritis*.

striae A line above or below tissue that differs in colour and texture from surrounding tissue.

stridor High-pitched, harsh inspiratory sound indicative of upper airway obstruction.

stroke (brain attack, cerebrovascular accident, CVA) A condition in which neurological deficits occur as a result of decreased blood flow to a focal (localised) area of brain tissue.

stroke volume (SV) The amount of blood pumped into the aorta with each contraction of the left ventricle.

subacute thyroiditis Inflammation of the thyroid gland.

subdural haematoma A localised mass of blood that collects between the dura mater and the arachnoid mater.

subluxation Partial separation (or dislocation) of the bones of a joint.

substance dependence A severe condition occurring when the use of a chemical substance is no longer under an individual's control for at least 3 months. Continued use of the substance usually persists despite adverse effects on the person's physical condition, psychological health and interpersonal relationships (used interchangeably with 'addiction').

substance-induced disorder A reversible substance-specific syndrome related to the type of drug used.

substance-related disorder Maladaptive patterns of substance use leading to clinically significant impairment or distress.

substance use The use of any chemical in a fashion inconsistent with medical or culturally defined social norms despite physical, psychological or socially adverse effects.

substance use disorder A medical condition in which the use of one or more substances leads to a clinically significant impairment characterised by a range of mental, physical and behavioural symptoms that often cause problems related to one's personal life, relationships and work, as well as increasingly hazardous use, tolerance and withdrawal.

sudden cardiac death (SCD) Unexpected death occurring within 1 hour of the onset of cardiovascular symptoms.

sundowning A behavioural change in Alzheimer's disease characterised by increased agitation, time disorientation and wandering during afternoon and evening hours.

superficial burn Burn involving only the epidermal layer of the skin; most often results from damage from sunburn, ultraviolet light, minor flash injury (from a sudden ignition or explosion) or mild radiation burn associated with cancer treatment.

surfactant A lipoprotein produced by the alveolar cells; interferes with adhesion of water molecules, reducing surface tension and helping to expand lungs.

surgery An invasive medical procedure performed to diagnose or treat illness, injury or deformity. Although surgery is a medical treatment, the nurse assumes an active role in caring for the person before, during and after surgery.

surgical debridement The process of excising a wound to the level of fascia (fascial excision) or sequentially removing thin slices of a burn wound to the level of viable tissue (sequential excision).

syndrome of inappropriate ADH secretion (SIADH) Characterised by high levels of antidiuretic hormone (ADH) in the absence of serum hypo-osmolality, and most often caused by the ectopic production of ADH by malignant tumours.

synovitis Inflammation of the synovial membrane lining the articular capsule of a joint.

syphilis A sexually transmitted infection caused by a spirochaete that may invade almost any body tissue or organ. It enters the body through a break in the skin or mucous membranes and can be transferred to the fetus through the placental circulation.

systemic lupus erythematosus (SLE) A chronic inflammatory immune complex connective tissue disease.

systolic blood pressure This arterial pressure wave produced by ventricular contraction (systole) averages 120 mmHg in healthy adults.

T lymphocytes (T cells) Type of lymphocyte that matures in the thymus gland.

tachypnoea Abnormally rapid respiratory rate.

telehealth A broad term that refers to the use of technology to contribute to the provision of healthcare, usually at a distance.

tendonitis Inflammation of a tendon.

tension pneumothorax A condition in which an injury to the chest allows air to enter but not escape the pleural cavity.

terrorism An action, or threat of action, that causes harm or interference, and is made with the intention of advancing a political, religious or ideological cause.

test sensitivity How specifically a test identifies (positive test result) individuals who are affected and/or who have a disease phenotype.

test specificity How specifically a test does not identify (negative test result) individuals who are unaffected or do not have a disease phenotype.

testicular torsion Twisting of the testes and spermatic cord.

testosterone Male hormone produced in the testes.

tetanus Disorder of the nervous system caused by a neurotoxin elaborated by *Clostridium tetani.*

tetany Tonic muscular spasms.

thalassaemia An inherited disorder of haemoglobin synthesis in which either the alpha or beta chains of the haemoglobin molecule are missing or defective.

therapeutic relationship A relationship that aims to empower the person with the knowledge and ability to recover from their illness.

third spacing The accumulation and sequestration of trapped extracellular fluid in an actual or potential body space as a result of disease or injury.

thoracentesis Invasive procedure in which fluid (or occasionally air) is removed from the pleural space with a needle.

thought content The actual content of what a person is thinking.

thrill Palpable vibration over the precordium or an artery.

thromboangiitis obliterans (Buerger's disease) An occlusive vascular disease involving inflammation, spasm and clot formation in small and medium-sized peripheral arteries.

thrombocytopenia A platelet count of less than 100,000 per millilitre of blood.

thromboembolus A thrombus that breaks loose from the arterial wall.

thrombus A blood clot that adheres to a vessel wall.

thyroid crisis An extreme state of hyperthyroidism that is rare today because of improved diagnosis and treatment methods. Also called thyroid storm.

thyroid gland A gland situated at the front of the throat which secretes thyroid hormones (thyroxine (T_4) and triiodothyronine (T_3)) to regulate the body's metabolic process.

thyroid storm *See thyroid crisis.*

thyroidectomy A procedure performed to treat cancer of the thyroid.

thyrotoxicosis See *hyperthyroidism*.

tidal volume (TV) The amount of air (approximately 500 mL) moved in and out of the lungs with each normal, quiet breath.

tinnitus Perception of sound such as ringing, buzzing or roaring in the ears.

titrate To determine the concentration of (a solution) by titration or perform the operation of titration.

tolerance A cumulative state in which a particular dose of a chemical elicits a smaller response than before. With increased tolerance, the individual needs higher and higher doses to obtain the desired effect.

tonsillitis Acute inflammation of the palatine tonsils.

tophi Small white nodules in subcutaneous tissue composed of urate deposits resulting from gout.

total gastrectomy Removal of the entire stomach.

total peripheral vascular resistance (TPVR) The opposing forces or impedance to blood flow as the arterial channels become more and more distant from the heart.

toxic multinodular goitre A tumour characterised by small, discrete, independently functioning nodules in the thyroid gland tissue that secrete excessive amounts of thyroid hormone.

trachoma A chronic conjunctivitis caused by *Chlamydia trachomatis*, and a significant preventable cause of blindness worldwide.

transdermal Medication absorbed through the skin without injection.

transdisciplinary Transdisciplinary approaches in health involve partnerships and strategies that cross many health and other professional discipline boundaries to create a holistic approach, addressing multiple influences.

transfusion An infusion of blood or blood components.

transient ischaemic attack (TIA) Brief period of localised cerebral ischaemia that causes neurological deficits lasting for less than 24 hours.

transjugular intrahepatic portosystemic shunt (TIPS) Used to relieve portal hypertension and its complications of oesophageal varices and ascites.

translocation The joining of a part of or a whole chromosome to another separate chromosome.

trauma An injury to human tissues and organs resulting from the transfer of energy from the environment.

traumatic brain injury (TBI) A traumatic insult to the brain capable of causing physical, intellectual, emotional, social and vocational changes.

tremor Rhythmic movement.

triage Means 'sorting'. Triage is the process by which all people presenting to an ED for care are assessed and their care prioritised according to actual or potential severity of illness or injury.

triage in regional and remote areas Clinical determination of the acuity of the presenting health problems for people seeking healthcare in regional and remote areas.

trichomoniasis A sexually transmitted infection caused by a parasite passed from person to person.

tricuspid valve A valve between the right atrium and ventricle of the heart; prevents blood from flowing backwards into the atrium.

trigeminal neuralgia (tic douloureux) A chronic disease of the trigeminal cranial nerve (cranial nerve V) that causes severe facial pain.

triglycerides Molecules of glycerol with fatty acids used to transport and store fats in body tissues.

trisomy Possessing three chromosomes instead of the usual two, as in trisomy 21 or Down syndrome.

Trousseau's sign Contraction of the hand and fingers in response to occlusion of the blood supply by a blood pressure cuff; caused by decreased blood calcium levels.

tuberculosis (TB) Chronic, recurrent infectious disease caused by *Mycobacterium tuberculosis*; usually affects the lungs, although any organ can be affected.

tumour marker A protein molecule detectable in serum or other body fluids. This marker is used as a biochemical indicator of the presence of a malignancy.

Turner's syndrome A chromosomal abnormality in which all or part of one of the sex chromosomes is absent.

twilight sedation Anaesthesia that provides analgesia and amnesia, but in which the person remains conscious. People are able to breathe independently and are cardiovascularly stable.

tympanoplasty Surgical reconstruction of the middle ear.

type 1 diabetes mellitus The result of pancreatic islet cell destruction and a total deficit of circulating insulin.

type 2 diabetes mellitus Results from insulin resistance with a defect in compensatory insulin secretion.

ulcer A lesion of the skin or mucous membranes.

ulcerative colitis Chronic inflammatory bowel disorder of the mucosa and submucosa of the colon and rectum.

ultrafiltration Removal of excess body water using a hydrostatic pressure gradient.

uraemia Literally, 'urine in the blood'; the syndrome or group of symptoms associated with end-stage kidney disease.

urea An end product of protein metabolism and, along with water, the main constituent of urine.

ureteral (or ureteric) stent Thin catheter inserted into the ureter to provide for urine flow and ureteral support.

ureteroplasty Surgical repair of a ureter.

urgency A sudden, compelling need to urinate.

urinary calculi Calculi or 'stones' in the urinary tract.

urinary diversion Procedure to provide for urine collection and drainage following cystectomy. The most common urinary diversion is the ileal conduit.

urinary drainage system The ureters, urinary bladder and urethra.

urinary incontinence Involuntary urination.

urinary retention Incomplete emptying of the bladder.

urticaria Hives.

vaccine Suspensions of whole or fractionated bacteria or viruses that have been treated to make them non-pathogenic.

Valsalva manoeuvre Closing the glottis and contracting the diaphragm and abdominal muscles to increase intra-abdominal pressure to facilitate expulsion of faeces.

valvular heart disease Interference of blood flow to, within and from the heart.

varicocoele Dilation of the pampiniform venous complex of the spermatic cord.

varicose veins Irregular, tortuous veins with incompetent valves.

vasoconstriction Smooth muscle contraction that narrows the vessel lumen.

vasodilation Smooth muscle relaxation that expands the vessel lumen.

vasogenic shock See *distributive shock*.

venous stasis Occurs when venous blood collects and stagnates in the lower leg.

venous thrombosis (thrombophlebitis) Blood clot (thrombus) formation on the wall of a vein, accompanied by inflammation of the vein wall and obstructed venous blood flow.

vertigo Sensation of whirling or rotation.

very-low-kilojoule diet (VLKD) A protein-sparing modified fast (1,700 to 3,500 kilojoules/day or less) under close medical supervision that may be used to treat significant obesity.

vital capacity The sum of TV (tidal volume) 1 IRV (inspiratory reserve volume) 1 ERV (expiratory reserve volume); approximately 4,500 mL in healthy people.

vitiligo Abnormal loss of melanin in patches.

volatile acids Acids eliminated from the body as a gas.

Volkmann's contracture A common complication of elbow fractures; can result from unresolved compartment syndrome. Arterial blood flow decreases, leading to ischaemia, degeneration and contracture of the muscle.

voluntary assisted dying (VAD) The assistance provided to a person by a health practitioner to end their life.

vomiting The forceful expulsion of the contents of the upper gastrointestinal tract resulting from contraction of muscles in the gut and abdominal wall.

warts (verrucae) Lesions of the skin caused by the human papillomavirus.

weaning Process of removing the person from ventilator support and re-establishing spontaneous, independent respirations.

wheeze Continuous, musical sound caused by narrowing of the lumen in a respiratory passage.

wild-type gene The most common type of gene; designated as normal.

withdrawal Cessation of use of a substance to which an individual has become addicted.

xenograft A transplant from an animal species to a human.

xerosis Dry skin.

xerostomia Excessive dryness of the mucous membranes (due to chemotherapy or radiation).

X-linked dominant Any gene found on the X chromosome or traits determined by such genes; also refers to the specific mode of inheritance of such genes. One altered gene on an X chromosome in a male can produce disease, such as haemophilia.

X-linked recessive The result of an altered gene on the X chromosome.

Zollinger–Ellison syndrome Peptic ulcer disease caused by a gastrinoma, or gastrin-secreting tumour of the pancreas, stomach or intestines.

Index

Page numbers in **bold** indicate definitions of key terms.

O

S